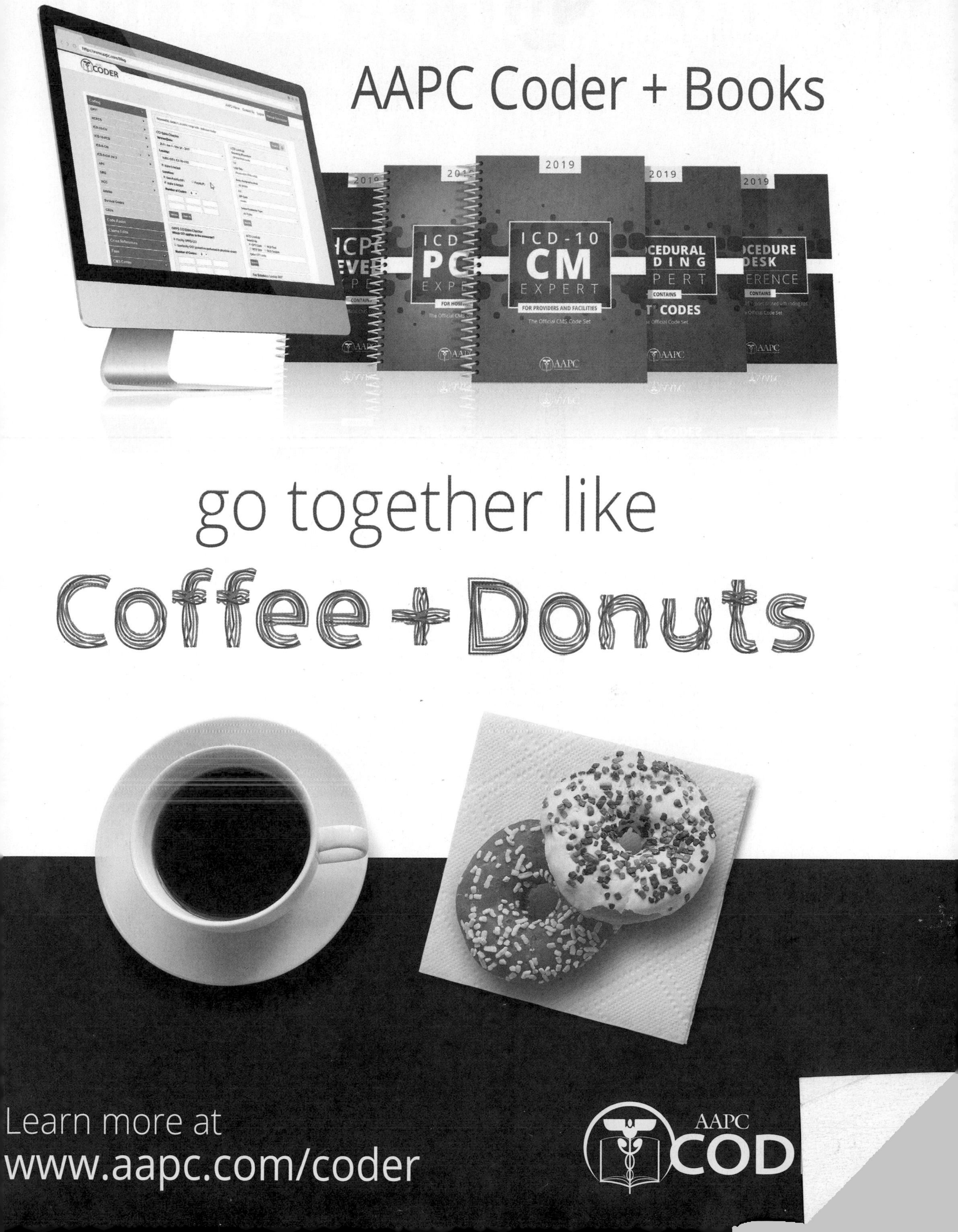
AAPC Coder + Books
go together like
Coffee + Donuts
Learn more at
www.aapc.com/coder

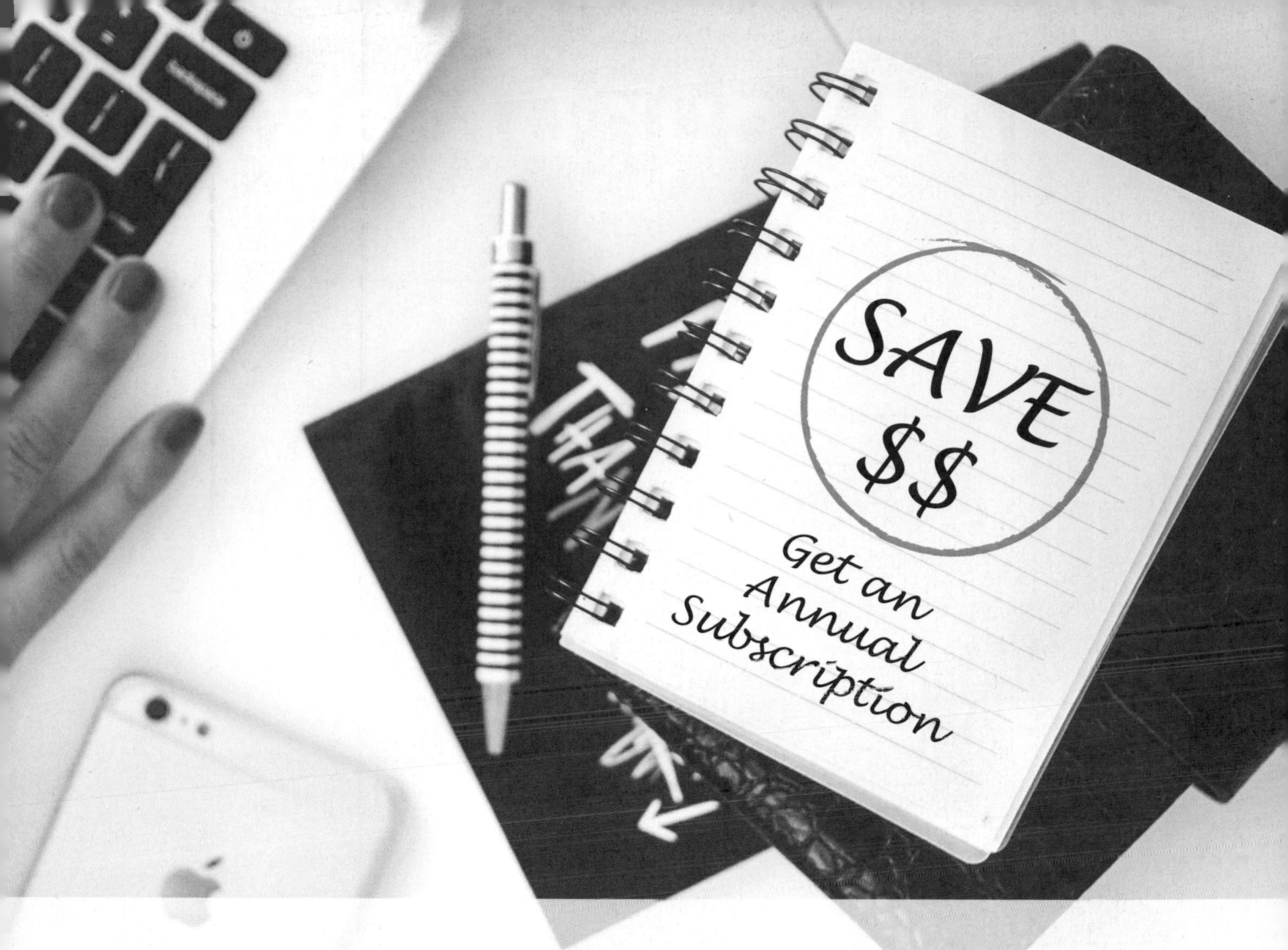
SAVE
$$
Get an
Annual
Subscription

- multiaxial- key attribute provides Framework For all other Structural attributes
- IPCS orginally completed 1998 - Updated in 2004 to include PICVA codes
- PCS preserves capacity to define past, present, Future procedures, using stable terminology in the form of characters & values
- PCS can easily be expanded w/o disrupting the structure of the system

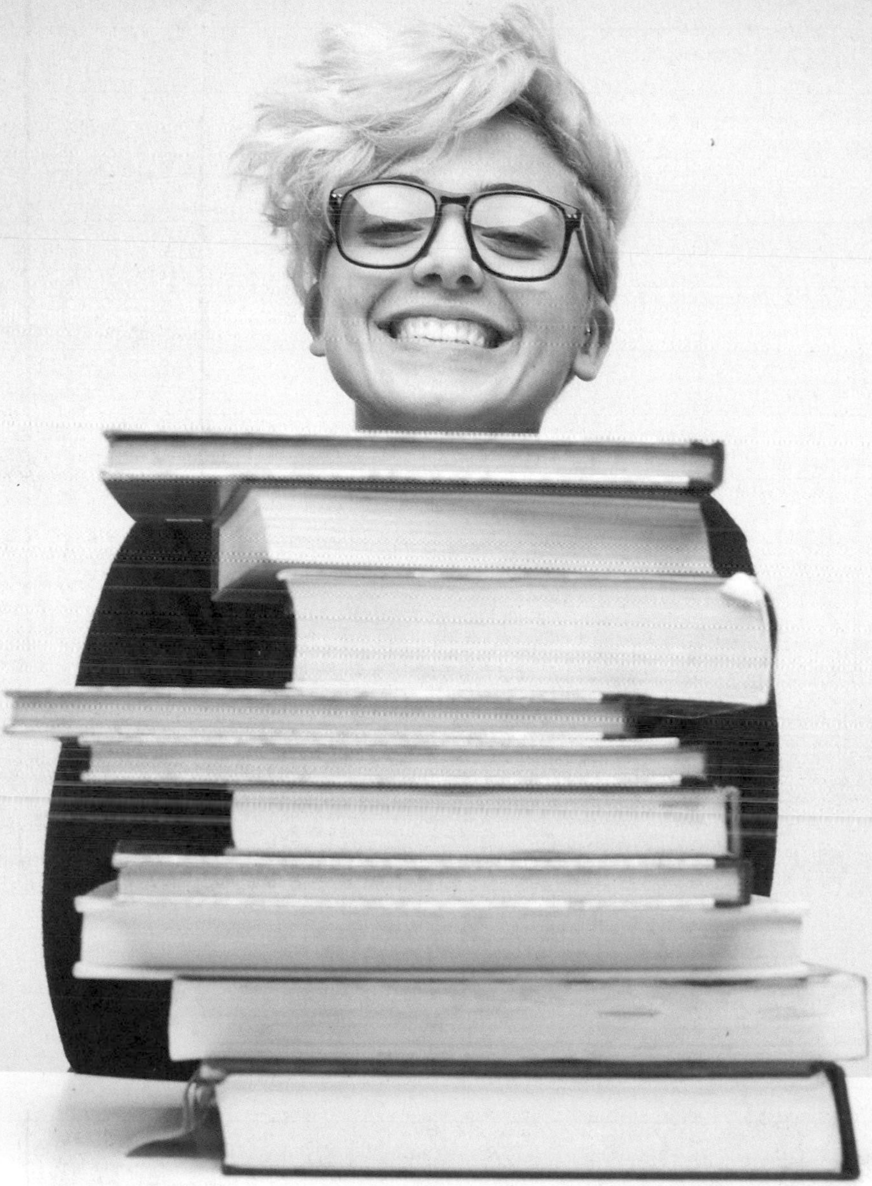

NOTES

2020

ICD-10 PCS EXPERT

The Official CMS Code Set

Inpatient Procedure Codes for Facilities

AAPC
Advancing the Business of Healthcare

AAPC'S COMMITMENT TO ACCURACY

This publisher is committed to providing our members accurate and reliable materials. However, codes and the guidelines by which they are applied change or are reinterpreted through the year. This book contains data from Medicare Code Edits (v. 36), MS-DRG v. 36.0 Definitions Manual, updates for CMS for symbols and Appendices, along with the 2020 PCS code set in the tables which was the latest information available at the time of printing. Check www.aapc.com periodically for updates. To report corrections and updates, please contact AAPC Customer Service via 1-800-626-2633 or, via email to code.books@aapc.com.

ACKNOWLEDGEMENT

Jaspal Singh Arora, Operations
Amit Gupta
Sandra Krokaugger
Lisa Meaney, BS
Harshita Sharma, PT, PhD
Sushanta Das, MBA
Leesa Israel, CPC, CUC, CEMC, CPPM, CMBS
Prashant Kumar, MBA
Sabyasachi Nath, MS
Rajendra Sharma, RN, CPC
Brad Ericson, MPC, CPC, COSC
Rahul Jain, MDSE
Beth Martin, BS, COC, CSM
Ganesh Prasad Sahoo
Patricia Zubritzky, BS, CRCE-I

Get Updates, Coding Tips, and Corrections for this book at www.aapc.com/codebook_updates.

Images/Illustrations by the following artists at shutterstock.com:

stockshoppe - 180896807, 99671552, 180896810, 187162193, 180896855, 180896738, 177790997, 177791516, 180896873 | Blamb - 786347626, 24129706 | Alila Medical Media - 76386163, 72231811, 149230337, 149230217, 228843253, 155445671, 147789479, 228843103, 88094230, 155445686, 101696095, 96426923, 97755608, 147943922, 147943910, 155445662, 147943874, 106263593, 106263560, 125891585, 228843262 | Designua - 430118209, 180938618, 135935735, 165084413 | Suwin - 405537832 | Vecton - 661087531 | Sakurra - 676139677 | stihii - 109588457, 129969767, 124562680, 121824442, 129804629, 225637774, 505306105, 505306069 | DeryaDraws - 557609659 | Naeblys - 650014342 | NatthapongSachan - 416973331, 452997697 | udaix - 502058023, 108531449 | ducu59us- 104022683, 125200733 | BlueRingMedia- 141161404, 141162229, 141161560 | joshya - 261971498 | Della_Liner- 324447776 | snapgalleria - 142194094 | okili77- 156466463 | lotan - 186878060 | Alexander_P - 404964388 | udaix - 1336924949

AAPC
Advancing the Business of Healthcare

ISBN: 978-1-626887-534

Table of Contents

Divided into 17 sections—numbers 0-9, letters B-D, F,H & X
Codes maintained & released by CMS

I of 34 values can be assigned to each character

Preface

Thank you for your purchase! We are pleased to offer you the 2020 ICD-10-PCS official code set in this book.

This manual goes beyond the basics to help you code accurately and efficiently. In addition to including the official Alphabetic Index, Tables, and ICD-10-PCS Official Guidelines, we've crafted a select set of bonus features based on requests from coders in the field as well as the recommendations of our core group of veteran coding educators.

Our goal was to apply our unique approach to focusing on the practical application of the codes to this procedure coding manual.

A few of the other features you'll benefit from page after page include the following:

- Updated and enhanced illustrations of body systems and disease processes at the front of the book so you don't have to search the manual for these large color images of body systems
- An Approach Table at the front of the book listing each approach, its definition, and examples
- Medicare Code Edits, including gender edits and edits for limited coverage, noncovered procedures, HAC-associated procedures, combination clusters, non-OR procedures affecting MS-DRG assignment, and questionable obstetric admission
- Intuitive color-coded symbols and alerts identify critical coding and reimbursement issues quickly
- List of non-OR procedures NOT affecting MS-DRG assignment
- Full list of adhesive tabs to label your book to quickly and easily find specific sections

See the complete List of Features to learn about everything this manual has to offer.

Rely on Our Combination of Official Sources and Experience

This manual includes the official ICD-10-PCS 2020 Alphabetic Index and Tables. We've also included the 2020 ICD-10-PCS Official Guidelines.

Additionally, our dedicated team drew on their years of experience using coding manuals to develop this manual's user-friendly symbols, color coding, and tabs, all designed to help you find the information you need quickly.

Let Us Know What You Think

Our goal for this manual is to support those involved in the business side of healthcare, helping them to do their jobs well. We'd appreciate your feedback, including your suggestions for what you'd like to see in an ICD-10-PCS resource, so we can be sure our manuals serve your needs. Thank you.

Changes for 2020

FY 2020 Update Summary

Change Summary Table

2019 Total	New Codes	Revised Titles	Deleted Codes	2020 Total
78,881	734	2	2,056	**77,559**

ICD-10-PCS Code FY 2020 Totals, By Section

Medical and Surgical	67,257
Obstetrics	302
Placement	861
Administration	1,332
Measurement and Monitoring	418
Extracorporeal or Systemic Assistance and Performance	48
Extracorporeal or Systemic Therapies	46
Osteopathic	100
Other Procedures	77
Chiropractic	90
Imaging	2,941
Nuclear Medicine	463
Radiation Therapy	2,019
Physical Rehabilitation and Diagnostic Audiology	1,380
Mental Health	30
Substance Abuse Treatment	59
New Technology	136
Total	**77,559**

List of FY 2020 Files

Note: All 2020 ICD-10-PCS data files can be found on the CMS website at: https://www.cms.gov/Medicare/Coding/ICD10/2020-ICD-10-PCS.html.

Descriptions of these data files are as follows:

2020 Official ICD-10-PCS Coding Guidelines

- New Guidelines D1.a, D1.b and D1.c added in response to public comment.
- Guidelines page 1, paragraph 3, A9, B2.1a, B3.1b, B3.2c, B3.5, B3.9, B4.1b, E1.a and E1.b revised in response to public comment and internal review.
- Downloadable PDF, file name **pcs_guidelines_2020.pdf**

2020 ICD-10-PCS Code Tables and Index (Zip file)

- Code tables for use beginning October 1, 2019.
- Downloadable PDF, file name is **pcs_2020.pdf**
- Downloadable xml files for developers, file names are **icd10pcs_tables_2020.xml, icd10pcs_index_2020.xml, icd10pcs_definitions_2020.xml**
- Accompanying schema for developers, file names are **icd10pcs_tables.xsd, icd10pcs_index.xsd, icd10pcs_definitions.xsd**

2020 ICD-10-PCS Codes File (Zip file)

- ICD-10-PCS Codes file is a simple format for non-technical uses, containing the valid FY 2020 ICD-10-PCS codes and their long titles.
- File is in text file format, file name is **icd10pcs_codes_2020.txt**
- Accompanying documentation for codes file, file name is **icd10pcsCodesFile.pdf**
- Codes file addenda in text format, file name is **codes_addenda_2020.txt**

2020 ICD-10-PCS Order File (Long and Abbreviated Titles) (Zip file)

- ICD-10-PCS order file is for developers, provides a unique five-digit "order number" for each ICD-10-PCS table and code, as well as a long and abbreviated code title.
- ICD-10-PCS order file name is **icd10pcs_order_2020.txt**
- Accompanying documentation for tabular order file, file name is **icd10pcsOrderFile.pdf**
- Tabular order file addenda in text format, file name is **order_addenda_2020.txt**

2020 ICD-10-PCS Final Addenda (Zip file)

- Addenda files in downloadable PDF, file names are **tables_addenda_2020.pdf, index_addenda_2020.pdf, definitions_addenda_2020.pdf**
- Addenda files also in machine readable text format for developers, file names are **tables_addenda_2020.txt, index_addenda_2020.txt, definitions_addenda_2020.txt**

2020 ICD-10-PCS Conversion Table (Zip file)

- ICD-10-PCS code conversion table is provided to assist users in data retrieval, in downloadable Excel spreadsheet, file name is **icd10pcs_conversion_table_2020.xlsx**
- Conversion table also in machine readable text format for developers, file name is **icd10pcs_conversion_table_2020.txt**
- Accompanying documentation for code conversion table, file name is **icd10pcsConversionTable.pdf**

Disclaimer: At the time of publication the CMS ICD-10-PCS Official Guidelines for Coding and Reporting 2020 did not contain section D1.c as stated above.

List of Features

ICD-10-PCS is essential to documenting medical necessity for services rendered, and accurate codes mean better outcomes for the patient, your claims, and your facility.

You can count on this manual to help you choose and report the right ICD-10-PCS code. Unique features, intuitive design, and expert details that coders developed assure this manual will keep your coding on target.

This manual includes the ICD-10-PCS Alphabetic Index and ICD-10-PCS Tables for procedures, effective October 1, 2019 (FY 2020 code set).

To help you make the most of this manual, we include the following features:

- ICD-10-PCS Official Conventions and additional conventions and symbols
- ICD-10-PCS Official Guidelines for Coding and Reporting, effective October 1, 2019 (FY 2020)
- Approach Table with each approach, definition, and example listed at the front of the book for quick reference
- Updated and enhanced color illustrations of body systems and disease processes at the front of the book for easy look-up
- Medicare Code Edits symbols, including gender edits and edits for limited coverage, noncovered procedures, hospital acquired conditions (HAC-) associated procedures, combination clusters, non-OR procedures affecting MS-DRG assignment, and questionable obstetric admission
- Intuitive color-coded symbols and alerts for quick identification of coding and reimbursement issues
- Adhesive tabs for specific sections of the book to find information more quickly and easily
- Appendices for root operations definitions in alphabetical order by Tables, body part key, device key and aggregation table, character meaning, substance key, combination clusters, and non-OR procedures not affecting MS-DRG assignment
- A user-friendly page design, including dictionary-style headers, colored bleed tabs, and legend keys

CMS - maintains inpt code set, released in 1998, (contracted) developed in 1993, updated yearly
agency responsible, 3M built classification system

Official Conventions and Additional Conventions Specific to This ICD-10-PCS Book

This manual includes the procedure code set from the International Classification of Diseases, 10th Revision, Procedure Coding System (ICD-10-PCS). Hospitals and third-party payers use these codes to classify inpatient procedures.

Official Conventions

Index

Refer to the ICD-10-PCS Index to access the Tables in the manual. The Index mirrors the structure of the Tables, so it follows a consistent pattern of organization and use of hierarchies. The Index is organized as an alphabetic lookup.

Two types of main terms are listed in the Index:

- Based on the value of the third character, such as a root operation (excision, insertion)
- Lists common procedure terms

Main Terms

For the Medical and Surgical and related sections, the root operation values are used as main terms in the Index. In other sections, the values representing the general type of procedure performed, such as nuclear medicine or imaging type, are listed as main terms.

For the Medical and Surgical and related sections, values such as Excision, Bypass, and Transplantation are included as main terms in the Index. The applicable body system entries are listed beneath the main term and refer to a specific table. For the ancillary sections, values such as Fluoroscopy and Positron Emission Tomography, are listed as main terms.

To find the code to cross-reference to the Tables, search for the root operation for the procedure in the Index, followed by the subterm for the anatomic site or the subterm that further describes the procedure. Locate the partial code, and cross-reference it to the Table that matches the first three characters of the code.

Tables

The Tables are organized in alphanumeric order in a series by Section, which is the first character of a code. Tables that begin with 0 to 9 are listed first, then tables beginning with B-D, then letters F-X, are listed next.

The same convention is followed within each table for the second through the seventh characters—numeric values in order first, followed by alphabetical values in order.

The Medical and Surgical section (first character 0) is organized by body system values. Each body system subdivision in the Medical and Surgical section contains tables that list the valid root operations for that body system. These are the root operation tables that form the system. These tables provide the valid choices of values available to construct a code.

The root operation tables consist of four columns and a varying number of rows, as in the following example of the root operation Insertion, in the Subcutaneous Tissue and Fascia body system.

The values for characters 1 through 3 are provided at the top of each table.

Character 1:	0: MEDICAL AND SURGICAL (Section) ← determines broad category or procedure or
Character 2:	J: SUBCUTANEOUS TISSUE AND FASCIA (Body System)
Character 3:	H: INSERTION: Putting in a nonbiological appliance that monitors, assists, performs, or prevents a physiological function but does not physically take the place of a body part (Root Operation)

Four columns contain the applicable values for characters 4 through 7, given the values in characters 1 through 3:

Body Part	Approach	Device	Qualifier
Character 4	Character 5	Character 6	Character 7
S Subcutaneous Tissue and Fascia, Head and Neck **V** Subcutaneous Tissue and Fascia, Upper Extremity **W** Subcutaneous Tissue and Fascia, Lower Extremity	**0** Open **3** Percutaneous	**1** Radioactive Element **3** Infusion Device **Y** Other Device	**Z** No Qualifier
T Subcutaneous Tissue and Fascia, Trunk	**0** Open **3** Percutaneous	**1** Radioactive Element **3** Infusion Device **V** Infusion Device, Pump **Y** Other Device	**Z** No Qualifier

A table may be separated into rows to specify the valid choices of values in characters 4 through 7. A code built using values from more than one row of a table is not a valid code.

Refer to the ICD-10-PCS Official Guidelines for Coding and Reporting in this manual for detailed guidance on assigning ICD-10-PCS codes.

See Reference

The See reference directs you to go elsewhere in the Index to find the root operation that you need.

Use Reference

The Use reference directs you to a character value selection as an additional reference.

Additional Conventions

Additional conventions that you will find in the Tables in this manual include Medicare Code Edits - Symbols and colored font.

Medicare Code Edits – Symbols Applied to 4th Characters

LC Limited Coverage

Procedures that are medically complex and serious in nature that incur extraordinary associated costs. Medicare limits coverage to a portion of the cost.

NC Noncovered

Procedures for which Medicare does not typically reimburse.

HAC HAC-associated Procedure

Procedures that are associated with hospital-acquired conditions (HAC).

CC Combination Cluster

The procedure is part of a procedure code combination, or cluster, listed in Appendix G of this manual. Medicare does not typically pay for these procedures unless you report them with other specific procedures.

DRG Non-OR-Affecting MS-DRG Assignment

Non-operating room procedures which affect MS-DRG assignment for claims reporting.

New/Revised Text in **Orange**

Procedure text was new or revised from the last version of the code set. For new codes, orange text will be shown for all characters in the code. New codes may be shown as their own row in a table and characters 4-7 may be shown in a row that is separate from other characters within that table.

♂ Male

Male procedure only

♀ Female

Female procedure only

QOA Questionable Obstetric Admission

Procedure codes for cesarean or vaginal delivery that are considered questionable unless reported with a corresponding secondary diagnosis describing the outcome of delivery.

Code Lists

Codes that are applicable to each type of symbol in the book are listed after each table.

Notes Pages

Notes pages are included between sections within the Tables.

maintained/released by CMS

ICD-10-PCS Official Guidelines for Coding and Reporting 2020

agency

The Centers for Medicare and Medicaid Services (CMS) and the National Center for Health Statistics (NCHS), two departments within the U.S. Federal Government's Department of Health and Human Services (DHHS) provide the following guidelines for coding and reporting using the International Classification of Diseases, 10th Revision, Procedure Coding System (ICD-10-PCS). These guidelines should be used as a companion document to the official version of the ICD-10-PCS as published on the CMS website. The ICD-10-PCS is a procedure classification published by the United States for classifying procedures performed in hospital inpatient health care settings.

These guidelines have been approved by the four organizations that make up the Cooperating Parties for the ICD-10-PCS: the American Hospital Association (AHA), the American Health Information Management Association (AHIMA), CMS, and NCHS.

These guidelines are a set of rules that have been developed to accompany and complement the official conventions and instructions provided within the ICD-10-PCS itself. They are intended to provide direction that is applicable in most circumstances. However, there may be unique circumstances where exceptions are applied. The instructions and conventions of the classification take precedence over guidelines. These guidelines are based on the coding and sequencing instructions in the Tables, Index and Definitions of ICD-10-PCS, but provide additional instruction.

Adherence to these guidelines when assigning ICD-10-PCS procedure codes is required under the Health Insurance Portability and Accountability Act (HIPAA). The procedure codes have been adopted under HIPAA for hospital inpatient healthcare settings.

WHO maintained ICD for recording death since 1893

A joint effort between the healthcare provider and the coder is essential to achieve complete and accurate documentation, code assignment, and reporting of diagnoses and procedures.

These guidelines have been developed to assist both the healthcare provider and the coder in identifying those procedures that are to be reported. The importance of consistent, complete documentation in the medical record cannot be overemphasized. Without such documentation accurate coding cannot be achieved.

Table of Contents

• 1st character in code determines the broad procedure category or section where the code is found

• Descriptions do not include eponyms or common procedure names

Conventions

A1
ICD-10-PCS codes are composed of seven characters. Each character is an axis of classification that specifies information about the procedure performed. Within a defined code range, a character specifies the same type of information in that axis of classification.

Example: The fifth axis of classification specifies the approach in sections 0 through 4 and 7 through 9 of the system.

A2
One of 34 possible values can be assigned to each axis of classification in the seven- character code: they are the numbers 0 through 9 and the alphabet (except I and O because they are easily confused with the numbers 1 and 0). The number of unique values used in an axis of classification differs as needed.

Example: Where the fifth axis of classification specifies the approach, seven different approach values are currently used to specify the approach.

A3
The valid values for an axis of classification can be added to as needed.

Example: If a significantly distinct type of device is used in a new procedure, a new device value can be added to the system.

A4
As with words in their context, the meaning of any single value is a combination of its axis of classification and any preceding values on which it may be dependent.

Example: The meaning of a body part value in the Medical and Surgical section is always dependent on the body system value. The body part value 0 in the Central Nervous body system specifies Brain and the body part value 0 in the Peripheral Nervous body system specifies Cervical Plexus.

A5
As the system is expanded to become increasingly detailed, over time more values will depend on preceding values for their meaning.

Example: In the Lower Joints body system, the device value 3 in the root operation Insertion specifies Infusion Device and the device value 3 in the root operation Replacement specifies Ceramic Synthetic Substitute.

A6
The purpose of the alphabetic index is to locate the appropriate table that contains all information necessary to construct a procedure code. The PCS Tables should always be consulted to find the most appropriate valid code.

A7
It is not required to consult the index first before proceeding to the tables to complete the code. A valid code may be chosen directly from the tables.

A8
All seven characters must be specified to be a valid code. If the documentation is incomplete for coding purposes, the physician should be queried for the necessary information.

A9
Within a PCS table, valid codes include all combinations of choices in characters 4 through 7 contained in the same row of the table. In the example below, 0JHT3VZ is a valid code, and 0JHW3VZ is *not* a valid code.

A10
"And," when used in a code description, means "and/or," except when used to describe a combination of multiple body parts for which separate values exist for each body part (e.g., Skin and Subcutaneous Tissue used as a qualifier, where there are separate body part values for "Skin" and "Subcutaneous Tissue").

Example: Lower Arm and Wrist Muscle means lower arm and/or wrist muscle.

A11
Many of the terms used to construct PCS codes are defined within the system. It is the coder's responsibility to determine what the documentation in the medical record equates to in the PCS definitions. The physician is not expected to use the terms used in PCS code descriptions, nor is the coder required to query the physician when the correlation between the documentation and the defined PCS terms is clear.

Example: When the physician documents "partial resection" the coder can independently correlate "partial resection" to the root operation Excision without querying the physician for clarification.

Section: 0 Medical and Surgical
Body System: J Subcutaneous Tissue and Fascia
Operation: H Insertion: Putting in a nonbiological appliance that monitors, assists, performs, or prevents a physiological function but does not physically take the place of a body part

Body Part	Approach	Device	Qualifier
S Subcutaneous Tissue and Fascia, Head and Neck V Subcutaneous Tissue and Fascia, Upper Extremity W Subcutaneous Tissue and Fascia, Lower Extremity	0 Open 3 Percutaneous	1 Radioactive Element 3 Infusion Device Y Other Device	Z No Qualifier
T Subcutaneous Tissue and Fascia, Trunk	0 Open 3 Percutaneous	1 Radioactive Element 3 Infusion Device V Infusion Pump Y Other Device	Z No Qualifier

34 possible values, no O or I
includes 0-9 & A-Z
have 7 characters

Medical and Surgical Section Guidelines (Section 0)
31 body systems recognized

B2. Body System

General guidelines

B2.1a
The procedure codes in Anatomical Regions, General, Anatomical Regions, Upper Extremities and Anatomical Regions, Lower Extremities can be used when the procedure is performed on an anatomical region rather than a specific body part, or on the rare occasion when no information is available to support assignment of a code to a specific body part.

Examples: Chest tube drainage of the pleural cavity is coded to the root operation Drainage found in the body system Anatomical Regions, General.

Suture repair of the abdominal wall is coded to the root operation Repair in the body system Anatomical Regions, General.

Amputation of the foot is coded to the root operation Detachment in the body system Anatomical Regions, Lower Extremities.

B2.1b
Where the general body part values "upper" and "lower" are provided as an option in the Upper Arteries, Lower Arteries, Upper Veins, Lower Veins, Muscles and Tendons body systems, "upper" or "lower "specifies body parts located above or below the diaphragm respectively.

Example: Vein body parts above the diaphragm are found in the Upper Veins body system; vein body parts below the diaphragm are found in the Lower Veins body system.

Based on intent, NOT on incisions made

B3. Root Operation
includes definition, explanation & examples

General guidelines
31 different root operation

B3.1a
In order to determine the appropriate root operation, the full definition of the root operation as contained in the PCS Tables must be applied. *Root operation determined by*

B3.1b
procedure actually performed, regardless if it works
Components of a procedure specified in the root operation definition or explanation as integral to that root operation are not coded separately. Procedural steps necessary to reach the operative site and close the operative site, including anastomosis of a tubular body part, are also not coded separately.

Examples: Resection of a joint as part of a joint replacement procedure is included in the root operation definition of Replacement and is not coded separately.

Laparotomy performed to reach the site of an open liver biopsy is not coded separately. In a resection of sigmoid colon with anastomosis of descending colon to rectum, the anastomosis is not coded separately.

Exceptions: Mastectomy followed by breast reconstruction, both resection and replacement of the breast are coded separately.

Multiple procedures

B3.2
During the same operative episode, multiple procedures are *OTTCO* coded if: *bilateral radical lymphadenectomy - only 1 code*

a. The same root operation is performed on different body parts as defined by distinct values of the body part character.

   Examples: Diagnostic excision of liver and pancreas are coded separately.

   Excision of lesion in the ascending colon and excision of lesion in the transverse colon are coded separately.

b. The same root operation is repeated in multiple body parts, and those body parts are separate and distinct body parts classified to a single ICD-10-PCS body part value.

   Examples: Excision of the sartorius muscle and excision of the gracilis muscle are both included in the upper leg muscle body part value, and multiple procedures are coded.

   Extraction of multiple toenails are coded separately.

c. Multiple root operations with distinct objectives are performed on the same body part.

   Example: Destruction of sigmoid lesion and bypass of sigmoid colon are coded separately.

d. The intended root operation is attempted using one approach but is converted to a different approach.

   Example: Laparoscopic cholecystectomy converted to an open cholecystectomy is coded as percutaneous endoscopic Inspection and open Resection.

Discontinued or incomplete procedures

B3.3
If the intended procedure is discontinued or otherwise not completed, code the procedure to the root operation performed. If a procedure is discontinued before any other root operation is performed, code the root operation Inspection of the body part or anatomical region inspected.

Example: A planned aortic valve replacement procedure is discontinued after the initial thoracotomy and before any incision is made in the heart muscle, when the patient becomes hemodynamically unstable. This procedure is coded as an open Inspection of the mediastinum.

Biopsy procedures
to use X - must be sent to pathology

B3.4a
Biopsy procedures are coded using the root operations Excision, Extraction, or Drainage and the qualifier Diagnostic. *pathology*

Examples: Fine needle aspiration biopsy of fluid in the lung is coded to the root operation Drainage with the qualifier Diagnostic.

Biopsy of bone marrow is coded to the root operation Extraction with the qualifier Diagnostic.

Lymph node sampling for biopsy is coded to the root operation Excision with the qualifier Diagnostic.

Do not confuse w/ diagnostic endoscopy or diagnostic laparoscopy

ollowed by more definitive treatment

iagnostic Excision, Extraction, or Drainage procedure (biopsy) ollowed by a more definitive procedure, such as Destruction, xcision or Resection at the same procedure site, both the biopsy and the more definitive treatment are coded.

Example: Biopsy of breast followed by partial mastectomy at the same procedure site, both the biopsy and the partial mastectomy procedure are coded.

Overlapping body layers

B3.5
If root operations such as Excision, Extraction, Repair or Inspection are performed on overlapping layers of the musculoskeletal system, the body part specifying the deepest layer is coded.

Example: Excisional debridement that includes skin and subcutaneous tissue and muscle is coded to the muscle body part.

Bypass procedures

SHUNT - do not use insertion for device

B3.6a   *non-coronary*
Bypass procedures are coded by identifying the body part bypassed "from" and the body part bypassed "to." The fourth character body part specifies the body part bypassed from, and the qualifier specifies the body part bypassed to.

Example: Bypass from stomach to jejunum, stomach is the body part and jejunum is the qualifier.

B3.6b
Coronary artery bypass procedures are coded differently than other bypass procedures as described in the previous guideline. Rather than identifying the body part bypassed from, the body part identifies the number of coronary arteries bypassed to, and the qualifier specifies the vessel bypassed from.

Example: Aortocoronary artery bypass of the left anterior descending coronary artery and the obtuse marginal coronary artery is classified in the body part axis of classification as two coronary arteries, and the qualifier specifies the aorta as the body part bypassed from.

B3.6c
If multiple coronary arteries are bypassed, a separate procedure is coded for each coronary artery that uses a different device and/or qualifier.

Example: Aortocoronary artery bypass and internal mammary coronary artery bypass are coded separately.

Control vs. more definitive root operations

B3.7
The root operation Control is defined as, "Stopping, or attempting to stop, postprocedural or other acute bleeding." If an attempt to stop postprocedural or other acute bleeding is unsuccessful, and to stop the bleeding requires performing a more definitive root operation, such as Bypass, Detachment, Excision, Extraction, Reposition, Replacement, or Resection, then the more definitive root operation is coded instead of Control.

Example: Resection of spleen to stop bleeding is coded to Resection instead of Control.

Excision vs. Resection   *use resection for anatomical subdivison of a body part*

B3.8
PCS contains specific body parts for anatomical subdivisions of a body part, such as lobes of the lungs or liver and regions of the intestine. Resection of the specific body part is coded whenever all of the body part is cut out or off, rather than coding Excision of a less specific body part.

Example: Left upper lung lobectomy is coded to Resection of Upper Lung Lobe, Left rather than Excision of Lung, Left.

Excision for graft

B3.9   *body part*
If an autograft is obtained from a different procedure site in order to complete the objective of the procedure, a separate procedure is coded, except when the seventh character qualifier value in the ICD-10-PCS table fully specifies the site from which the autograft was obtained.

Examples: Coronary bypass with excision of saphenous vein graft, excision of saphenous vein is coded separately.

Replacement of breast with autologous deep inferior epigastric artery perforator (DIEP) flap, excision of the DIEP flap is not coded separately. The seventh character qualifier value Deep Inferior Epigastric Artery Perforator Flap in the Replacement table fully specifies the site of the autograft harvest.

Fusion procedures of the spine

B3.10a
The body part coded for a spinal vertebral joint(s) rendered immobile by a spinal fusion procedure is classified by the level of the spine (e.g. thoracic). There are distinct body part values for a single vertebral joint and for multiple vertebral joints at each spinal level.

Example: Body part values specify Lumbar Vertebral Joint, Lumbar Vertebral Joints, 2 or More and Lumbosacral Vertebral Joint.

B3.10b
If multiple vertebral joints are fused, a separate procedure is coded for each vertebral joint that uses a different device and/or qualifier.

Example: Fusion of lumbar vertebral joint, posterior approach, anterior column and fusion of lumbar vertebral joint, posterior approach, posterior column are coded separately.

B3.10c
Combinations of devices and materials are often used on a vertebral joint to render the joint immobile. When combinations of devices are used on the same vertebral joint, the device value coded for the procedure is as follows:

- If an interbody fusion device is used to render the joint immobile (alone or containing other material like bone graft), the procedure is coded with the device value Interbody Fusion Device

- If bone graft is the *only* device used to render the joint immobile, the procedure is coded with the device value Nonautologous Tissue Substitute or Autologous Tissue Substitute
- If a mixture of autologous and nonautologous bone graft (with or without biological or synthetic extenders or binders) is used to render the joint immobile, code the procedure with the device value Autologous Tissue Substitute

Examples: Fusion of a vertebral joint using a cage style interbody fusion device containing morsellized bone graft is coded to the device Interbody Fusion Device.

Fusion of a vertebral joint using a bone dowel interbody fusion device made of cadaver bone and packed with a mixture of local morsellized bone and demineralized bone matrix is coded to the device Interbody Fusion Device.

Fusion of a vertebral joint using both autologous bone graft and bone bank bone graft is coded to the device Autologous Tissue Substitute.

Inspection procedures

B3.11a
Inspection of a body part(s) performed in order to achieve the objective of a procedure is not coded separately.

Example: Fiber optic bronchoscopy performed for irrigation of bronchus, only the irrigation procedure is coded.

B3.11b
If multiple tubular body parts are inspected, the most distal body part (the body part furthest from the starting point of the inspection) is coded. If multiple non-tubular body parts in a region are inspected, the body part that specifies the entire area inspected is coded.

Examples: Cystoureteroscopy with inspection of bladder and ureters is coded to the ureter body part value.

Exploratory laparotomy with general inspection of abdominal contents is coded to the peritoneal cavity body part value.

B3.11c
When both an Inspection procedure and another procedure are performed on the same body part during the same episode, if the Inspection procedure is performed using a different approach than the other procedure, the Inspection procedure is coded separately.

Example: Endoscopic Inspection of the duodenum is coded separately when open Excision of the duodenum is performed during the same procedural episode.

Occlusion vs. Restriction for vessel embolization procedures

B3.12
If the objective of an embolization procedure is to completely close a vessel, the root operation Occlusion is coded. If the objective of an embolization procedure is to narrow the lumen of a vessel, the root operation Restriction is coded.

Examples: Tumor embolization is coded to the root operation Occlusion, because the objective of the procedure is to cut off the blood supply to the vessel.

Embolization of a cerebral aneurysm is coded to the root operation Restriction, because the objective of the procedure is not to close off the vessel entirely, but to narrow the lumen of the vessel at the site of the aneurysm where it is abnormally wide.

Release procedures

B3.13
In the root operation Release, the body part value coded is the body part being freed and not the tissue being manipulated or cut to free the body part.

Example: Lysis of intestinal adhesions is coded to the specific intestine body part value.

Release vs. Division

B3.14
If the sole objective of the procedure is freeing a body part without cutting the body part, the root operation is Release. If the sole objective of the procedure is separating or transecting a body part, the root operation is Division.

Examples: Freeing a nerve root from surrounding scar tissue to relieve pain is coded to the root operation Release.

Severing a nerve root to relieve pain is coded to the root operation Division.

Reposition for fracture treatment

B3.15
Reduction of a displaced fracture is coded to the root operation Reposition and the application of a cast or splint in conjunction with the Reposition procedure is not coded separately. Treatment of a nondisplaced fracture is coded to the procedure performed.

Examples: Casting of a nondisplaced fracture is coded to the root operation Immobilization in the Placement section.

Putting a pin in a nondisplaced fracture is coded to the root operation Insertion.

Transplantation vs. Administration

B3.16
Putting in a mature and functioning living body part taken from another individual or animal is coded to the root operation Transplantation. Putting in autologous or nonautologous cells is coded to the Administration section.

Example: Putting in autologous or nonautologous bone marrow, pancreatic islet cells or stem cells is coded to the Administration section.

Transfer procedures using multiple tissue layers

B3.17
The root operation Transfer contains qualifiers that can be used to specify when a transfer flap is composed of more than one tissue layer, such as a musculocutaneous flap. For procedures involving

transfer of multiple tissue layers including skin, subcutaneous tissue, fascia or muscle, the procedure is coded to the body part value that describes the deepest tissue layer in the flap, and the qualifier can be used to describe the other tissue layer(s) in the transfer flap.

Example: A musculocutaneous flap transfer is coded to the appropriate body part value in the body system Muscles, and the qualifier is used to describe the additional tissue layer(s) in the transfer flap.

B4. Body Part

General guidelines

B4.1a
If a procedure is performed on a portion of a body part that does not have a separate body part value, code the body part value corresponding to the whole body part.

Example: A procedure performed on the alveolar process of the mandible is coded to the mandible body part.

B4.1b
If the prefix "peri" is combined with a body part to identify the site of the procedure, and the site of the procedure is not further specified, then the procedure is coded to the body part named. This guideline applies only when a more specific body part value is not available.

Examples: A procedure site identified as perirenal is coded to the kidney body part when the site of the procedure is not further specified.

A procedure site described in the documentation as peri-urethral, and the documentation also indicates that it is the vulvar tissue and not the urethral tissue that is the site of the procedure, then the procedure is coded to the vulva body part.

A procedure site documented as involving the periosteum is coded to the corresponding bone body part.

B4.1c
If a procedure is performed on a continuous section of a tubular body part, code the body part value corresponding to the furthest anatomical site from the point of entry.

Example: A procedure performed on a continuous section of artery from the femoral artery to the external iliac artery with the point of entry at the femoral artery is coded to the external iliac body part.

Branches of body parts

B4.2
Where a specific branch of a body part does not have its own body part value in PCS, the body part is typically coded to the closest proximal branch that has a specific body part value. In the cardiovascular body systems, if a general body part is available in the correct root operation table, and coding to a proximal branch would require assigning a code in a different body system, the procedure is coded using the general body part value.

Examples: A procedure performed on the mandibular branch of the trigeminal nerve is coded to the trigeminal nerve body part value.

Occlusion of the bronchial artery is coded to the body part value Upper Artery in the body system Upper Arteries, and not to the body part value Thoracic Aorta, Descending in the body system Heart and Great Vessels.

Bilateral body part values

B4.3
Bilateral body part values are available for a limited number of body parts. If the identical procedure is performed on contralateral body parts, and a bilateral body part value exists for that body part, a single procedure is coded using the bilateral body part value. If no bilateral body part value exists, each procedure is coded separately using the appropriate body part value.

Examples: The identical procedure performed on both fallopian tubes is coded once using the body part value Fallopian Tube, Bilateral.

The identical procedure performed on both knee joints is coded twice using the body part values Knee Joint, Right and Knee Joint, Left.

Coronary arteries

B4.4
The coronary arteries are classified as a single body part that is further specified by number of arteries treated. One procedure code specifying multiple arteries is used when the same procedure is performed, including the same device and qualifier values.

Examples: Angioplasty of two distinct coronary arteries with placement of two stents is coded as Dilation of Coronary Artery, Two Arteries with Two Intraluminal Devices.

Angioplasty of two distinct coronary arteries, one with stent placed and one without, is coded separately as Dilation of Coronary Artery, One Artery with Intraluminal Device, and Dilation of Coronary Artery, One Artery with no device.

Tendons, ligaments, bursae and fascia near a joint

B4.5
Procedures performed on tendons, ligaments, bursae and fascia supporting a joint are coded to the body part in the respective body system that is the focus of the procedure. Procedures performed on joint structures themselves are coded to the body part in the joint body systems.

Examples: Repair of the anterior cruciate ligament of the knee is coded to the knee bursa and ligament body part in the bursae and ligaments body system.

Knee arthroscopy with shaving of articular cartilage is coded to the knee joint body part in the Lower Joints body system.

Skin, subcutaneous tissue and fascia overlying a joint

B4.6
If a procedure is performed on the skin, subcutaneous tissue or fascia overlying a joint, the procedure is coded to the following body part:

- Shoulder is coded to Upper Arm
- Elbow is coded to Lower Arm
- Wrist is coded to Lower Arm
- Hip is coded to Upper Leg
- Knee is coded to Lower Leg
- Ankle is coded to Foot

Fingers and toes

B4.7
If a body system does not contain a separate body part value for fingers, procedures performed on the fingers are coded to the body part value for the hand. If a body system does not contain a separate body part value for toes, procedures performed on the toes are coded to the body part value for the foot.

Example: Excision of finger muscle is coded to one of the hand muscle body part values in the Muscles body system.

Upper and lower intestinal tract

B4.8
In the Gastrointestinal body system, the general body part values Upper Intestinal Tract and Lower Intestinal Tract are provided as an option for the root operations Change, Inspection, Removal and Revision. Upper Intestinal Tract includes the portion of the gastrointestinal tract from the esophagus down to and including the duodenum, and Lower Intestinal Tract includes the portion of the gastrointestinal tract from the jejunum down to and including the rectum and anus.

Example: In the root operation Change table, change of a device in the jejunum is coded using the body part Lower Intestinal Tract.

B5. Approach

Open approach with percutaneous endoscopic assistance

B5.2
Procedures performed using the open approach with percutaneous endoscopic assistance are coded to the approach Open.

Example: Laparoscopic-assisted sigmoidectomy is coded to the approach Open.

External approach

B5.3a
Procedures performed within an orifice on structures that are visible without the aid of any instrumentation are coded to the approach External.

Example: Resection of tonsils is coded to the approach External.

B5.3b
Procedures performed indirectly by the application of external force through the intervening body layers are coded to the approach External.

Example: Closed reduction of fracture is coded to the approach External.

Percutaneous procedure via device

B5.4
Procedures performed percutaneously via a device placed for the procedure are coded to the approach Percutaneous.

Example: Fragmentation of kidney stone performed via percutaneous nephrostomy is coded to the approach Percutaneous.

B6. Device

General guidelines

B6.1a
A device is coded only if a device remains after the procedure is completed. If no device remains, the device value No Device is coded. In limited root operations, the classification provides the qualifier values Temporary and Intraoperative, for specific procedures involving clinically significant devices, where the purpose of the device is to be utilized for a brief duration during the procedure or current inpatient stay. If a device that is intended to remain after the procedure is completed requires removal before the end of the operative episode in which it was inserted (for example, the device size is inadequate or a complication occurs), both the insertion and removal of the device should be coded.

B6.1b
Materials such as sutures, ligatures, radiological markers and temporary post-operative wound drains are considered integral to the performance of a procedure and are not coded as devices.

B6.1c
Procedures performed on a device only and not on a body part are specified in the root operations Change, Irrigation, Removal and Revision, and are coded to the procedure performed.

Example: Irrigation of percutaneous nephrostomy tube is coded to the root operation Irrigation of indwelling device in the Administration section.

Drainage device

B6.2
A separate procedure to put in a drainage device is coded to the root operation Drainage with the device value Drainage Device.

Obstetrics Section Guidelines (Section 1)

C. Obstetrics Section

Products of conception

C1
Procedures performed on the products of conception are coded to the Obstetrics section. Procedures performed on the pregnant female other than the products of conception are coded to the appropriate root operation in the Medical and Surgical section.

Example: Amniocentesis is coded to the products of conception body part in the Obstetrics section. Repair of obstetric urethral laceration is coded to the urethra body part in the Medical and Surgical section.

Procedures following delivery or abortion

C2
Procedures performed following a delivery or abortion for curettage of the endometrium or evacuation of retained products of conception are all coded in the Obstetrics section, to the root operation Extraction and the body part Products of Conception, Retained.

Diagnostic or therapeutic dilation and curettage performed during times other than the postpartum or post-abortion period are all coded in the Medical and Surgical section, to the root operation Extraction and the body part Endometrium.

Radiation Therapy Section Guidelines (Section D)

D. Radiation Therapy Section

Brachytherapy

D1.a
Brachytherapy is coded to the modality Brachytherapy in the Radiation Therapy section. When a radioactive brachytherapy source is left in the body at the end of the procedure, it is coded separately to the root operation Insertion with the device value Radioactive Element.

Example: Brachytherapy with implantation of a low dose rate brachytherapy source left in the body at the end of the procedure is coded to the applicable treatment site in section D, Radiation Therapy, with the modality Brachytherapy, the modality qualifier value Low Dose Rate, and the applicable isotope value and qualifier value. The implantation of the brachytherapy source is coded separately to the device value Radioactive Element in the appropriate Insertion table of the Medical and Surgical section. The Radiation Therapy section code identifies the specific modality and isotope of the brachytherapy, and the root operation Insertion code identifies the implantation of the brachytherapy source that remains in the body at the end of the procedure.

Exception: Implantation of Cesium-131 brachytherapy seeds embedded in a collagen matrix to the treatment site after resection of brain tumor is coded to the root operation Insertion with the device value Radioactive Element, Cesium-131 Collagen Implant. The procedure is coded to the root operation Insertion only, because the device value identifies both the implantation of the radioactive element and a specific brachytherapy isotope that is not included in the Radiation Therapy section tables.

D1.b
A separate procedure to place a temporary applicator for delivering the brachytherapy is coded to the root operation Insertion and the device value Other Device.

Examples: Intrauterine brachytherapy applicator placed as a separate procedure from the brachytherapy procedure is coded to Insertion of Other Device, and the brachytherapy is coded separately using the modality Brachytherapy in the Radiation Therapy section.

Intrauterine brachytherapy applicator placed concomitantly with delivery of the brachytherapy dose is coded with a single code using the modality Brachytherapy in the Radiation Therapy section.

New Technology Section Guidelines (Section X)

E. New Technology Section

General guidelines

E1.a
Section X codes fully represent the specific procedure described in the code title, and do not require additional codes from other sections of ICD-10-PCS. When section X contains a code title which fully describes a specific new technology procedure, and it is the only procedure performed, only the section X code is reported for the procedure.

There is no need to report an additional code in another section of ICD-10-PCS.

Example: XW04321 Introduction of Ceftazidime-Avibactam Anti-infective into Central Vein, Percutaneous Approach, New Technology Group 1, can be coded to indicate that Ceftazidime-Avibactam Anti-infective was administered via a central vein. A separate code from table 3E0 in the Administration section of ICD-10-PCS is not coded in addition to this code.

E1.b
When multiple procedures are performed, New Technology section X codes are coded following the multiple procedures guideline.

Examples: Dual filter cerebral embolic filtration used during transcatheter aortic valve replacement (TAVR), X2A5312 Cerebral Embolic Filtration, Dual Filter in Innominate Artery and Left Common Carotid Artery, Percutaneous Approach, New Technology Group 2, is coded for the cerebral embolic filtration, along with an ICD-10-PCS code for the TAVR procedure.

Magnetically controlled growth rod (MCGR) placed during a spinal fusion procedure, a code from table XNS, Reposition of the Bones is coded for the MCGR, along with an ICD-10-PCS code for the spinal fusion procedure.

F. Selection of Principal Procedure

The following instructions should be applied in the selection of principal procedure and clarification on the importance of the relation to the principal diagnosis when more than one procedure is performed:

1. Procedure performed for definitive treatment of both principal diagnosis and secondary diagnosis
   a. Sequence procedure performed for definitive treatment most related to principal diagnosis as principal procedure.
2. Procedure performed for definitive treatment and diagnostic procedures performed for both principal diagnosis and secondary diagnosis.
   a. Sequence procedure performed for definitive treatment most related to principal diagnosis as principal procedure
3. A diagnostic procedure was performed for the principal diagnosis and a procedure is performed for definitive treatment of a secondary diagnosis.
   a. Sequence diagnostic procedure as principal procedure, since the procedure most related to the principal diagnosis takes precedence.
4. No procedures performed that are related to principal diagnosis; procedures performed for definitive treatment and diagnostic procedures were performed for secondary diagnosis
   a. Sequence procedure performed for definitive treatment of secondary diagnosis as principal procedure, since there are no procedures (definitive or nondefinitive treatment) related to principal diagnosis.

This page intentionally left blank

Anatomical Illustrations

Circulatory System — Arteries and Veins

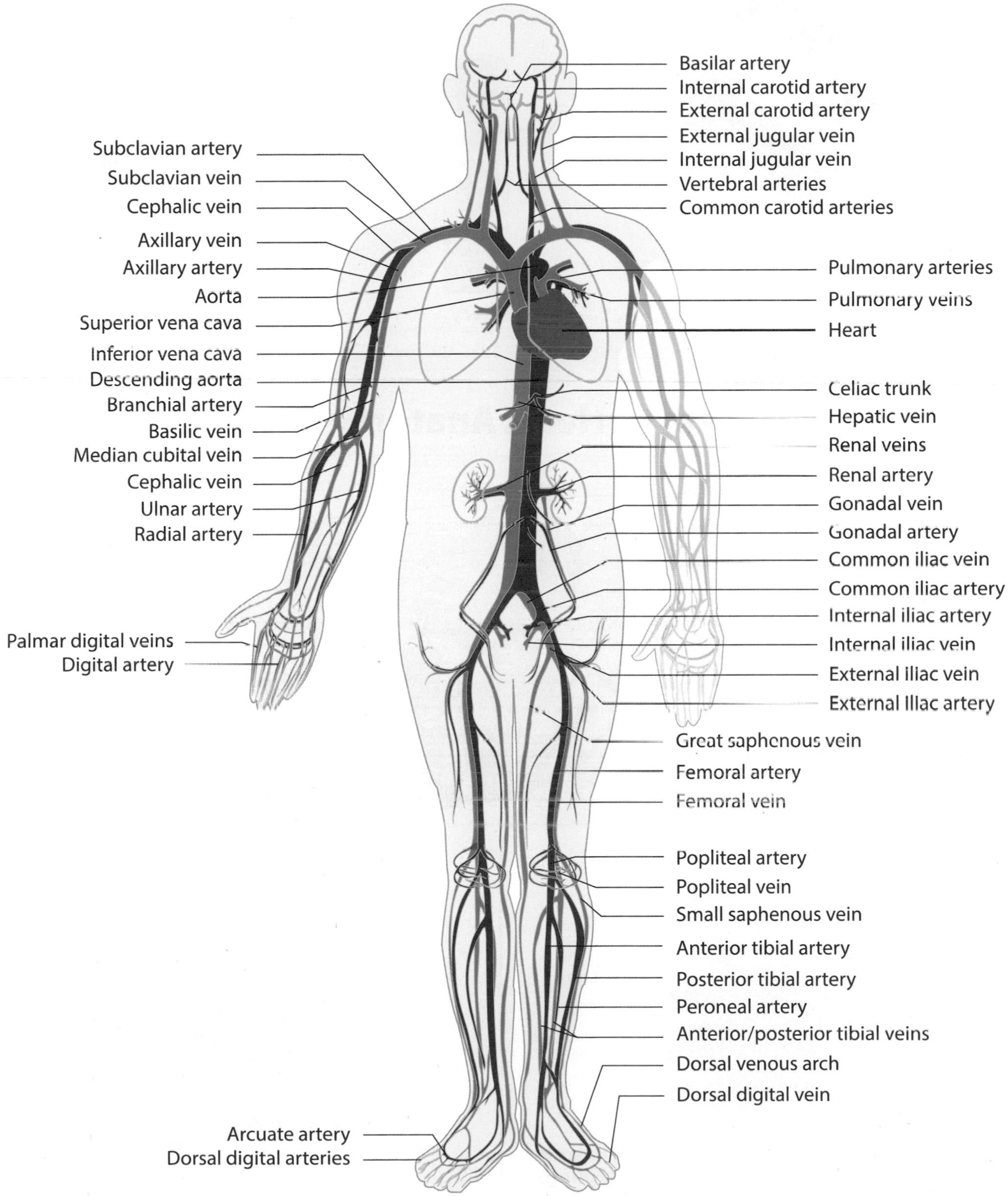

Basilar artery
Internal carotid artery
External carotid artery
External jugular vein
Internal jugular vein
Vertebral arteries
Common carotid arteries
Subclavian artery
Subclavian vein
Cephalic vein
Axillary vein
Axillary artery
Aorta
Superior vena cava
Inferior vena cava
Descending aorta
Branchial artery
Basilic vein
Median cubital vein
Cephalic vein
Ulnar artery
Radial artery
Pulmonary arteries
Pulmonary veins
Heart
Celiac trunk
Hepatic vein
Renal veins
Renal artery
Gonadal vein
Gonadal artery
Common iliac vein
Common iliac artery
Internal iliac artery
Internal iliac vein
External iliac vein
External Illac artery
Palmar digital veins
Digital artery
Great saphenous vein
Femoral artery
Femoral vein
Popliteal artery
Popliteal vein
Small saphenous vein
Anterior tibial artery
Posterior tibial artery
Peroneal artery
Anterior/posterior tibial veins
Dorsal venous arch
Dorsal digital vein
Arcuate artery
Dorsal digital arteries

Circulatory System — Artery and Vein Anatomy

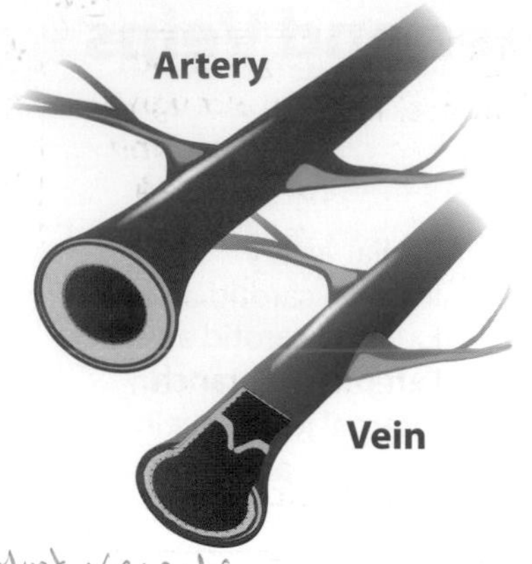

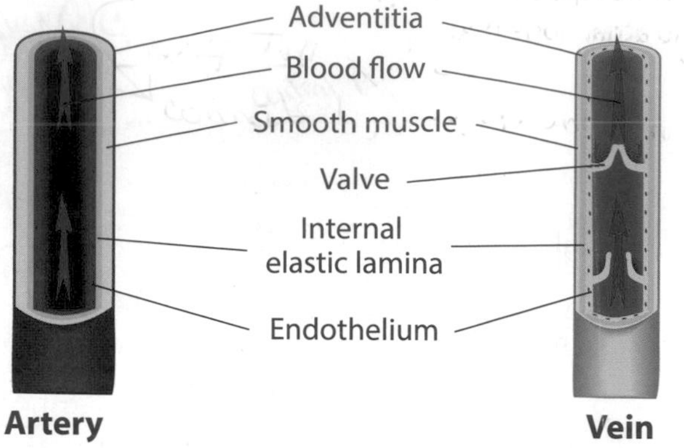

3 types blood vessels
1 arteries - blood away from heart
2. veins - carry blood to heart
3. capillaries - connect arteries to veins

Circulatory System — Heart Anatomy and Cardiac Cycle

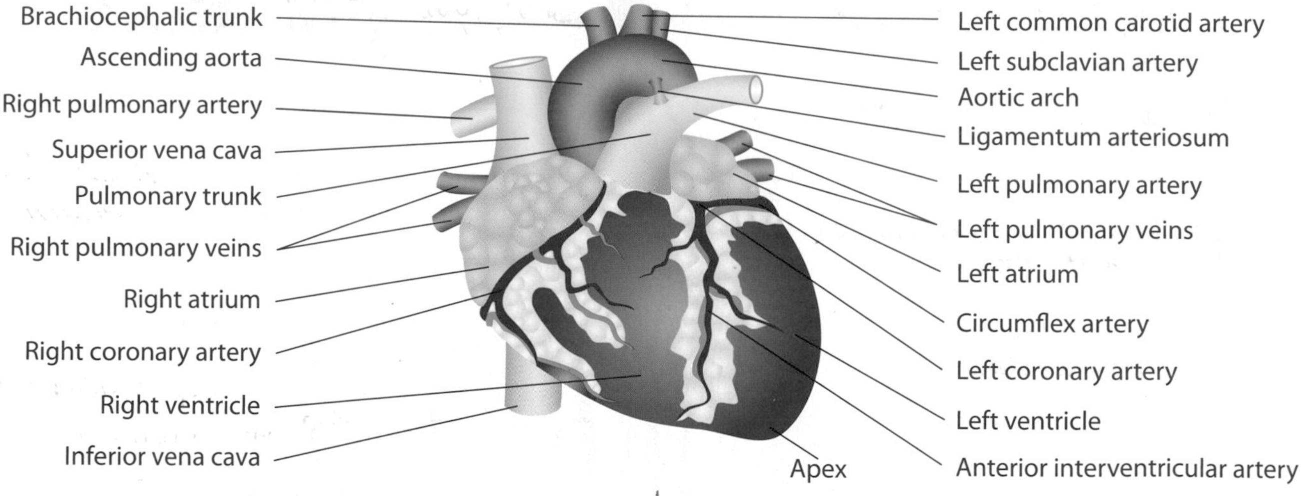

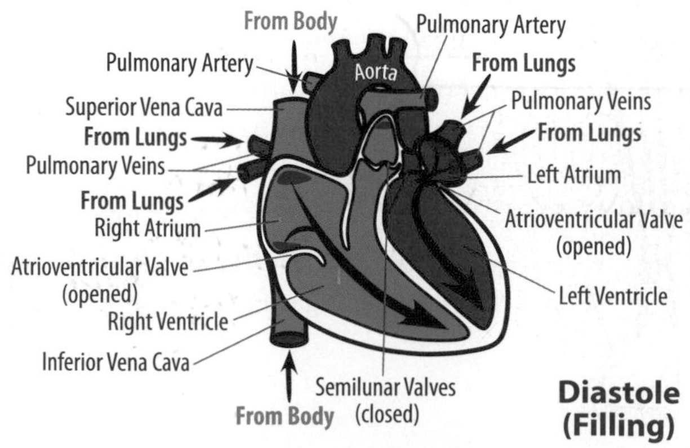

Diastole (Filling)

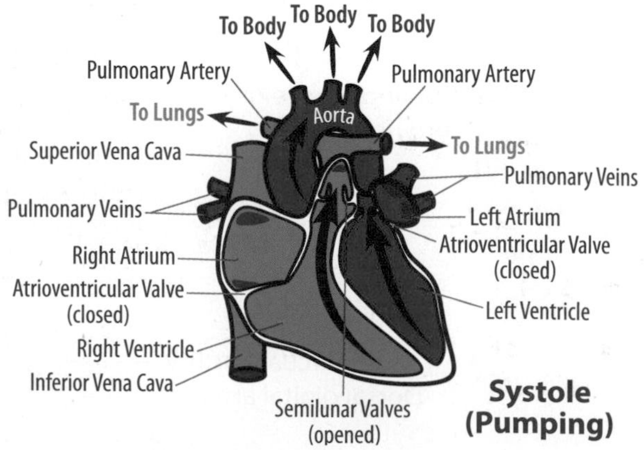

Systole (Pumping)

coronary arteries - branch off aorta

Cardiac

Electrical Conducting System of the Heart

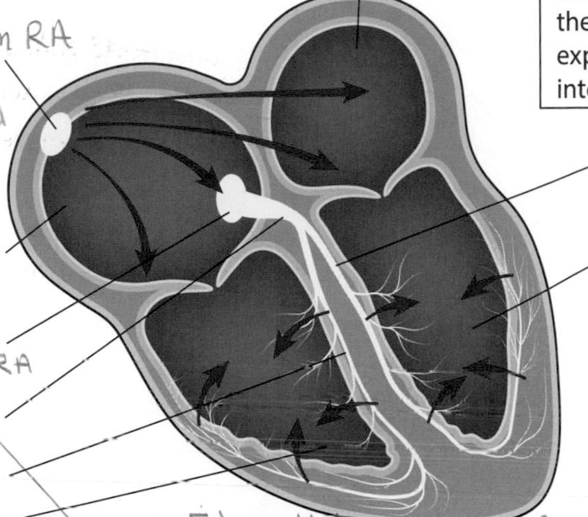

PATHWAY of pacemaker cells - conduction system
create impulse
1) SA node
2) AV node
3) HIS Bundle - muscle fibers
4) Purkinje fibers - end of bundle branches
impulses generated produce electrical currents,
detected by electrodes & record on ECG

Fibrous pericardium - outer layer
Serous pericardium - deepest layer
Serous further divided into parietal
& Viseral is AKA epicardium
Viseral

SA node fires & sends
the impulse from
the pacemaker through
the R & L atria
causing contraction

Left atrium

Electrical impulse spreads from sinus node throughout left and right atria causing the atria to contract and expelling its volume of blood into the ventricles

PACEMAKER in RA
Sino atrial node (SA)
Sets the pace of the heart generating electrical impulses between 60-100 times/minute

Right atrium

Left bundle branch

Left ventricle

Atrioventricular node (AV)
in lower septal wall of RA
slows the impulse conduction down between the atria & ventricles to allow time for the atria to fill w/ blood before the ventricles contract

Bundle of his

Right bundle branch

Right ventricle

muscle fibers that branch off to the left & right

Electrical impulse spreads from bundle branches throughout left and right ventricles which causes the ventricles to contract, forcing them to expel their volume of blood out into the general circulation

Purkinje fibers - cause the ventricles (2 lower chambers of the heart) to create synchronized contractions, located in the sub endocardium

The Pathway of Blood Flow Through the Heart

4 Heart Valves
- Atrioventricular Valves - AV
• mitral - AKA bi cuspid = Left AV
• tri cuspid = right AV
- Semilunar Valves SL
• aortic & • pulmonary
leave the heart - do not have chordae tendineae

upper chambers are atria & receive blood
lower chambers are ventricles & pump blood out
upper chambers = ATRIA
lower chambers = ventricles

between LV & aorta
LV aorta
aorta

pericardium - outside layer
inside is fibrous & serous pericardium
inside serous is parietal & Viseral
Viseral contacts w/ the heart, called epicardium

Aorta (to body)

Aortic valve

Left pulmonary artery (to left lung)

Superior vena cava (from upper body)

Right pulmonary artery (to right lung)

Left pulmonary veins (from left lung)

mitral valve between LA & LV
AKA
Left AV valve *AKA biscuspid between LV & aorta*

Left atrium

biscuspid/mitral opening of LV

tricuspid valve between RA & RV
AKA - RAV
mitral valve

pulmonary SL at beginning of PA

aorta SL at beginning of aorta

Right pulmonary veins (from right lung)

Right atrium

Right AV valve
AKA triscuspid

Inferior vena cava (from lower body)

Pulmonary valve

between RV & pulmonary artery

Right ventricle

Left ventricle *MAIN pumping chamber*

4 primary coronary arteries
1) R main
2) L main
3) L circumflex
4) LAD
may also include
5) Ramus Intermedius

L & R coronary arteries flow from the aorta. L coronary branches into L circumflex & LAD artery

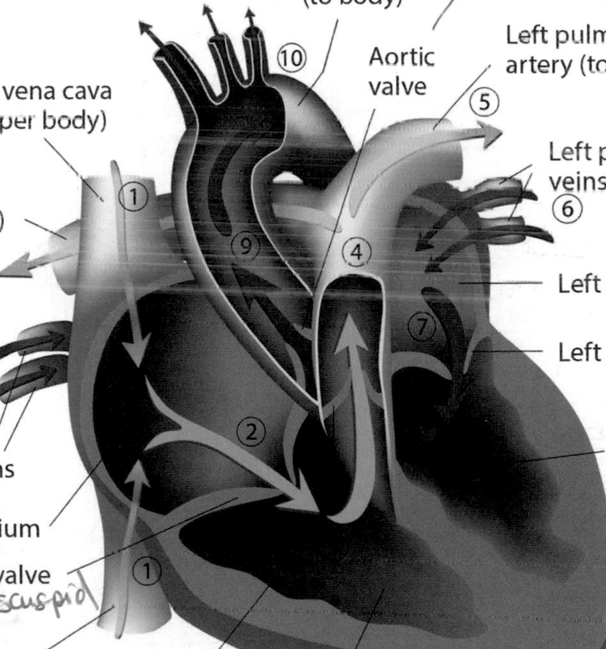

digestive tract - AKA Alimentary Canal
food moves by peristalsis

Digestive System Anatomy

peritoneal cavity —
space between
parietal peritoneum
(surrounds the abdominal
wall) + visceral peritoneum
that surrounds
the internal
organs

nasopharynx = epipharynx
oropharynx = mesopharynx
laryngopharynx = hypopharynx

part of digestive & respiratory
3 parts - nasopharynx,
oropharynx, laryngopharynx

connects by laryngopharynx

cholecyst —

in small intestine!
digestive enzymes
from pancreas &
gallbladder (bile)
mix together
enzymes break down proteins
bile emulsifies fat into micelles

Mouth
- Palate
- Uvula
- Tongue
- Teeth

Pharynx —
Esophagus

Liver
Gallbladder
Common bile duct

Stomach
Pancreas
Pancreatic duct

Small intestine
- Duodenum
- Jejunum
- Ileum

Large intestine
- Transverse colon
- Ascending colon
- Cecum
- Descending colon
- Sigmoid colon
- Rectum

Appendix
Anus

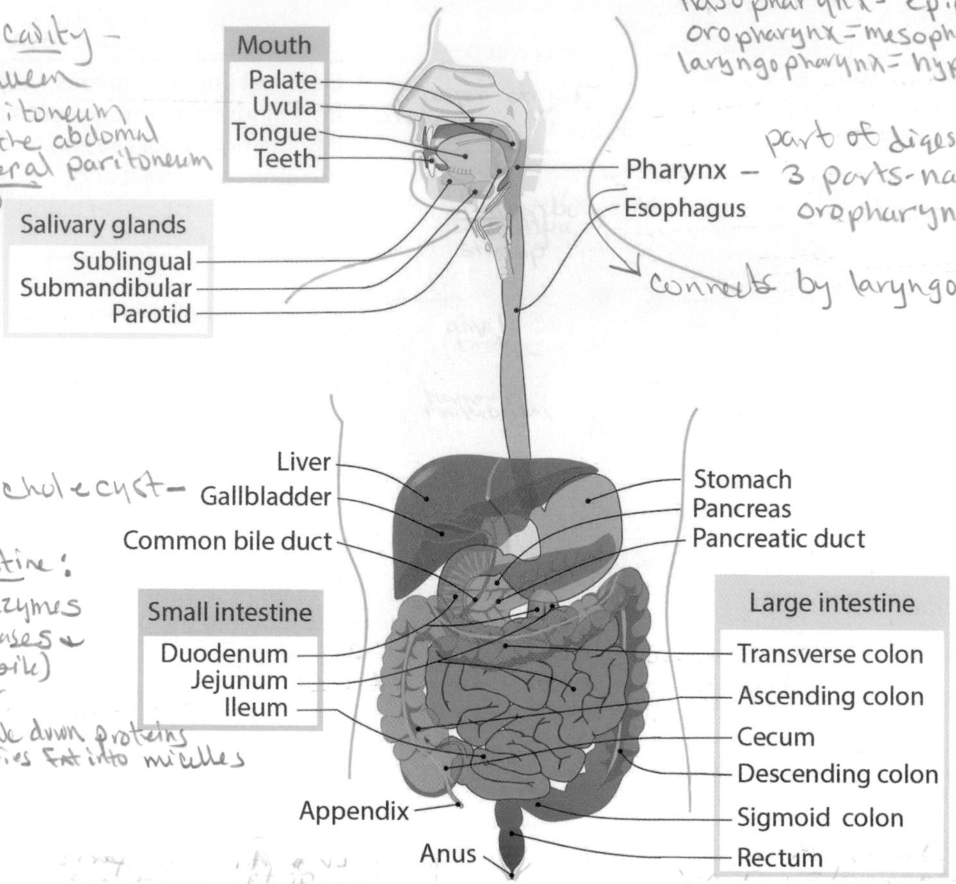

Title: Diagram of the gastrointestinal tract, **Author:** Mariana Ruiz (Lady of Hats), Jmarchn, **Source:** Own work, **License:** Public domain, **URL link:** https://en.wikiversity.org/wiki/File:Digestive_system_diagram_en.svg

Digestive System — Liver, Gallbladder, Pancreas

Liver
· makes bile
· stores/allows glucose into blood
· takes proteins/fats &
· turns it into glucose
· makes some fat & cholesterol
· metabolizes many things
· stores vitamins & minerals
· makes proteins

hemoglobin
proteins like insulin,
serum amyloid A,
ammonia, toxins

cholecyst

Pancreas
· releases substances through
cells called
islets of langerhans
· breaks down carbs, fats
& proteins
· releases hormones & enzymes
to aid digestion

Liver
Gallbladder

Right and left hepatic ducts
Cystic duct
Common hepatic duct
Bile duct
Accessory pancreatic duct
Pancreatic duct
Tail of pancreas
Body of pancreas
Head of pancreas

Minor duodenal papilla
Major duodenal papilla
Duodenum

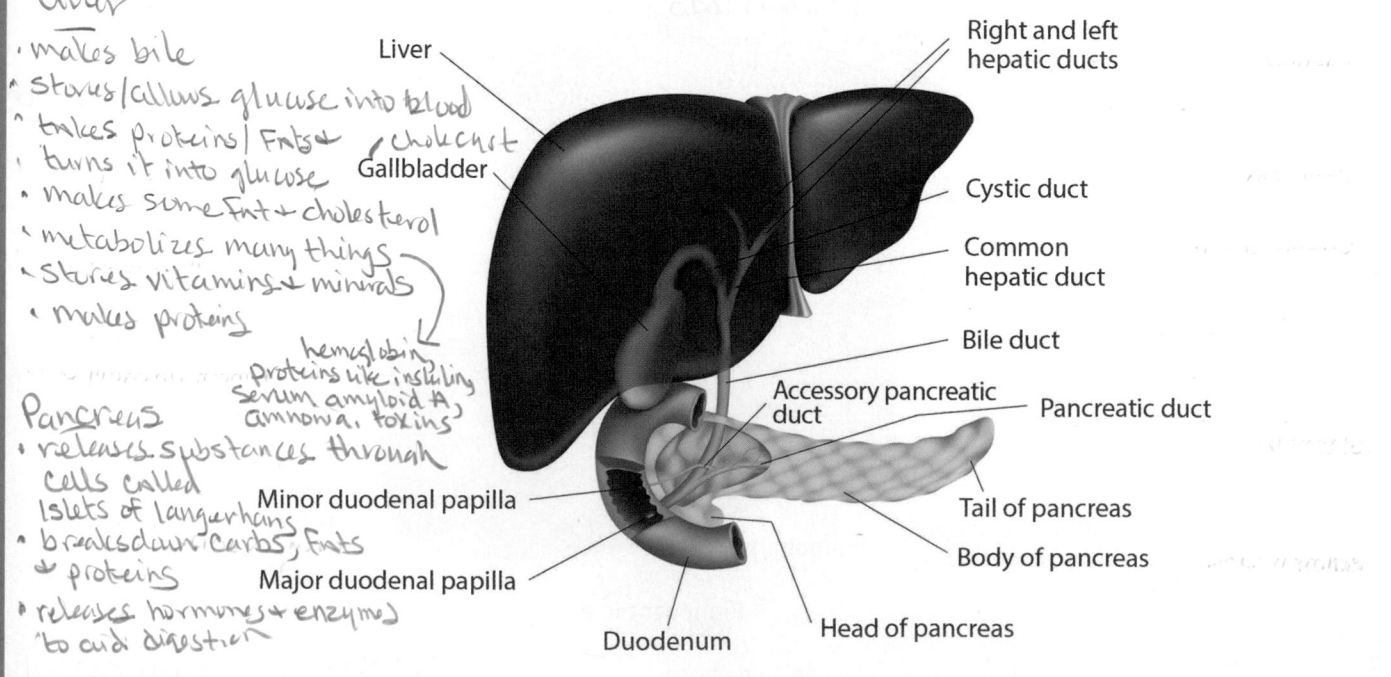

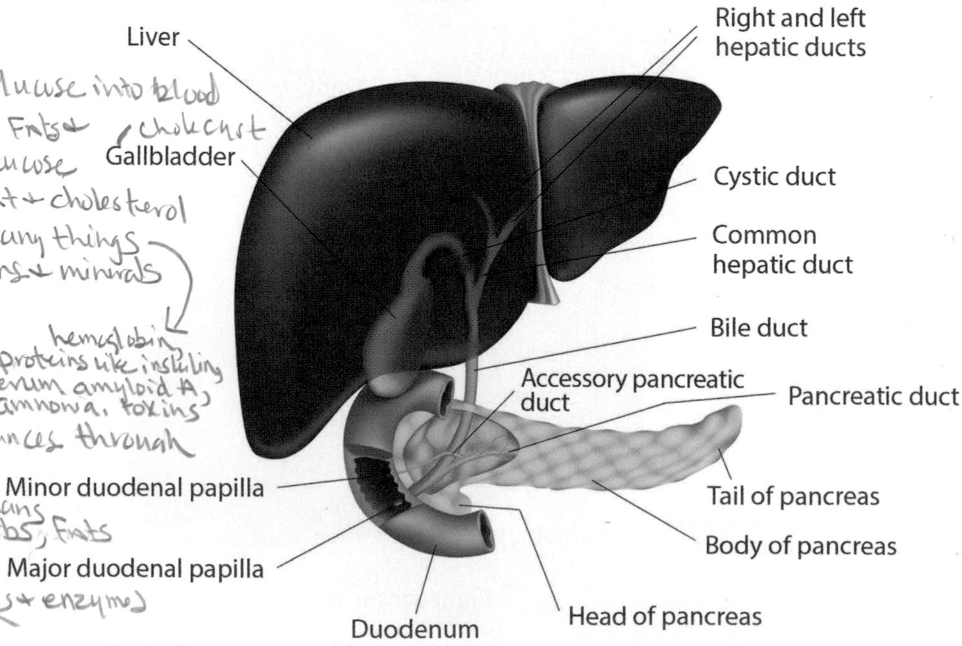

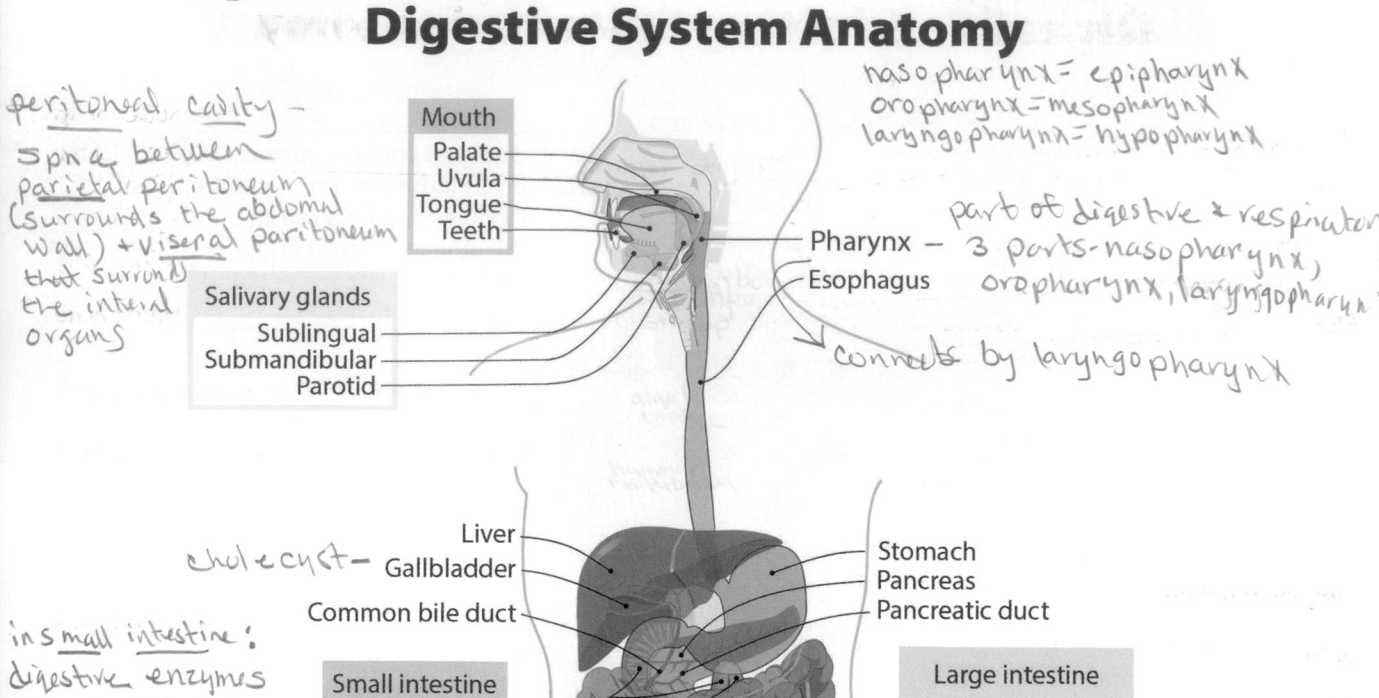

Digestive System — Mouth Anatomy

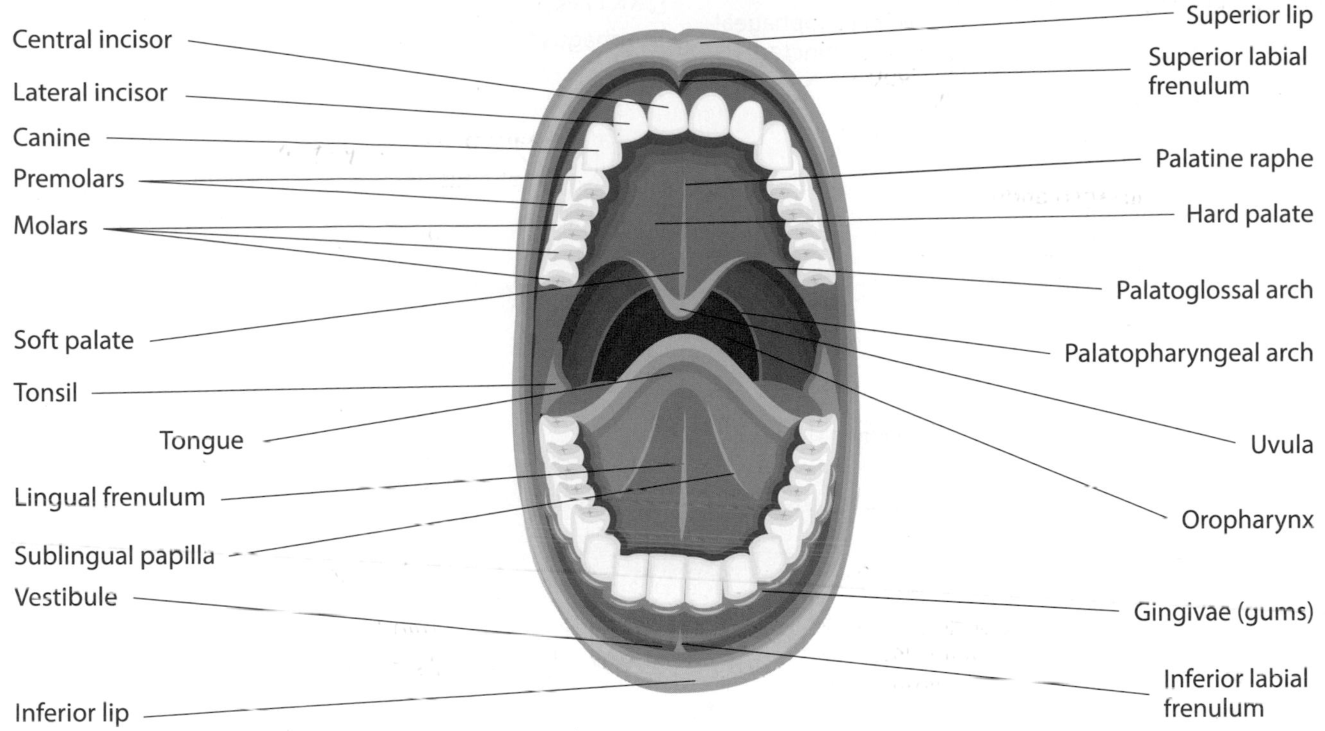

pharyngeal tonsils = adenoids

Digestive System — Tongue Anatomy

closes over glottis to prevent aspiration

pharyngeal tonsils - AKA adenoids in naso pharynx AKA epi pharynx

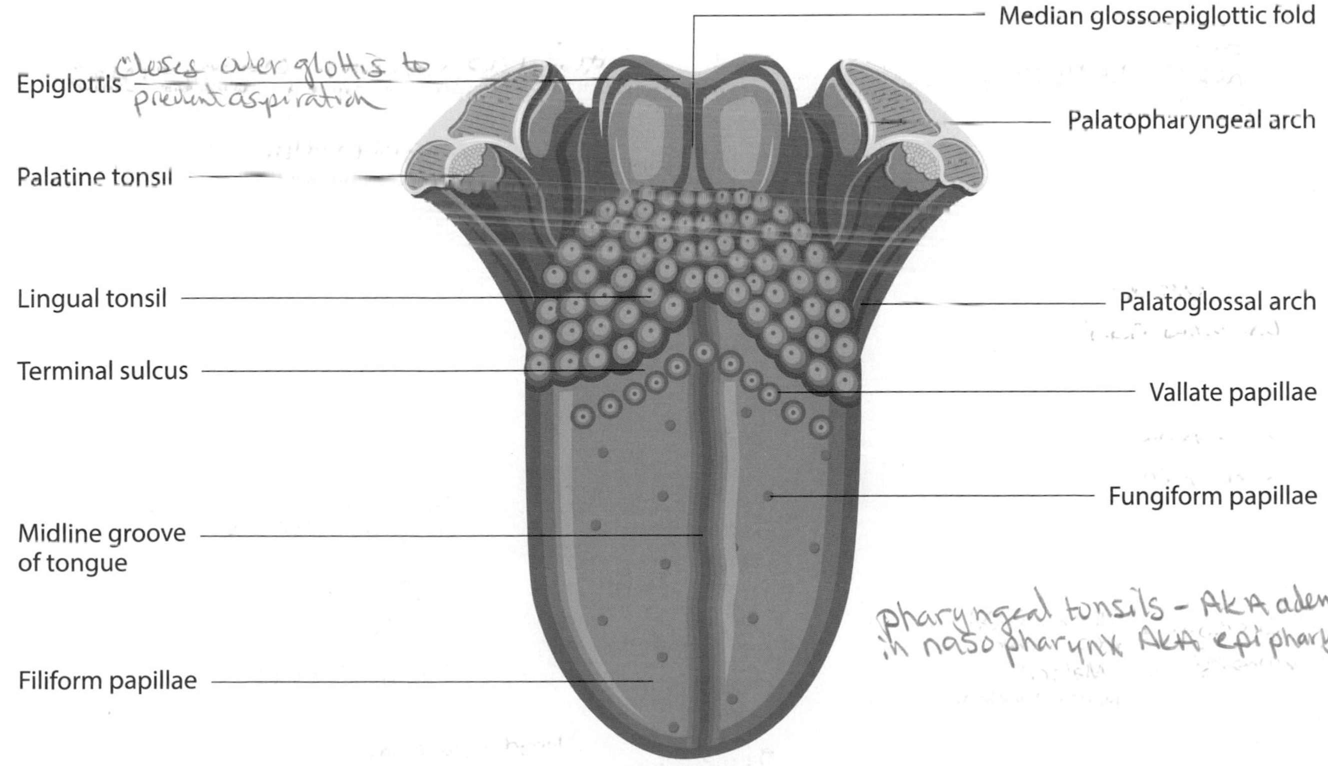

Digestive System — Stomach Anatomy

in stomach - enzymes mix w/Food into chyme

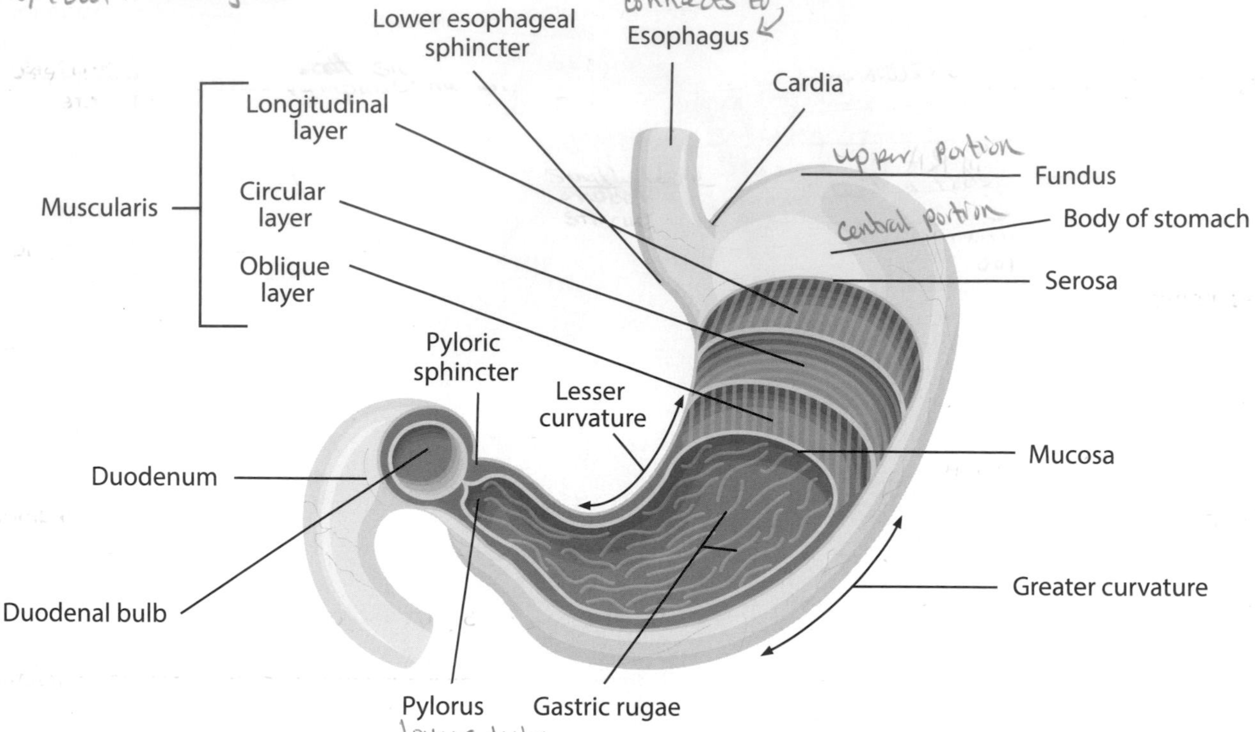

Digestive System — Small Intestine Anatomy

duodenum
jejunum
ileum

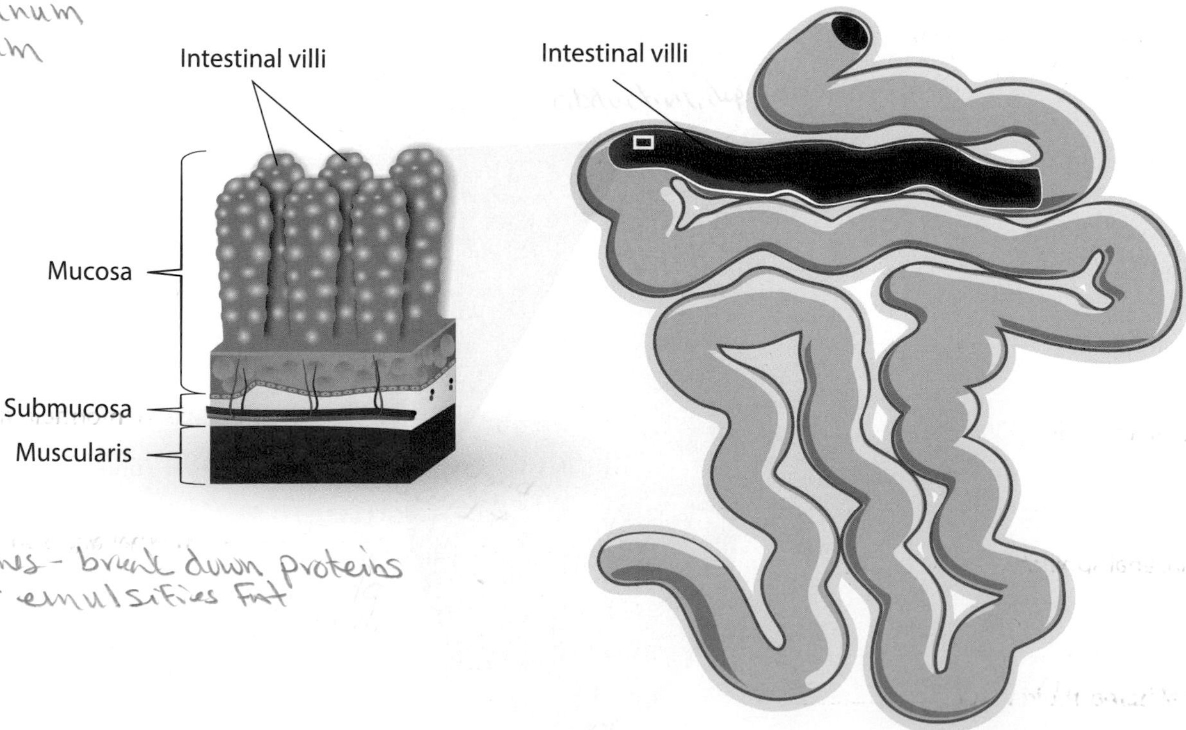

enzymes - break down proteins
bile - emulsifies Fat

also called colon - processes waste

Digestive System — Large Intestine Anatomy

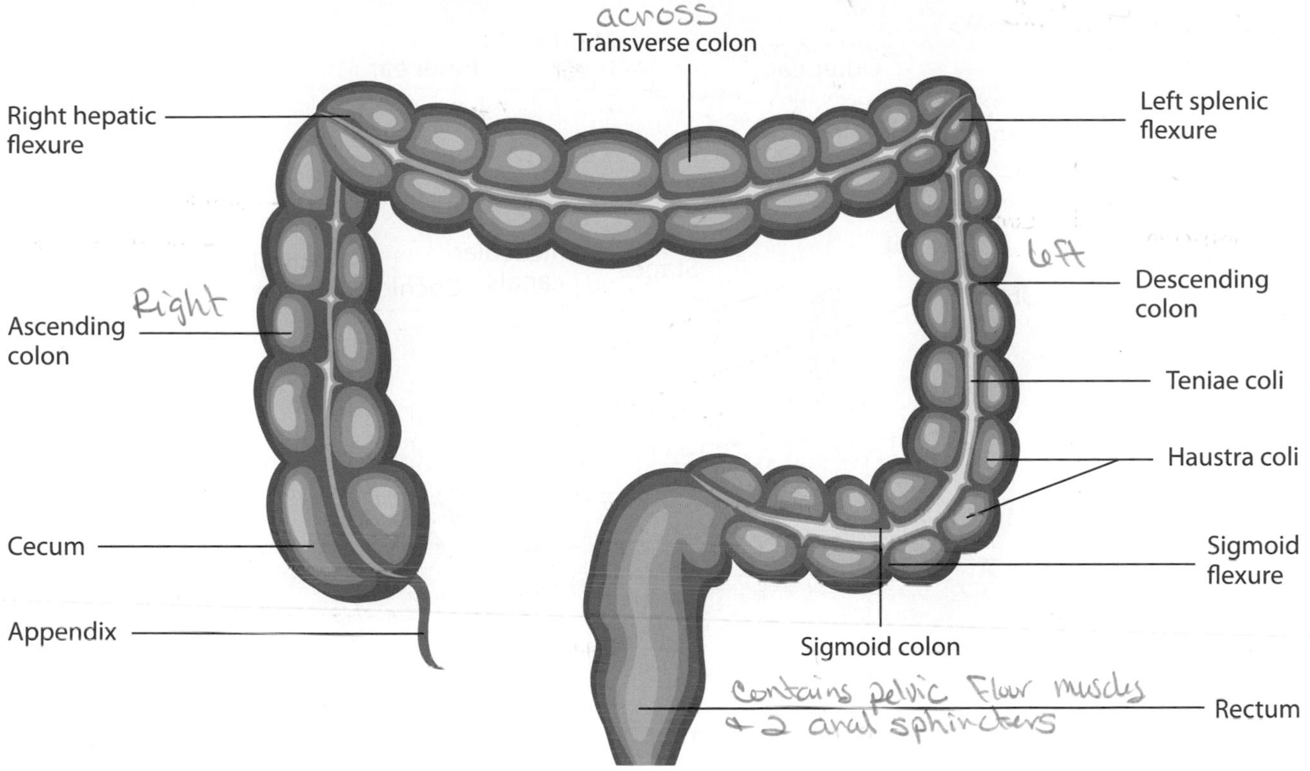

Digestive System — Rectum Anatomy

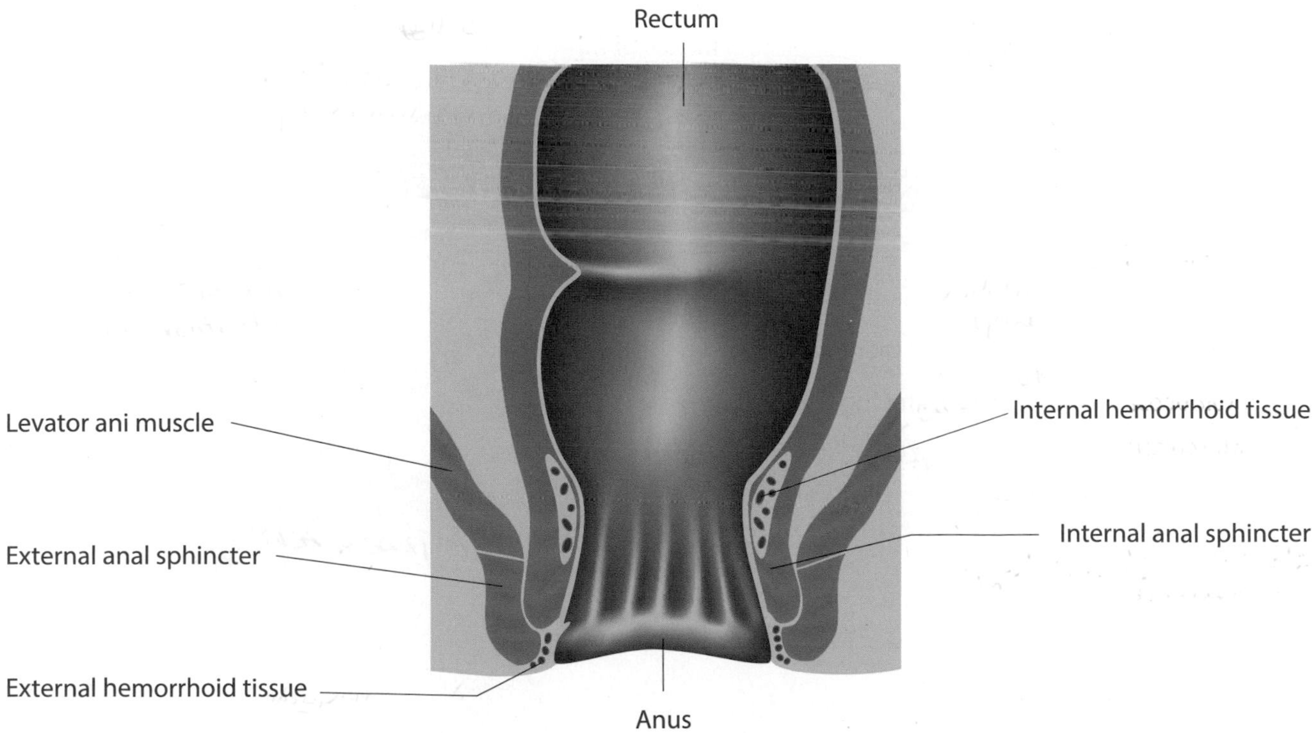

bones = ossicles

middle ear - air filled cavity behind tympanic membrane
opening of eustachian tube is in the middle ear

Ear Anatomy

tympanic membrane moves → malleus → incus → stapes footplate pushes on oval window causing movement of fluid w/in cochlea

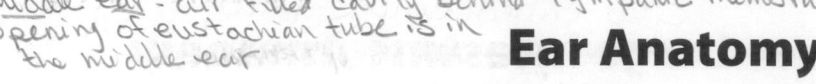

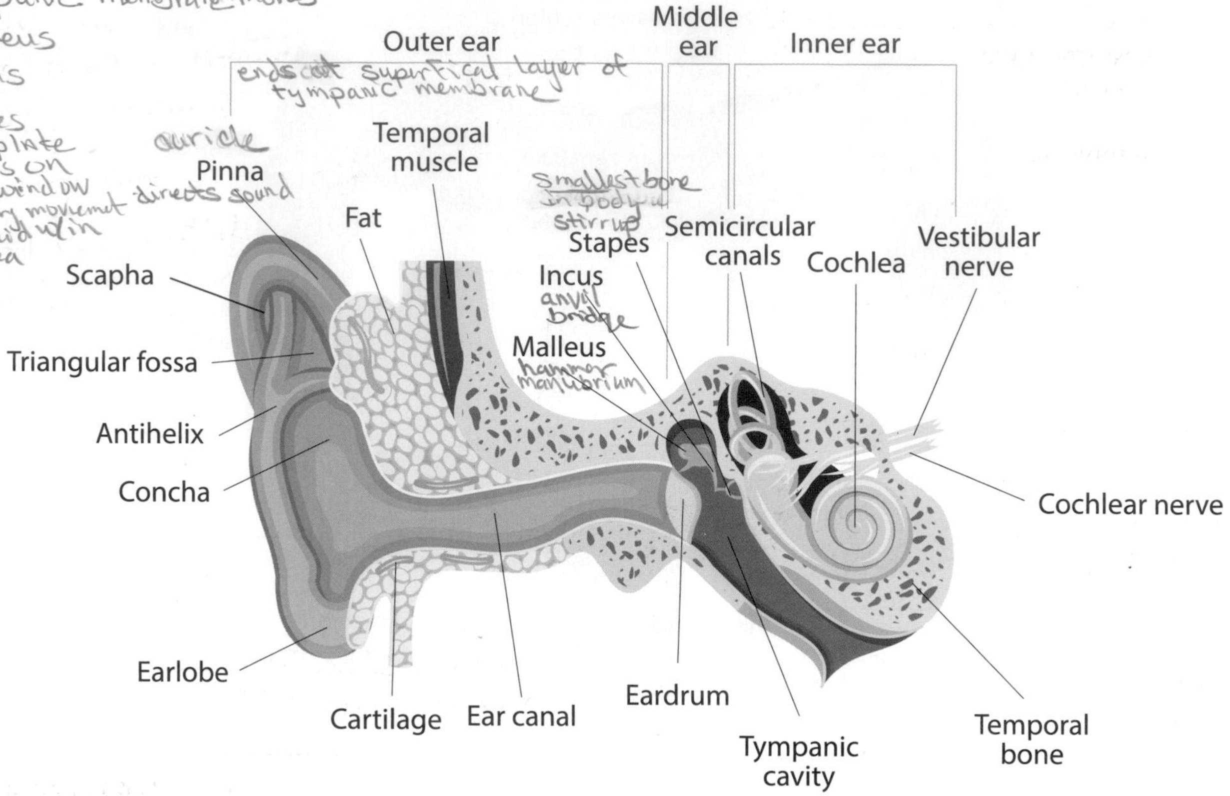

Ear Anatomy - Cochlea (Inner Ear)

attuned to the effects of gravity + motion

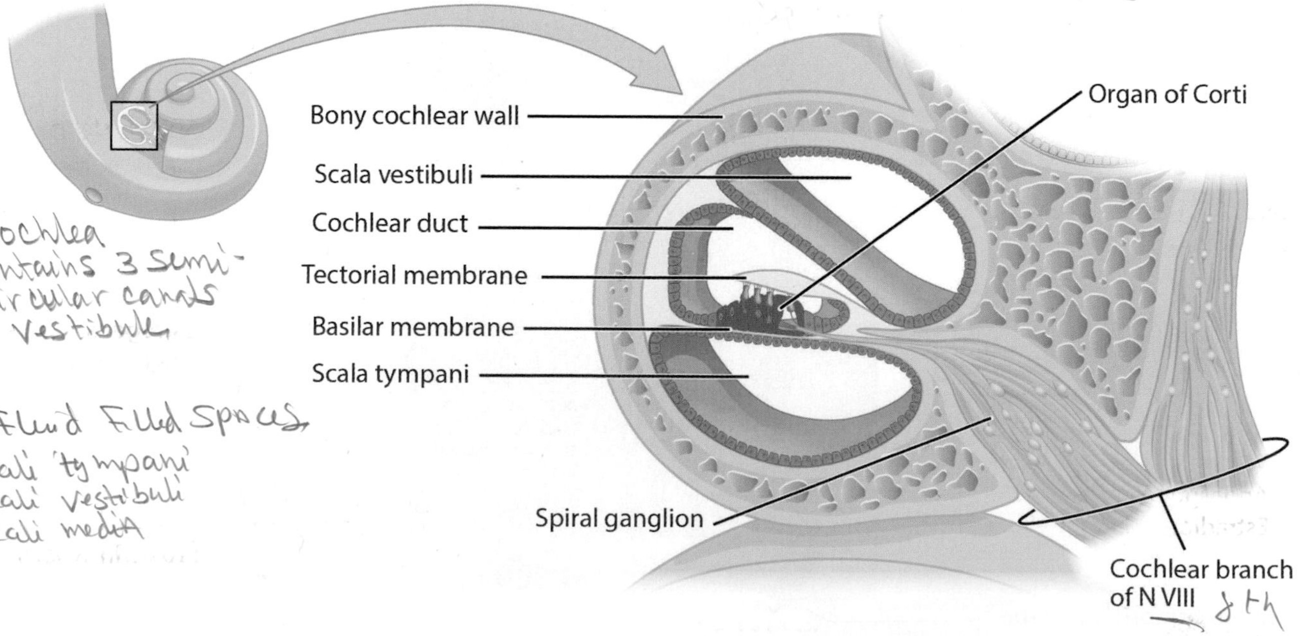

Cochlea contains 3 semi-circular canals + vestibule

3 fluid filled spaces
scali tympani
scali vestibuli
scali media

Title: 1406 Cochlea.jpg, **Author:** OpenStax, **Source:** https://cnx.org/contents/FPtK1zmh@8.25:fEI3C8Ot@10/Preface, **License/Permission:** This file is licensed under the Creative Commons Attribution 4.0 International license., **URL link:** https://en.wikiversity.org/wiki/File:1406_Cochlea.jpg

Endocrine System Anatomy and Hormones

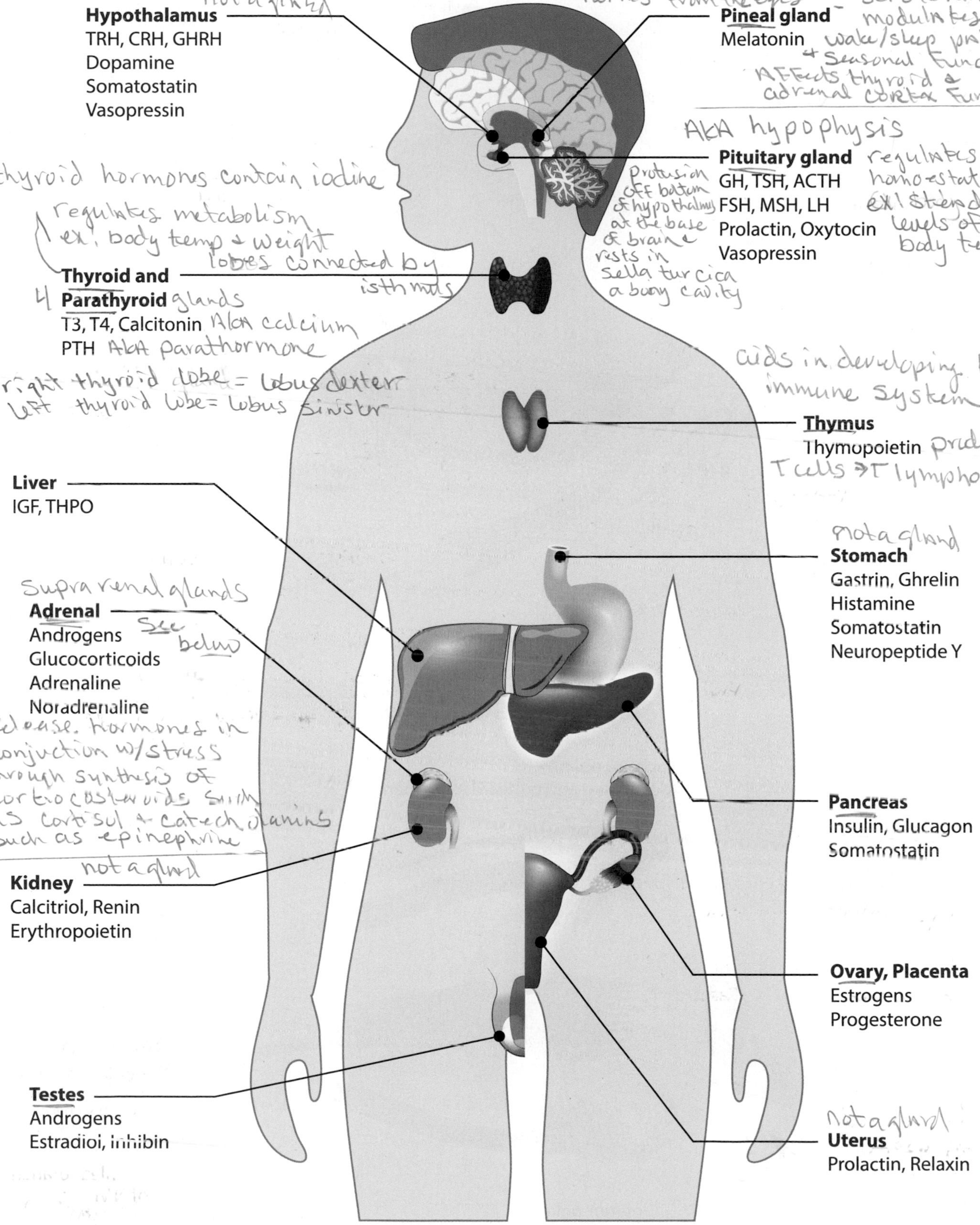
Hypothalamus
TRH, CRH, GHRH
Dopamine
Somatostatin
Vasopressin
Pineal gland
Melatonin
Pituitary gland
GH, TSH, ACTH
FSH, MSH, LH
Prolactin, Oxytocin
Vasopressin
Thyroid and Parathyroid
T3, T4, Calcitonin
PTH
Thymus
Thymopoietin
Liver
IGF, THPO
Stomach
Gastrin, Ghrelin
Histamine
Somatostatin
Neuropeptide Y
Adrenal
Androgens
Glucocorticoids
Adrenaline
Noradrenaline
Pancreas
Insulin, Glucagon
Somatostatin
Kidney
Calcitriol, Renin
Erythropoietin
Ovary, Placenta
Estrogens
Progesterone
Testes
Androgens
Estradiol, Inhibin
Uterus
Prolactin, Relaxin

diaphragm - regulates light intensity

Eye Anatomy

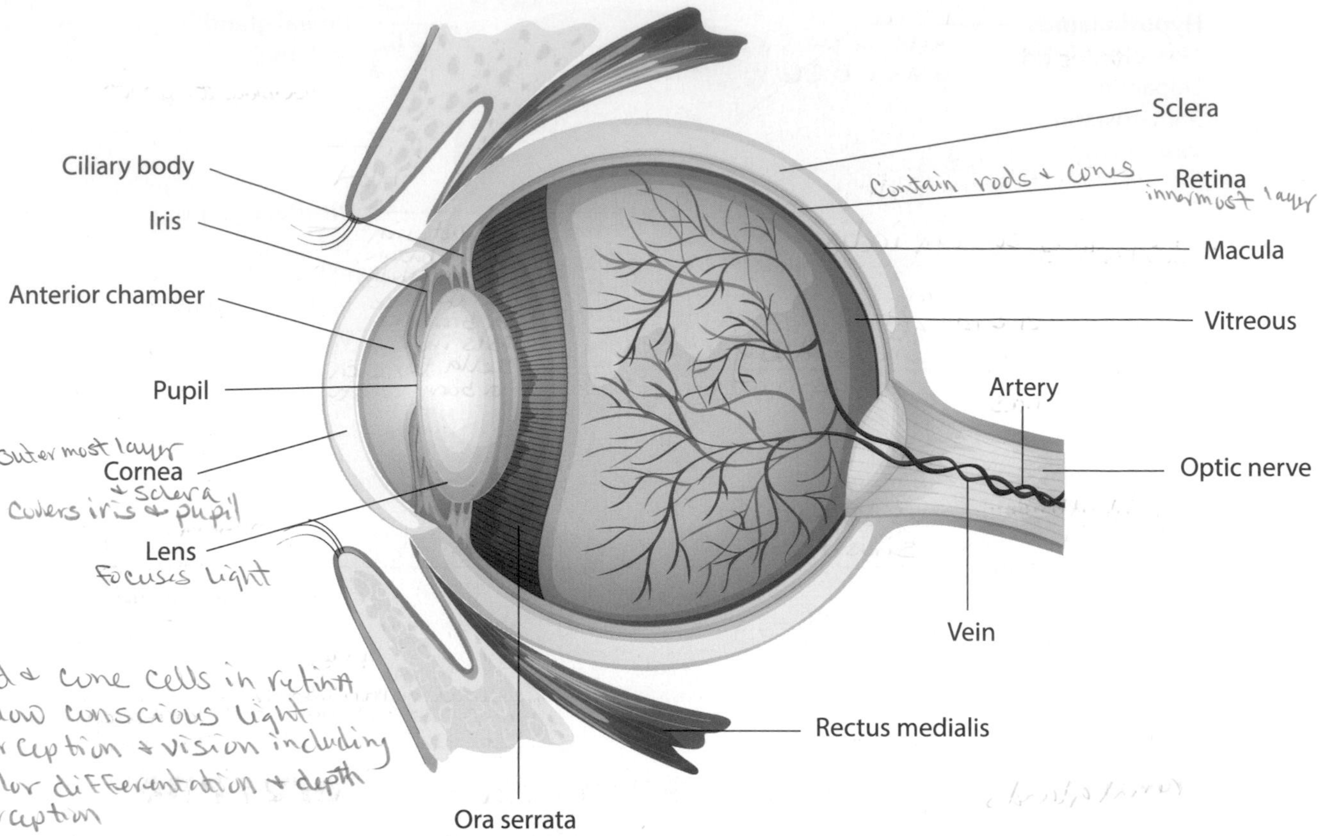

rod & cone cells in retina allow conscious light perception & vision including color differentation & depth perception

adduction - towards the midline

abduction - away from the midline of the body

Eye Musculature

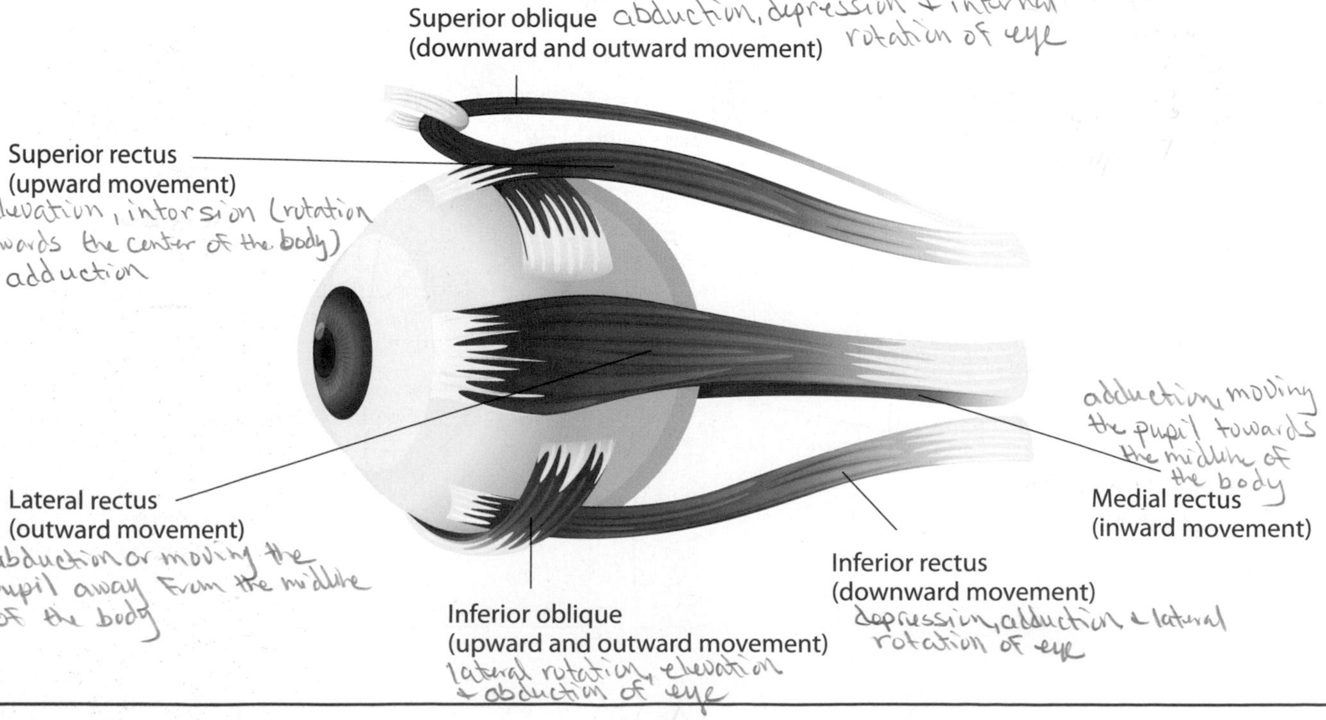

Female Reproductive System Anatomy

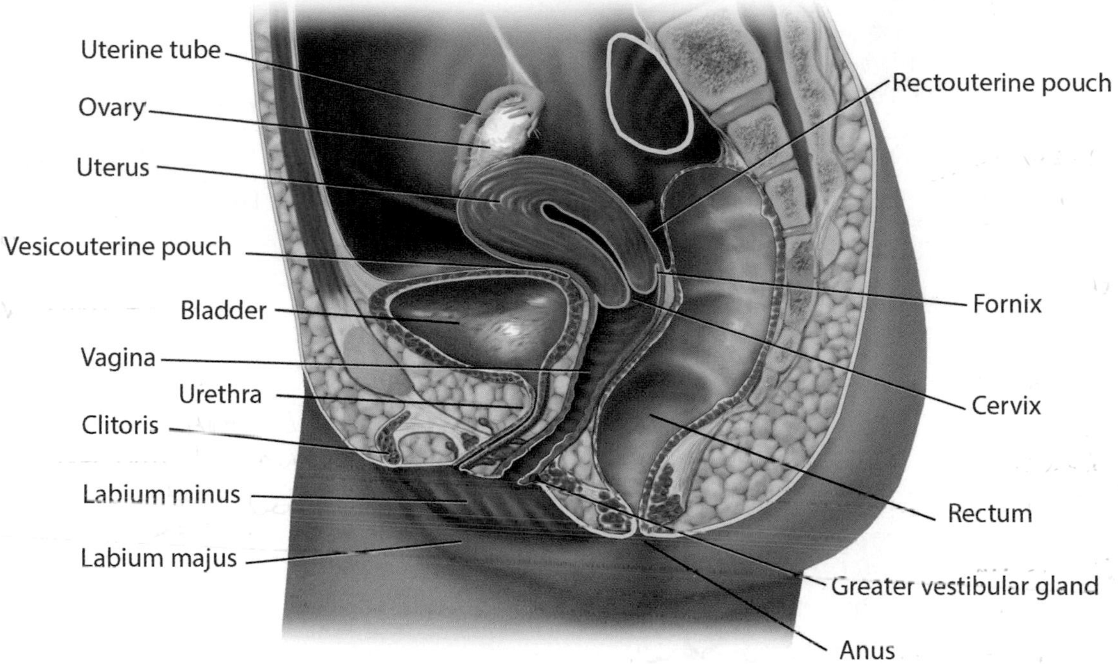

Title: Blausen 0400 FemaleReproSystem 02b.png, **Author:** BruceBlaus., **Source:** Blausen.com staff (2014). "Medical gallery of Blausen Medical 2014". *WikiJournal of Medicine* **1** (2). DOI:10.15347/wjm/2014.010. ISSN 2002-4436.Modified by User:ArnoldReinhold who released mods under CC0, **License/Permission:** This file is licensed under the Creative Commons Attribution 3.0 Unported license., **URL link:** https://commons.wikimedia.org/wiki/File:Blausen_0400_FemaleReproSystem_02b.png

Female Reproductive System — Uterus and Adnexa Anatomy

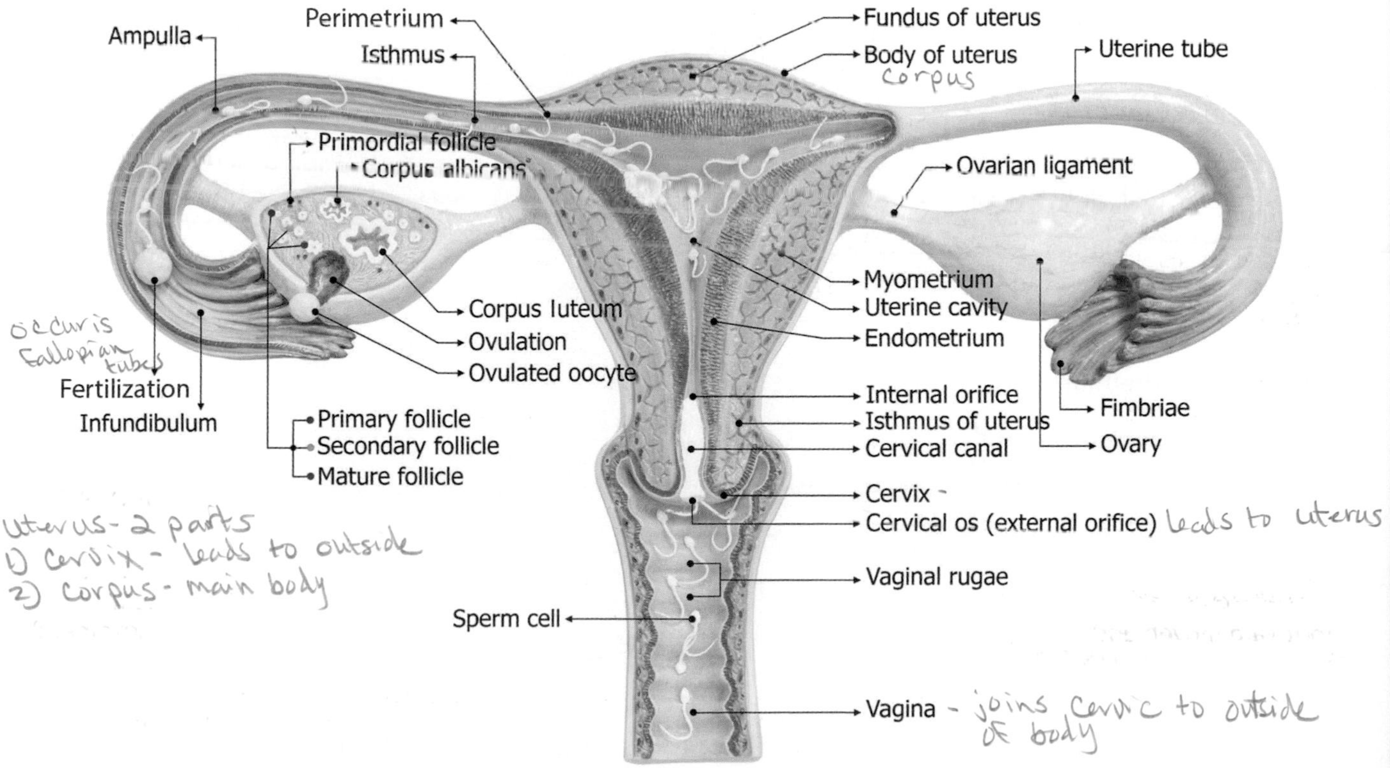

uterus - 2 parts
1) cervix - leads to outside
2) corpus - main body

Female Reproductive System — Breast Anatomy

Breasts are modified sweat glands

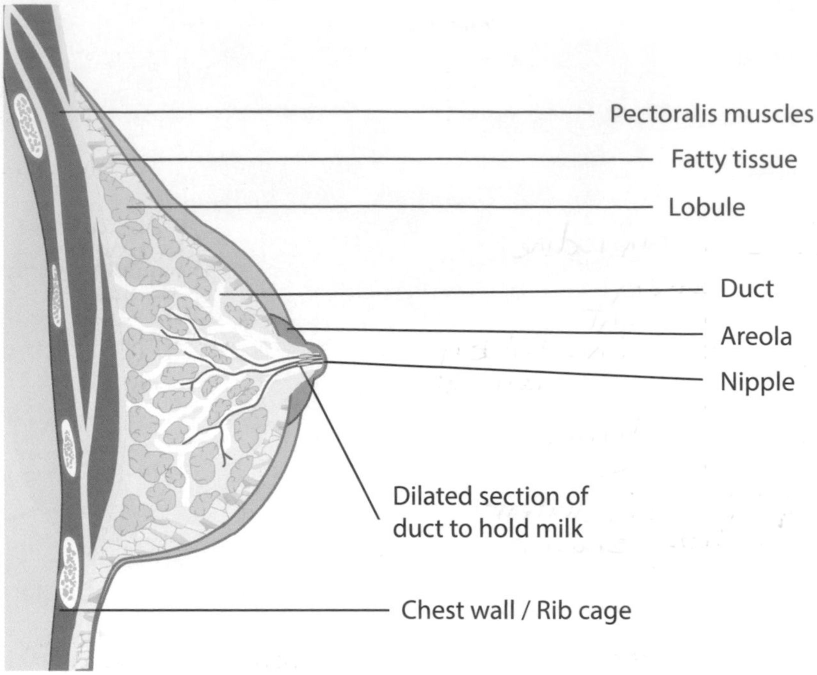

Female Reproductive System — Perineum Anatomy

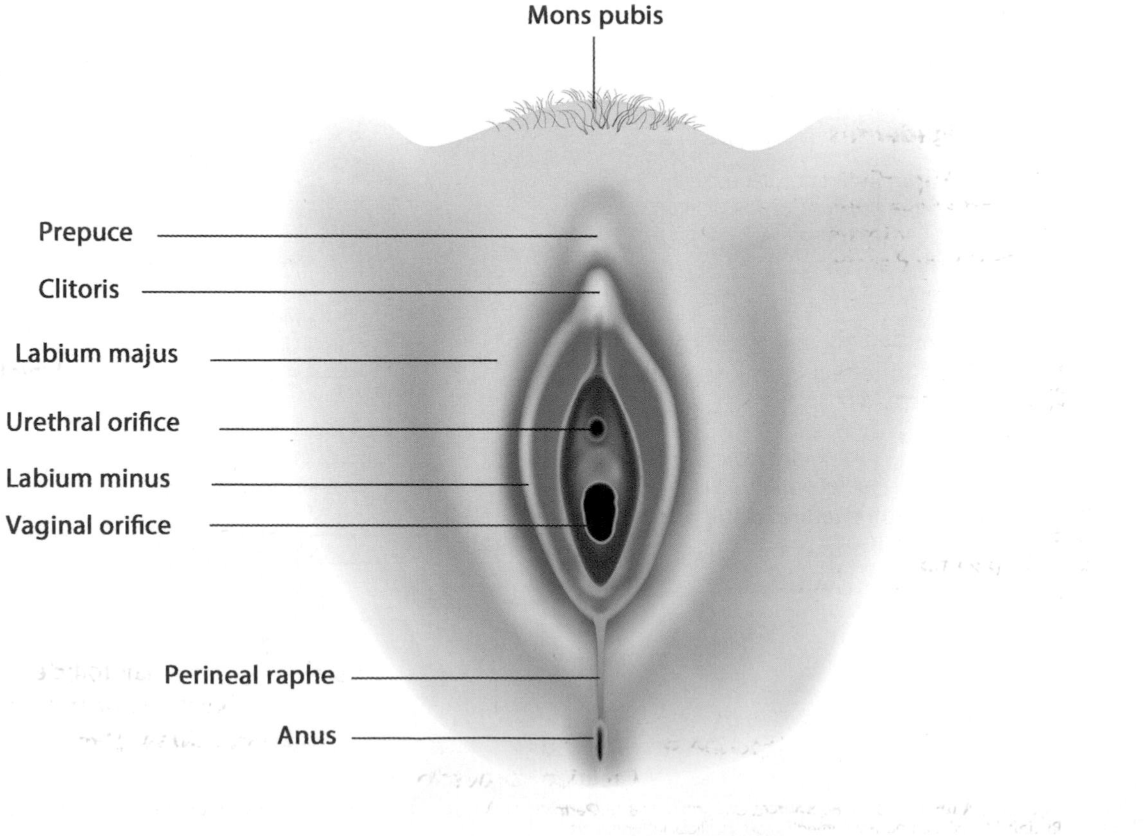

Largest Organ System in the body

Viseral fat in Peritoneal cavity

Integumentary System Anatomy

Functions!
- *protective barrier against outside invasion*
- *regulates body temperature*
- *synthesizes vitamin D*
- *contains touch & pressure receptors*

outermost layer

Epidermis — *contains 5 layers keratin & pre-keratin substances*

living part of skin

Dermis — *contains fibrous connective tissue, collagen & cells has hair bulbs, glands, nerve receptors*

Subcutaneous tissue — *fat storage contains loose connective tissue & faty large blood vessels & nerves*

Sweat pore

Hair shaft

Meissner's corpuscle

Sweat gland

Stratum corneum (horny cell layer)

Papillary layer

Sebaceous (oil) gland

Arrector pili muscle

Reticular layer

Nerve

Hair follicle

Vein

Artery

Pacinian corpuscle

Adipose (fat) tissue

Thick (hairless) skin

Thin (hairy) skin

Hair shaft

Opening of sweat duct

Dermal papillae

Epidermis

Superficial arteriovenous plexus

Papillary dermis

Dermis

Reticular dermis

Meissner's corpuscle

Sweat duct

Arrector pili muscle

Sebaceous gland

Subcutis/ hypodermis

Deep arteriovenous plexus

Subcutaneous fat

Dermal nerve fibres

Eccrine sweat gland

Pacinian corpuscle

Hair follicle

Eccrine sweat duct

Eccrine sweat gland

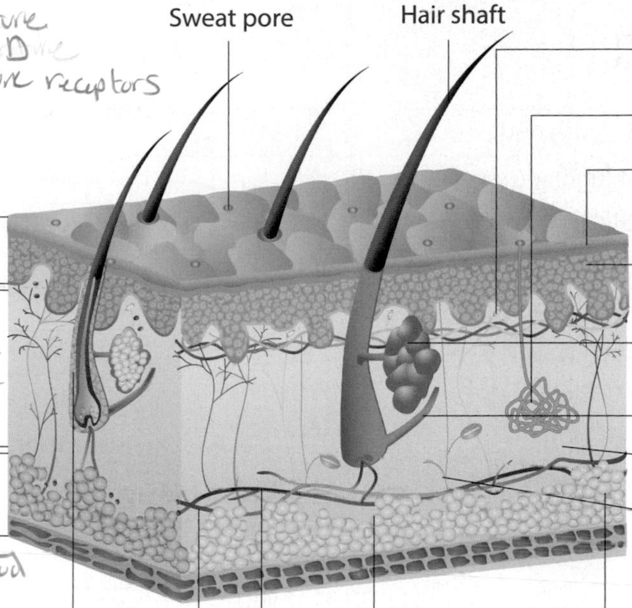

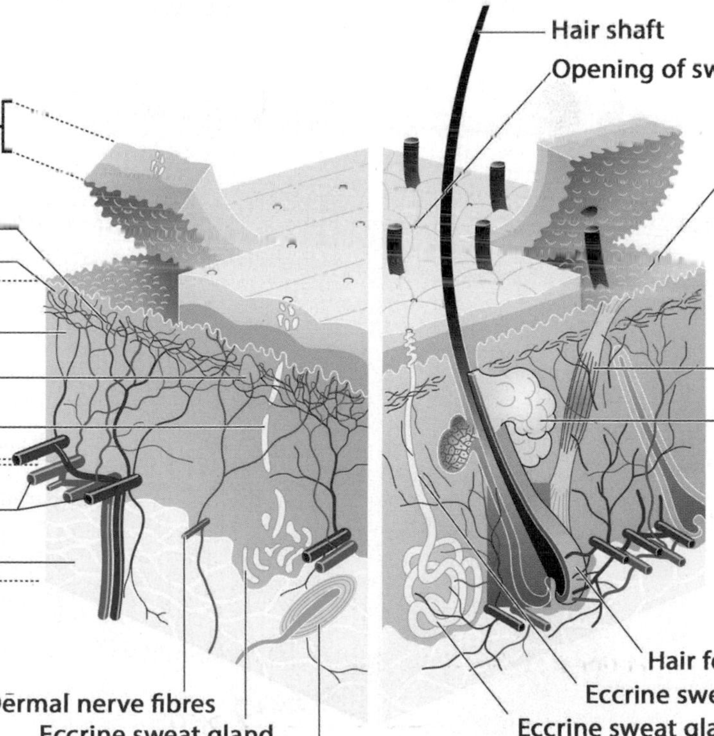

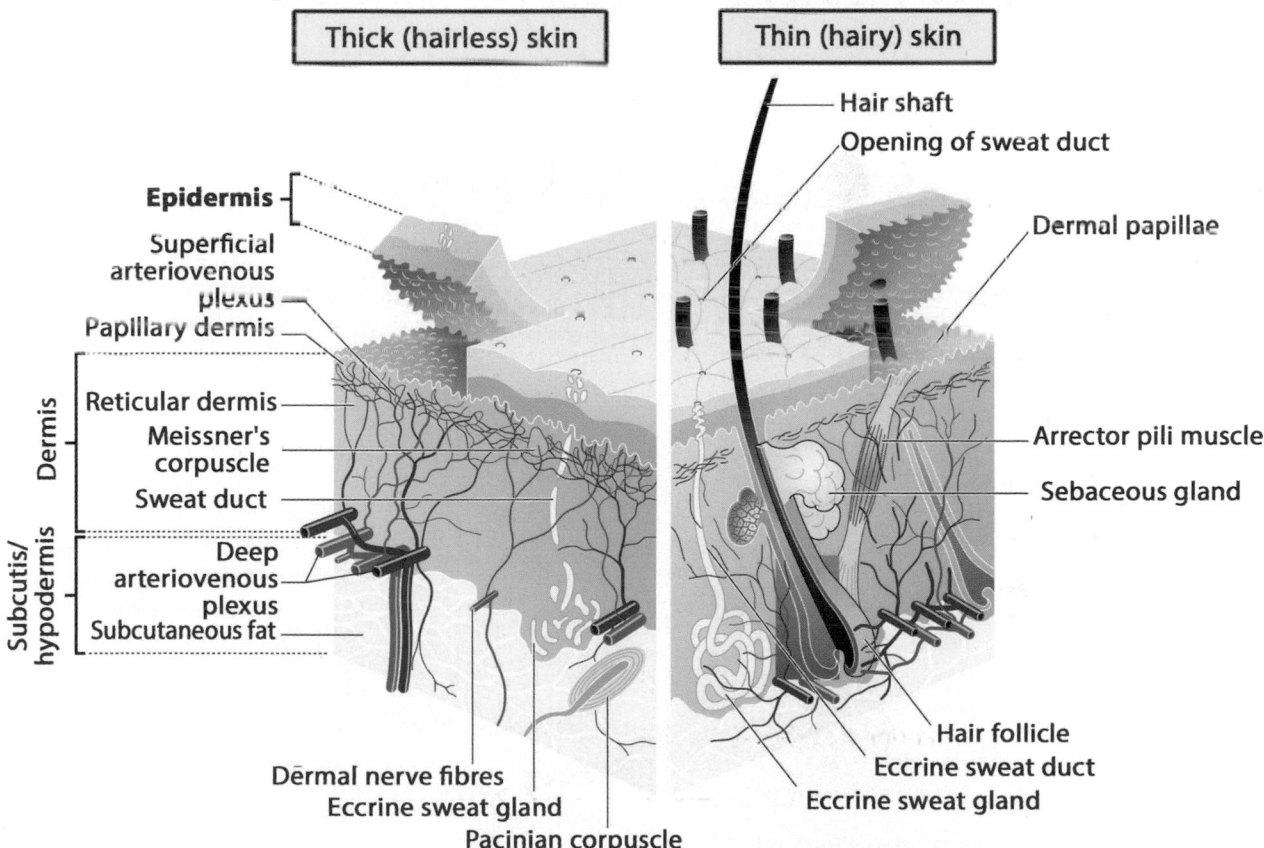

Lymph is carried towards the heart

Lymphatic System Anatomy

Produce lymphocytes
Spleen, thymus, bone marrow
lymphoid tissue associated w/digestive system

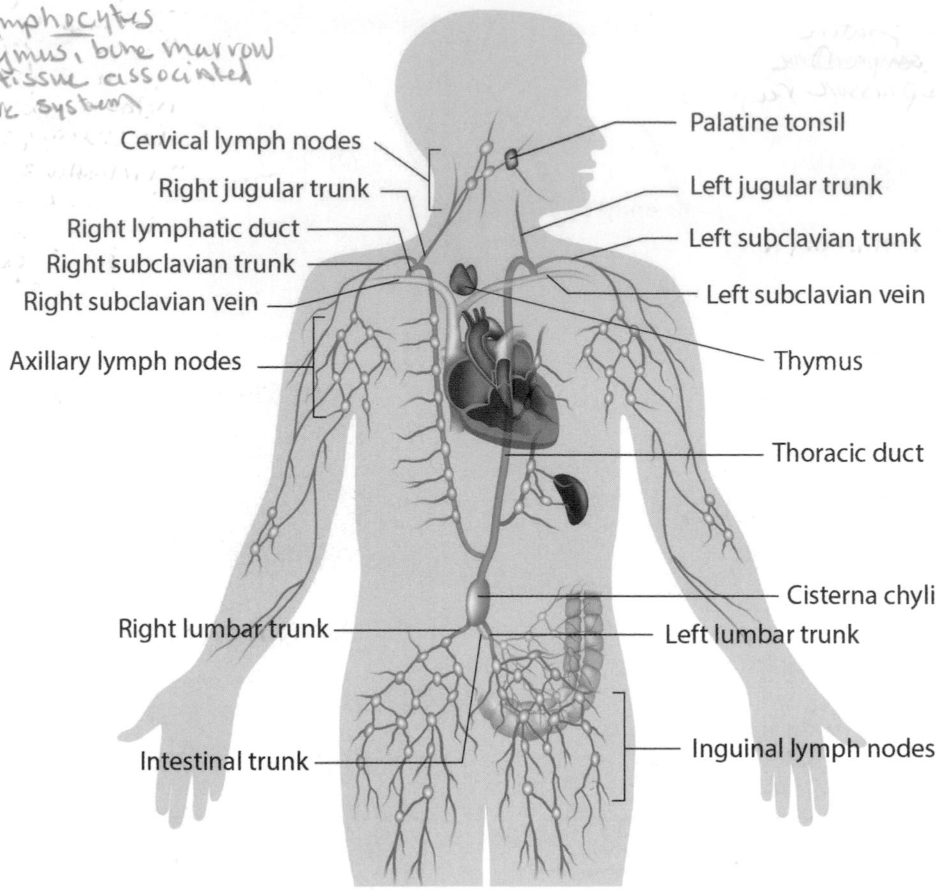

Lymph Nodes of the Head and Neck

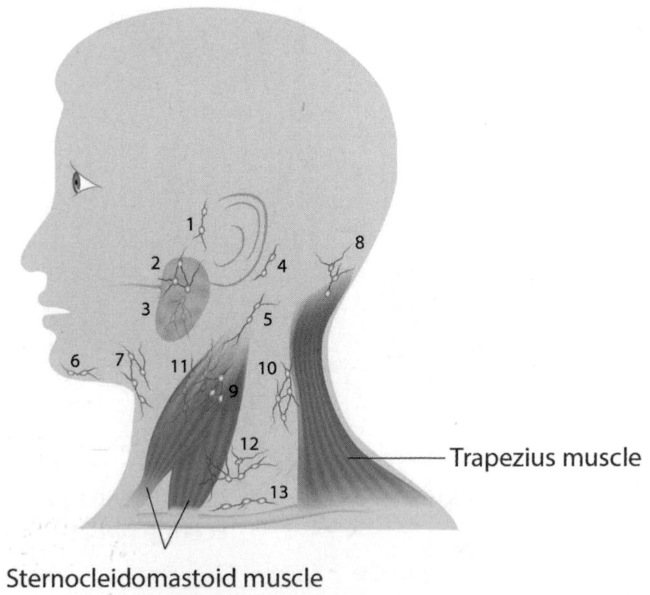

1. Preauricular
2. Superficial parotid
3. Deep parotid
4. Posterior auricular
5. Mastoid
6. Submental
7. Submandibular
8. Occipital
9. Superficial anterior cervical
10. Superficial posterior cervical
11. Superior deep cervical
12. Inferior deep cervical
13. Supraclavicular

Lymphatic System — Humoral Immunity

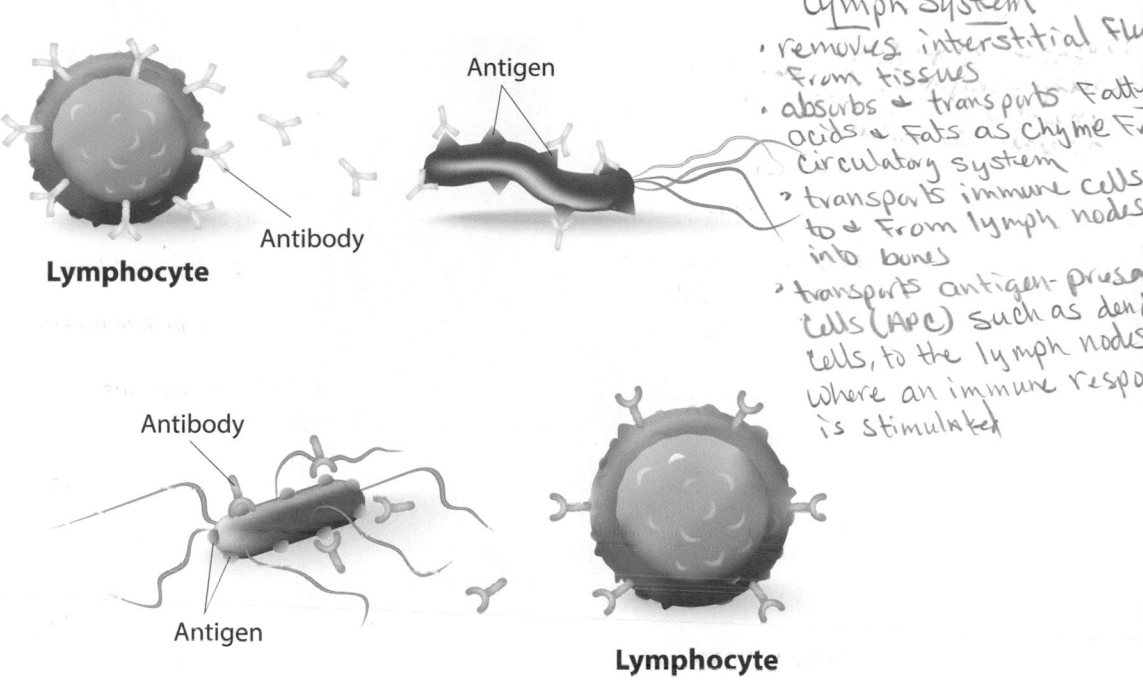

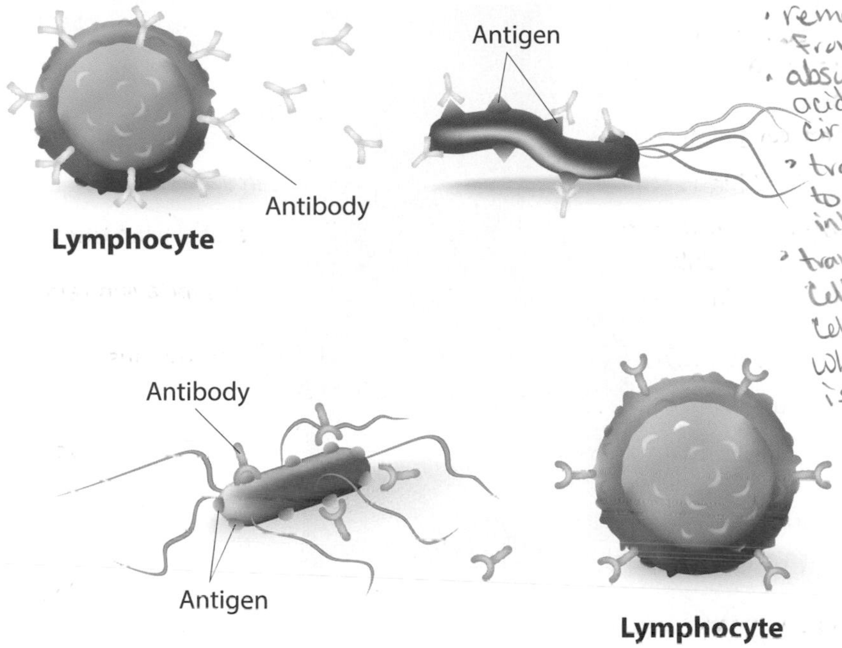

Lymph system
- removes interstitial fluid from tissues
- absorbs & transports fatty acids & fats as chyme from circulatory system
- transports immune cells to & from lymph nodes into bones
- transports antigen-presenting cells (APC) such as dendritic cells, to the lymph nodes where an immune response is stimulated

Lymph Node Anatomy

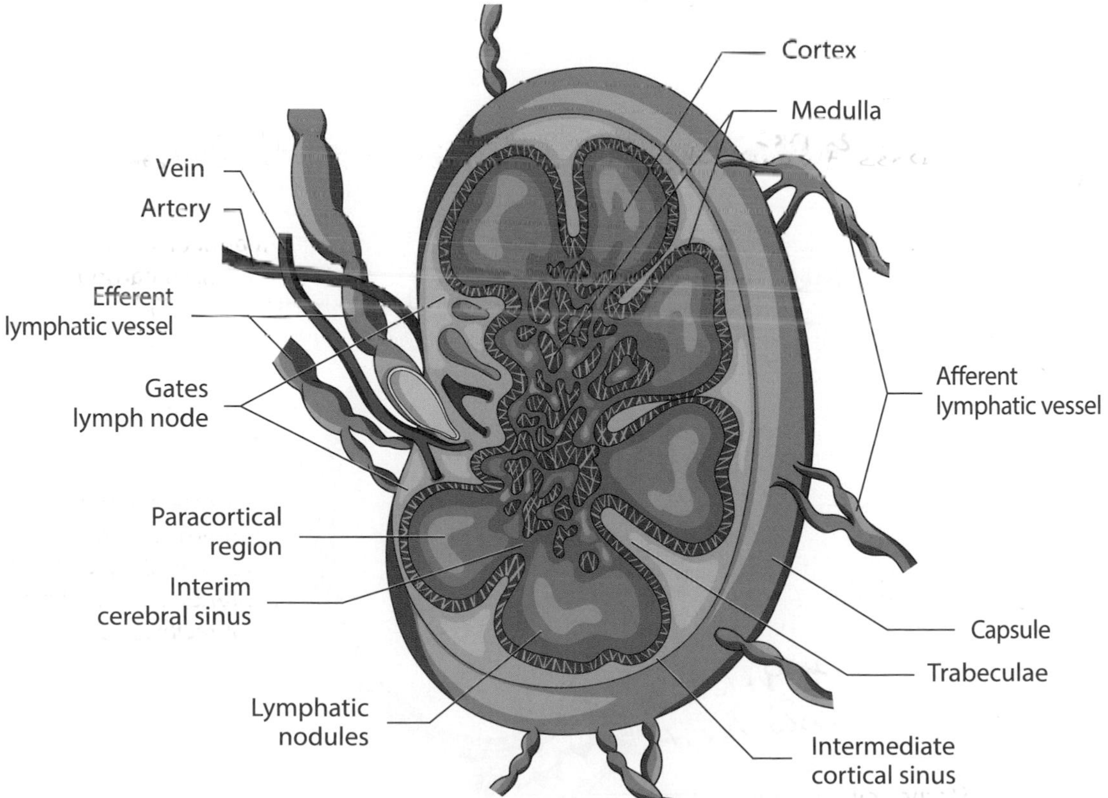

Male Reproductive System Anatomy

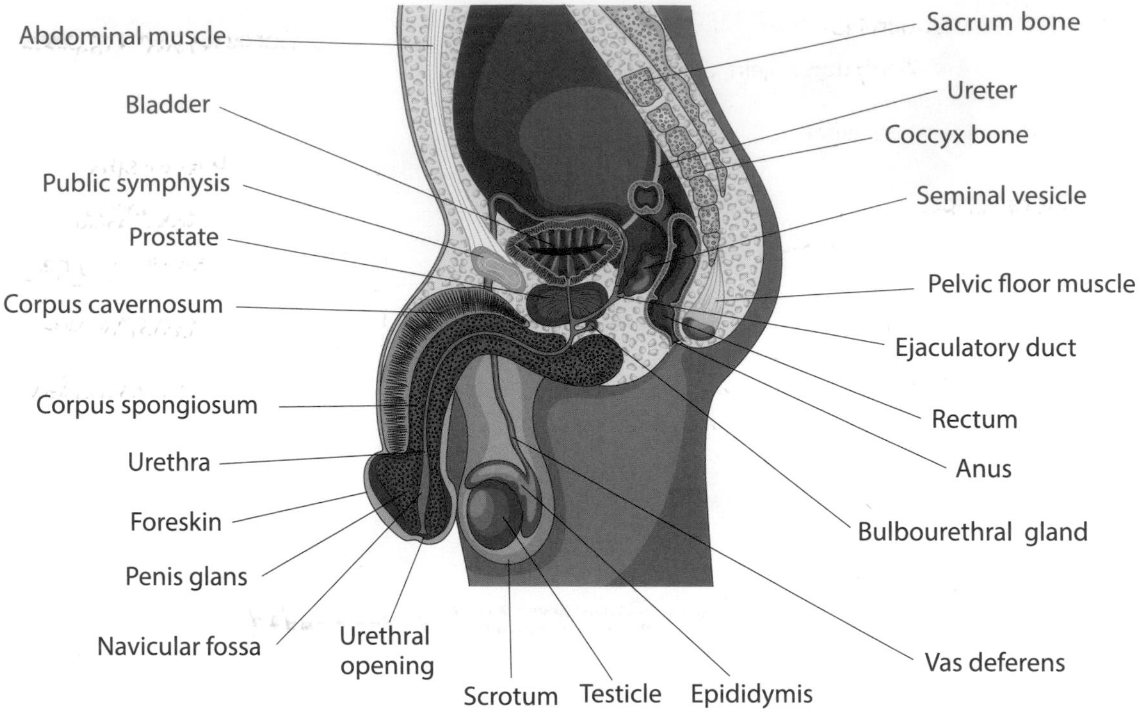

Male Reproductive System — Testicle

located in scrotum

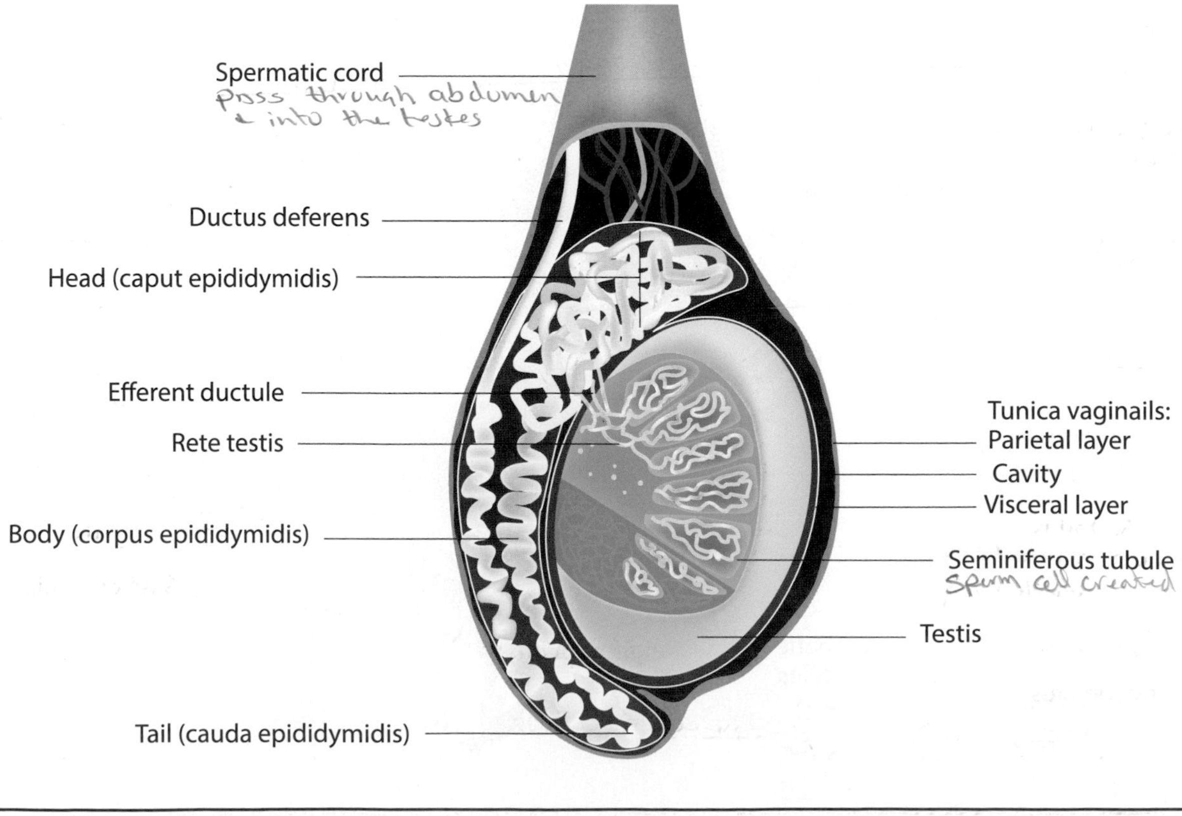

Male Reproductive System — Penis Anatomy

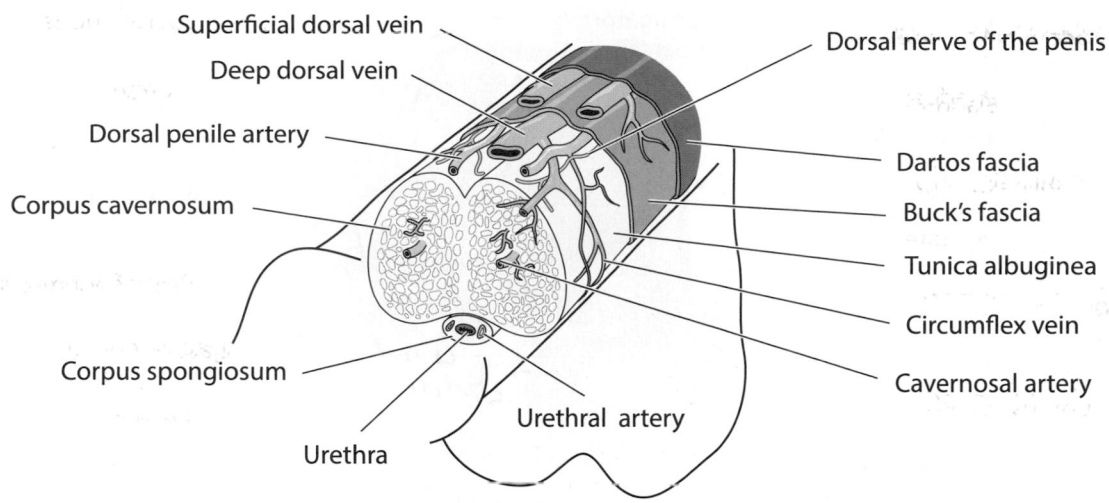

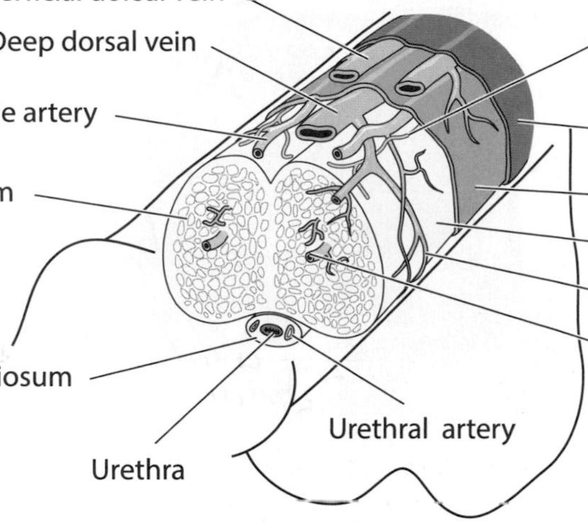
Superficial dorsal vein
Deep dorsal vein
Dorsal penile artery
Corpus cavernosum
Corpus spongiosum
Urethra
Urethral artery
Dorsal nerve of the penis
Dartos fascia
Buck's fascia
Tunica albuginea
Circumflex vein
Cavernosal artery

Muscular System Anatomy

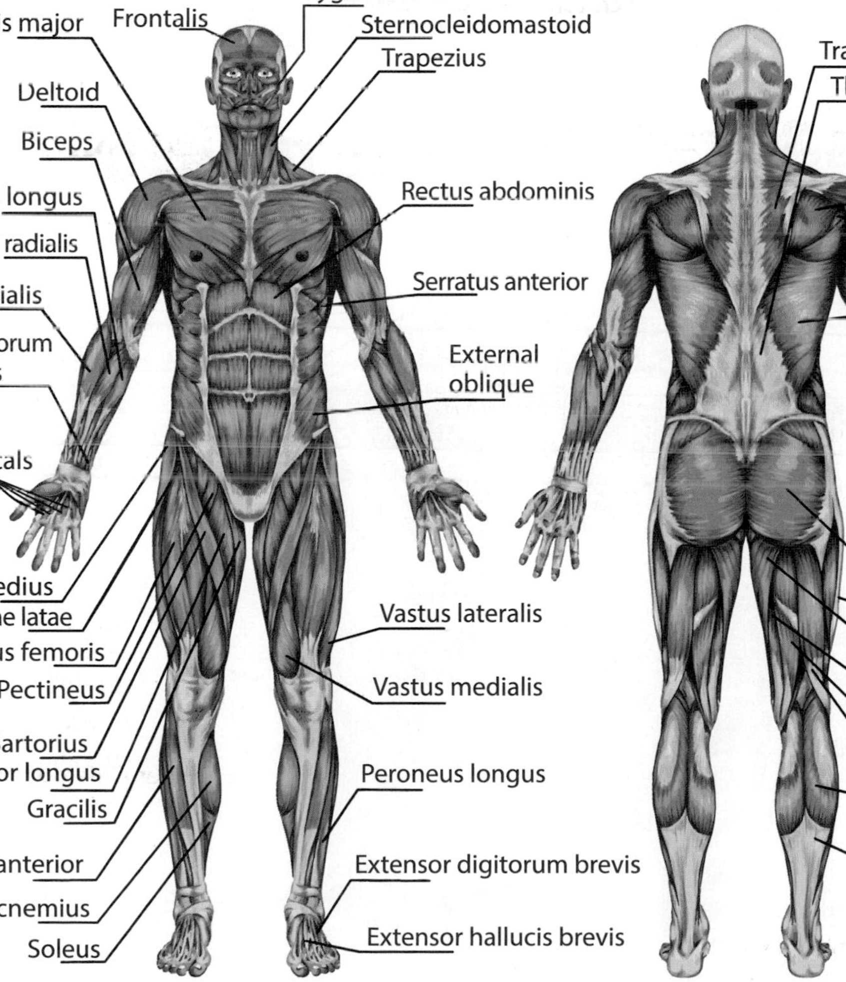
Pectoralis major
Frontalis
Zygomaticus
Sternocleidomastoid
Trapezius
Deltoid
Biceps
Palmaris longus
Flexor carpi radialis
Brachioradialis
Flexor digitorum superficialis
Lumbricals
Rectus abdominis
Serratus anterior
External oblique
Gluteus medius
Tensor faciae latae
Rectus femoris
Pectineus
Sartorius
Adductor longus
Gracilis
Tibialis anterior
Gastrocnemius
Soleus
Vastus lateralis
Vastus medialis
Peroneus longus
Extensor digitorum brevis
Extensor hallucis brevis
Trapezius
Thoraco-lumbar fascia
Deltoid
Rhomboid
Teres major
Triceps
Latissimus dorsi
Extensor carpi radialis
Extensor digitorum
Extensor carpi ulnaris
Extensor digiti minimi
Gluteus maximus
Vastus lateralis
Gracilis
Semimembranosus
Semitendinosus
Biceps femoris
Gastrocnemius
Soleus

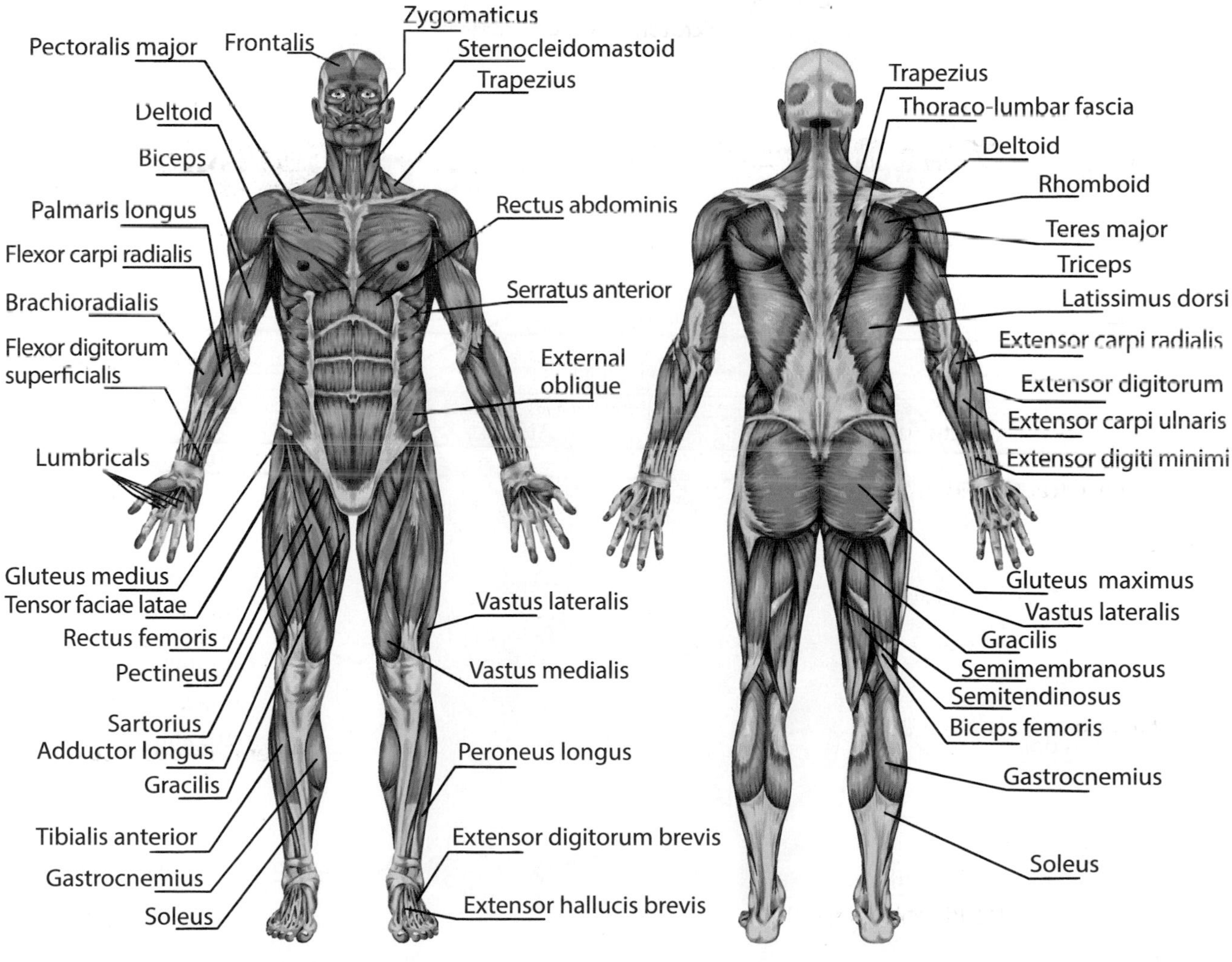

Fascia - deepest layer of fibrous tissue that permeates the human body
It is a connective tissue that surrounds muscles, blood vessels, nerves, binding the structures together.

layers of fascia
- superficial
- deep
- subserous - AKA visceral

fasciae - dense regular connective tissue, containing closely packed bundles of collagen fiber oriented in a wavy pattern parallel to the direction of pull

Muscular System — Face Muscles

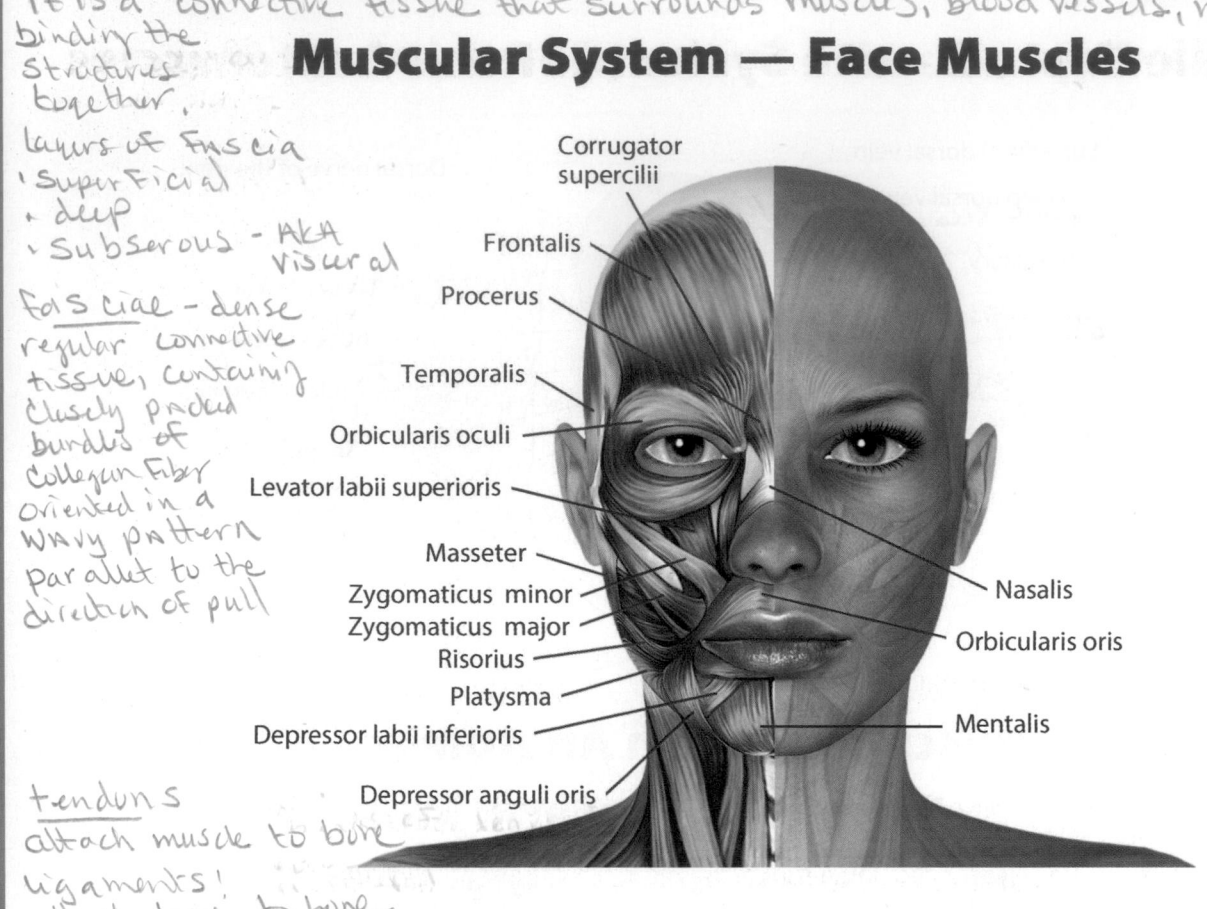

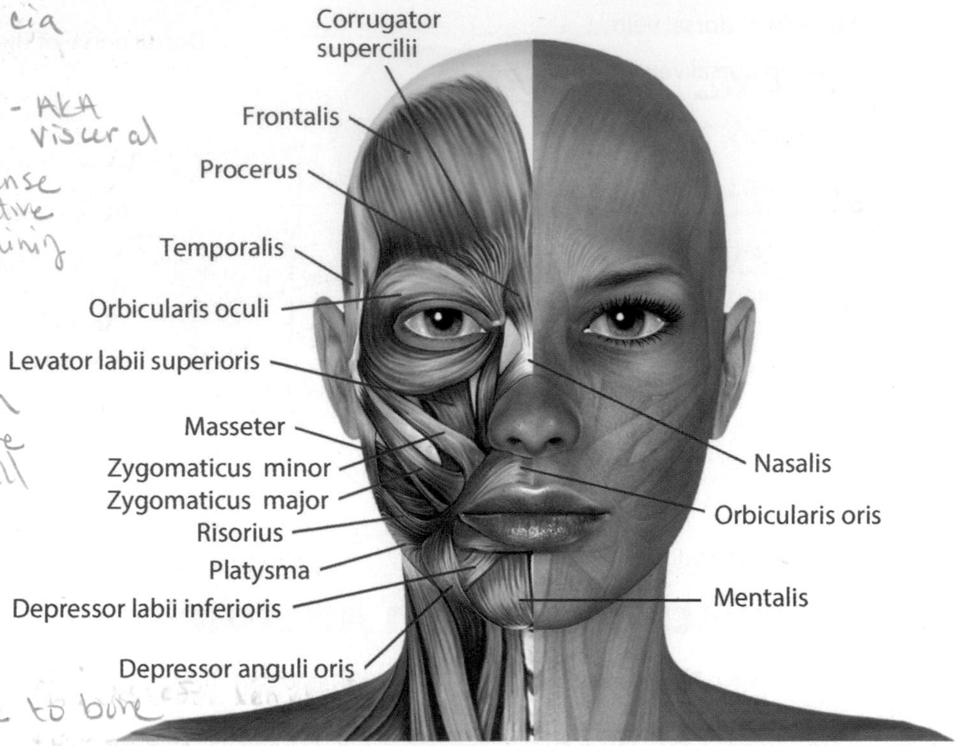

tendons
attach muscle to bone
ligaments:
attach bone to bone

Muscular System — Neck, Chest, Thorax Muscles

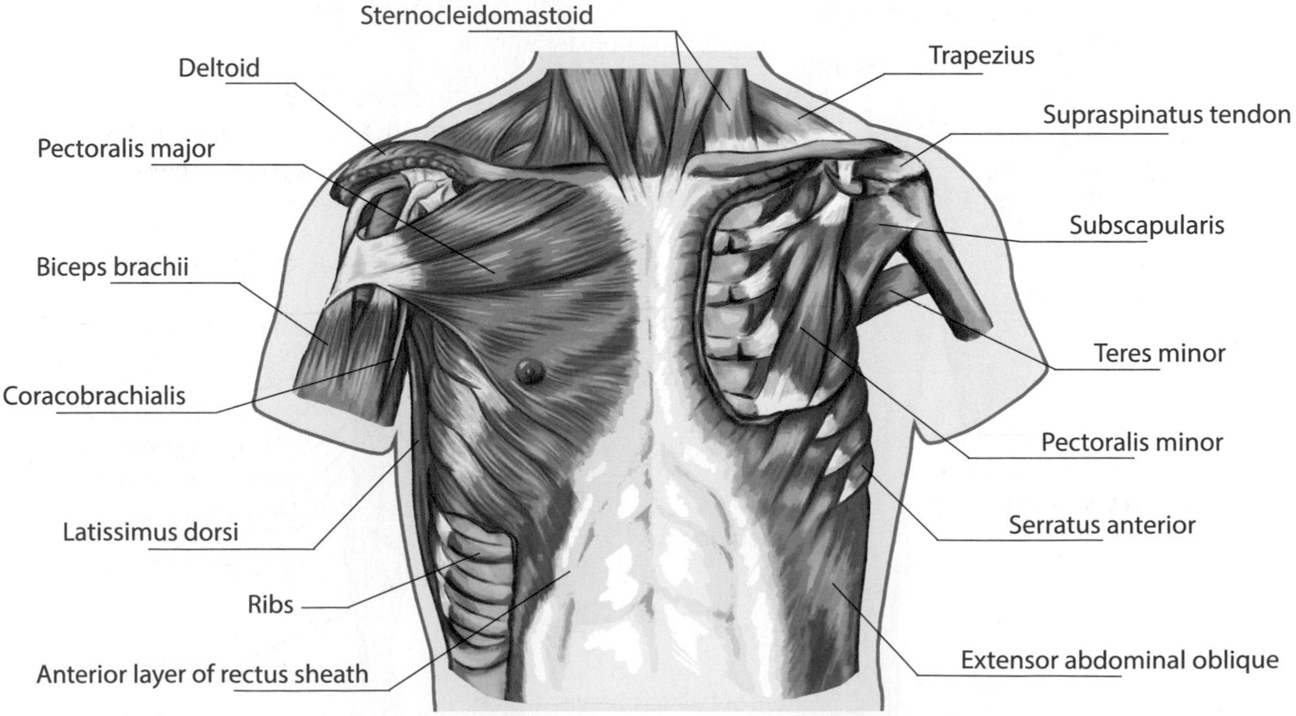

human body contains more than 650 muscles attached to the skeleton, keeps bones in place & provides pulling power needed for movement

Muscular System — Shoulder (Rotator Cuff) Muscles

3 types muscle tissues
1) skeletal
2) cardiac
3) smooth

most skeletal muscles are attached to bones by tendons

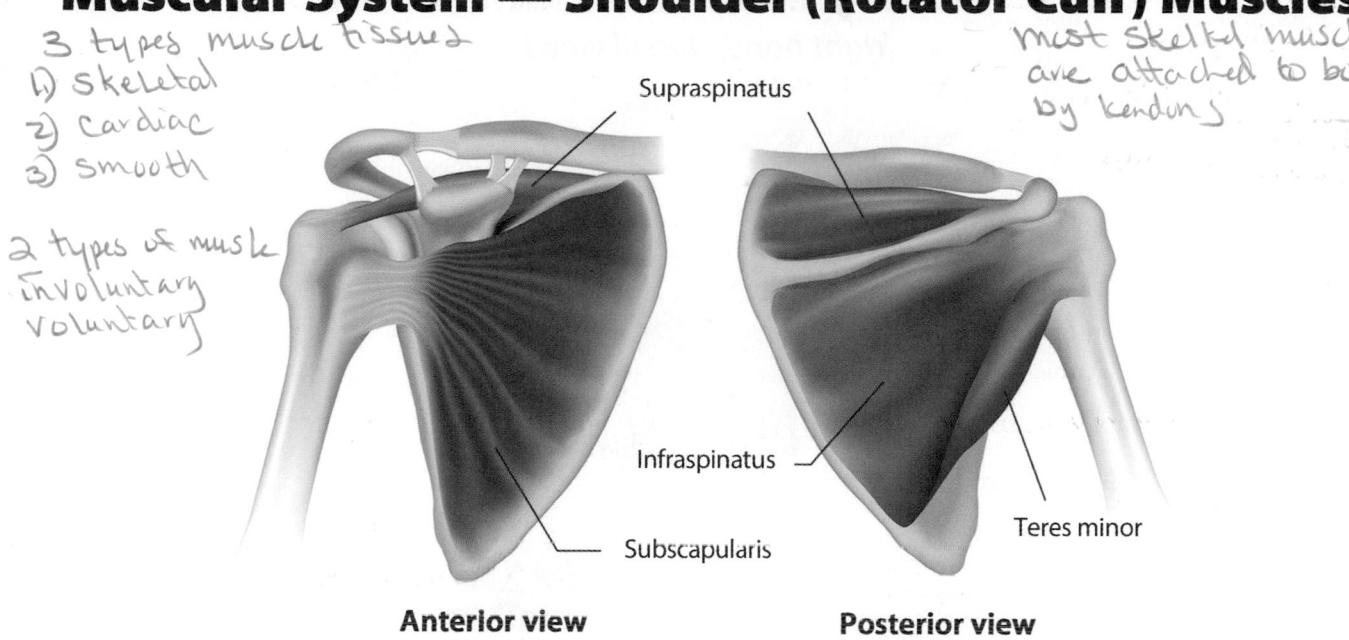

2 types of muscle
involuntary
voluntary

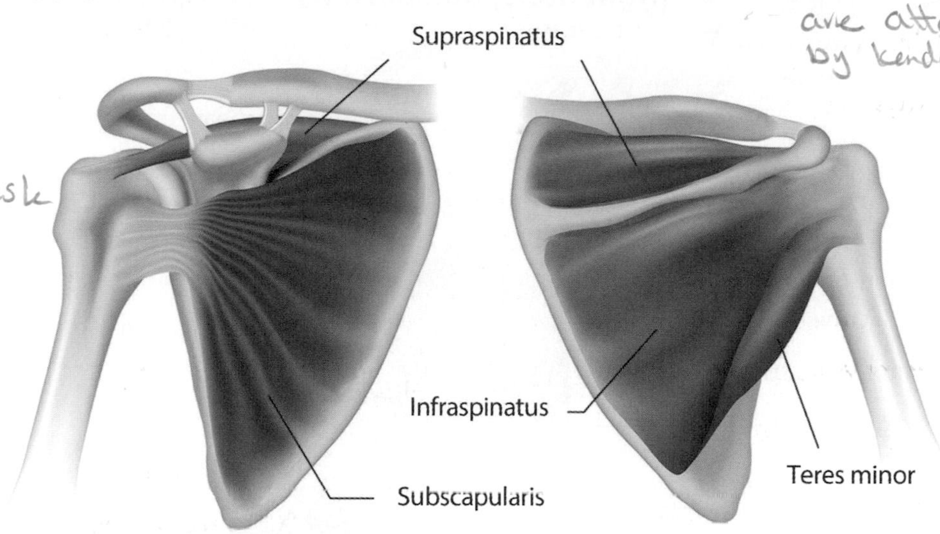

Anterior view **Posterior view**

Muscular System — Forearm Muscles (Right Arm, Posterior Compartment)

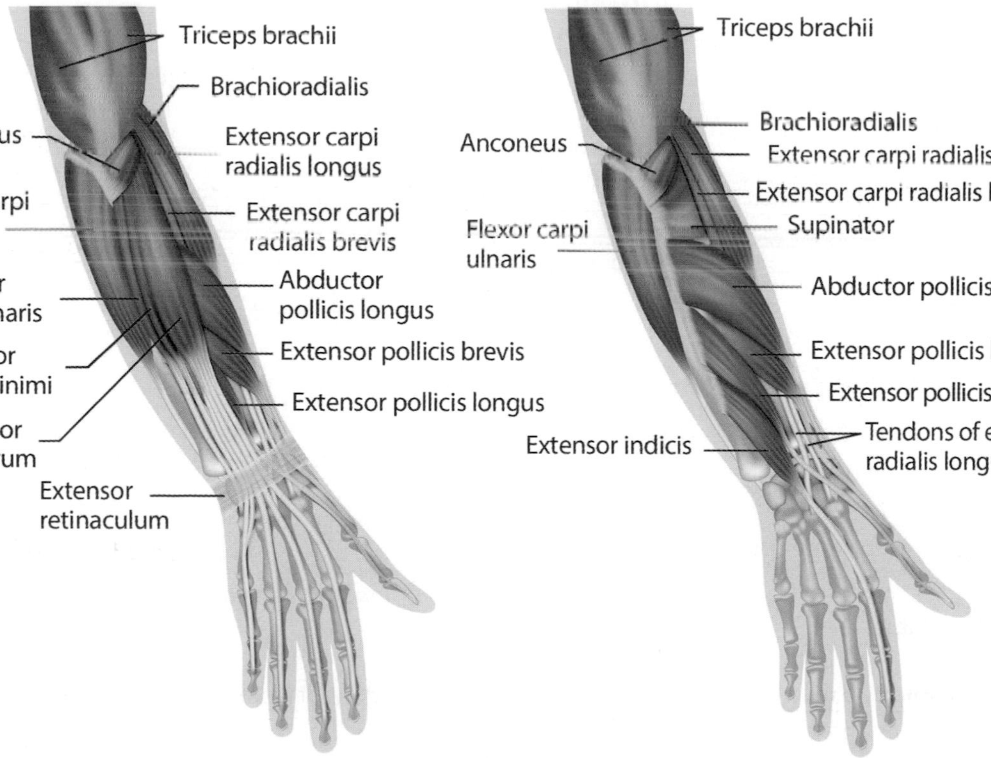

tendon - tough band of Fibrous connective tissue

tendons, ligament & Fasciae are made of collegan

Muscles of the Hand

(right hand, dorsal view)

tendon - enable movement
act as intermediaries
between the muscles
& the bones

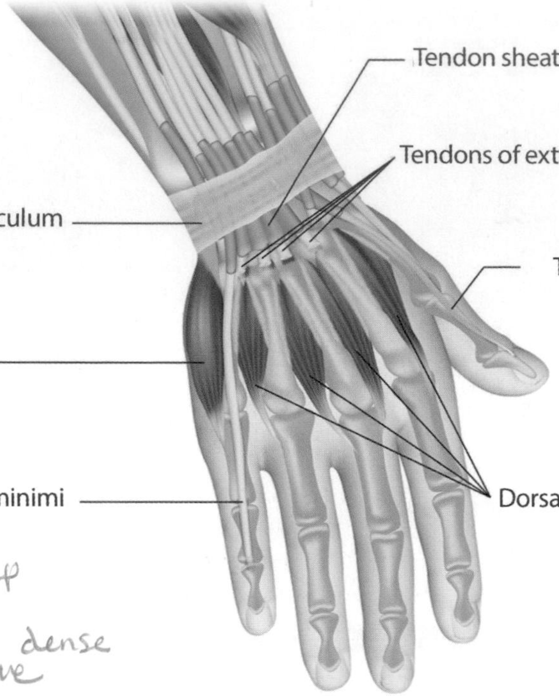

Ligaments -
* connect bone to bone & help to stabilize joints.
• composed of bands of dense regular connective tissue comprising attenuated collagenous Fiber

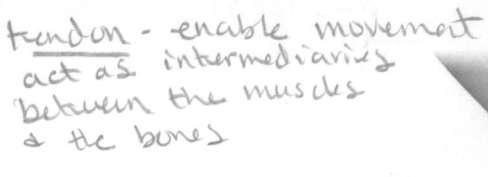

Muscles of the Hand

(right hand, palmar view)

Deep

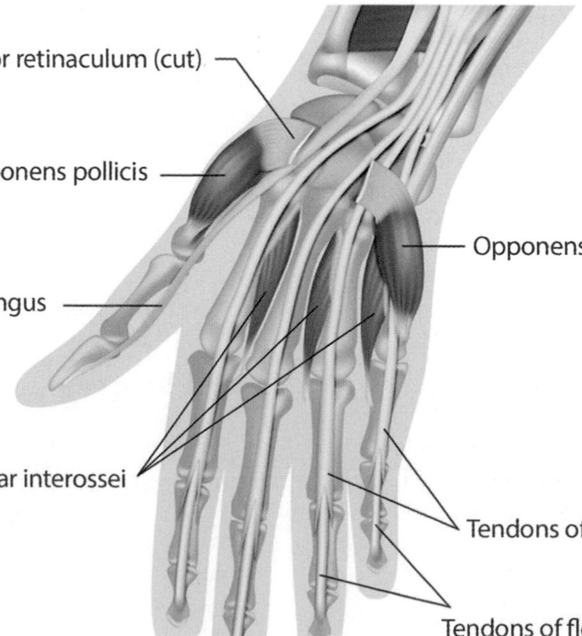

Bursa- Fluid Filled Sac Lined by Synovial membrane w/an inner capillary layer of Fluid that provides a cushion between bones & tendons and/or muscles around a joint, reduce Friction & allow Free movement

Muscular System — Leg Muscles

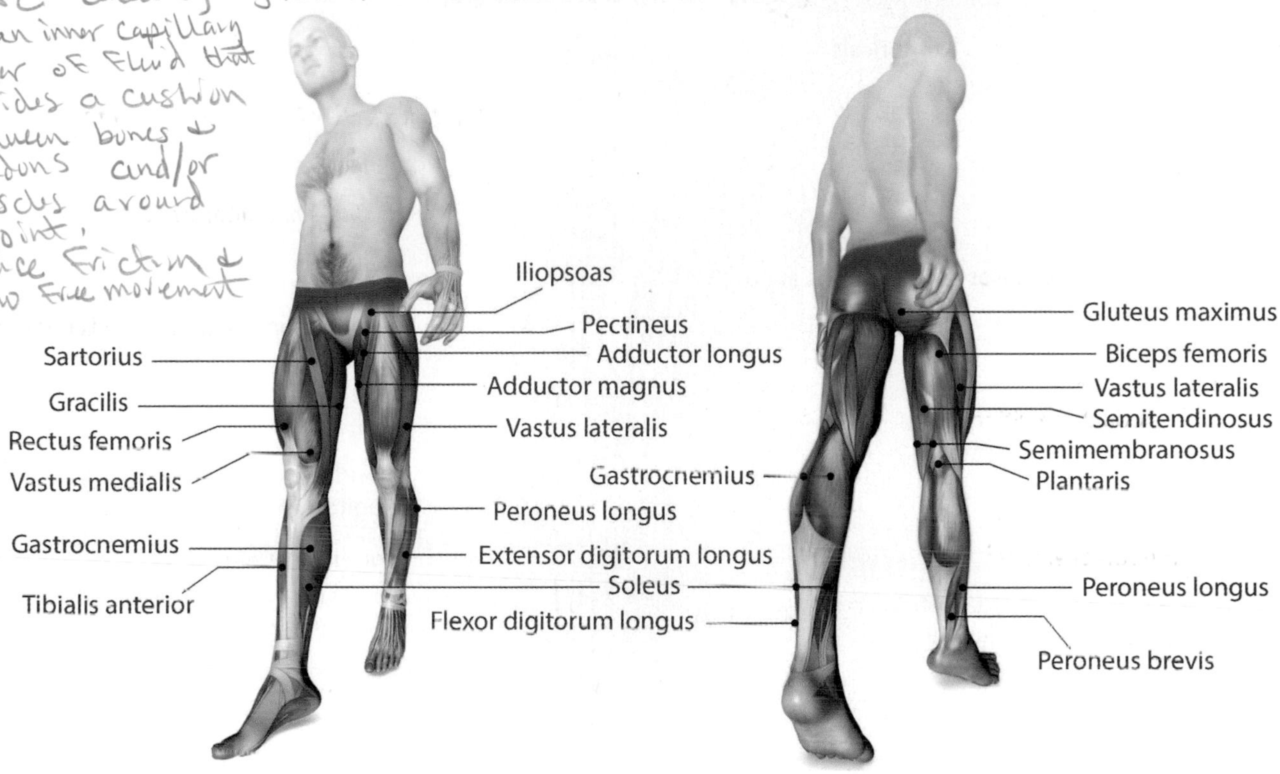

Muscular System — Knee and Leg

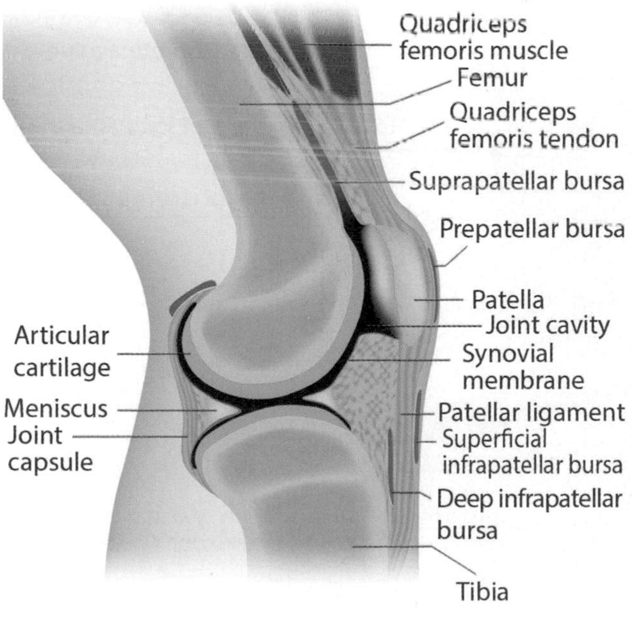

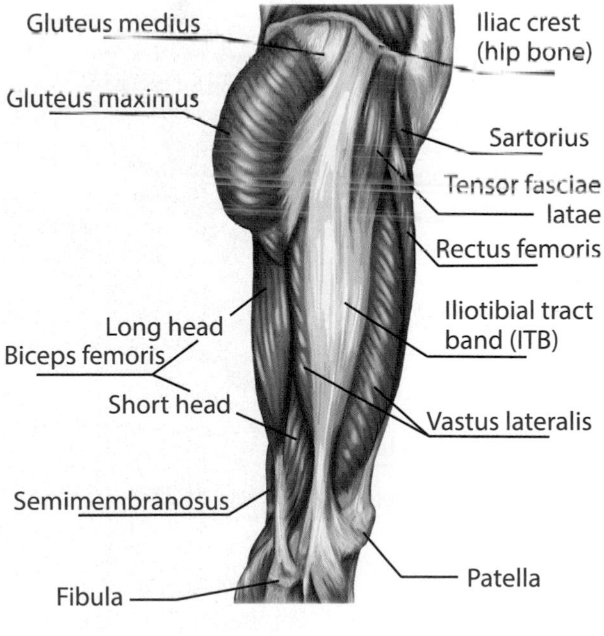

ANATOMICAL ILLUSTRATIONS

Muscular System — Foot Muscles

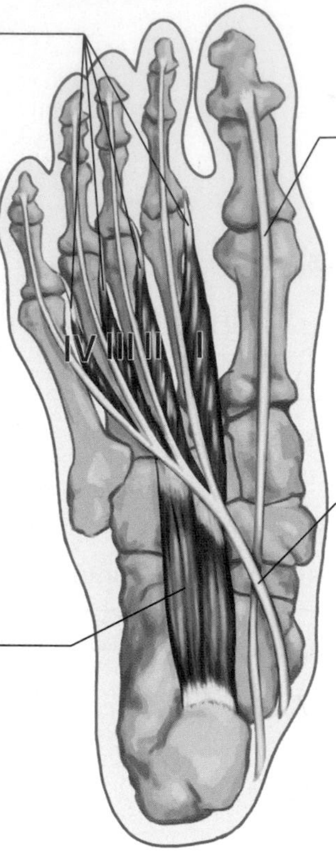

Lumbricals
Tendon of flexor hallucis longus
IV III II I
Tendon of flexor digitorum longus
Quadratus plantae

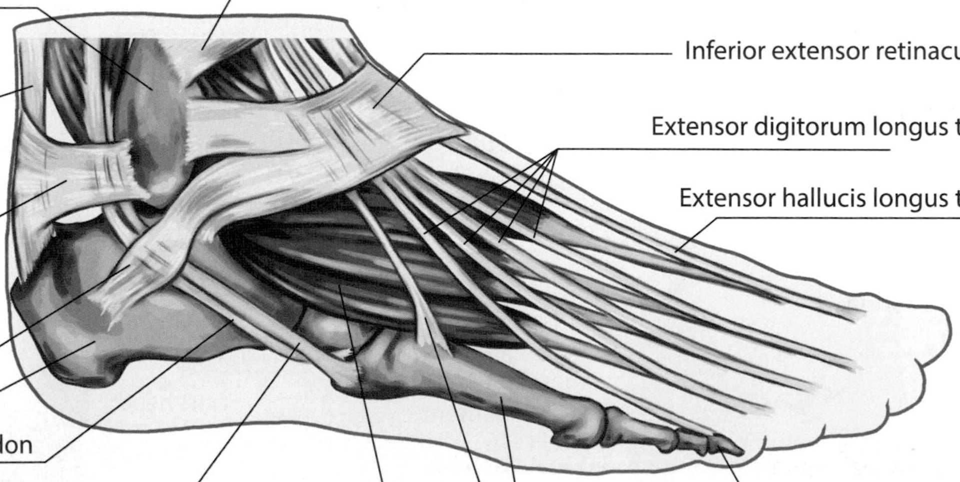

Superior extensor retinaculum
Fibula
Inferior extensor retinaculum
Achilles tendon
Extensor digitorum longus tendon
Superior peroneal retinaculum
Extensor hallucis longus tendon
Inferior peroneal retinaculum
Calcaneus
Peroneus longus tendon
Peroneus brevis tendon
V metatarsal bone
V distal bone
Extensor digitorum brevis
Peroneus tertius tendon

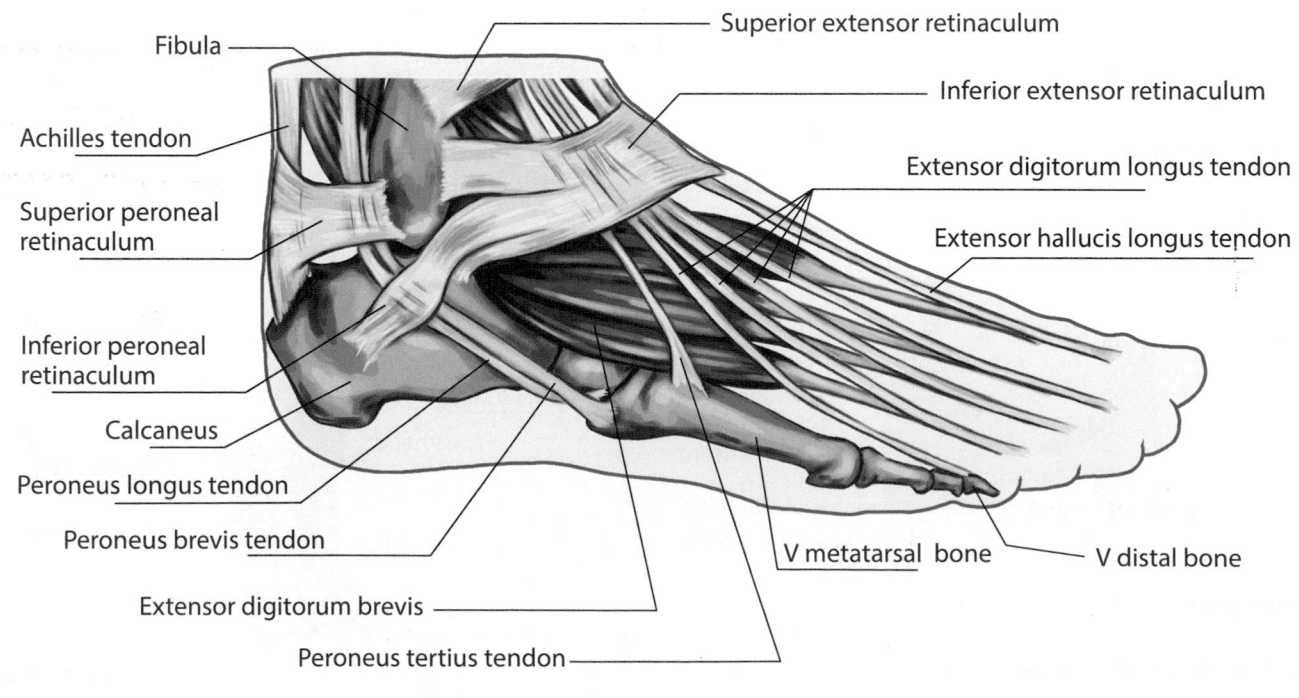

Musculoskeletal System — Shoulder Joint Structure

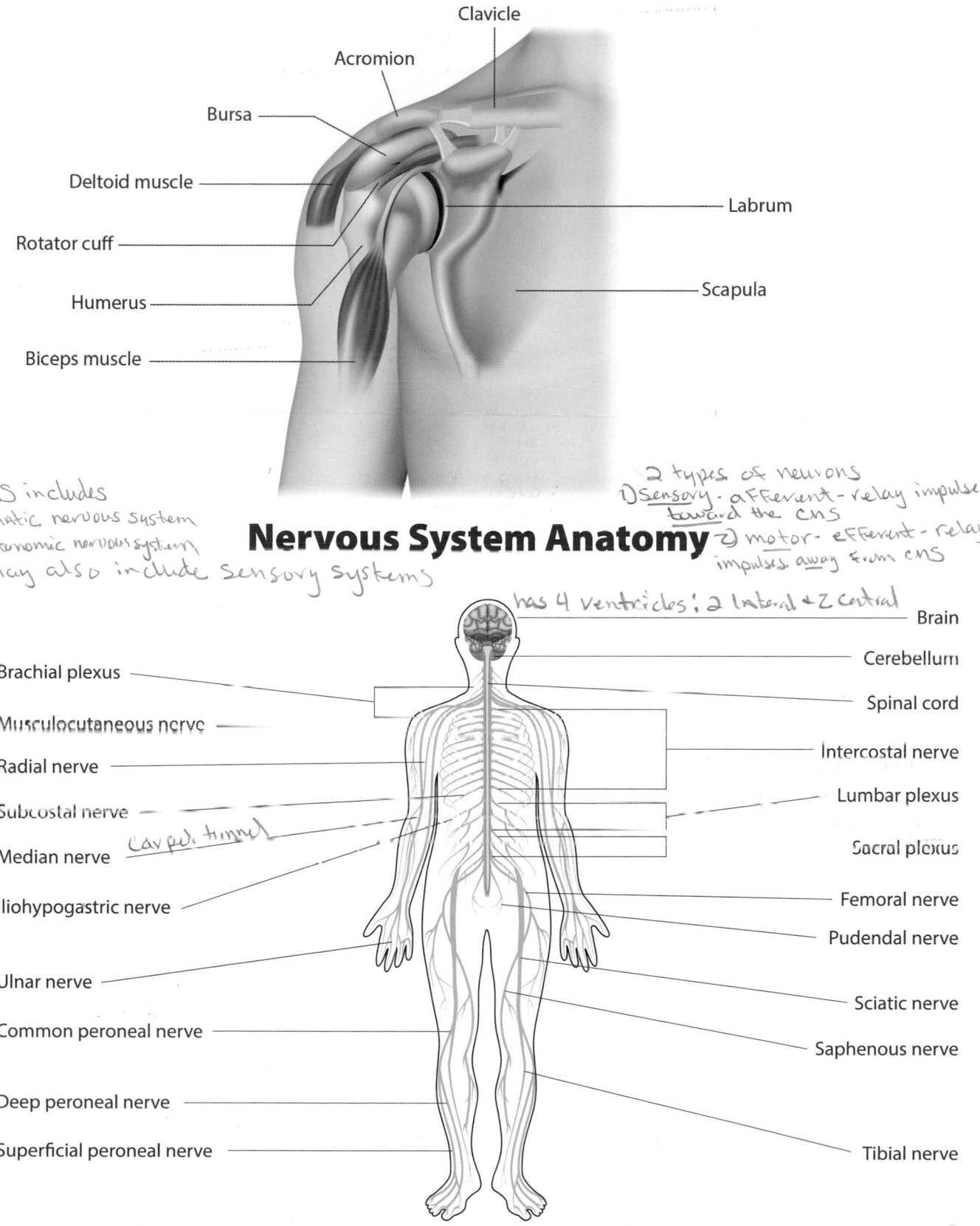

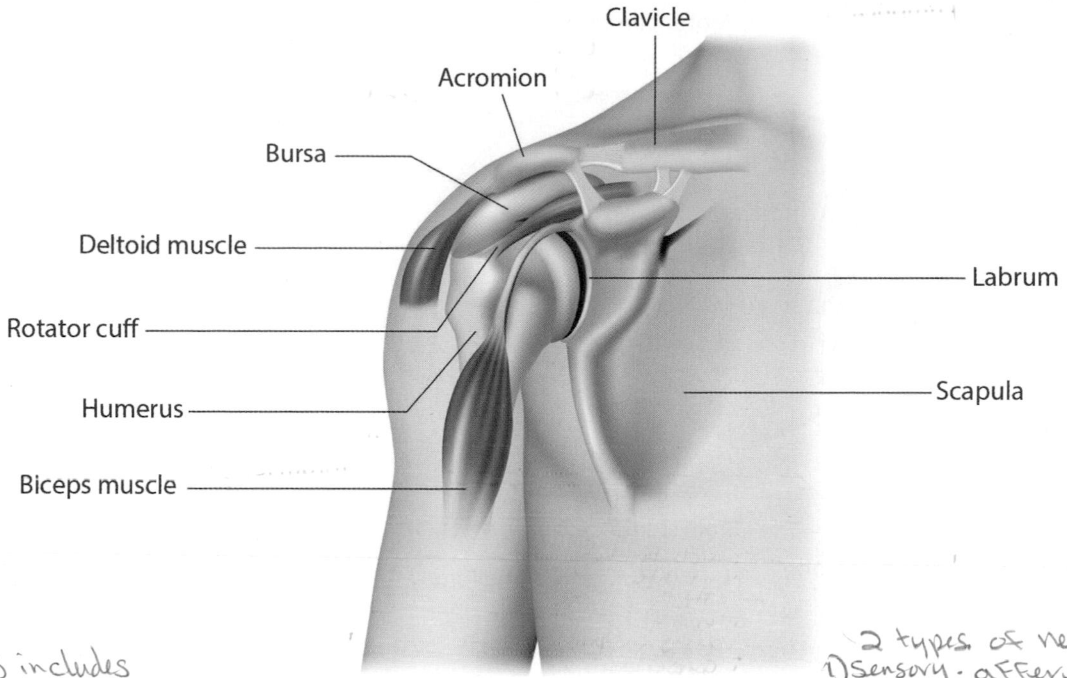

PNS includes
1) somatic nervous system
2) autonomic nervous system
may also include sensory systems

2 types of neurons
1) sensory - afferent - relay impulses toward the CNS
2) motor - efferent - relay impulses away from CNS

Nervous System Anatomy

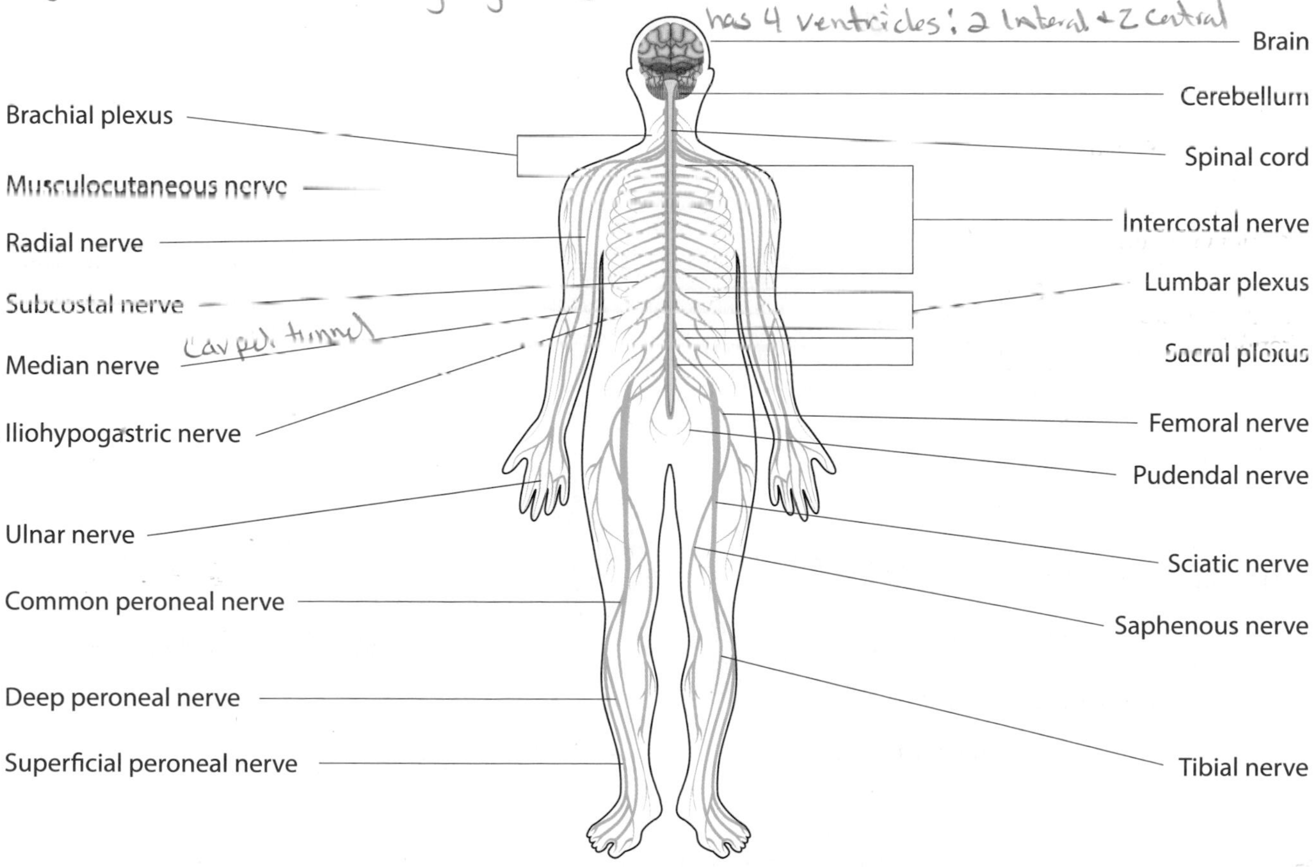

4 lobes - named after bones of skull that overlie them

Nervous System — Brain Anatomy

CNS in dorsal cavity
brain in cranial cavity
spinal cord in spinal cavity

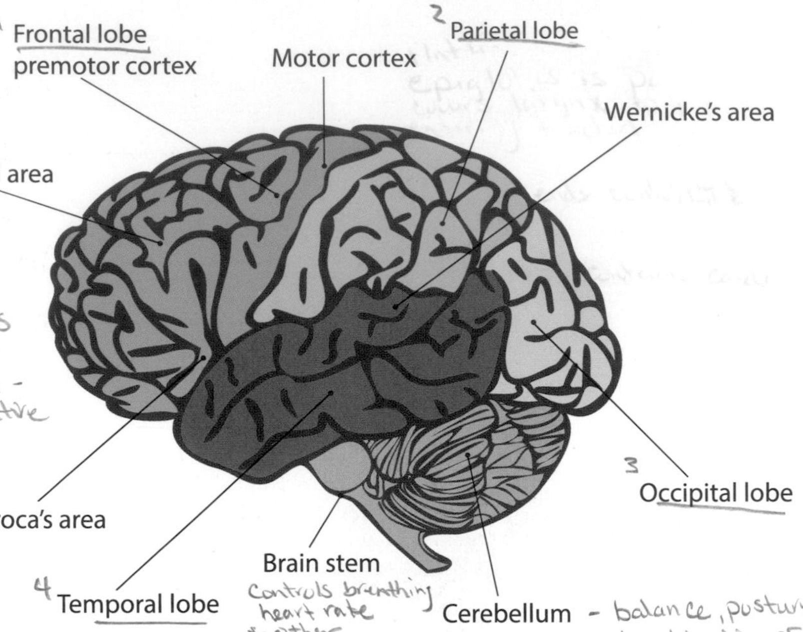

Spinal cord begins at occipital bone & extends to space between first & second lumbar vertebra - Does not extend to entire vertebral column.

Functions of spinal cord
1) conduit for motor information traveling down spinal cord
2) conduit for sensory information, traveling up the spinal cord
3) serves as center for coordinating certain reflexes

Brain stem: controls breathing, heart rate & other autonomic processes independent of conscious brain functions

Cerebellum - balance, posture & coordination of movement

Nervous System — Median Section of the Brain

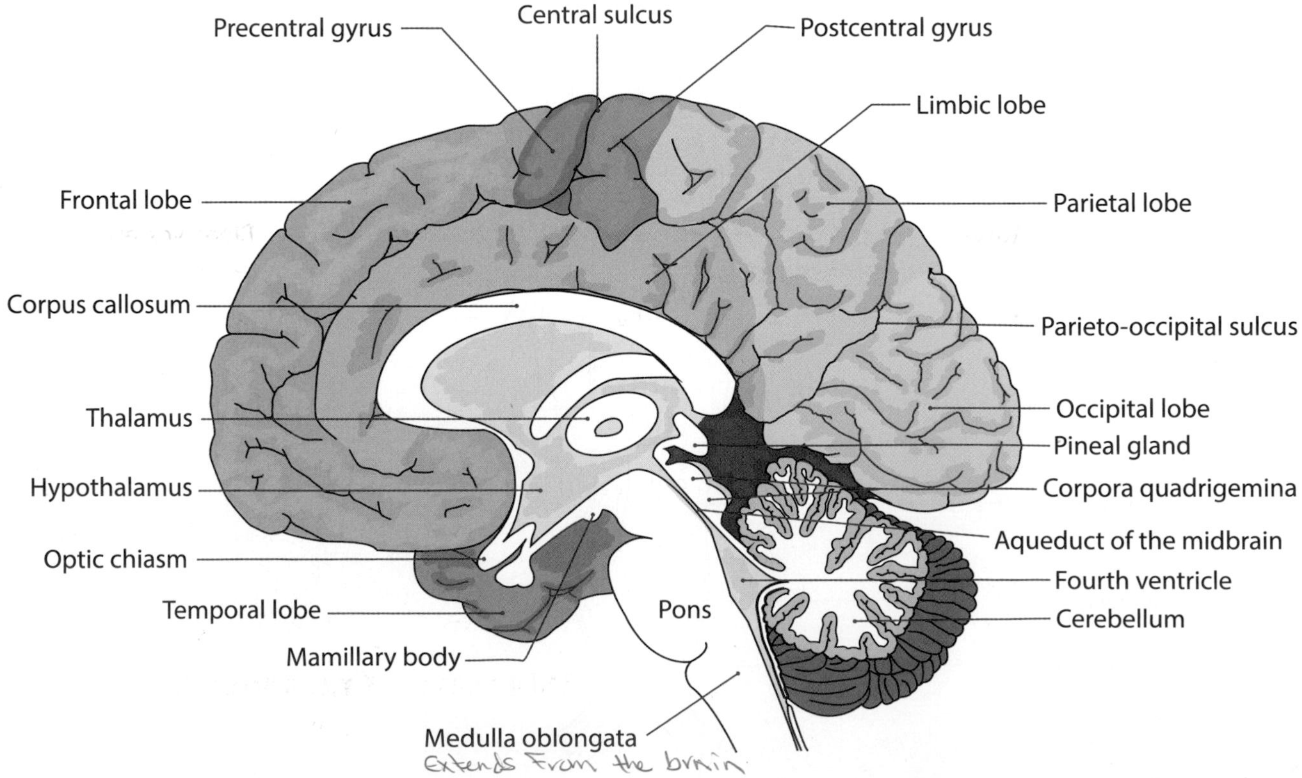

Medulla oblongata: Extends from the brain

Nervous System — Cranial Nerves - 12 pairs

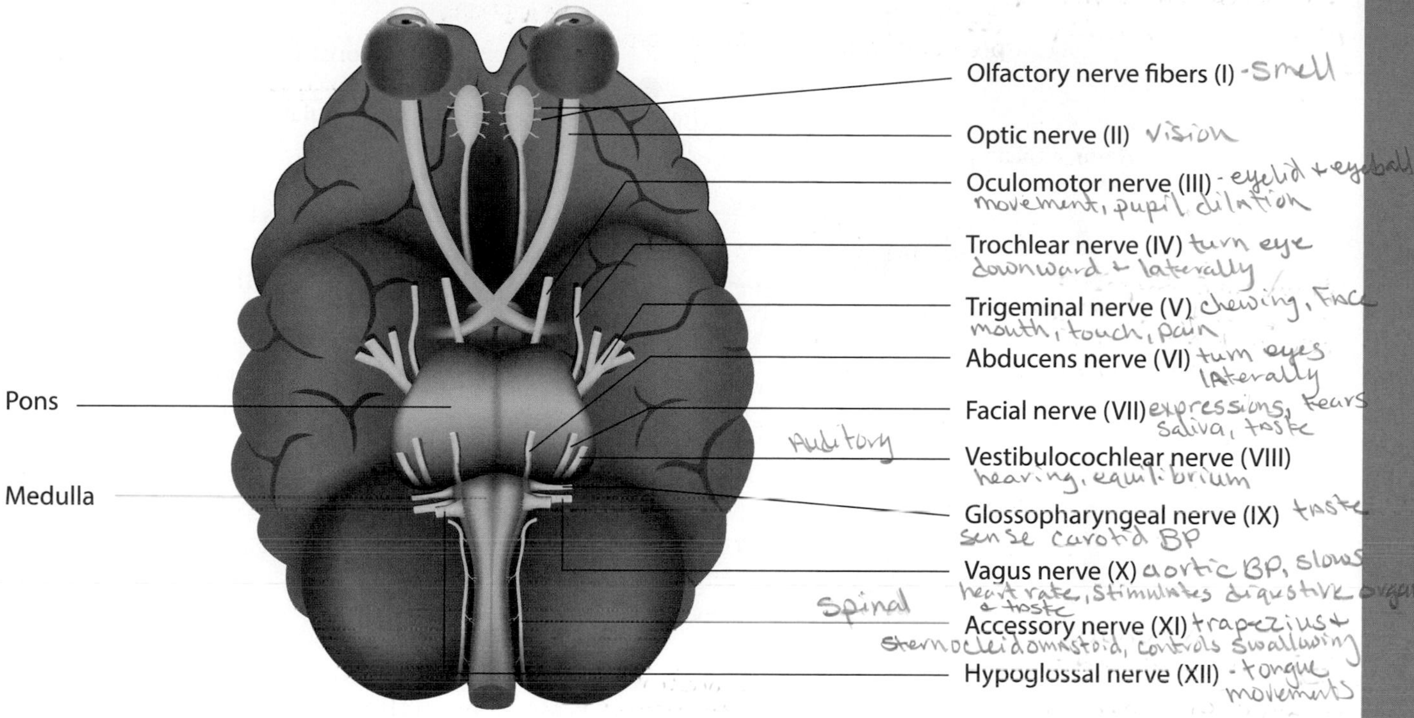
Olfactory nerve fibers (I) - smell
Optic nerve (II) vision
Oculomotor nerve (III) - eyelid + eyeball movement, pupil dilation
Trochlear nerve (IV) turn eye downward + laterally
Trigeminal nerve (V) chewing, face mouth, touch, pain
Abducens nerve (VI) turn eyes laterally
Pons
Facial nerve (VII) expressions, tears saliva, taste
Auditory
Vestibulocochlear nerve (VIII) hearing, equilibrium
Medulla
Glossopharyngeal nerve (IX) taste sense carotid BP
Vagus nerve (X) aortic BP, slows heart rate, stimulates digestive organs & taste
Spinal
Accessory nerve (XI) trapezius + sternocleidomastoid, controls swallowing
Hypoglossal nerve (XII) - tongue movements

Nervous System — Nerve Anatomy

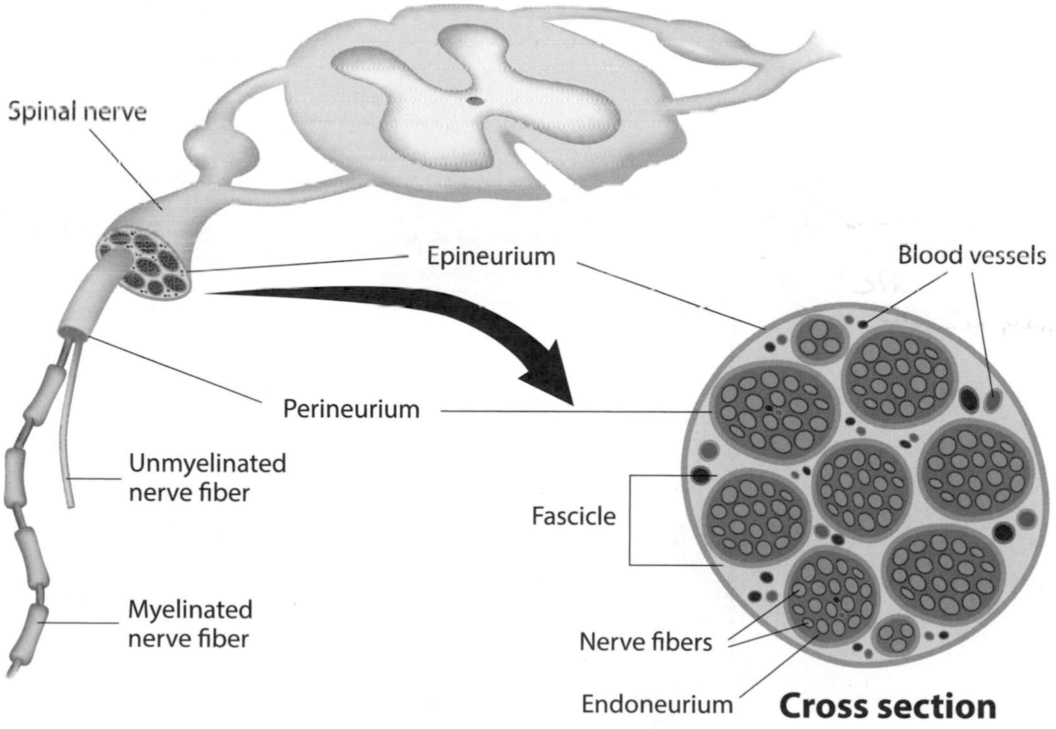
Spinal nerve
Epineurium
Blood vessels
Perineurium
Unmyelinated nerve fiber
Fascicle
Myelinated nerve fiber
Nerve fibers
Endoneurium
Cross section

Nervous System — Parasympathetic System Anatomy

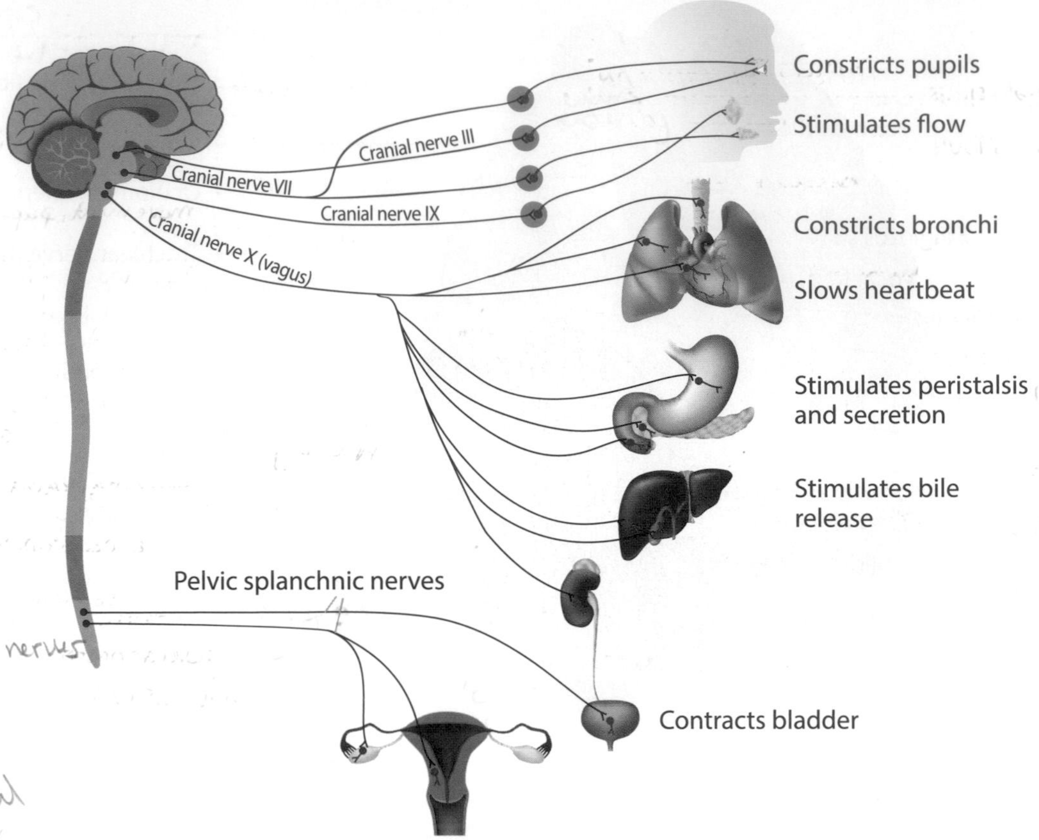

31 pr spinal nerves
8 cervical
12 thoracic
5 lumbar
5 sacral
1 coccygeal

Nervous System — Sympathetic System Anatomy

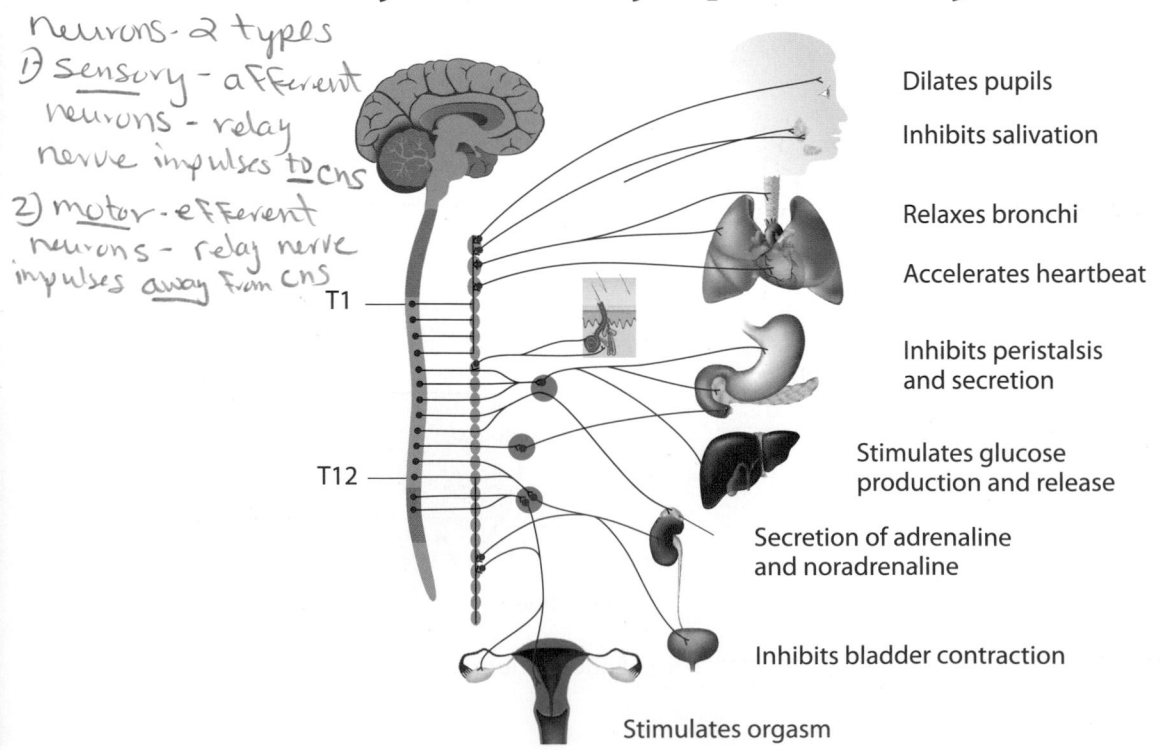

neurons - 2 types
1) Sensory - afferent neurons - relay nerve impulses to CNS
2) motor - efferent neurons - relay nerve impulses away from CNS

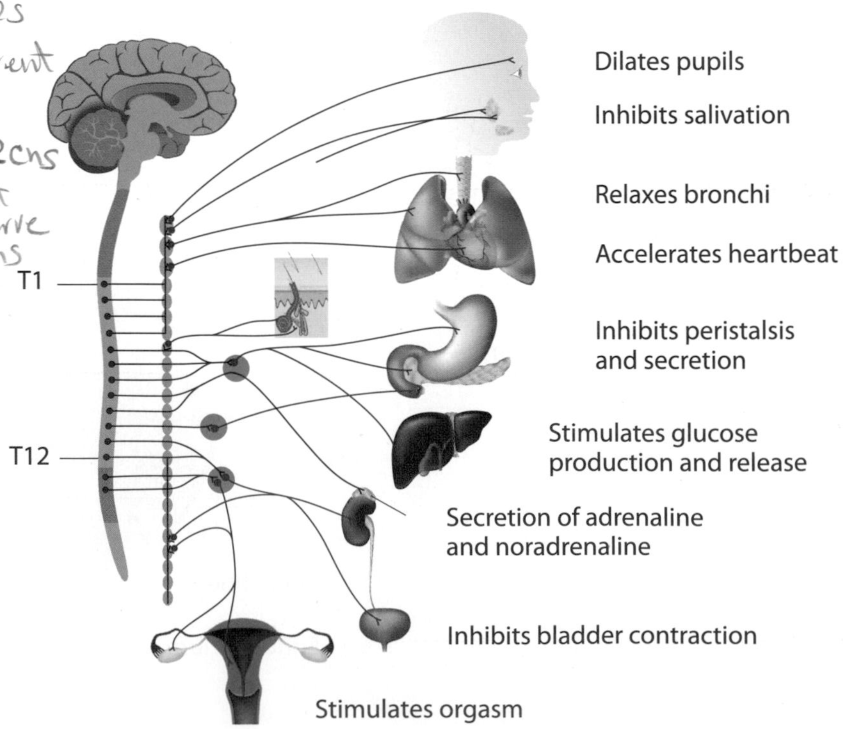

Respiratory System Anatomy

Exchange of gases O_2 + CO_2 by diffusion occurs in alveoli

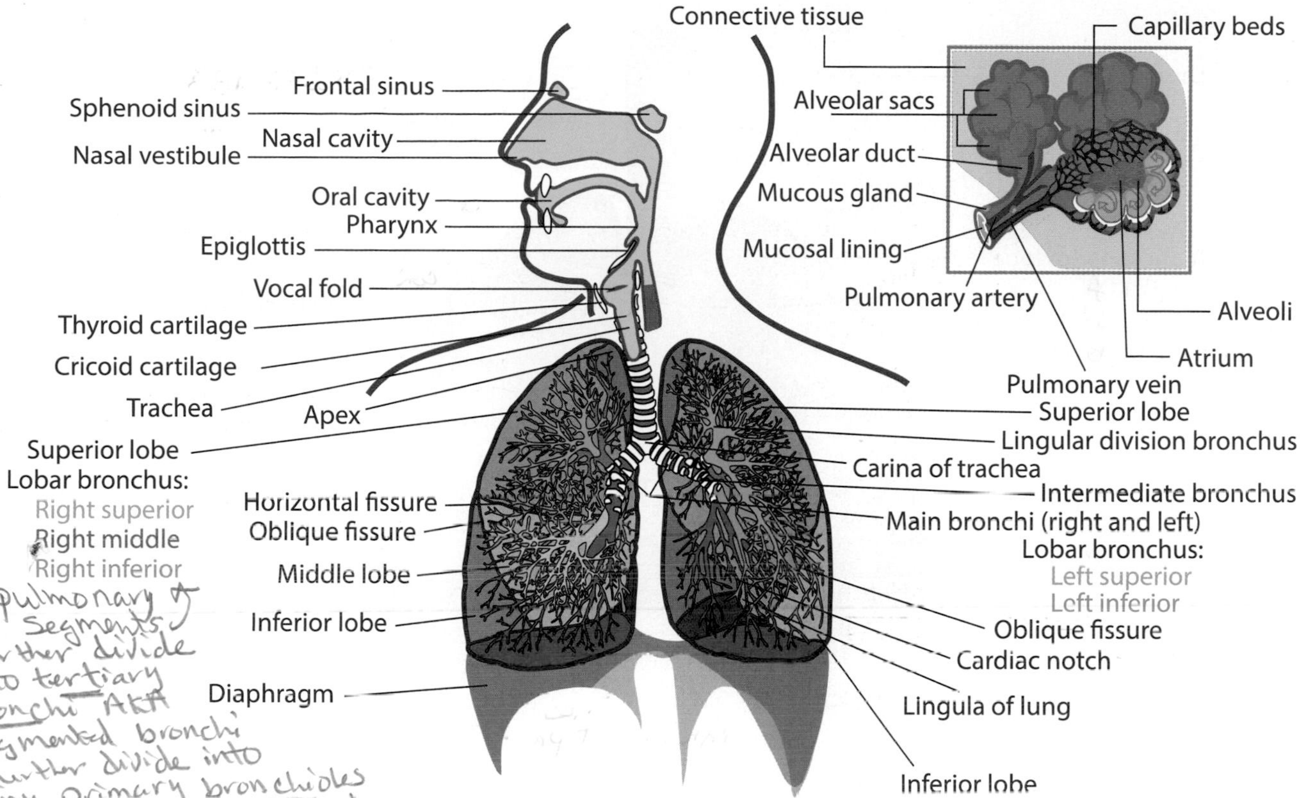

AKA pulmonary segments further divide into tertiary bronchi AKA segmented bronchi & further divide into many primary bronchioles & then divide into terminal bronchioles ⇒ alveolar ducts ⇒ alveolar sacs

Respiratory System — Larynx Anatomy

bronchioles are coded to bronchus
alveoli are coded to the lung

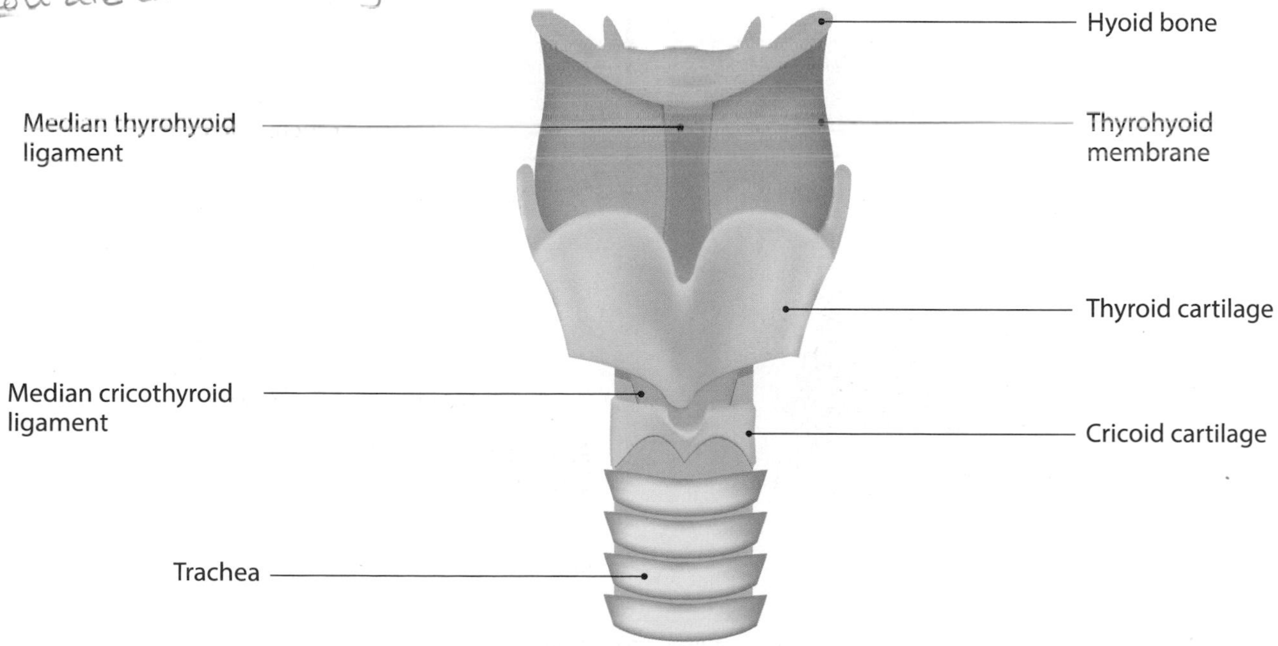

Respiratory System — Lung Anatomy

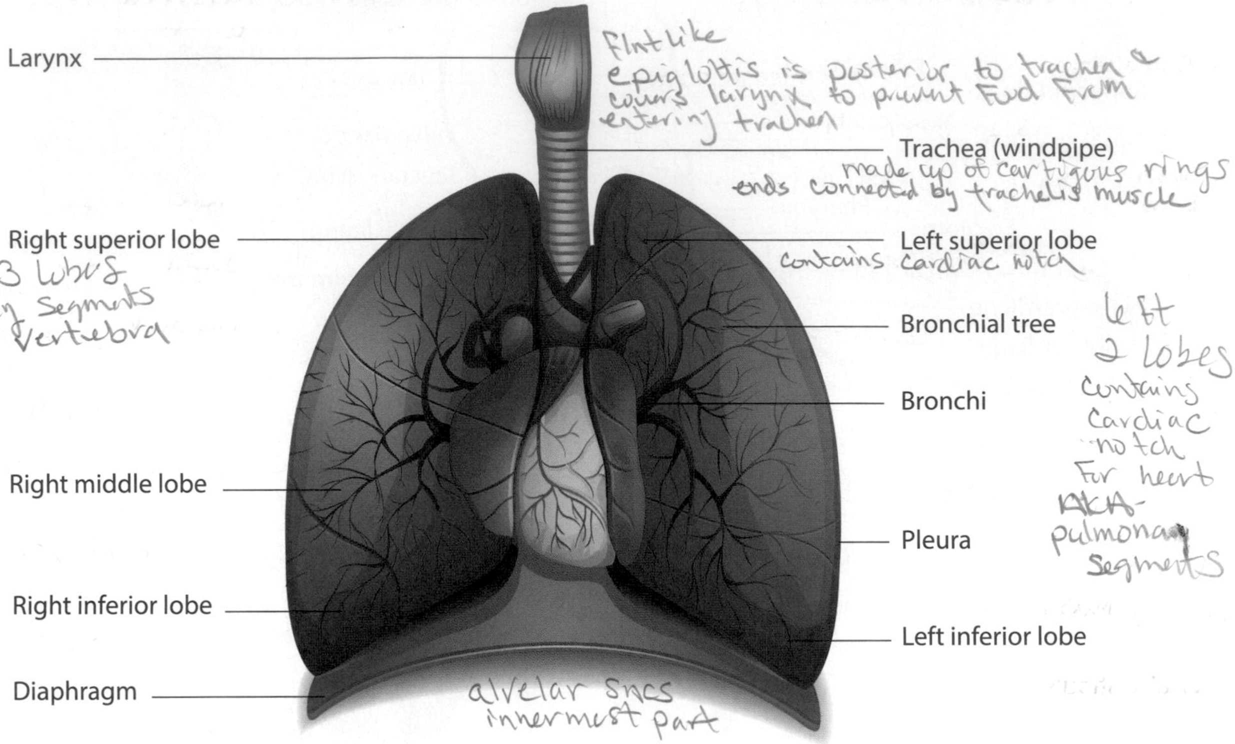

Larynx

flat like
epiglottis is posterior to trachea &
covers larynx to prevent food from
entering trachea

Trachea (windpipe)
made up of cartilagous rings
ends connected by trachelis muscle

Right superior lobe

Right 3 lobes
pulmonary segments
at T4 vertebra

Left superior lobe
contains cardiac notch

Bronchial tree

left
2 lobes
contains
cardiac
notch
for heart
AKA-
pulmonary
segments

Bronchi

Right middle lobe

Pleura

Right inferior lobe

Left inferior lobe

Diaphragm

alvelar snes
innermost part

Respiratory System Function

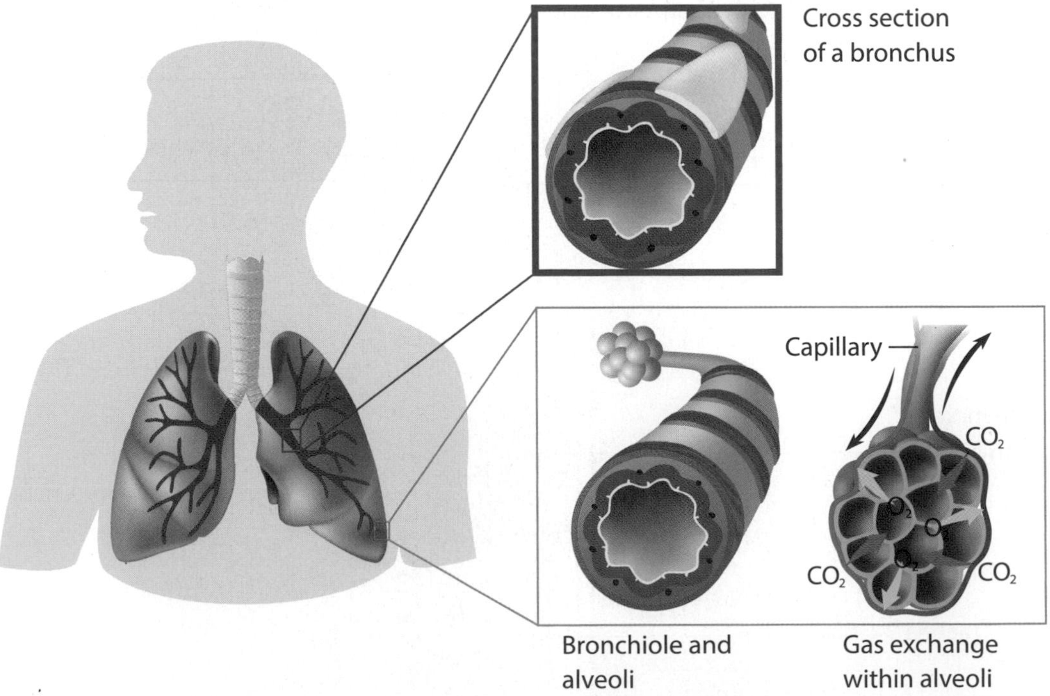

Cross section
of a bronchus

Capillary

CO_2

CO_2 CO_2

Bronchiole and
alveoli

Gas exchange
within alveoli

Respiratory System — Nose Anatomy

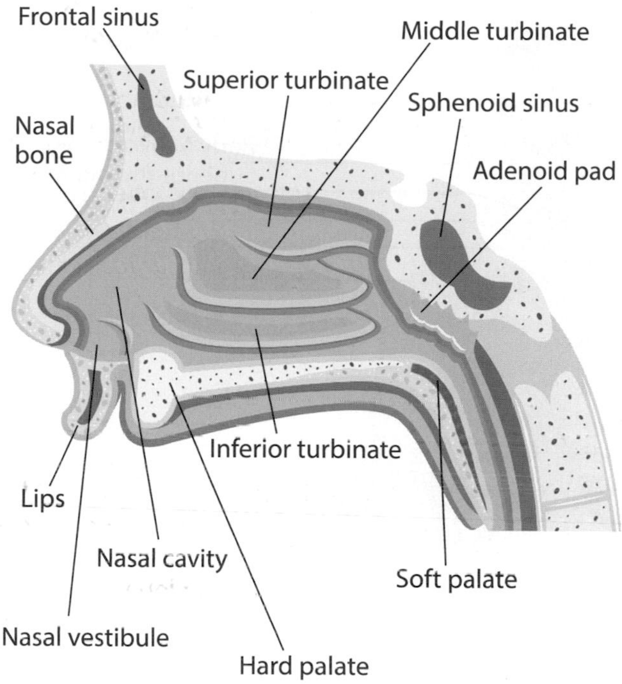

Respiratory System — Sinus Anatomy

- 4 groups paranasal sinuses

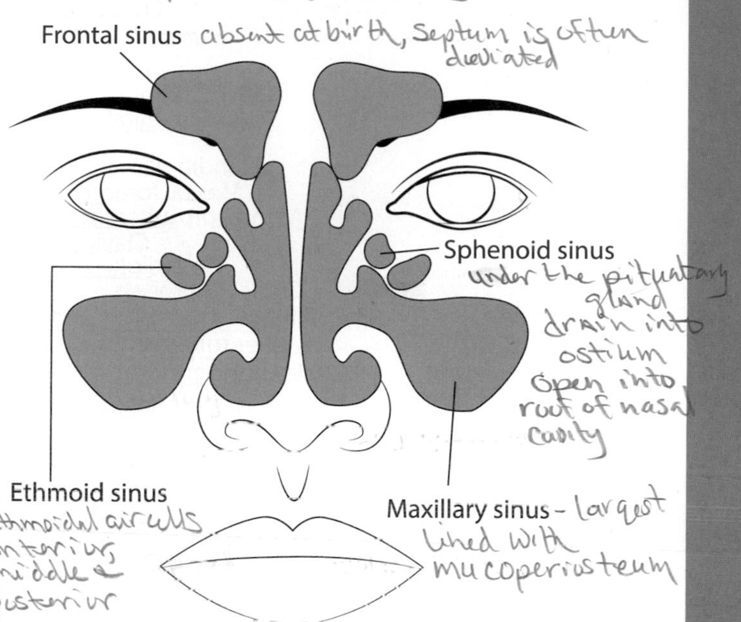

Respiratory System — Throat Anatomy

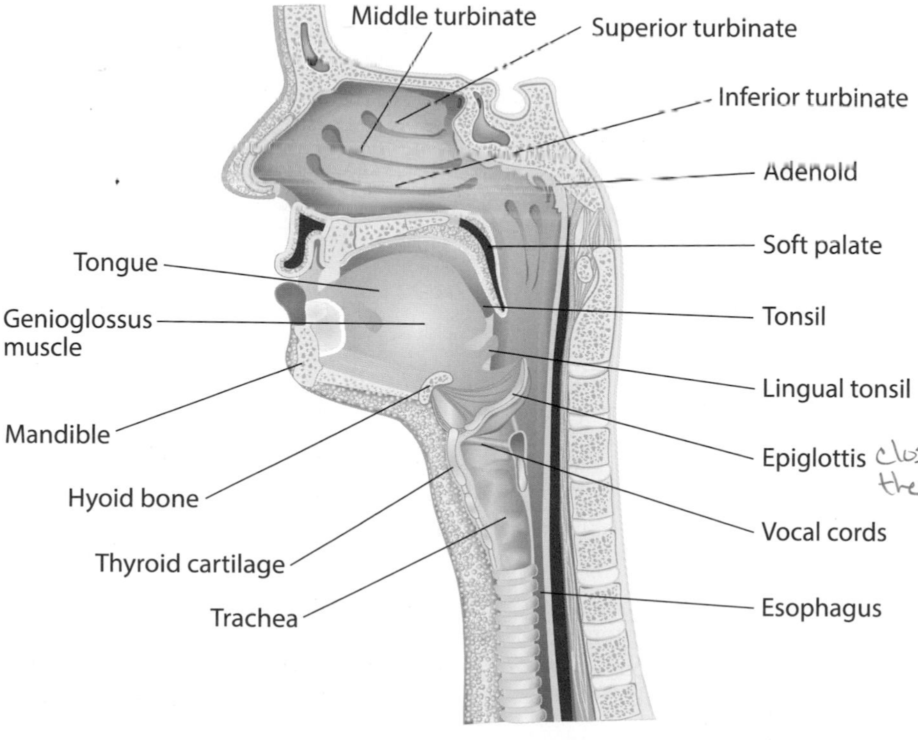

Skeletal System Anatomy

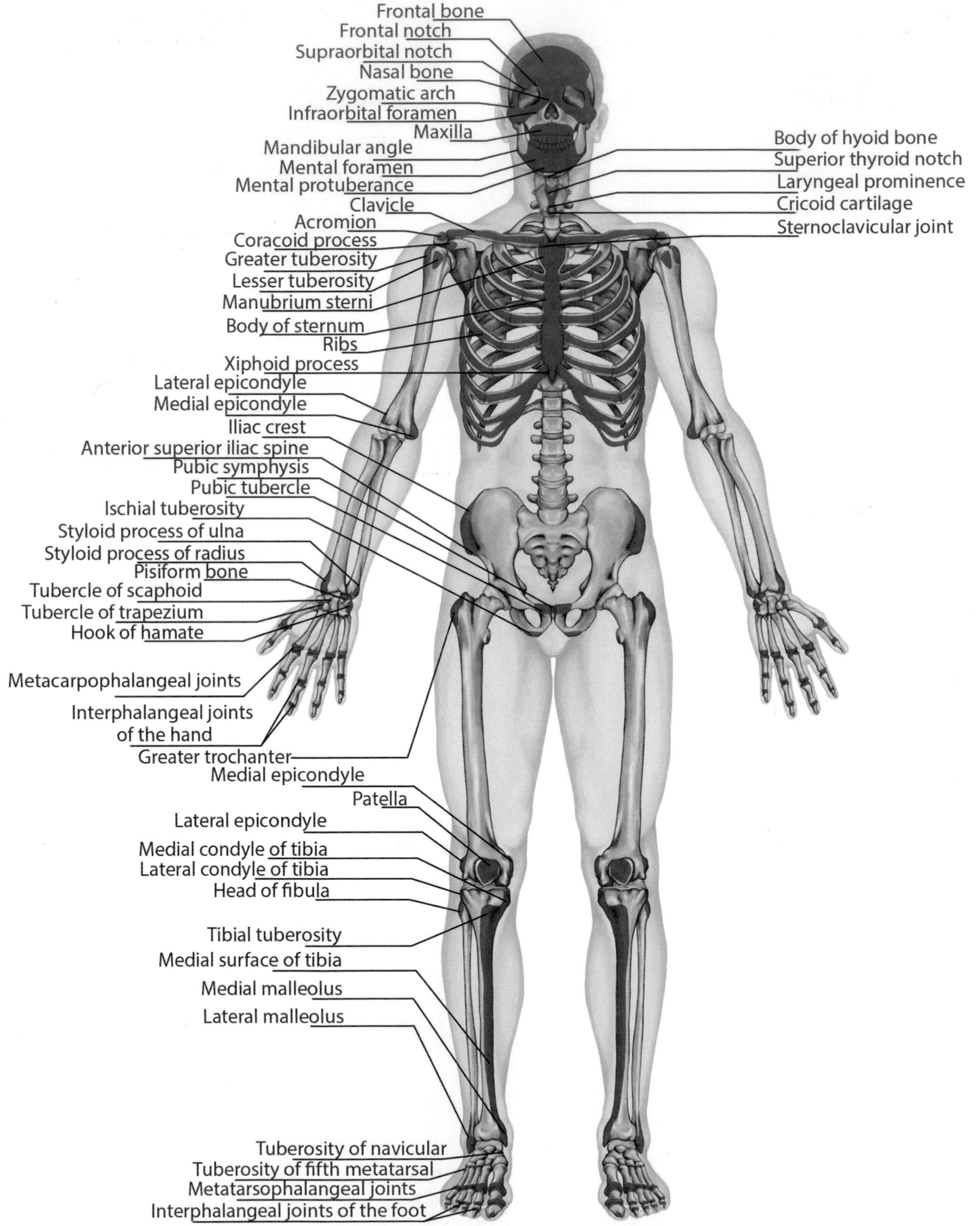
Frontal bone
Frontal notch
Supraorbital notch
Nasal bone
Zygomatic arch
Infraorbital foramen
Maxilla
Mandibular angle
Mental foramen
Mental protuberance
Clavicle
Acromion
Coracoid process
Greater tuberosity
Lesser tuberosity
Manubrium sterni
Body of sternum
Ribs
Xiphoid process
Lateral epicondyle
Medial epicondyle
Iliac crest
Anterior superior iliac spine
Pubic symphysis
Pubic tubercle
Ischial tuberosity
Styloid process of ulna
Styloid process of radius
Pisiform bone
Tubercle of scaphoid
Tubercle of trapezium
Hook of hamate
Metacarpophalangeal joints
Interphalangeal joints of the hand
Greater trochanter
Medial epicondyle
Patella
Lateral epicondyle
Medial condyle of tibia
Lateral condyle of tibia
Head of fibula
Tibial tuberosity
Medial surface of tibia
Medial malleolus
Lateral malleolus
Tuberosity of navicular
Tuberosity of fifth metatarsal
Metatarsophalangeal joints
Interphalangeal joints of the foot
Body of hyoid bone
Superior thyroid notch
Laryngeal prominence
Cricoid cartilage
Sternoclavicular joint

206 Bones in body, 80 are axial bones (head, facial, hyoid, auditory, trunk, ribs, sternum) - along the central axis of body
remaining 126 are appendicular bones (arms, shoulders, wrists, hands, legs, hips, ankles, feet)
related to movement & are appended to axial structure

Skeletal System — Bone Structure

Bones
4 categories
1) Long bones - longer than wide
& work as levers
Ex: upper/lower extremities
humerous, tibia, femur, ulna, metacarpel
2) Short bones
cube shaped found in wrist & ankles
3) Flat bones
broad surfaces to protect organs & attachment of muscles
Ex: ribs, cranial bones, bones of shoulder girdle
4) irregular bones
all others - ex: bones of vertebral & few in skull

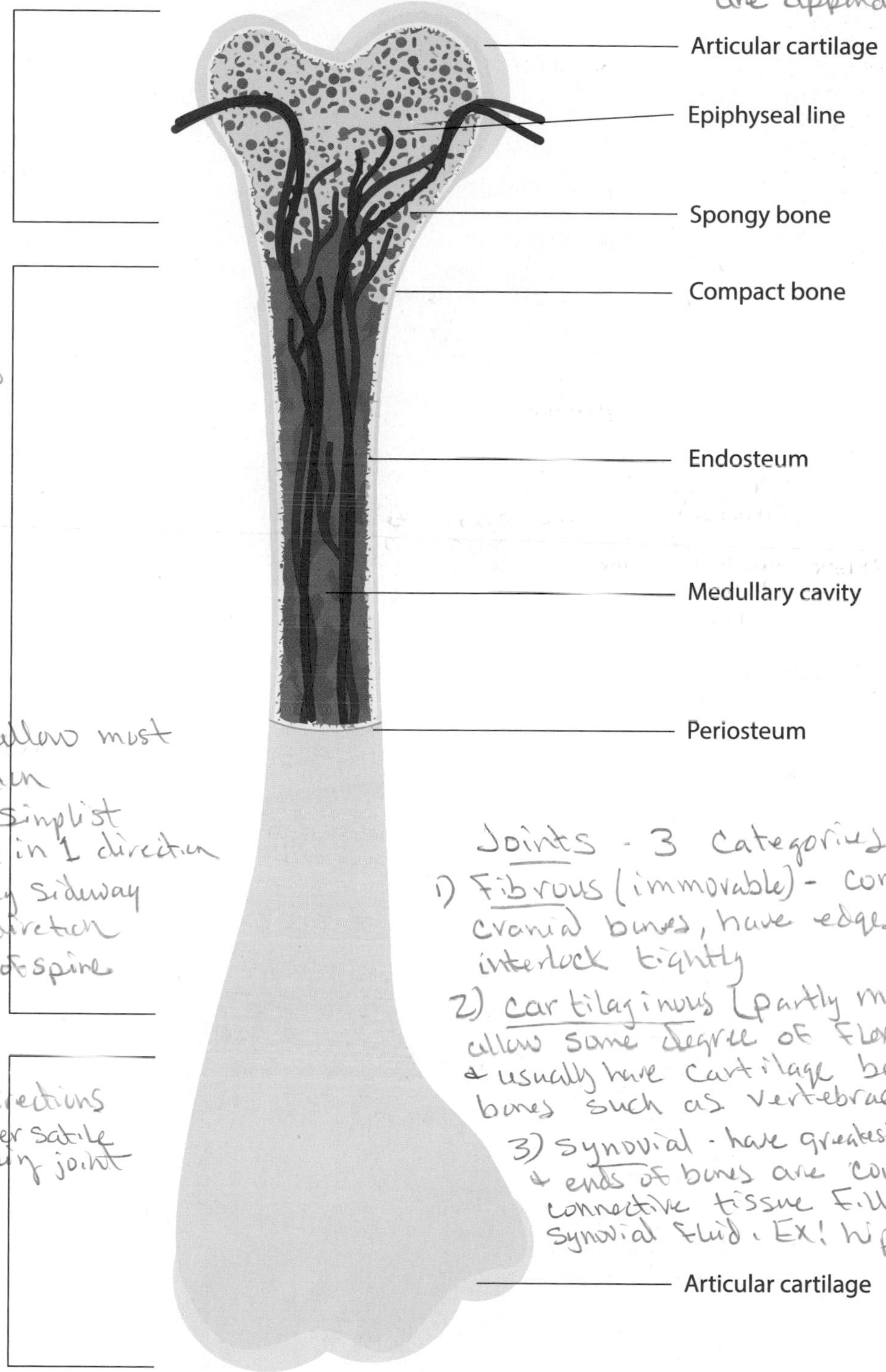

Joint Types
1) Ball & socket - allow most range of motion
2) Hinge - most simplist
allow movement in 1 direction
3) Gliding - mostly sideway movement & 1 direction
4) Pivot - near top of spine
& allow head to swivel & bend
5) Saddle - allow movement in 2 directions making it more versatile than hinge or gliding joint

Joints - 3 categories
1) Fibrous (immovable) - connect the cranial bones, have edges that interlock tightly
2) cartilaginous (partly movable)
allow some degree of flexibility & usually have cartilage between the bones such as vertebrae
3) Synovial - have greatest flexibility & ends of bones are covered with connective tissue filled with synovial fluid. Ex: hip

Skeletal System — Skull

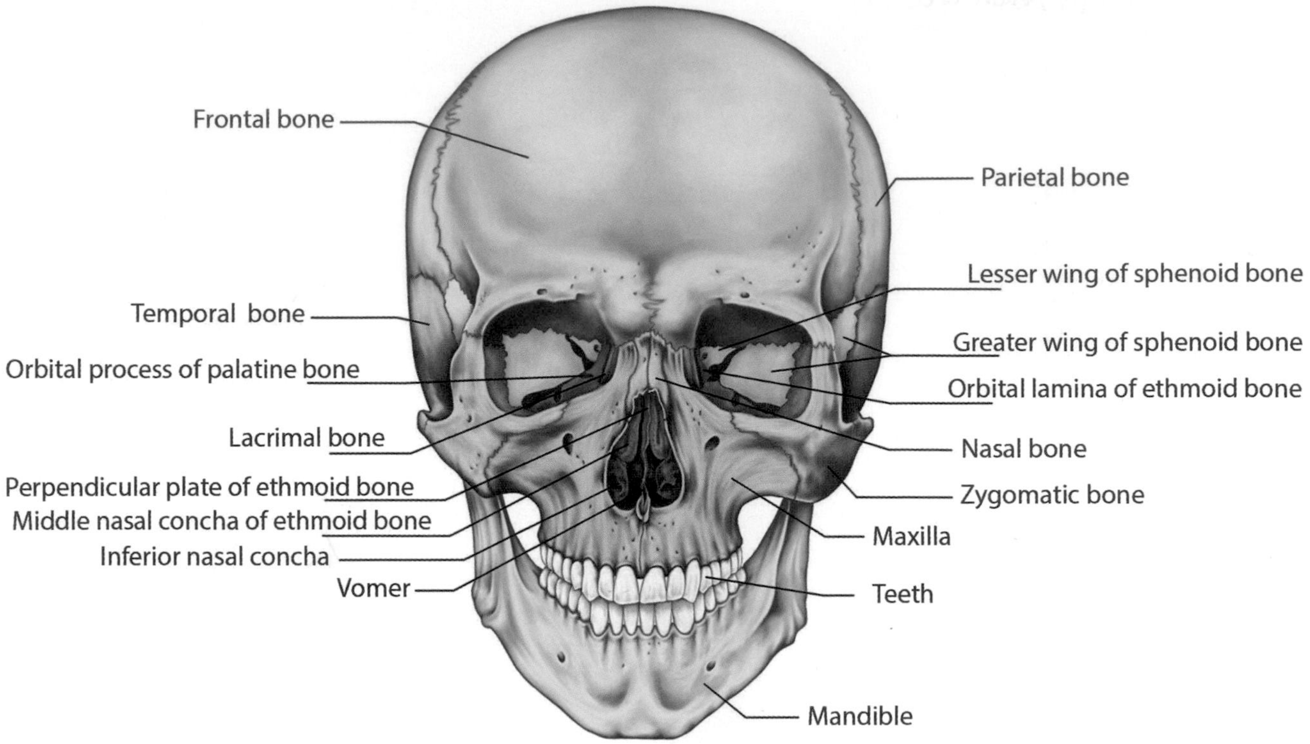
Frontal bone
Parietal bone
Lesser wing of sphenoid bone
Temporal bone
Greater wing of sphenoid bone
Orbital process of palatine bone
Orbital lamina of ethmoid bone
Lacrimal bone
Nasal bone
Perpendicular plate of ethmoid bone
Zygomatic bone
Middle nasal concha of ethmoid bone
Maxilla
Inferior nasal concha
Vomer
Teeth
Mandible

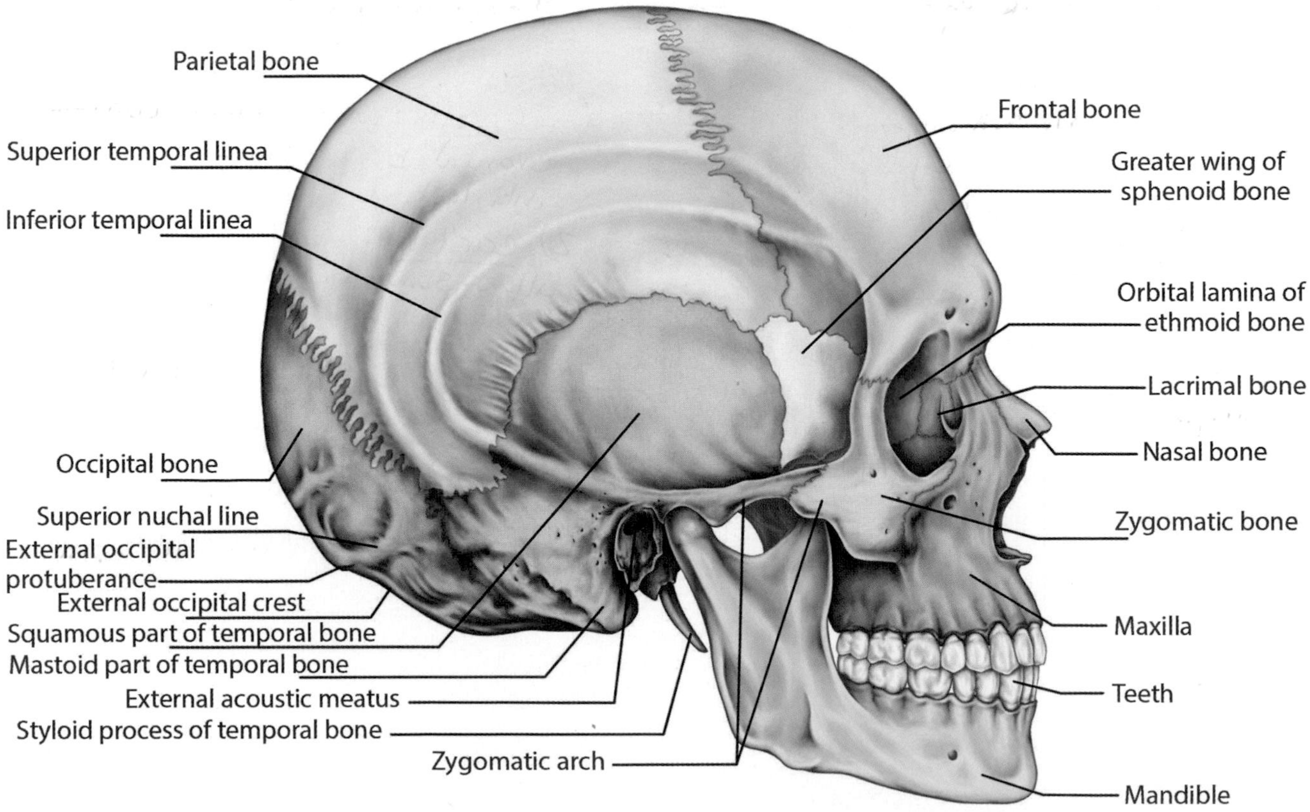
Parietal bone
Frontal bone
Superior temporal linea
Greater wing of sphenoid bone
Inferior temporal linea
Orbital lamina of ethmoid bone
Lacrimal bone
Occipital bone
Nasal bone
Superior nuchal line
Zygomatic bone
External occipital protuberance
External occipital crest
Maxilla
Squamous part of temporal bone
Mastoid part of temporal bone
Teeth
External acoustic meatus
Styloid process of temporal bone
Zygomatic arch
Mandible

Skeletal System — Cervical, Thoracic, and Lumbar Spine

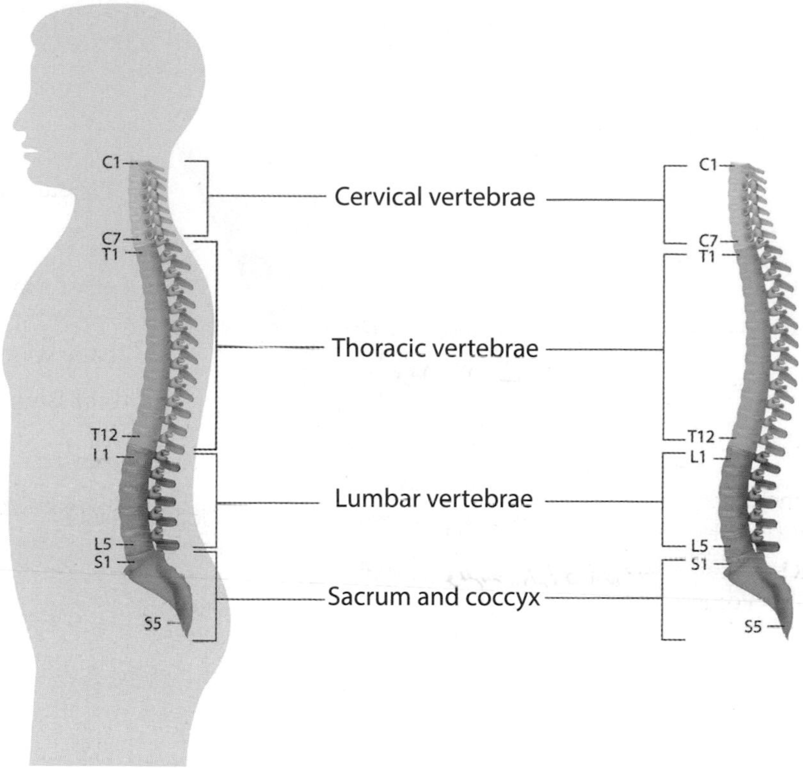

Skeletal System — Pelvic Girdle

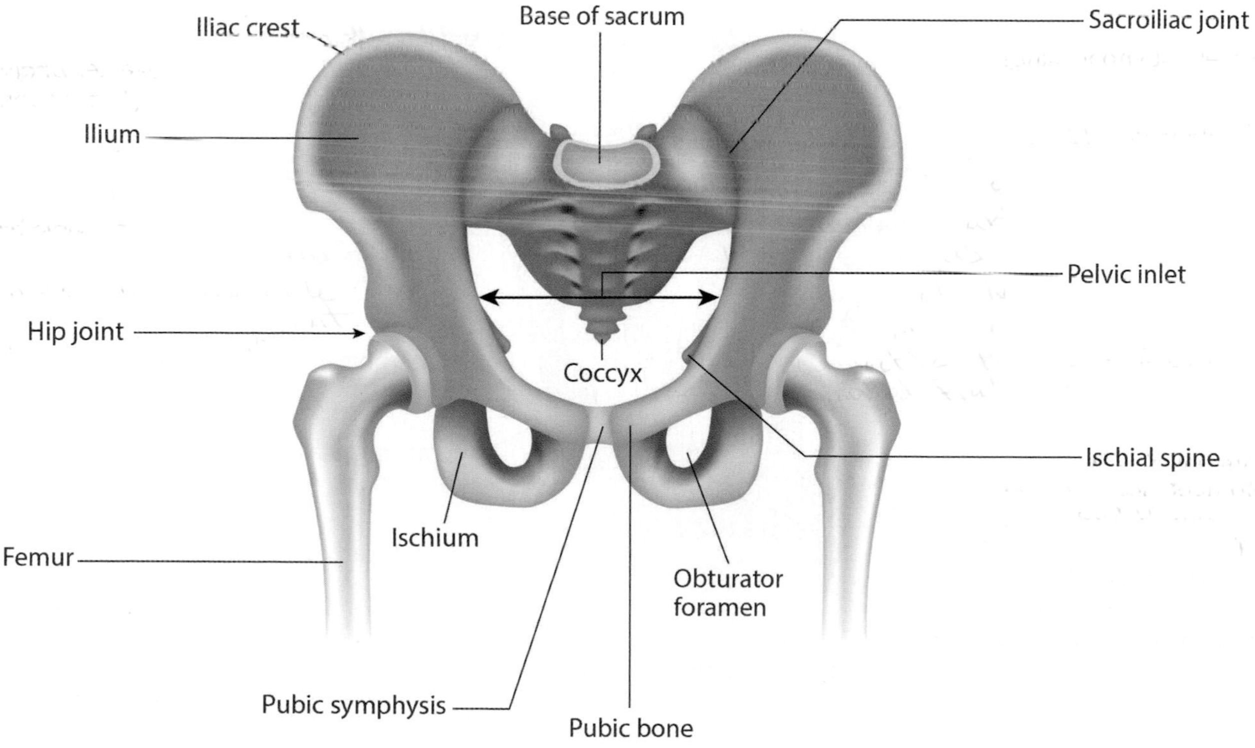

Skeletal System — Elbow Joint Structure

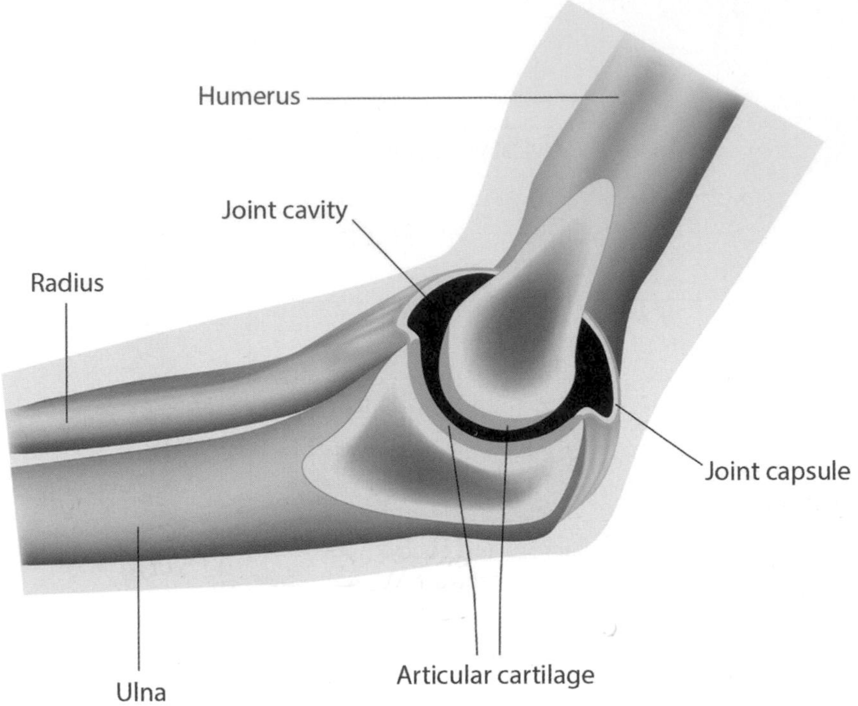

Skeletal System — Hand Bones

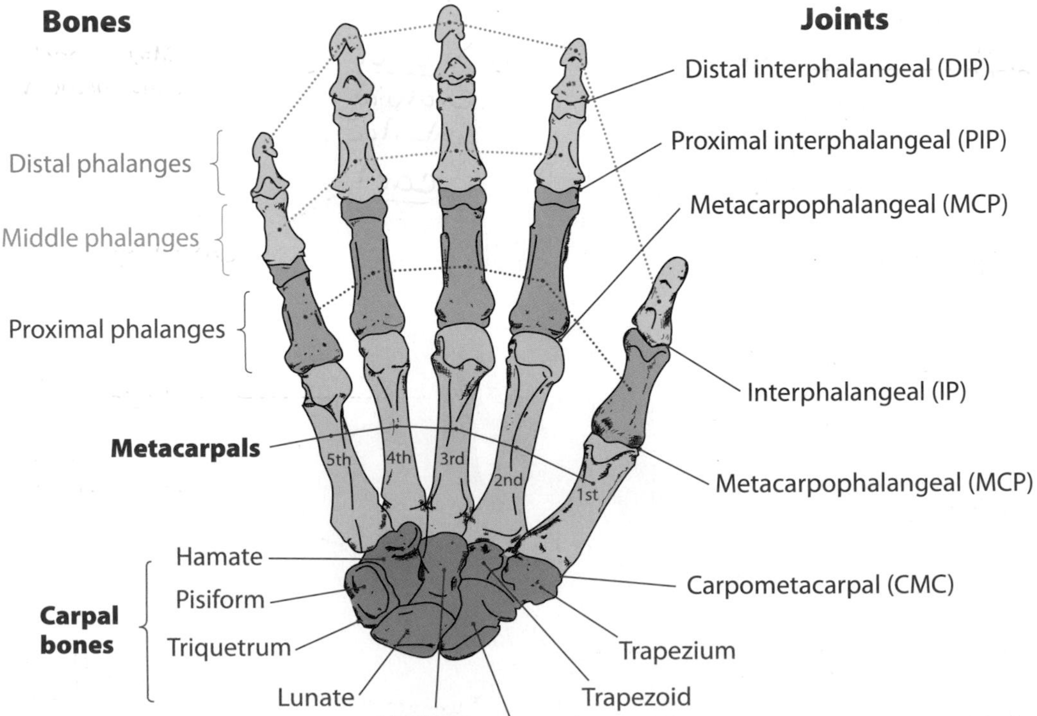

osteotomy of capitate = Division to shorten bone

Skeletal System — Foot Bones (Right Foot, Lateral View)

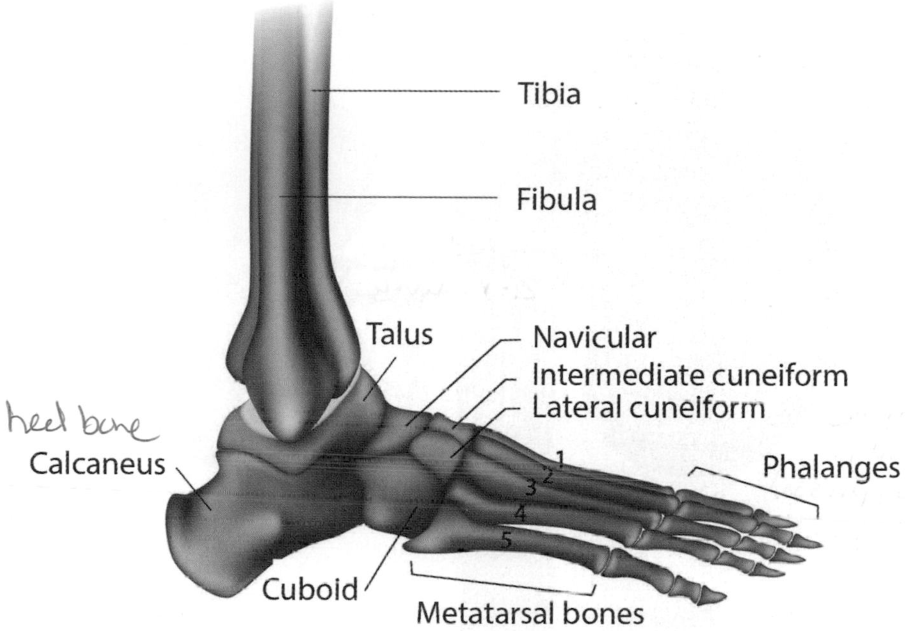

Urinary System Anatomy

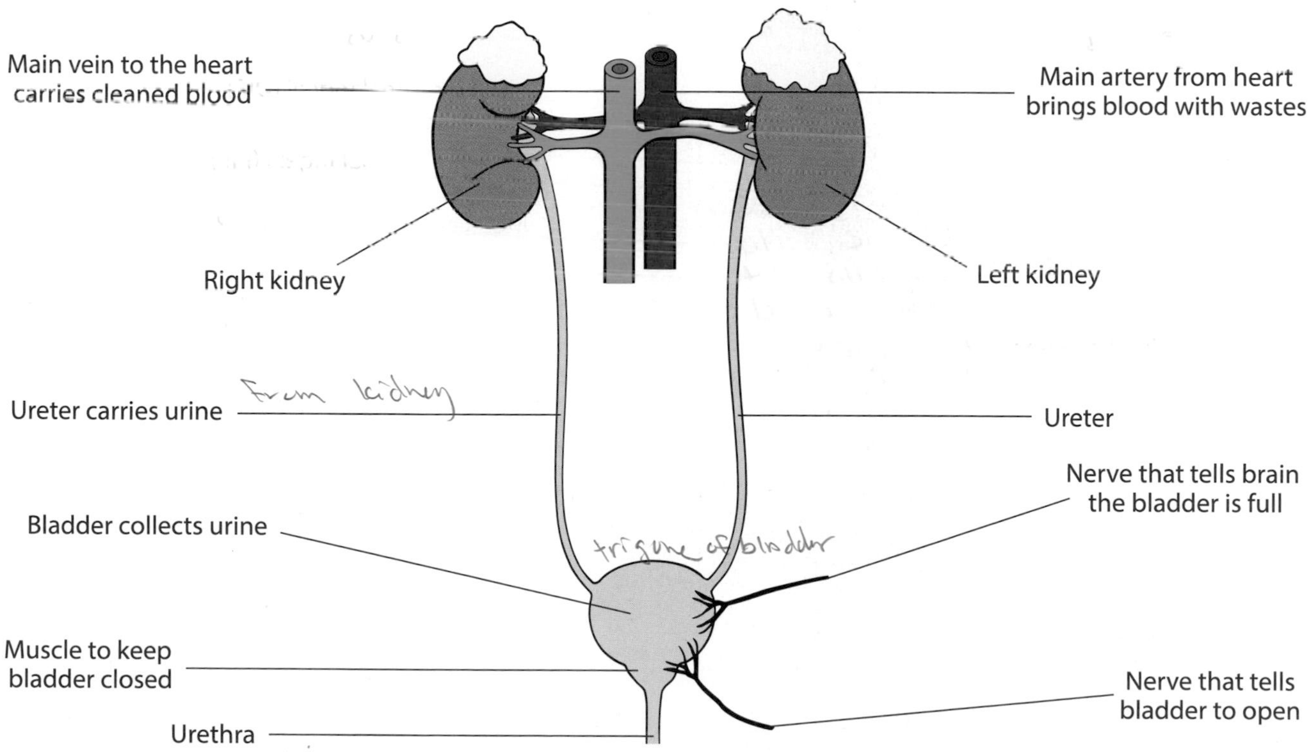

produces, stores & eliminates urine

Urinary System — Kidney Anatomy

includes 2 sphincter muscles

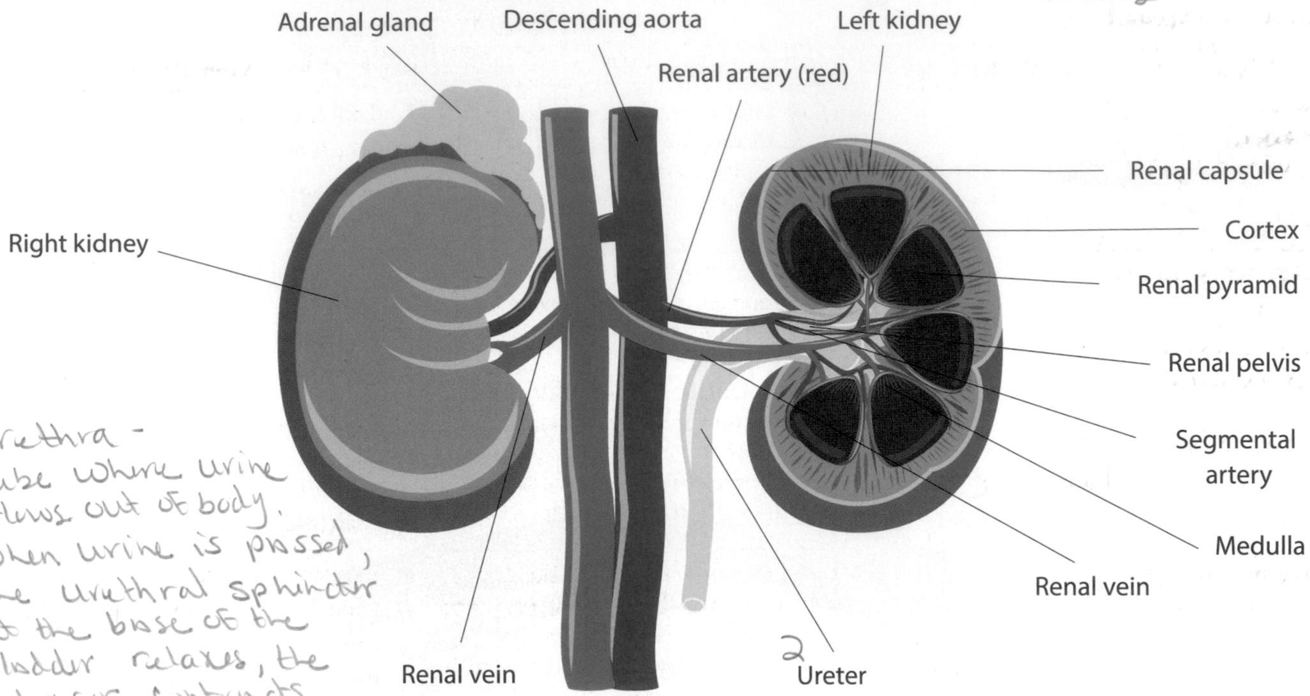

Urethra - tube where urine flows out of body. When urine is passed, the urethral sphincter at the base of the bladder relaxes, the detrusor contracts & urine is voided

Approach based on: access location, method, type of instrumentation

Approach Table - 7 approaches

Section 0 - Medical and Surgical
Character 5 - Approach technique used to reach site of procedure

Approach	5th Character	Definition	Examples
External mouth colostomy stoma	X	Procedures performed directly on the skin or mucous membrane and procedures performed indirectly by the application of external force through the skin or mucous membrane	• Cauterization of epistaxis • Reduction of a dislocated shoulder • Destruction of renal calculi with lithotripsy, skin excision closed reduction of fracture
Open puncture or minor incision is not open - it does not expose the site of the procedure AKA - otomy	0	Cutting through the skin or mucous membrane and any other body layers necessary to expose the site of the procedure may include percutaneous endoscopic assistance	• Open reduction and internal fixation of a fracture • Abdominal appendectomy • Open coronary artery bypass graft
Percutaneous AKA - endovascular	3	Entry, by puncture or minor incision, of instrumentation through the skin or mucous membrane and/or any other body layers necessary to reach the site of the procedure	• Percutaneous paracentesis • Tracheostomy formation with tracheostomy tube placement • Needle biopsy of breast mass
Percutaneous, Endoscopic - site must be visualized	4	Entry, by puncture or minor incision, of instrumentation through the skin or mucous membrane and/or any other body layers necessary to reach and visualize the site of the procedure	• Shoulder arthroscopy • Autograft nerve graft to right median nerve • Mapping of left cerebral hemisphere not liver biopsy
Via Natural or Artificial Opening	7	Entry of instrumentation through a natural or artificial external opening to reach the site of the procedure	• Placement of a Foley catheter • Endotracheal intubation • Transvaginal cervical cerclage
Via Natural or Artificial Opening, Endoscopic	8	Entry of instrumentation through a natural or artificial external opening to reach and visualize the site of the procedure	• Colonoscopy • Bronchoscopy • Esophagogastroduodenoscopy (EGD)
Via Natural or Artificial Opening, with Percutaneous Endoscopic Assistance	F	Entry of instrumentation through a natural or artificial external opening to reach and visualize the site of the procedure, and entry, by puncture or minor incision, of instrumentation through the skin or mucous membrane and any other body layers necessary to aid in the performance of the procedure	• Resections of the female reproductive system • Laparoscopic-assisted vaginal salpingo-oophorectomy and hysterectomy

endoscopic - not considered open because it does not expose the site of procedure
may have puncture or minor incision or through external opening

open w/percutaneous endoscopic assistance - code as open

Approach Table

This page intentionally left blank

main term can be body part, root operation, or common procedure/term
no eponyms

 alcohol detoxification HZ2ZZZZ

3

A

Aortography
see Plain Radiography, Upper Arteries B30
see Fluoroscopy, Upper Arteries B31
see Plain Radiography, Lower Arteries B40
see Fluoroscopy, Lower Arteries B41
Aortoplasty
see Repair, Aorta, Thoracic, Descending 02QW
see Repair, Aorta, Thoracic, Ascending/Arch 02QX
see Replacement, Aorta, Thoracic, Descending 02RW
see Replacement, Aorta, Thoracic, Ascending/Arch 02RX
see Supplement, Aorta, Thoracic, Descending 02UW
see Supplement, Aorta, Thoracic, Ascending/Arch 02UX
see Repair, Aorta, Abdominal 04Q0
see Replacement, Aorta, Abdominal 04R0
see Supplement, Aorta, Abdominal 04U0
Apalutamide Antineoplastic XW0DXJ5
Apical (subclavicular) lymph node
use Lymphatic, Right Axillary
use Lymphatic, Left Axillary
Apneustic center
use Pons
Appendectomy
see Excision, Appendix 0DBJ part
see Resection, Appendix 0DTJ all
Appendicolysis
see Release, Appendix 0DNJ
Appendicotomy
see Drainage, Appendix 0D9J
Application
see Introduction of substance in or on
Aquablation therapy, prostate XV508A4
Aquapheresis 6A550Z3
Aqueduct of Sylvius
use Cerebral Ventricle
Aqueous humour
use Anterior Chamber, Right
use Anterior Chamber, Left
Arachnoid mater, intracranial
use Cerebral Meninges
Arachnoid mater, spinal
use Spinal Meninges
Arcuate artery
use Foot Artery, Right
use Foot Artery, Left
Areola
use Nipple, Right
use Nipple, Left
AROM (artificial rupture of membranes) 10907ZC
Arterial canal (duct)
use Pulmonary Artery, Left
Arterial pulse tracing
see Measurement, Arterial 4A03
Arteriectomy
see Excision, Heart and Great Vessels 02B
see Excision, Upper Arteries 03B
see Excision, Lower Arteries 04B
Arteriography
see Plain Radiography, Heart B20
see Fluoroscopy, Heart B21
see Plain Radiography, Upper Arteries B30
see Fluoroscopy, Upper Arteries B31
see Plain Radiography, Lower Arteries B40
see Fluoroscopy, Lower Arteries B41
Arterioplasty
see Repair, Heart and Great Vessels 02Q
see Replacement, Heart and Great Vessels 02R
see Supplement, Heart and Great Vessels 02U
see Repair, Upper Arteries 03Q
Arterioplasty — *continued*
see Replacement, Upper Arteries 03R
see Supplement, Upper Arteries 03U
see Repair, Lower Arteries 04Q
see Replacement, Lower Arteries 04R
see Supplement, Lower Arteries 04U
Arteriorrhaphy
see Repair, Heart and Great Vessels 02Q
see Repair, Upper Arteries 03Q
see Repair, Lower Arteries 04Q
Arterioscopy
see Inspection, Great Vessel 02JY
see Inspection, Artery, Upper 03JY
see Inspection, Artery, Lower 04JY
Arthrectomy
see Excision, Upper Joints 0RB
see Resection, Upper Joints 0RT
see Excision, Lower Joints 0SB
see Resection, Lower Joints 0ST
Arthrocentesis
see Drainage, Upper Joints 0R9
see Drainage, Lower Joints 0S9
Arthrodesis see page 486
see Fusion, Upper Joints 0RG
see Fusion, Lower Joints 0SG
Arthrography
see Plain Radiography, Skull and Facial Bones BN0
see Plain Radiography, Non-Axial Upper Bones BP0
see Plain Radiography, Non-Axial Lower Bones BQ0
Arthrolysis
see Release, Upper Joints 0RN
see Release, Lower Joints 0SN
Arthropexy
see Repair, Upper Joints 0RQ
see Reposition, Upper Joints 0RS
see Repair, Lower Joints 0SQ
see Reposition, Lower Joints 0SS
Arthroplasty
see Repair, Upper Joints 0RQ
see Replacement, Upper Joints 0RR
see Supplement, Upper Joints 0RU
see Repair, Lower Joints 0SQ
see Replacement, Lower Joints 0SR
see Supplement, Lower Joints 0SU
Arthroplasty, radial head
see Replacement, Radius, Right 0PRH
see Replacement, Radius, Left 0PRJ
Arthroscopy
see Inspection, Upper Joints 0RJ
see Inspection, Lower Joints 0SJ knee
Arthrotomy
see Drainage, Upper Joints 0R9
see Drainage, Lower Joints 0S9
Articulating Spacer (Antibiotic)
use Articulating Spacer in Lower Joints
Artificial anal sphincter (AAS)
use Artificial Sphincter in Gastrointestinal System
Artificial bowel sphincter (neosphincter)
use Artificial Sphincter in Gastrointestinal System
Artificial Sphincter
Insertion of device in
Anus 0DHQ
Bladder 0THB
Bladder Neck 0THC
Urethra 0THD
Removal of device from
Anus 0DPQ
Bladder 0TPB
Urethra 0TPD
Revision of device in
Anus 0DWQ
Bladder 0TWB
Urethra 0TWD
Artificial urinary sphincter (AUS)
use Artificial Sphincter in Urinary System
Aryepiglottic fold
use Larynx
Arytenoid cartilage
use Larynx
Arytenoid muscle
use Neck Muscle, Right
use Neck Muscle, Left
Arytenoidectomy
see Excision, Larynx 0CBS
Arytenoidopexy
see Repair, Larynx 0CQS
Ascenda Intrathecal Catheter
use Infusion Device
Ascending aorta
use Thoracic Aorta, Ascending/Arch
Ascending palatine artery
use Face Artery
Ascending pharyngeal artery
use External Carotid Artery, Right
use External Carotid Artery, Left
Aspiration, fine needle
Fluid or gas *see* Drainage
Tissue biopsy
see Excision - thyroid gland FNA
see Extraction
Assessment
Activities of daily living *see* Activities of Daily Living Assessment, Rehabilitation F02
Hearing *see* Hearing Assessment, Diagnostic Audiology F13
Hearing aid *see* Hearing Aid Assessment, Diagnostic Audiology F14
Intravascular perfusion, using indocyanine green (ICG) dye *see* Monitoring, Physiological Systems 4A1
Motor function *see* Motor Function Assessment, Rehabilitation F01
Nerve function *see* Motor Function Assessment, Rehabilitation F01
Speech *see* Speech Assessment, Rehabilitation F00
Vestibular *see* Vestibular Assessment, Diagnostic Audiology F15
Vocational *see* Activities of Daily Living Treatment, Rehabilitation F08
Assistance
Cardiac
Continuous
Balloon Pump 5A02210
Impeller Pump 5A0221D
Other Pump 5A02216
Pulsatile Compression 5A02215
Intermittent
Balloon Pump 5A02110
Impeller Pump 5A0211D
Other Pump 5A02116
Pulsatile Compression 5A02115
Circulatory
Continuous
Hyperbaric 5A05221
Supersaturated 5A0522C
Intermittent
Hyperbaric 5A05121
Supersaturated 5A0512C
Respiratory
24-96 Consecutive Hours
Continuous Negative Airway Pressure 5A09459
Continuous Positive Airway Pressure 5A09457
Intermittent Negative Airway Pressure 5A0945B
Intermittent Positive Airway Pressure 5A09458

B

Bone Growth Stimulator - Bypass

Breast Implants - Alteration 0HD

CABG of LAD using LIMA 0210029

Capsulotomy - release

Choroidectomy
see Excision, Eye 08B
see Resection, Eye 08T
Ciliary body
use Eye, Right
use Eye, Left
Ciliary ganglion
use Head and Neck Sympathetic Nerve
Circle of Willis
use Intracranial Artery
Circumcision 0VTTXZZ
Circumflex iliac artery
use Femoral Artery, Right
use Femoral Artery, Left
CivaSheet®
use Radioactive Element
CivaSheet® Brachytherapy
see Brachytherapy with qualifier Unidirectional Source
see Insertion with device Radioactive Element
Clamp and rod internal fixation system (CRIF)
use Internal Fixation Device in Upper Bones
use Internal Fixation Device in Lower Bones
Clamping
see Occlusion
Claustrum
use Basal Ganglia
Claviculectomy
see Excision, Upper Bones 0PB
see Resection, Upper Bones 0PT
Claviculotomy
see Division, Upper Bones 0P8
see Drainage, Upper Bones 0P9
Clipping, aneurysm
see Occlusion using Extraluminal Device
see Restriction using Extraluminal Device
Clitorectomy, clitoridectomy
see Excision, Clitoris 0UBJ
see Resection, Clitoris 0UTJ
Clolar®
use Clofarabine
Closure
see Occlusion
see Repair
Clysis
see Introduction of substance in or on
Coagulation
see Destruction
Coagulation Factor Xa, Inactivated XW0
Coagulation Factor Xa, (Recombinant) Inactivated
use Coagulation Factor Xa, Inactivated
COALESCE® radiolucent interbody fusion device
use Interbody Fusion Device, Radiolucent Porous in New Technology
CoAxia NeuroFlo™ catheter
use Intraluminal Device
Cobalt/chromium head and polyethylene socket
use Synthetic Substitute, Metal on Polyethylene in 0SR
Cobalt/chromium head and socket
use Synthetic Substitute, Metal in 0SR
Coccygeal body
use Coccygeal Glomus
Coccygeus muscle
use Trunk Muscle, Right
use Trunk Muscle, Left
Cochlea
use Inner Ear, Right
use Inner Ear, Left
Cochlear implant (CI), multiple channel (electrode)
use Hearing Device, Multiple Channel Cochlear Prosthesis in 09H
Cochlear implant (CI), single channel (electrode)
use Hearing Device, Single Channel Cochlear Prosthesis in 09H
Cochlear Implant Treatment F0BZ0
Cochlear nerve
use Acoustic Nerve
COGNIS® CRT-D
use Cardiac Resynchronization Defibrillator Pulse Generator in 0JH
COHERE® radiolucent interbody fusion device
use Interbody Fusion Device, Radiolucent Porous in New Technology
Colectomy
see Excision, Gastrointestinal System 0DB
see Resection, Gastrointestinal System 0DT
Collapse
see Occlusion
Collection from
Breast, Breast Milk 8E0HX62
Indwelling Device
Circulatory System
Blood 8C02X6K
Other Fluid 8C02X6L
Nervous System
Cerebrospinal Fluid 8C01X6J
Other Fluid 8C01X6L
Integumentary System, Breast Milk 8E0HX62
Reproductive System, Male, Sperm 8E0VX63
Colocentesis
see Drainage, Gastrointestinal System 0D9
Colofixation
see Repair, Gastrointestinal System 0DQ
see Reposition, Gastrointestinal System 0DS
Cololysis
see Release, Gastrointestinal System 0DN
Colonic Z-Stent®
use Intraluminal Device
Colonoscopy 0DJD8ZZ
Colopexy
see Repair, Gastrointestinal System 0DQ
see Reposition, Gastrointestinal System 0DS
Coloplication
see Restriction, Gastrointestinal System 0DV
Coloproctectomy
see Excision, Gastrointestinal System 0DB
see Resection, Gastrointestinal System 0DT
Coloproctostomy
see Bypass, Gastrointestinal System 0D1
see Drainage, Gastrointestinal System 0D9
Colopuncture
see Drainage, Gastrointestinal System 0D9
Colorrhaphy
see Repair, Gastrointestinal System 0DQ
Colostomy
see Bypass, Gastrointestinal System 0D1
see Drainage, Gastrointestinal System 0D9
Colpectomy
see Excision, Vagina 0UBG
see Resection, Vagina 0UTG
Colpocentesis
see Drainage, Vagina 0U9G
Colpopexy
see Repair, Vagina 0UQG
see Reposition, Vagina 0USG
Colpoplasty
see Repair, Vagina 0UQG
see Supplement, Vagina 0UUG
Colporrhaphy
see Repair, Vagina 0UQG
Colposcopy 0UJH8ZZ
Columella
use Nasal Mucosa and Soft Tissue
Common digital vein
use Foot Vein, Right
use Foot Vein, Left
Common facial vein
use Face Vein, Right
use Face Vein, Left
Common fibular nerve
use Peroneal Nerve
Common hepatic artery
use Hepatic Artery
Common iliac (subaortic) lymph node
use Lymphatic, Pelvis
Common interosseous artery
use Ulnar Artery, Right
use Ulnar Artery, Left
Common peroneal nerve
use Peroneal Nerve
Complete® (SE) stent
use Intraluminal Device
Compression
see Restriction
Abdominal Wall 2W13X
Arm
Lower
Left 2W1DX
Right 2W1CX
Upper
Left 2W1BX
Right 2W1AX
Back 2W15X
Chest Wall 2W14X
Extremity
Lower
Left 2W1MX
Right 2W1LX
Upper
Left 2W19X
Right 2W18X
Face 2W11X
Finger
Left 2W1KX
Right 2W1JX
Foot
Left 2W1TX
Right 2W1SX
Hand
Left 2W1FX
Right 2W1EX
Head 2W10X
Inguinal Region
Left 2W17X
Right 2W16X
Leg
Lower
Left 2W1RX
Right 2W1QX
Upper
Left 2W1PX
Right 2W1NX
Neck 2W12X
Thumb
Left 2W1HX
Right 2W1GX
Toe
Left 2W1VX
Right 2W1UX
Computer Assisted Procedure
Extremity
Lower
No Qualifier 8E0YXBZ

Computer Assisted Procedure - Computerized Tomography (CT Scan)

ICD-10-PCS INDEX

Continuous Negative Airway Pressure
24-96 Consecutive Hours, Ventilation 5A09459
Greater than 96 Consecutive Hours, Ventilation 5A09559
Less than 24 Consecutive Hours, Ventilation 5A09359
Continuous Positive Airway Pressure
24-96 Consecutive Hours, Ventilation 5A09457
Greater than 96 Consecutive Hours, Ventilation 5A09557
Less than 24 Consecutive Hours, Ventilation 5A09357
Continuous renal replacement therapy (CRRT) 5A1D90Z
Contraceptive Device
Change device in, Uterus and Cervix 0U2DXHZ
Insertion of device in
Cervix 0UHC
Subcutaneous Tissue and Fascia
Abdomen 0JH8
Chest 0JH6
Lower Arm
Left 0JHH
Right 0JHG
Lower Leg
Left 0JHP
Right 0JHN
Upper Arm
Left 0JHF
Right 0JHD
Upper Leg
Left 0JHM
Right 0JHL
Uterus 0UH9 IUD
Removal of device from
Subcutaneous Tissue and Fascia
Lower Extremity 0JPW
Trunk 0JPT
Upper Extremity 0JPV
Uterus and Cervix 0UPD
Revision of device in
Subcutaneous Tissue and Fascia
Lower Extremity 0JWW
Trunk 0JWT
Upper Extremity 0JWV
Uterus and Cervix 0UWD
Contractility Modulation Device
Abdomen 0JH8
Chest 0JH6
Control, Epistaxis
see Control bleeding in, Nasal Mucosa and Soft Tissue 093K
Control bleeding in
Abdominal Wall 0W3F
Ankle Region
Left 0Y3L
Right 0Y3K
Arm
Lower
Left 0X3F
Right 0X3D
Upper
Left 0X39
Right 0X38
Axilla
Left 0X35
Right 0X34
Back
Lower 0W3L
Upper 0W3K
Buttock
Left 0Y31
Right 0Y30
Cavity, Cranial 0W31
Control bleeding in — *continued*
Chest Wall 0W38
Elbow Region
Left 0X3C
Right 0X3B
Extremity
Lower
Left 0Y3B
Right 0Y39
Upper
Left 0X37
Right 0X36
Face 0W32
Femoral Region
Left 0Y38
Right 0Y37
Foot
Left 0Y3N
Right 0Y3M
Gastrointestinal Tract 0W3P
Genitourinary Tract 0W3R
Hand
Left 0X3K
Right 0X3J
Head 0W30
Inguinal Region
Left 0Y36
Right 0Y35
Jaw
Lower 0W35
Upper 0W34
Knee Region
Left 0Y3G
Right 0Y3F
Leg
Lower
Left 0Y3J
Right 0Y3H
Upper
Left 0Y3D
Right 0Y3C
Mediastinum 0W3C
Nasal Mucosa and Soft Tissue 093K
Neck 0W36
Oral Cavity and Throat 0W33
Pelvic Cavity 0W3J
Pericardial Cavity 0W3D
Perineum
Female 0W3N
Male 0W3M
Peritoneal Cavity 0W3G
Pleural Cavity
Left 0W3B
Right 0W39
Respiratory Tract 0W3Q
Retroperitoneum 0W3H
Shoulder Region
Left 0X33
Right 0X32
Wrist Region
Left 0X3H
Right 0X3G
Conus arteriosus
use Ventricle, Right
Conus medullaris
use Lumbar Spinal Cord
Conversion
Cardiac rhythm 5A2204Z
Gastrostomy to jejunostomy feeding device *see* Insertion of device in, Jejunum 0DHA
Cook Biodesign® Fistula Plug(s)
use Nonautologous Tissue Substitute
Cook Biodesign® Hernia Graft(s)
use Nonautologous Tissue Substitute
Cook Biodesign® Layered Graft(s)
use Nonautologous Tissue Substitute
Cook Zenapro™ Layered Graft(s)
use Nonautologous Tissue Substitute
Cook Zenith™ AAA Endovascular Graft
use Intraluminal Device, Branched or Fenestrated, One or Two Arteries in 04V
use Intraluminal Device, Branched or Fenestrated, Three or More Arteries in 04V
use Intraluminal Device
Coracoacromial ligament
use Shoulder Bursa and Ligament, Right
use Shoulder Bursa and Ligament, Left
Coracobrachialis muscle
use Upper Arm Muscle, Right
use Upper Arm Muscle, Left
Coracoclavicular ligament
use Shoulder Bursa and Ligament, Right
use Shoulder Bursa and Ligament, Left
Coracohumeral ligament
use Shoulder Bursa and Ligament, Right
use Shoulder Bursa and Ligament, Left
Coracoid process
use Scapula, Right
use Scapula, Left
Cordotomy
see Division, Central Nervous System and Cranial Nerves 008
Core needle biopsy
see Excision with qualifier Diagnostic
CoreValve™ transcatheter aortic valve
use Zooplastic Tissue in Heart and Great Vessels
Cormet™ Hip Resurfacing System
use Resurfacing Device in Lower Joints
Corniculate cartilage
use Larynx
CoRoent® XL
use Interbody Fusion Device in Lower Joints
Coronary arteriography
see Plain Radiography, Heart B20
see Fluoroscopy, Heart B21
Corox® (OTW) Bipolar Lead
use Cardiac Lead, Pacemaker in 02H
use Cardiac Lead, Defibrillator in 02H
Corpus callosum
use Brain
Corpus cavernosum
use Penis
Corpus spongiosum
use Penis
Corpus striatum
use Basal Ganglia
Corrugator supercilii muscle
use Facial Muscle
Cortical strip neurostimulator lead
use Neurostimulator Lead in Central Nervous System and Cranial Nerves
Costatectomy
see Excision, Upper Bones 0PB
see Resection, Upper Bones 0PT
Costectomy
see Excision, Upper Bones 0PB
see Resection, Upper Bones 0PT
Costocervical trunk
use Subclavian Artery, Right
use Subclavian Artery, Left
Costochondrectomy
see Excision, Upper Bones 0PB
see Resection, Upper Bones 0PT
Costoclavicular ligament
use Shoulder Bursa and Ligament, Right
use Shoulder Bursa and Ligament, Left
Costosternoplasty
see Repair, Upper Bones 0PQ
see Replacement, Upper Bones 0PR
see Supplement, Upper Bones 0PU

D

Costotomy
 see Division, Upper Bones 0P8
 see Drainage, Upper Bones 0P9
Costotransverse joint
 use Thoracic Vertebral Joint
Costotransverse ligament
 use Rib(s) Bursa and Ligament
Costovertebral joint
 use Thoracic Vertebral Joint
Costoxiphoid ligament
 use Sternum Bursa and Ligament
Counseling
 Family, for substance abuse, Other Family
 Counseling HZ63ZZZ
 Group
 12-Step HZ43ZZZ
 Behavioral HZ41ZZZ
 Cognitive HZ40ZZZ
 Cognitive-Behavioral HZ42ZZZ
 Confrontational HZ48ZZZ
 Continuing Care HZ49ZZZ
 Infectious Disease
 Post-Test HZ4CZZZ
 Pre-Test HZ4CZZZ
 Interpersonal HZ44ZZZ
 Motivational Enhancement HZ47ZZZ
 Psychoeducation HZ46ZZZ
 Spiritual HZ4BZZZ
 Vocational HZ45ZZZ
 Individual
 12-Step HZ33ZZZ
 Behavioral HZ31ZZZ
 Cognitive HZ30ZZZ
 Cognitive-Behavioral HZ32ZZZ
 Confrontational HZ38ZZZ
 Continuing Care HZ39ZZZ
 Infectious Disease
 Post-Test HZ3CZZZ
 Pre-Test HZ3CZZZ
 Interpersonal HZ34ZZZ
 Motivational Enhancement HZ37ZZZ
 Psychoeducation HZ36ZZZ
 Spiritual HZ3BZZZ
 Vocational HZ35ZZZ
 Mental Health Services
 Educational GZ60ZZZ
 Other Counseling GZ63ZZZ
 Vocational GZ61ZZZ
Countershock, cardiac 5A2204Z
Cowper's (bulbourethral) gland
 use Urethra
CPAP (continuous positive airway pressure)
 see Assistance, Respiratory 5A09
Craniectomy
 see Resection, Head and Facial Bones 0NT
Cranioplasty
 see Repair, Head and Facial Bones 0NQ
 see Replacement, Head and Facial
 Bones 0NR
 see Supplement, Head and Facial
 Bones 0NU
Craniotomy
 see Drainage, Central Nervous System and
 Cranial Nerves 009
 see Division, Head and Facial Bones 0N8
 see Drainage, Head and Facial Bones 0N9
Creation
 Perineum
 Female 0W4N0
 Male 0W4M0
 Valve
 Aortic 024F0
 Mitral 024G0
 Tricuspid 024J0
Cremaster muscle
 use Perineum Muscle

Cribriform plate
 use Ethmoid Bone, Right
 use Ethmoid Bone, Left
Cricoid cartilage
 use Trachea
Cricoidectomy
 see Excision, Larynx 0CBS
Cricothyroid artery
 use Thyroid Artery, Right
 use Thyroid Artery, Left
Cricothyroid muscle
Crisis Intervention GZ2ZZZZ
CRRT (Continuous renal replacement therapy) 5A1D90Z
Crural fascia
 Upper Leg
 Upper Leg
Crushing, nerve
 Cranial *see* Destruction, Central Nervous
 System and Cranial Nerves 005
 Peripheral *see* Destruction, Peripheral
 Nervous System 015
Cryoablation
 see Destruction
Cryotherapy
 see Destruction
Cryptorchidectomy
 System 0VB
 see Resection, Male Reproductive
 System 0VT
Cryptorchiectomy
 System 0VB
 see Resection, Male Reproductive
 System 0VT
Cryptotomy
 see Division, Gastrointestinal System 0D8
 see Drainage, Gastrointestinal System 0D9
CT scan
 see Computerized Tomography (CT Scan)
CT sialogram
 see Computerized Tomography (CT Scan),
 Ear, Nose, Mouth and Throat B92
Cubital lymph node
 use Lymphatic, Right Upper Extremity
 use Lymphatic, Left Upper Extremity
Cubital nerve
 use Ulnar Nerve
Cuboid bone
 use Tarsal, Right
 use Tarsal, Left
Cuboideonavicular joint
 use Tarsal Joint, Right
 use Tarsal Joint, Left
Culdocentesis
 see Drainage, Cul-de-sac 0U9F
Culdoplasty
 see Repair, Cul-de-sac 0UQF
 see Supplement, Cul-de-sac 0UUF
Culdoscopy 0UJH8ZZ
Culdotomy
 see Drainage, Cul-de-sac 0U9F
Culmen
 use Cerebellum
Cultured epidermal cell autograft
 use Autologous Tissue Substitute
Cuneiform cartilage
 use Larynx
Cuneonavicular joint
 use Tarsal Joint, Right
 use Tarsal Joint, Left

Cuneonavicular ligament
Curettage
 see Excision
 see Extraction
Cutaneous (transverse) cervical nerve
 use Cervical Plexus
CVP (central venous pressure)
 see Measurement, Venous 4A04
Cyclodiathermy
 see Destruction, Eye 085
Cyclophotocoagulation
 see Destruction, Eye 085
CYPHER® Stent
 Heart and Great Vessels
Cystectomy
 see Excision, Bladder 0TBB
 see Resection, Bladder 0TTB
Cystocele repair *if w/ mesh = supplement*
 see Repair, Subcutaneous Tissue and Fascia,
 Pelvic Region 0JQC
Cystography
 see Plain Radiography, Urinary System BT0
 see Fluoroscopy, Urinary System BT1
Cystolithotomy
 see Extirpation, Bladder 0TCB
Cystopexy
 see Repair, Bladder 0TQB
 see Reposition, Bladder 0TSB
Cystoplasty
 see Repair, Bladder 0TQB
 see Replacement, Bladder 0TRB
 see Supplement, Bladder 0TUB
Cystorrhaphy
 see Repair, Bladder 0TQB
Cystoscopy 0TJB8ZZ *bladder*
Cystostomy
 see Bypass, Bladder 0T1B
Cystostomy tube
 use Drainage Device
Cystotomy
 see Drainage, Bladder 0T9B
Cystourethrography
 see Plain Radiography, Urinary System BT0
 see Fluoroscopy, Urinary System BT1
Cystourethroplasty
 see Repair, Urinary System 0TQ
 see Replacement, Urinary System 0TR
 see Supplement, Urinary System 0TU
Cytarabine and Daunorubicin Liposome Antineoplastic XW0

DBS lead
 use Neurostimulator Lead in Central
 Nervous System and Cranial Nerves
DeBakey Left Ventricular Assist Device
 Heart and Great Vessels
Debridement *articular OSBC*
 Excisional *see* Excision
 Non-excisional *see* Extraction
Decompression, Circulatory 6A15
Decortication, lung
 see Extirpation, Respiratory System 0BC
 see Release, Respiratory System 0BN
Deep brain neurostimulator lead
 use Neurostimulator Lead in Central
 Nervous System and Cranial Nerves
Deep cervical fascia
 Neck
 Neck

arrhythmogenic Focus A-V node Ø258

D + C = Extraction

E

Excision — *continued*
- Artery — *continued*
  - Pulmonary
    - Left 02BR
    - Right 02BQ
  - Pulmonary Trunk 02BP
  - Radial
    - Left 03BC
    - Right 03BB
  - Renal
    - Left 04BA
    - Right 04B9
  - Splenic 04B4
  - Subclavian
    - Left 03B4
    - Right 03B3
  - Superior Mesenteric 04B5
  - Temporal
    - Left 03BT
    - Right 03BS
  - Thyroid
    - Left 03BV
    - Right 03BU
  - Ulnar
    - Left 03BA
    - Right 03B9
  - Upper 03BY
  - Vertebral
    - Left 03BQ
    - Right 03BP
- Atrium
  - Left 02B7
  - Right 02B6
- Auditory Ossicle
  - Left 09BA
  - Right 09B9
- Axilla
  - Left 0XB5
  - Right 0XB4
- Back
  - Lower 0WBL
  - Upper 0WBK
- Basal Ganglia 00B8
- Bladder 0TBB
- Bladder Neck 0TBC
- Bone
  - Ethmoid
    - Left 0NBG
    - Right 0NBF
  - Frontal 0NB1
  - Hyoid 0NBX
  - Lacrimal
    - Left 0NBJ
    - Right 0NBH
  - Nasal 0NBB
  - Occipital 0NB7
  - Palatine
    - Left 0NBL
    - Right 0NBK
  - Parietal
    - Left 0NB4
    - Right 0NB3
  - Pelvic
    - Left 0QB3
    - Right 0QB2
  - Sphenoid 0NBC
  - Temporal
    - Left 0NB6
    - Right 0NB5
  - Zygomatic
    - Left 0NBN
    - Right 0NBM
- Brain 00B0
- Breast
  - Bilateral 0HBV
  - Left 0HBU
  - Right 0HBT
  - Supernumerary 0HBY

Excision — *continued*
- Bronchus
  - Lingula 0BB9
  - Lower Lobe
    - Left 0BBB
    - Right 0BB6
  - Main
    - Left 0BB7
    - Right 0BB3
  - Middle Lobe, Right 0BB5
  - Upper Lobe
    - Left 0BB8
    - Right 0BB4
- Buccal Mucosa 0CB4
- Bursa and Ligament
  - Abdomen
    - Left 0MBJ
    - Right 0MBH
  - Ankle
    - Left 0MBR
    - Right 0MBQ
  - Elbow
    - Left 0MB4
    - Right 0MB3
  - Foot
    - Left 0MBT
    - Right 0MBS
  - Hand
    - Left 0MB8
    - Right 0MB7
  - Head and Neck 0MB0
  - Hip
    - Left 0MBM
    - Right 0MBL
  - Knee
    - Left 0MBP
    - Right 0MBN
  - Lower Extremity
    - Left 0MBW
    - Right 0MBV
  - Perineum 0MBK
  - Rib(s) 0MBG
  - Shoulder
    - Left 0MB2
    - Right 0MB1
  - Spine
    - Lower 0MBD
    - Upper 0MBC
  - Sternum 0MBF
  - Upper Extremity
    - Left 0MBB
    - Right 0MB9
  - Wrist
    - Left 0MB6
    - Right 0MB5
- Buttock
  - Left 0YB1
  - Right 0YB0
- Carina 0BB2
- Carotid Bodies, Bilateral 0GB8
- Carotid Body
  - Left 0GB6
  - Right 0GB7
- Carpal
  - Left 0PBN
  - Right 0PBM
- Cecum 0DBH
- Cerebellum 00BC
- Cerebral Hemisphere 00B7
- Cerebral Meninges 00B1
- Cerebral Ventricle 00B6
- Cervix 0UBC
- Chest Wall 0WB8
- Chordae Tendineae 02B9
- Choroid
  - Left 08BB
  - Right 08BA

Excision — *continued*
- Cisterna Chyli 07BL
- Clavicle
  - Left 0PBB
  - Right 0PB9
- Clitoris 0UBJ
- Coccygeal Glomus 0GBB
- Coccyx 0QBS
- Colon
  - Ascending 0DBK
  - Descending 0DBM
  - Sigmoid 0DBN
  - Transverse 0DBL
- Conduction Mechanism 02B8
- Conjunctiva
  - Left 08BTXZ
  - Right 08BSXZ
- Cord
  - Bilateral 0VBH
  - Left 0VBG
  - Right 0VBF
- Cornea
  - Left 08B9XZ
  - Right 08B8XZ
- Cul-de-sac 0UBF
- Diaphragm 0BBT
- Disc
  - Cervical Vertebral 0RB3
  - Cervicothoracic Vertebral 0RB5
  - Lumbar Vertebral 0SB2
  - Lumbosacral 0SB4
  - Thoracic Vertebral 0RB9
  - Thoracolumbar Vertebral 0RBB
- Duct
  - Common Bile 0FB9
  - Cystic 0FB8
  - Hepatic
    - Common 0FB7
    - Left 0FB6
    - Right 0FB5
  - Lacrimal
    - Left 08BY
    - Right 08BX
  - Pancreatic 0FBD
    - Accessory 0FBF
  - Parotid
    - Left 0CBC
    - Right 0CBB
- Duodenum 0DB9
- Dura Mater 00B2
- Ear
  - External
    - Left 09B1
    - Right 09B0
  - External Auditory Canal
    - Left 09B4
    - Right 09B3
  - Inner
    - Left 09BE
    - Right 09BD
  - Middle
    - Left 09B6
    - Right 09B5
- Elbow Region
  - Left 0XBC
  - Right 0XBB
- Epididymis
  - Bilateral 0VBL
  - Left 0VBK
  - Right 0VBJ
- Epiglottis 0CBR
- Esophagogastric Junction 0DB4
- Esophagus 0DB5
  - Lower 0DB3
  - Middle 0DB2
  - Upper 0DB1

Explantation - take out resection or excision

Extensions F07

F

Flap closure = transfer

Fusion — *continued*
Knee
Left 0SGD
Right 0SGC
Lumbar Vertebral 0SG0
2 or more 0SG1
Interbody Fusion Device
Nanotextured Surface XRGC092
Radiolucent Porous XRGC0F3
Interbody Fusion Device
Nanotextured Surface XRGB092
Radiolucent Porous XRGB0F3
Lumbosacral 0SG3
Interbody Fusion Device
Nanotextured Surface XRGD092
Radiolucent Porous XRGD0F3
Metacarpophalangeal
Left 0RGV
Right 0RGU
Metatarsal-Phalangeal
Left 0SGN
Right 0SGM
Occipital-cervical 0RG0
Interbody Fusion Device
Nanotextured Surface XRG0092
Radiolucent Porous XRG00F3
Sacrococcygeal 0SG5 lower joint
Sacroiliac
Left 0SG8
Right 0SG7
Shoulder
Left 0RGK
Right 0RGJ
Sternoclavicular
Left 0RGF
Right 0RGE
Tarsal
Left 0SGJ
Right 0SGH
Tarsometatarsal
Left 0SGL
Right 0SGK
Temporomandibular
Left 0RGD
Right 0RGC
Thoracic Vertebral 0RG6
2 to 7 0RG7
Interbody Fusion Device
Nanotextured Surface XRG7092
Radiolucent Porous XRG70F3
8 or more 0RG8
Interbody Fusion Device
Nanotextured Surface XRG8092
Radiolucent Porous XRG80F3
Interbody Fusion Device
Nanotextured Surface XRG6092
Radiolucent Porous XRG60F3
Thoracolumbar Vertebral 0RGA
Interbody Fusion Device
Nanotextured Surface XRGA092
Radiolucent Porous XRGA0F3
Toe Phalangeal
Left 0SGQ
Right 0SGP
Wrist
Left 0RGP
Right 0RGN
Fusion screw (compression)(lag)(locking)
use Internal Fixation Device in Upper Joints
use Internal Fixation Device in Lower Joints

G

Gait training F07Z9
see Motor Treatment, Rehabilitation F07
Galea aponeurotica
use Subcutaneous Tissue and Fascia, Scalp
GammaTile™
use Radioactive Element, Cesium-131 Collagen Implant in 00H
Ganglion impar (ganglion of Walther)
use Sacral Sympathetic Nerve
Ganglionectomy
Destruction of lesion *see* Destruction
Excision of lesion *see* Excision
Gasserian ganglion
use Trigeminal Nerve
Gastrectomy
Partial *see* Excision, Stomach 0DB6
Total *see* Resection, Stomach 0DT6
Vertical (sleeve) *see* Excision, Stomach 0DB6
Gastric electrical stimulation (GES) lead
use Stimulator Lead in Gastrointestinal System
Gastric lymph node
use Lymphatic, Aortic
Gastric pacemaker lead
use Stimulator Lead in Gastrointestinal System
Gastric plexus
use Abdominal Sympathetic Nerve
Gastrocnemius muscle
use Lower Leg Muscle, Right
use Lower Leg Muscle, Left
Gastrocolic ligament
use Omentum
Gastrocolic omentum
use Omentum
Gastrocolostomy
see Bypass, Gastrointestinal System 0D1
see Drainage, Gastrointestinal System 0D9
Gastroduodenal artery
use Hepatic Artery
Gastroduodenectomy
see Excision, Gastrointestinal System 0DB
see Resection, Gastrointestinal System 0DT
Gastroduodenoscopy 0DJ08ZZ
Gastroenteroplasty
see Repair, Gastrointestinal System 0DQ
see Supplement, Gastrointestinal System 0DU
Gastroenterostomy
see Bypass, Gastrointestinal System 0D1
see Drainage, Gastrointestinal System 0D9
Gastroesophageal (GE) junction
use Esophagogastric Junction
Gastrogastrostomy
see Bypass, Stomach 0D16
see Drainage, Stomach 0D96
Gastrohepatic omentum
use Omentum
Gastrojejunostomy
see Bypass, Stomach 0D16
see Drainage, Stomach 0D96
Gastrolysis
see Release, Stomach 0DN6
Gastropexy
see Repair, Stomach 0DQ6
see Reposition, Stomach 0DS6
Gastrophrenic ligament
use Omentum
Gastroplasty
see Repair, Stomach 0DQ6
see Supplement, Stomach 0DU6
Gastroplication
see Restriction, Stomach 0DV6
Gastropylorectomy
see Excision, Gastrointestinal System 0DB
Gastrorrhaphy
see Repair, Stomach 0DQ6
Gastroscopy 0DJ68ZZ
Gastrosplenic ligament
use Omentum
Gastrostomy
see Bypass, Stomach 0D16
see Drainage, Stomach 0D96
Gastrotomy
see Drainage, Stomach 0D96
Gemellus muscle
use Hip Muscle, Right
use Hip Muscle, Left
Geniculate ganglion
use Facial Nerve
Geniculate nucleus
use Thalamus
Genioglossus muscle
use Tongue, Palate, Pharynx Muscle
Genioplasty
see Alteration, Jaw, Lower 0W05
Genitofemoral nerve
use Lumbar Plexus
GIAPREZA™
use Synthetic Human Angiotensin II
Gilteritinib Antineoplastic XW0DXV5
Gingivectomy
see Excision, Mouth and Throat 0CB
Gingivoplasty
see Repair, Mouth and Throat 0CQ
see Replacement, Mouth and Throat 0CR
see Supplement, Mouth and Throat 0CU
Glans penis
use Prepuce
Glenohumeral joint
use Shoulder Joint, Right
use Shoulder Joint, Left
Glenohumeral ligament
use Shoulder Bursa and Ligament, Right
use Shoulder Bursa and Ligament, Left
Glenoid fossa (of scapula)
use Glenoid Cavity, Right
use Glenoid Cavity, Left
Glenoid ligament (labrum)
use Shoulder Joint, Right
use Shoulder Joint, Left
Globus pallidus
use Basal Ganglia
Glomectomy
see Excision, Endocrine System 0GB
see Resection, Endocrine System 0GT
Glossectomy
see Excision, Tongue 0CB7
see Resection, Tongue 0CT7
Glossoepiglottic fold
use Epiglottis
Glossopexy
see Repair, Tongue 0CQ7
see Reposition, Tongue 0CS7
Glossoplasty
see Repair, Tongue 0CQ7
see Replacement, Tongue 0CR7
see Supplement, Tongue 0CU7
Glossorrhaphy
see Repair, Tongue 0CQ7
Glossotomy
see Drainage, Tongue 0C97
Glottis
use Larynx
Gluteal Artery Perforator Flap
Replacement
Bilateral 0HRV079
Left 0HRU079
Right 0HRT079
Transfer
Left 0KXG
Right 0KXF
Gluteal lymph node
use Lymphatic, Pelvis

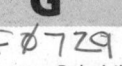

glottoplasty - repair larynx

Gluteal vein
use Hypogastric Vein, Right
use Hypogastric Vein, Left

Gluteus maximus muscle
use Hip Muscle, Right
use Hip Muscle, Left

Gluteus medius muscle
use Hip Muscle, Right
use Hip Muscle, Left

Gluteus minimus muscle
use Hip Muscle, Right
use Hip Muscle, Left

GORE EXCLUDER® AAA Endoprosthesis
use Intraluminal Device, Branched or Fenestrated, One or Two Arteries in 04V
use Intraluminal Device, Branched or Fenestrated, Three or More Arteries in 04V
use Intraluminal Device

GORE EXCLUDER® IBE Endoprosthesis
use Intraluminal Device, Branched or Fenestrated, One or Two Arteries in 04V

GORE TAG® Thoracic Endoprosthesis
use Intraluminal Device

GORE® DUALMESH®
use Synthetic Substitute

Gracilis muscle
use Upper Leg Muscle, Right
use Upper Leg Muscle, Left

Graft can be own skin
see Replacement
see Supplement

Great auricular nerve
use Cervical Plexus

Great cerebral vein
use Intracranial Vein

Great(er) saphenous vein
use Saphenous Vein, Right
use Saphenous Vein, Left

Greater alar cartilage
use Nasal Mucosa and Soft Tissue

Greater occipital nerve
use Cervical Nerve

Greater Omentum
use Omentum

Greater splanchnic nerve
use Thoracic Sympathetic Nerve

Greater superficial petrosal nerve
use Facial Nerve

Greater trochanter
use Upper Femur, Right
use Upper Femur, Left

Greater tuberosity
use Humeral Head, Right
use Humeral Head, Left

Greater vestibular (Bartholin's) gland
use Vestibular Gland

Greater wing
use Sphenoid Bone

Guedel airway
use Intraluminal Device, Airway in Mouth and Throat

Guidance, catheter placement
EKG *see* Measurement, Physiological Systems 4A0
Fluoroscopy *see* Fluoroscopy, Veins B51
Ultrasound *see* Ultrasonography, Veins B54

H

Hallux
use 1st Toe, Right
use 1st Toe, Left

Hamate bone
use Carpal, Right
use Carpal, Left

Hancock® Bioprosthesis (aortic) (mitral) valve
use Zooplastic Tissue in Heart and Great Vessels

Hancock® Bioprosthetic Valved Conduit
use Zooplastic Tissue in Heart and Great Vessels

Harvesting, stem cells
see Pheresis, Circulatory 6A55

Head of fibula
use Fibula, Right
use Fibula, Left

Hearing Aid Assessment F14Z

Hearing Assessment F13Z

Hearing Device
Bone Conduction
Left 09HE
Right 09HD
Insertion of device in
Left 0NH6
Right 0NH5
Multiple Channel Cochlear Prosthesis
Left 09HE
Right 09HD
Removal of device from, Skull 0NP0
Revision of device in, Skull 0NW0
Single Channel Cochlear Prosthesis
Left 09HE
Right 09HD

Hearing Treatment F09Z

Heart Assist System
Implantable
Insertion of device in, Heart 02HA
Removal of device from, Heart 02PA
Revision of device in, Heart 02WA
Short-term External
Insertion of device in, Heart 02HA
Removal of device from, Heart 02PA
Revision of device in, Heart 02WA

HeartMate 3™ LVAS
use Implantable Heart Assist System in Heart and Great Vessels

HeartMate II® Left Ventricular Assist Device (LVAD)
use Implantable Heart Assist System in Heart and Great Vessels

HeartMate XVE® Left Ventricular Assist Device (LVAD)
use Implantable Heart Assist System in Heart and Great Vessels

HeartMate® implantable heart assist system
see Insertion of device in, Heart 02HA

Helix
use External Ear, Right
use External Ear, Left
use External Ear, Bilateral

Hematopoietic cell transplant (HCT)
see Transfusion, Circulatory 302

Hemicolectomy
see Resection, Gastrointestinal System 0DT

Hemicystectomy
see Excision, Urinary System 0TB

Hemigastrectomy
see Excision, Gastrointestinal System 0DB

Hemiglossectomy
see Excision, Mouth and Throat 0CB

Hemilaminectomy
see Excision, Upper Bones 0PB
see Excision, Lower Bones 0QB

Hemilaminotomy
see Release, Central Nervous System and Cranial Nerves 00N
see Release, Peripheral Nervous System 01N
see Drainage, Upper Bones 0P9
see Excision, Upper Bones 0PB

Hemilaminotomy — *continued*
see Release, Upper Bones 0PN
see Drainage, Lower Bones 0Q9
see Excision, Lower Bones 0QB
see Release, Lower Bones 0QN

Hemilaryngectomy
see Excision, Larynx 0CBS

Hemimandibulectomy
see Excision, Head and Facial Bones 0NB

Hemimaxillectomy
see Excision, Head and Facial Bones 0NB

Hemipylorectomy
see Excision, Gastrointestinal System 0DB

Hemispherectomy
see Excision, Central Nervous System and Cranial Nerves 00B
see Resection, Central Nervous System and Cranial Nerves 00T

Hemithyroidectomy partial thyroidectomy
see Excision, Endocrine System 0GB
see Resection, Endocrine System 0GT Left or right lobe

Hemodialysis
see Performance, Urinary 5A1D

Hemolung® Respiratory Assist System (RAS) 5A0920Z

Hepatectomy
see Excision, Hepatobiliary System and Pancreas 0FB
see Resection, Hepatobiliary System and Pancreas 0FT

Hepatic artery proper
use Hepatic Artery

Hepatic flexure
use Transverse Colon

Hepatic lymph node
use Lymphatic, Aortic

Hepatic plexus
use Abdominal Sympathetic Nerve

Hepatic portal vein
use Portal Vein

Hepaticoduodenostomy
see Bypass, Hepatobiliary System and Pancreas 0F1
see Drainage, Hepatobiliary System and Pancreas 0F9

Hepaticotomy
see Drainage, Hepatobiliary System and Pancreas 0F9

Hepatocholedochostomy
see Drainage, Duct, Common Bile 0F99

Hepatogastric ligament
use Omentum

Hepatopancreatic ampulla
use Ampulla of Vater

Hepatopexy
see Repair, Hepatobiliary System and Pancreas 0FQ
see Reposition, Hepatobiliary System and Pancreas 0FS

Hepatorrhaphy
see Repair, Hepatobiliary System and Pancreas 0FQ

Hepatotomy
see Drainage, Hepatobiliary System and Pancreas 0F9

Herculink® (RX) Elite® Renal Stent System
use Intraluminal Device

Herniorrhaphy hernia repair
see Repair, Anatomical Regions, General 0WQ
see Repair, Anatomical Regions, Lower Extremities 0YQ
With synthetic substitute
see Supplement, Anatomical Regions, General 0WU
see Supplement, Anatomical Regions, Lower Extremities 0YU inguinal

I

Iliac fascia
use Subcutaneous Tissue and Fascia, Right Upper Leg
use Subcutaneous Tissue and Fascia, Left Upper Leg
Iliac lymph node
use Lymphatic, Pelvis
Iliacus muscle
use Hip Muscle, Right
use Hip Muscle, Left
Iliofemoral ligament
use Hip Bursa and Ligament, Right
use Hip Bursa and Ligament, Left
Iliohypogastric nerve
use Lumbar Plexus
Ilioinguinal nerve
use Lumbar Plexus
Iliolumbar artery
use Internal Iliac Artery, Right
use Internal Iliac Artery, Left
Iliolumbar ligament
use Lower Spine Bursa and Ligament
Iliotibial tract (band)
use Subcutaneous Tissue and Fascia, Right Upper Leg
use Subcutaneous Tissue and Fascia, Left Upper Leg
Ilium
use Pelvic Bone, Right
use Pelvic Bone, Left
Ilizarov external fixator
use External Fixation Device, Ring in 0PH
use External Fixation Device, Ring in 0PS
use External Fixation Device, Ring in 0QH
use External Fixation Device, Ring in 0QS
Ilizarov-Vecklich device
use External Fixation Device, Limb Lengthening in 0PH
use External Fixation Device, Limb Lengthening in 0QH
Imaging, diagnostic
see Plain Radiography
see Fluoroscopy
see Computerized Tomography (CT Scan)
see Magnetic Resonance Imaging (MRI)
see Ultrasonography
IMI/REL
use Imipenem-cilastatin-relebactam Anti-infective
Imipenem-cilastatin-relebactam Anti-infective XW0
Immobilization
Abdominal Wall 2W33X
Arm
Lower
Left 2W3DX
Right 2W3CX
Upper
Left 2W3BX
Right 2W3AX
Back 2W35X
Chest Wall 2W34X
Extremity
Lower
Left 2W3MX
Right 2W3LX
Upper
Left 2W39X
Right 2W38X
Face 2W31X
Finger
Left 2W3KX
Right 2W3JX
Foot
Left 2W3TX
Right 2W3SX
Immobilization — *continued*
Hand
Left 2W3FX
Right 2W3EX
Head 2W30X
Inguinal Region
Left 2W37X
Right 2W36X
Leg
Lower
Left 2W3RX
Right 2W3QX
Upper
Left 2W3PX
Right 2W3NX
Neck 2W32X
Thumb
Left 2W3HX
Right 2W3GX
Toe
Left 2W3VX
Right 2W3UX
Immunization
see Introduction of Serum, Toxoid, and Vaccine
Immunotherapy
see Introduction of Immunotherapeutic Substance
Immunotherapy, antineoplastic
Interferon *see* Introduction of Low-dose Interleukin-2
Interleukin-2, high-dose *see* Introduction of High-dose Interleukin-2
Interleukin-2, low-dose *see* Introduction of Low dose Interleukin-2
Monoclonal antibody *see* Introduction of Monoclonal Antibody
Proleukin, high-dose *see* Introduction of High-dose Interleukin-2
Proleukin, low-dose *see* Introduction of Low dose Interleukin-2
Impella® heart pump
use Short-term External Heart Assist System in Heart and Great Vessels
Impeller Pump
Continuous, Output 5A0221D
Intermittent, Output 5A0211D
Implantable cardioverter-defibrillator (ICD)
use Defibrillator Generator in 0JH
Implantable drug infusion pump (anti-spasmodic)(chemotherapy)(pain)
use Infusion Device, Pump in Subcutaneous Tissue and Fascia
Implantable glucose monitoring device
use Monitoring Device
Implantable hemodynamic monitor (IHM)
use Monitoring Device, Hemodynamic in 0JH
Implantable hemodynamic monitoring system (IHMS)
use Monitoring Device, Hemodynamic in 0JH
Implantable Miniature Telescope™ (IMT)
use Synthetic Substitute, Intraocular Telescope in 08R
Implantation
see Replacement
see Insertion
Implanted (venous)(access) port
use Vascular Access Device, Totally Implantable in Subcutaneous Tissue and Fascia
IMV (intermittent mandatory ventilation)
see Assistance, Respiratory 5A09
In Vitro Fertilization 8E0ZXY1
Incision, abscess
see Drainage
Incudectomy
see Excision, Ear, Nose, Sinus 09B
see Resection, Ear, Nose, Sinus 09T
Incudopexy
see Repair, Ear, Nose, Sinus 09Q
see Reposition, Ear, Nose, Sinus 09S
Incus
use Auditory Ossicle, Right
use Auditory Ossicle, Left
Induction of labor
Artificial rupture of membranes *see* Drainage, Pregnancy 109
Oxytocin *see* Introduction of Hormone
InDura®, intrathecal catheter (1P) (spinal)
use Infusion Device
Infection, Whole Blood Nucleic Acid-base Microbial Detection, Measurement XXE5XM5
Inferior cardiac nerve
use Thoracic Sympathetic Nerve
Inferior cerebellar vein
use Intracranial Vein
Inferior cerebral vein
use Intracranial Vein
Inferior epigastric artery
use External Iliac Artery, Right
use External Iliac Artery, Left
Inferior epigastric lymph node
use Lymphatic, Pelvis
Inferior genicular artery
use Popliteal Artery, Right
use Popliteal Artery, Left
Inferior gluteal artery
use Internal Iliac Artery, Right
use Internal Iliac Artery, Left
Inferior gluteal nerve
use Sacral Plexus
Inferior hypogastric plexus
use Abdominal Sympathetic Nerve
Inferior labial artery
use Face Artery
Inferior longitudinal muscle
use Tongue, Palate, Pharynx Muscle
Inferior mesenteric ganglion
use Abdominal Sympathetic Nerve
Inferior mesenteric lymph node
use Lymphatic, Mesenteric
Inferior mesenteric plexus
use Abdominal Sympathetic Nerve
Inferior oblique muscle
use Extraocular Muscle, Right
use Extraocular Muscle, Left
Inferior pancreaticoduodenal artery
use Superior Mesenteric Artery
Inferior phrenic artery
use Abdominal Aorta
Inferior rectus muscle
use Extraocular Muscle, Right
use Extraocular Muscle, Left
Inferior suprarenal artery
use Renal Artery, Right
use Renal Artery, Left
Inferior tarsal plate
use Lower Eyelid, Right
use Lower Eyelid, Left
Inferior thyroid vein
use Innominate Vein, Right
use Innominate Vein, Left
Inferior tibiofibular joint
use Ankle Joint, Right
use Ankle Joint, Left
Inferior turbinate
use Nasal Turbinate
Inferior ulnar collateral artery
use Brachial Artery, Right
use Brachial Artery, Left

implant breast 0H0 augmentation

Insertion of device in — *continued*
- Mandible
  - Left 0NHV
  - Right 0NHT
- Maxilla 0NHR
- Mediastinum 0WHC
- Metacarpal
  - Left 0PHQ
  - Right 0PHP
- Metatarsal
  - Left 0QHP
  - Right 0QHN
- Mouth and Throat 0CHY
- Muscle
  - Lower 0KHY
  - Upper 0KHX
- Nasal Mucosa and Soft Tissue 09HK
- Nasopharynx 09HN
- Neck 0WH6
- Nerve
  - Cranial 00HE
  - Peripheral 01HY
- Nipple
  - Left 0HHX
  - Right 0HHW
- Oral Cavity and Throat 0WH3
- Orbit
  - Left 0NHQ
  - Right 0NHP
- Ovary 0UH3
- Pancreas 0FHG
- Patella
  - Left 0QHF
  - Right 0QHD
- Pelvic Cavity 0WHJ
- Penis 0VHS
- Pericardial Cavity 0WHD
- Pericardium 02HN
- Perineum
  - Female 0WHN
  - Male 0WHM
- Peritoneal Cavity 0WHG
- Phalanx
  - Finger
    - Left 0PHV
    - Right 0PHT
  - Thumb
    - Left 0PHS
    - Right 0PHR
  - Toe
    - Left 0QHR
    - Right 0QHQ
- Pleura 0BHQ
- Pleural Cavity
  - Left 0WHB
  - Right 0WH9
- Prostate 0VH0
- Prostate and Seminal Vesicles 0VH4
- Radius
  - Left 0PHJ
  - Right 0PHH
- Rectum 0DHP
- Respiratory Tract 0WHQ
- Retroperitoneum 0WHH
- Ribs
  - 1 to 2 0PH1
  - 3 or More 0PH2
- Sacrum 0QH1
- Scapula
  - Left 0PH6
  - Right 0PH5
- Scrotum and Tunica Vaginalis 0VH8
- Shoulder Region
  - Left 0XH3
  - Right 0XH2
- Sinus 09HY
- Skin 0HHPXYZ

Insertion of device in — *continued*
- Skull 0NH0
- Spinal Canal 00HU
- Spinal Cord 00HV
- Spleen 07HP
- Sternum 0PH0
- Stomach 0DH6
- Subcutaneous Tissue and Fascia
  - Abdomen 0JH8
  - Back 0JH7
  - Buttock 0JH9
  - Wall Chest 0JH6 pocket for pacemaker
  - Face 0JH1
  - Foot
    - Left 0JHR
    - Right 0JHQ
  - Hand
    - Left 0JHK
    - Right 0JHJ
  - Head and Neck 0JHS
  - Lower Arm
    - Left 0JHH
    - Right 0JHG
  - Lower Extremity 0JHW
  - Lower Leg
    - Left 0JHP
    - Right 0JHN
  - Neck
    - Left 0JH5
    - Right 0JH4
  - Pelvic Region 0JHC
  - Perineum 0JHB
  - Scalp 0JH0
  - Trunk 0JHT
  - Upper Arm
    - Left 0JHF
    - Right 0JHD
  - Upper Extremity 0JHV
  - Upper Leg
    - Left 0JHM
    - Right 0JHL
- Tarsal
  - Left 0QHM
  - Right 0QHL
- Tendon
  - Lower 0LHY
  - Upper 0LHX
- Testis 0VHD
- Thymus 07HM
- Tibia
  - Left 0QHH
  - Right 0QHG
- Tongue 0CH7
- Trachea 0BH1
- Tracheobronchial Tree 0BH0
- Ulna
  - Left 0PHL
  - Right 0PHK
- Ureter 0TH9
- Urethra 0THD
- Uterus 0UH9 IUD
- Uterus and Cervix 0UHD
- Vagina 0UHG
- Vagina and Cul-de-sac 0UHH
- Vas Deferens 0VHR
- Vein
  - Axillary
    - Left 05H8
    - Right 05H7
  - Azygos 05H0
  - Basilic
    - Left 05HC
    - Right 05HB
  - Brachial
    - Left 05HA
    - Right 05H9

Insertion of device in — *continued*
- Vein — *continued*
  - Cephalic
    - Left 05HF
    - Right 05HD
  - Colic 06H7
  - Common Iliac
    - Left 06HD
    - Right 06HC
  - Coronary 02H4
  - Esophageal 06H3
  - External Iliac
    - Left 06HG
    - Right 06HF
  - External Jugular
    - Left 05HQ
    - Right 05HP
  - Face
    - Left 05HV
    - Right 05HT
  - Femoral
    - Left 06HN
    - Right 06HM
  - Foot
    - Left 06HV
    - Right 06HT
  - Gastric 06H2
  - Hand
    - Left 05HH
    - Right 05HG
  - Hemiazygos 05H1
  - Hepatic 06H4
  - Hypogastric
    - Left 06HJ
    - Right 06HH
  - Inferior Mesenteric 06H6
  - Innominate
    - Left 05H4
    - Right 05H3
  - Internal Jugular
    - Left 05HN
    - Right 05HM
  - Intracranial 05HL
  - Lower 06HY
  - Portal 06H8
  - Pulmonary
    - Left 02HT
    - Right 02HS
  - Renal
    - Left 06HB
    - Right 06H9
  - Saphenous
    - Left 06HQ
    - Right 06HP
  - Splenic 06H1
  - Subclavian
    - Left 05H6
    - Right 05H5
  - Superior Mesenteric 06H5
  - Upper 05HY
  - Vertebral
    - Left 05HS
    - Right 05HR
- Vena Cava
  - Inferior 06H0
  - Superior 02HV
- Ventricle
  - Left 02HL
  - Right 02HK
- Vertebra
  - Cervical 0PH3
  - Lumbar 0QH0
  - Thoracic 0PH4
- Wrist Region
  - Left 0XHH
  - Right 0XHG

Irrigation
- Biliary Tract, Irrigating Substance 3E1J
- Brain, Irrigating Substance 3E1Q38Z
- Cranial Cavity, Irrigating Substance 3E1Q38Z
- Ear, Irrigating Substance 3E1B
- Epidural Space, Irrigating Substance 3E1S38Z
- Eye, Irrigating Substance 3E1C
- Gastrointestinal Tract
  - Lower, Irrigating Substance 3E1H
  - Upper, Irrigating Substance 3E1G
- Genitourinary Tract, Irrigating Substance 3E1K
- Irrigating Substance 3C1ZX8Z
- Joint, Irrigating Substance 3E1U
- Mucous Membrane, Irrigating Substance 3E10
- Nose, Irrigating Substance 3E19
- Pancreatic Tract, Irrigating Substance 3E1J
- Pericardial Cavity, Irrigating Substance 3E1Y38Z
- Peritoneal Cavity
  - Dialysate 3E1M39Z
  - Irrigating Substance 3E1M38Z
- Pleural Cavity, Irrigating Substance 3E1L38Z
- Reproductive
  - Female, Irrigating Substance 3E1P
  - Male, Irrigating Substance 3E1N
- Respiratory Tract, Irrigating Substance 3E1F
- Skin, Irrigating Substance 3E10
- Spinal Canal, Irrigating Substance 3E1R38Z

Isavuconazole Anti-infective XW0

Ischiatic nerve
- *use* Sciatic Nerve

Ischiocavernosus muscle
- *use* Perineum Muscle

Ischiofemoral ligament
- *use* Hip Bursa and Ligament, Right
- *use* Hip Bursa and Ligament, Left

Ischium
- *use* Pelvic Bone, Right
- *use* Pelvic Bone, Left

Isolation 8E0ZXY6

Isotope Administration, Whole Body DWY5G

Itrel (3)(4) neurostimulator
- *use* Stimulator Generator, Single Array in 0JH

Isotonic muscle energy 7WØ

J

Jakafi®
- *use* Ruxolitinib

Jejunal artery
- *use* Superior Mesenteric Artery

Jejunectomy
- *see* Excision, Jejunum 0DBA
- *see* Resection, Jejunum 0DTA

Jejunocolostomy
- *see* Bypass, Gastrointestinal System 0D1
- *see* Drainage, Gastrointestinal System 0D9

Jejunopexy
- *see* Repair, Jejunum 0DQA
- *see* Reposition, Jejunum 0DSA

Jejunostomy
- *see* Bypass, Jejunum 0D1A
- *see* Drainage, Jejunum 0D9A

Jejunotomy
- *see* Drainage, Jejunum 0D9A

Joint fixation plate
- *use* Internal Fixation Device in Upper Joints
- *use* Internal Fixation Device in Lower Joints

Joint liner (insert)
- *use* Liner in Lower Joints

Joint spacer (antibiotic)
- *use* Spacer in Upper Joints
- *use* Spacer in Lower Joints

Jugular body
- *use* Glomus Jugulare

Jugular lymph node
- *use* Lymphatic, Right Neck
- *use* Lymphatic, Left Neck

K

Kappa®
- *use* Pacemaker, Dual Chamber in 0JH

Kcentra®
- *use* 4-Factor Prothrombin Complex Concentrate

Keratectomy, kerectomy
- *see* Excision, Eye 08B
- *see* Resection, Eye 08T

Keratocentesis
- *see* Drainage, Eye 089

Keratoplasty corneal transplant
- *see* Repair, Eye 08Q
- *see* Replacement, Eye 08R penetrating
- *see* Supplement, Eye 08U inlay + onlay

Keratotomy
- *see* Drainage, Eye 089
- *see* Repair, Eye 08Q

Keystone Heart TriGuard 3™ CEPD (cerebral embolic protection device) X2A6325

Kirschner wire (K-wire)
- *use* Internal Fixation Device in Head and Facial Bones
- *use* Internal Fixation Device in Upper Bones
- *use* Internal Fixation Device in Lower Bones
- *use* Internal Fixation Device in Upper Joints
- *use* Internal Fixation Device in Lower Joints

Knee (implant) insert
- *use* Liner in Lower Joints

KUB X-ray
- *see* Plain Radiography, Kidney, Ureter and Bladder BT04

Kuntscher nail
- *use* Internal Fixation Device, Intramedullary in Upper Bones
- *use* Internal Fixation Device, Intramedullary in Lower Bones

KYMRIAH™
- *use* Engineered Autologous Chimeric Antigen Receptor T-cell Immunotherapy

L

Labia majora
- *use* Vulva

Labia minora
- *use* Vulva

Labial gland
- *use* Upper Lip
- *use* Lower Lip

Labiectomy
- *see* Excision, Female Reproductive System 0UB
- *see* Resection, Female Reproductive System 0UT

Lacrimal canaliculus
- *use* Lacrimal Duct, Right
- *use* Lacrimal Duct, Left

Lacrimal punctum
- *use* Lacrimal Duct, Right
- *use* Lacrimal Duct, Left

Lacrimal sac
- *use* Lacrimal Duct, Right
- *use* Lacrimal Duct, Left

LAGB (laparoscopic adjustable gastric banding)
- Initial procedure 0DV64CZ
- Surgical correction *see* Revision of device in, Stomach 0DW6

Laminectomy
- *see* Release, Central Nervous System and Cranial Nerves 00N
- *see* Release, Peripheral Nervous System 01N
- *see* Excision, Upper Bones 0PB
- *see* Excision, Lower Bones 0QB

Laminotomy
- *see* Release, Central Nervous System and Cranial Nerves 00N
- *see* Release, Peripheral Nervous System 01N
- *see* Drainage, Upper Bones 0P9
- *see* Excision, Upper Bones 0PB
- *see* Release, Upper Bones 0PN
- *see* Drainage, Lower Bones 0Q9
- *see* Excision, Lower Bones 0QB
- *see* Release, Lower Bones 0QN

LAP-BAND® adjustable gastric banding system
- *use* Extraluminal Device

Laparoscopic-assisted transanal pull-through
- *see* Excision, Gastrointestinal System 0DB
- *see* Resection, Gastrointestinal System 0DT

Laparoscopy see page S30
- *see* Inspection

Laparotomy
- Drainage *see* Drainage, Peritoneal Cavity 0W9G
- Exploratory *see* Inspection, Peritoneal Cavity 0WJG

Laryngectomy
- *see* Excision, Larynx 0CBS
- *see* Resection, Larynx 0CTS

Laryngocentesis
- *see* Drainage, Larynx 0C9S

Laryngogram
- *see* Fluoroscopy, Larynx B91J

Laryngopexy
- *see* Repair, Larynx 0CQS

Laryngopharynx
- *use* Pharynx

Laryngoplasty
- *see* Repair, Larynx 0CQS
- *see* Replacement, Larynx 0CRS
- *see* Supplement, Larynx 0CUS

Laryngorrhaphy
- *see* Repair, Larynx 0CQS

Laryngoscopy 0CJS8ZZ

Laryngotomy
- *see* Drainage, Larynx 0C9S

Laser Interstitial Thermal Therapy
- Adrenal Gland DGY2KZZ
- Anus DDY8KZZ
- Bile Ducts DFY2KZZ
- Brain D0Y0KZZ
- Brain Stem D0Y1KZZ
- Breast
  - Left DMY0KZZ
  - Right DMY1KZZ
- Bronchus DBY1KZZ
- Chest Wall DBY7KZZ
- Colon DDY5KZZ
- Diaphragm DBY8KZZ
- Duodenum DDY2KZZ
- Esophagus DDY0KZZ
- Gallbladder DFY1KZZ

Laser Interstitial Thermal Therapy
— *continued*
Gland
Adrenal DGY2KZZ
Parathyroid DGY4KZZ
Pituitary DGY0KZZ
Thyroid DGY5KZZ
Ileum DDY4KZZ
Jejunum DDY3KZZ
Liver DFY0KZZ
Lung DBY2KZZ
Mediastinum DBY6KZZ
Nerve, Peripheral D0Y7KZZ
Pancreas DFY3KZZ
Parathyroid Gland DGY4KZZ
Pineal Body DGY1KZZ
Pituitary Gland DGY0KZZ
Pleura DBY5KZZ
Prostate DVY0KZZ
Rectum DDY7KZZ
Spinal Cord D0Y6KZZ
Stomach DDY1KZZ
Thyroid Gland DGY5KZZ
Trachea DBY0KZZ
Lateral (brachial) lymph node
use Lymphatic, Right Axillary
use Lymphatic, Left Axillary
Lateral canthus
use Upper Eyelid, Right
use Upper Eyelid, Left
Lateral collateral ligament (LCL)
use Knee Bursa and Ligament, Right
use Knee Bursa and Ligament, Left
Lateral condyle of femur
use Lower Femur, Right
use Lower Femur, Left
Lateral condyle of tibia
use Tibia, Right
use Tibia, Left
Lateral cuneiform bone
use Tarsal, Right
use Tarsal, Left
Lateral epicondyle of femur
use Lower Femur, Right
use Lower Femur, Left
Lateral epicondyle of humerus
use Humeral Shaft, Right
use Humeral Shaft, Left
Lateral femoral cutaneous nerve
use Lumbar Plexus
Lateral malleolus
use Fibula, Right
use Fibula, Left
Lateral meniscus
use Knee Joint, Right
use Knee Joint, Left
Lateral nasal cartilage
use Nasal Mucosa and Soft Tissue
Lateral plantar artery
use Foot Artery, Right
use Foot Artery, Left
Lateral plantar nerve
use Tibial Nerve
Lateral rectus muscle
use Extraocular Muscle, Right
use Extraocular Muscle, Left
Lateral sacral artery
use Internal Iliac Artery, Right
use Internal Iliac Artery, Left
Lateral sacral vein
use Hypogastric Vein, Right
use Hypogastric Vein, Left
Lateral sural cutaneous nerve
use Peroneal Nerve
Lateral tarsal artery
use Foot Artery, Right
use Foot Artery, Left
Lateral temporomandibular ligament
use Head and Neck Bursa and Ligament
Lateral thoracic artery
use Axillary Artery, Right
use Axillary Artery, Left
Latissimus dorsi muscle
use Trunk Muscle, Right
use Trunk Muscle, Left
Latissimus Dorsi Myocutaneous Flap
Replacement
Bilateral 0HRV075
Left 0HRU075
Right 0HRT075
Transfer
Left 0KXG
Right 0KXF
Lavage
see Irrigation
Bronchial alveolar, diagnostic *see* Drainage, Respiratory System 0B9
Least splanchnic nerve
use Thoracic Sympathetic Nerve
Left ascending lumbar vein
use Hemiazygos Vein
Left atrioventricular valve
use Mitral Valve
Left auricular appendix
use Atrium, Left
Left colic vein
use Colic Vein
Left coronary sulcus
use Heart, Left
Left gastric artery
use Gastric Artery
Left gastroepiploic artery
use Splenic Artery
Left gastroepiploic vein
use Splenic Vein
Left inferior phrenic vein
use Renal Vein, Left
Left inferior pulmonary vein
use Pulmonary Vein, Left
Left jugular trunk
use Thoracic Duct
Left lateral ventricle
use Cerebral Ventricle
Left ovarian vein
use Renal Vein, Left
Left second lumbar vein
use Renal Vein, Left
Left subclavian trunk
use Thoracic Duct
Left subcostal vein
use Hemiazygos Vein
Left superior pulmonary vein
use Pulmonary Vein, Left
Left suprarenal vein
use Renal Vein, Left
Left testicular vein
use Renal Vein, Left
Lengthening
Bone, with device *see* Insertion of Limb Lengthening Device
Muscle, by incision *see* Division, Muscles 0K8
Tendon, by incision *see* Division, Tendons 0L8
Leptomeninges, intracranial
use Cerebral Meninges
Leptomeninges, spinal
use Spinal Meninges
Lesser alar cartilage
use Nasal Mucosa and Soft Tissue
Lesser occipital nerve
use Cervical Plexus
Lesser Omentum
use Omentum
Lesser saphenous vein
use Saphenous Vein, Right
use Saphenous Vein, Left
Lesser splanchnic nerve
use Thoracic Sympathetic Nerve
Lesser trochanter
use Upper Femur, Right
use Upper Femur, Left
Lesser tuberosity
use Humeral Head, Right
use Humeral Head, Left
Lesser wing
use Sphenoid Bone
Leukopheresis, therapeutic
see Pheresis, Circulatory 6A55
Levator anguli oris muscle
use Facial Muscle
Levator ani muscle
use Perineum Muscle
Levator labii superioris alaeque nasi muscle
use Facial Muscle
Levator labii superioris muscle
use Facial Muscle
Levator palpebrae superioris muscle
use Upper Eyelid, Right
use Upper Eyelid, Left
Levator scapulae muscle
use Neck Muscle, Right
use Neck Muscle, Left
Levator veli palatini muscle
use Tongue, Palate, Pharynx Muscle
Levatores costarum muscle
use Thorax Muscle, Right
use Thorax Muscle, Left
LifeStent® (Flexstar)(XL) Vascular Stent System
use Intraluminal Device
Ligament of head of fibula
use Knee Bursa and Ligament, Right
use Knee Bursa and Ligament, Left
Ligament of the lateral malleolus
use Ankle Bursa and Ligament, Right
use Ankle Bursa and Ligament, Left
Ligamentum flavum, cervical
use Head and Neck Bursa and Ligament
Ligamentum flavum, lumbar
use Lower Spine Bursa and Ligament
Ligamentum flavum, thoracic
use Upper Spine Bursa and Ligament
Ligation
see Occlusion
Ligation, hemorrhoid
see Occlusion, Lower Veins, Hemorrhoidal Plexus
Light Therapy GZJZZZZ
Liner
Removal of device from
Hip
Left 0SPB09Z
Right 0SP909Z
Knee
Left 0SPD09Z
Right 0SPC09Z
Revision of device in
Hip
Left 0SWB09Z
Right 0SW909Z
Knee
Left 0SWD09Z
Right 0SWC09Z
Supplement
Hip
Left 0SUB09Z
Acetabular Surface 0SUE09Z
Femoral Surface 0SUS09Z

Lithotomy - Extirpation

Controlled mechanical Ventilation 5A19

N

near total thyroidectomy = Excision

Nail plate
  use Finger Nail
  use Toe Nail
nanoLOCK™ interbody fusion device
  use Interbody Fusion Device, Nanotextured Surface in New Technology
Narcosynthesis GZGZZZZ
Nasal cavity
  use Nasal Mucosa and Soft Tissue
Nasal concha
  use Nasal Turbinate
Nasalis muscle
  use Facial Muscle
Nasolacrimal duct
  use Lacrimal Duct, Right
  use Lacrimal Duct, Left
Nasopharyngeal airway (NPA)
  use Intraluminal Device, Airway in Ear, Nose, Sinus
Navicular bone
  use Tarsal, Right
  use Tarsal, Left
Near Infrared Spectroscopy, Circulatory System 8E023DZ
Neck of femur
  use Upper Femur, Right
  use Upper Femur, Left
Neck of humerus (anatomical)(surgical)
  use Humeral Head, Right
  use Humeral Head, Left
Nephrectomy
  see Excision, Urinary System 0TB
  see Resection, Urinary System 0TT
Nephrolithotomy
  see Extirpation, Urinary System 0TC
Nephrolysis
  see Release, Urinary System 0TN
Nephropexy
  see Repair, Urinary System 0TQ
  see Reposition, Urinary System 0TS
Nephroplasty
  see Repair, Urinary System 0TQ
  see Supplement, Urinary System 0TU
Nephropyeloureterostomy
  see Bypass, Urinary System 0T1
  see Drainage, Urinary System 0T9
Nephrorrhaphy
  see Repair, Urinary System 0TQ
Nephroscopy, transurethral 0TJ58ZZ
Nephrostomy
  see Bypass, Urinary System 0T1
  see Drainage, Urinary System 0T9
Nephrotomography
  see Plain Radiography, Urinary System BT0
  see Fluoroscopy, Urinary System BT1
Nephrotomy
  see Division, Urinary System 0T8
  see Drainage, Urinary System 0T9
Nerve conduction study
  see Measurement, Central Nervous 4A00
  see Measurement, Peripheral Nervous 4A01
Nerve Function Assessment F01
Nerve to the stapedius
  use Facial Nerve
Nesiritide
  use Human B-type Natriuretic Peptide
Neurectomy
  see Excision, Central Nervous System and Cranial Nerves 00B
  see Excision, Peripheral Nervous System 01B
Neurexeresis
  see Extraction, Central Nervous System and Cranial Nerves 00D
  see Extraction, Peripheral Nervous System 01D
Neurohypophysis
  use Pituitary Gland
Neurolysis
  see Release, Central Nervous System and Cranial Nerves 00N
  see Release, Peripheral Nervous System 01N
Neuromuscular electrical stimulation (NEMS) lead
  use Stimulator Lead in Muscles
Neurophysiologic monitoring
  see Monitoring, Central Nervous 4A10
Neuroplasty
  see Repair, Central Nervous System and Cranial Nerves 00Q
  see Supplement, Central Nervous System and Cranial Nerves 00U
  see Repair, Peripheral Nervous System 01Q
  see Supplement, Peripheral Nervous System 01U
Neurorrhaphy
  see Repair, Central Nervous System and Cranial Nerves 00Q
  see Repair, Peripheral Nervous System 01Q
Neurostimulator Generator
  Insertion of device in, Skull 0NH00NZ
  Removal of device from, Skull 0NP00NZ
  Revision of device in, Skull 0NW00NZ
Neurostimulator generator, multiple channel
  use Stimulator Generator, Multiple Array in 0JH
Neurostimulator generator, multiple channel rechargeable
  use Stimulator Generator, Multiple Array Rechargeable in 0JH
Neurostimulator generator, single channel
  use Stimulator Generator, Single Array in 0JH
Neurostimulator generator, single channel rechargeable
  use Stimulator Generator, Single Array Rechargeable in 0JH
Neurostimulator Lead
  Insertion of device in
    Brain 00H0
    Cerebral Ventricle 00H6
    Nerve
      Cranial 00HE
      Peripheral 01HY
    Spinal Canal 00HU
    Spinal Cord 00HV
    Vein
      Azygos 05H0
      Innominate
        Left 05H4
        Right 05H3
  Removal of device from
    Brain 00P0
    Cerebral Ventricle 00P6
    Nerve
      Cranial 00PE
      Peripheral 01PY
    Spinal Canal 00PU
    Spinal Cord 00PV
    Vein
      Azygos 05P0
      Innominate
        Left 05P4
        Right 05P3
  Revision of device in
    Brain 00W0
    Cerebral Ventricle 00W6
    Nerve
      Cranial 00WE
      Peripheral 01WY
Neurostimulator Lead — *continued*
  Revision of device in — *continued*
    Spinal Canal 00WU
    Spinal Cord 00WV
    Vein
      Azygos 05W0
      Innominate
        Left 05W4
        Right 05W3
Neurotomy
  see Division, Central Nervous System and Cranial Nerves 008
  see Division, Peripheral Nervous System 018
Neurotripsy
  see Destruction, Central Nervous System and Cranial Nerves 005
  see Destruction, Peripheral Nervous System 015
Neutralization plate
  use Internal Fixation Device in Head and Facial Bones
  use Internal Fixation Device in Upper Bones
  use Internal Fixation Device in Lower Bones
New Technology
  Apalutamide Antineoplastic XW0DXJ5
  Bezlotoxumab Monoclonal Antibody XW0
  Blinatumomab Antineoplastic Immunotherapy XW0
  Caplacizumab XW0
  Ceftazidime-Avibactam Anti-infective XW0
  Cerebral Embolic Filtration
    Dual Filter X2A5312
    Single Deflection Filter X2A6325
  Coagulation Factor Xa, Inactivated XW0
  Concentrated Bone Marrow Aspirate XK02303
  Cytarabine and Daunorubicin Liposome Antineoplastic XW0
  Defibrotide Sodium Anticoagulant XW0
  Destruction, Prostate, Robotic Waterjet Ablation XV508A4
  Dilation
    Anterior Tibial
      Left
        Sustained Release Drug-eluting Intraluminal Device X27Q385
        Four or More X27Q3C5
        Three X27Q3B5
        Two X27Q395
      Right
        Sustained Release Drug-eluting Intraluminal Device X27P385
        Four or More X27P3C5
        Three X27P3B5
        Two X27P395
    Femoral
      Left
        Sustained Release Drug-eluting Intraluminal Device X27J385
        Four or More X27J3C5
        Three X27J3B5
        Two X27J395
      Right
        Sustained Release Drug-eluting Intraluminal Device X27H385
        Four or More X27H3C5
        Three X27H3B5
        Two X27H395
    Peroneal
      Left
        Sustained Release Drug-eluting Intraluminal Device X27U385
        Four or More X27U3C5
        Three X27U3B5
        Two X27U395

O

 obstetric sonography = ultrasound

Occlusion — *continued*
Vein — *continued*
Face
Left 05LV
Right 05LT
Femoral
Left 06LN
Right 06LM
Foot
Left 06LV
Right 06LT
Gastric 06L2
Hand
Left 05LH
Right 05LG
Hemiazygos 05L1
Hepatic 06L4
Hypogastric
Left 06LJ
Right 06LH
Inferior Mesenteric 06L6
Innominate
Left 05L4
Right 05L3
Internal Jugular
Left 05LN
Right 05LM
Intracranial 05LL
Lower 06LY
Portal 06L8
Pulmonary
Left 02LT
Right 02LS
Renal
Left 06LB
Right 06L9
Saphenous
Left 06LQ
Right 06LP
Splenic 06L1
Subclavian
Left 05L6
Right 05L5
Superior Mesenteric 06L5
Upper 05LY
Vertebral
Left 05LS
Right 05LR
Vena Cava
Inferior 06L0
Superior 02LV
Occlusion, REBOA (resuscitative endovascular balloon occlusion of the aorta)
02LW3DJ
04L03DJ
Occupational therapy
see Activities of Daily Living Treatment, Rehabilitation F08
Odentectomy
see Excision, Mouth and Throat 0CB
see Resection, Mouth and Throat 0CT
Odontoid process
use Cervical Vertebra
Olecranon bursa
use Elbow Bursa and Ligament, Right
use Elbow Bursa and Ligament, Left
Olecranon process
use Ulna, Right
use Ulna, Left
Olfactory bulb
use Olfactory Nerve
Omentectomy, omentumectomy
see Excision, Gastrointestinal System 0DB
see Resection, Gastrointestinal System 0DT
Omentofixation
see Repair, Gastrointestinal System 0DQ
Omentoplasty
see Repair, Gastrointestinal System 0DQ
see Replacement, Gastrointestinal System 0DR
see Supplement, Gastrointestinal System 0DU
Omentorrhaphy
see Repair, Gastrointestinal System 0DQ
Omentotomy
see Drainage, Gastrointestinal System 0D9
Omnilink Elite® Vascular Balloon Expandable Stent System
use Intraluminal Device
Onychectomy
see Excision, Skin and Breast 0HB
see Resection, Skin and Breast 0HT
Onychoplasty
see Repair, Skin and Breast 0HQ
see Replacement, Skin and Breast 0HR
Onychotomy
see Drainage, Skin and Breast 0H9
Oophorectomy
see Excision, Female Reproductive System 0UB
see Resection, Female Reproductive System 0UT
Oophoropexy
see Repair, Female Reproductive System 0UQ
see Reposition, Female Reproductive System 0US
Oophoroplasty
see Repair, Female Reproductive System 0UQ
see Supplement, Female Reproductive System 0UU
Oophororrhaphy
see Repair, Female Reproductive System 0UQ
Oophorostomy
see Drainage, Female Reproductive System 0U9
Oophorotomy
see Division, Female Reproductive System 0U8
see Drainage, Female Reproductive System 0U9
Oophorrhaphy
see Repair, Female Reproductive System 0UQ
Open Pivot™ (mechanical) valve
use Synthetic Substitute
Open Pivot™ Aortic Valve Graft (AVG)
use Synthetic Substitute
Ophthalmic artery
use Intracranial Artery
Ophthalmic nerve
use Trigeminal Nerve
Ophthalmic vein
use Intracranial Vein
Opponensplasty
Tendon replacement *see* Replacement, Tendons 0LR
Tendon transfer *see* Transfer, Tendons 0LX
Optic chiasma
use Optic Nerve
Optic disc
use Retina, Right
use Retina, Left
Optic foramen
use Sphenoid Bone
Optical coherence tomography, intravascular
see Computerized Tomography (CT Scan)
Optimizer™ III implantable pulse generator
use Contractility Modulation Device in 0JH
Orbicularis oculi muscle
use Upper Eyelid, Right
use Upper Eyelid, Left
Orbicularis oris muscle
use Facial Muscle
Orbital Atherectomy Technology X2C
Orbital fascia
use Subcutaneous Tissue and Fascia, Face
Orbital portion of ethmoid bone
use Orbit, Right
use Orbit, Left
Orbital portion of frontal bone
use Orbit, Right
use Orbit, Left
Orbital portion of lacrimal bone
use Orbit, Right
use Orbit, Left
Orbital portion of maxilla
use Orbit, Right
use Orbit, Left
Orbital portion of palatine bone
use Orbit, Right
use Orbit, Left
Orbital portion of sphenoid bone
use Orbit, Right
use Orbit, Left
Orbital portion of zygomatic bone
use Orbit, Right
use Orbit, Left
Orchectomy, orchidectomy, orchiectomy
see Excision, Male Reproductive System 0VB
see Resection, Male Reproductive System 0VT
Orchidoplasty, orchioplasty
see Repair, Male Reproductive System 0VQ
see Replacement, Male Reproductive System 0VR
see Supplement, Male Reproductive System 0VU
Orchidorrhaphy, orchiorrhaphy
see Repair, Male Reproductive System 0VQ
Orchidotomy, orchiotomy, orchotomy
see Drainage, Male Reproductive System 0V9
Orchiopexy
see Repair, Male Reproductive System 0VQ
see Reposition, Male Reproductive System 0VS
Oropharyngeal airway (OPA)
use Intraluminal Device, Airway in Mouth and Throat
Oropharynx
use Pharynx
Ossiculectomy
see Excision, Ear, Nose, Sinus 09B
see Resection, Ear, Nose, Sinus 09T
Ossiculotomy
see Drainage, Ear, Nose, Sinus 099
Ostectomy
see Excision, Head and Facial Bones 0NB
see Resection, Head and Facial Bones 0NT
see Excision, Upper Bones 0PB
see Resection, Upper Bones 0PT
see Excision, Lower Bones 0QB
see Resection, Lower Bones 0QT
Osteoclasis
see Division, Head and Facial Bones 0N8
see Division, Upper Bones 0P8
see Division, Lower Bones 0Q8
Osteolysis
see Release, Head and Facial Bones 0NN
see Release, Upper Bones 0PN
see Release, Lower Bones 0QN
Osteopathic Treatment myofascial isotonic
Abdomen 7W09X
Cervical 7W01X

Osteopathic Treatment — *continued*
Extremity
Lower 7W06X
Upper 7W07X
Head 7W00X
Lumbar 7W03X
Pelvis 7W05X
Rib Cage 7W08X
Sacrum 7W04X
Thoracic 7W02X
Osteopexy
see Repair, Head and Facial Bones 0NQ
see Reposition, Head and Facial Bones 0NS
see Repair, Upper Bones 0PQ
see Reposition, Upper Bones 0PS
see Repair, Lower Bones 0QQ
see Reposition, Lower Bones 0QS
Osteoplasty
see Repair, Head and Facial Bones 0NQ
see Replacement, Head and Facial Bones 0NR
see Supplement, Head and Facial Bones 0NU
see Repair, Upper Bones 0PQ
see Replacement, Upper Bones 0PR
see Supplement, Upper Bones 0PU
see Repair, Lower Bones 0QQ
see Replacement, Lower Bones 0QR
see Supplement, Lower Bones 0QU
Osteorrhaphy
see Repair, Head and Facial Bones 0NQ
see Repair, Upper Bones 0PQ
see Repair, Lower Bones 0QQ
Osteotomy, ostotomy
see Division, Head and Facial Bones 0N8
see Drainage, Head and Facial Bones 0N9
see Division, Upper Bones 0P8
see Drainage, Upper Bones 0P9
see Division, Lower Bones 0Q8
see Drainage, Lower Bones 0Q9
Otic ganglion
use Head and Neck Sympathetic Nerve
Otoplasty
see Repair, Ear, Nose, Sinus 09Q
see Replacement, Ear, Nose, Sinus 09R
see Supplement, Ear, Nose, Sinus 09U
Otoscopy
see Inspection, Ear, Nose, Sinus 09J
Oval window
use Middle Ear, Right
use Middle Ear, Left
Ovarian artery
use Abdominal Aorta
Ovarian ligament
use Uterine Supporting Structure
Ovariectomy
see Excision, Female Reproductive System 0UB
see Resection, Female Reproductive System 0UT
Ovariocentesis
see Drainage, Female Reproductive System 0U9
Ovariopexy
see Repair, Female Reproductive System 0UQ
see Reposition, Female Reproductive System 0US
Ovariotomy
see Division, Female Reproductive System 0U8
see Drainage, Female Reproductive System 0U9
Ovatio™ CRT-D
use Cardiac Resynchronization Defibrillator Pulse Generator in 0JH
Oversewing
Gastrointestinal ulcer *see* Repair, Gastrointestinal System 0DQ
Pleural bleb *see* Repair, Respiratory System 0BQ
Oviduct
use Fallopian Tube, Right
use Fallopian Tube, Left
Oximetry, Fetal pulse 10H073Z
OXINIUM™
use Synthetic Substitute, Oxidized Zirconium on Polyethylene in 0SR
Oxygenation
Extracorporeal membrane (ECMO) *see* Performance, Circulatory 5A15
Hyperbaric *see* Assistance, Circulatory 5A05
Supersaturated *see* Assistance, Circulatory 5A05

P

Pacemaker
Dual Chamber
Abdomen 0JH8
Chest 0JH6
Intracardiac
Insertion of device in
Atrium
Left 02H7
Right 02H6
Vein, Coronary 02H4
Ventricle
Left 02HL
Right 02HK
Removal of device from, Heart 02PA
Revision of device in, Heart 02WA
Single Chamber
Abdomen 0JH8
Chest 0JH6
Single Chamber Rate Responsive
Abdomen 0JH8
Chest 0JH6
Packing
Abdominal Wall 2W43X5Z
Anorectal 2Y43X5Z
Arm
Lower
Left 2W4DX5Z
Right 2W4CX5Z
Upper
Left 2W4BX5Z
Right 2W4AX5Z
Back 2W45X5Z
Chest Wall 2W44X5Z
Ear 2Y42X5Z
Extremity
Lower
Left 2W4MX5Z
Right 2W4LX5Z
Upper
Left 2W49X5Z
Right 2W48X5Z
Face 2W41X5Z
Finger
Left 2W4KX5Z
Right 2W4JX5Z
Foot
Left 2W4TX5Z
Right 2W4SX5Z
Genital Tract, Female 2Y44X5Z
Hand
Left 2W4FX5Z
Right 2W4EX5Z
Head 2W40X5Z
Inguinal Region
Left 2W47X5Z
Right 2W46X5Z
Packing — *continued*
Leg
Lower
Left 2W4RX5Z
Right 2W4QX5Z
Upper
Left 2W4PX5Z
Right 2W4NX5Z
Mouth and Pharynx 2Y40X5Z
Nasal 2Y41X5Z
Neck 2W42X5Z
Thumb
Left 2W4HX5Z
Right 2W4GX5Z
Toe
Left 2W4VX5Z
Right 2W4UX5Z
Urethra 2Y45X5Z
Paclitaxel-eluting coronary stent
use Intraluminal Device, Drug-eluting in Heart and Great Vessels
Paclitaxel-eluting peripheral stent
use Intraluminal Device, Drug-eluting in Upper Arteries
use Intraluminal Device, Drug-eluting in Lower Arteries
Palatine gland
use Buccal Mucosa
Palatine tonsil
use Tonsils
Palatine uvula
use Uvula
Palatoglossal muscle
use Tongue, Palate, Pharynx Muscle
Palatopharyngeal muscle
use Tongue, Palate, Pharynx Muscle
Palatoplasty
see Repair, Mouth and Throat 0CQ
see Replacement, Mouth and Throat 0CR
see Supplement, Mouth and Throat 0CU
Palatorrhaphy
see Repair, Mouth and Throat 0CQ
Palmar (volar) digital vein
use Hand Vein, Right
use Hand Vein, Left
Palmar (volar) metacarpal vein
use Hand Vein, Right
use Hand Vein, Left
Palmar cutaneous nerve
use Median Nerve
use Radial Nerve
Palmar fascia (aponeurosis)
use Subcutaneous Tissue and Fascia, Right Hand
use Subcutaneous Tissue and Fascia, Left Hand
Palmar interosseous muscle
use Hand Muscle, Right
use Hand Muscle, Left
Palmar ulnocarpal ligament
use Wrist Bursa and Ligament, Right
use Wrist Bursa and Ligament, Left
Palmaris longus muscle
use Lower Arm and Wrist Muscle, Right
use Lower Arm and Wrist Muscle, Left
Pancreatectomy
see Excision, Pancreas 0FBG
see Resection, Pancreas 0FTG
Pancreatic artery
use Splenic Artery
Pancreatic plexus
use Abdominal Sympathetic Nerve
Pancreatic vein
use Splenic Vein

PCNL - percutaneous Nephrolithotomy - page 518

Pancreaticoduodenostomy
see Bypass, Hepatobiliary System and Pancreas 0F1
Pancreaticosplenic lymph node
use Lymphatic, Aortic
Pancreatogram, endoscopic retrograde
see Fluoroscopy, Pancreatic Duct BF18
Pancreatolithotomy
see Extirpation, Pancreas 0FCG
Pancreatotomy
see Division, Pancreas 0F8G
see Drainage, Pancreas 0F9G
Panniculectomy
see Excision, Skin, Abdomen 0HB7
see Excision, Subcutaneous Tissue and Fascia, Abdomen 0JB8
Paraaortic lymph node
use Lymphatic, Aortic
Paracentesis
Eye *see* Drainage, Eye 089
Peritoneal Cavity *see* Drainage, Peritoneal Cavity 0W9G
Tympanum *see* Drainage, Ear, Nose, Sinus 099
Pararectal lymph node
use Lymphatic, Mesenteric
Parasternal lymph node
use Lymphatic, Thorax
Parathyroidectomy
see Excision, Endocrine System 0GB
see Resection, Endocrine System 0GT
Paratracheal lymph node
use Lymphatic, Thorax
Paraurethral (Skene's) gland
use Vestibular Gland
Parenteral nutrition, total
see Introduction of Nutritional Substance
Parietal lobe
use Cerebral Hemisphere
Parotid lymph node
use Lymphatic, Head
Parotid plexus
use Facial Nerve
Parotidectomy
see Excision, Mouth and Throat 0CB
see Resection, Mouth and Throat 0CT
Pars flaccida
use Tympanic Membrane, Right
use Tympanic Membrane, Left
Partial joint replacement
Hip *see* Replacement, Lower Joints 0SR
Knee *see* Replacement, Lower Joints 0SR
Shoulder *see* Replacement, Upper Joints 0RR
Partially absorbable mesh
use Synthetic Substitute
Patch, blood, spinal 3E0R3GC
Patellapexy
see Repair, Lower Bones 0QQ
see Reposition, Lower Bones 0QS
Patellaplasty
see Repair, Lower Bones 0QQ
see Replacement, Lower Bones 0QR
see Supplement, Lower Bones 0QU
Patellar ligament
use Knee Bursa and Ligament, Right
use Knee Bursa and Ligament, Left
Patellar tendon
use Knee Tendon, Right
use Knee Tendon, Left
Patellectomy
see Excision, Lower Bones 0QB
see Resection, Lower Bones 0QT
Patellofemoral joint
use Knee Joint, Right
use Knee Joint, Left
use Knee Joint, Femoral Surface, Right
use Knee Joint, Femoral Surface, Left

Pectineus muscle
use Upper Leg Muscle, Right
use Upper Leg Muscle, Left
Pectoral (anterior) lymph node
use Lymphatic, Right Axillary
use Lymphatic, Left Axillary
Pectoral fascia
use Subcutaneous Tissue and Fascia, Chest
Pectoralis major muscle
use Thorax Muscle, Right
use Thorax Muscle, Left
Pectoralis minor muscle
use Thorax Muscle, Right
use Thorax Muscle, Left
Pedicle-based dynamic stabilization device
use Spinal Stabilization Device, Pedicle-Based in 0RH
use Spinal Stabilization Device, Pedicle-Based in 0SH
PEEP (positive end expiratory pressure)
see Assistance, Respiratory 5A09
PEG (percutaneous endoscopic gastrostomy) 0DH63UZ
PEJ (percutaneous endoscopic jejunostomy) 0DHA3UZ
Pelvic splanchnic nerve
use Abdominal Sympathetic Nerve
use Sacral Sympathetic Nerve
Penectomy
see Excision, Male Reproductive System 0VB
see Resection, Male Reproductive System 0VT
Penile urethra
use Urethra
Perceval sutureless valve
use Zooplastic Tissue, Rapid Deployment Technique in New Technology
Percutaneous endoscopic gastrojejunostomy (PEG/J) tube
use Feeding Device in Gastrointestinal System
Percutaneous endoscopic gastrostomy (PEG) tube
use Feeding Device in Gastrointestinal System
Percutaneous nephrostomy catheter
use Drainage Device
Percutaneous transluminal coronary angioplasty (PTCA)
see Dilation, Heart and Great Vessels 027
Performance
Biliary
Multiple, Filtration 5A1C60Z
Single, Filtration 5A1C00Z
Cardiac
Continuous
Output 5A1221Z
Pacing 5A1223Z
Intermittent, Pacing 5A1213Z
Single, Output, Manual 5A12012
Circulatory
Continuous
Central Membrane 5A1522F
Peripheral Veno-arterial Membrane 5A1522G
Peripheral Veno-venous Membrane 5A1522H
Intraoperative
Central Membrane 5A15A2F
Peripheral Veno-arterial Membrane 5A15A2G
Peripheral Veno-venous Membrane 5A15A2H
Respiratory
24-96 Consecutive Hours, Ventilation 5A1945Z CMV

Performance — *continued*
Respiratory — *continued*
Greater than 96 Consecutive Hours, Ventilation 5A1955Z
Less than 24 Consecutive Hours, Ventilation 5A1935Z
Single, Ventilation, Nonmechanical 5A19054
Urinary
Continuous, Greater than 18 hours per day, Filtration 5A1D90Z
Intermittent, Less than 6 Hours Per Day, Filtration 5A1D70Z
Prolonged Intermittent, 6-18 hours per day, Filtration 5A1D80Z
Perfusion
see Introduction of substance in or on
Perfusion, donor organ
Heart 6AB50BZ
Kidney(s) 6ABT0BZ
Liver 6ABF0BZ
Lung(s) 6ABB0BZ
Pericardiectomy
see Excision, Pericardium 02BN
see Resection, Pericardium 02TN
Pericardiocentesis
see Drainage, Pericardial Cavity 0W9D
Pericardiolysis
see Release, Pericardium 02NN
Pericardiophrenic artery
use Internal Mammary Artery, Right
use Internal Mammary Artery, Left
Pericardioplasty
see Repair, Pericardium 02QN
see Replacement, Pericardium 02RN
see Supplement, Pericardium 02UN
Pericardiorrhaphy
see Repair, Pericardium 02QN
Pericardiostomy
see Drainage, Pericardial Cavity 0W9D
Pericardiotomy
see Drainage, Pericardial Cavity 0W9D
Perimetrium
use Uterus
Peripheral parenteral nutrition
see Introduction of Nutritional Substance
Peripherally inserted central catheter (PICC)
use Infusion Device
Peritoneal dialysis 3E1M39Z
Peritoneocentesis
see Drainage, Peritoneum 0D9W
see Drainage, Peritoneal Cavity 0W9G
Peritoneoplasty
see Repair, Peritoneum 0DQW
see Replacement, Peritoneum 0DRW
see Supplement, Peritoneum 0DUW
Peritoneoscopy 0DJW4ZZ
Peritoneotomy
see Drainage, Peritoneum 0D9W
Peritoneumectomy
see Excision, Peritoneum 0DBW
Peroneus brevis muscle
use Lower Leg Muscle, Right
use Lower Leg Muscle, Left
Peroneus longus muscle
use Lower Leg Muscle, Right
use Lower Leg Muscle, Left
Pessary ring
use Intraluminal Device, Pessary in Female Reproductive System
PET scan
see Positron Emission Tomographic (PET) Imaging
Petrous part of temporal bone
use Temporal Bone, Right
use Temporal Bone, Left

Plain Radiography - Plaque Radiation
ICD-10-PCS Index
Plain Radiography - Plaque Radiation
ICD-10-PCS INDEX

- **Plain Radiography** — *continued*
  - Vein — *continued*
    - Epidural B500
    - Jugular
      - Bilateral B505
      - Left B504
      - Right B503
    - Lower Extremity
      - Bilateral B50D
      - Left B50C
      - Right B50B
    - Other B50V
    - Pelvic (Iliac)
      - Left B50G
      - Right B50F
    - Pelvic (Iliac) Bilateral B50H
    - Portal B50T
    - Pulmonary
      - Bilateral B50S
      - Left B50R
      - Right B50Q
    - Renal
      - Bilateral B50L
      - Left B50K
      - Right B50J
    - Splanchnic B50T
    - Subclavian
      - Left B507
      - Right B506
    - Upper Extremity
      - Bilateral B50P
      - Left B50N
      - Right B50M
  - Vena Cava
    - Inferior B509
    - Superior B508
  - Whole Body BW0KZZZ
    - Infant BW0MZZZ
  - Whole Skeleton BW0LZZZ
  - Wrist
    - Left BP0M
    - Right BP0L
- **Planar Nuclear Medicine Imaging**
  - Abdomen CW10
  - Abdomen and Chest CW14
  - Abdomen and Pelvis CW11
  - Anatomical Region, Other CW1ZZZZ
  - Anatomical Regions, Multiple CW1YYZZ
  - Bladder, Kidneys and Ureters CT13
  - Bladder and Ureters CT1H
  - Blood C713
  - Bone Marrow C710
  - Brain C010
  - Breast CH1YYZZ
    - Bilateral CH12
    - Left CH11
    - Right CH10
  - Bronchi and Lungs CB12
  - Central Nervous System C01YYZZ
  - Cerebrospinal Fluid C015
  - Chest CW13
  - Chest and Abdomen CW14
  - Chest and Neck CW16
  - Digestive System CD1YYZZ
  - Ducts, Lacrimal, Bilateral C819
  - Ear, Nose, Mouth and Throat C91YYZZ
  - Endocrine System CG1YYZZ
  - Extremity
    - Lower CW1D
      - Bilateral CP1F
      - Left CP1D
      - Right CP1C
    - Upper CW1M
      - Bilateral CP1B
      - Left CP19
      - Right CP18
  - Eye C81YYZZ
- **Planar Nuclear Medicine Imaging** — *continued*
  - Gallbladder CF14
  - Gastrointestinal Tract CD17
    - Upper CD15
  - Gland
    - Adrenal, Bilateral CG14
    - Parathyroid CG11
    - Thyroid CG12
  - Glands, Salivary, Bilateral C91B
  - Head and Neck CW1B
  - Heart C21YYZZ
    - Right and Left C216
  - Hepatobiliary System, All CF1C
  - Hepatobiliary System and Pancreas CF1YYZZ
  - Kidneys, Ureters and Bladder CT13
  - Liver CF15
  - Liver and Spleen CF16
  - Lungs and Bronchi CB12
  - Lymphatics
    - Head C71J
    - Head and Neck C715
    - Lower Extremity C71P
    - Neck C71K
    - Pelvic C71D
    - Trunk C71M
    - Upper Chest C71L
    - Upper Extremity C71N
  - Lymphatics and Hematologic System C71YYZZ
  - Musculoskeletal System
    - All CP1Z
    - Other CP1YYZZ
  - Myocardium C21G
  - Neck and Chest CW16
  - Neck and Head CW1B
  - Pancreas and Hepatobiliary System CF1YYZZ
  - Pelvic Region CW1J
  - Pelvis CP16
  - Pelvis and Abdomen CW11
  - Pelvis and Spine CP17
  - Reproductive System, Male CV1YYZZ
  - Respiratory System CB1YYZZ
  - Skin CH1YYZZ
  - Skull CP11
  - Spine CP15
  - Spine and Pelvis CP17
  - Spleen C712
  - Spleen and Liver CF16
  - Subcutaneous Tissue CH1YYZZ
  - Testicles, Bilateral CV19
  - Thorax CP14
  - Ureters, Kidneys and Bladder CT13
  - Ureters and Bladder CT1H
  - Urinary System CT1YYZZ
  - Veins C51YYZZ
    - Central C51R
    - Lower Extremity
      - Bilateral C51D
      - Left C51C
      - Right C51B
    - Upper Extremity
      - Bilateral C51Q
      - Left C51P
      - Right C51N
  - Whole Body CW1N
- **Plantar digital vein**
  - *use* Foot Vein, Right
  - *use* Foot Vein, Left
- **Plantar fascia (aponeurosis)**
  - *use* Subcutaneous Tissue and Fascia, Right Foot
  - *use* Subcutaneous Tissue and Fascia, Left Foot
- **Plantar metatarsal vein**
  - *use* Foot Vein, Right
  - *use* Foot Vein, Left
- **Plantar venous arch**
  - *use* Foot Vein, Right
  - *use* Foot Vein, Left
- **Plaque Radiation**
  - Abdomen DWY3FZZ
  - Adrenal Gland DGY2FZZ
  - Anus DDY8FZZ
  - Bile Ducts DFY2FZZ
  - Bladder DTY2FZZ
  - Bone, Other DPYCFZZ
  - Bone Marrow D7Y0FZZ
  - Brain D0Y0FZZ
  - Brain Stem D0Y1FZZ
  - Breast
    - Left DMY0FZZ
    - Right DMY1FZZ
  - Bronchus DBY1FZZ
  - Cervix DUY1FZZ
  - Chest DWY2FZZ
  - Chest Wall DBY7FZZ
  - Colon DDY5FZZ
  - Diaphragm DBY8FZZ
  - Duodenum DDY2FZZ
  - Ear D9Y0FZZ
  - Esophagus DDY0FZZ
  - Eye D8Y0FZZ
  - Femur DPY9FZZ
  - Fibula DPYBFZZ
  - Gallbladder DFY1FZZ
  - Gland
    - Adrenal DGY2FZZ
    - Parathyroid DGY4FZZ
    - Pituitary DGY0FZZ
    - Thyroid DGY5FZZ
  - Glands, Salivary D9Y6FZZ
  - Head and Neck DWY1FZZ
  - Hemibody DWY4FZZ
  - Humerus DPY6FZZ
  - Ileum DDY4FZZ
  - Jejunum DDY3FZZ
  - Kidney DTY0FZZ
  - Larynx D9YBFZZ
  - Liver DFY0FZZ
  - Lung DBY2FZZ
  - Lymphatics
    - Abdomen D7Y6FZZ
    - Axillary D7Y4FZZ
    - Inguinal D7Y8FZZ
    - Neck D7Y3FZZ
    - Pelvis D7Y7FZZ
    - Thorax D7Y5FZZ
  - Mandible DPY3FZZ
  - Maxilla DPY2FZZ
  - Mediastinum DBY6FZZ
  - Mouth D9Y4FZZ
  - Nasopharynx D9YDFZZ
  - Neck and Head DWY1FZZ
  - Nerve, Peripheral D0Y7FZZ
  - Nose D9Y1FZZ
  - Ovary DUY0FZZ
  - Palate
    - Hard D9Y8FZZ
    - Soft D9Y9FZZ
  - Pancreas DFY3FZZ
  - Parathyroid Gland DGY4FZZ
  - Pelvic Bones DPY8FZZ
  - Pelvic Region DWY6FZZ
  - Pharynx D9YCFZZ
  - Pineal Body DGY1FZZ
  - Pituitary Gland DGY0FZZ
  - Pleura DBY5FZZ
  - Prostate DVY0FZZ
  - Radius DPY7FZZ

PLIF - Posterior Lumbar Intebody Fusion = Fusion

Plaque Radiation — *continued*
- Rectum DDY7FZZ
- Rib DPY5FZZ
- Sinuses D9Y7FZZ
- Skin
  - Abdomen DHY8FZZ
  - Arm DHY4FZZ
  - Back DHY7FZZ
  - Buttock DHY9FZZ
  - Chest DHY6FZZ
  - Face DHY2FZZ
  - Foot DHYCFZZ
  - Hand DHY5FZZ
  - Leg DHYBFZZ
  - Neck DHY3FZZ
- Skull DPY0FZZ
- Spinal Cord D0Y6FZZ
- Spleen D7Y2FZZ
- Sternum DPY4FZZ
- Stomach DDY1FZZ
- Testis DVY1FZZ
- Thymus D7Y1FZZ
- Thyroid Gland DGY5FZZ
- Tibia DPYBFZZ
- Tongue D9Y5FZZ
- Trachea DBY0FZZ
- Ulna DPY7FZZ
- Ureter DTY1FZZ
- Urethra DTY3FZZ
- Uterus DUY2FZZ
- Whole Body DWY5FZZ

Plasmapheresis, therapeutic
- *see* Pheresis, Physiological Systems 6A5

Plateletpheresis, therapeutic
- *see* Pheresis, Physiological Systems 6A5

Platysma muscle
- *use* Neck Muscle, Right
- *use* Neck Muscle, Left

Plazomicin Anti-infective XW0

Pleurectomy
- *see* Excision, Respiratory System 0BB
- *see* Resection, Respiratory System 0BT

Pleurocentesis
- *see* Drainage, Anatomical Regions, General 0W9

Pleurodesis, pleurosclerosis
- Chemical injection *see* Introduction of substance in or on, Pleural Cavity 3E0L (talc)
- Surgical *see* Destruction, Respiratory System 0B5

Pleurolysis
- *see* Release, Respiratory System 0BN

Pleuroscopy 0BJQ4ZZ

Pleurotomy
- *see* Drainage, Respiratory System 0B9

Plica semilunaris
- *use* Conjunctiva, Right
- *use* Conjunctiva, Left

Plication
- *see* Restriction

Pneumectomy
- *see* Excision, Respiratory System 0BB
- *see* Resection, Respiratory System 0BT

Pneumocentesis
- *see* Drainage, Respiratory System 0B9

Pneumogastric nerve
- *use* Vagus Nerve

Pneumolysis
- *see* Release, Respiratory System 0BN

Pneumonectomy (lung entire)
- *see* Resection, Respiratory System 0BT

Pneumonolysis
- *see* Release, Respiratory System 0BN

Pneumonopexy
- *see* Repair, Respiratory System 0BQ
- *see* Reposition, Respiratory System 0BS

Pneumonorrhaphy
- *see* Repair, Respiratory System 0BQ

Pneumonotomy
- *see* Drainage, Respiratory System 0B9

Pneumotaxic center
- *use* Pons

Pneumotomy
- *see* Drainage, Respiratory System 0B9

Pollicization
- *see* Transfer, Anatomical Regions, Upper Extremities 0XX

Polyethylene socket
- *use* Synthetic Substitute, Polyethylene in 0SR

Polymethylmethacrylate (PMMA)
- *use* Synthetic Substitute

Polypectomy, gastrointestinal
- *see* Excision, Gastrointestinal System 0DB

Polypropylene mesh
- *use* Synthetic Substitute

Polysomnogram 4A1ZXQZ

Pontine tegmentum
- *use* Pons

Popliteal ligament
- *use* Knee Bursa and Ligament, Right
- *use* Knee Bursa and Ligament, Left

Popliteal lymph node
- *use* Lymphatic, Right Lower Extremity
- *use* Lymphatic, Left Lower Extremity

Popliteal vein
- *use* Femoral Vein, Right
- *use* Femoral Vein, Left

Popliteus muscle
- *use* Lower Leg Muscle, Right
- *use* Lower Leg Muscle, Left

Porcine (bioprosthetic) valve
- *use* Zooplastic Tissue in Heart and Great Vessels

Positive end expiratory pressure
- *see* Performance, Respiratory 5A19

Positron Emission Tomographic (PET) Imaging
- Brain C030
- Bronchi and Lungs CB32
- Central Nervous System C03YYZZ
- Heart C23YYZZ
- Lungs and Bronchi CB32
- Myocardium C23G
- Respiratory System CB3YYZZ
- Whole Body CW3NYZZ

Positron emission tomography
- *see* Positron Emission Tomographic (PET) Imaging

Postauricular (mastoid) lymph node
- *use* Lymphatic, Right Neck
- *use* Lymphatic, Left Neck

Postcava
- *use* Inferior Vena Cava

Posterior (subscapular) lymph node
- *use* Lymphatic, Right Axillary
- *use* Lymphatic, Left Axillary

Posterior auricular artery
- *use* External Carotid Artery, Right
- *use* External Carotid Artery, Left

Posterior auricular nerve
- *use* Facial Nerve

Posterior auricular vein
- *use* External Jugular Vein, Right
- *use* External Jugular Vein, Left

Posterior cerebral artery
- *use* Intracranial Artery

Posterior chamber
- *use* Eye, Right
- *use* Eye, Left

Posterior circumflex humeral artery
- *use* Axillary Artery, Right
- *use* Axillary Artery, Left

Posterior communicating artery
- *use* Intracranial Artery

Posterior cruciate ligament (PCL)
- *use* Knee Bursa and Ligament, Right
- *use* Knee Bursa and Ligament, Left

Posterior facial (retromandibular) vein
- *use* Face Vein, Right
- *use* Face Vein, Left

Posterior femoral cutaneous nerve
- *use* Sacral Plexus

Posterior inferior cerebellar artery (PICA)
- *use* Intracranial Artery

Posterior interosseous nerve
- *use* Radial Nerve

Posterior labial nerve
- *use* Pudendal Nerve

Posterior scrotal nerve
- *use* Pudendal Nerve

Posterior spinal artery
- *use* Vertebral Artery, Right
- *use* Vertebral Artery, Left

Posterior tibial recurrent artery
- *use* Anterior Tibial Artery, Right
- *use* Anterior Tibial Artery, Left

Posterior ulnar recurrent artery
- *use* Ulnar Artery, Right
- *use* Ulnar Artery, Left

Posterior vagal trunk
- *use* Vagus Nerve

PPN (peripheral parenteral nutrition)
- *see* Introduction of Nutritional Substance

Preauricular lymph node
- *use* Lymphatic, Head

Precava
- *use* Superior Vena Cava

PRECICE intramedullary limb lengthening system
- *use* Internal Fixation Device, Intramedullary Limb Lengthening in 0PH
- *use* Internal Fixation Device, Intramedullary Limb Lengthening in 0QH

Prepatellar bursa
- *use* Knee Bursa and Ligament, Right
- *use* Knee Bursa and Ligament, Left

Preputiotomy
- *see* Drainage, Male Reproductive System 0V9

Pressure support ventilation
- *see* Performance, Respiratory 5A19

PRESTIGE® Cervical Disc
- *use* Synthetic Substitute

Pretracheal fascia
- *use* Subcutaneous Tissue and Fascia, Right Neck
- *use* Subcutaneous Tissue and Fascia, Left Neck

Prevertebral fascia
- *use* Subcutaneous Tissue and Fascia, Right Neck
- *use* Subcutaneous Tissue and Fascia, Left Neck

PrimeAdvanced™ neurostimulator (SureScan)(MRI Safe)
- *use* Stimulator Generator, Multiple Array in 0JH

Princeps pollicis artery
- *use* Hand Artery, Right
- *use* Hand Artery, Left

Probing, duct
- Diagnostic *see* Inspection
- Dilation *see* Dilation

PROCEED™ Ventral Patch
- *use* Synthetic Substitute

Procerus muscle
- *use* Facial Muscle

Proctectomy
- *see* Excision, Rectum 0DBP
- *see* Resection, Rectum 0DTP

Q

 pulsative lavage F08

REBOA (resuscitative endovascular balloon occlusion of the aorta)
- 02LW3DJ
- 04L03DJ

Rebound HRD® (Hernia Repair Device)
- *use* Synthetic Substitute

RECELL® cell suspension autograft
- *see* Replacement, Skin and Breast 0HR

Recession
- *see* Repair
- *see* Reposition

Reclosure, disrupted abdominal wall 0WQFXZZ

Reconstruction
- *see* Repair
- *see* Replacement
- *see* Supplement

Rectectomy
- *see* Excision, Rectum 0DBP
- *see* Resection, Rectum 0DTP

Rectocele repair
- *see* Repair, Subcutaneous Tissue and Fascia, Pelvic Region 0JQC

Rectopexy
- *see* Repair, Gastrointestinal System 0DQ
- *see* Reposition, Gastrointestinal System 0DS

Rectoplasty
- *see* Repair, Gastrointestinal System 0DQ
- *see* Supplement, Gastrointestinal System 0DU

Rectorrhaphy
- *see* Repair, Gastrointestinal System 0DQ

Rectoscopy 0DJD8ZZ

Rectosigmoid junction
- *use* Sigmoid Colon

Rectosigmoidectomy
- *see* Excision, Gastrointestinal System 0DB
- *see* Resection, Gastrointestinal System 0DT

Rectostomy
- *see* Drainage, Rectum 0D9P

Rectotomy
- *see* Drainage, Rectum 0D9P

Rectus abdominis muscle
- *use* Abdomen Muscle, Right
- *use* Abdomen Muscle, Left

Rectus femoris muscle
- *use* Upper Leg Muscle, Right
- *use* Upper Leg Muscle, Left

Recurrent laryngeal nerve
- *use* Vagus Nerve

Reduction
- Dislocation *see* Reposition
- Fracture *see* Reposition
- Intussusception, intestinal *see* Reposition, Gastrointestinal System 0DS
- Mammoplasty *see* Excision, Skin and Breast 0HB
- Prolapse *see* Reposition
- Torsion *see* Reposition
- Volvulus, gastrointestinal *see* Reposition, Gastrointestinal System 0DS

Refusion
- *see* Fusion

Rehabilitation
- *see* Speech Assessment, Rehabilitation F00
- *see* Motor Function Assessment, Rehabilitation F01
- *see* Activities of Daily Living Assessment, Rehabilitation F02
- *see* Speech Treatment, Rehabilitation F06
- *see* Motor Treatment, Rehabilitation F07
- *see* Activities of Daily Living Treatment, Rehabilitation F08
- *see* Hearing Treatment, Rehabilitation F09
- *see* Cochlear Implant Treatment, Rehabilitation F0B

Rehabilitation — *continued*
- *see* Vestibular Treatment, Rehabilitation F0C
- *see* Device Fitting, Rehabilitation F0D
- *see* Caregiver Training, Rehabilitation F0F

Reimplantation
- *see* Reattachment
- *see* Reposition
- *see* Transfer

Reinforcement
- *see* Repair
- *see* Supplement

Relaxation, scar tissue
- *see* Release

Release
- Acetabulum
  - Left 0QN5
  - Right 0QN4
- Adenoids 0CNQ
- Ampulla of Vater 0FNC
- Anal Sphincter 0DNR
- Anterior Chamber
  - Left 08N33ZZ
  - Right 08N23ZZ
- Anus 0DNQ
- Aorta
  - Abdominal 04N0
  - Thoracic
    - Ascending/Arch 02NX
    - Descending 02NW
- Aortic Body 0GND
- Appendix 0DNJ
- Artery
  - Anterior Tibial
    - Left 04NQ
    - Right 04NP
  - Axillary
    - Left 03N6
    - Right 03N5
  - Brachial
    - Left 03N8
    - Right 03N7
  - Celiac 04N1
  - Colic
    - Left 04N7
    - Middle 04N8
    - Right 04N6
  - Common Carotid
    - Left 03NJ
    - Right 03NH
  - Common Iliac
    - Left 04ND
    - Right 04NC
  - Coronary
    - Four or More Arteries 02N3
    - One Artery 02N0
    - Three Arteries 02N2
    - Two Arteries 02N1
  - External Carotid
    - Left 03NN
    - Right 03NM
  - External Iliac
    - Left 04NJ
    - Right 04NH
  - Face 03NR
  - Femoral
    - Left 04NL
    - Right 04NK
  - Foot
    - Left 04NW
    - Right 04NV
  - Gastric 04N2
  - Hand
    - Left 03NF
    - Right 03ND
  - Hepatic 04N3
  - Inferior Mesenteric 04NB

Release — *continued*
- Artery — *continued*
  - Innominate 03N2
  - Internal Carotid
    - Left 03NL
    - Right 03NK
  - Internal Iliac
    - Left 04NF
    - Right 04NE
  - Internal Mammary
    - Left 03N1
    - Right 03N0
  - Intracranial 03NG
  - Lower 04NY
  - Peroneal
    - Left 04NU
    - Right 04NT
  - Popliteal
    - Left 04NN
    - Right 04NM
  - Posterior Tibial
    - Left 04NS
    - Right 04NR
  - Pulmonary
    - Left 02NR
    - Right 02NQ
  - Pulmonary Trunk 02NP
  - Radial
    - Left 03NC
    - Right 03NB
  - Renal
    - Left 04NA
    - Right 04N9
  - Splenic 04N4
  - Subclavian
    - Left 03N4
    - Right 03N3
  - Superior Mesenteric 04N5
  - Temporal
    - Left 03NT
    - Right 03NS
  - Thyroid
    - Left 03NV
    - Right 03NU
  - Ulnar
    - Left 03NA
    - Right 03N9
  - Upper 03NY
  - Vertebral
    - Left 03NQ
    - Right 03NP
- Atrium
  - Left 02N7
  - Right 02N6
- Auditory Ossicle
  - Left 09NA
  - Right 09N9
- Basal Ganglia 00N8
- Bladder 0TNB
- Bladder Neck 0TNC
- Bone
  - Ethmoid
    - Left 0NNG
    - Right 0NNF
  - Frontal 0NN1
  - Hyoid 0NNX
  - Lacrimal
    - Left 0NNJ
    - Right 0NNH
  - Nasal 0NNB
  - Occipital 0NN7
  - Palatine
    - Left 0NNL
    - Right 0NNK
  - Parietal
    - Left 0NN4
    - Right 0NN3

Replacement — *continued*
Vein — *continued*
Internal Jugular
Left 05RN
Right 05RM
Intracranial 05RL
Lower 06RY
Portal 06R8
Pulmonary
Left 02RT
Right 02RS
Renal
Left 06RB
Right 06R9
Saphenous
Left 06RQ
Right 06RP
Splenic 06R1
Subclavian
Left 05R6
Right 05R5
Superior Mesenteric 06R5
Upper 05RY
Vertebral
Left 05RS
Right 05RR
Vena Cava
Inferior 06R0
Superior 02RV
Ventricle
Left 02RL
Right 02RK
Vertebra
Cervical 0PR3
Lumbar 0QR0
Thoracic 0PR4
Vitreous
Left 08R53
Right 08R43
Vocal Cord
Left 0CRV
Right 0CRT
Zooplastic Tissue, Rapid Deployment Technique X2RF
Replacement, hip
Partial or total *see* Replacement, Lower Joints 0SR
Resurfacing only *see* Supplement, Lower Joints 0SU
Replantation
see Reposition
Replantation, scalp
see Reattachment, Skin, Scalp 0HM0
Reposition
Acetabulum
Left 0QS5
Right 0QS4
Ampulla of Vater 0FSC
Anus 0DSQ
Aorta
Abdominal 04S0
Thoracic
Ascending/Arch 02SX0ZZ
Descending 02SW0ZZ
Artery
Anterior Tibial
Left 04SQ
Right 04SP
Axillary
Left 03S6
Right 03S5
Brachial
Left 03S8
Right 03S7
Celiac 04S1
Colic
Left 04S7
Reposition — *continued*
Artery — *continued*
Middle 04S8
Right 04S6
Common Carotid
Left 03SJ
Right 03SH
Common Iliac
Left 04SD
Right 04SC
Coronary
One Artery 02S00ZZ
Two Arteries 02S10ZZ
External Carotid
Left 03SN
Right 03SM
External Iliac
Left 04SJ
Right 04SH
Face 03SR
Femoral
Left 04SL
Right 04SK
Foot
Left 04SW
Right 04SV
Gastric 04S2
Hand
Left 03SF
Right 03SD
Hepatic 04S3
Inferior Mesenteric 04SB
Innominate 03S2
Internal Carotid
Left 03SL
Right 03SK
Internal Iliac
Left 04SF
Right 04SE
Internal Mammary
Left 03S1
Right 03S0
Intracranial 03SG
Lower 04SY
Peroneal
Left 04SU
Right 04ST
Popliteal
Left 04SN
Right 04SM
Posterior Tibial
Left 04SS
Right 04SR
Pulmonary
Left 02SR0ZZ
Right 02SQ0ZZ
Pulmonary Trunk 02SP0ZZ
Radial
Left 03SC
Right 03SB
Renal
Left 04SA
Right 04S9
Splenic 04S4
Subclavian
Left 03S4
Right 03S3
Superior Mesenteric 04S5
Temporal
Left 03ST
Right 03SS
Thyroid
Left 03SV
Right 03SU
Ulnar
Left 03SA
Right 03S9
Reposition — *continued*
Artery — *continued*
Upper 03SY
Vertebral
Left 03SQ
Right 03SP
Auditory Ossicle
Left 09SA
Right 09S9
Bladder 0TSB
Bladder Neck 0TSC
Bone
Ethmoid
Left 0NSG
Right 0NSF
Frontal 0NS1
Hyoid 0NSX
Lacrimal
Left 0NSJ
Right 0NSH
Nasal 0NSB
Occipital 0NS7
Palatine
Left 0NSL
Right 0NSK
Parietal
Left 0NS4
Right 0NS3
Pelvic
Left 0QS3
Right 0QS2
Sphenoid 0NSC
Temporal
Left 0NS6
Right 0NS5
Zygomatic
Left 0NSN
Right 0NSM
Breast
Bilateral 0HSV0ZZ
Left 0HSU0ZZ
Right 0HST0ZZ
Bronchus
Lingula 0BS90ZZ
Lower Lobe
Left 0BSB0ZZ
Right 0BS60ZZ
Main
Left 0BS70ZZ
Right 0BS30ZZ
Middle Lobe, Right 0BS50ZZ
Upper Lobe
Left 0BS80ZZ
Right 0BS40ZZ
Bursa and Ligament
Abdomen
Left 0MSJ
Right 0MSH
Ankle
Left 0MSR
Right 0MSQ
Elbow
Left 0MS4
Right 0MS3
Foot
Left 0MST
Right 0MSS
Hand
Left 0MS8
Right 0MS7
Head and Neck 0MS0
Hip
Left 0MSM
Right 0MSL
Knee
Left 0MSP
Right 0MSN

- **Reposition** — *continued*
  - Bursa and Ligament — *continued*
    - Lower Extremity
      - Left 0MSW
      - Right 0MSV
    - Perineum 0MSK
    - Rib(s) 0MSG
    - Shoulder
      - Left 0MS2
      - Right 0MS1
    - Spine
      - Lower 0MSD
      - Upper 0MSC
    - Sternum 0MSF
    - Upper Extremity
      - Left 0MSB
      - Right 0MS9
    - Wrist
      - Left 0MS6
      - Right 0MS5
  - Carina 0BS20ZZ
  - Carpal capitate
    - Left 0PSN
    - Right 0PSM
  - Cecum 0DSH
  - Cervix 0USC
  - Clavicle
    - Left 0PSB
    - Right 0PS9
  - Coccyx 0QSS
  - Colon
    - Ascending 0DSK
    - Descending 0DSM
    - Sigmoid 0DSN
    - Transverse 0DSL
  - Cord
    - Bilateral 0VSH
    - Left 0VSG
    - Right 0VSF
  - Cul-de-sac 0USF
  - Diaphragm 0BST0ZZ
  - Duct
    - Common Bile 0FS9
    - Cystic 0FS8
    - Hepatic
      - Common 0FS7
      - Left 0FS6
      - Right 0FS5
    - Lacrimal
      - Left 08SY
      - Right 08SX
    - Pancreatic 0FSD
      - Accessory 0FSF
    - Parotid
      - Left 0CSC
      - Right 0CSB
  - Duodenum 0DS9
  - Ear
    - Bilateral 09S2
    - Left 09S1
    - Right 09S0
  - Epiglottis 0CSR
  - Esophagus 0DS5
  - Eustachian Tube
    - Left 09SG
    - Right 09SF
  - Eyelid
    - Lower
      - Left 08SR
      - Right 08SQ
    - Upper
      - Left 08SP
      - Right 08SN
  - Fallopian Tube
    - Left 0US6
    - Right 0US5
  - Fallopian Tubes, Bilateral 0US7

- **Reposition** — *continued*
  - Femoral Shaft lower bones
    - Left 0QS9
    - Right 0QS8
  - Femur
    - Lower
      - Left 0QSC
      - Right 0QSB
    - Upper Femoral neck
      - Left 0QS7
      - Right 0QS6
  - Fibula
    - Left 0QSK
    - Right 0QSJ
  - Gallbladder 0FS4
  - Gland
    - Adrenal
      - Left 0GS2
      - Right 0GS3
    - Lacrimal
      - Left 08SW
      - Right 08SV
  - Glenoid Cavity
    - Left 0PS8
    - Right 0PS7
  - Hair 0HSSXZZ
  - Humeral Head
    - Left 0PSD
    - Right 0PSC
  - Humeral Shaft
    - Left 0PSG
    - Right 0PSF
  - Ileum 0DSB
  - Intestine
    - Large 0DSE
    - Small 0DS8
  - Iris
    - Left 08SD3ZZ
    - Right 08SC3ZZ
  - Jejunum 0DSA
  - Joint
    - Acromioclavicular
      - Left 0RSH
      - Right 0RSG
    - Ankle
      - Left 0SSG
      - Right 0SSF
    - Carpal
      - Left 0RSR
      - Right 0RSQ
    - Carpometacarpal
      - Left 0RST
      - Right 0RSS
    - Cervical Vertebral 0RS1
    - Cervicothoracic Vertebral 0RS4
    - Coccygeal 0SS6
    - Elbow
      - Left 0RSM
      - Right 0RSL
    - Finger Phalangeal
      - Left 0RSX
      - Right 0RSW
    - Hip
      - Left 0SSB
      - Right 0SS9
    - Knee
      - Left 0SSD
      - Right 0SSC
    - Lumbar Vertebral 0SS0
    - Lumbosacral 0SS3
    - Metacarpophalangeal
      - Left 0RSV
      - Right 0RSU
    - Metatarsal-Phalangeal
      - Left 0SSN
      - Right 0SSM
    - Occipital-cervical 0RS0

- **Reposition** — *continued*
  - Joint — *continued*
    - Sacrococcygeal 0SS5
    - Sacroiliac
      - Left 0SS8
      - Right 0SS7
    - Shoulder
      - Left 0RSK
      - Right 0RSJ
    - Sternoclavicular
      - Left 0RSF
      - Right 0RSE
    - Tarsal
      - Left 0SSJ
      - Right 0SSH
    - Tarsometatarsal
      - Left 0SSL
      - Right 0SSK
    - Temporomandibular
      - Left 0RSD
      - Right 0RSC
    - Thoracic Vertebral 0RS6
    - Thoracolumbar Vertebral 0RSA
    - Toe Phalangeal
      - Left 0SSQ
      - Right 0SSP
    - Wrist
      - Left 0RSP
      - Right 0RSN
  - Kidney
    - Left 0TS1
    - Right 0TS0
  - Kidney Pelvis
    - Left 0TS4
    - Right 0TS3
  - Kidneys, Bilateral 0TS2
  - Lens
    - Left 08SK3ZZ
    - Right 08SJ3ZZ
  - Lip
    - Lower 0CS1
    - Upper 0CS0
  - Liver 0FS0
  - Lung
    - Left 0BSL0ZZ
    - Lower Lobe
      - Left 0BSJ0ZZ
      - Right 0BSF0ZZ
    - Middle Lobe, Right 0BSD0ZZ
    - Right 0BSK0ZZ
    - Upper Lobe
      - Left 0BSG0ZZ
      - Right 0BSC0ZZ
  - Lung Lingula 0BSH0ZZ
  - Mandible
    - Left 0NSV
    - Right 0NST
  - Maxilla 0NSR
  - Metacarpal
    - Left 0PSQ
    - Right 0PSP
  - Metatarsal
    - Left 0QSP
    - Right 0QSN
  - Muscle
    - Abdomen
      - Left 0KSL
      - Right 0KSK
    - Extraocular
      - Left 08SM
      - Right 08SL
    - Facial 0KS1
    - Foot
      - Left 0KSW
      - Right 0KSV
    - Hand
      - Left 0KSD
      - Right 0KSC

- **Reposition** — *continued*
  - Muscle — *continued*
    - Head 0KS0
    - Hip
      - Left 0KSP
      - Right 0KSN
    - Lower Arm and Wrist
      - Left 0KSB
      - Right 0KS9
    - Lower Leg
      - Left 0KST
      - Right 0KSS
    - Neck
      - Left 0KS3
      - Right 0KS2
    - Perineum 0KSM
    - Shoulder
      - Left 0KS6
      - Right 0KS5
    - Thorax
      - Left 0KSJ
      - Right 0KSH
    - Tongue, Palate, Pharynx 0KS4
    - Trunk
      - Left 0KSG
      - Right 0KSF
    - Upper Arm
      - Left 0KS8
      - Right 0KS7
    - Upper Leg
      - Left 0KSR
      - Right 0KSQ
  - Nasal Mucosa and Soft Tissue 09SK
  - Nerve
    - Abducens 00SL
    - Accessory 00SR
    - Acoustic 00SN
    - Brachial Plexus 01S3
    - Cervical 01S1
    - Cervical Plexus 01S0
    - Facial 00SM
    - Femoral 01SD
    - Glossopharyngeal 00SP
    - Hypoglossal 00SS
    - Lumbar 01SB
    - Lumbar Plexus 01S9
    - Lumbosacral Plexus 01SA
    - Median 01S5
    - Oculomotor 00SH
    - Olfactory 00SF
    - Optic 00SG
    - Peroneal 01SH
    - Phrenic 01S2
    - Pudendal 01SC
    - Radial 01S6
    - Sacral 01SR
    - Sacral Plexus 01SQ
    - Sciatic 01SF
    - Thoracic 01S8
    - Tibial 01SG
    - Trigeminal 00SK
    - Trochlear 00SJ
    - Ulnar 01S4
    - Vagus 00SQ
  - Nipple
    - Left 0HSXXZZ
    - Right 0HSWXZZ
  - Orbit
    - Left 0NSQ
    - Right 0NSP
  - Ovary
    - Bilateral 0US2
    - Left 0US1
    - Right 0US0
  - Palate
    - Hard 0CS2
    - Soft 0CS3

- **Reposition** — *continued*
  - Pancreas 0FSG
  - Parathyroid Gland 0GSR
    - Inferior
      - Left 0GSP
      - Right 0GSN
    - Multiple 0GSQ
    - Superior
      - Left 0GSM
      - Right 0GSL
  - Patella
    - Left 0QSF
    - Right 0QSD
  - Phalanx
    - Finger
      - Left 0PSV
      - Right 0PST
    - Thumb
      - Left 0PSS
      - Right 0PSR
    - Toe
      - Left 0QSR
      - Right 0QSQ
  - Products of Conception 10S0
    - Ectopic 10S2
  - Radius
    - Left 0PSJ
    - Right 0PSH
  - Rectum 0DSP
  - Retinal Vessel
    - Left 08SH3ZZ
    - Right 08SG3ZZ
  - Ribs
    - 1 to 2 0PS1
    - 3 or More 0PS2
  - Sacrum 0QS1
  - Scapula
    - Left 0PS6
    - Right 0PS5
  - Septum, Nasal 09SM
  - Sesamoid Bone(s) 1st Toe
    - *see* Reposition, Metatarsal, Right 0QSN
    - *see* Reposition, Metatarsal, Left 0QSP
  - Skull 0NS0
  - Spinal Cord
    - Cervical 00SW
    - Lumbar 00SY
    - Thoracic 00SX
  - Spleen 07SP0ZZ
  - Sternum 0PS0
  - Stomach 0DS6
  - Tarsal
    - Left 0QSM
    - Right 0QSL
  - Tendon
    - Abdomen
      - Left 0LSG
      - Right 0LSF
    - Ankle
      - Left 0LST
      - Right 0LSS
    - Foot
      - Left 0LSW
      - Right 0LSV
    - Hand
      - Left 0LS8
      - Right 0LS7
    - Head and Neck 0LS0
    - Hip
      - Left 0LSK
      - Right 0LSJ
    - Knee
      - Left 0LSR
      - Right 0LSQ
    - Lower Arm and Wrist
      - Left 0LS6
      - Right 0LS5

- **Reposition** — *continued*
  - Tendon — *continued*
    - Lower Leg
      - Left 0LSP
      - Right 0LSN
    - Perineum 0LSH
    - Shoulder
      - Left 0LS2
      - Right 0LS1
    - Thorax
      - Left 0LSD
      - Right 0LSC
    - Trunk
      - Left 0LSB
      - Right 0LS9
    - Upper Arm
      - Left 0LS4
      - Right 0LS3
    - Upper Leg
      - Left 0LSM
      - Right 0LSL
  - Testis
    - Bilateral 0VSC
    - Left 0VSB
    - Right 0VS9
  - Thymus 07SM0ZZ
  - Thyroid Gland
    - Left Lobe 0GSG
    - Right Lobe 0GSH
  - Tibia
    - Left 0QSH
    - Right 0QSG
  - Tongue 0CS7
  - Tooth
    - Lower 0CSX
    - Upper 0CSW
  - Trachea 0BS10ZZ
  - Turbinate, Nasal 09SL
  - Tympanic Membrane
    - Left 09S8
    - Right 09S7
  - Ulna
    - Left 0PSL
    - Right 0PSK
  - Ureter
    - Left 0TS7
    - Right 0TS6
  - Ureters, Bilateral 0TS8
  - Urethra 0TSD
  - Uterine Supporting Structure 0US4
  - Uterus 0US9
  - Uvula 0CSN
  - Vagina 0USG
  - Vein
    - Axillary
      - Left 05S8
      - Right 05S7
    - Azygos 05S0
    - Basilic
      - Left 05SC
      - Right 05SB
    - Brachial
      - Left 05SA
      - Right 05S9
    - Cephalic
      - Left 05SF
      - Right 05SD
    - Colic 06S7
    - Common Iliac
      - Left 06SD
      - Right 06SC
    - Esophageal 06S3
    - External Iliac
      - Left 06SG
      - Right 06SF
    - External Jugular
      - Left 05SQ
      - Right 05SP

Resection — *continued*
Ear — *continued*
Middle
Left 09T6
Right 09T5
Epididymis
Bilateral 0VTL
Left 0VTK
Right 0VTJ
Epiglottis 0CTR
Esophagogastric Junction 0DT4
Esophagus 0DT5
Lower 0DT3
Middle 0DT2
Upper 0DT1
Eustachian Tube
Left 09TG
Right 09TF
Eye
Left 08T1XZZ
Right 08T0XZZ
Eyelid
Lower
Left 08TR
Right 08TQ
Upper
Left 08TP
Right 08TN
Fallopian Tube
Left 0UT6
Right 0UT5
Fallopian Tubes, Bilateral 0UT7
Femoral Shaft
Left 0QT90ZZ
Right 0QT80ZZ
Femur
Lower
Left 0QTC0ZZ
Right 0QTB0ZZ
Upper
Left 0QT70ZZ
Right 0QT60ZZ
Fibula
Left 0QTK0ZZ
Right 0QTJ0ZZ
Finger Nail 0HTQXZZ
Gallbladder 0FT4 cholecystectomy
Gland
Adrenal
Bilateral 0GT4
Left 0GT2
Right 0GT3
Lacrimal
Left 08TW
Right 08TV
Minor Salivary 0CTJ0ZZ
Parotid
Left 0CT90ZZ
Right 0CT80ZZ
Pituitary 0GT0
Sublingual
Left 0CTF0ZZ
Right 0CTD0ZZ
Submaxillary
Left 0CTH0ZZ
Right 0CTG0ZZ
Vestibular 0UTL
Glenoid Cavity
Left 0PT80ZZ
Right 0PT70ZZ
Glomus Jugulare 0GTC
Humeral Head
Left 0PTD0ZZ
Right 0PTC0ZZ
Humeral Shaft
Left 0PTG0ZZ
Right 0PTF0ZZ

Resection — *continued*
Hymen 0UTK
Ileocecal Valve 0DTC
Ileum 0DTB
Intestine
Large 0DTE
Left 0DTG
Right 0DTF
Small 0DT8
Iris
Left 08TD3ZZ
Right 08TC3ZZ
Jejunum 0DTA
Joint
Acromioclavicular
Left 0RTH0ZZ
Right 0RTG0ZZ
Ankle
Left 0STG0ZZ
Right 0STF0ZZ
Carpal
Left 0RTR0ZZ
Right 0RTQ0ZZ
Carpometacarpal
Left 0RTT0ZZ
Right 0RTS0ZZ
Cervicothoracic Vertebral 0RT40ZZ
Coccygeal 0ST60ZZ
Elbow
Left 0RTM0ZZ
Right 0RTL0ZZ
Finger Phalangeal
Left 0RTX0ZZ
Right 0RTW0ZZ
Hip
Left 0STB0ZZ
Right 0ST90ZZ
Knee
Left 0STD0ZZ
Right 0STC0ZZ
Metacarpophalangeal
Left 0RTV0ZZ
Right 0RTU0ZZ
Metatarsal-Phalangeal
Left 0STN0ZZ
Right 0STM0ZZ
Sacrococcygeal 0ST50ZZ
Sacroiliac
Left 0ST80ZZ
Right 0ST70ZZ
Shoulder
Left 0RTK0ZZ
Right 0RTJ0ZZ
Sternoclavicular
Left 0RTF0ZZ
Right 0RTE0ZZ
Tarsal
Left 0STJ0ZZ
Right 0STH0ZZ
Tarsometatarsal
Left 0STL0ZZ
Right 0STK0ZZ
Temporomandibular
Left 0RTD0ZZ
Right 0RTC0ZZ
Toe Phalangeal
Left 0STQ0ZZ
Right 0STP0ZZ
Wrist
Left 0RTP0ZZ
Right 0RTN0ZZ
Kidney
Left 0TT1
Right 0TT0
Kidney Pelvis
Left 0TT4
Right 0TT3

Resection — *continued*
Kidneys, Bilateral 0TT2
Larynx 0CTS
Lens
Left 08TK3ZZ
Right 08TJ3ZZ
Lip
Lower 0CT1
Upper 0CT0
Liver 0FT0
Left Lobe 0FT2
Right Lobe 0FT1
Lung
Bilateral 0BTM
Left 0BTL
Lower Lobe
Left 0BTJ
Right 0BTF
Middle Lobe, Right 0BTD
Right 0BTK
Upper Lobe
Left 0BTG
Right 0BTC
Lung Lingula 0BTH
Lymphatic
Aortic 07TD
Axillary
Left 07T6
Right 07T5
Head 07T0
Inguinal
Left 07TJ
Right 07TH
Internal Mammary
Left 07T9
Right 07T8
Lower Extremity
Left 07TG
Right 07TF
Mesenteric 07TB
Neck
Left 07T2
Right 07T1
Pelvis 07TC
Thoracic Duct 07TK
Thorax 07T7
Upper Extremity
Left 07T4
Right 07T3
Mandible
Left 0NTV0ZZ
Right 0NTT0ZZ
Maxilla 0NTR0ZZ
Metacarpal
Left 0PTQ0ZZ
Right 0PTP0ZZ
Metatarsal
Left 0QTP0ZZ
Right 0QTN0ZZ
Muscle
Abdomen
Left 0KTL
Right 0KTK
Extraocular
Left 08TM
Right 08TL
Facial 0KT1
Foot
Left 0KTW
Right 0KTV
Hand
Left 0KTD
Right 0KTC
Head 0KT0
Hip
Left 0KTP
Right 0KTN

RRP = Radical Retropubic Prostatectomy
RPP = Radical Perineal Prostatectomy

S

Segmentectomy – excision

Skin lesion removal = excision
Skin Flap - transfer
Skin substitutes = replacement

Single plane imaging = planar nuclear medicine

supraglottoplasty ØCQS

Tissue Expander — *continued*
Insertion of device in — *continued*
Nipple
Left 0HHX
Right 0HHW
Subcutaneous Tissue and Fascia
Abdomen 0JH8
Back 0JH7
Buttock 0JH9
Chest 0JH6
Face 0JH1
Foot
Left 0JHR
Right 0JHQ
Hand
Left 0JHK
Right 0JHJ
Lower Arm
Left 0JHH
Right 0JHG
Lower Leg
Left 0JHP
Right 0JHN
Neck
Left 0JH5
Right 0JH4
Pelvic Region 0JHC
Perineum 0JHB
Scalp 0JH0
Upper Arm
Left 0JHF
Right 0JHD
Upper Leg
Left 0JHM
Right 0JHL
Removal of device from
Breast
Left 0HPU
Right 0HPT
Subcutaneous Tissue and Fascia
Head and Neck 0JPS
Lower Extremity 0JPW
Trunk 0JPT
Upper Extremity 0JPV
Revision of device in
Breast
Left 0HWU
Right 0HWT
Subcutaneous Tissue and Fascia
Head and Neck 0JWS
Lower Extremity 0JWW
Trunk 0JWT
Upper Extremity 0JWV
Tissue expander (inflatable)(injectable)
use Tissue Expander in Skin and Breast
use Tissue Expander in Subcutaneous Tissue and Fascia
Tissue Plasminogen Activator (tPA)(r-tPA)
use Other Thrombolytic
Titanium Sternal Fixation System (TSFS)
use Internal Fixation Device, Rigid Plate in 0PH
use Internal Fixation Device, Rigid Plate in 0PS
Tomographic (Tomo) Nuclear Medicine Imaging Tomosynthesis
Abdomen CW20
Abdomen and Chest CW24
Abdomen and Pelvis CW21
Anatomical Regions, Multiple CW2YYZZ
Bladder, Kidneys and Ureters CT23
Brain C020
Breast CH2YYZZ
Bilateral CH22
Left CH21
Right CH20
Bronchi and Lungs CB22
Tomographic (Tomo) Nuclear Medicine Imaging — *continued*
Central Nervous System C02YYZZ
Cerebrospinal Fluid C025
Chest CW23
Chest and Abdomen CW24
Chest and Neck CW26
Digestive System CD2YYZZ
Endocrine System CG2YYZZ
Extremity
Lower CW2D
Bilateral CP2F
Left CP2D
Right CP2C
Upper CW2M
Bilateral CP2B
Left CP29
Right CP28
Gallbladder CF24
Gastrointestinal Tract CD27
Gland, Parathyroid CG21
Head and Neck CW2B
Heart C22YYZZ
Right and Left C226
Hepatobiliary System and Pancreas CF2YYZZ
Kidneys, Ureters and Bladder CT23
Liver CF25
Liver and Spleen CF26
Lungs and Bronchi CB22
Lymphatics and Hematologic System C72YYZZ
Musculoskeletal System, Other CP2YYZZ
Myocardium C22G
Neck and Chest CW26
Neck and Head CW2B
Pancreas and Hepatobiliary System CF2YYZZ
Pelvic Region CW2J
Pelvis CP26
Pelvis and Abdomen CW21
Pelvis and Spine CP27
Respiratory System CB2YYZZ
Skin CH2YYZZ
Skull CP21
Skull and Cervical Spine CP23
Spine
Cervical CP22
Cervical and Skull CP23
Lumbar CP2H
Thoracic CP2G
Thoracolumbar CP2J
Spine and Pelvis CP27
Spleen C722
Spleen and Liver CF26
Subcutaneous Tissue CH2YYZZ
Thorax CP24
Ureters, Kidneys and Bladder CT23
Urinary System CT2YYZZ
Tomography, computerized
see Computerized Tomography (CT Scan)
Tongue, base of
use Pharynx
Tonometry 4A07XBZ
Tonsillectomy
see Excision, Mouth and Throat 0CB
see Resection, Mouth and Throat 0CT
Tonsillotomy
see Drainage, Mouth and Throat 0C9
Total Anomalous Pulmonary Venous Return (TAPVR) repair
see Bypass, Atrium, Left 0217
see Bypass, Vena Cava, Superior 021V
Total artificial (replacement) heart
use Synthetic Substitute
Total parenteral nutrition (TPN)
see Introduction of Nutritional Substance
Trachectomy
see Excision, Trachea 0BB1
see Resection, Trachea 0BT1
Trachelectomy
see Excision, Cervix 0UBC
see Resection, Cervix 0UTC
Trachelopexy
see Repair, Cervix 0UQC
see Reposition, Cervix 0USC
Tracheloplasty or restriction
see Repair, Cervix 0UQC
Trachelorrhaphy
see Repair, Cervix 0UQC
Trachelotomy
see Drainage, Cervix 0U9C
Tracheobronchial lymph node
use Lymphatic, Thorax
Tracheoesophageal fistulization 0B110D6
Tracheolysis
see Release, Respiratory System 0BN
Tracheoplasty
see Repair, Respiratory System 0BQ
see Supplement, Respiratory System 0BU
Tracheorrhaphy
see Repair, Respiratory System 0BQ
Tracheoscopy 0BJ18ZZ
Tracheostomy open airway
see Bypass, Respiratory System 0B1
Tracheostomy Device
Bypass, Trachea 0B11
Change device in, Trachea 0B21XFZ
Removal of device from, Trachea 0BP1
Revision of device in, Trachea 0BW1
Tracheostomy tube
use Tracheostomy Device in Respiratory System
Tracheotomy
see Drainage, Respiratory System 0B9
Traction
Abdominal Wall 2W63X
Arm
Lower
Left 2W6DX
Right 2W6CX
Upper
Left 2W6BX
Right 2W6AX
Back 2W65X
Chest Wall 2W64X
Extremity
Lower
Left 2W6MX
Right 2W6LX
Upper
Left 2W69X
Right 2W68X
Face 2W61X
Finger
Left 2W6KX
Right 2W6JX
Foot
Left 2W6TX
Right 2W6SX
Hand
Left 2W6FX
Right 2W6EX
Head 2W60X
Inguinal Region
Left 2W67X
Right 2W66X
Leg
Lower
Left 2W6RX
Right 2W6QX
Upper
Left 2W6PX
Right 2W6NX

Turbinectomy
see Excision, Ear, Nose, Sinus 09B
see Resection, Ear, Nose, Sinus 09T
Turbinoplasty
see Repair, Ear, Nose, Sinus 09Q
see Replacement, Ear, Nose, Sinus 09R
see Supplement, Ear, Nose, Sinus 09U
Turbinotomy
see Division, Ear, Nose, Sinus 098
see Drainage, Ear, Nose, Sinus 099
TURP (transurethral resection of prostate)
see Excision, Prostate 0VB0
see Resection, Prostate 0VT0
Twelfth cranial nerve
use Hypoglossal Nerve
Two lead pacemaker
use Pacemaker, Dual Chamber in 0JH
Tympanic cavity
use Middle Ear, Right
use Middle Ear, Left
Tympanic nerve
use Glossopharyngeal Nerve
Tympanic part of temporal bone
use Temporal Bone, Right
use Temporal Bone, Left
Tympanogram
see Hearing Assessment, Diagnostic Audiology F13
Tympanoplasty
see Repair, Ear, Nose, Sinus 09Q
see Replacement, Ear, Nose, Sinus 09R
see Supplement, Ear, Nose, Sinus 09U
Tympanosympathectomy
see Excision, Nerve, Head and Neck Sympathetic 01BK
Tympanotomy (middle ear)
see Drainage, Ear, Nose, Sinus 099
TYRX Antibacterial Envelope
use Anti-Infective Envelope

U

Ulnar collateral carpal ligament
use Wrist Bursa and Ligament, Right
use Wrist Bursa and Ligament, Left
Ulnar collateral ligament
use Elbow Bursa and Ligament, Right
use Elbow Bursa and Ligament, Left
Ulnar notch
use Radius, Right
use Radius, Left
Ulnar vein
use Brachial Vein, Right
use Brachial Vein, Left
Ultrafiltration
Hemodialysis *see* Performance, Urinary 5A1D
Therapeutic plasmapheresis *see* Pheresis, Circulatory 6A55
Ultraflex™ Precision Colonic Stent System
use Intraluminal Device
ULTRAPRO® Hernia System (UHS)
use Synthetic Substitute
ULTRAPRO® Partially Absorbable Lightweight Mesh
use Synthetic Substitute
ULTRAPRO® Plug
use Synthetic Substitute
Ultrasonic osteogenic stimulator
use Bone Growth Stimulator in Head and Facial Bones
use Bone Growth Stimulator in Upper Bones
use Bone Growth Stimulator in Lower Bones
Ultrasonography
Abdomen BW40ZZZ
Abdomen and Pelvis BW41ZZZ
Abdominal Wall BH49ZZZ
Aorta
Abdominal, Intravascular B440ZZ3
Thoracic, Intravascular B340ZZ3
Appendix BD48ZZZ
Artery
Brachiocephalic-Subclavian, Right, Intravascular B341ZZ3
Celiac and Mesenteric, Intravascular B44KZZ3
Common Carotid
Bilateral, Intravascular B345ZZ3
Left, Intravascular B344ZZ3
Right, Intravascular B343ZZ3
Coronary
Multiple B241YZZ
Intravascular B241ZZ3
Transesophageal B241ZZ4
Single B240YZZ
Intravascular B240ZZ3
Transesophageal B240ZZ4
Femoral, Intravascular B44LZZ3
Inferior Mesenteric, Intravascular B445ZZ3
Internal Carotid
Bilateral, Intravascular B348ZZ3
Left, Intravascular B347ZZ3
Right, Intravascular B346ZZ3
Intra-Abdominal, Other, Intravascular B44BZZ3
Intracranial, Intravascular B34RZZ3
Lower Extremity
Bilateral, Intravascular B44HZZ3
Left, Intravascular B44GZZ3
Right, Intravascular B44FZZ3
Mesenteric and Celiac, Intravascular B44KZZ3
Ophthalmic, Intravascular B34VZZ3
Penile, Intravascular B44NZZ3
Pulmonary
Left, Intravascular B34TZZ3
Right, Intravascular B34SZZ3
Renal
Bilateral, Intravascular B448ZZ3
Left, Intravascular B447ZZ3
Right, Intravascular B446ZZ3
Subclavian, Left, Intravascular B342ZZ3
Superior Mesenteric, Intravascular B444ZZ3
Upper Extremity
Bilateral, Intravascular B34KZZ3
Left, Intravascular B34JZZ3
Right, Intravascular B34HZZ3
Bile Duct BF40ZZZ
Bile Duct and Gallbladder BF43ZZZ
Bladder BT40ZZZ
and Kidney BT4JZZZ
Brain B040ZZZ
Breast
Bilateral BH42ZZZ
Left BH41ZZZ
Right BH40ZZZ
Chest Wall BH4BZZZ
Coccyx BR4FZZZ
Connective Tissue
Lower Extremity BL41ZZZ
Upper Extremity BL40ZZZ
Duodenum BD49ZZZ
Elbow
Left, Densitometry BP4HZZ1
Right, Densitometry BP4GZZ1
Esophagus BD41ZZZ
Extremity
Lower BH48ZZZ
Upper BH47ZZZ
Ultrasonography — *continued*
Eye
Bilateral B847ZZZ
Left B846ZZZ
Right B845ZZZ
Fallopian Tube
Bilateral BU42
Left BU41
Right BU40
Fetal Umbilical Cord BY47ZZZ
Fetus
First Trimester, Multiple Gestation BY4BZZZ
Second Trimester, Multiple Gestation BY4DZZZ
Single
First Trimester BY49ZZZ
Second Trimester BY4CZZZ
Third Trimester BY4FZZZ
Third Trimester, Multiple Gestation BY4GZZZ
Gallbladder BF42ZZZ
Gallbladder and Bile Duct BF43ZZZ
Gastrointestinal Tract BD47ZZZ
Gland
Adrenal
Bilateral BG42ZZZ
Left BG41ZZZ
Right BG40ZZZ
Parathyroid BG43ZZZ
Thyroid BG44ZZZ
Hand
Left, Densitometry BP4PZZ1
Right, Densitometry BP4NZZ1
Head and Neck BH4CZZZ
Heart
Left B245YZZ
Intravascular B245ZZ3
Transesophageal B245ZZ4
Pediatric B24DYZZ
Intravascular B24DZZ3
Transesophageal B24DZZ4
Right B244YZZ
Intravascular B244ZZ3
Transesophageal B244ZZ4
Right and Left B246YZZ
Intravascular B246ZZ3
Transesophageal B246ZZ4
Heart with Aorta B24BYZZ
Intravascular B24BZZ3
Transesophageal B24BZZ4
Hepatobiliary System, All BF4CZZZ
Hip
Bilateral BQ42ZZZ
Left BQ41ZZZ
Right BQ40ZZZ
Kidney
and Bladder BT4JZZZ
Bilateral BT43ZZZ
Left BT42ZZZ
Right BT41ZZZ
Transplant BT49ZZZ
Knee
Bilateral BQ49ZZZ
Left BQ48ZZZ
Right BQ47ZZZ
Liver BF45ZZZ
Liver and Spleen BF46ZZZ
Mediastinum BB4CZZZ
Neck BW4FZZZ
Ovary
Bilateral BU45
Left BU44
Right BU43
Ovary and Uterus BU4C
Pancreas BF47ZZZ
Pelvic Region BW4GZZZ

V

Vomer of nasal septum - Zyvox®
ICD-10-PCS Index

Vomer of nasal septum
use Nasal Bone
Voraxaze®
use Glucarpidase
Vulvectomy
see Excision, Female Reproductive System 0UB
see Resection, Female Reproductive System 0UT
VYXEOS™
use Cytarabine and Daunorubicin Liposome Antineoplastic

W

WALLSTENT® Endoprosthesis
use Intraluminal Device
Washing
see Irrigation
WavelinQ™ EndoAVF system
Radial Artery, Left 031C3ZF
Radial Artery, Right 031B3ZF
Ulnar Artery, Left 031A3ZF
Ulnar Artery, Right 03193ZF
Wedge resection, pulmonary
see Excision, Respiratory System 0BB
Window
see Drainage
Wiring, dental 2W31X9Z
Wounds management F08

X

X-ray
see Plain Radiography
X-STOP® Spacer
use Spinal Stabilization Device, Interspinous Process in 0RH
use Spinal Stabilization Device, Interspinous Process in 0SH
Xact® Carotid Stent System
use Intraluminal Device
Xenograft
use Zooplastic Tissue in Heart and Great Vessels
XIENCE™ Everolimus Eluting Coronary Stent System
use Intraluminal Device, Drug-eluting in Heart and Great Vessels
Xiphoid process
use Sternum
XLIF® System
use Interbody Fusion Device in Lower Joints
XOSPATA®
use Gilteritinib Antineoplastic

Y

Yoga Therapy 8E0ZXY4

Z

Z-plasty, skin for scar contracture
see Release, Skin and Breast 0HN
Zenith® AAA Endovascular Graft
use Intraluminal Device, Branched or Fenestrated, One or Two Arteries in 04V
use Intraluminal Device, Branched or Fenestrated, Three or More Arteries in 04V
use Intraluminal Device
Zenith Flex® AAA Endovascular Graft
use Intraluminal Device
Zenith TX2® TAA Endovascular Graft
use Intraluminal Device
Zenith® Renu™ AAA Ancillary Graft
use Intraluminal Device
Zilver® PTX® (paclitaxel) Drug-eluting Peripheral Stent
use Intraluminal Device, Drug-eluting in Upper Arteries
use Intraluminal Device, Drug-eluting in Lower Arteries
Zimmer® NexGen® LPS Mobile Bearing Knee
use Synthetic Substitute
Zimmer® NexGen® LPS-Flex Mobile Knee
use Synthetic Substitute
ZINPLAVA™
use Bezlotoxumab Monoclonal Antibody
Zonule of Zinn
use Lens, Right
use Lens, Left
Zooplastic Tissue, Rapid Deployment Technique, Replacement X2RF
Zotarolimus-eluting coronary stent
use Intraluminal Device, Drug-eluting in Heart and Great Vessels
Zygomatic process of frontal bone
use Frontal Bone
Zygomatic process of temporal bone
use Temporal Bone, Right
use Temporal Bone, Left
Zygomaticus muscle
use Facial Muscle
Zyvox®
use Oxazolidinones

Vomer of nasal septum - Zyvox®
ICD-10-PCS INDEX

ICD-10-PCS Tables

Medical and Surgical 001-0YW

Central Nervous System and Cranial Nerves 001-00X

0 Medical and Surgical
0 Central Nervous System and Cranial Nerves
1 Bypass: Altering the route of passage of the contents of a tubular body part

Body Part Character 4	Approach Character 5	Device Character 6	Qualifier Character 7
6 Cerebral Ventricle	0 Open 3 Percutaneous 4 Percutaneous Endoscopic	7 Autologous Tissue Substitute J Synthetic Substitute K Nonautologous Tissue Substitute	0 Nasopharynx 1 Mastoid Sinus 2 Atrium 3 Blood Vessel 4 Pleural Cavity 5 Intestine 6 Peritoneal Cavity 7 Urinary Tract 8 Bone Marrow A Subgaleal Space B Cerebral Cisterns
6 Cerebral Ventricle	0 Open 3 Percutaneous 4 Percutaneous Endoscopic	Z No Device	B Cerebral Cisterns
U Spinal Canal	0 Open 3 Percutaneous 4 Percutaneous Endoscopic	7 Autologous Tissue Substitute J Synthetic Substitute K Nonautologous Tissue Substitute	2 Atrium 4 Pleural Cavity 6 Peritoneal Cavity 7 Urinary Tract 9 Fallopian Tube

0 Medical and Surgical
0 Central Nervous System and Cranial Nerves
2 Change: Taking out or off a device from a body part and putting back an identical or similar device in or on the same body part without cutting or puncturing the skin or a mucous membrane

Body Part Character 4	Approach Character 5	Device Character 6	Qualifier Character 7
0 Brain E Cranial Nerve U Spinal Canal	X External	0 Drainage Device Y Other Device	Z No Qualifier

LC Limited Coverage NC Noncovered HAC HAC-associated Procedure CC Combination Cluster - See Appendix G for code lists
DRG Non-OR-Affecting MS-DRG Assignment New/Revised Text in **Orange** ♂ Male ♀ Female

0 Medical and Surgical
0 Central Nervous System and Cranial Nerves
5 Destruction: Physical eradication of all or a portion of a body part by the direct use of energy, force, or a destructive agent

Body Part Character 4	Approach Character 5	Device Character 6	Qualifier Character 7
0 Brain **1** Cerebral Meninges **2** Dura Mater **6** Cerebral Ventricle **7** Cerebral Hemisphere **8** Basal Ganglia **9** Thalamus **A** Hypothalamus **B** Pons **C** Cerebellum **D** Medulla Oblongata **F** Olfactory Nerve **G** Optic Nerve **H** Oculomotor Nerve **J** Trochlear Nerve **K** Trigeminal Nerve **L** Abducens Nerve **M** Facial Nerve **N** Acoustic Nerve **P** Glossopharyngeal Nerve **Q** Vagus Nerve **R** Accessory Nerve **S** Hypoglossal Nerve **T** Spinal Meninges **W** Cervical Spinal Cord **X** Thoracic Spinal Cord **Y** Lumbar Spinal Cord	**0** Open **3** Percutaneous **4** Percutaneous Endoscopic	**Z** No Device	**Z** No Qualifier

0 Medical and Surgical
0 Central Nervous System and Cranial Nerves
7 Dilation: Expanding an orifice or the lumen of a tubular body part

Body Part Character 4	Approach Character 5	Device Character 6	Qualifier Character 7
6 Cerebral Ventricle	**0** Open **3** Percutaneous **4** Percutaneous Endoscopic	**Z** No Device	**Z** No Qualifier

0 Medical and Surgical
0 Central Nervous System and Cranial Nerves
8 Division: Cutting into a body part, without draining fluids and/or gases from the body part, in order to separate or transect a body part

Body Part Character 4	Approach Character 5	Device Character 6	Qualifier Character 7
0 Brain **7** Cerebral Hemisphere **8** Basal Ganglia **F** Olfactory Nerve **G** Optic Nerve **H** Oculomotor Nerve **J** Trochlear Nerve **K** Trigeminal Nerve **L** Abducens Nerve **M** Facial Nerve **N** Acoustic Nerve **P** Glossopharyngeal Nerve **Q** Vagus Nerve **R** Accessory Nerve **S** Hypoglossal Nerve **W** Cervical Spinal Cord **X** Thoracic Spinal Cord **Y** Lumbar Spinal Cord	**0** Open **3** Percutaneous **4** Percutaneous Endoscopic	**Z** No Device	**Z** No Qualifier

0 Medical and Surgical
0 Central Nervous System and Cranial Nerves
9 Drainage: Taking or letting out fluids and/or gases from a body part

Body Part Character 4	Approach Character 5	Device Character 6	Qualifier Character 7
0 Brain **1** Cerebral Meninges **2** Dura Mater **3** Epidural Space, Intracranial **4** Subdural Space, Intracranial **5** Subarachnoid Space, Intracranial **6** Cerebral Ventricle **7** Cerebral Hemisphere **8** Basal Ganglia **9** Thalamus **A** Hypothalamus **B** Pons **C** Cerebellum **D** Medulla Oblongata **F** Olfactory Nerve **G** Optic Nerve **H** Oculomotor Nerve **J** Trochlear Nerve **K** Trigeminal Nerve **L** Abducens Nerve **M** Facial Nerve **N** Acoustic Nerve **P** Glossopharyngeal Nerve **Q** Vagus Nerve **R** Accessory Nerve **S** Hypoglossal Nerve **T** Spinal Meninges **U** Spinal Canal **W** Cervical Spinal Cord **X** Thoracic Spinal Cord **Y** Lumbar Spinal Cord	**0** Open **3** Percutaneous **4** Percutaneous Endoscopic	**0** Drainage Device	**Z** No Qualifier
0 Brain **1** Cerebral Meninges **2** Dura Mater **3** Epidural Space, Intracranial **4** Subdural Space, Intracranial **5** Subarachnoid Space, Intracranial **6** Cerebral Ventricle **7** Cerebral Hemisphere **8** Basal Ganglia **9** Thalamus **A** Hypothalamus **B** Pons **C** Cerebellum **D** Medulla Oblongata **F** Olfactory Nerve **G** Optic Nerve **H** Oculomotor Nerve **J** Trochlear Nerve **K** Trigeminal Nerve **L** Abducens Nerve **M** Facial Nerve **N** Acoustic Nerve **P** Glossopharyngeal Nerve **Q** Vagus Nerve **R** Accessory Nerve **S** Hypoglossal Nerve **T** Spinal Meninges **U** Spinal Canal **W** Cervical Spinal Cord **X** Thoracic Spinal Cord **Y** Lumbar Spinal Cord	**0** Open **3** Percutaneous **4** Percutaneous Endoscopic	**Z** No Device	**X** Diagnostic **Z** No Qualifier

0 Medical and Surgical
0 Central Nervous System and Cranial Nerves
B Excision: Cutting out or off, without replacement, a portion of a body part

Body Part Character 4	Approach Character 5	Device Character 6	Qualifier Character 7
0 Brain **1** Cerebral Meninges **2** Dura Mater **6** Cerebral Ventricle **7** Cerebral Hemisphere **8** Basal Ganglia **9** Thalamus **A** Hypothalamus **B** Pons **C** Cerebellum **D** Medulla Oblongata **F** Olfactory Nerve **G** Optic Nerve **H** Oculomotor Nerve **J** Trochlear Nerve **K** Trigeminal Nerve **L** Abducens Nerve **M** Facial Nerve **N** Acoustic Nerve **P** Glossopharyngeal Nerve **Q** Vagus Nerve **R** Accessory Nerve **S** Hypoglossal Nerve **T** Spinal Meninges **W** Cervical Spinal Cord **X** Thoracic Spinal Cord **Y** Lumbar Spinal Cord	**0** Open **3** Percutaneous **4** Percutaneous Endoscopic	**Z** No Device	**X** Diagnostic **Z** No Qualifier

0 Medical and Surgical
0 Central Nervous System and Cranial Nerves
C Extirpation: Taking or cutting out solid matter from a body part hematoma

Body Part Character 4	Approach Character 5	Device Character 6	Qualifier Character 7
0 Brain	**0** Open Craniotomy	**Z** No Device	**Z** No Qualifier
1 Cerebral Meninges	**3** Percutaneous - drill burr hole		
2 Dura Mater	**4** Percutaneous Endoscopic		
3 Epidural Space, Intracranial			
4 Subdural Space, Intracranial			
5 Subarachnoid Space, Intracranial			
6 Cerebral Ventricle			
7 Cerebral Hemisphere			
8 Basal Ganglia			
9 Thalamus			
A Hypothalamus			
B Pons			
C Cerebellum			
D Medulla Oblongata			
F Olfactory Nerve			
G Optic Nerve			
H Oculomotor Nerve			
J Trochlear Nerve			
K Trigeminal Nerve			
L Abducens Nerve			
M Facial Nerve			
N Acoustic Nerve			
P Glossopharyngeal Nerve			
Q Vagus Nerve			
R Accessory Nerve			
S Hypoglossal Nerve			
T Spinal Meninges			
U Spinal Canal			
W Cervical Spinal Cord			
X Thoracic Spinal Cord			
Y Lumbar Spinal Cord			

0 Medical and Surgical
0 Central Nervous System and Cranial Nerves
D Extraction: Pulling or stripping out or off all or a portion of a body part by the use of force

Body Part Character 4	Approach Character 5	Device Character 6	Qualifier Character 7
1 Cerebral Meninges	**0** Open	**Z** No Device	**Z** No Qualifier
2 Dura Mater	**3** Percutaneous		
F Olfactory Nerve	**4** Percutaneous Endoscopic		
G Optic Nerve			
H Oculomotor Nerve			
J Trochlear Nerve			
K Trigeminal Nerve			
L Abducens Nerve			
M Facial Nerve			
N Acoustic Nerve			
P Glossopharyngeal Nerve			
Q Vagus Nerve			
R Accessory Nerve			
S Hypoglossal Nerve			
T Spinal Meninges			

LC Limited Coverage NC Noncovered HAC HAC-associated Procedure CC Combination Cluster - See Appendix G for code lists
DRG Non-OR-Affecting MS-DRG Assignment New/Revised Text in **Orange** ♂ Male ♀ Female

0 Medical and Surgical
0 Central Nervous System and Cranial Nerves
F Fragmentation: Breaking solid matter in a body part into pieces

Body Part Character 4	Approach Character 5	Device Character 6	Qualifier Character 7
3 Epidural Space, Intracranial NC 4 Subdural Space, Intracranial NC 5 Subarachnoid Space, Intracranial NC 6 Cerebral Ventricle NC U Spinal Canal	0 Open 3 Percutaneous 4 Percutaneous Endoscopic X External	Z No Device	Z No Qualifier

NC 00F3XZZ 00F4XZZ 00F5XZZ 00F6XZZ

0 Medical and Surgical
0 Central Nervous System and Cranial Nerves
H Insertion: Putting in a nonbiological appliance that monitors, assists, performs, or prevents a physiological function but does not physically take the place of a body part can also code removal if replacing shunt

Body Part Character 4	Approach Character 5	Device Character 6	Qualifier Character 7
0 Brain DRG CC	0 Open	2 Monitoring Device 3 Infusion Device Shunt 4 Radioactive Element, Cesium-131 Collagen Implant M Neurostimulator Lead Y Other Device	Z No Qualifier
0 Brain CC	3 Percutaneous 4 Percutaneous Endoscopic	2 Monitoring Device 3 Infusion Device M Neurostimulator Lead Y Other Device	Z No Qualifier
6 Cerebral Ventricle CC E Cranial Nerve CC U Spinal Canal CC V Spinal Cord CC	0 Open 3 Percutaneous 4 Percutaneous Endoscopic	2 Monitoring Device 3 Infusion Device M Neurostimulator Lead Y Other Device	Z No Qualifier

DRG 00H004Z
CC 00H00MZ 00H03MZ 00H04MZ 00H60MZ 00H63MZ 00H64MZ 00HE0MZ 00HE3MZ 00HE4MZ 00HU0MZ 00HU3MZ 00HU4MZ 00HV0MZ 00HV3MZ 00HV4MZ

0 Medical and Surgical
0 Central Nervous System and Cranial Nerves
J Inspection: Visually and/or manually exploring a body part

Body Part Character 4	Approach Character 5	Device Character 6	Qualifier Character 7
0 Brain E Cranial Nerve U Spinal Canal V Spinal Cord	0 Open 3 Percutaneous 4 Percutaneous Endoscopic	Z No Device	Z No Qualifier

0 Medical and Surgical
0 Central Nervous System and Cranial Nerves
K Map: Locating the route of passage of electrical impulses and/or locating functional areas in a body part

Body Part Character 4	Approach Character 5	Device Character 6	Qualifier Character 7
0 Brain **7** Cerebral Hemisphere **8** Basal Ganglia **9** Thalamus **A** Hypothalamus **B** Pons **C** Cerebellum **D** Medulla Oblongata	**0** Open **3** Percutaneous **4** Percutaneous Endoscopic	**Z** No Device	**Z** No Qualifier

0 Medical and Surgical
0 Central Nervous System and Cranial Nerves
N Release: Freeing a body part from an abnormal physical constraint by cutting or by the use of force

Body Part Character 4	Approach Character 5	Device Character 6	Qualifier Character 7
0 Brain **1** Cerebral Meninges **2** Dura Mater **6** Cerebral Ventricle **7** Cerebral Hemisphere **8** Basal Ganglia **9** Thalamus **A** Hypothalamus **B** Pons **C** Cerebellum **D** Medulla Oblongata **F** Olfactory Nerve **G** Optic Nerve **H** Oculomotor Nerve **J** Trochlear Nerve **K** Trigeminal Nerve **L** Abducens Nerve **M** Facial Nerve **N** Acoustic Nerve **P** Glossopharyngeal Nerve **Q** Vagus Nerve **R** Accessory Nerve **S** Hypoglossal Nerve **T** Spinal Meninges **W** Cervical Spinal Cord **X** Thoracic Spinal Cord **Y** Lumbar Spinal Cord	**0** Open **3** Percutaneous **4** Percutaneous Endoscopic	**Z** No Device	**Z** No Qualifier

0 Medical and Surgical
0 Central Nervous System and Cranial Nerves
P Removal: Taking out or off a device from a body part

Body Part	Approach	Device	Qualifier
Character 4	**Character 5**	**Character 6**	**Character 7**
0 Brain **V** Spinal Cord	**0** Open **3** Percutaneous **4** Percutaneous Endoscopic	**0** Drainage Device **2** Monitoring Device **3** Infusion Device **7** Autologous Tissue Substitute **J** Synthetic Substitute **K** Nonautologous Tissue Substitute **M** Neurostimulator Lead **Y** Other Device	**Z** No Qualifier
0 Brain **V** Spinal Cord	**X** External	**0** Drainage Device **2** Monitoring Device **3** Infusion Device **M** Neurostimulator Lead	**Z** No Qualifier
6 Cerebral Ventricle **U** Spinal Canal	**0** Open **3** Percutaneous **4** Percutaneous Endoscopic	**0** Drainage Device **2** Monitoring Device **3** Infusion Device **J** Synthetic Substitute Shunt **M** Neurostimulator Lead **Y** Other Device	**Z** No Qualifier
6 Cerebral Ventricle **U** Spinal Canal	**X** External	**0** Drainage Device **2** Monitoring Device **3** Infusion Device **M** Neurostimulator Lead	**Z** No Qualifier
E Cranial Nerve	**0** Open **3** Percutaneous **4** Percutaneous Endoscopic	**0** Drainage Device **2** Monitoring Device **3** Infusion Device **7** Autologous Tissue Substitute **M** Neurostimulator Lead **Y** Other Device	**Z** No Qualifier
E Cranial Nerve	**X** External	**0** Drainage Device **2** Monitoring Device **3** Infusion Device **M** Neurostimulator Lead	**Z** No Qualifier

0 Medical and Surgical
0 Central Nervous System and Cranial Nerves
Q Repair: Restoring, to the extent possible, a body part to its normal anatomic structure and function

Body Part	Approach	Device	Qualifier
Character 4	**Character 5**	**Character 6**	**Character 7**
0 Brain **1** Cerebral Meninges **2** Dura Mater **6** Cerebral Ventricle **7** Cerebral Hemisphere **8** Basal Ganglia **9** Thalamus **A** Hypothalamus **B** Pons **C** Cerebellum **D** Medulla Oblongata **F** Olfactory Nerve **G** Optic Nerve **H** Oculomotor Nerve **J** Trochlear Nerve **K** Trigeminal Nerve **L** Abducens Nerve **M** Facial Nerve **N** Acoustic Nerve **P** Glossopharyngeal Nerve **Q** Vagus Nerve **R** Accessory Nerve **S** Hypoglossal Nerve **T** Spinal Meninges **W** Cervical Spinal Cord **X** Thoracic Spinal Cord **Y** Lumbar Spinal Cord	**0** Open **3** Percutaneous **4** Percutaneous Endoscopic	**Z** No Device	**Z** No Qualifier

0 Medical and Surgical
0 Central Nervous System and Cranial Nerves
R Replacement: Putting in or on biological or synthetic material that physically takes the place and/or function of all or a portion of a body part

Body Part	Approach	Device	Qualifier
Character 4	**Character 5**	**Character 6**	**Character 7**
1 Cerebral Meninges **2** Dura Mater **6** Cerebral Ventricle **F** Olfactory Nerve **G** Optic Nerve **H** Oculomotor Nerve **J** Trochlear Nerve **K** Trigeminal Nerve **L** Abducens Nerve **M** Facial Nerve **N** Acoustic Nerve **P** Glossopharyngeal Nerve **Q** Vagus Nerve **R** Accessory Nerve **S** Hypoglossal Nerve **T** Spinal Meninges	**0** Open **4** Percutaneous Endoscopic	**7** Autologous Tissue Substitute **J** Synthetic Substitute **K** Nonautologous Tissue Substitute	**Z** No Qualifier

LC Limited Coverage NC Noncovered HAC HAC-associated Procedure CC Combination Cluster - See Appendix G for code lists
DRG Non-OR-Affecting MS-DRG Assignment New/Revised Text in **Orange** ♂ Male ♀ Female

2020 ICD-10-PCS 179

0 Medical and Surgical
0 Central Nervous System and Cranial Nerves
S Reposition: Moving to its normal location, or other suitable location, all or a portion of a body part

Body Part Character 4	Approach Character 5	Device Character 6	Qualifier Character 7
F Olfactory Nerve **G** Optic Nerve **H** Oculomotor Nerve **J** Trochlear Nerve **K** Trigeminal Nerve **L** Abducens Nerve **M** Facial Nerve **N** Acoustic Nerve **P** Glossopharyngeal Nerve **Q** Vagus Nerve **R** Accessory Nerve **S** Hypoglossal Nerve **W** Cervical Spinal Cord **X** Thoracic Spinal Cord **Y** Lumbar Spinal Cord	**0** Open **3** Percutaneous **4** Percutaneous Endoscopic	**Z** No Device	**Z** No Qualifier

0 Medical and Surgical
0 Central Nervous System and Cranial Nerves
T Resection: Cutting out or off, without replacement, all of a body part

Body Part Character 4	Approach Character 5	Device Character 6	Qualifier Character 7
7 Cerebral Hemisphere	**0** Open **3** Percutaneous **4** Percutaneous Endoscopic	**Z** No Device	**Z** No Qualifier

0 Medical and Surgical
0 Central Nervous System and Cranial Nerves
U Supplement: Putting in or on biological or synthetic material that physically reinforces and/or augments the function of a portion of a body part

Body Part Character 4	Approach Character 5	Device Character 6	Qualifier Character 7
1 Cerebral Meninges **2** Dura Mater **6** Cerebral Ventricle **F** Olfactory Nerve **G** Optic Nerve **H** Oculomotor Nerve **J** Trochlear Nerve **K** Trigeminal Nerve **L** Abducens Nerve **M** Facial Nerve **N** Acoustic Nerve **P** Glossopharyngeal Nerve **Q** Vagus Nerve **R** Accessory Nerve **S** Hypoglossal Nerve **T** Spinal Meninges	**0** Open **3** Percutaneous **4** Percutaneous Endoscopic	**7** Autologous Tissue Substitute **J** Synthetic Substitute **K** Nonautologous Tissue Substitute	**Z** No Qualifier

0 Medical and Surgical
0 Central Nervous System and Cranial Nerves
W Revision: Correcting, to the extent possible, a portion of a malfunctioning device or the position of a displaced device

Body Part Character 4	Approach Character 5	Device Character 6	Qualifier Character 7
0 Brain V Spinal Cord	0 Open 3 Percutaneous 4 Percutaneous Endoscopic	0 Drainage Device 2 Monitoring Device 3 Infusion Device 7 Autologous Tissue Substitute J Synthetic Substitute K Nonautologous Tissue Substitute M Neurostimulator Lead Y Other Device	Z No Qualifier
0 Brain V Spinal Cord	X External	0 Drainage Device 2 Monitoring Device 3 Infusion Device 7 Autologous Tissue Substitute J Synthetic Substitute K Nonautologous Tissue Substitute M Neurostimulator Lead	Z No Qualifier
6 Cerebral Ventricle U Spinal Canal	0 Open 3 Percutaneous 4 Percutaneous Endoscopic	0 Drainage Device 2 Monitoring Device 3 Infusion Device J Synthetic Substitute M Neurostimulator Lead Y Other Device	Z No Qualifier
6 Cerebral Ventricle U Spinal Canal	X External	0 Drainage Device 2 Monitoring Device 3 Infusion Device J Synthetic Substitute M Neurostimulator Lead	Z No Qualifier
E Cranial Nerve	0 Open 3 Percutaneous 4 Percutaneous Endoscopic	0 Drainage Device 2 Monitoring Device 3 Infusion Device 7 Autologous Tissue Substitute M Neurostimulator Lead Y Other Device	Z No Qualifier
E Cranial Nerve	X External	0 Drainage Device 2 Monitoring Device 3 Infusion Device 7 Autologous Tissue Substitute M Neurostimulator Lead	Z No Qualifier

0 Medical and Surgical
0 Central Nervous System and Cranial Nerves
X Transfer: Moving, without taking out, all or a portion of a body part to another location to take over the function of all or a portion of a body part

Body Part Character 4	Approach Character 5	Device Character 6	Qualifier Character 7
F Olfactory Nerve G Optic Nerve H Oculomotor Nerve J Trochlear Nerve K Trigeminal Nerve L Abducens Nerve M Facial Nerve N Acoustic Nerve P Glossopharyngeal Nerve Q Vagus Nerve R Accessory Nerve S Hypoglossal Nerve	0 Open 4 Percutaneous Endoscopic	Z No Device	F Olfactory Nerve G Optic Nerve H Oculomotor Nerve J Trochlear Nerve K Trigeminal Nerve L Abducens Nerve M Facial Nerve N Acoustic Nerve P Glossopharyngeal Nerve Q Vagus Nerve R Accessory Nerve S Hypoglossal Nerve

LC Limited Coverage NC Noncovered HAC HAC-associated Procedure CC Combination Cluster - See Appendix G for code lists
DRG Non-OR-Affecting MS-DRG Assignment New/Revised Text in **Orange** ♂ Male ♀ Female

3 pieces of shunt
1) cerebral ventricular catheter (brain)
2) peritoneal catheter
3) valve

NOTES

CSF shunt - device is synthetic substitute <u>not</u> drainage

Revision - 1 or more shunt components are replaced due to malfunction

Bypass - when all of the shunt needs replaced, also code for removal

Peripheral Nervous System 012-01X

includes carpal tunnel, nerve transfer, CSF shunts

0 Medical and Surgical
1 Peripheral Nervous System
2 Change: Taking out or off a device from a body part and putting back an identical or similar device in or on the same body part without cutting or puncturing the skin or a mucous membrane

Body Part	Approach	Device	Qualifier
Character 4	**Character 5**	**Character 6**	**Character 7**
Y Peripheral Nerve	**X** External	**0** Drainage Device **Y** Other Device	**Z** No Qualifier

0 Medical and Surgical
1 Peripheral Nervous System
5 Destruction: Physical eradication of all or a portion of a body part by the direct use of energy, force, or a destructive agent

Body Part	Approach	Device	Qualifier
Character 4	**Character 5**	**Character 6**	**Character 7**
0 Cervical Plexus **1** Cervical Nerve **2** Phrenic Nerve **3** Brachial Plexus **4** Ulnar Nerve **5** Median Nerve **6** Radial Nerve **8** Thoracic Nerve **9** Lumbar Plexus **A** Lumbosacral Plexus **B** Lumbar Nerve **C** Pudendal Nerve **D** Femoral Nerve **F** Sciatic Nerve **G** Tibial Nerve **H** Peroneal Nerve **K** Head and Neck Sympathetic Nerve **L** Thoracic Sympathetic Nerve **M** Abdominal Sympathetic Nerve **N** Lumbar Sympathetic Nerve **P** Sacral Sympathetic Nerve **Q** Sacral Plexus **R** Sacral Nerve	**0** Open **3** Percutaneous **4** Percutaneous Endoscopic	**Z** No Device	**Z** No Qualifier

Sclerotherapy of brachial plexus lesion w/ alcohol injection Ø15322

0 Medical and Surgical
1 Peripheral Nervous System
8 Division: Cutting into a body part, without draining fluids and/or gases from the body part, in order to separate or transect a body part

Body Part Character 4	Approach Character 5	Device Character 6	Qualifier Character 7
0 Cervical Plexus **1** Cervical Nerve **2** Phrenic Nerve **3** Brachial Plexus **4** Ulnar Nerve **5** Median Nerve **6** Radial Nerve **8** Thoracic Nerve **9** Lumbar Plexus **A** Lumbosacral Plexus **B** Lumbar Nerve **C** Pudendal Nerve **D** Femoral Nerve **F** Sciatic Nerve **G** Tibial Nerve **H** Peroneal Nerve **K** Head and Neck Sympathetic Nerve **L** Thoracic Sympathetic Nerve **M** Abdominal Sympathetic Nerve **N** Lumbar Sympathetic Nerve **P** Sacral Sympathetic Nerve **Q** Sacral Plexus **R** Sacral Nerve	**0** Open **3** Percutaneous **4** Percutaneous Endoscopic	**Z** No Device	**Z** No Qualifier

0 Medical and Surgical
1 Peripheral Nervous System
9 Drainage: Taking or letting out fluids and/or gases from a body part

Body Part Character 4	Approach Character 5	Device Character 6	Qualifier Character 7
0 Cervical Plexus **1** Cervical Nerve **2** Phrenic Nerve **3** Brachial Plexus **4** Ulnar Nerve **5** Median Nerve **6** Radial Nerve **8** Thoracic Nerve **9** Lumbar Plexus **A** Lumbosacral Plexus **B** Lumbar Nerve **C** Pudendal Nerve **D** Femoral Nerve **F** Sciatic Nerve **G** Tibial Nerve **H** Peroneal Nerve **K** Head and Neck Sympathetic Nerve **L** Thoracic Sympathetic Nerve **M** Abdominal Sympathetic Nerve **N** Lumbar Sympathetic Nerve **P** Sacral Sympathetic Nerve **Q** Sacral Plexus **R** Sacral Nerve	**0** Open **3** Percutaneous **4** Percutaneous Endoscopic	**0** Drainage Device	**Z** No Qualifier

019 continued on next page

0 **Medical and Surgical**
1 **Peripheral Nervous System**
9 **Drainage:** Taking or letting out fluids and/or gases from a body part

019 continued from previous page

Body Part Character 4	Approach Character 5	Device Character 6	Qualifier Character 7
0 Cervical Plexus **1** Cervical Nerve **2** Phrenic Nerve **3** Brachial Plexus **4** Ulnar Nerve **5** Median Nerve **6** Radial Nerve **8** Thoracic Nerve **9** Lumbar Plexus **A** Lumbosacral Plexus **B** Lumbar Nerve **C** Pudendal Nerve **D** Femoral Nerve **F** Sciatic Nerve **G** Tibial Nerve **H** Peroneal Nerve **K** Head and Neck Sympathetic Nerve **L** Thoracic Sympathetic Nerve **M** Abdominal Sympathetic Nerve **N** Lumbar Sympathetic Nerve **P** Sacral Sympathetic Nerve **Q** Sacral Plexus **R** Sacral Nerve	**0** Open **3** Percutaneous **4** Percutaneous Endoscopic	**Z** No Device	**X** Diagnostic **Z** No Qualifier

0 **Medical and Surgical**
1 **Peripheral Nervous System**
B **Excision:** Cutting out or off, without replacement, a portion of a body part

Body Part Character 4	Approach Character 5	Device Character 6	Qualifier Character 7
0 Cervical Plexus **1** Cervical Nerve **2** Phrenic Nerve **3** Brachial Plexus **4** Ulnar Nerve **5** Median Nerve **6** Radial Nerve **8** Thoracic Nerve **9** Lumbar Plexus **A** Lumbosacral Plexus **B** Lumbar Nerve **C** Pudendal Nerve **D** Femoral Nerve **F** Sciatic Nerve **G** Tibial Nerve **H** Peroneal Nerve **K** Head and Neck Sympathetic Nerve **L** Thoracic Sympathetic Nerve **M** Abdominal Sympathetic Nerve **N** Lumbar Sympathetic Nerve **P** Sacral Sympathetic Nerve **Q** Sacral Plexus **R** Sacral Nerve	**0** Open **3** Percutaneous **4** Percutaneous Endoscopic	**Z** No Device	**X** Diagnostic **Z** No Qualifier

LC Limited Coverage NC Noncovered HAC HAC-associated Procedure CC Combination Cluster - See Appendix G for code lists
DRG Non-OR-Affecting MS-DRG Assignment New/Revised Text in **Orange** ♂ Male ♀ Female

0 Medical and Surgical
1 Peripheral Nervous System
C Extirpation: Taking or cutting out solid matter from a body part

Body Part Character 4	Approach Character 5	Device Character 6	Qualifier Character 7
0 Cervical Plexus 1 Cervical Nerve 2 Phrenic Nerve 3 Brachial Plexus 4 Ulnar Nerve 5 Median Nerve 6 Radial Nerve 8 Thoracic Nerve 9 Lumbar Plexus A Lumbosacral Plexus B Lumbar Nerve C Pudendal Nerve D Femoral Nerve F Sciatic Nerve G Tibial Nerve H Peroneal Nerve K Head and Neck Sympathetic Nerve L Thoracic Sympathetic Nerve M Abdominal Sympathetic Nerve N Lumbar Sympathetic Nerve P Sacral Sympathetic Nerve Q Sacral Plexus R Sacral Nerve	0 Open 3 Percutaneous 4 Percutaneous Endoscopic	Z No Device	Z No Qualifier

0 Medical and Surgical
1 Peripheral Nervous System
D Extraction: Pulling or stripping out or off all or a portion of a body part by the use of force

Body Part Character 4	Approach Character 5	Device Character 6	Qualifier Character 7
0 Cervical Plexus 1 Cervical Nerve 2 Phrenic Nerve 3 Brachial Plexus 4 Ulnar Nerve 5 Median Nerve 6 Radial Nerve 8 Thoracic Nerve 9 Lumbar Plexus A Lumbosacral Plexus B Lumbar Nerve C Pudendal Nerve D Femoral Nerve F Sciatic Nerve G Tibial Nerve H Peroneal Nerve K Head and Neck Sympathetic Nerve L Thoracic Sympathetic Nerve M Abdominal Sympathetic Nerve N Lumbar Sympathetic Nerve P Sacral Sympathetic Nerve Q Sacral Plexus R Sacral Nerve	0 Open 3 Percutaneous 4 Percutaneous Endoscopic	Z No Device	Z No Qualifier

0 Medical and Surgical
1 Peripheral Nervous System
H Insertion: Putting in a nonbiological appliance that monitors, assists, performs, or prevents a physiological function but does not physically take the place of a body part

Body Part Character 4	Approach Character 5	Device Character 6	Qualifier Character 7
Y Peripheral Nerve CC	**0** Open **3** Percutaneous **4** Percutaneous Endoscopic	**2** Monitoring Device **M** Neurostimulator Lead **Y** Other Device	**Z** No Qualifier

CC 01HY0MZ 01HY3MZ 01HY4MZ

0 Medical and Surgical
1 Peripheral Nervous System
J Inspection: Visually and/or manually exploring a body part

Body Part Character 4	Approach Character 5	Device Character 6	Qualifier Character 7
Y Peripheral Nerve	**0** Open **3** Percutaneous **4** Percutaneous Endoscopic	**Z** No Device	**Z** No Qualifier

0 Medical and Surgical
1 Peripheral Nervous System
N Release: Freeing a body part from an abnormal physical constraint by cutting or by the use of force

Body Part Character 4	Approach Character 5	Device Character 6	Qualifier Character 7
0 Cervical Plexus **1** Cervical Nerve **2** Phrenic Nerve **3** Brachial Plexus **4** Ulnar Nerve **5** Median Nerve - CTS - divide transfer carpel ligament **6** Radial Nerve **8** Thoracic Nerve **9** Lumbar Plexus **A** Lumbosacral Plexus **B** Lumbar Nerve **C** Pudendal Nerve **D** Femoral Nerve **F** Sciatic Nerve **G** Tibial Nerve **H** Peroneal Nerve **K** Head and Neck Sympathetic Nerve **L** Thoracic Sympathetic Nerve **M** Abdominal Sympathetic Nerve **N** Lumbar Sympathetic Nerve **P** Sacral Sympathetic Nerve **Q** Sacral Plexus **R** Sacral Nerve	**0** Open **3** Percutaneous **4** Percutaneous Endoscopic may use synovial elevator	**Z** No Device	**Z** No Qualifier Carpel tunnel release CTS Ø1N5ØZZ

0 Medical and Surgical
1 Peripheral Nervous System
P Removal: Taking out or off a device from a body part

Body Part Character 4	Approach Character 5	Device Character 6	Qualifier Character 7
Y Peripheral Nerve	**0** Open **3** Percutaneous **4** Percutaneous Endoscopic	**0** Drainage Device **2** Monitoring Device **7** Autologous Tissue Substitute **M** Neurostimulator Lead **Y** Other Device	**Z** No Qualifier
Y Peripheral Nerve	**X** External	**0** Drainage Device **2** Monitoring Device **M** Neurostimulator Lead	**Z** No Qualifier

LC Limited Coverage NC Noncovered HAC HAC-associated Procedure CC Combination Cluster - See Appendix G for code lists
DRG Non-OR-Affecting MS-DRG Assignment New/Revised Text in **Orange** ♂ Male ♀ Female

digital nerve laceration

0 Medical and Surgical
1 Peripheral Nervous System
Q Repair: Restoring, to the extent possible, a body part to its normal anatomic structure and function

Body Part Character 4	Approach Character 5	Device Character 6	Qualifier Character 7
0 Cervical Plexus **1** Cervical Nerve **2** Phrenic Nerve **3** Brachial Plexus **4** Ulnar Nerve - may be digit **5** Median Nerve **6** Radial Nerve **8** Thoracic Nerve **9** Lumbar Plexus **A** Lumbosacral Plexus **B** Lumbar Nerve **C** Pudendal Nerve **D** Femoral Nerve **F** Sciatic Nerve **G** Tibial Nerve **H** Peroneal Nerve **K** Head and Neck Sympathetic Nerve **L** Thoracic Sympathetic Nerve **M** Abdominal Sympathetic Nerve **N** Lumbar Sympathetic Nerve **P** Sacral Sympathetic Nerve **Q** Sacral Plexus **R** Sacral Nerve	**0** Open **3** Percutaneous **4** Percutaneous Endoscopic	**Z** No Device	**Z** No Qualifier

0 Medical and Surgical
1 Peripheral Nervous System
R Replacement: Putting in or on biological or synthetic material that physically takes the place and/or function of all or a portion of a body part

Body Part Character 4	Approach Character 5	Device Character 6	Qualifier Character 7
1 Cervical Nerve **2** Phrenic Nerve **4** Ulnar Nerve **5** Median Nerve **6** Radial Nerve **8** Thoracic Nerve **B** Lumbar Nerve **C** Pudendal Nerve **D** Femoral Nerve **F** Sciatic Nerve **G** Tibial Nerve **H** Peroneal Nerve **R** Sacral Nerve	**0** Open **4** Percutaneous Endoscopic	**7** Autologous Tissue Substitute **J** Synthetic Substitute **K** Nonautologous Tissue Substitute	**Z** No Qualifier

0 Medical and Surgical
1 Peripheral Nervous System
S Reposition: Moving to its normal location, or other suitable location, all or a portion of a body part

Body Part Character 4	Approach Character 5	Device Character 6	Qualifier Character 7
0 Cervical Plexus **1** Cervical Nerve **2** Phrenic Nerve **3** Brachial Plexus **4** Ulnar Nerve **5** Median Nerve **6** Radial Nerve **8** Thoracic Nerve **9** Lumbar Plexus **A** Lumbosacral Plexus **B** Lumbar Nerve **C** Pudendal Nerve **D** Femoral Nerve **F** Sciatic Nerve **G** Tibial Nerve **H** Peroneal Nerve **Q** Sacral Plexus **R** Sacral Nerve	**0** Open **3** Percutaneous **4** Percutaneous Endoscopic	**Z** No Device	**Z** No Qualifier

0 Medical and Surgical
1 Peripheral Nervous System
U Supplement: Putting in or on biological or synthetic material that physically reinforces and/or augments the function of a portion of a body part

Body Part Character 4	Approach Character 5	Device Character 6	Qualifier Character 7
1 Cervical Nerve **2** Phrenic Nerve **4** Ulnar Nerve **5** Median Nerve **6** Radial Nerve **8** Thoracic Nerve **B** Lumbar Nerve **C** Pudendal Nerve **D** Femoral Nerve **F** Sciatic Nerve **G** Tibial Nerve **H** Peroneal Nerve **R** Sacral Nerve	**0** Open **3** Percutaneous **4** Percutaneous Endoscopic	**7** Autologous Tissue Substitute **J** Synthetic Substitute **K** Nonautologous Tissue Substitute	**Z** No Qualifier

0 Medical and Surgical
1 Peripheral Nervous System
W Revision: Correcting, to the extent possible, a portion of a malfunctioning device or the position of a displaced device

Body Part Character 4	Approach Character 5	Device Character 6	Qualifier Character 7
Y Peripheral Nerve	**0** Open **3** Percutaneous **4** Percutaneous Endoscopic	**0** Drainage Device **2** Monitoring Device **7** Autologous Tissue Substitute **M** Neurostimulator Lead **Y** Other Device	**Z** No Qualifier
Y Peripheral Nerve	**X** External	**0** Drainage Device **2** Monitoring Device **7** Autologous Tissue Substitute **M** Neurostimulator Lead	**Z** No Qualifier

0 Medical and Surgical
1 Peripheral Nervous System
X Transfer: Moving, without taking out, all or a portion of a body part to another location to take over the function of all or a portion of a body part

Body Part Character 4	Approach Character 5	Device Character 6	Qualifier Character 7
1 Cervical Nerve **2** Phrenic Nerve	**0** Open **4** Percutaneous Endoscopic	**Z** No Device	**1** Cervical Nerve **2** Phrenic Nerve
4 Ulnar Nerve **5** Median Nerve **6** Radial Nerve	**0** Open **4** Percutaneous Endoscopic	**Z** No Device	**4** Ulnar Nerve **5** Median Nerve **6** Radial Nerve
8 Thoracic Nerve	**0** Open **4** Percutaneous Endoscopic	**Z** No Device	**8** Thoracic Nerve
B Lumbar Nerve **C** Pudendal Nerve	**0** Open **4** Percutaneous Endoscopic	**Z** No Device	**B** Lumbar Nerve **C** Perineal Nerve
D Femoral Nerve **F** Sciatic Nerve **G** Tibial Nerve **H** Peroneal Nerve	**0** Open **4** Percutaneous Endoscopic	**Z** No Device	**D** Femoral Nerve **F** Sciatic Nerve **G** Tibial Nerve **H** Peroneal Nerve

pacemaker + defibrillator - include pulse generator & electrodes
use subclavian or jugular vein to cannulate
pulse generator placed in subQ pocket

NOTES

- heart receives blood from coronary arteries
- 2 major coronary arteries branch off from the aorta near the point where the aorta & the left ventricle meet. These arteries & their branches supply the heart w/ blood

Left main coronary artery AKA left main trunk
↓ branches into
circumflex artery & left anterior descending artery LAD

Left cornary arteries supply:

- circumflex artery - supplies blood to the LA, side & back of LV
- left LAD - supplies front & bottom of LV & front of septum

Right coronary Artery (RAC) branches into:

- right marginal artery
- posterior descending artery

RAC supplies: RA, RV, bottom portion of both ventricles & back of septum

main portion of RCA provides blood to right side of heart, which pumps blood to the lungs. The rest of the RCA & its main branch, the posterior DA, together w/ the branches of the circumflex artery, run across the surface of the hearts underside, supplying the bottom portion of the LV & back of the septum

coronary veins - take O_2 poor (deoxygenated) blood back to RA

Coronary - branches off aorta
conduit = qualifier = healthy vessel

NOTES

LIM - left internal mammary
~~PTCA - Percutaneous Transluminal Coronary Angioplasty~~

0210029
CABG of LAD using LIMA w/ the pt off bypass. 1 conduit is used & placed

See B3.6b page 10
body part - IDs how many coronary arteries are bypassed to (what is being bypassed)
qualifier - specifies the vessel bypassed from

If all bypasses use same graft material (6th) only 1 code is needed

If CABG uses different grafts - code each. Ex: ① LIMA & ② saphenous vein
Thus code for each graft created

Open aortocoronary bypass graft of 2 coronary arteries using 2 sections of saphenous vein from left leg harvested endoscopically
021109W & 06BQ4ZZ for graft excision
Blood is bypassed from aorta (W) to 2 coronary arteries (1)

- Cardiac cath that are therapeutic use Ø medical & surgical
- Cardiac cath than are diagnostic use "4" for imaging, measuring & monitoring
- When coding for insertion of pacemaker/defibrillator, code each device separate
  When devices are removed code removal of each device
  defibrillator = AICD = automatic implantable cardioverter defibrillator

How to code CABG - need to know:
- How many coronary artery sites are bypassed
- How many different devices (veins, arteries, autologous, non-autologous, synthetic) are used - Character 6
- How many different qualifiers (point of origin for new blood supply to heart, ex: the aorta) are used?
- Was the pt on cardiopulmonary bypass?
- Was an autologous vein and/or artery harvested? From what site?

- Swan Ganz - AKA pulmonary artery catheterization
  - goes into pulmonary artery - purpose is diagnostic
  - Detects: heart failure, sepsis, monitor therapy, evaluates effects of drugs
- Bi-ventricular pacing - for CHF pumps blood

Mapping done during left heart cath = map, section 02

Stent insertion = dilation
angioplasty = dilation, device value Z - no device
measurement & monitoring - main left heart cath
imaging - cardiac arteries & existing bypass grafts

Heart and Great Vessels 021-02Y

0 Medical and Surgical
2 Heart and Great Vessels
1 Bypass: Altering the route of passage of the contents of a tubular body part

Body Part Character 4	Approach Character 5	Device Character 6	Qualifier Character 7
0 Coronary Artery, One Artery HAC **1** Coronary Artery, Two Arteries HAC **2** Coronary Artery, Three Arteries HAC **3** Coronary Artery, Four or More Arteries HAC	**0** Open	**8** Zooplastic Tissue **9** Autologous Venous Tissue **A** Autologous Arterial Tissue **J** Synthetic Substitute **K** Nonautologous Tissue Substitute	**3** Coronary Artery **8** Internal Mammary, Right **9** Internal Mammary, Left **C** Thoracic Artery **F** Abdominal Artery **W** Aorta
0 Coronary Artery, One Artery HAC **1** Coronary Artery, Two Arteries HAC **2** Coronary Artery, Three Arteries HAC **3** Coronary Artery, Four or More Arteries HAC	**0** Open	**Z** No Device	**3** Coronary Artery **8** Internal Mammary, Right **9** Internal Mammary, Left **C** Thoracic Artery **F** Abdominal Artery
0 Coronary Artery, One Artery **1** Coronary Artery, Two Arteries **2** Coronary Artery, Three Arteries **3** Coronary Artery, Four or More Arteries	**3** Percutaneous	**4** Intraluminal Device, Drug-eluting **D** Intraluminal Device	**4** Coronary Vein
0 Coronary Artery, One Artery **1** Coronary Artery, Two Arteries **2** Coronary Artery, Three Arteries **3** Coronary Artery, Four or More Arteries	**4** Percutaneous Endoscopic	**4** Intraluminal Device, Drug-eluting **D** Intraluminal Device	**4** Coronary Vein
0 Coronary Artery, One Artery HAC **1** Coronary Artery, Two Arteries HAC **2** Coronary Artery, Three Arteries HAC **3** Coronary Artery, Four or More Arteries HAC	**4** Percutaneous Endoscopic	**8** Zooplastic Tissue **9** Autologous Venous Tissue **A** Autologous Arterial Tissue **J** Synthetic Substitute **K** Nonautologous Tissue Substitute	**3** Coronary Artery **8** Internal Mammary, Right **9** Internal Mammary, Left **C** Thoracic Artery **F** Abdominal Artery **W** Aorta
0 Coronary Artery, One Artery HAC **1** Coronary Artery, Two Arteries HAC **2** Coronary Artery, Three Arteries HAC **3** Coronary Artery, Four or More Arteries HAC	**4** Percutaneous Endoscopic	**Z** No Device	**3** Coronary Artery **8** Internal Mammary, Right **9** Internal Mammary, Left **C** Thoracic Artery **F** Abdominal Artery
6 Atrium, Right	**0** Open **4** Percutaneous Endoscopic	**8** Zooplastic Tissue **9** Autologous Venous Tissue **A** Autologous Arterial Tissue **J** Synthetic Substitute **K** Nonautologous Tissue Substitute	**P** Pulmonary Trunk **Q** Pulmonary Artery, Right **R** Pulmonary Artery, Left
6 Atrium, Right	**0** Open **4** Percutaneous Endoscopic	**Z** No Device	**7** Atrium, Left **P** Pulmonary Trunk **Q** Pulmonary Artery, Right **R** Pulmonary Artery, Left

021 continued on next page

LC Limited Coverage NC Noncovered HAC HAC-associated Procedure CC Combination Cluster - See Appendix G for code lists
DRG Non-OR-Affecting MS-DRG Assignment New/Revised Text in **Orange** ♂ Male ♀ Female

0 Medical and Surgical
2 Heart and Great Vessels
1 Bypass: Altering the route of passage of the contents of a tubular body part

021 continued from previous page

healthy vessel = conduit

Body Part Character 4	Approach Character 5	Device Character 6	Qualifier Character 7
6 Atrium, Right	3 Percutaneous	Z No Device	7 Atrium, Left
7 Atrium, Left V Superior Vena Cava	0 Open 4 Percutaneous Endoscopic	8 Zooplastic Tissue 9 Autologous Venous Tissue A Autologous Arterial Tissue J Synthetic Substitute K Nonautologous Tissue Substitute Z No Device	P Pulmonary Trunk Q Pulmonary Artery, Right R Pulmonary Artery, Left S Pulmonary Vein, Right T Pulmonary Vein, Left U Pulmonary Vein, Confluence
K Ventricle, Right L Ventricle, Left	0 Open 4 Percutaneous Endoscopic	8 Zooplastic Tissue 9 Autologous Venous Tissue A Autologous Arterial Tissue J Synthetic Substitute K Nonautologous Tissue Substitute	P Pulmonary Trunk Q Pulmonary Artery, Right R Pulmonary Artery, Left
K Ventricle, Right L Ventricle, Left	0 Open 4 Percutaneous Endoscopic	Z No Device	5 Coronary Circulation 8 Internal Mammary, Right 9 Internal Mammary, Left C Thoracic Artery F Abdominal Artery P Pulmonary Trunk Q Pulmonary Artery, Right R Pulmonary Artery, Left W Aorta
P Pulmonary Trunk Q Pulmonary Artery, Right R Pulmonary Artery, Left	0 Open 4 Percutaneous Endoscopic	8 Zooplastic Tissue 9 Autologous Venous Tissue A Autologous Arterial Tissue J Synthetic Substitute K Nonautologous Tissue Substitute Z No Device	A Innominate Artery B Subclavian D Carotid
W Thoracic Aorta, Descending	0 Open	8 Zooplastic Tissue 9 Autologous Venous Tissue A Autologous Arterial Tissue J Synthetic Substitute K Nonautologous Tissue Substitute	A Innominate Artery B Subclavian D Carotid F Abdominal Artery G Axillary Artery H Brachial Artery P Pulmonary Trunk Q Pulmonary Artery, Right R Pulmonary Artery, Left V Lower Extremity Artery
W Thoracic Aorta, Descending	0 Open	Z No Device	A Innominate Artery B Subclavian D Carotid P Pulmonary Trunk Q Pulmonary Artery, Right R Pulmonary Artery, Left

021 continued on next page

0 Medical and Surgical
2 Heart and Great Vessels
1 Bypass: Altering the route of passage of the contents of a tubular body part

021 continued from previous page

Body Part	Approach	Device	Qualifier
Character 4	Character 5	Character 6	Character 7
W Thoracic Aorta, Descending	**4** Percutaneous Endoscopic	**8** Zooplastic Tissue **9** Autologous Venous Tissue **A** Autologous Arterial Tissue **J** Synthetic Substitute **K** Nonautologous Tissue Substitute **Z** No Device	**A** Innominate Artery **B** Subclavian **D** Carotid **P** Pulmonary Trunk **Q** Pulmonary Artery, Right **R** Pulmonary Artery, Left
X Thoracic Aorta, Ascending/Arch	**0** Open **4** Percutaneous Endoscopic	**8** Zooplastic Tissue **9** Autologous Venous Tissue **A** Autologous Arterial Tissue **J** Synthetic Substitute **K** Nonautologous Tissue Substitute **Z** No Device	**A** Innominate Artery **B** Subclavian **D** Carotid **P** Pulmonary Trunk **Q** Pulmonary Artery, Right **R** Pulmonary Artery, Left

HAC 0210083 0210088 0210089 021008C 021008F 021008W 0210093 0210098 0210099 021009C 021009F 021009W 02100A3
02100A8 02100A9 02100AC 02100AF 02100AW 02100J3 02100J8 02100J9 02100JC 02100JF 02100JW 02100K3 02100K8
02100K9 02100KC 02100KF 02100KW 02100Z3 02100Z8 02100Z9 02100ZC 02100ZF 0210483 0210488 0210489 021048C
021048F 021048W 0210493 0210498 0210499 021049C 021049F 021049W 02104A3 02104A8 02104A9 02104AC 02104AF
02104AW 02104J3 02104J8 02104J9 02104JC 02104JF 02104JW 02104K3 02104K8 02104K9 02104KC 02104KF 02104KW
02104Z3 02104Z8 02104Z9 02104ZC 02104ZF 0211083 0211088 0211089 021108C 021108F 021108W 0211093 0211098
0211099 021109C 021109F 021109W 02110A3 02110A8 02110A9 02110AC 02110AF 02110AW 02110J3 02110J8 02110J9
02110JC 02110JF 02110JW 02110K3 02110K8 02110K9 02110KC 02110KF 02110KW 02110Z3 02110Z8 02110Z9 02110ZC
02110ZF 0211483 0211488 0211489 021148C 021148F 021148W 0211493 0211498 0211499 021149C 021149F 021149W
02114A3 02114A8 02114A9 02114AC 02114AF 02114AW 02114J3 02114J8 02114J9 02114JC 02114JF 02114JW 02114K3
02114K8 02114K9 02114KC 02114KF 02114KW 02114Z3 02114Z8 02114Z9 02114ZC 02114ZF 0212083 0212088 0212089
021208C 021208F 021208W 0212093 0212098 0212099 021209C 021209F 021209W 02120A3 02120A8 02120A9 02120AC
02120AF 02120AW 02120J3 02120J8 02120J9 02120JC 02120JF 02120JW 02120K3 02120K8 02120K9 02120KC 02120KF
02120KW 02120Z3 02120Z8 02120Z9 02120ZC 02120ZF 0212483 0212488 0212489 021248C 021248F 021248W 0212493
0212498 0212499 021249C 021249F 021249W 02124A3 02124A8 02124A9 02124AC 02124AF 02124AW 02124J3 02124J8
02124J9 02124JC 02124JF 02124JW 02124K3 02124K8 02124K9 02124KC 02124KF 02124KW 02124Z3 02124Z8 02124Z9
02124ZC 02124ZF 0213083 0213088 0213089 021308C 021308F 021308W 0213093 0213098 0213099 021309C 021309F
021309W 02130A3 02130A8 02130A9 02130AC 02130AF 02130AW 02130J3 02130J8 02130J9 02130JC 02130JF 02130JW
02130K3 02130K8 02130K9 02130KC 02130KF 02130KW 02130Z3 02130Z8 02130Z9 02130ZC 02130ZF 0213483 0213488
0213489 021348C 021348F 021348W 0213493 0213498 0213499 021349C 021349F 021349W 02134A3 02134A8 02134A9
02134AC 02134AF 02134AW 02134J3 02134J8 02134J9 02134JC 02134JF 02134JW 02134K3 02134K8 02134K9 02134KC
02134KF 02134KW 02134Z3 02134Z8 02134Z9 02134ZC 02134ZF
Surgical site Infection, mediastinitis, following coronary artery bypass graft (CABG) and secondary diagnosis J98.51, J98.59.

0 Medical and Surgical
2 Heart and Great Vessels
4 Creation: Putting in or on biological or synthetic material to form a new body part that to the extent possible replicates the anatomic structure or function of an absent body part

Body Part	Approach	Device	Qualifier
Character 4	Character 5	Character 6	Character 7
F Aortic Valve	**0** Open	**7** Autologous Tissue Substitute **8** Zooplastic Tissue **J** Synthetic Substitute **K** Nonautologous Tissue Substitute	**J** Truncal Valve
G Mitral Valve **J** Tricuspid Valve	**0** Open	**7** Autologous Tissue Substitute **8** Zooplastic Tissue **J** Synthetic Substitute **K** Nonautologous Tissue Substitute	**2** Common Atrioventricular Valve

0 Medical and Surgical
2 Heart and Great Vessels
5 Destruction: Physical eradication of all or a portion of a body part by the direct use of energy, force, or a destructive agent

Body Part Character 4	Approach Character 5	Device Character 6	Qualifier Character 7
4 Coronary Vein 5 Atrial Septum 6 Atrium, Right 8 Conduction Mechanism 9 Chordae Tendineae D Papillary Muscle F Aortic Valve G Mitral Valve H Pulmonary Valve J Tricuspid Valve K Ventricle, Right L Ventricle, Left M Ventricular Septum N Pericardium P Pulmonary Trunk Q Pulmonary Artery, Right R Pulmonary Artery, Left S Pulmonary Vein, Right T Pulmonary Vein, Left V Superior Vena Cava W Thoracic Aorta, Descending X Thoracic Aorta, Ascending/Arch	0 Open 3 Percutaneous 4 Percutaneous Endoscopic arrhythmogenic focus of A-V node includes heart cath	Z No Device	Z No Qualifier
7 Atrium, Left DRG	0 Open 3 Percutaneous 4 Percutaneous Endoscopic	Z No Device	K Left Atrial Appendage Z No Qualifier

DRG 02570ZK 02573ZK 02574ZK

lazer destruction of arrhythmogenic focus on AV node
left heart cath done percutaneous unless otherwise stated
ablution of AV node 02583ZZ
radio frequency destroys tissue that is causing rapid or irregular heartbeat

0 Medical and Surgical
2 Heart and Great Vessels
7 Dilation: Expanding an orifice or the lumen of a tubular body part

drug eluting stents & angioplasty

Body Part	Approach	Device	Qualifier
Character 4	**Character 5**	**Character 6**	**Character 7**
0 Coronary Artery, One Artery LAD **1** Coronary Artery, Two Arteries **2** Coronary Artery, Three Arteries **3** Coronary Artery, Four or More Arteries	**0** Open **3** Percutaneous **4** Percutaneous Endoscopic	**4** Intraluminal Device, Drug-eluting **5** Intraluminal Device, Drug-eluting, Two **6** Intraluminal Device, Drug-eluting, Three **7** Intraluminal Device, Drug-eluting, Four or More **D** Intraluminal Device no drug **E** Intraluminal Device, Two **F** Intraluminal Device, Three **G** Intraluminal Device, Four or More **T** Intraluminal Device, Radioactive **Z** No Device - angioplasty	**6** Bifurcation **Z** No Qualifier
F Aortic Valve **G** Mitral Valve **H** Pulmonary Valve **J** Tricuspid Valve **K** Ventricle, Right **L** Ventricle, Left **P** Pulmonary Trunk **Q** Pulmonary Artery, Right **S** Pulmonary Vein, Right **T** Pulmonary Vein, Left **V** Superior Vena Cava **W** Thoracic Aorta, Descending **X** Thoracic Aorta, Ascending/Arch	**0** Open **3** Percutaneous **4** Percutaneous Endoscopic	**4** Intraluminal Device, Drug-eluting **D** Intraluminal Device **Z** No Device - angioplasty	**Z** No Qualifier
R Pulmonary Artery, Left	**0** Open **3** Percutaneous **4** Percutaneous Endoscopic	**4** Intraluminal Device, Drug-eluting **D** Intraluminal Device **Z** No Device	**T** Ductus Arteriosus **Z** No Qualifier

insert drug eluting stent into LAD artery percutaneous 027034Z
assign 1 code for total # of arteries w/a drug eluting stent & 1 code for total # of arteries using a bare metal stent

0 Medical and Surgical
2 Heart and Great Vessels
8 Division: Cutting into a body part, without draining fluids and/or gases from the body part, in order to separate or transect a body part

Body Part	Approach	Device	Qualifier
Character 4	Character 5	Character 6	Character 7
8 Conduction Mechanism **9** Chordae Tendineae **D** Papillary Muscle	**0** Open **3** Percutaneous **4** Percutaneous Endoscopic	**Z** No Device	**Z** No Qualifier

0 Medical and Surgical
2 Heart and Great Vessels
B Excision: Cutting out or off, without replacement, a portion of a body part

Body Part	Approach	Device	Qualifier
Character 4	Character 5	Character 6	Character 7
4 Coronary Vein **5** Atrial Septum **6** Atrium, Right **8** Conduction Mechanism **9** Chordae Tendineae **D** Papillary Muscle **F** Aortic Valve **G** Mitral Valve **H** Pulmonary Valve **J** Tricuspid Valve **K** Ventricle, Right NC **L** Ventricle, Left NC **M** Ventricular Septum **N** Pericardium **P** Pulmonary Trunk **Q** Pulmonary Artery, Right **R** Pulmonary Artery, Left **S** Pulmonary Vein, Right **T** Pulmonary Vein, Left **V** Superior Vena Cava **W** Thoracic Aorta, Descending **X** Thoracic Aorta, Ascending/Arch	**0** Open **3** Percutaneous **4** Percutaneous Endoscopic	**Z** No Device	**X** Diagnostic **Z** No Qualifier
7 Atrium, Left DRG	**0** Open **3** Percutaneous **4** Percutaneous Endoscopic	**Z** No Device	**K** Left Atrial Appendage **X** Diagnostic **Z** No Qualifier

NC 02BK0ZZ 02BK3ZZ 02BK4ZZ 02BL0ZZ 02BL3ZZ 02BL4ZZ
DRG 02B70ZK 02B73ZK 02B74ZK

0 Medical and Surgical
2 Heart and Great Vessels
C Extirpation: Taking or cutting out solid matter from a body part

Body Part Character 4	Approach Character 5	Device Character 6	Qualifier Character 7
0 Coronary Artery, One Artery **1** Coronary Artery, Two Arteries **2** Coronary Artery, Three Arteries **3** Coronary Artery, Four or More Arteries	**0** Open **3** Percutaneous **4** Percutaneous Endoscopic	**Z** No Device	**6** Bifurcation **Z** No Qualifier
4 Coronary Vein **5** Atrial Septum **6** Atrium, Right **7** Atrium, Left **8** Conduction Mechanism **9** Chordae Tendineae **D** Papillary Muscle **F** Aortic Valve **G** Mitral Valve **H** Pulmonary Valve **J** Tricuspid Valve **K** Ventricle, Right **L** Ventricle, Left **M** Ventricular Septum **N** Pericardium **P** Pulmonary Trunk **Q** Pulmonary Artery, Right **R** Pulmonary Artery, Left **S** Pulmonary Vein, Right **T** Pulmonary Vein, Left **V** Superior Vena Cava **W** Thoracic Aorta, Descending **X** Thoracic Aorta, Ascending/Arch	**0** Open **3** Percutaneous **4** Percutaneous Endoscopic	**Z** No Device	**Z** No Qualifier

0 Medical and Surgical
2 Heart and Great Vessels
F Fragmentation: Breaking solid matter in a body part into pieces

Body Part Character 4	Approach Character 5	Device Character 6	Qualifier Character 7
N Pericardium NC	**0** Open **3** Percutaneous **4** Percutaneous Endoscopic **X** External	**Z** No Device	**Z** No Qualifier

NC 02FNXZZ

LC Limited Coverage NC Noncovered HAC HAC-associated Procedure CC Combination Cluster - See Appendix G for code lists
DRG Non-OR-Affecting MS-DRG Assignment New/Revised Text in **Orange** ♂ Male ♀ Female

Swan Ganz - measures heart failure or sepsis, monitor therapy + evaluate effects of drugs. Simultaneously measures processes in: RA, RV, pulmonary artery + filling pressure of LA. To report actual measurement + monitoring, use monitoring

0 Medical and Surgical
2 Heart and Great Vessels
H Insertion: Putting in a nonbiological appliance that monitors, assists, performs, or prevents a physiological function but does not physically take the place of a body part   Swan Ganz, insert leads + pulse generator

Body Part Character 4 (Final destination)	Approach Character 5	Device Character 6	Qualifier Character 7
0 Coronary Artery, One Artery **1** Coronary Artery, Two Arteries **2** Coronary Artery, Three Arteries **3** Coronary Artery, Four or More Arteries	**0** Open **3** Percutaneous - groin or neck **4** Percutaneous Endoscopic	**D** Intraluminal Device **Y** Other Device	**Z** No Qualifier
4 Coronary Vein DRG HAC CC **6** Atrium, Right DRG HAC CC **7** Atrium, Left DRG HAC CC **K** Ventricle, Right DRG HAC CC **L** Ventricle, Left DRG HAC CC	**0** Open **3** Percutaneous **4** Percutaneous Endoscopic heart cath are percutaneous unless otherwise noted	**0** Monitoring Device, Pressure Sensor **2** Monitoring Device cardiac pressure (wedge) in RA **3** Infusion Device **D** Intraluminal Device **J** Cardiac Lead, Pacemaker **K** Cardiac Lead, Defibrillator **M** Cardiac Lead **N** Intracardiac Pacemaker **Y** Other Device	**Z** No Qualifier
A Heart LC NC	**0** Open **3** Percutaneous **4** Percutaneous Endoscopic	**Q** Implantable Heart Assist System **Y** Other Device	**Z** No Qualifier
A Heart CC	**0** Open **3** Percutaneous **4** Percutaneous Endoscopic	**R** Short term External Heart Assist System	**J** Intraoperative **S** Biventricular **Z** No Qualifier
N Pericardium DRG HAC CC	**0** Open **3** Percutaneous **4** Percutaneous Endoscopic	**0** Monitoring Device, Pressure Sensor **2** Monitoring Device **J** Cardiac Lead, Pacemaker **K** Cardiac Lead, Defibrillator **M** Cardiac Lead **Y** Other Device	**Z** No Qualifier
P Pulmonary Trunk **Q** Pulmonary Artery, Right **R** Pulmonary Artery, Left **S** Pulmonary Vein, Right HAC **T** Pulmonary Vein, Left HAC **V** Superior Vena Cava HAC **W** Thoracic Aorta, Descending	**0** Open **3** Percutaneous Swan Ganz **4** Percutaneous Endoscopic	**0** Monitoring Device, Pressure Sensor **2** Monitoring Device Swan Ganz catheter maybe pressure assessment **3** Infusion Device PICC **D** Intraluminal Device **Y** Other Device	**Z** No Qualifier Fluoroscopic Guidance PICC vena cava B5182ZA
X Thoracic Aorta, Ascending/Arch	**0** Open **3** Percutaneous **4** Percutaneous Endoscopic	**0** Monitoring Device, Pressure Sensor **2** Monitoring Device **3** Infusion Device **D** Intraluminal Device	**Z** No Qualifier

LC 02HA0QZ

NC 02HA3QZ 02HA4QZ

DRG 02H40JZ 02H40MZ 02H43JZ 02H43MZ 02H44JZ 02H44MZ 02H60JZ 02H60MZ 02H63JZ 02H63MZ 02H64JZ 02H64MZ 02H70JZ 02H70MZ 02H73JZ 02H73MZ 02H74JZ 02H74MZ 02HK0JZ 02HK0MZ 02HK32Z 02HK3JZ 02HK3MZ 02HK4JZ 02HK4MZ 02HL0JZ 02HL0MZ 02HL3JZ 02HL3MZ 02HL4JZ 02HL4MZ 02HN0JZ 02HN0MZ 02HN3JZ 02HN3MZ 02HN4JZ 02HN4MZ

HAC 02H43JZ 02H43KZ 02H43MZ 02H63JZ 02H63MZ 02H73JZ 02H73MZ 02HK3JZ 02HL3JZ 02HN0JZ 02HN0MZ 02HN3JZ 02HN3MZ 02HN4JZ 02HN4MZ
Surgical site infection (SSI) following cardiac implantable electronic device (CIED) procedures and secondary diagnosis K68.11, T81.40XA, T81.41XA, T81.42XA, T81.43XA, T81.44XA, T81.49XA, T82.6XXA, T82.7XXA.

HAC 02H633Z 02HK33Z 02HS33Z 02HS43Z 02HT33Z 02HT43Z 02HV33Z 02HV43Z
Iatrogenic pneumothorax w/ venous catheterization procedures and secondary diagnosis J95.811.

CC 02H40JZ 02H40KZ 02H40MZ 02H43JZ 02H43KZ 02H43MZ 02H44JZ 02H44KZ 02H44MZ 02H60JZ 02H60KZ 02H60MZ 02H63JZ 02H63KZ 02H63MZ 02H64JZ 02H64KZ 02H64MZ 02H70JZ 02H70KZ 02H70MZ 02H73JZ 02H73KZ 02H73MZ 02H74JZ 02H74KZ 02H74MZ 02HA0RS 02HA0RZ 02HA3RS 02HA4RS 02HA4RZ 02HK0JZ 02HK0KZ 02HK0MZ 02HK3JZ 02HK3KZ 02HK3MZ 02HK4JZ 02HK4KZ 02HK4MZ 02HL0JZ 02HL0KZ 02HL0MZ 02HL3JZ 02HL3KZ 02HL3MZ 02HL4JZ 02HL4KZ 02HL4MZ 02HN0JZ 02HN0KZ 02HN0MZ 02HN3JZ 02HN3KZ 02HN3MZ 02HN4JZ 02HN4KZ 02HN4MZ

Ex: insert 2 leads 1 in RA + 1 right Ventricular + then creates pocket for pacemaker pulse generator - 3 codes
02H63JZ, 02HK3JZ, 0JH606Z

LC Limited Coverage NC Noncovered HAC HAC-associated Procedure CC Combination Cluster - See Appendix G for code lists
DRG Non-OR-Affecting MS-DRG Assignment New/Revised Text in **Orange** ♂ Male ♀ Female

0 Medical and Surgical
2 Heart and Great Vessels
J Inspection: Visually and/or manually exploring a body part

Body Part Character 4	Approach Character 5	Device Character 6	Qualifier Character 7
A Heart **Y** Great Vessel	**0** Open **3** Percutaneous **4** Percutaneous Endoscopic	**Z** No Device	**Z** No Qualifier

0 Medical and Surgical
2 Heart and Great Vessels
K Map: Locating the route of passage of electrical impulses and/or locating functional areas in a body part

Body Part Character 4	Approach Character 5	Device Character 6	Qualifier Character 7
8 Conduction Mechanism DRG	**0** Open **3** Percutaneous **4** Percutaneous Endoscopic	**Z** No Device	**Z** No Qualifier

DRG 02K80ZZ 02K83ZZ 02K84ZZ

0 Medical and Surgical
2 Heart and Great Vessels
L Occlusion: Completely closing an orifice or the lumen of a tubular body part

Body Part Character 4	Approach Character 5	Device Character 6	Qualifier Character 7
7 Atrium, Left DRG	**0** Open **3** Percutaneous **4** Percutaneous Endoscopic	**C** Extraluminal Device **D** Intraluminal Device **Z** No Device	**K** Left Atrial Appendage
H Pulmonary Valve **P** Pulmonary Trunk **Q** Pulmonary Artery, Right **S** Pulmonary Vein, Right **T** Pulmonary Vein, Left **V** Superior Vena Cava	**0** Open **3** Percutaneous **4** Percutaneous Endoscopic	**C** Extraluminal Device **D** Intraluminal Device **Z** No Device	**Z** No Qualifier
R Pulmonary Artery, Left	**0** Open **3** Percutaneous **4** Percutaneous Endoscopic	**C** Extraluminal Device **D** Intraluminal Device **Z** No Device	**T** Ductus Arteriosus **Z** No Qualifier
W Thoracic Aorta, Descending	**3** Percutaneous	**D** Intraluminal Device	**J** Temporary

DRG 02L70CK 02L70DK 02L70ZK 02L73CK 02L73DK 02L73ZK 02L74CK 02L74DK 02L74ZK

0 **Medical and Surgical**
2 **Heart and Great Vessels**
N **Release:** Freeing a body part from an abnormal physical constraint by cutting or by the use of force

Body Part Character 4	Approach Character 5	Device Character 6	Qualifier Character 7
0 Coronary Artery, One Artery 1 Coronary Artery, Two Arteries 2 Coronary Artery, Three Arteries 3 Coronary Artery, Four or More Arteries 4 Coronary Vein 5 Atrial Septum 6 Atrium, Right 7 Atrium, Left 8 Conduction Mechanism 9 Chordae Tendineae D Papillary Muscle F Aortic Valve G Mitral Valve H Pulmonary Valve J Tricuspid Valve K Ventricle, Right L Ventricle, Left M Ventricular Septum N Pericardium P Pulmonary Trunk Q Pulmonary Artery, Right R Pulmonary Artery, Left S Pulmonary Vein, Right T Pulmonary Vein, Left V Superior Vena Cava W Thoracic Aorta, Descending X Thoracic Aorta, Ascending/Arch	0 Open 3 Percutaneous 4 Percutaneous Endoscopic	Z No Device	Z No Qualifier

0 Medical and Surgical
2 Heart and Great Vessels
P Removal: Taking out or off a device from a body part

Body Part Character 4	Approach Character 5	Device Character 6	Qualifier Character 7
A Heart HAC	**0** Open **3** Percutaneous **4** Percutaneous Endoscopic	**2** Monitoring Device **3** Infusion Device **7** Autologous Tissue Substitute **8** Zooplastic Tissue **C** Extraluminal Device **D** Intraluminal Device **J** Synthetic Substitute **K** Nonautologous Tissue Substitute **M** Cardiac Lead **N** Intracardiac Pacemaker **Q** Implantable Heart Assist System **Y** Other Device	**Z** No Qualifier
A Heart CC	**0** Open **3** Percutaneous **4** Percutaneous Endoscopic	**R** Short-term External Heart Assist System	**S** Biventricular **Z** No Qualifier
A Heart	**X** External	**2** Monitoring Device **3** Infusion Device **D** Intraluminal Device **M** Cardiac Lead	**Z** No Qualifier
Y Great Vessel	**0** Open **3** Percutaneous **4** Percutaneous Endoscopic	**2** Monitoring Device **3** Infusion Device **7** Autologous Tissue Substitute **8** Zooplastic Tissue **C** Extraluminal Device **D** Intraluminal Device **J** Synthetic Substitute **K** Nonautologous Tissue Substitute **Y** Other Device	**Z** No Qualifier
Y Great Vessel	**X** External	**2** Monitoring Device **3** Infusion Device **D** Intraluminal Device	**Z** No Qualifier

HAC 02PA0MZ 02PA3MZ 02PA4MZ 02PAXMZ
Surgical site Infection (SSI) following cardiac implantable electronic device (CIED) procedures and secondary diagnosis K68.11, T81.40XA, T81.41XA, T81.42XA, T81.43XA, T81.44XA, T81.49XA, T82.6XXA, T82.7XXA.

CC 02PA0RZ 02PA3RZ 02PA4RZ

LC Limited Coverage NC Noncovered HAC HAC-associated Procedure CC Combination Cluster - See Appendix G for code lists
DRG Non-OR-Affecting MS-DRG Assignment New/Revised Text in **Orange** ♂ Male ♀ Female

0 Medical and Surgical
2 Heart and Great Vessels
Q Repair: Restoring, to the extent possible, a body part to its normal anatomic structure and function

Body Part Character 4	Approach Character 5	Device Character 6	Qualifier Character 7
0 Coronary Artery, One Artery **1** Coronary Artery, Two Arteries **2** Coronary Artery, Three Arteries **3** Coronary Artery, Four or More Arteries **4** Coronary Vein **5** Atrial Septum **6** Atrium, Right **7** Atrium, Left **8** Conduction Mechanism **9** Chordae Tendineae **A** Heart **B** Heart, Right **C** Heart, Left **D** Papillary Muscle **H** Pulmonary Valve **K** Ventricle, Right **L** Ventricle, Left **M** Ventricular Septum **N** Pericardium **P** Pulmonary Trunk **Q** Pulmonary Artery, Right **R** Pulmonary Artery, Left **S** Pulmonary Vein, Right **T** Pulmonary Vein, Left **V** Superior Vena Cava **W** Thoracic Aorta, Descending **X** Thoracic Aorta, Ascending/Arch	**0** Open **3** Percutaneous **4** Percutaneous Endoscopic	**Z** No Device	**Z** No Qualifier
F Aortic Valve	**0** Open **3** Percutaneous **4** Percutaneous Endoscopic	**Z** No Device	**J** Truncal Valve **Z** No Qualifier
G Mitral Valve	**0** Open **3** Percutaneous **4** Percutaneous Endoscopic	**Z** No Device	**E** Atrioventricular Valve, Left **Z** No Qualifier
J Tricuspid Valve	**0** Open **3** Percutaneous **4** Percutaneous Endoscopic	**Z** No Device	**G** Atrioventricular Valve, Right **Z** No Qualifier

used w/ mitral valve prolapse MVP

0 Medical and Surgical
2 Heart and Great Vessels - do not code removal, integral to procedure
R Replacement: Putting in or on biological or synthetic material that physically takes the place and/or function of all or a portion of a body part

Body Part Character 4	Approach Character 5	Device Character 6	Qualifier Character 7
5 Atrial Septum **6** Atrium, Right **7** Atrium, Left **9** Chordae Tendineae **D** Papillary Muscle **K** Ventricle, Right [LC] [CC] **L** Ventricle, Left [LC] [CC] **M** Ventricular Septum **N** Pericardium **P** Pulmonary Trunk **Q** Pulmonary Artery, Right **R** Pulmonary Artery, Left **S** Pulmonary Vein, Right **T** Pulmonary Vein, Left **V** Superior Vena Cava **W** Thoracic Aorta, Descending **X** Thoracic Aorta, Ascending/Arch	**0** Open **4** Percutaneous Endoscopic	**7** Autologous Tissue Substitute **8** Zooplastic Tissue - porpine **J** Synthetic Substitute **K** Nonautologous Tissue Substitute	**Z** No Qualifier
F Aortic Valve **G** Mitral Valve **H** Pulmonary Valve **J** Tricuspid Valve	**0** Open **4** Percutaneous Endoscopic	**7** Autologous Tissue Substitute **8** Zooplastic Tissue **J** Synthetic Substitute artifical prostetic **K** Nonautologous Tissue Substitute	**Z** No Qualifier
F Aortic Valve **G** Mitral Valve **H** Pulmonary Valve **J** Tricuspid Valve	**3** Percutaneous	**7** Autologous Tissue Substitute **8** Zooplastic Tissue **J** Synthetic Substitute **K** Nonautologous Tissue Substitute	**H** Transapical **Z** No Qualifier

[LC] 02RK0JZ with 02RL0JZ
The procedures shown above are identified as limited coverage procedures when combined with diagnosis code Z00.6.
[NC] 02RK0JZ or 02RL0JZ with 02RL0JZ
Noncovered except when combined with diagnosis code Z00.6.
[CC] 02RK0JZ 02RL0JZ

0 Medical and Surgical
2 Heart and Great Vessels
S Reposition: Moving to its normal location, or other suitable location, all or a portion of a body part

Body Part Character 4	Approach Character 5	Device Character 6	Qualifier Character 7
0 Coronary Artery, One Artery **1** Coronary Artery, Two Arteries **P** Pulmonary Trunk **Q** Pulmonary Artery, Right **R** Pulmonary Artery, Left **S** Pulmonary Vein, Right **T** Pulmonary Vein, Left **V** Superior Vena Cava **W** Thoracic Aorta, Descending **X** Thoracic Aorta, Ascending/Arch	**0** Open	**Z** No Device	**Z** No Qualifier

[LC] Limited Coverage [NC] Noncovered [HAC] HAC-associated Procedure [CC] Combination Cluster - See Appendix G for code lists
[DRG] Non-OR-Affecting MS-DRG Assignment New/Revised Text in **Orange** ♂ Male ♀ Female

0 Medical and Surgical
2 Heart and Great Vessels
T Resection: Cutting out or off, without replacement, all of a body part

Body Part Character 4	Approach Character 5	Device Character 6	Qualifier Character 7
5 Atrial Septum **8** Conduction Mechanism **9** Chordae Tendineae **D** Papillary Muscle **H** Pulmonary Valve **M** Ventricular Septum **N** Pericardium	**0** Open **3** Percutaneous **4** Percutaneous Endoscopic	**Z** No Device	**Z** No Qualifier

0 Medical and Surgical
2 Heart and Great Vessels
U Supplement: Putting in or on biological or synthetic material that physically reinforces and/or augments the function of a portion of a body part

Body Part Character 4	Approach Character 5	Device Character 6	Qualifier Character 7
0 Coronary Artery, One Artery **1** Coronary Artery, Two Arteries **2** Coronary Artery, Three Arteries **3** Coronary Artery, Four or More Arteries **5** Atrial Septum **6** Atrium, Right **7** Atrium, Left DRG **9** Chordae Tendineae **A** Heart **D** Papillary Muscle **H** Pulmonary Valve **K** Ventricle, Right **L** Ventricle, Left **M** Ventricular Septum **N** Pericardium **P** Pulmonary Trunk **Q** Pulmonary Artery, Right **R** Pulmonary Artery, Left **S** Pulmonary Vein, Right **T** Pulmonary Vein, Left **V** Superior Vena Cava **W** Thoracic Aorta, Descending **X** Thoracic Aorta, Ascending/Arch	**0** Open **3** Percutaneous **4** Percutaneous Endoscopic	**7** Autologous Tissue Substitute **8** Zooplastic Tissue **J** Synthetic Substitute **K** Nonautologous Tissue Substitute	**Z** No Qualifier
F Aortic Valve	**0** Open **3** Percutaneous **4** Percutaneous Endoscopic	**7** Autologous Tissue Substitute **8** Zooplastic Tissue **J** Synthetic Substitute **K** Nonautologous Tissue Substitute	**J** Truncal Valve **Z** No Qualifier
G Mitral Valve	**0** Open **3** Percutaneous **4** Percutaneous Endoscopic	**7** Autologous Tissue Substitute **8** Zooplastic Tissue **J** Synthetic Substitute **K** Nonautologous Tissue Substitute	**E** Atrioventricular Valve, Left **Z** No Qualifier
J Tricuspid Valve	**0** Open **3** Percutaneous **4** Percutaneous Endoscopic	**7** Autologous Tissue Substitute **8** Zooplastic Tissue **J** Synthetic Substitute **K** Nonautologous Tissue Substitute	**G** Atrioventricular Valve, Right **Z** No Qualifier

DRG 02U73JZ 02U74JZ

0 Medical and Surgical
2 Heart and Great Vessels
V Restriction: Partially closing an orifice or the lumen of a tubular body part

Body Part Character 4	Approach Character 5	Device Character 6	Qualifier Character 7
A Heart	**0** Open **3** Percutaneous **4** Percutaneous Endoscopic	**C** Extraluminal Device **Z** No Device	**Z** No Qualifier
G Mitral Valve	**0** Open **3** Percutaneous **4** Percutaneous Endoscopic	**Z** No Device	**Z** No Qualifier
P Pulmonary Trunk **Q** Pulmonary Artery, Right **S** Pulmonary Vein, Right **T** Pulmonary Vein, Left **V** Superior Vena Cava	**0** Open **3** Percutaneous **4** Percutaneous Endoscopic	**C** Extraluminal Device **D** Intraluminal Device **Z** No Device	**Z** No Qualifier
R Pulmonary Artery, Left	**0** Open **3** Percutaneous **4** Percutaneous Endoscopic	**C** Extraluminal Device **D** Intraluminal Device **Z** No Device	**T** Ductus Arteriosus **Z** No Qualifier
W Thoracic Aorta, Descending **X** Thoracic Aorta, Ascending/Arch	**0** Open **3** Percutaneous **4** Percutaneous Endoscopic	**C** Extraluminal Device **D** Intraluminal Device **E** Intraluminal Device, Branched or Fenestrated, One or Two Arteries **F** Intraluminal Device, Branched or Fenestrated, Three or More Arteries **Z** No Device	**Z** No Qualifier

For Devices, not body parts, use reposition for body parts
ex: adjust pacemaker lead in LV = 02WA3MZ

0 Medical and Surgical
2 Heart and Great Vessels
W Revision: Correcting, to the extent possible, a portion of a malfunctioning device or the position of a displaced device

Body Part Character 4	Approach Character 5	Device Character 6	Qualifier Character 7
5 Atrial Septum **M** Ventricular Septum	**0** Open **4** Percutaneous Endoscopic	**J** Synthetic Substitute	**Z** No Qualifier
A Heart LC NC HAC CC	**0** Open **3** Percutaneous **4** Percutaneous Endoscopic	**2** Monitoring Device **3** Infusion Device **7** Autologous Tissue Substitute **8** Zooplastic Tissue **C** Extraluminal Device **D** Intraluminal Device **J** Synthetic Substitute **K** Nonautologous Tissue Substitute **M** Cardiac Lead • pacemaker lead **N** Intracardiac Pacemaker **Q** Implantable Heart Assist System **Y** Other Device	**Z** No Qualifier
A Heart CC	**0** Open **3** Percutaneous **4** Percutaneous Endoscopic	**R** Short-term External Heart Assist System	**S** Biventricular **Z** No Qualifier
A Heart LC	**X** External	**2** Monitoring Device **3** Infusion Device **7** Autologous Tissue Substitute **8** Zooplastic Tissue **C** Extraluminal Device **D** Intraluminal Device **J** Synthetic Substitute **K** Nonautologous Tissue Substitute **M** Cardiac Lead **N** Intracardiac Pacemaker **Q** Implantable Heart Assist System	**Z** No Qualifier
A Heart	**X** External	**R** Short-term External Heart Assist System	**S** Biventricular **Z** No Qualifier

02W continued on next page

LC Limited Coverage   NC Noncovered   HAC HAC-associated Procedure   CC Combination Cluster - See Appendix G for code lists
DRG Non-OR-Affecting MS-DRG Assignment   New/Revised Text in **Orange**   ♂ Male   ♀ Female

02W continued from previous page

0 Medical and Surgical
2 Heart and Great Vessels
W Revision: Correcting, to the extent possible, a portion of a malfunctioning device or the position of a displaced device

Body Part Character 4	Approach Character 5	Device Character 6	Qualifier Character 7
F Aortic Valve **G** Mitral Valve **H** Pulmonary Valve **J** Tricuspid Valve	**0** Open **3** Percutaneous **4** Percutaneous Endoscopic	**7** Autologous Tissue Substitute **8** Zooplastic Tissue **J** Synthetic Substitute **K** Nonautologous Tissue Substitute	**Z** No Qualifier
Y Great Vessel	**0** Open **3** Percutaneous **4** Percutaneous Endoscopic	**2** Monitoring Device **3** Infusion Device **7** Autologous Tissue Substitute **8** Zooplastic Tissue **C** Extraluminal Device **D** Intraluminal Device **J** Synthetic Substitute **K** Nonautologous Tissue Substitute **Y** Other Device	**Z** No Qualifier
Y Great Vessel	**X** External	**2** Monitoring Device **3** Infusion Device **7** Autologous Tissue Substitute **8** Zooplastic Tissue **C** Extraluminal Device **D** Intraluminal Device **J** Synthetic Substitute **K** Nonautologous Tissue Substitute	**Z** No Qualifier

LC 02WA0JZ 02WA0QZ
NC 02WA3QZ 02WA4QZ
HAC 02WA0MZ 02WA3MZ 02WA4MZ
Surgical site infection (SSI) following cardiac implantable electronic device (CIED) procedures and secondary diagnosis K68.11, T81.40XA, T81.41XA, T81.42XA, T81.43XA, T81.44XA, T81.49XA, T82.6XXA, T82.7XXA.
CC 02WA0QZ 02WA0RZ 02WA3QZ 02WA3RZ 02WA4QZ 02WA4RZ

0 Medical and Surgical
2 Heart and Great Vessels
Y Transplantation: Putting in or on all or a portion of a living body part taken from another individual or animal to physically take the place and/or function of all or a portion of a similar body part

Body Part Character 4	Approach Character 5	Device Character 6	Qualifier Character 7
A Heart LC	**0** Open	**Z** No Device	**0** Allogeneic **1** Syngeneic **2** Zooplastic

LC 02YA0Z0 02YA0Z1 02YA0Z2

NOTES

NOTES

Upper Arteries 031-03W

0 Medical and Surgical
3 Upper Arteries
1 Bypass: Altering the route of passage of the contents of a tubular body part

Body Part Character 4	Approach Character 5	Device Character 6	Qualifier Character 7
2 Innominate Artery	**0** Open	**9** Autologous Venous Tissue **A** Autologous Arterial Tissue **J** Synthetic Substitute **K** Nonautologous Tissue Substitute **Z** No Device	**0** Upper Arm Artery, Right **1** Upper Arm Artery, Left **2** Upper Arm Artery, Bilateral **3** Lower Arm Artery, Right **4** Lower Arm Artery, Left **5** Lower Arm Artery, Bilateral **6** Upper Leg Artery, Right **7** Upper Leg Artery, Left **8** Upper Leg Artery, Bilateral **9** Lower Leg Artery, Right **B** Lower Leg Artery, Left **C** Lower Leg Artery, Bilateral **D** Upper Arm Vein **F** Lower Arm Vein **J** Extracranial Artery, Right **K** Extracranial Artery, Left **W** Lower Extremity Vein
3 Subclavian Artery, Right **4** Subclavian Artery, Left	**0** Open	**9** Autologous Venous Tissue **A** Autologous Arterial Tissue **J** Synthetic Substitute **K** Nonautologous Tissue Substitute **Z** No Device	**0** Upper Arm Artery, Right **1** Upper Arm Artery, Left **2** Upper Arm Artery, Bilateral **3** Lower Arm Artery, Right **4** Lower Arm Artery, Left **5** Lower Arm Artery, Bilateral **6** Upper Leg Artery, Right **7** Upper Leg Artery, Left **8** Upper Leg Artery, Bilateral **9** Lower Leg Artery, Right **B** Lower Leg Artery, Left **C** Lower Leg Artery, Bilateral **D** Upper Arm Vein **F** Lower Arm Vein **J** Extracranial Artery, Right **K** Extracranial Artery, Left **M** Pulmonary Artery, Right **N** Pulmonary Artery, Left **W** Lower Extremity Vein
5 Axillary Artery, Right **6** Axillary Artery, Left	**0** Open	**9** Autologous Venous Tissue **A** Autologous Arterial Tissue **J** Synthetic Substitute **K** Nonautologous Tissue Substitute **Z** No Device	**0** Upper Arm Artery, Right **1** Upper Arm Artery, Left **2** Upper Arm Artery, Bilateral **3** Lower Arm Artery, Right **4** Lower Arm Artery, Left **5** Lower Arm Artery, Bilateral **6** Upper Leg Artery, Right **7** Upper Leg Artery, Left **8** Upper Leg Artery, Bilateral **9** Lower Leg Artery, Right **B** Lower Leg Artery, Left **C** Lower Leg Artery, Bilateral **D** Upper Arm Vein **F** Lower Arm Vein **J** Extracranial Artery, Right **K** Extracranial Artery, Left **T** Abdominal Artery **V** Superior Vena Cava **W** Lower Extremity Vein

031 continued on next page

0 Medical and Surgical
3 Upper Arteries
1 Bypass: Altering the route of passage of the contents of a tubular body part

031 continued from previous page

Body Part Character 4	Approach Character 5	Device Character 6	Qualifier Character 7
7 Brachial Artery, Right	0 Open	9 Autologous Venous Tissue A Autologous Arterial Tissue J Synthetic Substitute K Nonautologous Tissue Substitute Z No Device	0 Upper Arm Artery, Right 3 Lower Arm Artery, Right D Upper Arm Vein F Lower Arm Vein V Superior Vena Cava W Lower Extremity Vein
8 Brachial Artery, Left	0 Open	9 Autologous Venous Tissue A Autologous Arterial Tissue J Synthetic Substitute K Nonautologous Tissue Substitute Z No Device	1 Upper Arm Artery, Left 4 Lower Arm Artery, Left D Upper Arm Vein F Lower Arm Vein V Superior Vena Cava W Lower Extremity Vein
9 Ulnar Artery, Right B Radial Artery, Right	0 Open	9 Autologous Venous Tissue A Autologous Arterial Tissue J Synthetic Substitute K Nonautologous Tissue Substitute Z No Device	3 Lower Arm Artery, Right F Lower Arm Vein
9 Ulnar Artery, Right B Radial Artery, Right	3 Percutaneous	Z No Device	F Lower Arm Vein
A Ulnar Artery, Left C Radial Artery, Left	0 Open	9 Autologous Venous Tissue A Autologous Arterial Tissue J Synthetic Substitute K Nonautologous Tissue Substitute Z No Device	4 Lower Arm Artery, Left F Lower Arm Vein
A Ulnar Artery, Left C Radial Artery, Left	3 Percutaneous	Z No Device	F Lower Arm Vein
G Intracranial Artery S Temporal Artery, Right T Temporal Artery, Left	0 Open	9 Autologous Venous Tissue A Autologous Arterial Tissue J Synthetic Substitute K Nonautologous Tissue Substitute Z No Device	G Intracranial Artery
H Common Carotid Artery, Right J Common Carotid Artery, Left	0 Open	9 Autologous Venous Tissue A Autologous Arterial Tissue J Synthetic Substitute K Nonautologous Tissue Substitute Z No Device	G Intracranial Artery J Extracranial Artery, Right K Extracranial Artery, Left Y Upper Artery
K Internal Carotid Artery, Right L Internal Carotid Artery, Left M External Carotid Artery, Right N External Carotid Artery, Left	0 Open	9 Autologous Venous Tissue A Autologous Arterial Tissue J Synthetic Substitute K Nonautologous Tissue Substitute Z No Device	J Extracranial Artery, Right K Extracranial Artery, Left

0 Medical and Surgical
3 Upper Arteries
5 Destruction: Physical eradication of all or a portion of a body part by the direct use of energy, force, or a destructive agent

Body Part Character 4	Approach Character 5	Device Character 6	Qualifier Character 7
0 Internal Mammary Artery, Right **1** Internal Mammary Artery, Left **2** Innominate Artery **3** Subclavian Artery, Right **4** Subclavian Artery, Left **5** Axillary Artery, Right **6** Axillary Artery, Left **7** Brachial Artery, Right **8** Brachial Artery, Left **9** Ulnar Artery, Right **A** Ulnar Artery, Left **B** Radial Artery, Right **C** Radial Artery, Left **D** Hand Artery, Right **F** Hand Artery, Left **G** Intracranial Artery **H** Common Carotid Artery, Right **J** Common Carotid Artery, Left **K** Internal Carotid Artery, Right **L** Internal Carotid Artery, Left **M** External Carotid Artery, Right **N** External Carotid Artery, Left **P** Vertebral Artery, Right **Q** Vertebral Artery, Left **R** Face Artery **S** Temporal Artery, Right **T** Temporal Artery, Left **U** Thyroid Artery, Right **V** Thyroid Artery, Left **Y** Upper Artery	**0** Open **3** Percutaneous **4** Percutaneous Endoscopic	**Z** No Device	**Z** No Qualifier

0 Medical and Surgical
3 Upper Arteries
7 Dilation: Expanding an orifice or the lumen of a tubular body part

Body Part Character 4	Approach Character 5	Device Character 6	Qualifier Character 7
0 Internal Mammary Artery, Right **1** Internal Mammary Artery, Left **2** Innominate Artery **3** Subclavian Artery, Right **4** Subclavian Artery, Left **5** Axillary Artery, Right **6** Axillary Artery, Left **7** Brachial Artery, Right **8** Brachial Artery, Left **9** Ulnar Artery, Right **A** Ulnar Artery, Left **B** Radial Artery, Right **C** Radial Artery, Left	**0** Open **3** Percutaneous **4** Percutaneous Endoscopic	**4** Intraluminal Device, Drug-eluting **5** Intraluminal Device, Drug-eluting, Two **6** Intraluminal Device, Drug-eluting, Three **7** Intraluminal Device, Drug-eluting, Four or More **E** Intraluminal Device, Two **F** Intraluminal Device, Three **G** Intraluminal Device, Four or More	**Z** No Qualifier
0 Internal Mammary Artery, Right **1** Internal Mammary Artery, Left **2** Innominate Artery **3** Subclavian Artery, Right **4** Subclavian Artery, Left **5** Axillary Artery, Right **6** Axillary Artery, Left **7** Brachial Artery, Right **8** Brachial Artery, Left **9** Ulnar Artery, Right **A** Ulnar Artery, Left **B** Radial Artery, Right **C** Radial Artery, Left	**0** Open **3** Percutaneous **4** Percutaneous Endoscopic	**D** Intraluminal Device **Z** No Device	**1** Drug-Coated Balloon **Z** No Qualifier
D Hand Artery, Right **F** Hand Artery, Left **G** Intracranial Artery NC **H** Common Carotid Artery, Right **J** Common Carotid Artery, Left **K** Internal Carotid Artery, Right **L** Internal Carotid Artery, Left **M** External Carotid Artery, Right **N** External Carotid Artery, Left **P** Vertebral Artery, Right **Q** Vertebral Artery, Left **R** Face Artery **S** Temporal Artery, Right **T** Temporal Artery, Left **U** Thyroid Artery, Right **V** Thyroid Artery, Left **Y** Upper Artery	**0** Open **3** Percutaneous **4** Percutaneous Endoscopic	**4** Intraluminal Device, Drug-eluting **5** Intraluminal Device, Drug-eluting, Two **6** Intraluminal Device, Drug-eluting, Three **7** Intraluminal Device, Drug-eluting, Four or More **D** Intraluminal Device **E** Intraluminal Device, Two **F** Intraluminal Device, Three **G** Intraluminal Device, Four or More **Z** No Device	**Z** No Qualifier

NC 037G3ZZ 037G4ZZ

0 Medical and Surgical
3 Upper Arteries
9 Drainage: Taking or letting out fluids and/or gases from a body part

Body Part Character 4	Approach Character 5	Device Character 6	Qualifier Character 7
0 Internal Mammary Artery, Right **1** Internal Mammary Artery, Left **2** Innominate Artery **3** Subclavian Artery, Right **4** Subclavian Artery, Left **5** Axillary Artery, Right **6** Axillary Artery, Left **7** Brachial Artery, Right **8** Brachial Artery, Left **9** Ulnar Artery, Right **A** Ulnar Artery, Left **B** Radial Artery, Right **C** Radial Artery, Left **D** Hand Artery, Right **F** Hand Artery, Left **G** Intracranial Artery **H** Common Carotid Artery, Right **J** Common Carotid Artery, Left **K** Internal Carotid Artery, Right **L** Internal Carotid Artery, Left **M** External Carotid Artery, Right **N** External Carotid Artery, Left **P** Vertebral Artery, Right **Q** Vertebral Artery, Left **R** Face Artery **S** Temporal Artery, Right **T** Temporal Artery, Left **U** Thyroid Artery, Right **V** Thyroid Artery, Left **Y** Upper Artery	**0** Open **3** Percutaneous **4** Percutaneous Endoscopic	**0** Drainage Device	**Z** No Qualifier
0 Internal Mammary Artery, Right **1** Internal Mammary Artery, Left **2** Innominate Artery **3** Subclavian Artery, Right **4** Subclavian Artery, Left **5** Axillary Artery, Right **6** Axillary Artery, Left **7** Brachial Artery, Right **8** Brachial Artery, Left **9** Ulnar Artery, Right **A** Ulnar Artery, Left **B** Radial Artery, Right **C** Radial Artery, Left **D** Hand Artery, Right **F** Hand Artery, Left **G** Intracranial Artery **H** Common Carotid Artery, Right **J** Common Carotid Artery, Left **K** Internal Carotid Artery, Right **L** Internal Carotid Artery, Left **M** External Carotid Artery, Right **N** External Carotid Artery, Left **P** Vertebral Artery, Right **Q** Vertebral Artery, Left **R** Face Artery **S** Temporal Artery, Right **T** Temporal Artery, Left **U** Thyroid Artery, Right **V** Thyroid Artery, Left **Y** Upper Artery	**0** Open **3** Percutaneous **4** Percutaneous Endoscopic	**Z** No Device	**X** Diagnostic **Z** No Qualifier

0 Medical and Surgical
3 Upper Arteries
B Excision: Cutting out or off, without replacement, a portion of a body part

Body Part Character 4	Approach Character 5	Device Character 6	Qualifier Character 7
0 Internal Mammary Artery, Right **1** Internal Mammary Artery, Left **2** Innominate Artery **3** Subclavian Artery, Right **4** Subclavian Artery, Left **5** Axillary Artery, Right **6** Axillary Artery, Left **7** Brachial Artery, Right **8** Brachial Artery, Left **9** Ulnar Artery, Right **A** Ulnar Artery, Left **B** Radial Artery, Right **C** Radial Artery, Left **D** Hand Artery, Right **F** Hand Artery, Left **G** Intracranial Artery **H** Common Carotid Artery, Right **J** Common Carotid Artery, Left **K** Internal Carotid Artery, Right **L** Internal Carotid Artery, Left **M** External Carotid Artery, Right **N** External Carotid Artery, Left **P** Vertebral Artery, Right **Q** Vertebral Artery, Left **R** Face Artery **S** Temporal Artery, Right **T** Temporal Artery, Left **U** Thyroid Artery, Right **V** Thyroid Artery, Left **Y** Upper Artery	**0** Open **3** Percutaneous **4** Percutaneous Endoscopic	**Z** No Device	**X** Diagnostic **Z** No Qualifier

0 Medical and Surgical
3 Upper Arteries
C Extirpation: Taking or cutting out solid matter from a body part

Body Part Character 4	Approach Character 5	Device Character 6	Qualifier Character 7
0 Internal Mammary Artery, Right **1** Internal Mammary Artery, Left **2** Innominate Artery **3** Subclavian Artery, Right **4** Subclavian Artery, Left **5** Axillary Artery, Right **6** Axillary Artery, Left **7** Brachial Artery, Right **8** Brachial Artery, Left **9** Ulnar Artery, Right **A** Ulnar Artery, Left **B** Radial Artery, Right **C** Radial Artery, Left **D** Hand Artery, Right **F** Hand Artery, Left **R** Face Artery **S** Temporal Artery, Right **T** Temporal Artery, Left **U** Thyroid Artery, Right **V** Thyroid Artery, Left **Y** Upper Artery	**0** Open **3** Percutaneous **4** Percutaneous Endoscopic	**Z** No Device	**Z** No Qualifier
G Intracranial Artery **H** Common Carotid Artery, Right **J** Common Carotid Artery, Left **K** Internal Carotid Artery, Right **L** Internal Carotid Artery, Left **M** External Carotid Artery, Right **N** External Carotid Artery, Left **P** Vertebral Artery, Right **Q** Vertebral Artery, Left	**0** Open **4** Percutaneous Endoscopic	**Z** No Device	**Z** No Qualifier
G Intracranial Artery **H** Common Carotid Artery, Right **J** Common Carotid Artery, Left **K** Internal Carotid Artery, Right **L** Internal Carotid Artery, Left **M** External Carotid Artery, Right **N** External Carotid Artery, Left **P** Vertebral Artery, Right **Q** Vertebral Artery, Left	**3** Percutaneous	**Z** No Device	**7** Stent Retriever **Z** No Qualifier

0 Medical and Surgical
3 Upper Arteries
H Insertion: Putting in a nonbiological appliance that monitors, assists, performs, or prevents a physiological function but does not physically take the place of a body part

Body Part Character 4	Approach Character 5	Device Character 6	Qualifier Character 7
0 Internal Mammary Artery, Right **1** Internal Mammary Artery, Left **2** Innominate Artery **3** Subclavian Artery, Right **4** Subclavian Artery, Left **5** Axillary Artery, Right **6** Axillary Artery, Left **7** Brachial Artery, Right **8** Brachial Artery, Left **9** Ulnar Artery, Right **A** Ulnar Artery, Left **B** Radial Artery, Right **C** Radial Artery, Left **D** Hand Artery, Right **F** Hand Artery, Left **G** Intracranial Artery **H** Common Carotid Artery, Right **J** Common Carotid Artery, Left **M** External Carotid Artery, Right **N** External Carotid Artery, Left **P** Vertebral Artery, Right **Q** Vertebral Artery, Left **R** Face Artery **S** Temporal Artery, Right **T** Temporal Artery, Left **U** Thyroid Artery, Right **V** Thyroid Artery, Left	**0** Open **3** Percutaneous **4** Percutaneous Endoscopic	**3** Infusion Device **D** Intraluminal Device	**Z** No Qualifier
K Internal Carotid Artery, Right **L** Internal Carotid Artery, Left	**0** Open **3** Percutaneous **4** Percutaneous Endoscopic	**3** Infusion Device **D** Intraluminal Device **M** Stimulator Lead	**Z** No Qualifier
Y Upper Artery	**0** Open **3** Percutaneous **4** Percutaneous Endoscopic	**2** Monitoring Device **3** Infusion Device **D** Intraluminal Device **Y** Other Device	**Z** No Qualifier

0 Medical and Surgical
3 Upper Arteries
J Inspection: Visually and/or manually exploring a body part

Body Part Character 4	Approach Character 5	Device Character 6	Qualifier Character 7
Y Upper Artery	**0** Open **3** Percutaneous **4** Percutaneous Endoscopic **X** External	**Z** No Device	**Z** No Qualifier

0 Medical and Surgical
3 Upper Arteries
L Occlusion: Completely closing an orifice or the lumen of a tubular body part , cut off blood supply to tumor or meningioma

Body Part Character 4	Approach Character 5	Device Character 6	Qualifier Character 7
0 Internal Mammary Artery, Right **1** Internal Mammary Artery, Left **2** Innominate Artery **3** Subclavian Artery, Right **4** Subclavian Artery, Left **5** Axillary Artery, Right **6** Axillary Artery, Left **7** Brachial Artery, Right **8** Brachial Artery, Left **9** Ulnar Artery, Right **A** Ulnar Artery, Left **B** Radial Artery, Right **C** Radial Artery, Left **D** Hand Artery, Right **F** Hand Artery, Left **R** Face Artery **S** Temporal Artery, Right **T** Temporal Artery, Left **U** Thyroid Artery, Right **V** Thyroid Artery, Left **Y** Upper Artery	**0** Open **3** Percutaneous **4** Percutaneous Endoscopic	**C** Extraluminal Device **D** Intraluminal Device **Z** No Device	**Z** No Qualifier
G Intracranial Artery **H** Common Carotid Artery, Right **J** Common Carotid Artery, Left **K** Internal Carotid Artery, Right **L** Internal Carotid Artery, Left **M** External Carotid Artery, Right **N** External Carotid Artery, Left **P** Vertebral Artery, Right **Q** Vertebral Artery, Left	**0** Open **3** Percutaneous **4** Percutaneous Endoscopic	**B** Intraluminal Device, Bioactive **C** Extraluminal Device **D** Intraluminal Device **Z** No Device	**Z** No Qualifier

0 Medical and Surgical
3 Upper Arteries
N Release: Freeing a body part from an abnormal physical constraint by cutting or by the use of force

Body Part Character 4	Approach Character 5	Device Character 6	Qualifier Character 7
0 Internal Mammary Artery, Right **1** Internal Mammary Artery, Left **2** Innominate Artery **3** Subclavian Artery, Right **4** Subclavian Artery, Left **5** Axillary Artery, Right **6** Axillary Artery, Left **7** Brachial Artery, Right **8** Brachial Artery, Left **9** Ulnar Artery, Right **A** Ulnar Artery, Left **B** Radial Artery, Right **C** Radial Artery, Left **D** Hand Artery, Right **F** Hand Artery, Left **G** Intracranial Artery **H** Common Carotid Artery, Right **J** Common Carotid Artery, Left **K** Internal Carotid Artery, Right **L** Internal Carotid Artery, Left **M** External Carotid Artery, Right **N** External Carotid Artery, Left **P** Vertebral Artery, Right **Q** Vertebral Artery, Left **R** Face Artery **S** Temporal Artery, Right **T** Temporal Artery, Left **U** Thyroid Artery, Right **V** Thyroid Artery, Left **Y** Upper Artery	**0** Open **3** Percutaneous **4** Percutaneous Endoscopic	**Z** No Device	**Z** No Qualifier

0 Medical and Surgical
3 Upper Arteries
P Removal: Taking out or off a device from a body part

Body Part Character 4	Approach Character 5	Device Character 6	Qualifier Character 7
Y Upper Artery	**0** Open **3** Percutaneous **4** Percutaneous Endoscopic	**0** Drainage Device **2** Monitoring Device **3** Infusion Device **7** Autologous Tissue Substitute **C** Extraluminal Device **D** Intraluminal Device **J** Synthetic Substitute **K** Nonautologous Tissue Substitute **M** Stimulator Lead **Y** Other Device	**Z** No Qualifier
Y Upper Artery	**X** External	**0** Drainage Device **2** Monitoring Device **3** Infusion Device **D** Intraluminal Device **M** Stimulator Lead	**Z** No Qualifier

0 Medical and Surgical
3 Upper Arteries
Q Repair: Restoring, to the extent possible, a body part to its normal anatomic structure and function

Body Part Character 4	Approach Character 5	Device Character 6	Qualifier Character 7
0 Internal Mammary Artery, Right **1** Internal Mammary Artery, Left **2** Innominate Artery **3** Subclavian Artery, Right **4** Subclavian Artery, Left **5** Axillary Artery, Right **6** Axillary Artery, Left **7** Brachial Artery, Right **8** Brachial Artery, Left **9** Ulnar Artery, Right **A** Ulnar Artery, Left **B** Radial Artery, Right **C** Radial Artery, Left **D** Hand Artery, Right **F** Hand Artery, Left **G** Intracranial Artery **H** Common Carotid Artery, Right **J** Common Carotid Artery, Left **K** Internal Carotid Artery, Right **L** Internal Carotid Artery, Left **M** External Carotid Artery, Right **N** External Carotid Artery, Left **P** Vertebral Artery, Right **Q** Vertebral Artery, Left **R** Face Artery **S** Temporal Artery, Right **T** Temporal Artery, Left **U** Thyroid Artery, Right **V** Thyroid Artery, Left **Y** Upper Artery	**0** Open **3** Percutaneous **4** Percutaneous Endoscopic	**Z** No Device	**Z** No Qualifier

0 Medical and Surgical
3 Upper Arteries
R Replacement: Putting in or on biological or synthetic material that physically takes the place and/or function of all or a portion of a body part

Body Part	Approach	Device	Qualifier
Character 4	**Character 5**	**Character 6**	**Character 7**
0 Internal Mammary Artery, Right **1** Internal Mammary Artery, Left **2** Innominate Artery **3** Subclavian Artery, Right **4** Subclavian Artery, Left **5** Axillary Artery, Right **6** Axillary Artery, Left **7** Brachial Artery, Right **8** Brachial Artery, Left **9** Ulnar Artery, Right **A** Ulnar Artery, Left **B** Radial Artery, Right **C** Radial Artery, Left **D** Hand Artery, Right **F** Hand Artery, Left **G** Intracranial Artery **H** Common Carotid Artery, Right **J** Common Carotid Artery, Left **K** Internal Carotid Artery, Right **L** Internal Carotid Artery, Left **M** External Carotid Artery, Right **N** External Carotid Artery, Left **P** Vertebral Artery, Right **Q** Vertebral Artery, Left **R** Face Artery **S** Temporal Artery, Right **T** Temporal Artery, Left **U** Thyroid Artery, Right **V** Thyroid Artery, Left **Y** Upper Artery	**0** Open **4** Percutaneous Endoscopic	**7** Autologous Tissue Substitute **J** Synthetic Substitute **K** Nonautologous Tissue Substitute	**Z** No Qualifier

0 Medical and Surgical
3 Upper Arteries
S Reposition: Moving to its normal location, or other suitable location, all or a portion of a body part

Body Part Character 4	Approach Character 5	Device Character 6	Qualifier Character 7
0 Internal Mammary Artery, Right **1** Internal Mammary Artery, Left **2** Innominate Artery **3** Subclavian Artery, Right **4** Subclavian Artery, Left **5** Axillary Artery, Right **6** Axillary Artery, Left **7** Brachial Artery, Right **8** Brachial Artery, Left **9** Ulnar Artery, Right **A** Ulnar Artery, Left **B** Radial Artery, Right **C** Radial Artery, Left **D** Hand Artery, Right **F** Hand Artery, Left **G** Intracranial Artery **H** Common Carotid Artery, Right **J** Common Carotid Artery, Left **K** Internal Carotid Artery, Right **L** Internal Carotid Artery, Left **M** External Carotid Artery, Right **N** External Carotid Artery, Left **P** Vertebral Artery, Right **Q** Vertebral Artery, Left **R** Face Artery **S** Temporal Artery, Right **T** Temporal Artery, Left **U** Thyroid Artery, Right **V** Thyroid Artery, Left **Y** Upper Artery	**0** Open **3** Percutaneous **4** Percutaneous Endoscopic	**Z** No Device	**Z** No Qualifier

LC Limited Coverage NC Noncovered HAC HAC-associated Procedure CC Combination Cluster - See Appendix G for code lists
DRG Non-OR-Affecting MS-DRG Assignment New/Revised Text in **Orange** ♂ Male ♀ Female
2020 ICD-10-PCS 223

0 Medical and Surgical
3 Upper Arteries
U Supplement: Putting in or on biological or synthetic material that physically reinforces and/or augments the function of a portion of a body part

Body Part Character 4	Approach Character 5	Device Character 6	Qualifier Character 7
0 Internal Mammary Artery, Right **1** Internal Mammary Artery, Left **2** Innominate Artery **3** Subclavian Artery, Right **4** Subclavian Artery, Left **5** Axillary Artery, Right **6** Axillary Artery, Left **7** Brachial Artery, Right **8** Brachial Artery, Left **9** Ulnar Artery, Right **A** Ulnar Artery, Left **B** Radial Artery, Right **C** Radial Artery, Left **D** Hand Artery, Right **F** Hand Artery, Left **G** Intracranial Artery **H** Common Carotid Artery, Right **J** Common Carotid Artery, Left **K** Internal Carotid Artery, Right **L** Internal Carotid Artery, Left **M** External Carotid Artery, Right **N** External Carotid Artery, Left **P** Vertebral Artery, Right **Q** Vertebral Artery, Left **R** Face Artery **S** Temporal Artery, Right **T** Temporal Artery, Left **U** Thyroid Artery, Right **V** Thyroid Artery, Left **Y** Upper Artery	**0** Open **3** Percutaneous **4** Percutaneous Endoscopic	**7** Autologous Tissue Substitute **J** Synthetic Substitute **K** Nonautologous Tissue Substitute	**Z** No Qualifier

0 Medical and Surgical
3 Upper Arteries
V Restriction: Partially closing an orifice or the lumen of a tubular body part

Body Part Character 4	Approach Character 5	Device Character 6	Qualifier Character 7
0 Internal Mammary Artery, Right **1** Internal Mammary Artery, Left **2** Innominate Artery **3** Subclavian Artery, Right **4** Subclavian Artery, Left **5** Axillary Artery, Right **6** Axillary Artery, Left **7** Brachial Artery, Right **8** Brachial Artery, Left **9** Ulnar Artery, Right **A** Ulnar Artery, Left **B** Radial Artery, Right **C** Radial Artery, Left **D** Hand Artery, Right **F** Hand Artery, Left **R** Face Artery **S** Temporal Artery, Right **T** Temporal Artery, Left **U** Thyroid Artery, Right **V** Thyroid Artery, Left **Y** Upper Artery	**0** Open **3** Percutaneous **4** Percutaneous Endoscopic	**C** Extraluminal Device **D** Intraluminal Device **Z** No Device	**Z** No Qualifier
G Intracranial Artery **H** Common Carotid Artery, Right **J** Common Carotid Artery, Left **K** Internal Carotid Artery, Right **L** Internal Carotid Artery, Left **M** External Carotid Artery, Right **N** External Carotid Artery, Left **P** Vertebral Artery, Right **Q** Vertebral Artery, Left	**0** Open **3** Percutaneous **4** Percutaneous Endoscopic	**B** Intraluminal Device, Bioactive **C** Extraluminal Device **D** Intraluminal Device **H** Intraluminal Device, Flow Diverter **Z** No Device	**Z** No Qualifier

0 Medical and Surgical
3 Upper Arteries
W Revision: Correcting, to the extent possible, a portion of a malfunctioning device or the position of a displaced device

Body Part Character 4	Approach Character 5	Device Character 6	Qualifier Character 7
Y Upper Artery	**0** Open **3** Percutaneous **4** Percutaneous Endoscopic	**0** Drainage Device **2** Monitoring Device **3** Infusion Device **7** Autologous Tissue Substitute **C** Extraluminal Device **D** Intraluminal Device **J** Synthetic Substitute **K** Nonautologous Tissue Substitute **M** Stimulator Lead **Y** Other Device	**Z** No Qualifier
Y Upper Artery	**X** External	**0** Drainage Device **2** Monitoring Device **3** Infusion Device **7** Autologous Tissue Substitute **C** Extraluminal Device **D** Intraluminal Device **J** Synthetic Substitute **K** Nonautologous Tissue Substitute **M** Stimulator Lead	**Z** No Qualifier

NOTES

Lower Arteries 041-04W

0 Medical and Surgical
4 Lower Arteries
1 Bypass: Altering the route of passage of the contents of a tubular body part

Body Part Character 4	Approach Character 5	Device Character 6	Qualifier Character 7
0 Abdominal Aorta **C** Common Iliac Artery, Right **D** Common Iliac Artery, Left	**0** Open **4** Percutaneous Endoscopic	**9** Autologous Venous Tissue **A** Autologous Arterial Tissue **J** Synthetic Substitute **K** Nonautologous Tissue Substitute **Z** No Device	**0** Abdominal Aorta **1** Celiac Artery **2** Mesenteric Artery **3** Renal Artery, Right **4** Renal Artery, Left **5** Renal Artery, Bilateral **6** Common Iliac Artery, Right **7** Common Iliac Artery, Left **8** Common Iliac Arteries, Bilateral **9** Internal Iliac Artery, Right **B** Internal Iliac Artery, Left **C** Internal Iliac Arteries, Bilateral **D** External Iliac Artery, Right **F** External Iliac Artery, Left **G** External Iliac Arteries, Bilateral **H** Femoral Artery, Right **J** Femoral Artery, Left **K** Femoral Arteries, Bilateral **Q** Lower Extremity Artery **R** Lower Artery
3 Hepatic Artery **4** Splenic Artery	**0** Open **4** Percutaneous Endoscopic	**9** Autologous Venous Tissue **A** Autologous Arterial Tissue **J** Synthetic Substitute **K** Nonautologous Tissue Substitute **Z** No Device	**3** Renal Artery, Right **4** Renal Artery, Left **5** Renal Artery, Bilateral
E Internal Iliac Artery, Right **F** Internal Iliac Artery, Left **H** External Iliac Artery, Right **J** External Iliac Artery, Left	**0** Open **4** Percutaneous Endoscopic	**9** Autologous Venous Tissue **A** Autologous Arterial Tissue **J** Synthetic Substitute **K** Nonautologous Tissue Substitute **Z** No Device	**9** Internal Iliac Artery, Right **B** Internal Iliac Artery, Left **C** Internal Iliac Arteries, Bilateral **D** External Iliac Artery, Right **F** External Iliac Artery, Left **G** External Iliac Arteries, Bilateral **H** Femoral Artery, Right **J** Femoral Artery, Left **K** Femoral Arteries, Bilateral **P** Foot Artery **Q** Lower Extremity Artery
K Femoral Artery, Right **L** Femoral Artery, Left	**0** Open **4** Percutaneous Endoscopic	**9** Autologous Venous Tissue **A** Autologous Arterial Tissue **J** Synthetic Substitute **K** Nonautologous Tissue Substitute **Z** No Device	**H** Femoral Artery, Right **J** Femoral Artery, Left **K** Femoral Arteries, Bilateral **L** Popliteal Artery **M** Peroneal Artery **N** Posterior Tibial Artery **P** Foot Artery **Q** Lower Extremity Artery **S** Lower Extremity Vein
K Femoral Artery, Right **L** Femoral Artery, Left	**3** Percutaneous	**J** Synthetic Substitute	**Q** Lower Extremity Artery **S** Lower Extremity Vein
M Popliteal Artery, Right **N** Popliteal Artery, Left	**0** Open **4** Percutaneous Endoscopic	**9** Autologous Venous Tissue **A** Autologous Arterial Tissue **J** Synthetic Substitute **K** Nonautologous Tissue Substitute **Z** No Device	**L** Popliteal Artery **M** Peroneal Artery **P** Foot Artery **Q** Lower Extremity Artery **S** Lower Extremity Vein
M Popliteal Artery, Right **N** Popliteal Artery, Left	**3** Percutaneous	**J** Synthetic Substitute	**Q** Lower Extremity Artery **S** Lower Extremity Vein

041 continued on next page

041 continued from previous page

0 Medical and Surgical
4 Lower Arteries
1 Bypass: Altering the route of passage of the contents of a tubular body part

Body Part Character 4	Approach Character 5	Device Character 6	Qualifier Character 7
P Anterior Tibial Artery, Right **Q** Anterior Tibial Artery, Left **R** Posterior Tibial Artery, Right **S** Posterior Tibial Artery	**0** Open **3** Percutaneous **4** Percutaneous Endoscopic	**J** Synthetic Substitute	**Q** Lower Extremity Artery **S** Lower Extremity Vein
T Peroneal Artery, Right **U** Peroneal Artery, Left **V** Foot Artery, Right **W** Foot Artery, Left	**0** Open **4** Percutaneous Endoscopic	**9** Autologous Venous Tissue **A** Autologous Arterial Tissue **J** Synthetic Substitute **K** Nonautologous Tissue Substitute **Z** No Device	**P** Foot Artery **Q** Lower Extremity Artery **S** Lower Extremity Vein
T Peroneal Artery, Right **U** Peroneal Artery, Left **V** Foot Artery, Right **W** Foot Artery, Left	**3** Percutaneous	**J** Synthetic Substitute	**Q** Lower Extremity Artery **S** Lower Extremity Vein

0 Medical and Surgical
4 Lower Arteries
5 Destruction: Physical eradication of all or a portion of a body part by the direct use of energy, force, or a destructive agent

Body Part Character 4	Approach Character 5	Device Character 6	Qualifier Character 7
0 Abdominal Aorta **1** Celiac Artery **2** Gastric Artery **3** Hepatic Artery **4** Splenic Artery **5** Superior Mesenteric Artery **6** Colic Artery, Right **7** Colic Artery, Left **8** Colic Artery, Middle **9** Renal Artery, Right **A** Renal Artery, Left **B** Inferior Mesenteric Artery **C** Common Iliac Artery, Right **D** Common Iliac Artery, Left **E** Internal Iliac Artery, Right **F** Internal Iliac Artery, Left **H** External Iliac Artery, Right **J** External Iliac Artery, Left **K** Femoral Artery, Right **L** Femoral Artery, Left **M** Popliteal Artery, Right **N** Popliteal Artery, Left **P** Anterior Tibial Artery, Right **Q** Anterior Tibial Artery, Left **R** Posterior Tibial Artery, Right **S** Posterior Tibial Artery, Left **T** Peroneal Artery, Right **U** Peroneal Artery, Left **V** Foot Artery, Right **W** Foot Artery, Left **Y** Lower Artery	**0** Open **3** Percutaneous **4** Percutaneous Endoscopic	**Z** No Device	**Z** No Qualifier

0 Medical and Surgical
4 Lower Arteries
7 Dilation: Expanding an orifice or the lumen of a tubular body part

Body Part Character 4	Approach Character 5	Device Character 6	Qualifier Character 7
0 Abdominal Aorta **1** Celiac Artery **2** Gastric Artery **3** Hepatic Artery **4** Splenic Artery **5** Superior Mesenteric Artery **6** Colic Artery, Right **7** Colic Artery, Left **8** Colic Artery, Middle **9** Renal Artery, Right **A** Renal Artery, Left **B** Inferior Mesenteric Artery **C** Common Iliac Artery, Right **D** Common Iliac Artery, Left **E** Internal Iliac Artery, Right **F** Internal Iliac Artery, Left **H** External Iliac Artery, Right **J** External Iliac Artery, Left **K** Femoral Artery, Right **L** Femoral Artery, Left **M** Popliteal Artery, Right **N** Popliteal Artery, Left **P** Anterior Tibial Artery, Right **Q** Anterior Tibial Artery, Left **R** Posterior Tibial Artery, Right **S** Posterior Tibial Artery, Left **T** Peroneal Artery, Right **U** Peroneal Artery, Left **V** Foot Artery, Right **W** Foot Artery, Left **Y** Lower Artery	**0** Open **3** Percutaneous **4** Percutaneous Endoscopic	**4** Intraluminal Device, Drug-eluting **D** Intraluminal Device **Z** No Device	**1** Drug-Coated Balloon **Z** No Qualifier
0 Abdominal Aorta **1** Celiac Artery **2** Gastric Artery **3** Hepatic Artery **4** Splenic Artery **5** Superior Mesenteric Artery **6** Colic Artery, Right **7** Colic Artery, Left **8** Colic Artery, Middle **9** Renal Artery, Right **A** Renal Artery, Left **B** Inferior Mesenteric Artery **C** Common Iliac Artery, Right **D** Common Iliac Artery, Left **E** Internal Iliac Artery, Right **F** Internal Iliac Artery, Left **H** External Iliac Artery, Right **J** External Iliac Artery, Left **K** Femoral Artery, Right **L** Femoral Artery, Left **M** Popliteal Artery, Right **N** Popliteal Artery, Left **P** Anterior Tibial Artery, Right **Q** Anterior Tibial Artery, Left **R** Posterior Tibial Artery, Right **S** Posterior Tibial Artery, Left **T** Peroneal Artery, Right **U** Peroneal Artery, Left **V** Foot Artery, Right **W** Foot Artery, Left **Y** Lower Artery	**0** Open **3** Percutaneous **4** Percutaneous Endoscopic	**5** Intraluminal Device, Drug-eluting, Two **6** Intraluminal Device, Drug-eluting, Three **7** Intraluminal Device, Drug-eluting, Four or More **E** Intraluminal Device, Two **F** Intraluminal Device, Three **G** Intraluminal Device, Four or More	**Z** No Qualifier

0 Medical and Surgical
4 Lower Arteries
9 Drainage: Taking or letting out fluids and/or gases from a body part

Body Part Character 4	Approach Character 5	Device Character 6	Qualifier Character 7
0 Abdominal Aorta 1 Celiac Artery 2 Gastric Artery 3 Hepatic Artery 4 Splenic Artery 5 Superior Mesenteric Artery 6 Colic Artery, Right 7 Colic Artery, Left 8 Colic Artery, Middle 9 Renal Artery, Right A Renal Artery, Left B Inferior Mesenteric Artery C Common Iliac Artery, Right D Common Iliac Artery, Left E Internal Iliac Artery, Right F Internal Iliac Artery, Left H External Iliac Artery, Right J External Iliac Artery, Left K Femoral Artery, Right L Femoral Artery, Left M Popliteal Artery, Right N Popliteal Artery, Left P Anterior Tibial Artery, Right Q Anterior Tibial Artery, Left R Posterior Tibial Artery, Right S Posterior Tibial Artery, Left T Peroneal Artery, Right U Peroneal Artery, Left V Foot Artery, Right W Foot Artery, Left Y Lower Artery	0 Open 3 Percutaneous 4 Percutaneous Endoscopic	0 Drainage Device	Z No Qualifier
0 Abdominal Aorta 1 Celiac Artery 2 Gastric Artery 3 Hepatic Artery 4 Splenic Artery 5 Superior Mesenteric Artery 6 Colic Artery, Right 7 Colic Artery, Left 8 Colic Artery, Middle 9 Renal Artery, Right A Renal Artery, Left B Inferior Mesenteric Artery C Common Iliac Artery, Right D Common Iliac Artery, Left E Internal Iliac Artery, Right F Internal Iliac Artery, Left H External Iliac Artery, Right J External Iliac Artery, Left K Femoral Artery, Right L Femoral Artery, Left M Popliteal Artery, Right N Popliteal Artery, Left P Anterior Tibial Artery, Right Q Anterior Tibial Artery, Left R Posterior Tibial Artery, Right S Posterior Tibial Artery, Left T Peroneal Artery, Right U Peroneal Artery, Left V Foot Artery, Right W Foot Artery, Left Y Lower Artery	0 Open 3 Percutaneous 4 Percutaneous Endoscopic	Z No Device	X Diagnostic Z No Qualifier

0 Medical and Surgical
4 Lower Arteries
B Excision: Cutting out or off, without replacement, a portion of a body part

Body Part Character 4	Approach Character 5	Device Character 6	Qualifier Character 7
0 Abdominal Aorta **1** Celiac Artery **2** Gastric Artery **3** Hepatic Artery **4** Splenic Artery **5** Superior Mesenteric Artery **6** Colic Artery, Right **7** Colic Artery, Left **8** Colic Artery, Middle **9** Renal Artery, Right **A** Renal Artery, Left **B** Inferior Mesenteric Artery **C** Common Iliac Artery, Right **D** Common Iliac Artery, Left **E** Internal Iliac Artery, Right **F** Internal Iliac Artery, Left **H** External Iliac Artery, Right **J** External Iliac Artery, Left **K** Femoral Artery, Right **L** Femoral Artery, Left **M** Popliteal Artery, Right **N** Popliteal Artery, Left **P** Anterior Tibial Artery, Right **Q** Anterior Tibial Artery, Left **R** Posterior Tibial Artery, Right **S** Posterior Tibial Artery, Left **T** Peroneal Artery, Right **U** Peroneal Artery, Left **V** Foot Artery, Right **W** Foot Artery, Left **Y** Lower Artery	**0** Open **3** Percutaneous **4** Percutaneous Endoscopic	**Z** No Device	**X** Diagnostic **Z** No Qualifier

0 Medical and Surgical
4 Lower Arteries
C Extirpation: Taking or cutting out solid matter from a body part

Body Part Character 4	Approach Character 5	Device Character 6	Qualifier Character 7
0 Abdominal Aorta **1** Celiac Artery **2** Gastric Artery **3** Hepatic Artery **4** Splenic Artery **5** Superior Mesenteric Artery **6** Colic Artery, Right **7** Colic Artery, Left **8** Colic Artery, Middle **9** Renal Artery, Right **A** Renal Artery, Left **B** Inferior Mesenteric Artery **C** Common Iliac Artery, Right **D** Common Iliac Artery, Left **E** Internal Iliac Artery, Right **F** Internal Iliac Artery, Left **H** External Iliac Artery, Right **J** External Iliac Artery, Left **K** Femoral Artery, Right **L** Femoral Artery, Left **M** Popliteal Artery, Right **N** Popliteal Artery, Left **P** Anterior Tibial Artery, Right **Q** Anterior Tibial Artery, Left **R** Posterior Tibial Artery, Right **S** Posterior Tibial Artery, Left **T** Peroneal Artery, Right **U** Peroneal Artery, Left **V** Foot Artery, Right **W** Foot Artery, Left **Y** Lower Artery	**0** Open **3** Percutaneous **4** Percutaneous Endoscopic	**Z** No Device	**Z** No Qualifier

0 Medical and Surgical
4 Lower Arteries
H Insertion: Putting in a nonbiological appliance that monitors, assists, performs, or prevents a physiological function but does not physically take the place of a body part

Body Part Character 4	Approach Character 5	Device Character 6	Qualifier Character 7
0 Abdominal Aorta	0 Open 3 Percutaneous 4 Percutaneous Endoscopic	2 Monitoring Device 3 Infusion Device D Intraluminal Device	Z No Qualifier
1 Celiac Artery 2 Gastric Artery 3 Hepatic Artery 4 Splenic Artery 5 Superior Mesenteric Artery 6 Colic Artery, Right 7 Colic Artery, Left 8 Colic Artery, Middle 9 Renal Artery, Right A Renal Artery, Left B Inferior Mesenteric Artery C Common Iliac Artery, Right D Common Iliac Artery, Left E Internal Iliac Artery, Right F Internal Iliac Artery, Left H External Iliac Artery, Right J External Iliac Artery, Left K Femoral Artery, Right L Femoral Artery, Left M Popliteal Artery, Right N Popliteal Artery, Left P Anterior Tibial Artery, Right Q Anterior Tibial Artery, Left R Posterior Tibial Artery, Right S Posterior Tibial Artery, Left T Peroneal Artery, Right U Peroneal Artery, Left V Foot Artery, Right W Foot Artery, Left	0 Open 3 Percutaneous 4 Percutaneous Endoscopic	3 Infusion Device D Intraluminal Device	Z No Qualifier
Y Lower Artery	0 Open 3 Percutaneous 4 Percutaneous Endoscopic	2 Monitoring Device 3 Infusion Device D Intraluminal Device Y Other Device	Z No Qualifier

0 Medical and Surgical
4 Lower Arteries
J Inspection: Visually and/or manually exploring a body part

Body Part Character 4	Approach Character 5	Device Character 6	Qualifier Character 7
Y Lower Artery	0 Open 3 Percutaneous 4 Percutaneous Endoscopic X External	Z No Device	Z No Qualifier

0 **Medical and Surgical**
4 **Lower Arteries**
L **Occlusion:** Completely closing an orifice or the lumen of a tubular body part

Body Part Character 4	Approach Character 5	Device Character 6	Qualifier Character 7
0 Abdominal Aorta	**0** Open **4** Percutaneous Endoscopic	**C** Extraluminal Device **D** Intraluminal Device **Z** No Device	**Z** No Qualifier
0 Abdominal Aorta	**3** Percutaneous	**C** Extraluminal Device **Z** No Device	**Z** No Qualifier
0 Abdominal Aorta	**3** Percutaneous	**D** Intraluminal Device	**J** Temporary **Z** No Qualifier
1 Celiac Artery **2** Gastric Artery **3** Hepatic Artery **4** Splenic Artery **5** Superior Mesenteric Artery **6** Colic Artery, Right **7** Colic Artery, Left **8** Colic Artery, Middle **9** Renal Artery, Right **A** Renal Artery, Left **B** Inferior Mesenteric Artery **C** Common Iliac Artery, Right **D** Common Iliac Artery, Left **H** External Iliac Artery, Right **J** External Iliac Artery, Left **K** Femoral Artery, Right **L** Femoral Artery, Left **M** Popliteal Artery, Right **N** Popliteal Artery, Left **P** Anterior Tibial Artery, Right **Q** Anterior Tibial Artery, Left **R** Posterior Tibial Artery, Right **S** Posterior Tibial Artery, Left **T** Peroneal Artery, Right **U** Peroneal Artery, Left **V** Foot Artery, Right **W** Foot Artery, Left **Y** Lower Artery	**0** Open **3** Percutaneous **4** Percutaneous Endoscopic	**C** Extraluminal Device **D** Intraluminal Device **Z** No Device	**Z** No Qualifier
E Internal Iliac Artery, Right ♀	**0** Open **3** Percutaneous **4** Percutaneous Endoscopic	**C** Extraluminal Device **D** Intraluminal Device **Z** No Device	**T** Uterine Artery, Right **Z** No Qualifier
F Internal Iliac Artery, Left ♀	**0** Open **3** Percutaneous **4** Percutaneous Endoscopic	**C** Extraluminal Device **D** Intraluminal Device **Z** No Device	**U** Uterine Artery, Left **Z** No Qualifier

♀ 04LE0CT 04LE0DT 04LE0ZT 04LE3CT 04LE3DT 04LE3ZT 04LE4CT 04LE4DT 04LE4ZT 04LF0CU 04LF0DU 04LF0ZU 04LF3CU 04LF3DU 04LF3ZU 04LF4CU 04LF4DU 04LF4ZU

LC Limited Coverage NC Noncovered HAC HAC-associated Procedure CC Combination Cluster - See Appendix G for code lists
DRG Non-OR-Affecting MS-DRG Assignment New/Revised Text in **Orange** ♂ Male ♀ Female
234 2020 ICD-10-PCS

0 Medical and Surgical
4 Lower Arteries
N Release: Freeing a body part from an abnormal physical constraint by cutting or by the use of force

Body Part Character 4	Approach Character 5	Device Character 6	Qualifier Character 7
0 Abdominal Aorta **1** Celiac Artery **2** Gastric Artery **3** Hepatic Artery **4** Splenic Artery **5** Superior Mesenteric Artery **6** Colic Artery, Right **7** Colic Artery, Left **8** Colic Artery, Middle **9** Renal Artery, Right **A** Renal Artery, Left **B** Inferior Mesenteric Artery **C** Common Iliac Artery, Right **D** Common Iliac Artery, Left **E** Internal Iliac Artery, Right **F** Internal Iliac Artery, Left **H** External Iliac Artery, Right **J** External Iliac Artery, Left **K** Femoral Artery, Right **L** Femoral Artery, Left **M** Popliteal Artery, Right **N** Popliteal Artery, Left **P** Anterior Tibial Artery, Right **Q** Anterior Tibial Artery, Left **R** Posterior Tibial Artery, Right **S** Posterior Tibial Artery, Left **T** Peroneal Artery, Right **U** Peroneal Artery, Left **V** Foot Artery, Right **W** Foot Artery, Left **Y** Lower Artery	**0** Open **3** Percutaneous **4** Percutaneous Endoscopic	**Z** No Device	**Z** No Qualifier

0 Medical and Surgical
4 Lower Arteries
P Removal: Taking out or off a device from a body part

Body Part Character 4	Approach Character 5	Device Character 6	Qualifier Character 7
Y Lower Artery	**0** Open **3** Percutaneous **4** Percutaneous Endoscopic	**0** Drainage Device **2** Monitoring Device **3** Infusion Device **7** Autologous Tissue Substitute **C** Extraluminal Device **D** Intraluminal Device **J** Synthetic Substitute **K** Nonautologous Tissue Substitute **Y** Other Device	**Z** No Qualifier
Y Lower Artery	**X** External	**0** Drainage Device **1** Radioactive Element **2** Monitoring Device **3** Infusion Device **D** Intraluminal Device	**Z** No Qualifier

0 Medical and Surgical
4 Lower Arteries
Q Repair: Restoring, to the extent possible, a body part to its normal anatomic structure and function

Body Part Character 4	Approach Character 5	Device Character 6	Qualifier Character 7
0 Abdominal Aorta **1** Celiac Artery **2** Gastric Artery **3** Hepatic Artery **4** Splenic Artery **5** Superior Mesenteric Artery **6** Colic Artery, Right **7** Colic Artery, Left **8** Colic Artery, Middle **9** Renal Artery, Right **A** Renal Artery, Left **B** Inferior Mesenteric Artery **C** Common Iliac Artery, Right **D** Common Iliac Artery, Left **E** Internal Iliac Artery, Right **F** Internal Iliac Artery, Left **H** External Iliac Artery, Right **J** External Iliac Artery, Left **K** Femoral Artery, Right **L** Femoral Artery, Left **M** Popliteal Artery, Right **N** Popliteal Artery, Left **P** Anterior Tibial Artery, Right **Q** Anterior Tibial Artery, Left **R** Posterior Tibial Artery, Right **S** Posterior Tibial Artery, Left **T** Peroneal Artery, Right **U** Peroneal Artery, Left **V** Foot Artery, Right **W** Foot Artery, Left **Y** Lower Artery	**0** Open **3** Percutaneous **4** Percutaneous Endoscopic	**Z** No Device	**Z** No Qualifier

0 Medical and Surgical
4 Lower Arteries
R Replacement: Putting in or on biological or synthetic material that physically takes the place and/or function of all or a portion of a body part

Body Part Character 4	Approach Character 5	Device Character 6	Qualifier Character 7
0 Abdominal Aorta **1** Celiac Artery **2** Gastric Artery **3** Hepatic Artery **4** Splenic Artery **5** Superior Mesenteric Artery **6** Colic Artery, Right **7** Colic Artery, Left **8** Colic Artery, Middle **9** Renal Artery, Right **A** Renal Artery, Left **B** Inferior Mesenteric Artery **C** Common Iliac Artery, Right **D** Common Iliac Artery, Left **E** Internal Iliac Artery, Right **F** Internal Iliac Artery, Left **H** External Iliac Artery, Right **J** External Iliac Artery, Left **K** Femoral Artery, Right **L** Femoral Artery, Left **M** Popliteal Artery, Right **N** Popliteal Artery, Left **P** Anterior Tibial Artery, Right **Q** Anterior Tibial Artery, Left **R** Posterior Tibial Artery, Right **S** Posterior Tibial Artery, Left **T** Peroneal Artery, Right **U** Peroneal Artery, Left **V** Foot Artery, Right **W** Foot Artery, Left **Y** Lower Artery	**0** Open **4** Percutaneous Endoscopic	**7** Autologous Tissue Substitute **J** Synthetic Substitute **K** Nonautologous Tissue Substitute	**Z** No Qualifier

0 Medical and Surgical
4 Lower Arteries
S Reposition: Moving to its normal location, or other suitable location, all or a portion of a body part

Body Part Character 4	Approach Character 5	Device Character 6	Qualifier Character 7
0 Abdominal Aorta **1** Celiac Artery **2** Gastric Artery **3** Hepatic Artery **4** Splenic Artery **5** Superior Mesenteric Artery **6** Colic Artery, Right **7** Colic Artery, Left **8** Colic Artery, Middle **9** Renal Artery, Right **A** Renal Artery, Left **B** Inferior Mesenteric Artery **C** Common Iliac Artery, Right **D** Common Iliac Artery, Left **E** Internal Iliac Artery, Right **F** Internal Iliac Artery, Left **H** External Iliac Artery, Right **J** External Iliac Artery, Left **K** Femoral Artery, Right **L** Femoral Artery, Left **M** Popliteal Artery, Right **N** Popliteal Artery, Left **P** Anterior Tibial Artery, Right **Q** Anterior Tibial Artery, Left **R** Posterior Tibial Artery, Right **S** Posterior Tibial Artery, Left **T** Peroneal Artery, Right **U** Peroneal Artery, Left **V** Foot Artery, Right **W** Foot Artery, Left **Y** Lower Artery	**0** Open **3** Percutaneous **4** Percutaneous Endoscopic	**Z** No Device	**Z** No Qualifier

0 Medical and Surgical
4 Lower Arteries
U Supplement: Putting in or on biological or synthetic material that physically reinforces and/or augments the function of a portion of a body part

Body Part Character 4	Approach Character 5	Device Character 6	Qualifier Character 7
0 Abdominal Aorta **1** Celiac Artery **2** Gastric Artery **3** Hepatic Artery **4** Splenic Artery **5** Superior Mesenteric Artery **6** Colic Artery, Right **7** Colic Artery, Left **8** Colic Artery, Middle **9** Renal Artery, Right **A** Renal Artery, Left **B** Inferior Mesenteric Artery **C** Common Iliac Artery, Right **D** Common Iliac Artery, Left **E** Internal Iliac Artery, Right **F** Internal Iliac Artery, Left **H** External Iliac Artery, Right **J** External Iliac Artery, Left **K** Femoral Artery, Right **L** Femoral Artery, Left **M** Popliteal Artery, Right **N** Popliteal Artery, Left **P** Anterior Tibial Artery, Right **Q** Anterior Tibial Artery, Left **R** Posterior Tibial Artery, Right **S** Posterior Tibial Artery, Left **T** Peroneal Artery, Right **U** Peroneal Artery, Left **V** Foot Artery, Right **W** Foot Artery, Left **Y** Lower Artery	**0** Open **3** Percutaneous **4** Percutaneous Endoscopic	**7** Autologous Tissue Substitute **J** Synthetic Substitute **K** Nonautologous Tissue Substitute	**Z** No Qualifier

0 Medical and Surgical
4 Lower Arteries
V Restriction: Partially closing an orifice or the lumen of a tubular body part

Body Part Character 4	Approach Character 5	Device Character 6	Qualifier Character 7
0 Abdominal Aorta	**0** Open **3** Percutaneous **4** Percutaneous Endoscopic	**C** Extraluminal Device **E** Intraluminal Device, Branched or Fenestrated, One or Two Arteries **F** Intraluminal Device, Branched or Fenestrated, Three or More Arteries **Z** No Device	**Z** No Qualifier
0 Abdominal Aorta	**0** Open **3** Percutaneous **4** Percutaneous Endoscopic	**D** Intraluminal Device	**J** Temporary **Z** No Qualifier
1 Celiac Artery **2** Gastric Artery **3** Hepatic Artery **4** Splenic Artery **5** Superior Mesenteric Artery **6** Colic Artery, Right **7** Colic Artery, Left **8** Colic Artery, Middle **9** Renal Artery, Right **A** Renal Artery, Left **B** Inferior Mesenteric Artery **E** Internal Iliac Artery, Right **F** Internal Iliac Artery, Left **H** External Iliac Artery, Right **J** External Iliac Artery, Left **K** Femoral Artery, Right **L** Femoral Artery, Left **M** Popliteal Artery, Right **N** Popliteal Artery, Left **P** Anterior Tibial Artery, Right **Q** Anterior Tibial Artery, Left **R** Posterior Tibial Artery, Right **S** Posterior Tibial Artery, Left **T** Peroneal Artery, Right **U** Peroneal Artery, Left **V** Foot Artery, Right **W** Foot Artery, Left **Y** Lower Artery	**0** Open **3** Percutaneous **4** Percutaneous Endoscopic	**C** Extraluminal Device **D** Intraluminal Device **Z** No Device	**Z** No Qualifier
C Common Iliac Artery, Right **D** Common Iliac Artery, Left	**0** Open **3** Percutaneous **4** Percutaneous Endoscopic	**C** Extraluminal Device **D** Intraluminal Device **E** Intraluminal Device, Branched or Fenestrated, One or Two Arteries **Z** No Device	**Z** No Qualifier

0 Medical and Surgical
4 Lower Arteries
W Revision: Correcting, to the extent possible, a portion of a malfunctioning device or the position of a displaced device

Body Part	Approach	Device	Qualifier
Character 4	**Character 5**	**Character 6**	**Character 7**
Y Lower Artery	**0** Open **3** Percutaneous **4** Percutaneous Endoscopic	**0** Drainage Device **2** Monitoring Device **3** Infusion Device **7** Autologous Tissue Substitute **C** Extraluminal Device **D** Intraluminal Device **J** Synthetic Substitute **K** Nonautologous Tissue Substitute **Y** Other Device	**Z** No Qualifier
Y Lower Artery	**X** External	**0** Drainage Device **2** Monitoring Device **3** Infusion Device **7** Autologous Tissue Substitute **C** Extraluminal Device **D** Intraluminal Device **J** Synthetic Substitute **K** Nonautologous Tissue Substitute	**Z** No Qualifier

NOTES

Upper Veins 051-05W

0 Medical and Surgical
5 Upper Veins
1 Bypass: Altering the route of passage of the contents of a tubular body part

Body Part Character 4	Approach Character 5	Device Character 6	Qualifier Character 7
0 Azygos Vein **1** Hemiazygos Vein **3** Innominate Vein, Right **4** Innominate Vein, Left **5** Subclavian Vein, Right **6** Subclavian Vein, Left **7** Axillary Vein, Right **8** Axillary Vein, Left **9** Brachial Vein, Right **A** Brachial Vein, Left **B** Basilic Vein, Right **C** Basilic Vein, Left **D** Cephalic Vein, Right **F** Cephalic Vein, Left **G** Hand Vein, Right **H** Hand Vein, Left **L** Intracranial Vein **M** Internal Jugular Vein, Right **N** Internal Jugular Vein, Left **P** External Jugular Vein, Right **Q** External Jugular Vein, Left **R** Vertebral Vein, Right **S** Vertebral Vein, Left **T** Face Vein, Right **V** Face Vein, Left	**0** Open **4** Percutaneous Endoscopic	**7** Autologous Tissue Substitute **9** Autologous Venous Tissue **A** Autologous Arterial Tissue **J** Synthetic Substitute **K** Nonautologous Tissue Substitute **Z** No Device	**Y** Upper Vein

0 Medical and Surgical
5 Upper Veins
5 Destruction: Physical eradication of all or a portion of a body part by the direct use of energy, force, or a destructive agent

Body Part Character 4	Approach Character 5	Device Character 6	Qualifier Character 7
0 Azygos Vein **1** Hemiazygos Vein **3** Innominate Vein, Right **4** Innominate Vein, Left **5** Subclavian Vein, Right **6** Subclavian Vein, Left **7** Axillary Vein, Right **8** Axillary Vein, Left **9** Brachial Vein, Right **A** Brachial Vein, Left **B** Basilic Vein, Right **C** Basilic Vein, Left **D** Cephalic Vein, Right **F** Cephalic Vein, Left **G** Hand Vein, Right **H** Hand Vein, Left **L** Intracranial Vein **M** Internal Jugular Vein, Right **N** Internal Jugular Vein, Left **P** External Jugular Vein, Right **Q** External Jugular Vein, Left **R** Vertebral Vein, Right **S** Vertebral Vein, Left **T** Face Vein, Right **V** Face Vein, Left **Y** Upper Vein	**0** Open **3** Percutaneous **4** Percutaneous Endoscopic	**Z** No Device	**Z** No Qualifier

0 Medical and Surgical
5 Upper Veins
7 Dilation: Expanding an orifice or the lumen of a tubular body part

Body Part Character 4	Approach Character 5	Device Character 6	Qualifier Character 7
0 Azygos Vein **1** Hemiazygos Vein **G** Hand Vein, Right **H** Hand Vein, Left **L** Intracranial Vein NC **M** Internal Jugular Vein, Right **N** Internal Jugular Vein, Left **P** External Jugular Vein, Right **Q** External Jugular Vein, Left **R** Vertebral Vein, Right **S** Vertebral Vein, Left **T** Face Vein, Right **V** Face Vein, Left **Y** Upper Vein	**0** Open **3** Percutaneous **4** Percutaneous Endoscopic	**D** Intraluminal Device **Z** No Device	**Z** No Qualifier
3 Innominate Vein, Right **4** Innominate Vein, Left **5** Subclavian Vein, Right **6** Subclavian Vein, Left **7** Axillary Vein, Right **8** Axillary Vein, Left **9** Brachial Vein, Right **A** Brachial Vein, Left **B** Basilic Vein, Right **C** Basilic Vein, Left **D** Cephalic Vein, Right **F** Cephalic Vein, Left	**0** Open **3** Percutaneous **4** Percutaneous Endoscopic	**D** Intraluminal Device **Z** No Device	**1** Drug-Coated Balloon **Z** No Qualifier

NC 057L3ZZ 057L4ZZ

0 Medical and Surgical
5 Upper Veins
9 Drainage: Taking or letting out fluids and/or gases from a body part

Body Part Character 4	Approach Character 5	Device Character 6	Qualifier Character 7
0 Azygos Vein **1** Hemiazygos Vein **3** Innominate Vein, Right **4** Innominate Vein, Left **5** Subclavian Vein, Right **6** Subclavian Vein, Left **7** Axillary Vein, Right **8** Axillary Vein, Left **9** Brachial Vein, Right **A** Brachial Vein, Left **B** Basilic Vein, Right **C** Basilic Vein, Left **D** Cephalic Vein, Right **F** Cephalic Vein, Left **G** Hand Vein, Right **H** Hand Vein, Left **L** Intracranial Vein **M** Internal Jugular Vein, Right **N** Internal Jugular Vein, Left **P** External Jugular Vein, Right **Q** External Jugular Vein, Left **R** Vertebral Vein, Right **S** Vertebral Vein, Left **T** Face Vein, Right **V** Face Vein, Left **Y** Upper Vein	**0** Open **3** Percutaneous **4** Percutaneous Endoscopic	**0** Drainage Device	**Z** No Qualifier
0 Azygos Vein **1** Hemiazygos Vein **3** Innominate Vein, Right **4** Innominate Vein, Left **5** Subclavian Vein, Right **6** Subclavian Vein, Left **7** Axillary Vein, Right **8** Axillary Vein, Left **9** Brachial Vein, Right **A** Brachial Vein, Left **B** Basilic Vein, Right **C** Basilic Vein, Left **D** Cephalic Vein, Right **F** Cephalic Vein, Left **G** Hand Vein, Right **H** Hand Vein, Left **L** Intracranial Vein **M** Internal Jugular Vein, Right **N** Internal Jugular Vein, Left **P** External Jugular Vein, Right **Q** External Jugular Vein, Left **R** Vertebral Vein, Right **S** Vertebral Vein, Left **T** Face Vein, Right **V** Face Vein, Left **Y** Upper Vein	**0** Open **3** Percutaneous **4** Percutaneous Endoscopic	**Z** No Device	**X** Diagnostic **Z** No Qualifier

0 Medical and Surgical
5 Upper Veins
B Excision: Cutting out or off, without replacement, a portion of a body part

Body Part Character 4	Approach Character 5	Device Character 6	Qualifier Character 7
0 Azygos Vein 1 Hemiazygos Vein 3 Innominate Vein, Right 4 Innominate Vein, Left 5 Subclavian Vein, Right 6 Subclavian Vein, Left 7 Axillary Vein, Right 8 Axillary Vein, Left 9 Brachial Vein, Right A Brachial Vein, Left B Basilic Vein, Right C Basilic Vein, Left D Cephalic Vein, Right F Cephalic Vein, Left G Hand Vein, Right H Hand Vein, Left L Intracranial Vein M Internal Jugular Vein, Right N Internal Jugular Vein, Left P External Jugular Vein, Right Q External Jugular Vein, Left R Vertebral Vein, Right S Vertebral Vein, Left T Face Vein, Right V Face Vein, Left Y Upper Vein	0 Open 3 Percutaneous 4 Percutaneous Endoscopic	Z No Device	X Diagnostic Z No Qualifier

0 Medical and Surgical
5 Upper Veins
C Extirpation: Taking or cutting out solid matter from a body part

Body Part Character 4	Approach Character 5	Device Character 6	Qualifier Character 7
0 Azygos Vein 1 Hemiazygos Vein 3 Innominate Vein, Right 4 Innominate Vein, Left 5 Subclavian Vein, Right 6 Subclavian Vein, Left 7 Axillary Vein, Right 8 Axillary Vein, Left 9 Brachial Vein, Right A Brachial Vein, Left B Basilic Vein, Right C Basilic Vein, Left D Cephalic Vein, Right F Cephalic Vein, Left G Hand Vein, Right H Hand Vein, Left L Intracranial Vein M Internal Jugular Vein, Right N Internal Jugular Vein, Left P External Jugular Vein, Right Q External Jugular Vein, Left R Vertebral Vein, Right S Vertebral Vein, Left T Face Vein, Right V Face Vein, Left Y Upper Vein	0 Open 3 Percutaneous 4 Percutaneous Endoscopic	Z No Device	Z No Qualifier

0 Medical and Surgical
5 Upper Veins
D Extraction: Pulling or stripping out or off all or a portion of a body part by the use of force

Body Part Character 4	Approach Character 5	Device Character 6	Qualifier Character 7
9 Brachial Vein, Right **A** Brachial Vein, Left **B** Basilic Vein, Right **C** Basilic Vein, Left **D** Cephalic Vein, Right **F** Cephalic Vein, Left **G** Hand Vein, Right **H** Hand Vein, Left **Y** Upper Vein	**0** Open **3** Percutaneous	**Z** No Device	**Z** No Qualifier

0 Medical and Surgical
5 Upper Veins
H Insertion: Putting in a nonbiological appliance that monitors, assists, performs, or prevents a physiological function but does not physically take the place of a body part

Body Part Character 4	Approach Character 5	Device Character 6	Qualifier Character 7
0 Azygos Vein HAC CC	**0** Open **3** Percutaneous **4** Percutaneous Endoscopic	**2** Monitoring Device **3** Infusion Device **D** Intraluminal Device **M** Neurostimulator Lead	**Z** No Qualifier
1 Hemiazygos Vein HAC **5** Subclavian Vein, Right HAC **6** Subclavian Vein, Left HAC **7** Axillary Vein, Right **8** Axillary Vein, Left **9** Brachial Vein, Right **A** Brachial Vein, Left **B** Basilic Vein, Right **C** Basilic Vein, Left **D** Cephalic Vein, Right **F** Cephalic Vein, Left **G** Hand Vein, Right **H** Hand Vein, Left **L** Intracranial Vein **M** Internal Jugular Vein, Right HAC **N** Internal Jugular Vein, Left HAC **P** External Jugular Vein, Right HAC **Q** External Jugular Vein, Left HAC **R** Vertebral Vein, Right **S** Vertebral Vein, Left **T** Face Vein, Right **V** Face Vein, Left	**0** Open **3** Percutaneous **4** Percutaneous Endoscopic	**3** Infusion Device **D** Intraluminal Device	**Z** No Qualifier
3 Innominate Vein, Right HAC CC **4** Innominate Vein, Left HAC CC	**0** Open **3** Percutaneous **4** Percutaneous Endoscopic	**3** Infusion Device **D** Intraluminal Device **M** Neurostimulator Lead	**Z** No Qualifier
Y Upper Vein	**0** Open **3** Percutaneous **4** Percutaneous Endoscopic	**2** Monitoring Device **3** Infusion Device **D** Intraluminal Device **Y** Other Device	**Z** No Qualifier

HAC 05H033Z 05H043Z 05H133Z 05H143Z 05H333Z 05H343Z 05H433Z 05H443Z 05H533Z 05H543Z 05H633Z 05H643Z 05HM33Z 05HN33Z 05HP33Z 05HQ33Z
Iatrogenic pneumothorax w/ venous catheterization procedures and secondary diagnosis J95.811.
CC 05H00MZ 05H03MZ 05H04MZ 05H30MZ 05H33MZ 05H34MZ 05H40MZ 05H43MZ 05H44MZ

0 Medical and Surgical
5 Upper Veins
J Inspection: Visually and/or manually exploring a body part

Body Part	Approach	Device	Qualifier
Character 4	**Character 5**	**Character 6**	**Character 7**
Y Upper Vein	**0** Open **3** Percutaneous **4** Percutaneous Endoscopic **X** External	**Z** No Device	**Z** No Qualifier

0 Medical and Surgical
5 Upper Veins
L Occlusion: Completely closing an orifice or the lumen of a tubular body part

Body Part	Approach	Device	Qualifier
Character 4	**Character 5**	**Character 6**	**Character 7**
0 Azygos Vein **1** Hemiazygos Vein **3** Innominate Vein, Right **4** Innominate Vein, Left **5** Subclavian Vein, Right **6** Subclavian Vein, Left **7** Axillary Vein, Right **8** Axillary Vein, Left **9** Brachial Vein, Right **A** Brachial Vein, Left **B** Basilic Vein, Right **C** Basilic Vein, Left **D** Cephalic Vein, Right **F** Cephalic Vein, Left **G** Hand Vein, Right **H** Hand Vein, Left **L** Intracranial Vein **M** Internal Jugular Vein, Right **N** Internal Jugular Vein, Left **P** External Jugular Vein, Right **Q** External Jugular Vein, Left **R** Vertebral Vein, Right **S** Vertebral Vein, Left **T** Face Vein, Right **V** Face Vein, Left **Y** Upper Vein	**0** Open **3** Percutaneous **4** Percutaneous Endoscopic	**C** Extraluminal Device **D** Intraluminal Device **Z** No Device	**Z** No Qualifier

0 Medical and Surgical
5 Upper Veins
N Release: Freeing a body part from an abnormal physical constraint by cutting or by the use of force

Body Part Character 4	Approach Character 5	Device Character 6	Qualifier Character 7
0 Azygos Vein **1** Hemiazygos Vein **3** Innominate Vein, Right **4** Innominate Vein, Left **5** Subclavian Vein, Right **6** Subclavian Vein, Left **7** Axillary Vein, Right **8** Axillary Vein, Left **9** Brachial Vein, Right **A** Brachial Vein, Left **B** Basilic Vein, Right **C** Basilic Vein, Left **D** Cephalic Vein, Right **F** Cephalic Vein, Left **G** Hand Vein, Right **H** Hand Vein, Left **L** Intracranial Vein **M** Internal Jugular Vein, Right **N** Internal Jugular Vein, Left **P** External Jugular Vein, Right **Q** External Jugular Vein, Left **R** Vertebral Vein, Right **S** Vertebral Vein, Left **T** Face Vein, Right **V** Face Vein, Left **Y** Upper Vein	**0** Open **3** Percutaneous **4** Percutaneous Endoscopic	**Z** No Device	**Z** No Qualifier

0 Medical and Surgical
5 Upper Veins
P Removal: Taking out or off a device from a body part

Body Part Character 4	Approach Character 5	Device Character 6	Qualifier Character 7
0 Azygos Vein	**0** Open **3** Percutaneous **4** Percutaneous Endoscopic **X** External	**2** Monitoring Device **M** Neurostimulator Lead	**Z** No Qualifier
3 Innominate Vein, Right **4** Innominate Vein, Left	**0** Open **3** Percutaneous **4** Percutaneous Endoscopic **X** External	**M** Neurostimulator Lead	**Z** No Qualifier
Y Upper Vein Subclavian Vein	**0** Open **3** Percutaneous **4** Percutaneous Endoscopic	**0** Drainage Device **2** Monitoring Device **3** Infusion Device - chemo **7** Autologous Tissue Substitute **C** Extraluminal Device **D** Intraluminal Device **J** Synthetic Substitute **K** Nonautologous Tissue Substitute **Y** Other Device	**Z** No Qualifier
Y Upper Vein	**X** External	**0** Drainage Device **2** Monitoring Device **3** Infusion Device **D** Intraluminal Device	**Z** No Qualifier

0 Medical and Surgical
5 Upper Veins
Q Repair: Restoring, to the extent possible, a body part to its normal anatomic structure and function

Body Part Character 4	Approach Character 5	Device Character 6	Qualifier Character 7
0 Azygos Vein **1** Hemiazygos Vein **3** Innominate Vein, Right **4** Innominate Vein, Left **5** Subclavian Vein, Right **6** Subclavian Vein, Left **7** Axillary Vein, Right **8** Axillary Vein, Left **9** Brachial Vein, Right **A** Brachial Vein, Left **B** Basilic Vein, Right **C** Basilic Vein, Left **D** Cephalic Vein, Right **F** Cephalic Vein, Left **G** Hand Vein, Right **H** Hand Vein, Left **L** Intracranial Vein **M** Internal Jugular Vein, Right **N** Internal Jugular Vein, Left **P** External Jugular Vein, Right **Q** External Jugular Vein, Left **R** Vertebral Vein, Right **S** Vertebral Vein, Left **T** Face Vein, Right **V** Face Vein, Left **Y** Upper Vein	**0** Open **3** Percutaneous **4** Percutaneous Endoscopic	**Z** No Device	**Z** No Qualifier

0 Medical and Surgical
5 Upper Veins
R Replacement: Putting in or on biological or synthetic material that physically takes the place and/or function of all or a portion of a body part

Body Part Character 4	Approach Character 5	Device Character 6	Qualifier Character 7
0 Azygos Vein **1** Hemiazygos Vein **3** Innominate Vein, Right **4** Innominate Vein, Left **5** Subclavian Vein, Right **6** Subclavian Vein, Left **7** Axillary Vein, Right **8** Axillary Vein, Left **9** Brachial Vein, Right **A** Brachial Vein, Left **B** Basilic Vein, Right **C** Basilic Vein, Left **D** Cephalic Vein, Right **F** Cephalic Vein, Left **G** Hand Vein, Right **H** Hand Vein, Left **L** Intracranial Vein **M** Internal Jugular Vein, Right **N** Internal Jugular Vein, Left **P** External Jugular Vein, Right **Q** External Jugular Vein, Left **R** Vertebral Vein, Right **S** Vertebral Vein, Left **T** Face Vein, Right **V** Face Vein, Left **Y** Upper Vein	**0** Open **4** Percutaneous Endoscopic	**7** Autologous Tissue Substitute **J** Synthetic Substitute **K** Nonautologous Tissue Substitute	**Z** No Qualifier

0 **Medical and Surgical**
5 **Upper Veins**
S **Reposition:** Moving to its normal location, or other suitable location, all or a portion of a body part

Body Part Character 4	Approach Character 5	Device Character 6	Qualifier Character 7
0 Azygos Vein **1** Hemiazygos Vein **3** Innominate Vein, Right **4** Innominate Vein, Left **5** Subclavian Vein, Right **6** Subclavian Vein, Left **7** Axillary Vein, Right **8** Axillary Vein, Left **9** Brachial Vein, Right **A** Brachial Vein, Left **B** Basilic Vein, Right **C** Basilic Vein, Left **D** Cephalic Vein, Right **F** Cephalic Vein, Left **G** Hand Vein, Right **H** Hand Vein, Left **L** Intracranial Vein **M** Internal Jugular Vein, Right **N** Internal Jugular Vein, Left **P** External Jugular Vein, Right **Q** External Jugular Vein, Left **R** Vertebral Vein, Right **S** Vertebral Vein, Left **T** Face Vein, Right **V** Face Vein, Left **Y** Upper Vein	**0** Open **3** Percutaneous **4** Percutaneous Endoscopic	**Z** No Device	**Z** No Qualifier

0 **Medical and Surgical**
5 **Upper Veins**
U **Supplement:** Putting in or on biological or synthetic material that physically reinforces and/or augments the function of a portion of a body part

Body Part Character 4	Approach Character 5	Device Character 6	Qualifier Character 7
0 Azygos Vein **1** Hemiazygos Vein **3** Innominate Vein, Right **4** Innominate Vein, Left **5** Subclavian Vein, Right **6** Subclavian Vein, Left **7** Axillary Vein, Right **8** Axillary Vein, Left **9** Brachial Vein, Right **A** Brachial Vein, Left **B** Basilic Vein, Right **C** Basilic Vein, Left **D** Cephalic Vein, Right **F** Cephalic Vein, Left **G** Hand Vein, Right **H** Hand Vein, Left **L** Intracranial Vein **M** Internal Jugular Vein, Right **N** Internal Jugular Vein, Left **P** External Jugular Vein, Right **Q** External Jugular Vein, Left **R** Vertebral Vein, Right **S** Vertebral Vein, Left **T** Face Vein, Right **V** Face Vein, Left **Y** Upper Vein	**0** Open **3** Percutaneous **4** Percutaneous Endoscopic	**7** Autologous Tissue Substitute **J** Synthetic Substitute **K** Nonautologous Tissue Substitute	**Z** No Qualifier

0 Medical and Surgical
5 Upper Veins
V Restriction: Partially closing an orifice or the lumen of a tubular body part

Body Part Character 4	Approach Character 5	Device Character 6	Qualifier Character 7
0 Azygos Vein **1** Hemiazygos Vein **3** Innominate Vein, Right **4** Innominate Vein, Left **5** Subclavian Vein, Right **6** Subclavian Vein, Left **7** Axillary Vein, Right **8** Axillary Vein, Left **9** Brachial Vein, Right **A** Brachial Vein, Left **B** Basilic Vein, Right **C** Basilic Vein, Left **D** Cephalic Vein, Right **F** Cephalic Vein, Left **G** Hand Vein, Right **H** Hand Vein, Left **L** Intracranial Vein **M** Internal Jugular Vein, Right **N** Internal Jugular Vein, Left **P** External Jugular Vein, Right **Q** External Jugular Vein, Left **R** Vertebral Vein, Right **S** Vertebral Vein, Left **T** Face Vein, Right **V** Face Vein, Left **Y** Upper Vein	**0** Open **3** Percutaneous **4** Percutaneous Endoscopic	**C** Extraluminal Device **D** Intraluminal Device **Z** No Device	**Z** No Qualifier

0 Medical and Surgical
5 Upper Veins
W Revision: Correcting, to the extent possible, a portion of a malfunctioning device or the position of a displaced device

Body Part Character 4	Approach Character 5	Device Character 6	Qualifier Character 7
0 Azygos Vein	**0** Open **3** Percutaneous **4** Percutaneous Endoscopic **X** External	**2** Monitoring Device **M** Neurostimulator Lead	**Z** No Qualifier
3 Innominate Vein, Right **4** Innominate Vein, Left	**0** Open **3** Percutaneous **4** Percutaneous Endoscopic **X** External	**M** Neurostimulator Lead	**Z** No Qualifier
Y Upper Vein	**0** Open **3** Percutaneous **4** Percutaneous Endoscopic	**0** Drainage Device **2** Monitoring Device **3** Infusion Device **7** Autologous Tissue Substitute **C** Extraluminal Device **D** Intraluminal Device **J** Synthetic Substitute **K** Nonautologous Tissue Substitute **Y** Other Device	**Z** No Qualifier
Y Upper Vein	**X** External	**0** Drainage Device **2** Monitoring Device **3** Infusion Device **7** Autologous Tissue Substitute **C** Extraluminal Device **D** Intraluminal Device **J** Synthetic Substitute **K** Nonautologous Tissue Substitute	**Z** No Qualifier

NOTES

NOTES

Lower Veins 061-06W

0 Medical and Surgical
6 Lower Veins
1 Bypass: Altering the route of passage of the contents of a tubular body part

Body Part Character 4	Approach Character 5	Device Character 6	Qualifier Character 7
0 Inferior Vena Cava	**0** Open **4** Percutaneous Endoscopic	**7** Autologous Tissue Substitute **9** Autologous Venous Tissue **A** Autologous Arterial Tissue **J** Synthetic Substitute **K** Nonautologous Tissue Substitute **Z** No Device	**5** Superior Mesenteric Vein **6** Inferior Mesenteric Vein **P** Pulmonary Trunk **Q** Pulmonary Artery, Right **R** Pulmonary Artery, Left **Y** Lower Vein
1 Splenic Vein	**0** Open **4** Percutaneous Endoscopic	**7** Autologous Tissue Substitute **9** Autologous Venous Tissue **A** Autologous Arterial Tissue **J** Synthetic Substitute **K** Nonautologous Tissue Substitute **Z** No Device	**9** Renal Vein, Right **B** Renal Vein, Left **Y** Lower Vein
2 Gastric Vein **3** Esophageal Vein **4** Hepatic Vein **5** Superior Mesenteric Vein **6** Inferior Mesenteric Vein **7** Colic Vein **9** Renal Vein, Right **B** Renal Vein, Left **C** Common Iliac Vein, Right **D** Common Iliac Vein, Left **F** External Iliac Vein, Right **G** External Iliac Vein, Left **H** Hypogastric Vein, Right **J** Hypogastric Vein, Left **M** Femoral Vein, Right **N** Femoral Vein, Left **P** Saphenous Vein, Right **Q** Saphenous Vein, Left **T** Foot Vein, Right **V** Foot Vein, Left	**0** Open **4** Percutaneous Endoscopic	**7** Autologous Tissue Substitute **9** Autologous Venous Tissue **A** Autologous Arterial Tissue **J** Synthetic Substitute **K** Nonautologous Tissue Substitute **Z** No Device	**Y** Lower Vein
8 Portal Vein	**0** Open	**7** Autologous Tissue Substitute **9** Autologous Venous Tissue **A** Autologous Arterial Tissue **J** Synthetic Substitute **K** Nonautologous Tissue Substitute **Z** No Device	**9** Renal Vein, Right **B** Renal Vein, Left **Y** Lower Vein
8 Portal Vein	**3** Percutaneous	**J** Synthetic Substitute	**4** Hepatic Vein **Y** Lower Vein
8 Portal Vein	**4** Percutaneous Endoscopic	**7** Autologous Tissue Substitute **9** Autologous Venous Tissue **A** Autologous Arterial Tissue **K** Nonautologous Tissue Substitute **Z** No Device	**9** Renal Vein, Right **B** Renal Vein, Left **Y** Lower Vein
8 Portal Vein	**4** Percutaneous Endoscopic	**J** Synthetic Substitute	**4** Hepatic Vein **9** Renal Vein, Right **B** Renal Vein, Left **Y** Lower Vein

0 Medical and Surgical
6 Lower Veins
5 Destruction: Physical eradication of all or a portion of a body part by the direct use of energy, force, or a destructive agent

Body Part Character 4	Approach Character 5	Device Character 6	Qualifier Character 7
0 Inferior Vena Cava **1** Splenic Vein **2** Gastric Vein **3** Esophageal Vein **4** Hepatic Vein **5** Superior Mesenteric Vein **6** Inferior Mesenteric Vein **7** Colic Vein **8** Portal Vein **9** Renal Vein, Right **B** Renal Vein, Left **C** Common Iliac Vein, Right **D** Common Iliac Vein, Left **F** External Iliac Vein, Right **G** External Iliac Vein, Left **H** Hypogastric Vein, Right **J** Hypogastric Vein, Left **M** Femoral Vein, Right **N** Femoral Vein, Left **P** Saphenous Vein, Right **Q** Saphenous Vein, Left **T** Foot Vein, Right **V** Foot Vein, Left	**0** Open **3** Percutaneous **4** Percutaneous Endoscopic	**Z** No Device	**Z** No Qualifier
Y Lower Vein	**0** Open **3** Percutaneous **4** Percutaneous Endoscopic	**Z** No Device	**C** Hemorrhoidal Plexus **Z** No Qualifier

0 Medical and Surgical
6 Lower Veins
7 Dilation: Expanding an orifice or the lumen of a tubular body part

Body Part Character 4	Approach Character 5	Device Character 6	Qualifier Character 7
0 Inferior Vena Cava **1** Splenic Vein **2** Gastric Vein **3** Esophageal Vein **4** Hepatic Vein **5** Superior Mesenteric Vein **6** Inferior Mesenteric Vein **7** Colic Vein **8** Portal Vein **9** Renal Vein, Right **B** Renal Vein, Left **C** Common Iliac Vein, Right **D** Common Iliac Vein, Left **F** External Iliac Vein, Right **G** External Iliac Vein, Left **H** Hypogastric Vein, Right **J** Hypogastric Vein, Left **M** Femoral Vein, Right **N** Femoral Vein, Left **P** Saphenous Vein, Right **Q** Saphenous Vein, Left **T** Foot Vein, Right **V** Foot Vein, Left **Y** Lower Vein	**0** Open **3** Percutaneous **4** Percutaneous Endoscopic	**D** Intraluminal Device **Z** No Device	**Z** No Qualifier

0 Medical and Surgical
6 Lower Veins
9 Drainage: Taking or letting out fluids and/or gases from a body part

Body Part Character 4	Approach Character 5	Device Character 6	Qualifier Character 7
0 Inferior Vena Cava **1** Splenic Vein **2** Gastric Vein **3** Esophageal Vein **4** Hepatic Vein **5** Superior Mesenteric Vein **6** Inferior Mesenteric Vein **7** Colic Vein **8** Portal Vein **9** Renal Vein, Right **B** Renal Vein, Left **C** Common Iliac Vein, Right **D** Common Iliac Vein, Left **F** External Iliac Vein, Right **G** External Iliac Vein, Left **H** Hypogastric Vein, Right **J** Hypogastric Vein, Left **M** Femoral Vein, Right **N** Femoral Vein, Left **P** Saphenous Vein, Right **Q** Saphenous Vein, Left **T** Foot Vein, Right **V** Foot Vein, Left **Y** Lower Vein	**0** Open **3** Percutaneous **4** Percutaneous Endoscopic	**0** Drainage Device	**Z** No Qualifier
0 Inferior Vena Cava **1** Splenic Vein **2** Gastric Vein **3** Esophageal Vein **4** Hepatic Vein **5** Superior Mesenteric Vein **6** Inferior Mesenteric Vein **7** Colic Vein **8** Portal Vein **9** Renal Vein, Right **B** Renal Vein, Left **C** Common Iliac Vein, Right **D** Common Iliac Vein, Left **F** External Iliac Vein, Right **G** External Iliac Vein, Left **H** Hypogastric Vein, Right **J** Hypogastric Vein, Left **M** Femoral Vein, Right **N** Femoral Vein, Left **P** Saphenous Vein, Right **Q** Saphenous Vein, Left **T** Foot Vein, Right **V** Foot Vein, Left **Y** Lower Vein	**0** Open **3** Percutaneous **4** Percutaneous Endoscopic	**Z** No Device	**X** Diagnostic **Z** No Qualifier

0 Medical and Surgical
6 Lower Veins
B Excision: Cutting out or off, without replacement, a portion of a body part

Body Part Character 4	Approach Character 5	Device Character 6	Qualifier Character 7
0 Inferior Vena Cava **1** Splenic Vein **2** Gastric Vein **3** Esophageal Vein **4** Hepatic Vein **5** Superior Mesenteric Vein **6** Inferior Mesenteric Vein **7** Colic Vein **8** Portal Vein **9** Renal Vein, Right **B** Renal Vein, Left **C** Common Iliac Vein, Right **D** Common Iliac Vein, Left **F** External Iliac Vein, Right **G** External Iliac Vein, Left **H** Hypogastric Vein, Right **J** Hypogastric Vein, Left **M** Femoral Vein, Right **N** Femoral Vein, Left **P** Saphenous Vein, Right **Q** Saphenous Vein, Left **T** Foot Vein, Right **V** Foot Vein, Left	**0** Open **3** Percutaneous **4** Percutaneous Endoscopic	**Z** No Device	**X** Diagnostic **Z** No Qualifier
Y Lower Vein	**0** Open **3** Percutaneous **4** Percutaneous Endoscopic	**Z** No Device	**C** Hemorrhoidal Plexus **X** Diagnostic **Z** No Qualifier

0 Medical and Surgical
6 Lower Veins
C Extirpation: Taking or cutting out solid matter from a body part

Body Part Character 4	Approach Character 5	Device Character 6	Qualifier Character 7
0 Inferior Vena Cava **1** Splenic Vein **2** Gastric Vein **3** Esophageal Vein **4** Hepatic Vein **5** Superior Mesenteric Vein **6** Inferior Mesenteric Vein **7** Colic Vein **8** Portal Vein **9** Renal Vein, Right **B** Renal Vein, Left **C** Common Iliac Vein, Right **D** Common Iliac Vein, Left **F** External Iliac Vein, Right **G** External Iliac Vein, Left **H** Hypogastric Vein, Right **J** Hypogastric Vein, Left **M** Femoral Vein, Right **N** Femoral Vein, Left **P** Saphenous Vein, Right **Q** Saphenous Vein, Left **T** Foot Vein, Right **V** Foot Vein, Left **Y** Lower Vein	**0** Open **3** Percutaneous **4** Percutaneous Endoscopic	**Z** No Device	**Z** No Qualifier

0 Medical and Surgical
6 Lower Veins
D Extraction: Pulling or stripping out or off all or a portion of a body part by the use of force

Body Part Character 4	Approach Character 5	Device Character 6	Qualifier Character 7
M Femoral Vein, Right **N** Femoral Vein, Left **P** Saphenous Vein, Right **Q** Saphenous Vein, Left **T** Foot Vein, Right **V** Foot Vein, Left **Y** Lower Vein	**0** Open **3** Percutaneous **4** Percutaneous Endoscopic	**Z** No Device	**Z** No Qualifier

0 Medical and Surgical
6 Lower Veins
H Insertion: Putting in a nonbiological appliance that monitors, assists, performs, or prevents a physiological function but does not physically take the place of a body part

Body Part Character 4	Approach Character 5	Device Character 6	Qualifier Character 7
0 Inferior Vena Cava	**0** Open **3** Percutaneous	**3** Infusion Device	**T** Via Umbilical Vein **Z** No Qualifier
0 Inferior Vena Cava	**0** Open **3** Percutaneous	**D** Intraluminal Device	**Z** No Qualifier
0 Inferior Vena Cava	**4** Percutaneous Endoscopic	**3** Infusion Device **D** Intraluminal Device	**Z** No Qualifier
1 Splenic Vein **2** Gastric Vein **3** Esophageal Vein **4** Hepatic Vein **5** Superior Mesenteric Vein **6** Inferior Mesenteric Vein **7** Colic Vein **8** Portal Vein **9** Renal Vein, Right **B** Renal Vein, Left **C** Common Iliac Vein, Right **D** Common Iliac Vein, Left **F** External Iliac Vein, Right **G** External Iliac Vein, Left **H** Hypogastric Vein, Right **J** Hypogastric Vein, Left **M** Femoral Vein, Right **N** Femoral Vein, Left **P** Saphenous Vein, Right **Q** Saphenous Vein, Left **T** Foot Vein, Right **V** Foot Vein, Left	**0** Open **3** Percutaneous **4** Percutaneous Endoscopic	**3** Infusion Device **D** Intraluminal Device	**Z** No Qualifier
Y Lower Vein	**0** Open **3** Percutaneous **4** Percutaneous Endoscopic	**2** Monitoring Device **3** Infusion Device **D** Intraluminal Device **Y** Other Device	**Z** No Qualifier

LC Limited Coverage NC Noncovered HAC HAC-associated Procedure CC Combination Cluster - See Appendix G for code lists
DRG Non-OR-Affecting MS-DRG Assignment New/Revised Text in **Orange** ♂ Male ♀ Female

2020 ICD-10-PCS

259

0 Medical and Surgical
6 Lower Veins
J Inspection: Visually and/or manually exploring a body part

Body Part Character 4	Approach Character 5	Device Character 6	Qualifier Character 7
Y Lower Vein	**0** Open **3** Percutaneous **4** Percutaneous Endoscopic **X** External	**Z** No Device	**Z** No Qualifier

0 Medical and Surgical
6 Lower Veins
L Occlusion: Completely closing an orifice or the lumen of a tubular body part

Body Part Character 4	Approach Character 5	Device Character 6	Qualifier Character 7
0 Inferior Vena Cava **1** Splenic Vein **4** Hepatic Vein **5** Superior Mesenteric Vein **6** Inferior Mesenteric Vein **7** Colic Vein **8** Portal Vein **9** Renal Vein, Right **B** Renal Vein, Left **C** Common Iliac Vein, Right **D** Common Iliac Vein, Left **F** External Iliac Vein, Right **G** External Iliac Vein, Left **H** Hypogastric Vein, Right **J** Hypogastric Vein, Left **M** Femoral Vein, Right **N** Femoral Vein, Left **P** Saphenous Vein, Right **Q** Saphenous Vein, Left **T** Foot Vein, Right **V** Foot Vein, Left	**0** Open **3** Percutaneous **4** Percutaneous Endoscopic	**C** Extraluminal Device **D** Intraluminal Device **Z** No Device	**Z** No Qualifier
2 Gastric Vein **3** Esophageal Vein	**0** Open **3** Percutaneous **4** Percutaneous Endoscopic **7** Via Natural or Artificial Opening **8** Via Natural or Artificial Opening Endoscopic	**C** Extraluminal Device **D** Intraluminal Device **Z** No Device	**Z** No Qualifier
Y Lower Vein	**0** Open **3** Percutaneous **4** Percutaneous Endoscopic	**C** Extraluminal Device **D** Intraluminal Device **Z** No Device	**C** Hemorrhoidal Plexus **Z** No Qualifier

0 Medical and Surgical
6 Lower Veins
N Release: Freeing a body part from an abnormal physical constraint by cutting or by the use of force

Body Part Character 4	Approach Character 5	Device Character 6	Qualifier Character 7
0 Inferior Vena Cava **1** Splenic Vein **2** Gastric Vein **3** Esophageal Vein **4** Hepatic Vein **5** Superior Mesenteric Vein **6** Inferior Mesenteric Vein **7** Colic Vein **8** Portal Vein **9** Renal Vein, Right **B** Renal Vein, Left **C** Common Iliac Vein, Right **D** Common Iliac Vein, Left **F** External Iliac Vein, Right **G** External Iliac Vein, Left **H** Hypogastric Vein, Right **J** Hypogastric Vein, Left **M** Femoral Vein, Right **N** Femoral Vein, Left **P** Saphenous Vein, Right **Q** Saphenous Vein, Left **T** Foot Vein, Right **V** Foot Vein, Left **Y** Lower Vein	**0** Open **3** Percutaneous **4** Percutaneous Endoscopic	**Z** No Device	**Z** No Qualifier

0 Medical and Surgical
6 Lower Veins
P Removal: Taking out or off a device from a body part

Body Part Character 4	Approach Character 5	Device Character 6	Qualifier Character 7
Y Lower Vein	**0** Open **3** Percutaneous **4** Percutaneous Endoscopic	**0** Drainage Device **2** Monitoring Device **3** Infusion Device **7** Autologous Tissue Substitute **C** Extraluminal Device **D** Intraluminal Device **J** Synthetic Substitute **K** Nonautologous Tissue Substitute **Y** Other Device	**Z** No Qualifier
Y Lower Vein	**X** External	**0** Drainage Device **2** Monitoring Device **3** Infusion Device **D** Intraluminal Device	**Z** No Qualifier

0 Medical and Surgical
6 Lower Veins
Q Repair: Restoring, to the extent possible, a body part to its normal anatomic structure and function

Body Part Character 4	Approach Character 5	Device Character 6	Qualifier Character 7
0 Inferior Vena Cava **1** Splenic Vein **2** Gastric Vein **3** Esophageal Vein **4** Hepatic Vein **5** Superior Mesenteric Vein **6** Inferior Mesenteric Vein **7** Colic Vein **8** Portal Vein **9** Renal Vein, Right **B** Renal Vein, Left **C** Common Iliac Vein, Right **D** Common Iliac Vein, Left **F** External Iliac Vein, Right **G** External Iliac Vein, Left **H** Hypogastric Vein, Right **J** Hypogastric Vein, Left **M** Femoral Vein, Right **N** Femoral Vein, Left **P** Saphenous Vein, Right **Q** Saphenous Vein, Left **T** Foot Vein, Right **V** Foot Vein, Left **Y** Lower Vein	**0** Open **3** Percutaneous **4** Percutaneous Endoscopic	**Z** No Device	**Z** No Qualifier

0 Medical and Surgical
6 Lower Veins
R Replacement: Putting in or on biological or synthetic material that physically takes the place and/or function of all or a portion of a body part

Body Part Character 4	Approach Character 5	Device Character 6	Qualifier Character 7
0 Inferior Vena Cava **1** Splenic Vein **2** Gastric Vein **3** Esophageal Vein **4** Hepatic Vein **5** Superior Mesenteric Vein **6** Inferior Mesenteric Vein **7** Colic Vein **8** Portal Vein **9** Renal Vein, Right **B** Renal Vein, Left **C** Common Iliac Vein, Right **D** Common Iliac Vein, Left **F** External Iliac Vein, Right **G** External Iliac Vein, Left **H** Hypogastric Vein, Right **J** Hypogastric Vein, Left **M** Femoral Vein, Right **N** Femoral Vein, Left **P** Saphenous Vein, Right **Q** Saphenous Vein, Left **T** Foot Vein, Right **V** Foot Vein, Left **Y** Lower Vein	**0** Open **4** Percutaneous Endoscopic	**7** Autologous Tissue Substitute **J** Synthetic Substitute **K** Nonautologous Tissue Substitute	**Z** No Qualifier

0 Medical and Surgical
6 Lower Veins
S Reposition: Moving to its normal location, or other suitable location, all or a portion of a body part

Body Part Character 4	Approach Character 5	Device Character 6	Qualifier Character 7
0 Inferior Vena Cava 1 Splenic Vein 2 Gastric Vein 3 Esophageal Vein 4 Hepatic Vein 5 Superior Mesenteric Vein 6 Inferior Mesenteric Vein 7 Colic Vein 8 Portal Vein 9 Renal Vein, Right B Renal Vein, Left C Common Iliac Vein, Right D Common Iliac Vein, Left F External Iliac Vein, Right G External Iliac Vein, Left H Hypogastric Vein, Right J Hypogastric Vein, Left M Femoral Vein, Right N Femoral Vein, Left P Saphenous Vein, Right Q Saphenous Vein, Left T Foot Vein, Right V Foot Vein, Left Y Lower Vein	0 Open 3 Percutaneous 4 Percutaneous Endoscopic	Z No Device	Z No Qualifier

0 Medical and Surgical
6 Lower Veins
U Supplement: Putting in or on biological or synthetic material that physically reinforces and/or augments the function of a portion of a body part

Body Part Character 4	Approach Character 5	Device Character 6	Qualifier Character 7
0 Inferior Vena Cava 1 Splenic Vein 2 Gastric Vein 3 Esophageal Vein 4 Hepatic Vein 5 Superior Mesenteric Vein 6 Inferior Mesenteric Vein 7 Colic Vein 8 Portal Vein 9 Renal Vein, Right B Renal Vein, Left C Common Iliac Vein, Right D Common Iliac Vein, Left F External Iliac Vein, Right G External Iliac Vein, Left H Hypogastric Vein, Right J Hypogastric Vein, Left M Femoral Vein, Right N Femoral Vein, Left P Saphenous Vein, Right Q Saphenous Vein, Left T Foot Vein, Right V Foot Vein, Left Y Lower Vein	0 Open 3 Percutaneous 4 Percutaneous Endoscopic	7 Autologous Tissue Substitute J Synthetic Substitute K Nonautologous Tissue Substitute	Z No Qualifier

0 Medical and Surgical
6 Lower Veins
V Restriction: Partially closing an orifice or the lumen of a tubular body part

Body Part Character 4	Approach Character 5	Device Character 6	Qualifier Character 7
0 Inferior Vena Cava **1** Splenic Vein **2** Gastric Vein **3** Esophageal Vein **4** Hepatic Vein **5** Superior Mesenteric Vein **6** Inferior Mesenteric Vein **7** Colic Vein **8** Portal Vein **9** Renal Vein, Right **B** Renal Vein, Left **C** Common Iliac Vein, Right **D** Common Iliac Vein, Left **F** External Iliac Vein, Right **G** External Iliac Vein, Left **H** Hypogastric Vein, Right **J** Hypogastric Vein, Left **M** Femoral Vein, Right **N** Femoral Vein, Left **P** Saphenous Vein, Right **Q** Saphenous Vein, Left **T** Foot Vein, Right **V** Foot Vein, Left **Y** Lower Vein	**0** Open **3** Percutaneous **4** Percutaneous Endoscopic	**C** Extraluminal Device **D** Intraluminal Device **Z** No Device	**Z** No Qualifier

0 Medical and Surgical
6 Lower Veins
W Revision: Correcting, to the extent possible, a portion of a malfunctioning device or the position of a displaced device

Body Part Character 4	Approach Character 5	Device Character 6	Qualifier Character 7
Y Lower Vein	**0** Open **3** Percutaneous **4** Percutaneous Endoscopic	**0** Drainage Device **2** Monitoring Device **3** Infusion Device **7** Autologous Tissue Substitute **C** Extraluminal Device **D** Intraluminal Device **J** Synthetic Substitute **K** Nonautologous Tissue Substitute **Y** Other Device	**Z** No Qualifier
Y Lower Vein	**X** External	**0** Drainage Device **2** Monitoring Device **3** Infusion Device **7** Autologous Tissue Substitute **C** Extraluminal Device **D** Intraluminal Device **J** Synthetic Substitute **K** Nonautologous Tissue Substitute	**Z** No Qualifier

NOTES

NOTES

Lymphatic and Hemic Systems 072-07Y

0 Medical and Surgical
7 Lymphatic and Hemic Systems
2 Change: Taking out or off a device from a body part and putting back an identical or similar device in or on the same body part without cutting or puncturing the skin or a mucous membrane

Body Part	Approach	Device	Qualifier
Character 4	**Character 5**	**Character 6**	**Character 7**
K Thoracic Duct **L** Cisterna Chyli **M** Thymus **N** Lymphatic **P** Spleen **T** Bone Marrow	**X** External	**0** Drainage Device **Y** Other Device	**Z** No Qualifier

0 Medical and Surgical
7 Lymphatic and Hemic Systems
5 Destruction: Physical eradication of all or a portion of a body part by the direct use of energy, force, or a destructive agent

Body Part	Approach	Device	Qualifier
Character 4	**Character 5**	**Character 6**	**Character 7**
0 Lymphatic, Head **1** Lymphatic, Right Neck **2** Lymphatic, Left Neck **3** Lymphatic, Right Upper Extremity **4** Lymphatic, Left Upper Extremity **5** Lymphatic, Right Axillary **6** Lymphatic, Left Axillary **7** Lymphatic, Thorax **8** Lymphatic, Internal Mammary, Right **9** Lymphatic, Internal Mammary, Left **B** Lymphatic, Mesenteric **C** Lymphatic, Pelvis **D** Lymphatic, Aortic **F** Lymphatic, Right Lower Extremity **G** Lymphatic, Left Lower Extremity **H** Lymphatic, Right Inguinal **J** Lymphatic, Left Inguinal **K** Thoracic Duct **L** Cisterna Chyli **M** Thymus **P** Spleen	**0** Open **3** Percutaneous **4** Percutaneous Endoscopic	**Z** No Device	**Z** No Qualifier

0 Medical and Surgical
7 Lymphatic and Hemic Systems
9 Drainage: Taking or letting out fluids and/or gases from a body part

Body Part Character 4	Approach Character 5	Device Character 6	Qualifier Character 7
0 Lymphatic, Head **1** Lymphatic, Right Neck **2** Lymphatic, Left Neck **3** Lymphatic, Right Upper Extremity **4** Lymphatic, Left Upper Extremity **5** Lymphatic, Right Axillary **6** Lymphatic, Left Axillary **7** Lymphatic, Thorax **8** Lymphatic, Internal Mammary, Right **9** Lymphatic, Internal Mammary, Left **B** Lymphatic, Mesenteric **C** Lymphatic, Pelvis **D** Lymphatic, Aortic **F** Lymphatic, Right Lower Extremity **G** Lymphatic, Left Lower Extremity **H** Lymphatic, Right Inguinal **J** Lymphatic, Left Inguinal **K** Thoracic Duct **L** Cisterna Chyli	**0** Open **3** Percutaneous **4** Percutaneous Endoscopic **8** Via Natural or Artificial Opening Endoscopic	**0** Drainage Device	**Z** No Qualifier
0 Lymphatic, Head **1** Lymphatic, Right Neck **2** Lymphatic, Left Neck **3** Lymphatic, Right Upper Extremity **4** Lymphatic, Left Upper Extremity **5** Lymphatic, Right Axillary **6** Lymphatic, Left Axillary **7** Lymphatic, Thorax **8** Lymphatic, Internal Mammary, Right **9** Lymphatic, Internal Mammary, Left **B** Lymphatic, Mesenteric **C** Lymphatic, Pelvis **D** Lymphatic, Aortic **F** Lymphatic, Right Lower Extremity **G** Lymphatic, Left Lower Extremity **H** Lymphatic, Right Inguinal **J** Lymphatic, Left Inguinal **K** Thoracic Duct **L** Cisterna Chyli	**0** Open **3** Percutaneous **4** Percutaneous Endoscopic **8** Via Natural or Artificial Opening Endoscopic	**Z** No Device	**X** Diagnostic · pathology **Z** No Qualifier
M Thymus **P** Spleen **T** Bone Marrow	**0** Open **3** Percutaneous **4** Percutaneous Endoscopic	**0** Drainage Device	**Z** No Qualifier
M Thymus **P** Spleen **T** Bone Marrow	**0** Open **3** Percutaneous **4** Percutaneous Endoscopic	**Z** No Device	**X** Diagnostic **Z** No Qualifier

0 Medical and Surgical
7 Lymphatic and Hemic Systems
B Excision: Cutting out or off, without replacement, a portion of a body part

Body Part Character 4	Approach Character 5	Device Character 6	Qualifier Character 7
0 Lymphatic, Head	**0** Open	**Z** No Device	**X** Diagnostic
1 Lymphatic, Right Neck	**3** Percutaneous		**Z** No Qualifier
2 Lymphatic, Left Neck	**4** Percutaneous Endoscopic		
3 Lymphatic, Right Upper Extremity			
4 Lymphatic, Left Upper Extremity			
5 Lymphatic, Right Axillary			
6 Lymphatic, Left Axillary			
7 Lymphatic, Thorax			
8 Lymphatic, Internal Mammary, Right			
9 Lymphatic, Internal Mammary, Left			
B Lymphatic, Mesenteric			
C Lymphatic, Pelvis			
D Lymphatic, Aortic			
F Lymphatic, Right Lower Extremity			
G Lymphatic, Left Lower Extremity			
H Lymphatic, Right Inguinal CC			
J Lymphatic, Left Inguinal CC			
K Thoracic Duct			
L Cisterna Chyli			
M Thymus			
P Spleen			

CC 07BH0ZZ 07BH4ZZ 07BJ0ZZ 07BJ4ZZ

0 Medical and Surgical
7 Lymphatic and Hemic Systems
C Extirpation: Taking or cutting out solid matter from a body part

Body Part Character 4	Approach Character 5	Device Character 6	Qualifier Character 7
0 Lymphatic, Head	**0** Open	**Z** No Device	**Z** No Qualifier
1 Lymphatic, Right Neck	**3** Percutaneous		
2 Lymphatic, Left Neck	**4** Percutaneous Endoscopic		
3 Lymphatic, Right Upper Extremity			
4 Lymphatic, Left Upper Extremity			
5 Lymphatic, Right Axillary			
6 Lymphatic, Left Axillary			
7 Lymphatic, Thorax			
8 Lymphatic, Internal Mammary, Right			
9 Lymphatic, Internal Mammary, Left			
B Lymphatic, Mesenteric			
C Lymphatic, Pelvis			
D Lymphatic, Aortic			
F Lymphatic, Right Lower Extremity			
G Lymphatic, Left Lower Extremity			
H Lymphatic, Right Inguinal			
J Lymphatic, Left Inguinal			
K Thoracic Duct			
L Cisterna Chyli			
M Thymus			
P Spleen			

0 Medical and Surgical
7 Lymphatic and Hemic Systems
D Extraction: Pulling or stripping out or off all or a portion of a body part by the use of force

Body Part Character 4	Approach Character 5	Device Character 6	Qualifier Character 7
0 Lymphatic, Head **1** Lymphatic, Right Neck **2** Lymphatic, Left Neck **3** Lymphatic, Right Upper Extremity **4** Lymphatic, Left Upper Extremity **5** Lymphatic, Right Axillary **6** Lymphatic, Left Axillary **7** Lymphatic, Thorax **8** Lymphatic, Internal Mammary, Right **9** Lymphatic, Internal Mammary, Left **B** Lymphatic, Mesenteric **C** Lymphatic, Pelvis **D** Lymphatic, Aortic **F** Lymphatic, Right Lower Extremity **G** Lymphatic, Left Lower Extremity **H** Lymphatic, Right Inguinal **J** Lymphatic, Left Inguinal **K** Thoracic Duct **L** Cisterna Chyli	**3** Percutaneous **4** Percutaneous Endoscopic **8** Via Natural or Artificial Opening Endoscopic	**Z** No Device	**X** Diagnostic
M Thymus **P** Spleen	**3** Percutaneous **4** Percutaneous Endoscopic	**Z** No Device	**X** Diagnostic
Q Bone Marrow, Sternum **R** Bone Marrow, Iliac **S** Bone Marrow, Vertebral	**0** Open **3** Percutaneous kelly, trephine needle	**Z** No Device	**X** Diagnostic **Z** No Qualifier

0 Medical and Surgical
7 Lymphatic and Hemic Systems
H Insertion: Putting in a nonbiological appliance that monitors, assists, performs, or prevents a physiological function but does not physically take the place of a body part

Body Part Character 4	Approach Character 5	Device Character 6	Qualifier Character 7
K Thoracic Duct **L** Cisterna Chyli **M** Thymus **N** Lymphatic **P** Spleen	**0** Open **3** Percutaneous **4** Percutaneous Endoscopic	**3** Infusion Device **Y** Other Device	**Z** No Qualifier

0 Medical and Surgical
7 Lymphatic and Hemic Systems
J Inspection: Visually and/or manually exploring a body part

Body Part Character 4	Approach Character 5	Device Character 6	Qualifier Character 7
K Thoracic Duct **L** Cisterna Chyli **M** Thymus **T** Bone Marrow	**0** Open **3** Percutaneous **4** Percutaneous Endoscopic	**Z** No Device	**Z** No Qualifier
N Lymphatic	**0** Open **3** Percutaneous **4** Percutaneous Endoscopic **8** Via Natural or Artificial Opening Endoscopic **X** External	**Z** No Device	**Z** No Qualifier
P Spleen	**0** Open **3** Percutaneous **4** Percutaneous Endoscopic **X** External	**Z** No Device	**Z** No Qualifier

0 Medical and Surgical
7 Lymphatic and Hemic Systems
L Occlusion: Completely closing an orifice or the lumen of a tubular body part

Body Part Character 4	Approach Character 5	Device Character 6	Qualifier Character 7
0 Lymphatic, Head **1** Lymphatic, Right Neck **2** Lymphatic, Left Neck **3** Lymphatic, Right Upper Extremity **4** Lymphatic, Left Upper Extremity **5** Lymphatic, Right Axillary **6** Lymphatic, Left Axillary **7** Lymphatic, Thorax **8** Lymphatic, Internal Mammary, Right **9** Lymphatic, Internal Mammary, Left **B** Lymphatic, Mesenteric **C** Lymphatic, Pelvis **D** Lymphatic, Aortic **F** Lymphatic, Right Lower Extremity **G** Lymphatic, Left Lower Extremity **H** Lymphatic, Right Inguinal **J** Lymphatic, Left Inguinal **K** Thoracic Duct **L** Cisterna Chyli	**0** Open **3** Percutaneous **4** Percutaneous Endoscopic	**C** Extraluminal Device **D** Intraluminal Device **Z** No Device	**Z** No Qualifier

LC Limited Coverage NC Noncovered HAC HAC-associated Procedure CC Combination Cluster - See Appendix G for code lists
DRG Non-OR-Affecting MS-DRG Assignment New/Revised Text in **Orange** ♂ Male ♀ Female
2020 ICD-10-PCS
271

0 Medical and Surgical
7 Lymphatic and Hemic Systems
N Release: Freeing a body part from an abnormal physical constraint by cutting or by the use of force

Body Part	Approach	Device	Qualifier
Character 4	**Character 5**	**Character 6**	**Character 7**
0 Lymphatic, Head **1** Lymphatic, Right Neck **2** Lymphatic, Left Neck **3** Lymphatic, Right Upper Extremity **4** Lymphatic, Left Upper Extremity **5** Lymphatic, Right Axillary **6** Lymphatic, Left Axillary **7** Lymphatic, Thorax **8** Lymphatic, Internal Mammary, Right **9** Lymphatic, Internal Mammary, Left **B** Lymphatic, Mesenteric **C** Lymphatic, Pelvis **D** Lymphatic, Aortic **F** Lymphatic, Right Lower Extremity **G** Lymphatic, Left Lower Extremity **H** Lymphatic, Right Inguinal **J** Lymphatic, Left Inguinal **K** Thoracic Duct **L** Cisterna Chyli **M** Thymus **P** Spleen	**0** Open **3** Percutaneous **4** Percutaneous Endoscopic	**Z** No Device	**Z** No Qualifier

0 Medical and Surgical
7 Lymphatic and Hemic Systems
P Removal: Taking out or off a device from a body part

Body Part	Approach	Device	Qualifier
Character 4	**Character 5**	**Character 6**	**Character 7**
K Thoracic Duct **L** Cisterna Chyli **N** Lymphatic	**0** Open **3** Percutaneous **4** Percutaneous Endoscopic	**0** Drainage Device **3** Infusion Device **7** Autologous Tissue Substitute **C** Extraluminal Device **D** Intraluminal Device **J** Synthetic Substitute **K** Nonautologous Tissue Substitute **Y** Other Device	**Z** No Qualifier
K Thoracic Duct **L** Cisterna Chyli **N** Lymphatic	**X** External	**0** Drainage Device **3** Infusion Device **D** Intraluminal Device	**Z** No Qualifier
M Thymus **P** Spleen	**0** Open **3** Percutaneous **4** Percutaneous Endoscopic	**0** Drainage Device **3** Infusion Device **Y** Other Device	**Z** No Qualifier
M Thymus **P** Spleen	**X** External	**0** Drainage Device **3** Infusion Device	**Z** No Qualifier
T Bone Marrow	**0** Open **3** Percutaneous **4** Percutaneous Endoscopic **X** External	**0** Drainage Device	**Z** No Qualifier

0 Medical and Surgical
7 Lymphatic and Hemic Systems
Q Repair: Restoring, to the extent possible, a body part to its normal anatomic structure and function

Body Part Character 4	Approach Character 5	Device Character 6	Qualifier Character 7
0 Lymphatic, Head **1** Lymphatic, Right Neck **2** Lymphatic, Left Neck **3** Lymphatic, Right Upper Extremity **4** Lymphatic, Left Upper Extremity **5** Lymphatic, Right Axillary **6** Lymphatic, Left Axillary **7** Lymphatic, Thorax **8** Lymphatic, Internal Mammary, Right **9** Lymphatic, Internal Mammary, Left **B** Lymphatic, Mesenteric **C** Lymphatic, Pelvis **D** Lymphatic, Aortic **F** Lymphatic, Right Lower Extremity **G** Lymphatic, Left Lower Extremity **H** Lymphatic, Right Inguinal **J** Lymphatic, Left Inguinal **K** Thoracic Duct **L** Cisterna Chyli	**0** Open **3** Percutaneous **4** Percutaneous Endoscopic **8** Via Natural or Artificial Opening Endoscopic	**Z** No Device	**Z** No Qualifier
M Thymus **P** Spleen	**0** Open **3** Percutaneous **4** Percutaneous Endoscopic	**Z** No Device	**Z** No Qualifier

0 Medical and Surgical
7 Lymphatic and Hemic Systems
S Reposition: Moving to its normal location, or other suitable location, all or a portion of a body part

Body Part Character 4	Approach Character 5	Device Character 6	Qualifier Character 7
M Thymus **P** Spleen	**0** Open	**Z** No Device	**Z** No Qualifier

0 Medical and Surgical
7 Lymphatic and Hemic Systems
T Resection: Cutting out or off, without replacement, all of a body part

Body Part Character 4	Approach Character 5	Device Character 6	Qualifier Character 7
0 Lymphatic, Head	**0** Open	**Z** No Device	**Z** No Qualifier
1 Lymphatic, Right Neck	**4** Percutaneous Endoscopic		
2 Lymphatic, Left Neck			
3 Lymphatic, Right Upper Extremity			
4 Lymphatic, Left Upper Extremity			
5 Lymphatic, Right Axillary CC			
6 Lymphatic, Left Axillary CC			
7 Lymphatic, Thorax CC			
8 Lymphatic, Internal Mammary, Right CC			
9 Lymphatic, Internal Mammary, Left CC			
B Lymphatic, Mesenteric			
C Lymphatic, Pelvis - iliac, may be bilateral			
D Lymphatic, Aortic			
F Lymphatic, Right Lower Extremity			
G Lymphatic, Left Lower Extremity			
H Lymphatic, Right Inguinal			
J Lymphatic, Left Inguinal			
K Thoracic Duct			
L Cisterna Chyli			
M Thymus			
P Spleen			

CC 07T50ZZ 07T60ZZ 07T70ZZ 07T80ZZ 07T90ZZ

0 Medical and Surgical
7 Lymphatic and Hemic Systems
U Supplement: Putting in or on biological or synthetic material that physically reinforces and/or augments the function of a portion of a body part

Body Part Character 4	Approach Character 5	Device Character 6	Qualifier Character 7
0 Lymphatic, Head	**0** Open	**7** Autologous Tissue Substitute	**Z** No Qualifier
1 Lymphatic, Right Neck	**4** Percutaneous Endoscopic	**J** Synthetic Substitute	
2 Lymphatic, Left Neck		**K** Nonautologous Tissue Substitute	
3 Lymphatic, Right Upper Extremity			
4 Lymphatic, Left Upper Extremity			
5 Lymphatic, Right Axillary			
6 Lymphatic, Left Axillary			
7 Lymphatic, Thorax			
8 Lymphatic, Internal Mammary, Right			
9 Lymphatic, Internal Mammary, Left			
B Lymphatic, Mesenteric			
C Lymphatic, Pelvis			
D Lymphatic, Aortic			
F Lymphatic, Right Lower Extremity			
G Lymphatic, Left Lower Extremity			
H Lymphatic, Right Inguinal			
J Lymphatic, Left Inguinal			
K Thoracic Duct			
L Cisterna Chyli			

0 Medical and Surgical
7 Lymphatic and Hemic Systems
V Restriction: Partially closing an orifice or the lumen of a tubular body part

Body Part Character 4	Approach Character 5	Device Character 6	Qualifier Character 7
0 Lymphatic, Head **1** Lymphatic, Right Neck **2** Lymphatic, Left Neck **3** Lymphatic, Right Upper Extremity **4** Lymphatic, Left Upper Extremity **5** Lymphatic, Right Axillary **6** Lymphatic, Left Axillary **7** Lymphatic, Thorax **8** Lymphatic, Internal Mammary, Right **9** Lymphatic, Internal Mammary, Left **B** Lymphatic, Mesenteric **C** Lymphatic, Pelvis **D** Lymphatic, Aortic **F** Lymphatic, Right Lower Extremity **G** Lymphatic, Left Lower Extremity **H** Lymphatic, Right Inguinal **J** Lymphatic, Left Inguinal **K** Thoracic Duct **L** Cisterna Chyli	**0** Open **3** Percutaneous **4** Percutaneous Endoscopic	**C** Extraluminal Device **D** Intraluminal Device **Z** No Device	**Z** No Qualifier

0 Medical and Surgical
7 Lymphatic and Hemic Systems
W Revision: Correcting, to the extent possible, a portion of a malfunctioning device or the position of a displaced device

Body Part Character 4	Approach Character 5	Device Character 6	Qualifier Character 7
K Thoracic Duct **L** Cisterna Chyli **N** Lymphatic	**0** Open **3** Percutaneous **4** Percutaneous Endoscopic	**0** Drainage Device **3** Infusion Device **7** Autologous Tissue Substitute **C** Extraluminal Device **D** Intraluminal Device **J** Synthetic Substitute **K** Nonautologous Tissue Substitute **Y** Other Device	**Z** No Qualifier
K Thoracic Duct **L** Cisterna Chyli **N** Lymphatic	**X** External	**0** Drainage Device **3** Infusion Device **7** Autologous Tissue Substitute **C** Extraluminal Device **D** Intraluminal Device **J** Synthetic Substitute **K** Nonautologous Tissue Substitute	**Z** No Qualifier
M Thymus **P** Spleen	**0** Open **3** Percutaneous **4** Percutaneous Endoscopic	**0** Drainage Device **3** Infusion Device **Y** Other Device	**Z** No Qualifier
M Thymus **P** Spleen	**X** External	**0** Drainage Device **3** Infusion Device	**Z** No Qualifier
T Bone Marrow	**0** Open **3** Percutaneous **4** Percutaneous Endoscopic **X** External	**0** Drainage Device	**Z** No Qualifier

0 **Medical and Surgical**
7 **Lymphatic and Hemic Systems**
Y **Transplantation:** Putting in or on all or a portion of a living body part taken from another individual or animal to physically take the place and/or function of all or a portion of a similar body part

Body Part	Approach	Device	Qualifier
Character 4	Character 5	Character 6	Character 7
M Thymus P Spleen	0 Open	Z No Device	*human* 0 Allogeneic *same species* 1 Syngeneic *- generally similar* 2 Zooplastic

NOTES

nonautogous = human cadaver (K) - donor matched
autograft = autologous tissue substitute (7), use pts own

NOTES

Phacoemulsification - cataract surgery on lens
If intraocular lens is inserted = replacement
If lens is not replaced, aspiration only = extraction

Keratoplasty - cornea transplant
done percutaneous
1) penetrating - cornea replaced w/ human cadaver - Full transplant = replacement
2) Lamellar = partial transplant - 2 types: inlay + onlay = supplement - augment
onlay = external approach
onlay
leaves descement membrane + endothelium

Cataract - clouding in crystalline lens of eye or in its envelope
senile = occurs in the elderly, age-related
morgagnian - senile, cortex liquefies over time to form milky white fluid
can cause phacomorphic glaucoma

Eye 080-08X

0 Medical and Surgical
8 Eye
0 Alteration: Modifying the anatomic structure of a body part without affecting the function of the body part

Body Part	Approach	Device	Qualifier
Character 4	**Character 5**	**Character 6**	**Character 7**
N Upper Eyelid, Right **P** Upper Eyelid, Left **Q** Lower Eyelid, Right **R** Lower Eyelid, Left	**0** Open **3** Percutaneous **X** External	**7** Autologous Tissue Substitute **J** Synthetic Substitute **K** Nonautologous Tissue Substitute **Z** No Device	**Z** No Qualifier

0 Medical and Surgical
8 Eye
1 Bypass: Altering the route of passage of the contents of a tubular body part

Body Part	Approach	Device	Qualifier
Character 4	**Character 5**	**Character 6**	**Character 7**
2 Anterior Chamber, Right **3** Anterior Chamber, Left	**3** Percutaneous	**J** Synthetic Substitute **K** Nonautologous Tissue Substitute **Z** No Device	**4** Sclera
X Lacrimal Duct, Right **Y** Lacrimal Duct, Left	**0** Open **3** Percutaneous	**J** Synthetic Substitute **K** Nonautologous Tissue Substitute **Z** No Device	**3** Nasal Cavity

0 Medical and Surgical
8 Eye
2 Change: Taking out or off a device from a body part and putting back an identical or similar device in or on the same body part without cutting or puncturing the skin or a mucous membrane

Body Part	Approach	Device	Qualifier
Character 4	**Character 5**	**Character 6**	**Character 7**
0 Eye, Right **1** Eye, Left	**X** External	**0** Drainage Device **Y** Other Device	**Z** No Qualifier

0 Medical and Surgical
8 Eye
5 Destruction: Physical eradication of all or a portion of a body part by the direct use of energy, force, or a destructive agent

Body Part Character 4	Approach Character 5	Device Character 6	Qualifier Character 7
0 Eye, Right **1** Eye, Left **6** Sclera, Right **7** Sclera, Left **8** Cornea, Right **9** Cornea, Left **S** Conjunctiva, Right **T** Conjunctiva, Left	**X** External	**Z** No Device	**Z** No Qualifier
2 Anterior Chamber, Right **3** Anterior Chamber, Left **4** Vitreous, Right **5** Vitreous, Left **C** Iris, Right **D** Iris, Left **E** Retina, Right **F** Retina, Left **G** Retinal Vessel, Right **H** Retinal Vessel, Left **J** Lens, Right **K** Lens, Left	**3** Percutaneous	**Z** No Device	**Z** No Qualifier
A Choroid, Right **B** Choroid, Left **L** Extraocular Muscle, Right **M** Extraocular Muscle, Left **V** Lacrimal Gland, Right **W** Lacrimal Gland, Left	**0** Open **3** Percutaneous	**Z** No Device	**Z** No Qualifier
N Upper Eyelid, Right **P** Upper Eyelid, Left **Q** Lower Eyelid, Right **R** Lower Eyelid, Left	**0** Open **3** Percutaneous **X** External	**Z** No Device	**Z** No Qualifier
X Lacrimal Duct, Right **Y** Lacrimal Duct, Left	**0** Open **3** Percutaneous **7** Via Natural or Artificial Opening **8** Via Natural or Artificial Opening Endoscopic	**Z** No Device	**Z** No Qualifier

0 Medical and Surgical
8 Eye
7 Dilation: Expanding an orifice or the lumen of a tubular body part

Body Part Character 4	Approach Character 5	Device Character 6	Qualifier Character 7
X Lacrimal Duct, Right **Y** Lacrimal Duct, Left	**0** Open **3** Percutaneous **7** Via Natural or Artificial Opening **8** Via Natural or Artificial Opening Endoscopic	**D** Intraluminal Device **Z** No Device	**Z** No Qualifier

0 **Medical and Surgical**
8 **Eye**
9 **Drainage:** Taking or letting out fluids and/or gases from a body part

Body Part Character 4	Approach Character 5	Device Character 6	Qualifier Character 7
0 Eye, Right **1** Eye, Left **6** Sclera, Right **7** Sclera, Left **8** Cornea, Right **9** Cornea, Left **S** Conjunctiva, Right **T** Conjunctiva, Left	**X** External	**0** Drainage Device	**Z** No Qualifier
0 Eye, Right **1** Eye, Left **6** Sclera, Right **7** Sclera, Left **8** Cornea, Right **9** Cornea, Left **S** Conjunctiva, Right **T** Conjunctiva, Left	**X** External	**Z** No Device	**X** Diagnostic **Z** No Qualifier
2 Anterior Chamber, Right **3** Anterior Chamber, Left **4** Vitreous, Right **5** Vitreous, Left **C** Iris, Right **D** Iris, Left **E** Retina, Right **F** Retina, Left **G** Retinal Vessel, Right **H** Retinal Vessel, Left **J** Lens, Right **K** Lens, Left	**3** Percutaneous	**0** Drainage Device	**Z** No Qualifier
2 Anterior Chamber, Right **3** Anterior Chamber, Left **4** Vitreous, Right **5** Vitreous, Left **C** Iris, Right **D** Iris, Left **E** Retina, Right **F** Retina, Left **G** Retinal Vessel, Right **H** Retinal Vessel, Left **J** Lens, Right **K** Lens, Left	**3** Percutaneous	**Z** No Device	**X** Diagnostic **Z** No Qualifier
A Choroid, Right **B** Choroid, Left **L** Extraocular Muscle, Right **M** Extraocular Muscle, Left **V** Lacrimal Gland, Right **W** Lacrimal Gland, Left	**0** Open **3** Percutaneous	**0** Drainage Device	**Z** No Qualifier
A Choroid, Right **B** Choroid, Left **L** Extraocular Muscle, Right **M** Extraocular Muscle, Left **V** Lacrimal Gland, Right **W** Lacrimal Gland, Left	**0** Open **3** Percutaneous	**Z** No Device	**X** Diagnostic **Z** No Qualifier
N Upper Eyelid, Right **P** Upper Eyelid, Left **Q** Lower Eyelid, Right **R** Lower Eyelid, Left	**0** Open **3** Percutaneous **X** External	**0** Drainage Device	**Z** No Qualifier

089 continued on next page

LC Limited Coverage NC Noncovered HAC HAC-associated Procedure CC Combination Cluster - See Appendix G for code lists
DRG Non-OR-Affecting MS-DRG Assignment New/Revised Text in **Orange** ♂ Male ♀ Female

2020 ICD-10-PCS **281**

089 EYE 080-08X

089 continued from previous page

0 Medical and Surgical
8 Eye
9 Drainage: Taking or letting out fluids and/or gases from a body part

Body Part Character 4	Approach Character 5	Device Character 6	Qualifier Character 7
N Upper Eyelid, Right **P** Upper Eyelid, Left **Q** Lower Eyelid, Right **R** Lower Eyelid, Left	**0** Open **3** Percutaneous **X** External	**Z** No Device	**X** Diagnostic **Z** No Qualifier
X Lacrimal Duct, Right **Y** Lacrimal Duct, Left	**0** Open **3** Percutaneous **7** Via Natural or Artificial Opening **8** Via Natural or Artificial Opening Endoscopic	**0** Drainage Device	**Z** No Qualifier
X Lacrimal Duct, Right **Y** Lacrimal Duct, Left	**0** Open **3** Percutaneous **7** Via Natural or Artificial Opening **8** Via Natural or Artificial Opening Endoscopic	**Z** No Device	**X** Diagnostic **Z** No Qualifier

0 Medical and Surgical
8 Eye
B Excision: Cutting out or off, without replacement, a portion of a body part

Body Part Character 4	Approach Character 5	Device Character 6	Qualifier Character 7
0 Eye, Right **1** Eye, Left **N** Upper Eyelid, Right **P** Upper Eyelid, Left **Q** Lower Eyelid, Right **R** Lower Eyelid, Left	**0** Open **3** Percutaneous **X** External	**Z** No Device	**X** Diagnostic **Z** No Qualifier
4 Vitreous, Right **5** Vitreous, Left **C** Iris, Right **D** Iris, Left **E** Retina, Right **F** Retina, Left **J** Lens, Right **K** Lens, Left	**3** Percutaneous	**Z** No Device	**X** Diagnostic **Z** No Qualifier
6 Sclera, Right **7** Sclera, Left **8** Cornea, Right **9** Cornea, Left **S** Conjunctiva, Right **T** Conjunctiva, Left	**X** External	**Z** No Device	**X** Diagnostic **Z** No Qualifier
A Choroid, Right **B** Choroid, Left **L** Extraocular Muscle, Right **M** Extraocular Muscle, Left **V** Lacrimal Gland, Right **W** Lacrimal Gland, Left	**0** Open **3** Percutaneous	**Z** No Device	**X** Diagnostic **Z** No Qualifier
X Lacrimal Duct, Right **Y** Lacrimal Duct, Left	**0** Open **3** Percutaneous **7** Via Natural or Artificial Opening **8** Via Natural or Artificial Opening Endoscopic	**Z** No Device	**X** Diagnostic **Z** No Qualifier

0 Medical and Surgical
8 Eye
C Extirpation: Taking or cutting out solid matter from a body part

Body Part Character 4	Approach Character 5	Device Character 6	Qualifier Character 7
0 Eye, Right **1** Eye, Left **6** Sclera, Right **7** Sclera, Left **8** Cornea, Right **9** Cornea, Left **S** Conjunctiva, Right **T** Conjunctiva, Left	**X** External	**Z** No Device	**Z** No Qualifier
2 Anterior Chamber, Right **3** Anterior Chamber, Left **4** Vitreous, Right **5** Vitreous, Left **C** Iris, Right **D** Iris, Left **E** Retina, Right **F** Retina, Left **G** Retinal Vessel, Right **H** Retinal Vessel, Left **J** Lens, Right **K** Lens, Left	**3** Percutaneous **X** External	**Z** No Device	**Z** No Qualifier
A Choroid, Right **B** Choroid, Left **L** Extraocular Muscle, Right **M** Extraocular Muscle, Left **N** Upper Eyelid, Right **P** Upper Eyelid, Left **Q** Lower Eyelid, Right **R** Lower Eyelid, Left **V** Lacrimal Gland, Right **W** Lacrimal Gland, Left	**0** Open **3** Percutaneous **X** External	**Z** No Device	**Z** No Qualifier
X Lacrimal Duct, Right **Y** Lacrimal Duct, Left	**0** Open **3** Percutaneous **7** Via Natural or Artificial Opening **8** Via Natural or Artificial Opening Endoscopic	**Z** No Device	**Z** No Qualifier

0 Medical and Surgical
8 Eye
D Extraction: Pulling or stripping out or off all or a portion of a body part by the use of force

Body Part Character 4	Approach Character 5	Device Character 6	Qualifier Character 7
8 Cornea, Right **9** Cornea, Left	**X** External	**Z** No Device	**X** Diagnostic **Z** No Qualifier
J Lens, Right **K** Lens, Left cataract phacoemulsification no replacement	**3** Percutaneous	**Z** No Device	**Z** No Qualifier

0 Medical and Surgical
8 Eye
F Fragmentation: Breaking solid matter in a body part into pieces

Body Part Character 4	Approach Character 5	Device Character 6	Qualifier Character 7
4 Vitreous, Right NC **5** Vitreous, Left NC	**3** Percutaneous **X** External	**Z** No Device	**Z** No Qualifier

NC 08F4XZZ 08F5XZZ

0 Medical and Surgical
8 Eye
H Insertion: Putting in a nonbiological appliance that monitors, assists, performs, or prevents a physiological function but does not physically take the place of a body part

Body Part Character 4	Approach Character 5	Device Character 6	Qualifier Character 7
0 Eye, Right **1** Eye, Left	**0** Open	**5** Epiretinal Visual Prosthesis **Y** Other Device	**Z** No Qualifier
0 Eye, Right **1** Eye, Left	**3** Percutaneous	**1** Radioactive Element **3** Infusion Device **Y** Other Device	**Z** No Qualifier
0 Eye, Right **1** Eye, Left	**7** Via Natural or Artificial Opening **8** Via Natural or Artificial Opening Endoscopic	**Y** Other Device	**Z** No Qualifier
0 Eye, Right **1** Eye, Left	**X** External	**1** Radioactive Element **3** Infusion Device	**Z** No Qualifier

0 Medical and Surgical
8 Eye
J Inspection: Visually and/or manually exploring a body part

Body Part Character 4	Approach Character 5	Device Character 6	Qualifier Character 7
0 Eye, Right **1** Eye, Left **J** Lens, Right **K** Lens, Left	**X** External	**Z** No Device	**Z** No Qualifier
L Extraocular Muscle, Right **M** Extraocular Muscle, Left	**0** Open **X** External	**Z** No Device	**Z** No Qualifier

0 Medical and Surgical
8 Eye
L Occlusion: Completely closing an orifice or the lumen of a tubular body part

Body Part Character 4	Approach Character 5	Device Character 6	Qualifier Character 7
X Lacrimal Duct, Right **Y** Lacrimal Duct, Left	**0** Open **3** Percutaneous	**C** Extraluminal Device **D** Intraluminal Device **Z** No Device	**Z** No Qualifier
X Lacrimal Duct, Right **Y** Lacrimal Duct, Left	**7** Via Natural or Artificial Opening **8** Via Natural or Artificial Opening Endoscopic	**D** Intraluminal Device **Z** No Device	**Z** No Qualifier

0 Medical and Surgical
8 Eye
M Reattachment: Putting back in or on all or a portion of a separated body part to its normal location or other suitable location

Body Part Character 4	Approach Character 5	Device Character 6	Qualifier Character 7
N Upper Eyelid, Right **P** Upper Eyelid, Left **Q** Lower Eyelid, Right **R** Lower Eyelid, Left	**X** External	**Z** No Device	**Z** No Qualifier

EYE 080-08X
LC Limited Coverage NC Noncovered HAC HAC-associated Procedure CC Combination Cluster - See Appendix G for code lists
DRG Non-OR-Affecting MS-DRG Assignment New/Revised Text in **Orange** ♂ Male ♀ Female
284
2020 ICD-10-PCS

0 Medical and Surgical
8 Eye
N Release: Freeing a body part from an abnormal physical constraint by cutting or by the use of force

Body Part Character 4	Approach Character 5	Device Character 6	Qualifier Character 7
0 Eye, Right 1 Eye, Left 6 Sclera, Right 7 Sclera, Left 8 Cornea, Right 9 Cornea, Left S Conjunctiva, Right T Conjunctiva, Left	X External	Z No Device	Z No Qualifier
2 Anterior Chamber, Right 3 Anterior Chamber, Left 4 Vitreous, Right 5 Vitreous, Left C Iris, Right D Iris, Left E Retina, Right F Retina, Left G Retinal Vessel, Right H Retinal Vessel, Left J Lens, Right K Lens, Left	3 Percutaneous	Z No Device	Z No Qualifier
A Choroid, Right B Choroid, Left L Extraocular Muscle, Right M Extraocular Muscle, Left V Lacrimal Gland, Right W Lacrimal Gland, Left	0 Open 3 Percutaneous	Z No Device	Z No Qualifier
N Upper Eyelid, Right P Upper Eyelid, Left Q Lower Eyelid, Right R Lower Eyelid, Left	0 Open 3 Percutaneous X External	Z No Device	Z No Qualifier
X Lacrimal Duct, Right Y Lacrimal Duct, Left	0 Open 3 Percutaneous 7 Via Natural or Artificial Opening 8 Via Natural or Artificial Opening Endoscopic	Z No Device	Z No Qualifier

0 **Medical and Surgical**
8 **Eye**
P **Removal:** Taking out or off a device from a body part

Body Part Character 4	Approach Character 5	Device Character 6	Qualifier Character 7
0 Eye, Right **1** Eye, Left	**0** Open **3** Percutaneous **7** Via Natural or Artificial Opening **8** Via Natural or Artificial Opening Endoscopic	**0** Drainage Device **1** Radioactive Element **3** Infusion Device **7** Autologous Tissue Substitute **C** Extraluminal Device **D** Intraluminal Device **J** Synthetic Substitute **K** Nonautologous Tissue Substitute **Y** Other Device	**Z** No Qualifier
0 Eye, Right **1** Eye, Left	**X** External	**0** Drainage Device **1** Radioactive Element **3** Infusion Device **7** Autologous Tissue Substitute **C** Extraluminal Device **D** Intraluminal Device **J** Synthetic Substitute **K** Nonautologous Tissue Substitute	**Z** No Qualifier
J Lens, Right **K** Lens, Left	**3** Percutaneous	**J** Synthetic Substitute **Y** Other Device	**Z** No Qualifier
L Extraocular Muscle, Right **M** Extraocular Muscle, Left	**0** Open **3** Percutaneous	**0** Drainage Device **7** Autologous Tissue Substitute **J** Synthetic Substitute **K** Nonautologous Tissue Substitute **Y** Other Device	**Z** No Qualifier

LC Limited Coverage NC Noncovered HAC HAC-associated Procedure CC Combination Cluster - See Appendix G for code lists
DRG Non-OR-Affecting MS-DRG Assignment New/Revised Text in **Orange** ♂ Male ♀ Female

EYE 080-08X

286 2020 ICD-10-PCS

0 Medical and Surgical
8 Eye
Q Repair: Restoring, to the extent possible, a body part to its normal anatomic structure and function

Body Part Character 4	Approach Character 5	Device Character 6	Qualifier Character 7
0 Eye, Right **1** Eye, Left **6** Sclera, Right **7** Sclera, Left **8** Cornea, Right NC **9** Cornea, Left NC **S** Conjunctiva, Right **T** Conjunctiva, Left	**X** External	**Z** No Device	**Z** No Qualifier
2 Anterior Chamber, Right **3** Anterior Chamber, Left **4** Vitreous, Right **5** Vitreous, Left **C** Iris, Right **D** Iris, Left **E** Retina, Right **F** Retina, Left **G** Retinal Vessel, Right **H** Retinal Vessel, Left **J** Lens, Right **K** Lens, Left	**3** Percutaneous	**Z** No Device	**Z** No Qualifier
A Choroid, Right **B** Choroid, Left **L** Extraocular Muscle, Right **M** Extraocular Muscle, Left **V** Lacrimal Gland, Right **W** Lacrimal Gland, Left	**0** Open **3** Percutaneous	**Z** No Device	**Z** No Qualifier
N Upper Eyelid, Right **P** Upper Eyelid, Left **Q** Lower Eyelid, Right **R** Lower Eyelid, Left	**0** Open **3** Percutaneous **X** External	**Z** No Device	**Z** No Qualifier
X Lacrimal Duct, Right **Y** Lacrimal Duct, Left	**0** Open **3** Percutaneous **7** Via Natural or Artificial Opening **8** Via Natural or Artificial Opening Endoscopic	**Z** No Device	**Z** No Qualifier

NC 08Q8XZZ 08Q9XZZ

If no lens is replaced, code only extraction

0 Medical and Surgical
8 Eye
R Replacement: Putting in or on biological or synthetic material that physically takes the place and/or function of all or a portion of a body part

Body Part Character 4	Approach Character 5	Device Character 6	Qualifier Character 7
0 Eye, Right **1** Eye, Left **A** Choroid, Right **B** Choroid, Left	**0** Open **3** Percutaneous	**7** Autologous Tissue Substitute **J** Synthetic Substitute - prosthetic **K** Nonautologous Tissue Substitute - donor	**Z** No Qualifier
4 Vitreous, Right **5** Vitreous, Left **C** Iris, Right **D** Iris, Left **G** Retinal Vessel, Right **H** Retinal Vessel, Left	**3** Percutaneous	**7** Autologous Tissue Substitute **J** Synthetic Substitute - prostetic **K** Nonautologous Tissue Substitute	**Z** No Qualifier
6 Sclera, Right **7** Sclera, Left **S** Conjunctiva, Right **T** Conjunctiva, Left	**X** External	**7** Autologous Tissue Substitute **J** Synthetic Substitute **K** Nonautologous Tissue Substitute	**Z** No Qualifier
8 Cornea, Right > keratoplasty **9** Cornea, Left > penetrating full thickness	**3** Percutaneous **X** External	**7** Autologous Tissue Substitute **J** Synthetic Substitute **K** Nonautologous Tissue Substitute cadavar, donor	**Z** No Qualifier
J Lens, Right > cataract **K** Lens, Left phacoemulsification w/introcular lens replaced	**3** Percutaneous	**0** Synthetic Substitute, Intraocular Telescope IOL **7** Autologous Tissue Substitute -self **J** Synthetic Substitute prosthetic IOL - acrylic **K** Nonautologous Tissue Substitute - donor	**Z** No Qualifier
N Upper Eyelid, Right **P** Upper Eyelid, Left **Q** Lower Eyelid, Right **R** Lower Eyelid, Left	**0** Open **3** Percutaneous **X** External	**7** Autologous Tissue Substitute **J** Synthetic Substitute **K** Nonautologous Tissue Substitute	**Z** No Qualifier
X Lacrimal Duct, Right **Y** Lacrimal Duct, Left	**0** Open **3** Percutaneous **7** Via Natural or Artificial Opening **8** Via Natural or Artificial Opening Endoscopic	**7** Autologous Tissue Substitute **J** Synthetic Substitute **K** Nonautologous Tissue Substitute	**Z** No Qualifier

LC Limited Coverage NC Noncovered HAC HAC-associated Procedure CC Combination Cluster - See Appendix G for code lists
DRG Non-OR-Affecting MS-DRG Assignment New/Revised Text in **Orange** ♂ Male ♀ Female

288 2020 ICD-10-PCS

08R
EYE 080-08X

0 **Medical and Surgical**
8 **Eye**
S **Reposition:** Moving to its normal location, or other suitable location, all or a portion of a body part

Body Part Character 4	Approach Character 5	Device Character 6	Qualifier Character 7
C Iris, Right **D** Iris, Left **G** Retinal Vessel, Right **H** Retinal Vessel, Left **J** Lens, Right **K** Lens, Left	**3** Percutaneous	**Z** No Device	**Z** No Qualifier
L Extraocular Muscle, Right **M** Extraocular Muscle, Left **V** Lacrimal Gland, Right **W** Lacrimal Gland, Left	**0** Open **3** Percutaneous	**Z** No Device	**Z** No Qualifier
N Upper Eyelid, Right **P** Upper Eyelid, Left **Q** Lower Eyelid, Right **R** Lower Eyelid, Left	**0** Open **3** Percutaneous **X** External	**Z** No Device	**Z** No Qualifier
X Lacrimal Duct, Right **Y** Lacrimal Duct, Left	**0** Open **3** Percutaneous **7** Via Natural or Artificial Opening **8** Via Natural or Artificial Opening Endoscopic	**Z** No Device	**Z** No Qualifier

0 **Medical and Surgical**
8 **Eye**
T **Resection:** Cutting out or off, without replacement, all of a body part

Body Part Character 4	Approach Character 5	Device Character 6	Qualifier Character 7
0 Eye, Right **1** Eye, Left **8** Cornea, Right **9** Cornea, Left	**X** External	**Z** No Device	**Z** No Qualifier
4 Vitreous, Right **5** Vitreous, Left **C** Iris, Right **D** Iris, Left **J** Lens, Right **K** Lens, Left	**3** Percutaneous	**Z** No Device	**Z** No Qualifier
L Extraocular Muscle, Right **M** Extraocular Muscle, Left **V** Lacrimal Gland, Right **W** Lacrimal Gland, Left	**0** Open **3** Percutaneous	**Z** No Device	**Z** No Qualifier
N Upper Eyelid, Right **P** Upper Eyelid, Left **Q** Lower Eyelid, Right **R** Lower Eyelid, Left	**0** Open **X** External	**Z** No Device	**Z** No Qualifier
X Lacrimal Duct, Right **Y** Lacrimal Duct, Left	**0** Open **3** Percutaneous **7** Via Natural or Artificial Opening **8** Via Natural or Artificial Opening Endoscopic	**Z** No Device	**Z** No Qualifier

0 Medical and Surgical
8 Eye
U Supplement: Putting in or on biological or synthetic material that physically reinforces and/or augments the function of a portion of a body part

Body Part Character 4	Approach Character 5	Device Character 6	Qualifier Character 7
0 Eye, Right **1** Eye, Left **C** Iris, Right **D** Iris, Left **E** Retina, Right **F** Retina, Left **G** Retinal Vessel, Right **H** Retinal Vessel, Left **L** Extraocular Muscle, Right **M** Extraocular Muscle, Left	**0** Open **3** Percutaneous	**7** Autologous Tissue Substitute **J** Synthetic Substitute **K** Nonautologous Tissue Substitute	**Z** No Qualifier
8 Cornea, Right NC **9** Cornea, Left NC **N** Upper Eyelid, Right **P** Upper Eyelid, Left **Q** Lower Eyelid, Right **R** Lower Eyelid, Left	**0** Open **3** Percutaneous **X** External	**7** Autologous Tissue Substitute **J** Synthetic Substitute **K** Nonautologous Tissue Substitute	**Z** No Qualifier
X Lacrimal Duct, Right **Y** Lacrimal Duct, Left	**0** Open **3** Percutaneous **7** Via Natural or Artificial Opening **8** Via Natural or Artificial Opening Endoscopic	**7** Autologous Tissue Substitute **J** Synthetic Substitute **K** Nonautologous Tissue Substitute	**Z** No Qualifier

NC 08U80KZ 08U83KZ 08U8XKZ 08U90KZ 08U93KZ 08U9XKZ

0 Medical and Surgical
8 Eye
V Restriction: Partially closing an orifice or the lumen of a tubular body part

Body Part Character 4	Approach Character 5	Device Character 6	Qualifier Character 7
X Lacrimal Duct, Right **Y** Lacrimal Duct, Left	**0** Open **3** Percutaneous	**C** Extraluminal Device **D** Intraluminal Device **Z** No Device	**Z** No Qualifier
X Lacrimal Duct, Right **Y** Lacrimal Duct, Left	**7** Via Natural or Artificial Opening **8** Via Natural or Artificial Opening Endoscopic	**D** Intraluminal Device **Z** No Device	**Z** No Qualifier

0 Medical and Surgical
8 Eye
W Revision: Correcting, to the extent possible, a portion of a malfunctioning device or the position of a displaced device

Body Part Character 4	Approach Character 5	Device Character 6	Qualifier Character 7
0 Eye, Right **1** Eye, Left	**0** Open **3** Percutaneous **7** Via Natural or Artificial Opening **8** Via Natural or Artificial Opening Endoscopic	**0** Drainage Device **3** Infusion Device **7** Autologous Tissue Substitute **C** Extraluminal Device **D** Intraluminal Device **J** Synthetic Substitute **K** Nonautologous Tissue Substitute **Y** Other Device	**Z** No Qualifier
0 Eye, Right **1** Eye, Left	**X** External	**0** Drainage Device **3** Infusion Device **7** Autologous Tissue Substitute **C** Extraluminal Device **D** Intraluminal Device **J** Synthetic Substitute **K** Nonautologous Tissue Substitute	**Z** No Qualifier
J Lens, Right **K** Lens, Left	**3** Percutaneous	**J** Synthetic Substitute **Y** Other Device	**Z** No Qualifier
J Lens, Right **K** Lens, Left	**X** External	**J** Synthetic Substitute	**Z** No Qualifier
L Extraocular Muscle, Right **M** Extraocular Muscle, Left	**0** Open **3** Percutaneous	**0** Drainage Device **7** Autologous Tissue Substitute **J** Synthetic Substitute **K** Nonautologous Tissue Substitute **Y** Other Device	**Z** No Qualifier

0 Medical and Surgical
8 Eye
X Transfer: Moving, without taking out, all or a portion of a body part to another location to take over the function of all or a portion of a body part

Body Part Character 4	Approach Character 5	Device Character 6	Qualifier Character 7
L Extraocular Muscle, Right **M** Extraocular Muscle, Left	**0** Open **3** Percutaneous	**Z** No Device	**Z** No Qualifier

NOTES

tympanotomy w/ myringotomy tubes for otitis media = drainage middle ear

Ear, Nose, Sinus 090-09W

0 Medical and Surgical
9 Ear, Nose, Sinus
0 Alteration: Modifying the anatomic structure of a body part without affecting the function of the body part

Body Part Character 4	Approach Character 5	Device Character 6	Qualifier Character 7
0 External Ear, Right **1** External Ear, Left **2** External Ear, Bilateral **K** Nasal Mucosa and Soft Tissue nose	**0** Open **3** Percutaneous **4** Percutaneous Endoscopic **X** External	**7** Autologous Tissue Substitute **J** Synthetic Substitute **K** Nonautologous Tissue Substitute **Z** No Device	**Z** No Qualifier local tissue graft

0 Medical and Surgical
9 Ear, Nose, Sinus
1 Bypass: Altering the route of passage of the contents of a tubular body part

Body Part Character 4	Approach Character 5	Device Character 6	Qualifier Character 7
D Inner Ear, Right **E** Inner Ear, Left	**0** Open	**7** Autologous Tissue Substitute **J** Synthetic Substitute **K** Nonautologous Tissue Substitute **Z** No Device	**0** Endolymphatic

0 Medical and Surgical
9 Ear, Nose, Sinus
2 Change: Taking out or off a device from a body part and putting back an identical or similar device in or on the same body part without cutting or puncturing the skin or a mucous membrane

Body Part Character 4	Approach Character 5	Device Character 6	Qualifier Character 7
H Ear, Right **J** Ear, Left **K** Nasal Mucosa and Soft Tissue **Y** Sinus	**X** External	**0** Drainage Device **Y** Other Device	**Z** No Qualifier

0 Medical and Surgical
9 Ear, Nose, Sinus
3 Control: Stopping, or attempting to stop, postprocedural or other acute bleeding

Body Part Character 4	Approach Character 5	Device Character 6	Qualifier Character 7
K Nasal Mucosa and Soft Tissue	**7** Via Natural or Artificial Opening **8** Via Natural or Artificial Opening Endoscopic	**Z** No Device	**Z** No Qualifier

0 Medical and Surgical
9 Ear, Nose, Sinus
5 Destruction: Physical eradication of all or a portion of a body part by the direct use of energy, force, or a destructive agent

Body Part Character 4	Approach Character 5	Device Character 6	Qualifier Character 7
0 External Ear, Right **1** External Ear, Left	**0** Open **3** Percutaneous **4** Percutaneous Endoscopic **X** External	**Z** No Device	**Z** No Qualifier
3 External Auditory Canal, Right **4** External Auditory Canal, Left	**0** Open **3** Percutaneous **4** Percutaneous Endoscopic **7** Via Natural or Artificial Opening **8** Via Natural or Artificial Opening Endoscopic **X** External	**Z** No Device	**Z** No Qualifier
5 Middle Ear, Right **6** Middle Ear, Left **9** Auditory Ossicle, Right **A** Auditory Ossicle, Left **D** Inner Ear, Right **E** Inner Ear, Left	**0** Open **8** Via Natural or Artificial Opening Endoscopic	**Z** No Device	**Z** No Qualifier
7 Tympanic Membrane, Right **8** Tympanic Membrane, Left **F** Eustachian Tube, Right **G** Eustachian Tube, Left **L** Nasal Turbinate **N** Nasopharynx	**0** Open **3** Percutaneous **4** Percutaneous Endoscopic **7** Via Natural or Artificial Opening **8** Via Natural or Artificial Opening Endoscopic	**Z** No Device	**Z** No Qualifier
B Mastoid Sinus, Right **C** Mastoid Sinus, Left **M** Nasal Septum **P** Accessory Sinus **Q** Maxillary Sinus, Right **R** Maxillary Sinus, Left **S** Frontal Sinus, Right **T** Frontal Sinus, Left **U** Ethmoid Sinus, Right **V** Ethmoid Sinus, Left **W** Sphenoid Sinus, Right **X** Sphenoid Sinus, Left	**0** Open **3** Percutaneous **4** Percutaneous Endoscopic **8** Via Natural or Artificial Opening Endoscopic	**Z** No Device	**Z** No Qualifier
K Nasal Mucosa and Soft Tissue	**0** Open **3** Percutaneous **4** Percutaneous Endoscopic **8** Via Natural or Artificial Opening Endoscopic **X** External	**Z** No Device	**Z** No Qualifier

0 Medical and Surgical
9 Ear, Nose, Sinus
7 Dilation: Expanding an orifice or the lumen of a tubular body part

Body Part Character 4	Approach Character 5	Device Character 6	Qualifier Character 7
F Eustachian Tube, Right **G** Eustachian Tube, Left	**0** Open **7** Via Natural or Artificial Opening **8** Via Natural or Artificial Opening Endoscopic	**D** Intraluminal Device **Z** No Device	**Z** No Qualifier
F Eustachian Tube, Right **G** Eustachian Tube, Left	**3** Percutaneous **4** Percutaneous Endoscopic	**Z** No Device	**Z** No Qualifier

0 Medical and Surgical
9 Ear, Nose, Sinus
8 Division: Cutting into a body part, without draining fluids and/or gases from the body part, in order to separate or transect a body part

Body Part Character 4	Approach Character 5	Device Character 6	Qualifier Character 7
L Nasal Turbinate	**0** Open **3** Percutaneous **4** Percutaneous Endoscopic **7** Via Natural or Artificial Opening **8** Via Natural or Artificial Opening Endoscopic	**Z** No Device	**Z** No Qualifier

0 Medical and Surgical
9 Ear, Nose, Sinus
9 Drainage: Taking or letting out fluids and/or gases from a body part

myringotomy
tympanotomy - insert myringotomy tubes in middle ear. do not code cutting hole

Body Part Character 4	Approach Character 5	Device Character 6	Qualifier Character 7
0 External Ear, Right **1** External Ear, Left	**0** Open **3** Percutaneous **4** Percutaneous Endoscopic **X** External	**0** Drainage Device	**Z** No Qualifier
0 External Ear, Right **1** External Ear, Left	**0** Open **3** Percutaneous **4** Percutaneous Endoscopic **X** External	**Z** No Device	**X** Diagnostic **Z** No Qualifier
3 External Auditory Canal, Right **4** External Auditory Canal, Left **K** Nasal Mucosa and Soft Tissue	**0** Open **3** Percutaneous **4** Percutaneous Endoscopic **7** Via Natural or Artificial Opening **8** Via Natural or Artificial Opening Endoscopic **X** External	**0** Drainage Device	**Z** No Qualifier
3 External Auditory Canal, Right **4** External Auditory Canal, Left **K** Nasal Mucosa and Soft Tissue	**0** Open **3** Percutaneous **4** Percutaneous Endoscopic **7** Via Natural or Artificial Opening **8** Via Natural or Artificial Opening Endoscopic **X** External	**Z** No Device	**X** Diagnostic **Z** No Qualifier
5 Middle Ear, Right > tympanotomy See below **6** Middle Ear, Left **9** Auditory Ossicle, Right **A** Auditory Ossicle, Left **D** Inner Ear, Right **E** Inner Ear, Left	**0** Open - no endoscope method - may use microscope **7** Via Natural or Artificial Opening **8** Via Natural or Artificial Opening Endoscopic	**0** Drainage Device myringotomy tube ventilation device	**Z** No Qualifier
5 Middle Ear, Right **6** Middle Ear, Left **9** Auditory Ossicle, Right **A** Auditory Ossicle, Left **D** Inner Ear, Right **E** Inner Ear, Left	**0** Open **7** Via Natural or Artificial Opening **8** Via Natural or Artificial Opening Endoscopic	**Z** No Device	**X** Diagnostic **Z** No Qualifier

tube may be placed w/in tympanic membrane to drain mucopurulent debris w/in middle ear cleft - if so use middle ear as that is where drainage is need. Do not code also the insertion of tubes myringotomy
tympanotomy - hole made in tymphanic membrane

099 continued on next page

percutaneous endoscopic - small puncture made through the ethmoid bone to get into ethmoid sinus

099 continued from previous page

0 Medical and Surgical
9 Ear, Nose, Sinus
9 Drainage: Taking or letting out fluids and/or gases from a body part antrostomy

Body Part Character 4	Approach Character 5	Device Character 6	Qualifier Character 7
7 Tympanic Membrane, Right **8** Tympanic Membrane, Left **B** Mastoid Sinus, Right **C** Mastoid Sinus, Left **F** Eustachian Tube, Right **G** Eustachian Tube, Left **L** Nasal Turbinate **M** Nasal Septum **N** Nasopharynx **P** Accessory Sinus **Q** Maxillary Sinus, Right **R** Maxillary Sinus, Left ? antrostomy **S** Frontal Sinus, Right **T** Frontal Sinus, Left **U** Ethmoid Sinus, Right **V** Ethmoid Sinus, Left **W** Sphenoid Sinus, Right **X** Sphenoid Sinus, Left	**0** Open **3** Percutaneous **4** Percutaneous Endoscopic **7** Via Natural or Artificial Opening **8** Via Natural or Artificial Opening Endoscopic · nasal	**0** Drainage Device – must be left in place	**Z** No Qualifier
7 Tympanic Membrane, Right **8** Tympanic Membrane, Left **B** Mastoid Sinus, Right **C** Mastoid Sinus, Left **F** Eustachian Tube, Right **G** Eustachian Tube, Left **L** Nasal Turbinate **M** Nasal Septum **N** Nasopharynx **P** Accessory Sinus **Q** Maxillary Sinus, Right **R** Maxillary Sinus, Left **S** Frontal Sinus, Right **T** Frontal Sinus, Left **U** Ethmoid Sinus, Right **V** Ethmoid Sinus, Left **W** Sphenoid Sinus, Right **X** Sphenoid Sinus, Left	**0** Open **3** Percutaneous - puncture **4** Percutaneous Endoscopic **7** Via Natural or Artificial Opening **8** Via Natural or Artificial Opening Endoscopic	**Z** No Device	**X** Diagnostic **Z** No Qualifier

0 Medical and Surgical
9 Ear, Nose, Sinus
B Excision: Cutting out or off, without replacement, a portion of a body part

Body Part Character 4	Approach Character 5	Device Character 6	Qualifier Character 7
0 External Ear, Right **1** External Ear, Left	**0** Open **3** Percutaneous **4** Percutaneous Endoscopic **X** External	**Z** No Device	**X** Diagnostic **Z** No Qualifier
3 External Auditory Canal, Right **4** External Auditory Canal, Left	**0** Open **3** Percutaneous **4** Percutaneous Endoscopic **7** Via Natural or Artificial Opening **8** Via Natural or Artificial Opening Endoscopic **X** External	**Z** No Device	**X** Diagnostic **Z** No Qualifier
5 Middle Ear, Right **6** Middle Ear, Left **9** Auditory Ossicle, Right **A** Auditory Ossicle, Left **D** Inner Ear, Right **E** Inner Ear, Left	**0** Open **8** Via Natural or Artificial Opening Endoscopic	**Z** No Device	**X** Diagnostic **Z** No Qualifier
7 Tympanic Membrane, Right **8** Tympanic Membrane, Left **F** Eustachian Tube, Right **G** Eustachian Tube, Left **L** Nasal Turbinate **N** Nasopharynx	**0** Open **3** Percutaneous **4** Percutaneous Endoscopic **7** Via Natural or Artificial Opening **8** Via Natural or Artificial Opening Endoscopic	**Z** No Device	**X** Diagnostic **Z** No Qualifier
B Mastoid Sinus, Right **C** Mastoid Sinus, Left **M** Nasal Septum **P** Accessory Sinus **Q** Maxillary Sinus, Right **R** Maxillary Sinus, Left **S** Frontal Sinus, Right **T** Frontal Sinus, Left **U** Ethmoid Sinus, Right **V** Ethmoid Sinus, Left **W** Sphenoid Sinus, Right **X** Sphenoid Sinus, Left	**0** Open **3** Percutaneous **4** Percutaneous Endoscopic **8** Via Natural or Artificial Opening Endoscopic	**Z** No Device	**X** Diagnostic **Z** No Qualifier
K Nasal Mucosa and Soft Tissue	**0** Open **3** Percutaneous **4** Percutaneous Endoscopic **8** Via Natural or Artificial Opening Endoscopic **X** External	**Z** No Device	**X** Diagnostic **Z** No Qualifier

0 Medical and Surgical
9 Ear, Nose, Sinus
C Extirpation: Taking or cutting out solid matter from a body part

Body Part Character 4	Approach Character 5	Device Character 6	Qualifier Character 7
0 External Ear, Right **1** External Ear, Left	**0** Open **3** Percutaneous **4** Percutaneous Endoscopic **X** External	**Z** No Device	**Z** No Qualifier
3 External Auditory Canal, Right **4** External Auditory Canal, Left	**0** Open **3** Percutaneous **4** Percutaneous Endoscopic **7** Via Natural or Artificial Opening **8** Via Natural or Artificial Opening Endoscopic **X** External	**Z** No Device	**Z** No Qualifier
5 Middle Ear, Right **6** Middle Ear, Left **9** Auditory Ossicle, Right **A** Auditory Ossicle, Left **D** Inner Ear, Right **E** Inner Ear, Left	**0** Open **8** Via Natural or Artificial Opening Endoscopic	**Z** No Device	**Z** No Qualifier
7 Tympanic Membrane, Right **8** Tympanic Membrane, Left **F** Eustachian Tube, Right **G** Eustachian Tube, Left **L** Nasal Turbinate **N** Nasopharynx	**0** Open **3** Percutaneous **4** Percutaneous Endoscopic **7** Via Natural or Artificial Opening **8** Via Natural or Artificial Opening Endoscopic	**Z** No Device	**Z** No Qualifier
B Mastoid Sinus, Right **C** Mastoid Sinus, Left **M** Nasal Septum **P** Accessory Sinus **Q** Maxillary Sinus, Right **R** Maxillary Sinus, Left **S** Frontal Sinus, Right **T** Frontal Sinus, Left **U** Ethmoid Sinus, Right **V** Ethmoid Sinus, Left **W** Sphenoid Sinus, Right **X** Sphenoid Sinus, Left	**0** Open **3** Percutaneous **4** Percutaneous Endoscopic **8** Via Natural or Artificial Opening Endoscopic	**Z** No Device	**Z** No Qualifier
K Nasal Mucosa and Soft Tissue nostril	**0** Open **3** Percutaneous **4** Percutaneous Endoscopic **8** Via Natural or Artificial Opening Endoscopic **X** External - use forceps	**Z** No Device	**Z** No Qualifier

LC Limited Coverage NC Noncovered HAC HAC-associated Procedure CC Combination Cluster - See Appendix G for code lists
DRG Non-OR-Affecting MS-DRG Assignment New/Revised Text in **Orange** ♂ Male ♀ Female

0 Medical and Surgical
9 Ear, Nose, Sinus
D Extraction: Pulling or stripping out or off all or a portion of a body part by the use of force

Body Part Character 4	Approach Character 5	Device Character 6	Qualifier Character 7
7 Tympanic Membrane, Right 8 Tympanic Membrane, Left L Nasal Turbinate	0 Open 3 Percutaneous 4 Percutaneous Endoscopic 7 Via Natural or Artificial Opening 8 Via Natural or Artificial Opening Endoscopic	Z No Device	Z No Qualifier
9 Auditory Ossicle, Right A Auditory Ossicle, Left	0 Open	Z No Device	Z No Qualifier
B Mastoid Sinus, Right C Mastoid Sinus, Left M Nasal Septum P Accessory Sinus Q Maxillary Sinus, Right R Maxillary Sinus, Left S Frontal Sinus, Right T Frontal Sinus, Left U Ethmoid Sinus, Right V Ethmoid Sinus, Left W Sphenoid Sinus, Right X Sphenoid Sinus, Left	0 Open 3 Percutaneous 4 Percutaneous Endoscopic	Z No Device	Z No Qualifier

0 Medical and Surgical
9 Ear, Nose, Sinus
H Insertion: Putting in a nonbiological appliance that monitors, assists, performs, or prevents a physiological function but does not physically take the place of a body part cochlear implant

Body Part Character 4	Approach Character 5	Device Character 6	Qualifier Character 7
D Inner Ear, Right E Inner Ear, Left — cochlear	0 Open 3 Percutaneous 4 Percutaneous Endoscopic	4 Hearing Device, Bone Conduction 5 Hearing Device, Single Channel Cochlear Prosthesis 6 Hearing Device, Multiple Channel Cochlear Prosthesis S Hearing Device	Z No Qualifier
H Ear, Right J Ear, Left K Nasal Mucosa and Soft Tissue Y Sinus	0 Open 3 Percutaneous 4 Percutaneous Endoscopic 7 Via Natural or Artificial Opening 8 Via Natural or Artificial Opening Endoscopic	Y Other Device	Z No Qualifier
N Nasopharynx	7 Via Natural or Artificial Opening 8 Via Natural or Artificial Opening Endoscopic	B Intraluminal Device, Airway	Z No Qualifier

0 Medical and Surgical
9 Ear, Nose, Sinus
J Inspection: Visually and/or manually exploring a body part

Body Part Character 4	Approach Character 5	Device Character 6	Qualifier Character 7
7 Tympanic Membrane, Right 8 Tympanic Membrane, Left H Ear, Right J Ear, Left	0 Open 3 Percutaneous 4 Percutaneous Endoscopic 7 Via Natural or Artificial Opening 8 Via Natural or Artificial Opening Endoscopic X External	Z No Device	Z No Qualifier
D Inner Ear, Right E Inner Ear, Left K Nasal Mucosa and Soft tissue Y Sinus	0 Open 3 Percutaneous 4 Percutaneous Endoscopic 8 Via Natural or Artificial Opening Endoscopic X External	Z No Device	Z No Qualifier

0 Medical and Surgical
9 Ear, Nose, Sinus
M Reattachment: Putting back in or on all or a portion of a separated body part to its normal location or other suitable location

Body Part Character 4	Approach Character 5	Device Character 6	Qualifier Character 7
0 External Ear, Right **1** External Ear, Left **K** Nasal Mucosa and Soft Tissue	**X** External	**Z** No Device	**Z** No Qualifier

0 Medical and Surgical
9 Ear, Nose, Sinus
N Release: Freeing a body part from an abnormal physical constraint by cutting or by the use of force

Body Part Character 4	Approach Character 5	Device Character 6	Qualifier Character 7
0 External Ear, Right **1** External Ear, Left	**0** Open **3** Percutaneous **4** Percutaneous Endoscopic **X** External	**Z** No Device	**Z** No Qualifier
3 External Auditory Canal, Right **4** External Auditory Canal, Left	**0** Open **3** Percutaneous **4** Percutaneous Endoscopic **7** Via Natural or Artificial Opening **8** Via Natural or Artificial Opening Endoscopic **X** External	**Z** No Device	**Z** No Qualifier
5 Middle Ear, Right **6** Middle Ear, Left **9** Auditory Ossicle, Right **A** Auditory Ossicle, Left **D** Inner Ear, Right **E** Inner Ear, Left	**0** Open **8** Via Natural or Artificial Opening Endoscopic	**Z** No Device	**Z** No Qualifier
7 Tympanic Membrane, Right **8** Tympanic Membrane, Left **F** Eustachian Tube, Right **G** Eustachian Tube, Left **L** Nasal Turbinate **N** Nasopharynx	**0** Open **3** Percutaneous **4** Percutaneous Endoscopic **7** Via Natural or Artificial Opening **8** Via Natural or Artificial Opening Endoscopic	**Z** No Device	**Z** No Qualifier
B Mastoid Sinus, Right **C** Mastoid Sinus, Left **M** Nasal Septum **P** Accessory Sinus **Q** Maxillary Sinus, Right **R** Maxillary Sinus, Left **S** Frontal Sinus, Right **T** Frontal Sinus, Left **U** Ethmoid Sinus, Right **V** Ethmoid Sinus, Left **W** Sphenoid Sinus, Right **X** Sphenoid Sinus, Left	**0** Open **3** Percutaneous **4** Percutaneous Endoscopic **8** Via Natural or Artificial Opening Endoscopic	**Z** No Device	**Z** No Qualifier
K Nasal Mucosa and Soft Tissue	**0** Open **3** Percutaneous **4** Percutaneous Endoscopic **8** Via Natural or Artificial Opening Endoscopic **X** External	**Z** No Device	**Z** No Qualifier

0 Medical and Surgical
9 Ear, Nose, Sinus
P Removal: Taking out or off a device from a body part

Body Part Character 4	Approach Character 5	Device Character 6	Qualifier Character 7
7 Tympanic Membrane, Right **8** Tympanic Membrane, Left	**0** Open **7** Via Natural or Artificial Opening **8** Via Natural or Artificial Opening Endoscopic **X** External	**0** Drainage Device	**Z** No Qualifier
D Inner Ear, Right **E** Inner Ear, Left	**0** Open **7** Via Natural or Artificial Opening **8** Via Natural or Artificial Opening Endoscopic	**S** Hearing Device	**Z** No Qualifier
H Ear, Right **J** Ear, Left **K** Nasal Mucosa and Soft Tissue	**0** Open **3** Percutaneous **4** Percutaneous Endoscopic **7** Via Natural or Artificial Opening **8** Via Natural or Artificial Opening Endoscopic	**0** Drainage Device **7** Autologous Tissue Substitute **D** Intraluminal Device **J** Synthetic Substitute **K** Nonautologous Tissue Substitute **Y** Other Device	**Z** No Qualifier
H Ear, Right **J** Ear, Left **K** Nasal Mucosa and Soft Tissue	**X** External	**0** Drainage Device **7** Autologous Tissue Substitute **D** Intraluminal Device **J** Synthetic Substitute **K** Nonautologous Tissue Substitute	**Z** No Qualifier
Y Sinus	**0** Open **3** Percutaneous **4** Percutaneous Endoscopic	**0** Drainage Device **Y** Other Device	**Z** No Qualifier
Y Sinus	**7** Via Natural or Artificial Opening **8** Via Natural or Artificial Opening Endoscopic	**Y** Other Device	**Z** No Qualifier
Y Sinus	**X** External	**0** Drainage Device	**Z** No Qualifier

0 Medical and Surgical
9 Ear, Nose, Sinus
Q Repair: Restoring, to the extent possible, a body part to its normal anatomic structure and function

Body Part	Approach	Device	Qualifier
Character 4	**Character 5**	**Character 6**	**Character 7**
0 External Ear, Right **1** External Ear, Left **2** External Ear, Bilateral	**0** Open **3** Percutaneous **4** Percutaneous Endoscopic **X** External	**Z** No Device	**Z** No Qualifier
3 External Auditory Canal, Right **4** External Auditory Canal, Left **F** Eustachian Tube, Right **G** Eustachian Tube, Left	**0** Open **3** Percutaneous **4** Percutaneous Endoscopic **7** Via Natural or Artificial Opening **8** Via Natural or Artificial Opening Endoscopic **X** External	**Z** No Device	**Z** No Qualifier
5 Middle Ear, Right **6** Middle Ear, Left **9** Auditory Ossicle, Right **A** Auditory Ossicle, Left **D** Inner Ear, Right **E** Inner Ear, Left	**0** Open **8** Via Natural or Artificial Opening Endoscopic	**Z** No Device	**Z** No Qualifier
7 Tympanic Membrane, Right **8** Tympanic Membrane, Left **L** Nasal Turbinate **N** Nasopharynx	**0** Open **3** Percutaneous **4** Percutaneous Endoscopic **7** Via Natural or Artificial Opening **8** Via Natural or Artificial Opening Endoscopic	**Z** No Device	**Z** No Qualifier
B Mastoid Sinus, Right **C** Mastoid Sinus, Left **M** Nasal Septum Septoplasty **P** Accessory Sinus **Q** Maxillary Sinus, Right **R** Maxillary Sinus, Left **S** Frontal Sinus, Right **T** Frontal Sinus, Left **U** Ethmoid Sinus, Right **V** Ethmoid Sinus, Left **W** Sphenoid Sinus, Right **X** Sphenoid Sinus, Left	**0** Open submucous **3** Percutaneous **4** Percutaneous Endoscopic **8** Via Natural or Artificial Opening Endoscopic	**Z** No Device	**Z** No Qualifier
K Nasal Mucosa and Soft Tissue	**0** Open **3** Percutaneous **4** Percutaneous Endoscopic **8** Via Natural or Artificial Opening Endoscopic **X** External	**Z** No Device	**Z** No Qualifier

nasal septoplasty 09QM0ZZ

0 Medical and Surgical
9 Ear, Nose, Sinus
R Replacement: Putting in or on biological or synthetic material that physically takes the place and/or function of all or a portion of a body part

Body Part Character 4	Approach Character 5	Device Character 6	Qualifier Character 7
0 External Ear, Right **1** External Ear, Left **2** External Ear, Bilateral **K** Nasal Mucosa and Soft Tissue	**0** Open **X** External	**7** Autologous Tissue Substitute **J** Synthetic Substitute **K** Nonautologous Tissue Substitute	**Z** No Qualifier
5 Middle Ear, Right **6** Middle Ear, Left **9** Auditory Ossicle, Right **A** Auditory Ossicle, Left **D** Inner Ear, Right **E** Inner Ear, Left	**0** Open	**7** Autologous Tissue Substitute **J** Synthetic Substitute **K** Nonautologous Tissue Substitute	**Z** No Qualifier
7 Tympanic Membrane, Right **8** Tympanic Membrane, Left **N** Nasopharynx	**0** Open **7** Via Natural or Artificial Opening **8** Via Natural or Artificial Opening Endoscopic	**7** Autologous Tissue Substitute **J** Synthetic Substitute **K** Nonautologous Tissue Substitute	**Z** No Qualifier
L Nasal Turbinate	**0** Open **3** Percutaneous **4** Percutaneous Endoscopic **7** Via Natural or Artificial Opening **8** Via Natural or Artificial Opening Endoscopic	**7** Autologous Tissue Substitute **J** Synthetic Substitute **K** Nonautologous Tissue Substitute	**Z** No Qualifier
M Nasal Septum	**0** Open **3** Percutaneous **4** Percutaneous Endoscopic	**7** Autologous Tissue Substitute **J** Synthetic Substitute **K** Nonautologous Tissue Substitute	**Z** No Qualifier

0 Medical and Surgical
9 Ear, Nose, Sinus
S Reposition: Moving to its normal location, or other suitable location, all or a portion of a body part

Body Part Character 4	Approach Character 5	Device Character 6	Qualifier Character 7
0 External Ear, Right **1** External Ear, Left **2** External Ear, Bilateral **K** Nasal Mucosa and Soft Tissue	**0** Open **4** Percutaneous Endoscopic **X** External	**Z** No Device	**Z** No Qualifier
7 Tympanic Membrane, Right **8** Tympanic Membrane, Left **F** Eustachian Tube, Right **G** Eustachian Tube, Left **L** Nasal Turbinate	**0** Open **4** Percutaneous Endoscopic **7** Via Natural or Artificial Opening **8** Via Natural or Artificial Opening Endoscopic	**Z** No Device	**Z** No Qualifier
9 Auditory Ossicle, Right **A** Auditory Ossicle, Left **M** Nasal Septum	**0** Open **4** Percutaneous Endoscopic	**Z** No Device	**Z** No Qualifier

0 Medical and Surgical
9 Ear, Nose, Sinus
T Resection: Cutting out or off, without replacement, all of a body part

Body Part Character 4	Approach Character 5	Device Character 6	Qualifier Character 7
0 External Ear, Right **1** External Ear, Left	**0** Open **4** Percutaneous Endoscopic **X** External	**Z** No Device	**Z** No Qualifier
5 Middle Ear, Right **6** Middle Ear, Left **9** Auditory Ossicle, Right **A** Auditory Ossicle, Left **D** Inner Ear, Right **E** Inner Ear, Left	**0** Open **8** Via Natural or Artificial Opening Endoscopic	**Z** No Device	**Z** No Qualifier
7 Tympanic Membrane, Right **8** Tympanic Membrane, Left **F** Eustachian Tube, Right **G** Eustachian Tube, Left **L** Nasal Turbinate **N** Nasopharynx	**0** Open **4** Percutaneous Endoscopic **7** Via Natural or Artificial Opening **8** Via Natural or Artificial Opening Endoscopic	**Z** No Device	**Z** No Qualifier
B Mastoid Sinus, Right **C** Mastoid Sinus, Left **M** Nasal Septum **P** Accessory Sinus **Q** Maxillary Sinus, Right **R** Maxillary Sinus, Left **S** Frontal Sinus, Right **T** Frontal Sinus, Left **U** Ethmoid Sinus, Right **V** Ethmoid Sinus, Left **W** Sphenoid Sinus, Right **X** Sphenoid Sinus, Left	**0** Open - submuchous **4** Percutaneous Endoscopic **8** Via Natural or Artificial Opening Endoscopic complete submucuous septectomy nasal	**Z** No Device	**Z** No Qualifier
K Nasal Mucosa and Soft Tissue	**0** Open **4** Percutaneous Endoscopic **8** Via Natural or Artificial Opening Endoscopic **X** External	**Z** No Device	**Z** No Qualifier

submucous septectomy 09TM0ZZ

0 Medical and Surgical
9 Ear, Nose, Sinus
U Supplement: Putting in or on biological or synthetic material that physically reinforces and/or augments the function of a portion of a body part

Body Part Character 4	Approach Character 5	Device Character 6	Qualifier Character 7
0 External Ear, Right **1** External Ear, Left **2** External Ear, Bilateral	**0** Open **X** External	**7** Autologous Tissue Substitute **J** Synthetic Substitute **K** Nonautologous Tissue Substitute	**Z** No Qualifier
5 Middle Ear, Right **6** Middle Ear, Left **9** Auditory Ossicle, Right **A** Auditory Ossicle, Left **D** Inner Ear, Right **E** Inner Ear, Left	**0** Open **8** Via Natural or Artificial Opening Endoscopic	**7** Autologous Tissue Substitute **J** Synthetic Substitute **K** Nonautologous Tissue Substitute	**Z** No Qualifier
7 Tympanic Membrane, Right **8** Tympanic Membrane, Left **N** Nasopharynx	**0** Open **7** Via Natural or Artificial Opening **8** Via Natural or Artificial Opening Endoscopic	**7** Autologous Tissue Substitute **J** Synthetic Substitute **K** Nonautologous Tissue Substitute	**Z** No Qualifier
B Mastoid Sinus, Right **C** Mastoid Sinus, Left **L** Nasal Turbinate **P** Accessory Sinus **Q** Maxillary Sinus, Right **R** Maxillary Sinus, Left **S** Frontal Sinus, Right **T** Frontal Sinus, Left **U** Ethmoid Sinus, Right **V** Ethmoid Sinus, Left **W** Sphenoid Sinus, Right **X** Sphenoid Sinus, Left	**0** Open **3** Percutaneous **4** Percutaneous Endoscopic **7** Via Natural or Artificial Opening **8** Via Natural or Artificial Opening Endoscopic	**7** Autologous Tissue Substitute **J** Synthetic Substitute **K** Nonautologous Tissue Substitute	**Z** No Qualifier
K Nasal Mucosa and Soft Tissue	**0** Open **8** Via Natural or Artificial Opening Endoscopic **X** External	**7** Autologous Tissue Substitute **J** Synthetic Substitute **K** Nonautologous Tissue Substitute	**Z** No Qualifier
M Nasal Septum	**0** Open **3** Percutaneous **4** Percutaneous Endoscopic **8** Via Natural or Artificial Opening Endoscopic	**7** Autologous Tissue Substitute **J** Synthetic Substitute **K** Nonautologous Tissue Substitute	**Z** No Qualifier

0 Medical and Surgical
9 Ear, Nose, Sinus
W Revision: Correcting, to the extent possible, a portion of a malfunctioning device or the position of a displaced device

Body Part Character 4	Approach Character 5	Device Character 6	Qualifier Character 7
7 Tympanic Membrane, Right **8** Tympanic Membrane, Left **9** Auditory Ossicle, Right **A** Auditory Ossicle, Left	**0** Open **7** Via Natural or Artificial Opening **8** Via Natural or Artificial Opening Endoscopic	**7** Autologous Tissue Substitute **J** Synthetic Substitute **K** Nonautologous Tissue Substitute	**Z** No Qualifier
D Inner Ear, Right **E** Inner Ear, Left	**0** Open **7** Via Natural or Artificial Opening **8** Via Natural or Artificial Opening Endoscopic	**S** Hearing Device	**Z** No Qualifier
H Ear, Right **J** Ear, Left **K** Nasal Mucosa and Soft Tissue	**0** Open **3** Percutaneous **4** Percutaneous Endoscopic **7** Via Natural or Artificial Opening **8** Via Natural or Artificial Opening Endoscopic	**0** Drainage Device **7** Autologous Tissue Substitute **D** Intraluminal Device **J** Synthetic Substitute **K** Nonautologous Tissue Substitute **Y** Other Device	**Z** No Qualifier
H Ear, Right **J** Ear, Left **K** Nasal Mucosa and Soft Tissue	**X** External	**0** Drainage Device **7** Autologous Tissue Substitute **D** Intraluminal Device **J** Synthetic Substitute **K** Nonautologous Tissue Substitute	**Z** No Qualifier
Y Sinus	**0** Open **3** Percutaneous **4** Percutaneous Endoscopic	**0** Drainage Device **Y** Other Device	**Z** No Qualifier
Y Sinus	**7** Via Natural or Artificial Opening **8** Via Natural or Artificial Opening Endoscopic	**Y** Other Device	**Z** No Qualifier
Y Sinus	**X** External	**0** Drainage Device	**Z** No Qualifier

NOTES

NOTES

Respiratory System 0B1-0BY

0 Medical and Surgical
B Respiratory System
1 Bypass: Altering the route of passage of the contents of a tubular body part

Body Part Character 4	Approach Character 5	Device Character 6	Qualifier Character 7
1 Trachea	**0** Open	**D** Intraluminal Device	**6** Esophagus
1 Trachea	**0** Open	**F** Tracheostomy Device **Z** No Device	**4** Cutaneous
1 Trachea DRG	**3** Percutaneous **4** Percutaneous Endoscopic	**F** Tracheostomy Device **Z** No Device	**4** Cutaneous

DRG 0B113F4 0B113Z4

0 Medical and Surgical
B Respiratory System
2 Change: Taking out or off a device from a body part and putting back an identical or similar device in or on the same body part without cutting or puncturing the skin or a mucous membrane

Body Part Character 4	Approach Character 5	Device Character 6	Qualifier Character 7
0 Tracheobronchial Tree **K** Lung, Right **L** Lung, Left **Q** Pleura **T** Diaphragm	**X** External	**0** Drainage Device **Y** Other Device	**Z** No Qualifier
1 Trachea tracheostomy tube exchange	**X** External	**0** Drainage Device **E** Intraluminal Device, Endotracheal Airway **F** Tracheostomy Device trach tube **Y** Other Device	**Z** No Qualifier

0 Medical and Surgical
B Respiratory System
5 Destruction: Physical eradication of all or a portion of a body part by the direct use of energy, force, or a destructive agent

Body Part Character 4	Approach Character 5	Device Character 6	Qualifier Character 7
1 Trachea **2** Carina **3** Main Bronchus, Right **4** Upper Lobe Bronchus, Right **5** Middle Lobe Bronchus, Right **6** Lower Lobe Bronchus, Right **7** Main Bronchus, Left **8** Upper Lobe Bronchus, Left **9** Lingula Bronchus **B** Lower Lobe Bronchus, Left **C** Upper Lung Lobe, Right **D** Middle Lung Lobe, Right **F** Lower Lung Lobe, Right **G** Upper Lung Lobe, Left **H** Lung Lingula **J** Lower Lung Lobe, Left **K** Lung, Right **L** Lung, Left **M** Lungs, Bilateral	**0** Open **3** Percutaneous **4** Percutaneous Endoscopic **7** Via Natural or Artificial Opening **8** Via Natural or Artificial Opening Endoscopic	**Z** No Device	**Z** No Qualifier
N Pleura, Right **P** Pleura, Left **T** Diaphragm	**0** Open **3** Percutaneous **4** Percutaneous Endoscopic	**Z** No Device	**Z** No Qualifier

LC Limited Coverage NC Noncovered HAC HAC-associated Procedure CC Combination Cluster - See Appendix G for code lists
DRG Non-OR-Affecting MS-DRG Assignment New/Revised Text in **Orange** ♂ Male ♀ Female

2020 ICD-10-PCS **309**

0 Medical and Surgical
B Respiratory System
7 Dilation: Expanding an orifice or the lumen of a tubular body part

Body Part Character 4	Approach Character 5	Device Character 6	Qualifier Character 7
1 Trachea **2** Carina **3** Main Bronchus, Right **4** Upper Lobe Bronchus, Right **5** Middle Lobe Bronchus, Right **6** Lower Lobe Bronchus, Right **7** Main Bronchus, Left **8** Upper Lobe Bronchus, Left **9** Lingula Bronchus **B** Lower Lobe Bronchus, Left	**0** Open **3** Percutaneous **4** Percutaneous Endoscopic **7** Via Natural or Artificial Opening **8** Via Natural or Artificial Opening Endoscopic	**D** Intraluminal Device **Z** No Device	**Z** No Qualifier

0 Medical and Surgical
B Respiratory System
9 Drainage: Taking or letting out fluids and/or gases from a body part

Body Part Character 4	Approach Character 5	Device Character 6	Qualifier Character 7
1 Trachea **2** Carina **3** Main Bronchus, Right **4** Upper Lobe Bronchus, Right **5** Middle Lobe Bronchus, Right **6** Lower Lobe Bronchus, Right **7** Main Bronchus, Left **8** Upper Lobe Bronchus, Left **9** Lingula Bronchus **B** Lower Lobe Bronchus, Left **C** Upper Lung Lobe, Right **D** Middle Lung Lobe, Right **F** Lower Lung Lobe, Right **G** Upper Lung Lobe, Left **H** Lung Lingula **J** Lower Lung Lobe, Left **K** Lung, Right **L** Lung, Left **M** Lungs, Bilateral	**0** Open **3** Percutaneous **4** Percutaneous Endoscopic **7** Via Natural or Artificial Opening **8** Via Natural or Artificial Opening Endoscopic	**0** Drainage Device	**Z** No Qualifier
1 Trachea **2** Carina **3** Main Bronchus, Right **4** Upper Lobe Bronchus, Right **5** Middle Lobe Bronchus, Right **6** Lower Lobe Bronchus, Right **7** Main Bronchus, Left **8** Upper Lobe Bronchus, Left **9** Lingula Bronchus **B** Lower Lobe Bronchus, Left **C** Upper Lung Lobe, Right **D** Middle Lung Lobe, Right **F** Lower Lung Lobe, Right **G** Upper Lung Lobe, Left **H** Lung Lingula **J** Lower Lung Lobe, Left **K** Lung, Right **L** Lung, Left **M** Lungs, Bilateral	**0** Open **3** Percutaneous **4** Percutaneous Endoscopic **7** Via Natural or Artificial Opening **8** Via Natural or Artificial Opening Endoscopic	**Z** No Device	**X** Diagnostic **Z** No Qualifier

0B9 continued on next page

Segmentectomy - 4 - puncture chest wall & use endoscopic technique/may use thorascope

0B9 continued from previous page

0 Medical and Surgical
B Respiratory System
9 Drainage: Taking or letting out fluids and/or gases from a body part

Body Part Character 4	Approach Character 5	Device Character 6	Qualifier Character 7
N Pleura, Right **P** Pleura, Left	**0** Open **3** Percutaneous **4** Percutaneous Endoscopic **8** Via Natural or Artificial Opening Endoscopic	**0** Drainage Device	**Z** No Qualifier
N Pleura, Right **P** Pleura, Left	**0** Open **3** Percutaneous **4** Percutaneous Endoscopic **8** Via Natural or Artificial Opening Endoscopic	**Z** No Device	**X** Diagnostic **Z** No Qualifier
T Diaphragm	**0** Open **3** Percutaneous **4** Percutaneous Endoscopic	**0** Drainage Device	**Z** No Qualifier
T Diaphragm	**0** Open **3** Percutaneous **4** Percutaneous Endoscopic	**Z** No Device	**X** Diagnostic **Z** No Qualifier

0 Medical and Surgical
B Respiratory System
B Excision: Cutting out or off, without replacement, a portion of a body part may be wedge or Segmentectomy

Body Part Character 4	Approach Character 5	Device Character 6	Qualifier Character 7
1 Trachea **2** Carina **3** Main Bronchus, Right **4** Upper Lobe Bronchus, Right **5** Middle Lobe Bronchus, Right **6** Lower Lobe Bronchus, Right **7** Main Bronchus, Left **8** Upper Lobe Bronchus, Left **9** Lingula Bronchus **B** Lower Lobe Bronchus, Left **C** Upper Lung Lobe, Right **D** Middle Lung Lobe, Right **F** Lower Lung Lobe, Right **G** Upper Lung Lobe, Left **H** Lung Lingula **J** Lower Lung Lobe, Left **K** Lung, Right **L** Lung, Left **M** Lungs, Bilateral	**0** Open **3** Percutaneous **4** Percutaneous Endoscopic - puncture chest wall **7** Via Natural or Artificial Opening **8** Via Natural or Artificial Opening Endoscopic mouth - Bronchoscopy	**Z** No Device	**X** Diagnostic **Z** No Qualifier - use if pt already has cancer - no biopsy needed
N Pleura, Right **P** Pleura, Left	**0** Open **3** Percutaneous **4** Percutaneous Endoscopic **8** Via Natural or Artificial Opening Endoscopic	**Z** No Device	**X** Diagnostic **Z** No Qualifier
T Diaphragm	**0** Open **3** Percutaneous **4** Percutaneous Endoscopic	**Z** No Device	**X** Diagnostic **Z** No Qualifier

0 Medical and Surgical
B Respiratory System
C Extirpation: Taking or cutting out solid matter from a body part

Body Part Character 4	Approach Character 5	Device Character 6	Qualifier Character 7
1 Trachea **2** Carina **3** Main Bronchus, Right **4** Upper Lobe Bronchus, Right **5** Middle Lobe Bronchus, Right **6** Lower Lobe Bronchus, Right **7** Main Bronchus, Left **8** Upper Lobe Bronchus, Left **9** Lingula Bronchus **B** Lower Lobe Bronchus, Left **C** Upper Lung Lobe, Right **D** Middle Lung Lobe, Right **F** Lower Lung Lobe, Right **G** Upper Lung Lobe, Left **H** Lung Lingula **J** Lower Lung Lobe, Left **K** Lung, Right **L** Lung, Left **M** Lungs, Bilateral	**0** Open **3** Percutaneous **4** Percutaneous Endoscopic **7** Via Natural or Artificial Opening **8** Via Natural or Artificial Opening Endoscopic	**Z** No Device	**Z** No Qualifier
N Pleura, Right **P** Pleura, Left **T** Diaphragm	**0** Open **3** Percutaneous **4** Percutaneous Endoscopic	**Z** No Device	**Z** No Qualifier

0 Medical and Surgical
B Respiratory System
D Extraction: Pulling or stripping out or off all or a portion of a body part by the use of force

Body Part Character 4	Approach Character 5	Device Character 6	Qualifier Character 7
1 Trachea **2** Carina **3** Main Bronchus, Right **4** Upper Lobe Bronchus, Right **5** Middle Lobe Bronchus, Right **6** Lower Lobe Bronchus, Right **7** Main Bronchus, Left **8** Upper Lobe Bronchus, Left **9** Lingula Bronchus **B** Lower Lobe Bronchus, Left **C** Upper Lung Lobe, Right **D** Middle Lung Lobe, Right **F** Lower Lung Lobe, Right **G** Upper Lung Lobe, Left **H** Lung Lingula **J** Lower Lung Lobe, Left **K** Lung, Right **L** Lung, Left **M** Lungs, Bilateral	**4** Percutaneous Endoscopic **8** Via Natural or Artificial Opening Endoscopic	**Z** No Device	**X** Diagnostic
N Pleura, Right **P** Pleura, Left	**0** Open **3** Percutaneous **4** Percutaneous Endoscopic	**Z** No Device	**X** Diagnostic **Z** No Qualifier

LC Limited Coverage **NC** Noncovered **HAC** HAC-associated Procedure **CC** Combination Cluster - See Appendix G for code lists
non-OR Non-OR-Affecting MS-DRG Assignment New/Revised Text in **Orange** ♂ Male ♀ Female

312

2020 ICD-10-PCS

0 Medical and Surgical
B Respiratory System
F Fragmentation: Breaking solid matter in a body part into pieces

Body Part Character 4	Approach Character 5	
1 Trachea NC **2** Carina NC **3** Main Bronchus, Right NC **4** Upper Lobe Bronchus, Right NC **5** Middle Lobe Bronchus, Right NC **6** Lower Lobe Bronchus, Right NC **7** Main Bronchus, Left NC **8** Upper Lobe Bronchus, Left NC **9** Lingula Bronchus NC **B** Lower Lobe Bronchus, Left NC	**0** Open **3** Percutaneous **4** Percutaneous Endoscopic **7** Via Natural or Artificial Opening **8** Via Natural or Artificial Opening Endoscopic **X** External	**Z** No

NC 0BF1XZZ 0BF2XZZ 0BF3XZZ 0BF4XZZ 0BF5XZZ 0BF6XZZ 0BF7XZZ 0BF8XZZ 0BF9XZZ 0BFBXZZ

0 Medical and Surgical
B Respiratory System
H Insertion: Putting in a nonbiological appliance that monitors, assists, performs, or prevents a physiological function but does not physica... place of a body part

Body Part Character 4	Approach Character 5	Device Character 6	Qualifier Character 7
0 Tracheobronchial Tree	**0** Open **3** Percutaneous **4** Percutaneous Endoscopic **7** Via Natural or Artificial Opening **8** Via Natural or Artificial Opening Endoscopic	**1** Radioactive Element **2** Monitoring Device **3** Infusion Device **D** Intraluminal Device **Y** Other Device	**Z** No Qualifier
1 Trachea	**0** Open	**2** Monitoring Device **D** Intraluminal Device **Y** Other Device	**Z** No Qualifier
1 Trachea	**3** Percutaneous	**D** Intraluminal Device **E** Intraluminal Device, Endotracheal Airway **Y** Other Device	**Z** No Qualifier
1 Trachea	**4** Percutaneous Endoscopic	**D** Intraluminal Device **Y** Other Device	**Z** No Qualifier
1 Trachea	**7** Via Natural or Artificial Opening **8** Via Natural or Artificial Opening Endoscopic	**2** Monitoring Device **D** Intraluminal Device **E** Intraluminal Device, Endotracheal Airway **Y** Other Device	**Z** No Qualifier
3 Main Bronchus, Right **4** Upper Lobe Bronchus, Right **5** Middle Lobe Bronchus, Right **6** Lower Lobe Bronchus, Right **7** Main Bronchus, Left **8** Upper Lobe Bronchus, Left **9** Lingula Bronchus **B** Lower Lobe Bronchus, Left	**0** Open **3** Percutaneous **4** Percutaneous Endoscopic **7** Via Natural or Artificial Opening **8** Via Natural or Artificial Opening Endoscopic	**G** Intraluminal Device, Endobronchial Valve	**Z** No Qualifier
K Lung, Right **L** Lung, Left	**0** Open **3** Percutaneous **4** Percutaneous Endoscopic **7** Via Natural or Artificial Opening **8** Via Natural or Artificial Opening Endoscopic	**1** Radioactive Element **2** Monitoring Device **3** Infusion Device **Y** Other Device	**Z** No Qualifier

0BH continued on next page

0BH continued from previous page

pliance that monitors, assists, performs, or prevents a physiological function but does not physically take the

	Approach Character 5	Device Character 6	Qualifier Character 7
	0 Open 3 Percutaneous 4 Percutaneous Endoscopic 7 Via Natural or Artificial Opening 8 Via Natural or Artificial Opening Endoscopic	Y Other Device	Z No Qualifier
	0 Open 3 Percutaneous 4 Percutaneous Endoscopic	2 Monitoring Device M Diaphragmatic Pacemaker Lead Y Other Device	Z No Qualifier
n	7 Via Natural or Artificial Opening 8 Via Natural or Artificial Opening Endoscopic	Y Other Device	Z No Qualifier

cal and Surgical
iratory System
pection: Visually and/or manually exploring a body part diagnostic bronchoscopy - part of tracheobronchial tree

Body Part Character 4	Approach Character 5	Device Character 6	Qualifier Character 7
0 Tracheobronchial Tree bronchus 1 Trachea K Lung, Right L Lung, Left Q Pleura T Diaphragm	0 Open 3 Percutaneous 4 Percutaneous Endoscopic 7 Via Natural or Artificial Opening 8 Via Natural or Artificial Opening Endoscopic bronchoscopy X External	Z No Device	Z No Qualifier

0 Medical and Surgical
B Respiratory System
L Occlusion: Completely closing an orifice or the lumen of a tubular body part

Body Part Character 4	Approach Character 5	Device Character 6	Qualifier Character 7
1 Trachea 2 Carina 3 Main Bronchus, Right 4 Upper Lobe Bronchus, Right 5 Middle Lobe Bronchus, Right 6 Lower Lobe Bronchus, Right 7 Main Bronchus, Left 8 Upper Lobe Bronchus, Left 9 Lingula Bronchus B Lower Lobe Bronchus, Left	0 Open 3 Percutaneous 4 Percutaneous Endoscopic	C Extraluminal Device D Intraluminal Device Z No Device	Z No Qualifier
1 Trachea 2 Carina 3 Main Bronchus, Right 4 Upper Lobe Bronchus, Right 5 Middle Lobe Bronchus, Right 6 Lower Lobe Bronchus, Right 7 Main Bronchus, Left 8 Upper Lobe Bronchus, Left 9 Lingula Bronchus B Lower Lobe Bronchus, Left	7 Via Natural or Artificial Opening 8 Via Natural or Artificial Opening Endoscopic	D Intraluminal Device Z No Device	Z No Qualifier

0 Medical and Surgical
B Respiratory System
M Reattachment: Putting back in or on all or a portion of a separated body part to its normal location or other suitable location

Body Part Character 4	Approach Character 5	Device Character 6	Qualifier Character 7
1 Trachea **2** Carina **3** Main Bronchus, Right **4** Upper Lobe Bronchus, Right **5** Middle Lobe Bronchus, Right **6** Lower Lobe Bronchus, Right **7** Main Bronchus, Left **8** Upper Lobe Bronchus, Left **9** Lingula Bronchus **B** Lower Lobe Bronchus, Left **C** Upper Lung Lobe, Right **D** Middle Lung Lobe, Right **F** Lower Lung Lobe, Right **G** Upper Lung Lobe, Left **H** Lung Lingula **J** Lower Lung Lobe, Left **K** Lung, Right **L** Lung, Left **T** Diaphragm	**0** Open	**Z** No Device	**Z** No Qualifier

0 Medical and Surgical
B Respiratory System
N Release: Freeing a body part from an abnormal physical constraint by cutting or by the use of force

Body Part Character 4	Approach Character 5	Device Character 6	Qualifier Character 7
1 Trachea **2** Carina **3** Main Bronchus, Right **4** Upper Lobe Bronchus, Right **5** Middle Lobe Bronchus, Right **6** Lower Lobe Bronchus, Right **7** Main Bronchus, Left **8** Upper Lobe Bronchus, Left **9** Lingula Bronchus **B** Lower Lobe Bronchus, Left **C** Upper Lung Lobe, Right **D** Middle Lung Lobe, Right **F** Lower Lung Lobe, Right **G** Upper Lung Lobe, Left **H** Lung Lingula **J** Lower Lung Lobe, Left **K** Lung, Right **L** Lung, Left **M** Lungs, Bilateral	**0** Open **3** Percutaneous **4** Percutaneous Endoscopic **7** Via Natural or Artificial Opening **8** Via Natural or Artificial Opening Endoscopic	**Z** No Device	**Z** No Qualifier
N Pleura, Right **P** Pleura, Left **T** Diaphragm	**0** Open **3** Percutaneous **4** Percutaneous Endoscopic	**Z** No Device	**Z** No Qualifier

0 Medical and Surgical
B Respiratory System
P Removal: Taking out or off a device from a body part

Body Part Character 4	Approach Character 5	Device Character 6	Qualifier Character 7
0 Tracheobronchial Tree	**0** Open **3** Percutaneous **4** Percutaneous Endoscopic **7** Via Natural or Artificial Opening **8** Via Natural or Artificial Opening Endoscopic	**0** Drainage Device **1** Radioactive Element **2** Monitoring Device **3** Infusion Device **7** Autologous Tissue Substitute **C** Extraluminal Device **D** Intraluminal Device *tube, nose or mouth* **J** Synthetic Substitute **K** Nonautologous Tissue Substitute **Y** Other Device	**Z** No Qualifier
0 Tracheobronchial Tree	**X** External	**0** Drainage Device **1** Radioactive Element **2** Monitoring Device **3** Infusion Device **D** Intraluminal Device	**Z** No Qualifier
1 Trachea *extubation*	**0** Open **3** Percutaneous **4** Percutaneous Endoscopic **7** Via Natural or Artificial Opening **8** Via Natural or Artificial Opening Endoscopic	**0** Drainage Device **2** Monitoring Device **7** Autologous Tissue Substitute **C** Extraluminal Device **D** Intraluminal Device *endotrachel tube* **F** Tracheostomy Device *– tube in neck* **J** Synthetic Substitute **K** Nonautologous Tissue Substitute	**Z** No Qualifier
1 Trachea *extubation*	**X** External	**0** Drainage Device **2** Monitoring Device **D** Intraluminal Device *endo trach tube* **F** Tracheostomy Device	**Z** No Qualifier
K Lung, Right **L** Lung, Left	**0** Open **3** Percutaneous **4** Percutaneous Endoscopic **7** Via Natural or Artificial Opening **8** Via Natural or Artificial Opening Endoscopic	**0** Drainage Device **1** Radioactive Element **2** Monitoring Device **3** Infusion Device **Y** Other Device	**Z** No Qualifier
K Lung, Right **L** Lung, Left	**X** External	**0** Drainage Device **1** Radioactive Element **2** Monitoring Device **3** Infusion Device	**Z** No Qualifier
Q Pleura	**0** Open **3** Percutaneous **4** Percutaneous Endoscopic **7** Via Natural or Artificial Opening **8** Via Natural or Artificial Opening Endoscopic	**0** Drainage Device **1** Radioactive Element **2** Monitoring Device **Y** Other Device	**Z** No Qualifier
Q Pleura	**X** External	**0** Drainage Device **1** Radioactive Element **2** Monitoring Device	**Z** No Qualifier
T Diaphragm	**0** Open **3** Percutaneous **4** Percutaneous Endoscopic **7** Via Natural or Artificial Opening **8** Via Natural or Artificial Opening Endoscopic	**0** Drainage Device **2** Monitoring Device **7** Autologous Tissue Substitute **J** Synthetic Substitute **K** Nonautologous Tissue Substitute **M** Diaphragmatic Pacemaker Lead **Y** Other Device	**Z** No Qualifier
T Diaphragm	**X** External	**0** Drainage Device **2** Monitoring Device **M** Diaphragmatic Pacemaker Lead	**Z** No Qualifier

0 Medical and Surgical
B Respiratory System
Q Repair: Restoring, to the extent possible, a body part to its normal anatomic structure and function

Body Part Character 4	Approach Character 5	Device Character 6	Qualifier Character 7
1 Trachea **2** Carina **3** Main Bronchus, Right **4** Upper Lobe Bronchus, Right **5** Middle Lobe Bronchus, Right **6** Lower Lobe Bronchus, Right **7** Main Bronchus, Left **8** Upper Lobe Bronchus, Left **9** Lingula Bronchus **B** Lower Lobe Bronchus, Left **C** Upper Lung Lobe, Right **D** Middle Lung Lobe, Right **F** Lower Lung Lobe, Right **G** Upper Lung Lobe, Left **H** Lung Lingula **J** Lower Lung Lobe, Left **K** Lung, Right **L** Lung, Left **M** Lungs, Bilateral	**0** Open **3** Percutaneous **4** Percutaneous Endoscopic **7** Via Natural or Artificial Opening **8** Via Natural or Artificial Opening Endoscopic	**Z** No Device	**Z** No Qualifier
N Pleura, Right **P** Pleura, Left **T** Diaphragm	**0** Open **3** Percutaneous **4** Percutaneous Endoscopic	**Z** No Device	**Z** No Qualifier

0 Medical and Surgical
B Respiratory System
R Replacement: Putting in or on biological or synthetic material that physically takes the place and/or function of all or a portion of a body part

Body Part Character 4	Approach Character 5	Device Character 6	Qualifier Character 7
1 Trachea **2** Carina **3** Main Bronchus, Right **4** Upper Lobe Bronchus, Right **5** Middle Lobe Bronchus, Right **6** Lower Lobe Bronchus, Right **7** Main Bronchus, Left **8** Upper Lobe Bronchus, Left **9** Lingula Bronchus **B** Lower Lobe Bronchus, Left **T** Diaphragm	**0** Open **4** Percutaneous Endoscopic	**7** Autologous Tissue Substitute **J** Synthetic Substitute tube **K** Nonautologous Tissue Substitute · cadivar	**Z** No Qualifier

0 Medical and Surgical
B Respiratory System
S Reposition: Moving to its normal location, or other suitable location, all or a portion of a body part

Body Part Character 4	Approach Character 5	Device Character 6	Qualifier Character 7
1 Trachea **2** Carina **3** Main Bronchus, Right **4** Upper Lobe Bronchus, Right **5** Middle Lobe Bronchus, Right **6** Lower Lobe Bronchus, Right **7** Main Bronchus, Left **8** Upper Lobe Bronchus, Left **9** Lingula Bronchus **B** Lower Lobe Bronchus, Left **C** Upper Lung Lobe, Right **D** Middle Lung Lobe, Right **F** Lower Lung Lobe, Right **G** Upper Lung Lobe, Left **H** Lung Lingula **J** Lower Lung Lobe, Left **K** Lung, Right **L** Lung, Left **T** Diaphragm	**0** Open	**Z** No Device	**Z** No Qualifier

0 Medical and Surgical
B Respiratory System
T Resection: Cutting out or off, without replacement, all of a body part

Body Part Character 4	Approach Character 5	Device Character 6	Qualifier Character 7
1 Trachea **2** Carina **3** Main Bronchus, Right **4** Upper Lobe Bronchus, Right **5** Middle Lobe Bronchus, Right **6** Lower Lobe Bronchus, Right **7** Main Bronchus, Left **8** Upper Lobe Bronchus, Left **9** Lingula Bronchus **B** Lower Lobe Bronchus, Left **C** Upper Lung Lobe, Right **D** Middle Lung Lobe, Right **F** Lower Lung Lobe, Right **G** Upper Lung Lobe, Left **H** Lung Lingula **J** Lower Lung Lobe, Left **K** Lung, Right pneumonectomy **L** Lung, Left **M** Lungs, Bilateral **T** Diaphragm	**0** Open **4** Percutaneous Endoscopic	**Z** No Device	**Z** No Qualifier

0 Medical and Surgical
B Respiratory System
U Supplement: Putting in or on biological or synthetic material that physically reinforces and/or augments the function of a portion of a body part

Body Part Character 4	Approach Character 5	Device Character 6	Qualifier Character 7
1 Trachea **2** Carina **3** Main Bronchus, Right **4** Upper Lobe Bronchus, Right **5** Middle Lobe Bronchus, Right **6** Lower Lobe Bronchus, Right **7** Main Bronchus, Left **8** Upper Lobe Bronchus, Left **9** Lingula Bronchus **B** Lower Lobe Bronchus, Left	**0** Open **4** Percutaneous Endoscopic **8** Via Natural or Artificial Opening Endoscopic	**7** Autologous Tissue Substitute **J** Synthetic Substitute **K** Nonautologous Tissue Substitute	**Z** No Qualifier
T Diaphragm	**0** Open **4** Percutaneous Endoscopic	**7** Autologous Tissue Substitute **J** Synthetic Substitute **K** Nonautologous Tissue Substitute	**Z** No Qualifier

0 Medical and Surgical
B Respiratory System
V Restriction: Partially closing an orifice or the lumen of a tubular body part

Body Part Character 4	Approach Character 5	Device Character 6	Qualifier Character 7
1 Trachea **2** Carina **3** Main Bronchus, Right **4** Upper Lobe Bronchus, Right **5** Middle Lobe Bronchus, Right **6** Lower Lobe Bronchus, Right **7** Main Bronchus, Left **8** Upper Lobe Bronchus, Left **9** Lingula Bronchus **B** Lower Lobe Bronchus, Left	**0** Open **3** Percutaneous **4** Percutaneous Endoscopic	**C** Extraluminal Device **D** Intraluminal Device **Z** No Device	**Z** No Qualifier
1 Trachea **2** Carina **3** Main Bronchus, Right **4** Upper Lobe Bronchus, Right **5** Middle Lobe Bronchus, Right **6** Lower Lobe Bronchus, Right **7** Main Bronchus, Left **8** Upper Lobe Bronchus, Left **9** Lingula Bronchus **B** Lower Lobe Bronchus, Left	**7** Via Natural or Artificial Opening **8** Via Natural or Artificial Opening Endoscopic	**D** Intraluminal Device **Z** No Device	**Z** No Qualifier

LC Limited Coverage NC Noncovered HAC HAC-associated Procedure CC Combination Cluster - See Appendix G for code lists
DRG Non-OR-Affecting MS-DRG Assignment New/Revised Text in **Orange** ♂ Male ♀ Female

2020 ICD-10-PCS	319

0 **Medical and Surgical**
B **Respiratory System**
W **Revision:** Correcting, to the extent possible, a portion of a malfunctioning device or the position of a displaced device

Body Part Character 4	Approach Character 5	Device Character 6	Qualifier Character 7
0 Tracheobronchial Tree	**0** Open **3** Percutaneous **4** Percutaneous Endoscopic **7** Via Natural or Artificial Opening **8** Via Natural or Artificial Opening Endoscopic	**0** Drainage Device **2** Monitoring Device **3** Infusion Device **7** Autologous Tissue Substitute **C** Extraluminal Device **D** Intraluminal Device **J** Synthetic Substitute **K** Nonautologous Tissue Substitute **Y** Other Device	**Z** No Qualifier
0 Tracheobronchial Tree	**X** External	**0** Drainage Device **2** Monitoring Device **3** Infusion Device **7** Autologous Tissue Substitute **C** Extraluminal Device **D** Intraluminal Device **J** Synthetic Substitute **K** Nonautologous Tissue Substitute	**Z** No Qualifier
1 Trachea	**0** Open **3** Percutaneous **4** Percutaneous Endoscopic **7** Via Natural or Artificial Opening **8** Via Natural or Artificial Opening Endoscopic **X** External	**0** Drainage Device **2** Monitoring Device **7** Autologous Tissue Substitute **C** Extraluminal Device **D** Intraluminal Device **F** Tracheostomy Device **J** Synthetic Substitute **K** Nonautologous Tissue Substitute	**Z** No Qualifier
K Lung, Right **L** Lung, Left	**0** Open **3** Percutaneous **4** Percutaneous Endoscopic **7** Via Natural or Artificial Opening **8** Via Natural or Artificial Opening Endoscopic	**0** Drainage Device **2** Monitoring Device **3** Infusion Device **Y** Other Device	**Z** No Qualifier
K Lung, Right **L** Lung, Left	**X** External	**0** Drainage Device **2** Monitoring Device **3** Infusion Device	**Z** No Qualifier
Q Pleura	**0** Open **3** Percutaneous **4** Percutaneous Endoscopic **7** Via Natural or Artificial Opening **8** Via Natural or Artificial Opening Endoscopic	**0** Drainage Device **2** Monitoring Device **Y** Other Device	**Z** No Qualifier
Q Pleura	**X** External	**0** Drainage Device **2** Monitoring Device	**Z** No Qualifier
T Diaphragm	**0** Open **3** Percutaneous **4** Percutaneous Endoscopic **7** Via Natural or Artificial Opening **8** Via Natural or Artificial Opening Endoscopic	**0** Drainage Device **2** Monitoring Device **7** Autologous Tissue Substitute **J** Synthetic Substitute **K** Nonautologous Tissue Substitute **M** Diaphragmatic Pacemaker Lead **Y** Other Device	**Z** No Qualifier
T Diaphragm	**X** External	**0** Drainage Device **2** Monitoring Device **7** Autologous Tissue Substitute **J** Synthetic Substitute **K** Nonautologous Tissue Substitute **M** Diaphragmatic Pacemaker Lead	**Z** No Qualifier

0 Medical and Surgical
B Respiratory System
Y Transplantation: Putting in or on all or a portion of a living body part taken from another individual or animal to physically take the place and/or function of all or a portion of a similar body part

Body Part Character 4	Approach Character 5	Device Character 6	Qualifier Character 7
C Upper Lung Lobe, Right LC **D** Middle Lung Lobe, Right LC **F** Lower Lung Lobe, Right LC **G** Upper Lung Lobe, Left LC **H** Lung Lingula LC **J** Lower Lung Lobe, Left LC **K** Lung, Right LC **L** Lung, Left LC **M** Lungs, Bilateral LC	**0** Open	**Z** No Device	**0** Allogeneic **1** Syngeneic **2** Zooplastic

LC 0BYC0Z0 0BYC0Z1 0BYC0Z2 0BYD0Z0 0BYD0Z1 0BYD0Z2 0BYF0Z0 0BYF0Z1 0BYF0Z2 0BYG0Z0 0BYG0Z1 0BYG0Z2 0BYH0Z0 0BYH0Z1 0BYH0Z2 0BYJ0Z0 0BYJ0Z1 0BYJ0Z2 0BYK0Z0 0BYK0Z1 0BYK0Z2 0BYL0Z0 0BYL0Z1 0BYL0Z2 0BYM0Z0 0BYM0Z1 0BYM0Z2

NOTES

Mouth and Throat 0C0-0CX

0 Medical and Surgical
C Mouth and Throat
0 Alteration: Modifying the anatomic structure of a body part without affecting the function of the body part

Body Part Character 4	Approach Character 5	Device Character 6	Qualifier Character 7
0 Upper Lip **1** Lower Lip	**X** External	**7** Autologous Tissue Substitute **J** Synthetic Substitute **K** Nonautologous Tissue Substitute **Z** No Device	**Z** No Qualifier

0 Medical and Surgical
C Mouth and Throat
2 Change: Taking out or off a device from a body part and putting back an identical or similar device in or on the same body part without cutting or puncturing the skin or a mucous membrane

Body Part Character 4	Approach Character 5	Device Character 6	Qualifier Character 7
A Salivary Gland **S** Larynx **Y** Mouth and Throat	**X** External	**0** Drainage Device **Y** Other Device	**Z** No Qualifier

0 Medical and Surgical
C Mouth and Throat RFA- radio Frequency Ablation
5 Destruction: Physical eradication of all or a portion of a body part by the direct use of energy, force, or a destructive agent

Body Part Character 4	Approach Character 5	Device Character 6	Qualifier Character 7
0 Upper Lip **1** Lower Lip **2** Hard Palate **3** Soft Palate **4** Buccal Mucosa **5** Upper Gingiva **6** Lower Gingiva **7** Tongue **N** Uvula **P** Tonsils **Q** Adenoids	**0** Open **3** Percutaneous **X** External	**Z** No Device	**Z** No Qualifier
8 Parotid Gland, Right **9** Parotid Gland, Left **B** Parotid Duct, Right **C** Parotid Duct, Left **D** Sublingual Gland, Right **F** Sublingual Gland, Left **G** Submaxillary Gland, Right **H** Submaxillary Gland, Left **J** Minor Salivary Gland	**0** Open **3** Percutaneous	**Z** No Device	**Z** No Qualifier
M Pharynx **R** Epiglottis **S** Larynx **T** Vocal Cord, Right Lesion **V** Vocal Cord, Left	**0** Open **3** Percutaneous **4** Percutaneous Endoscopic **7** Via Natural or Artificial Opening **8** Via Natural or Artificial Opening Endoscopic	**Z** No Device	**Z** No Qualifier
W Upper Tooth **X** Lower Tooth	**0** Open **X** External	**Z** No Device	**0** Single **1** Multiple **2** All

LC Limited Coverage NC Noncovered HAC HAC-associated Procedure CC Combination Cluster - See Appendix G for code lists
DRG Non-OR-Affecting MS-DRG Assignment New/Revised Text in **Orange** ♂ Male ♀ Female

0 Medical and Surgical
C Mouth and Throat
7 Dilation: Expanding an orifice or the lumen of a tubular body part

Body Part Character 4	Approach Character 5	Device Character 6	Qualifier Character 7
B Parotid Duct, Right **C** Parotid Duct, Left	**0** Open **3** Percutaneous **7** Via Natural or Artificial Opening	**D** Intraluminal Device **Z** No Device	**Z** No Qualifier
M Pharynx	**7** Via Natural or Artificial Opening **8** Via Natural or Artificial Opening Endoscopic	**D** Intraluminal Device **Z** No Device	**Z** No Qualifier
S Larynx	**0** Open **3** Percutaneous **4** Percutaneous Endoscopic **7** Via Natural or Artificial Opening **8** Via Natural or Artificial Opening Endoscopic	**D** Intraluminal Device **Z** No Device	**Z** No Qualifier

0 Medical and Surgical
C Mouth and Throat
9 Drainage: Taking or letting out fluids and/or gases from a body part

Body Part Character 4	Approach Character 5	Device Character 6	Qualifier Character 7
0 Upper Lip **1** Lower Lip **2** Hard Palate **3** Soft Palate **4** Buccal Mucosa **5** Upper Gingiva **6** Lower Gingiva **7** Tongue **N** Uvula **P** Tonsils **Q** Adenoids	**0** Open **3** Percutaneous **X** External	**0** Drainage Device	**Z** No Qualifier
0 Upper Lip **1** Lower Lip **2** Hard Palate **3** Soft Palate **4** Buccal Mucosa **5** Upper Gingiva **6** Lower Gingiva **7** Tongue **N** Uvula **P** Tonsils **Q** Adenoids	**0** Open **3** Percutaneous **X** External	**Z** No Device	**X** Diagnostic **Z** No Qualifier
8 Parotid Gland, Right **9** Parotid Gland, Left **B** Parotid Duct, Right **C** Parotid Duct, Left **D** Sublingual Gland, Right **F** Sublingual Gland, Left **G** Submaxillary Gland, Right **H** Submaxillary Gland, Left **J** Minor Salivary Gland	**0** Open **3** Percutaneous	**0** Drainage Device	**Z** No Qualifier

0C9 continued on next page

0C9 continued from previous page

0 Medical and Surgical
C Mouth and Throat
9 Drainage: Taking or letting out fluids and/or gases from a body part

Body Part Character 4	Approach Character 5	Device Character 6	Qualifier Character 7
8 Parotid Gland, Right **9** Parotid Gland, Left **B** Parotid Duct, Right **C** Parotid Duct, Left **D** Sublingual Gland, Right **F** Sublingual Gland, Left **G** Submaxillary Gland, Right **H** Submaxillary Gland, Left **J** Minor Salivary Gland	**0** Open **3** Percutaneous	**Z** No Device	**X** Diagnostic **Z** No Qualifier
M Pharynx **R** Epiglottis **S** Larynx **T** Vocal Cord, Right **V** Vocal Cord, Left	**0** Open **3** Percutaneous **4** Percutaneous Endoscopic **7** Via Natural or Artificial Opening **8** Via Natural or Artificial Opening Endoscopic	**0** Drainage Device	**Z** No Qualifier
M Pharynx **R** Epiglottis **S** Larynx **T** Vocal Cord, Right **V** Vocal Cord, Left	**0** Open **3** Percutaneous **4** Percutaneous Endoscopic **7** Via Natural or Artificial Opening **8** Via Natural or Artificial Opening Endoscopic	**Z** No Device	**X** Diagnostic **Z** No Qualifier
W Upper Tooth **X** Lower Tooth	**0** Open **X** External	**0** Drainage Device **Z** No Device	**0** Single **1** Multiple **2** All

0 Medical and Surgical
C Mouth and Throat
B Excision: Cutting out or off, without replacement, a portion of a body part

Body Part Character 4	Approach Character 5	Device Character 6	Qualifier Character 7
0 Upper Lip **1** Lower Lip **2** Hard Palate **3** Soft Palate **4** Buccal Mucosa **5** Upper Gingiva **6** Lower Gingiva **7** Tongue **N** Uvula **P** Tonsils **Q** Adenoids	**0** Open **3** Percutaneous **X** External	**Z** No Device	**X** Diagnostic **Z** No Qualifier
8 Parotid Gland, Right **9** Parotid Gland, Left **B** Parotid Duct, Right **C** Parotid Duct, Left **D** Sublingual Gland, Right **F** Sublingual Gland, Left **G** Submaxillary Gland, Right **H** Submaxillary Gland, Left **J** Minor Salivary Gland	**0** Open **3** Percutaneous	**Z** No Device	**X** Diagnostic **Z** No Qualifier
M Pharynx **R** Epiglottis **S** Larynx **T** Vocal Cord, Right **V** Vocal Cord, Left	**0** Open **3** Percutaneous **4** Percutaneous Endoscopic **7** Via Natural or Artificial Opening **8** Via Natural or Artificial Opening Endoscopic	**Z** No Device	**X** Diagnostic **Z** No Qualifier
W Upper Tooth **X** Lower Tooth	**0** Open **X** External	**Z** No Device	**0** Single **1** Multiple **2** All

0 Medical and Surgical
C Mouth and Throat
C Extirpation: Taking or cutting out solid matter from a body part

Body Part Character 4	Approach Character 5	Device Character 6	Qualifier Character 7
0 Upper Lip **1** Lower Lip **2** Hard Palate **3** Soft Palate **4** Buccal Mucosa **5** Upper Gingiva **6** Lower Gingiva **7** Tongue **N** Uvula **P** Tonsils **Q** Adenoids	**0** Open **3** Percutaneous **X** External	**Z** No Device	**Z** No Qualifier
8 Parotid Gland, Right **9** Parotid Gland, Left **B** Parotid Duct, Right **C** Parotid Duct, Left **D** Sublingual Gland, Right **F** Sublingual Gland, Left **G** Submaxillary Gland, Right **H** Submaxillary Gland, Left **J** Minor Salivary Gland	**0** Open **3** Percutaneous	**Z** No Device	**Z** No Qualifier
M Pharynx **R** Epiglottis **S** Larynx **T** Vocal Cord, Right **V** Vocal Cord, Left	**0** Open **3** Percutaneous **4** Percutaneous Endoscopic **7** Via Natural or Artificial Opening **8** Via Natural or Artificial Opening Endoscopic	**Z** No Device	**Z** No Qualifier
W Upper Tooth **X** Lower Tooth	**0** Open **X** External	**Z** No Device	**0** Single **1** Multiple **2** All

0 Medical and Surgical
C Mouth and Throat
D Extraction: Pulling or stripping out or off all or a portion of a body part by the use of force

Body Part Character 4	Approach Character 5	Device Character 6	Qualifier Character 7
T Vocal Cord, Right **V** Vocal Cord, Left	**0** Open **3** Percutaneous **4** Percutaneous Endoscopic **7** Via Natural or Artificial Opening **8** Via Natural or Artificial Opening Endoscopic	**Z** No Device	**Z** No Qualifier
W Upper Tooth **X** Lower Tooth	**X** External	**Z** No Device	**0** Single **1** Multiple **2** All

0 Medical and Surgical
C Mouth and Throat
F Fragmentation: Breaking solid matter in a body part into pieces

Body Part Character 4	Approach Character 5	Device Character 6	Qualifier Character 7
B Parotid Duct, Right NC **C** Parotid Duct, Left NC	**0** Open **3** Percutaneous **7** Via Natural or Artificial Opening **X** External	**Z** No Device	**Z** No Qualifier

NC 0CFBXZZ 0CFCXZZ

0 Medical and Surgical
C Mouth and Throat
H Insertion: Putting in a nonbiological appliance that monitors, assists, performs, or prevents a physiological function but does not physically take the place of a body part

Body Part Character 4	Approach Character 5	Device Character 6	Qualifier Character 7
7 Tongue	0 Open 3 Percutaneous X External	1 Radioactive Element	Z No Qualifier
A Salivary Gland S Larynx	0 Open 3 Percutaneous 7 Via Natural or Artificial Opening 8 Via Natural or Artificial Opening Endoscopic	Y Other Device	Z No Qualifier
Y Mouth and Throat	0 Open 3 Percutaneous	Y Other Device	Z No Qualifier
Y Mouth and Throat	7 Via Natural or Artificial Opening 8 Via Natural or Artificial Opening Endoscopic	B Intraluminal Device, Airway Y Other Device	Z No Qualifier

0 Medical and Surgical
C Mouth and Throat
J Inspection: Visually and/or manually exploring a body part

Body Part Character 4	Approach Character 5	Device Character 6	Qualifier Character 7
A Salivary Gland	0 Open 3 Percutaneous X External	Z No Device	Z No Qualifier
S Larynx Y Mouth and Throat	0 Open 3 Percutaneous 4 Percutaneous Endoscopic 7 Via Natural or Artificial Opening 8 Via Natural or Artificial Opening Endoscopic X External	Z No Device	Z No Qualifier

0 Medical and Surgical
C Mouth and Throat
L Occlusion: Completely closing an orifice or the lumen of a tubular body part

Body Part Character 4	Approach Character 5	Device Character 6	Qualifier Character 7
B Parotid Duct, Right C Parotid Duct, Left	0 Open 3 Percutaneous 4 Percutaneous Endoscopic	C Extraluminal Device D Intraluminal Device Z No Device	Z No Qualifier
B Parotid Duct, Right C Parotid Duct, Left	7 Via Natural or Artificial Opening 8 Via Natural or Artificial Opening Endoscopic	D Intraluminal Device Z No Device	Z No Qualifier

0 Medical and Surgical
C Mouth and Throat
M Reattachment: Putting back in or on all or a portion of a separated body part to its normal location or other suitable location

Body Part Character 4	Approach Character 5	Device Character 6	Qualifier Character 7
0 Upper Lip 1 Lower Lip 3 Soft Palate 7 Tongue N Uvula	0 Open	Z No Device	Z No Qualifier
W Upper Tooth X Lower Tooth	0 Open X External	Z No Device	0 Single 1 Multiple 2 All

0 Medical and Surgical
C Mouth and Throat
N Release: Freeing a body part from an abnormal physical constraint by cutting or by the use of force

Body Part Character 4	Approach Character 5	Device Character 6	Qualifier Character 7
0 Upper Lip **1** Lower Lip **2** Hard Palate **3** Soft Palate **4** Buccal Mucosa **5** Upper Gingiva **6** Lower Gingiva **7** Tongue **N** Uvula **P** Tonsils **Q** Adenoids	**0** Open **3** Percutaneous **X** External	**Z** No Device	**Z** No Qualifier
8 Parotid Gland, Right **9** Parotid Gland, Left **B** Parotid Duct, Right **C** Parotid Duct, Left **D** Sublingual Gland, Right **F** Sublingual Gland, Left **G** Submaxillary Gland, Right **H** Submaxillary Gland, Left **J** Minor Salivary Gland	**0** Open **3** Percutaneous	**Z** No Device	**Z** No Qualifier
M Pharynx **R** Epiglottis **S** Larynx **T** Vocal Cord, Right **V** Vocal Cord, Left	**0** Open **3** Percutaneous **4** Percutaneous Endoscopic **7** Via Natural or Artificial Opening **8** Via Natural or Artificial Opening Endoscopic	**Z** No Device	**Z** No Qualifier
W Upper Tooth **X** Lower Tooth	**0** Open **X** External	**Z** No Device	**0** Single **1** Multiple **2** All

0 Medical and Surgical
C Mouth and Throat
P Removal: Taking out or off a device from a body part

Body Part Character 4	Approach Character 5	Device Character 6	Qualifier Character 7
A Salivary Gland	**0** Open **3** Percutaneous	**0** Drainage Device **C** Extraluminal Device **Y** Other Device	**Z** No Qualifier
A Salivary Gland	**7** Via Natural or Artificial Opening **8** Via Natural or Artificial Opening Endoscopic	**Y** Other Device	**Z** No Qualifier
S Larynx	**0** Open **3** Percutaneous **7** Via Natural or Artificial Opening **8** Via Natural or Artificial Opening Endoscopic	**0** Drainage Device **7** Autologous Tissue Substitute **D** Intraluminal Device **J** Synthetic Substitute **K** Nonautologous Tissue Substitute **Y** Other Device	**Z** No Qualifier
S Larynx	**X** External	**0** Drainage Device **7** Autologous Tissue Substitute **D** Intraluminal Device **J** Synthetic Substitute **K** Nonautologous Tissue Substitute	**Z** No Qualifier

0CP continued on next page

0CP continued from previous page

0 Medical and Surgical
C Mouth and Throat
P Removal: Taking out or off a device from a body part

Body Part Character 4	Approach Character 5	Device Character 6	Qualifier Character 7
Y Mouth and Throat	**0** Open **3** Percutaneous **7** Via Natural or Artificial Opening **8** Via Natural or Artificial Opening Endoscopic	**0** Drainage Device **1** Radioactive Element **7** Autologous Tissue Substitute **D** Intraluminal Device **J** Synthetic Substitute **K** Nonautologous Tissue Substitute **Y** Other Device	**Z** No Qualifier
Y Mouth and Throat	**X** External	**0** Drainage Device **1** Radioactive Element **7** Autologous Tissue Substitute **D** Intraluminal Device **J** Synthetic Substitute **K** Nonautologous Tissue Substitute	**Z** No Qualifier

0 Medical and Surgical
C Mouth and Throat
Q Repair: Restoring, to the extent possible, a body part to its normal anatomic structure and function

Body Part Character 4	Approach Character 5	Device Character 6	Qualifier Character 7
0 Upper Lip **1** Lower Lip **2** Hard Palate **3** Soft Palate **4** Buccal Mucosa **5** Upper Gingiva **6** Lower Gingiva **7** Tongue **N** Uvula **P** Tonsils **Q** Adenoids	**0** Open **3** Percutaneous **X** External	**Z** No Device	**Z** No Qualifier
8 Parotid Gland, Right **9** Parotid Gland, Left **B** Parotid Duct, Right **C** Parotid Duct, Left **D** Sublingual Gland, Right **F** Sublingual Gland, Left **G** Submaxillary Gland, Right **H** Submaxillary Gland, Left **J** Minor Salivary Gland	**0** Open **3** Percutaneous	**Z** No Device	**Z** No Qualifier
M Pharynx **R** Epiglottis **S** Larynx Supraglottis **T** Vocal Cord, Right **V** Vocal Cord, Left	**0** Open **3** Percutaneous **4** Percutaneous Endoscopic **7** Via Natural or Artificial Opening **8** Via Natural or Artificial Opening Endoscopic larynxscope in nose	**Z** No Device	**Z** No Qualifier
W Upper Tooth **X** Lower Tooth	**0** Open **X** External	**Z** No Device	**0** Single **1** Multiple **2** All

0 Medical and Surgical
C Mouth and Throat
R Replacement: Putting in or on biological or synthetic material that physically takes the place and/or function of all or a portion of a body part

Body Part Character 4	Approach Character 5	Device Character 6	Qualifier Character 7
0 Upper Lip **1** Lower Lip **2** Hard Palate **3** Soft Palate **4** Buccal Mucosa **5** Upper Gingiva **6** Lower Gingiva **7** Tongue **N** Uvula	**0** Open **3** Percutaneous **X** External	**7** Autologous Tissue Substitute **J** Synthetic Substitute **K** Nonautologous Tissue Substitute	**Z** No Qualifier
B Parotid Duct, Right **C** Parotid Duct, Left	**0** Open **3** Percutaneous	**7** Autologous Tissue Substitute **J** Synthetic Substitute **K** Nonautologous Tissue Substitute	**Z** No Qualifier
M Pharynx **R** Epiglottis **S** Larynx **T** Vocal Cord, Right **V** Vocal Cord, Left	**0** Open **7** Via Natural or Artificial Opening **8** Via Natural or Artificial Opening Endoscopic	**7** Autologous Tissue Substitute **J** Synthetic Substitute **K** Nonautologous Tissue Substitute	**Z** No Qualifier
W Upper Tooth **X** Lower Tooth	**0** Open **X** External	**7** Autologous Tissue Substitute **J** Synthetic Substitute **K** Nonautologous Tissue Substitute	**0** Single **1** Multiple **2** All

0 Medical and Surgical
C Mouth and Throat
S Reposition: Moving to its normal location, or other suitable location, all or a portion of a body part

Body Part Character 4	Approach Character 5	Device Character 6	Qualifier Character 7
0 Upper Lip **1** Lower Lip **2** Hard Palate **3** Soft Palate **7** Tongue **N** Uvula	**0** Open **X** External	**Z** No Device	**Z** No Qualifier
B Parotid Duct, Right **C** Parotid Duct, Left	**0** Open **3** Percutaneous	**Z** No Device	**Z** No Qualifier
R Epiglottis **T** Vocal Cord, Right **V** Vocal Cord, Left	**0** Open **7** Via Natural or Artificial Opening **8** Via Natural or Artificial Opening Endoscopic	**Z** No Device	**Z** No Qualifier
W Upper Tooth **X** Lower Tooth	**0** Open **X** External	**5** External Fixation Device **Z** No Device	**0** Single **1** Multiple **2** All

0 Medical and Surgical
C Mouth and Throat
T Resection: Cutting out or off, without replacement, all of a body part

Body Part Character 4	Approach Character 5	Device Character 6	Qualifier Character 7
0 Upper Lip **1** Lower Lip **2** Hard Palate **3** Soft Palate **7** Tongue **N** Uvula **P** Tonsils **Q** Adenoids	**0** Open **X** External – visable w/o aid of instrumentation	**Z** No Device	**Z** No Qualifier
8 Parotid Gland, Right **9** Parotid Gland, Left **B** Parotid Duct, Right **C** Parotid Duct, Left **D** Sublingual Gland, Right **F** Sublingual Gland, Left **G** Submaxillary Gland, Right **H** Submaxillary Gland, Left **J** Minor Salivary Gland	**0** Open	**Z** No Device	**Z** No Qualifier
M Pharynx **R** Epiglottis **S** Larynx **T** Vocal Cord, Right **V** Vocal Cord, Left	**0** Open **4** Percutaneous Endoscopic **7** Via Natural or Artificial Opening **8** Via Natural or Artificial Opening Endoscopic	**Z** No Device	**Z** No Qualifier
W Upper Tooth **X** Lower Tooth	**0** Open	**Z** No Device	**0** Single **1** Multiple **2** All

0 Medical and Surgical
C Mouth and Throat
U Supplement: Putting in or on biological or synthetic material that physically reinforces and/or augments the function of a portion of a body part

Body Part Character 4	Approach Character 5	Device Character 6	Qualifier Character 7
0 Upper Lip **1** Lower Lip **2** Hard Palate **3** Soft Palate **4** Buccal Mucosa **5** Upper Gingiva **6** Lower Gingiva **7** Tongue **N** Uvula	**0** Open **3** Percutaneous **X** External	**7** Autologous Tissue Substitute **J** Synthetic Substitute **K** Nonautologous Tissue Substitute	**Z** No Qualifier
M Pharynx **R** Epiglottis **S** Larynx **T** Vocal Cord, Right **V** Vocal Cord, Left	**0** Open **7** Via Natural or Artificial Opening **8** Via Natural or Artificial Opening Endoscopic	**7** Autologous Tissue Substitute **J** Synthetic Substitute **K** Nonautologous Tissue Substitute	**Z** No Qualifier

0 Medical and Surgical
C Mouth and Throat
V Restriction: Partially closing an orifice or the lumen of a tubular body part

Body Part Character 4	Approach Character 5	Device Character 6	Qualifier Character 7
B Parotid Duct, Right **C** Parotid Duct, Left	**0** Open **3** Percutaneous	**C** Extraluminal Device **D** Intraluminal Device **Z** No Device	**Z** No Qualifier
B Parotid Duct, Right **C** Parotid Duct, Left	**7** Via Natural or Artificial Opening **8** Via Natural or Artificial Opening Endoscopic	**D** Intraluminal Device **Z** No Device	**Z** No Qualifier

0 Medical and Surgical
C Mouth and Throat
W Revision: Correcting, to the extent possible, a portion of a malfunctioning device or the position of a displaced device

Body Part Character 4	Approach Character 5	Device Character 6	Qualifier Character 7
A Salivary Gland	**0** Open **3** Percutaneous	**0** Drainage Device **C** Extraluminal Device **Y** Other Device	**Z** No Qualifier
A Salivary Gland	**7** Via Natural or Artificial Opening **8** Via Natural or Artificial Opening Endoscopic	**Y** Other Device	**Z** No Qualifier
A Salivary Gland	**X** External	**0** Drainage Device **C** Extraluminal Device	**Z** No Qualifier
S Larynx	**0** Open **3** Percutaneous **7** Via Natural or Artificial Opening **8** Via Natural or Artificial Opening Endoscopic	**0** Drainage Device **7** Autologous Tissue Substitute **D** Intraluminal Device **J** Synthetic Substitute **K** Nonautologous Tissue Substitute **Y** Other Device	**Z** No Qualifier
S Larynx	**X** External	**0** Drainage Device **7** Autologous Tissue Substitute **D** Intraluminal Device **J** Synthetic Substitute **K** Nonautologous Tissue Substitute	**Z** No Qualifier
Y Mouth and Throat	**0** Open **3** Percutaneous **7** Via Natural or Artificial Opening **8** Via Natural or Artificial Opening Endoscopic	**0** Drainage Device **1** Radioactive Element **7** Autologous Tissue Substitute **D** Intraluminal Device **J** Synthetic Substitute **K** Nonautologous Tissue Substitute **Y** Other Device	**Z** No Qualifier
Y Mouth and Throat	**X** External	**0** Drainage Device **1** Radioactive Element **7** Autologous Tissue Substitute **D** Intraluminal Device **J** Synthetic Substitute **K** Nonautologous Tissue Substitute	**Z** No Qualifier

0 Medical and Surgical
C Mouth and Throat
X Transfer: Moving, without taking out, all or a portion of a body part to another location to take over the function of all or a portion of a body part

Body Part Character 4	Approach Character 5	Device Character 6	Qualifier Character 7
0 Upper Lip **1** Lower Lip **3** Soft Palate **4** Buccal Mucosa **5** Upper Gingiva **6** Lower Gingiva **7** Tongue	**0** Open **X** External	**Z** No Device	**Z** No Qualifier

NOTES

NOTES

Gastrointestinal System 0D1-0DY

0 Medical and Surgical
D Gastrointestinal System
1 Bypass: Altering the route of passage of the contents of a tubular body part

Body Part Character 4	Approach Character 5	Device Character 6	Qualifier Character 7
1 Esophagus, Upper **2** Esophagus, Middle **3** Esophagus, Lower **5** Esophagus	**0** Open **4** Percutaneous Endoscopic **8** Via Natural or Artificial Opening Endoscopic	**7** Autologous Tissue Substitute **J** Synthetic Substitute **K** Nonautologous Tissue Substitute **Z** No Device	**4** Cutaneous **6** Stomach **9** Duodenum **A** Jejunum **B** Ileum
1 Esophagus, Upper **2** Esophagus, Middle **3** Esophagus, Lower **5** Esophagus	**3** Percutaneous	**J** Synthetic Substitute	**4** Cutaneous
6 Stomach HAC **9** Duodenum	**0** Open **4** Percutaneous Endoscopic **8** Via Natural or Artificial Opening Endoscopic	**7** Autologous Tissue Substitute **J** Synthetic Substitute **K** Nonautologous Tissue Substitute **Z** No Device	**4** Cutaneous **9** Duodenum **A** Jejunum **B** Ileum **L** Transverse Colon
6 Stomach **9** Duodenum	**3** Percutaneous	**J** Synthetic Substitute	**4** Cutaneous
8 Small Intestine	**0** Open **4** Percutaneous Endoscopic **8** Via Natural or Artificial Opening Endoscopic	**7** Autologous Tissue Substitute **J** Synthetic Substitute **K** Nonautologous Tissue Substitute **Z** No Device	**4** Cutaneous **8** Small Intestine **H** Cecum **K** Ascending Colon **L** Transverse Colon **M** Descending Colon **N** Sigmoid Colon **P** Rectum **Q** Anus
A Jejunum	**0** Open **4** Percutaneous Endoscopic **8** Via Natural or Artificial Opening Endoscopic	**7** Autologous Tissue Substitute **J** Synthetic Substitute **K** Nonautologous Tissue Substitute **Z** No Device	**4** Cutaneous **A** Jejunum **B** Ileum **H** Cecum **K** Ascending Colon **L** Transverse Colon **M** Descending Colon **N** Sigmoid Colon **P** Rectum **Q** Anus
A Jejunum	**3** Percutaneous	**J** Synthetic Substitute	**4** Cutaneous
B Ileum	**0** Open **4** Percutaneous Endoscopic **8** Via Natural or Artificial Opening Endoscopic	**7** Autologous Tissue Substitute **J** Synthetic Substitute **K** Nonautologous Tissue Substitute **Z** No Device	**4** Cutaneous **B** Ileum **H** Cecum **K** Ascending Colon **L** Transverse Colon **M** Descending Colon **N** Sigmoid Colon **P** Rectum **Q** Anus
B Ileum	**3** Percutaneous	**J** Synthetic Substitute	**4** Cutaneous
E Large Intestine	**0** Open **4** Percutaneous Endoscopic **8** Via Natural or Artificial Opening Endoscopic	**7** Autologous Tissue Substitute **J** Synthetic Substitute **K** Nonautologous Tissue Substitute **Z** No Device	**4** Cutaneous **E** Large Intestine **P** Rectum

0D1 continued on next page

0 Medical and Surgical
D Gastrointestinal System
1 Bypass: Altering the route of passage of the contents of a tubular body part

0D1 continued from previous page

Body Part	Approach	Device	Qualifier
Character 4	Character 5	Character 6	Character 7
H Cecum	**0** Open **4** Percutaneous Endoscopic **8** Via Natural or Artificial Opening Endoscopic	**7** Autologous Tissue Substitute **J** Synthetic Substitute **K** Nonautologous Tissue Substitute **Z** No Device	**4** Cutaneous **H** Cecum **K** Ascending Colon **L** Transverse Colon **M** Descending Colon **N** Sigmoid Colon **P** Rectum
H Cecum	**3** Percutaneous	**J** Synthetic Substitute	**4** Cutaneous
K Ascending Colon	**0** Open **4** Percutaneous Endoscopic **8** Via Natural or Artificial Opening Endoscopic	**7** Autologous Tissue Substitute **J** Synthetic Substitute **K** Nonautologous Tissue Substitute **Z** No Device	**4** Cutaneous **K** Ascending Colon **L** Transverse Colon **M** Descending Colon **N** Sigmoid Colon **P** Rectum
K Ascending Colon	**3** Percutaneous	**J** Synthetic Substitute	**4** Cutaneous
L Transverse Colon	**0** Open **4** Percutaneous Endoscopic **8** Via Natural or Artificial Opening Endoscopic	**7** Autologous Tissue Substitute **J** Synthetic Substitute **K** Nonautologous Tissue Substitute **Z** No Device	**4** Cutaneous **L** Transverse Colon **M** Descending Colon **N** Sigmoid Colon **P** Rectum
L Transverse Colon	**3** Percutaneous	**J** Synthetic Substitute	**4** Cutaneous
M Descending Colon	**0** Open **4** Percutaneous Endoscopic **8** Via Natural or Artificial Opening Endoscopic	**7** Autologous Tissue Substitute **J** Synthetic Substitute **K** Nonautologous Tissue Substitute **Z** No Device	**4** Cutaneous **M** Descending Colon **N** Sigmoid Colon **P** Rectum
M Descending Colon	**3** Percutaneous	**J** Synthetic Substitute	**4** Cutaneous
N Sigmoid Colon	**0** Open **4** Percutaneous Endoscopic **8** Via Natural or Artificial Opening Endoscopic	**7** Autologous Tissue Substitute **J** Synthetic Substitute **K** Nonautologous Tissue Substitute **Z** No Device	**4** Cutaneous **N** Sigmoid Colon **P** Rectum
N Sigmoid Colon	**3** Percutaneous	**J** Synthetic Substitute	**4** Cutaneous

HAC 0D16079 0D1607A 0D1607B 0D1607L 0D160J9 0D160JA 0D160JB 0D160JL 0D160K9 0D160KA 0D160KB 0D160KL 0D160Z9 0D160ZA 0D160ZB 0D160ZL 0D16479 0D1647A 0D1647B 0D1647L 0D164J9 0D164JA 0D164JB 0D164JL 0D164K9 0D164KA 0D164KB 0D164KL 0D164Z9 0D164ZA 0D164ZB 0D164ZL 0D16879 0D1687A 0D1687B 0D1687L 0D168J9 0D168JA 0D168JB 0D168JL 0D168K9 0D168KA 0D168KB 0D168KL 0D168Z9 0D168ZA 0D168ZB 0D168ZL
Surgical site infection following bariatric surgery procedures and principal diagnoses E66.01 and secondary diagnoses K68.11, K95.01, K95.81, T81.40XA, T81.41XA, T81.42XA, T81.43XA, T81.44XA, T81.49XA.

0 Medical and Surgical
D Gastrointestinal System
2 Change: Taking out or off a device from a body part and putting back an identical or similar device in or on the same body part without cutting or puncturing the skin or a mucous membrane

Body Part	Approach	Device	Qualifier
Character 4	Character 5	Character 6	Character 7
0 Upper Intestinal Tract **D** Lower Intestinal Tract	**X** External	**0** Drainage Device **U** Feeding Device **Y** Other Device	**Z** No Qualifier
U Omentum **V** Mesentery **W** Peritoneum	**X** External	**0** Drainage Device **Y** Other Device	**Z** No Qualifier

0 Medical and Surgical
D Gastrointestinal System
5 Destruction: Physical eradication of all or a portion of a body part by the direct use of energy, force, or a destructive agent Snare

Body Part Character 4	Approach Character 5	Device Character 6	Qualifier Character 7
1 Esophagus, Upper **2** Esophagus, Middle **3** Esophagus, Lower **4** Esophagogastric Junction **5** Esophagus **6** Stomach **7** Stomach, Pylorus **8** Small Intestine **9** Duodenum **A** Jejunum **B** Ileum **C** Ileocecal Valve **E** Large Intestine **F** Large Intestine, Right **G** Large Intestine, Left **H** Cecum **J** Appendix **K** Ascending Colon **L** Transverse Colon **M** Descending Colon **N** Sigmoid Colon **P** Rectum	**0** Open **3** Percutaneous **4** Percutaneous Endoscopic **7** Via Natural or Artificial Opening **8** Via Natural or Artificial Opening Endoscopic	**Z** No Device	**Z** No Qualifier
Q Anus	**0** Open **3** Percutaneous **4** Percutaneous Endoscopic **7** Via Natural or Artificial Opening **8** Via Natural or Artificial Opening Endoscopic **X** External	**Z** No Device	**Z** No Qualifier
R Anal Sphincter **U** Omentum **V** Mesentery **W** Peritoneum	**0** Open **3** Percutaneous **4** Percutaneous Endoscopic	**Z** No Device	**Z** No Qualifier

0 Medical and Surgical
D Gastrointestinal System
7 Dilation: Expanding an orifice or the lumen of a tubular body part

Body Part Character 4	Approach Character 5	Device Character 6	Qualifier Character 7
1 Esophagus, Upper **2** Esophagus, Middle **3** Esophagus, Lower **4** Esophagogastric Junction **5** Esophagus **6** Stomach **7** Stomach, Pylorus **8** Small Intestine **9** Duodenum **A** Jejunum **B** Ileum **C** Ileocecal Valve **E** Large Intestine **F** Large Intestine, Right **G** Large Intestine, Left **H** Cecum **K** Ascending Colon **L** Transverse Colon **M** Descending Colon **N** Sigmoid Colon **P** Rectum **Q** Anus	**0** Open **3** Percutaneous **4** Percutaneous Endoscopic **7** Via Natural or Artificial Opening **8** Via Natural or Artificial Opening Endoscopic	**D** Intraluminal Device **Z** No Device	**Z** No Qualifier

0 Medical and Surgical
D Gastrointestinal System
8 Division: Cutting into a body part, without draining fluids and/or gases from the body part, in order to separate or transect a body part

Body Part Character 4	Approach Character 5	Device Character 6	Qualifier Character 7
4 Esophagogastric Junction **7** Stomach, Pylorus	**0** Open **3** Percutaneous **4** Percutaneous Endoscopic **7** Via Natural or Artificial Opening **8** Via Natural or Artificial Opening Endoscopic	**Z** No Device	**Z** No Qualifier
R Anal Sphincter	**0** Open **3** Percutaneous	**Z** No Device	**Z** No Qualifier

0 Medical and Surgical
D Gastrointestinal System
9 Drainage: Taking or letting out fluids and/or gases from a body part

Body Part Character 4	Approach Character 5	Device Character 6	Qualifier Character 7
1 Esophagus, Upper 2 Esophagus, Middle 3 Esophagus, Lower 4 Esophagogastric Junction 5 Esophagus 6 Stomach 7 Stomach, Pylorus 8 Small Intestine 9 Duodenum A Jejunum B Ileum C Ileocecal Valve E Large Intestine F Large Intestine, Right G Large Intestine, Left H Cecum J Appendix K Ascending Colon L Transverse Colon M Descending Colon N Sigmoid Colon P Rectum	0 Open 3 Percutaneous 4 Percutaneous Endoscopic 7 Via Natural or Artificial Opening 8 Via Natural or Artificial Opening Endoscopic	0 Drainage Device	Z No Qualifier
1 Esophagus, Upper 2 Esophagus, Middle 3 Esophagus, Lower 4 Esophagogastric Junction 5 Esophagus 6 Stomach 7 Stomach, Pylorus 8 Small Intestine 9 Duodenum A Jejunum B Ileum C Ileocecal Valve E Large Intestine F Large Intestine, Right G Large Intestine, Left H Cecum J Appendix K Ascending Colon L Transverse Colon M Descending Colon N Sigmoid Colon P Rectum	0 Open 3 Percutaneous 4 Percutaneous Endoscopic 7 Via Natural or Artificial Opening 8 Via Natural or Artificial Opening Endoscopic	Z No Device	X Diagnostic Z No Qualifier
Q Anus	0 Open 3 Percutaneous 4 Percutaneous Endoscopic 7 Via Natural or Artificial Opening 8 Via Natural or Artificial Opening Endoscopic X External	0 Drainage Device	Z No Qualifier
Q Anus	0 Open 3 Percutaneous 4 Percutaneous Endoscopic 7 Via Natural or Artificial Opening 8 Via Natural or Artificial Opening Endoscopic X External	Z No Device	X Diagnostic Z No Qualifier

0D9 continued on next page

LC Limited Coverage NC Noncovered HAC HAC-associated Procedure CC Combination Cluster - See Appendix G for code lists
DRG Non-OR-Affecting MS-DRG Assignment New/Revised Text in **Orange** ♂ Male ♀ Female

0D9 continued from previous page

0 Medical and Surgical
D Gastrointestinal System
9 Drainage: Taking or letting out fluids and/or gases from a body part

Body Part Character 4	Approach Character 5	Device Character 6	Qualifier Character 7
R Anal Sphincter **U** Omentum **V** Mesentery **W** Peritoneum	**0** Open **3** Percutaneous **4** Percutaneous Endoscopic	**0** Drainage Device	**Z** No Qualifier
R Anal Sphincter **U** Omentum **V** Mesentery **W** Peritoneum	**0** Open **3** Percutaneous **4** Percutaneous Endoscopic	**Z** No Device	**X** Diagnostic **Z** No Qualifier

0 Medical and Surgical
D Gastrointestinal System
B Excision: Cutting out or off, without replacement, a portion of a body part

Body Part Character 4	Approach Character 5	Device Character 6	Qualifier Character 7
1 Esophagus, Upper **2** Esophagus, Middle **3** Esophagus, Lower **4** Esophagogastric Junction **5** Esophagus **7** Stomach, Pylorus **8** Small Intestine **9** Duodenum **A** Jejunum **B** Ileum **C** Ileocecal Valve **E** Large Intestine **F** Large Intestine, Right **H** Cecum **J** Appendix **K** Ascending Colon **P** Rectum	**0** Open **3** Percutaneous **4** Percutaneous Endoscopic **7** Via Natural or Artificial Opening **8** Via Natural or Artificial Opening Endoscopic EGD	**Z** No Device	**X** Diagnostic **Z** No Qualifier
6 Stomach EGD w/ biopsy 0DB6	**0** Open **3** Percutaneous **4** Percutaneous Endoscopic **7** Via Natural or Artificial Opening **8** Via Natural or Artificial Opening Endoscopic EGD, colonscopy	**Z** No Device	**3** Vertical **X** Diagnostic - if sent to pathology CLOTEST **Z** No Qualifier
G Large Intestine, Left **L** Transverse Colon **M** Descending Colon **N** Sigmoid Colon - snare polypectomy or cold forceps	**0** Open **3** Percutaneous **4** Percutaneous Endoscopic **7** Via Natural or Artificial Opening **8** Via Natural or Artificial Opening Endoscopic sigmoidscopy	**Z** No Device	**X** Diagnostic - if sent to patholog **Z** No Qualifier
G Large Intestine, Left **L** Transverse Colon **M** Descending Colon **N** Sigmoid Colon	**F** Via Natural or Artificial Opening With Percutaneous Endoscopic Assistance	**Z** No Device	**Z** No Qualifier
Q Anus	**0** Open **3** Percutaneous **4** Percutaneous Endoscopic **7** Via Natural or Artificial Opening **8** Via Natural or Artificial Opening Endoscopic **X** External	**Z** No Device	**X** Diagnostic **Z** No Qualifier

0DB continued on next page

0DB continued from previous page

0 Medical and Surgical
D Gastrointestinal System
B Excision: Cutting out or off, without replacement, a portion of a body part Biopsy

Body Part	Approach	Device	Qualifier
Character 4	**Character 5**	**Character 6**	**Character 7**
R Anal Sphincter **U** Omentum **V** Mesentery **W** Peritoneum	**0** Open **3** Percutaneous **4** Percutaneous Endoscopic	**Z** No Device	**X** Diagnostic **Z** No Qualifier

0 Medical and Surgical
D Gastrointestinal System
C Extirpation: Taking or cutting out solid matter from a body part

Body Part	Approach	Device	Qualifier
Character 4	**Character 5**	**Character 6**	**Character 7**
1 Esophagus, Upper **2** Esophagus, Middle **3** Esophagus, Lower **4** Esophagogastric Junction GE **5** Esophagus **6** Stomach **7** Stomach, Pylorus **8** Small Intestine **9** Duodenum **A** Jejunum **B** Ileum **C** Ileocecal Valve **E** Large Intestine **F** Large Intestine, Right **G** Large Intestine, Left **H** Cecum **J** Appendix **K** Ascending Colon **L** Transverse Colon **M** Descending Colon **N** Sigmoid Colon **P** Rectum	**0** Open laparotomy **3** Percutaneous **4** Percutaneous Endoscopic **7** Via Natural or Artificial Opening **8** Via Natural or Artificial Opening Endoscopic EGD	**Z** No Device	**Z** No Qualifier
Q Anus	**0** Open **3** Percutaneous **4** Percutaneous Endoscopic **7** Via Natural or Artificial Opening **8** Via Natural or Artificial Opening Endoscopic **X** External	**Z** No Device	**Z** No Qualifier
R Anal Sphincter **U** Omentum **V** Mesentery **W** Peritoneum	**0** Open **3** Percutaneous **4** Percutaneous Endoscopic	**Z** No Device	**Z** No Qualifier

LC Limited Coverage NC Noncovered HAC HAC-associated Procedure CC Combination Cluster - See Appendix G for code lists
DRG Non-OR-Affecting MS-DRG Assignment New/Revised Text in **Orange** ♂ Male ♀ Female

0 Medical and Surgical
D Gastrointestinal System
D Extraction: Pulling or stripping out or off all or a portion of a body part by the use of force

Body Part Character 4	Approach Character 5	Device Character 6	Qualifier Character 7
1 Esophagus, Upper **2** Esophagus, Middle **3** Esophagus, Lower **4** Esophagogastric Junction **5** Esophagus **6** Stomach **7** Stomach, Pylorus **8** Small Intestine **9** Duodenum **A** Jejunum **B** Ileum **C** Ileocecal Valve **E** Large Intestine **F** Large Intestine, Right **G** Large Intestine, Left **H** Cecum **J** Appendix **K** Ascending Colon **L** Transverse Colon **M** Descending Colon **N** Sigmoid Colon **P** Rectum	**3** Percutaneous **4** Percutaneous Endoscopic **8** Via Natural or Artificial Opening Endoscopic	**Z** No Device	**X** Diagnostic
Q Anus	**3** Percutaneous **4** Percutaneous Endoscopic **8** Via Natural or Artificial Opening Endoscopic **X** External	**Z** No Device	**X** Diagnostic

0 Medical and Surgical
D Gastrointestinal System
F Fragmentation: Breaking solid matter in a body part into pieces

Body Part Character 4	Approach Character 5	Device Character 6	Qualifier Character 7
5 Esophagus NC **6** Stomach NC **8** Small Intestine NC **9** Duodenum NC **A** Jejunum NC **B** Ileum NC **E** Large Intestine NC **F** Large Intestine, Right NC **G** Large Intestine, Left NC **H** Cecum NC **J** Appendix NC **K** Ascending Colon NC **L** Transverse Colon NC **M** Descending Colon NC **N** Sigmoid Colon NC **P** Rectum NC **Q** Anus NC	**0** Open **3** Percutaneous **4** Percutaneous Endoscopic **7** Via Natural or Artificial Opening **8** Via Natural or Artificial Opening Endoscopic **X** External	**Z** No Device	**Z** No Qualifier

NC 0DF5XZZ 0DF6XZZ 0DF8XZZ 0DF9XZZ 0DFAXZZ 0DFBXZZ 0DFEXZZ 0DFFXZZ 0DFGXZZ 0DFHXZZ 0DFJXZZ 0DFKXZZ 0DFLXZZ 0DFMXZZ 0DFNXZZ 0DFPXZZ 0DFQXZZ

0 Medical and Surgical
D Gastrointestinal System
H Insertion: Putting in a nonbiological appliance that monitors, assists, performs, or prevents a physiological function but does not physically take the place of a body part

Body Part Character 4	Approach Character 5	Device Character 6	Qualifier Character 7
0 Upper Intestinal Tract **D** Lower Intestinal Tract	**0** Open **3** Percutaneous **4** Percutaneous Endoscopic **7** Via Natural or Artificial Opening **8** Via Natural or Artificial Opening Endoscopic	**Y** Other Device	**Z** No Qualifier
5 Esophagus	**0** Open **3** Percutaneous **4** Percutaneous Endoscopic	**1** Radioactive Element **2** Monitoring Device **3** Infusion Device **D** Intraluminal Device **U** Feeding Device **Y** Other Device	**Z** No Qualifier
5 Esophagus	**7** Via Natural or Artificial Opening **8** Via Natural or Artificial Opening Endoscopic	**1** Radioactive Element **2** Monitoring Device **3** Infusion Device **B** Intraluminal Device, Airway **D** Intraluminal Device **U** Feeding Device **Y** Other Device	**Z** No Qualifier
6 Stomach CC	**0** Open **3** Percutaneous **4** Percutaneous Endoscopic	**2** Monitoring Device **3** Infusion Device **D** Intraluminal Device **M** Stimulator Lead **U** Feeding Device **Y** Other Device	**Z** No Qualifier
6 Stomach	**7** Via Natural or Artificial Opening **8** Via Natural or Artificial Opening Endoscopic	**2** Monitoring Device **3** Infusion Device **D** Intraluminal Device **U** Feeding Device **Y** Other Device	**Z** No Qualifier
8 Small Intestine **9** Duodenum **A** Jejunum **B** Ileum	**0** Open **3** Percutaneous **4** Percutaneous Endoscopic **7** Via Natural or Artificial Opening **8** Via Natural or Artificial Opening Endoscopic	**2** Monitoring Device **3** Infusion Device **D** Intraluminal Device **U** Feeding Device	**Z** No Qualifier
E Large Intestine	**0** Open **3** Percutaneous **4** Percutaneous Endoscopic **7** Via Natural or Artificial Opening **8** Via Natural or Artificial Opening Endoscopic	**D** Intraluminal Device	**Z** No Qualifier
P Rectum	**0** Open **3** Percutaneous **4** Percutaneous Endoscopic **7** Via Natural or Artificial Opening **8** Via Natural or Artificial Opening Endoscopic	**1** Radioactive Element **D** Intraluminal Device	**Z** No Qualifier
Q Anus	**0** Open **3** Percutaneous **4** Percutaneous Endoscopic	**D** Intraluminal Device **L** Artificial Sphincter	**Z** No Qualifier
Q Anus	**7** Via Natural or Artificial Opening **8** Via Natural or Artificial Opening Endoscopic	**D** Intraluminal Device	**Z** No Qualifier
R Anal Sphincter	**0** Open **3** Percutaneous **4** Percutaneous Endoscopic	**M** Stimulator Lead	**Z** No Qualifier

CC 0DH60MZ 0DH63MZ 0DH64MZ

0 Medical and Surgical
D Gastrointestinal System
J Inspection: Visually and/or manually exploring a body part

Body Part Character 4	Approach Character 5	Device Character 6	Qualifier Character 7
0 Upper Intestinal Tract **6** Stomach gastroscopy **D** Lower Intestinal Tract — Sigmoid	**0** Open **3** Percutaneous **4** Percutaneous Endoscopic **7** Via Natural or Artificial Opening **8** Via Natural or Artificial Opening Endoscopic gastroscopy **X** External	**Z** No Device	**Z** No Qualifier
U Omentum **V** Mesentery **W** Peritoneum	**0** Open **3** Percutaneous **4** Percutaneous Endoscopic **X** External	**Z** No Device	**Z** No Qualifier

0 Medical and Surgical
D Gastrointestinal System
L Occlusion: Completely closing an orifice or the lumen of a tubular body part

Body Part Character 4	Approach Character 5	Device Character 6	Qualifier Character 7
1 Esophagus, Upper **2** Esophagus, Middle **3** Esophagus, Lower **4** Esophagogastric Junction **5** Esophagus **6** Stomach **7** Stomach, Pylorus **8** Small Intestine **9** Duodenum **A** Jejunum **B** Ileum **C** Ileocecal Valve **E** Large Intestine **F** Large Intestine, Right **G** Large Intestine, Left **H** Cecum **K** Ascending Colon **L** Transverse Colon **M** Descending Colon **N** Sigmoid Colon **P** Rectum	**0** Open **3** Percutaneous **4** Percutaneous Endoscopic	**C** Extraluminal Device **D** Intraluminal Device **Z** No Device	**Z** No Qualifier
1 Esophagus, Upper **2** Esophagus, Middle **3** Esophagus, Lower **4** Esophagogastric Junction **5** Esophagus **6** Stomach **7** Stomach, Pylorus **8** Small Intestine **9** Duodenum **A** Jejunum **B** Ileum **C** Ileocecal Valve **E** Large Intestine **F** Large Intestine, Right **G** Large Intestine, Left **H** Cecum **K** Ascending Colon **L** Transverse Colon **M** Descending Colon **N** Sigmoid Colon **P** Rectum	**7** Via Natural or Artificial Opening **8** Via Natural or Artificial Opening Endoscopic	**D** Intraluminal Device **Z** No Device	**Z** No Qualifier

0DL continued on next page

0DL continued from previous page

0 Medical and Surgical
D Gastrointestinal System
L Occlusion: Completely closing an orifice or the lumen of a tubular body part

Body Part Character 4	Approach Character 5	Device Character 6	Qualifier Character 7
Q Anus	**0** Open **3** Percutaneous **4** Percutaneous Endoscopic **X** External	**C** Extraluminal Device **D** Intraluminal Device **Z** No Device	**Z** No Qualifier
Q Anus	**7** Via Natural or Artificial Opening **8** Via Natural or Artificial Opening Endoscopic	**D** Intraluminal Device **Z** No Device	**Z** No Qualifier

0 Medical and Surgical
D Gastrointestinal System
M Reattachment: Putting back in or on all or a portion of a separated body part to its normal location or other suitable location

Body Part Character 4	Approach Character 5	Device Character 6	Qualifier Character 7
5 Esophagus **6** Stomach **8** Small Intestine **9** Duodenum **A** Jejunum **B** Ileum **E** Large Intestine **F** Large Intestine, Right **G** Large Intestine, Left **H** Cecum **K** Ascending Colon **L** Transverse Colon **M** Descending Colon **N** Sigmoid Colon **P** Rectum	**0** Open **4** Percutaneous Endoscopic	**Z** No Device	**Z** No Qualifier

0 Medical and Surgical
D Gastrointestinal System
N Release: Freeing a body part from an abnormal physical constraint by cutting or by the use of force

Body Part Character 4	Approach Character 5	Device Character 6	Qualifier Character 7
1 Esophagus, Upper **2** Esophagus, Middle **3** Esophagus, Lower **4** Esophagogastric Junction **5** Esophagus **6** Stomach **7** Stomach, Pylorus **8** Small Intestine **9** Duodenum **A** Jejunum **B** Ileum **C** Ileocecal Valve **E** Large Intestine **F** Large Intestine, Right **G** Large Intestine, Left **H** Cecum **J** Appendix **K** Ascending Colon **L** Transverse Colon **M** Descending Colon **N** Sigmoid Colon **P** Rectum	**0** Open **3** Percutaneous **4** Percutaneous Endoscopic **7** Via Natural or Artificial Opening **8** Via Natural or Artificial Opening Endoscopic	**Z** No Device	**Z** No Qualifier

0DN continued on next page

0DN continued from previous page

0 Medical and Surgical
D Gastrointestinal System
N Release: Freeing a body part from an abnormal physical constraint by cutting or by the use of force

Body Part Character 4	Approach Character 5	Device Character 6	Qualifier Character 7
Q Anus	**0** Open **3** Percutaneous **4** Percutaneous Endoscopic **7** Via Natural or Artificial Opening **8** Via Natural or Artificial Opening Endoscopic **X** External	**Z** No Device	**Z** No Qualifier
R Anal Sphincter **U** Omentum **V** Mesentery **W** Peritoneum	**0** Open **3** Percutaneous **4** Percutaneous Endoscopic	**Z** No Device	**Z** No Qualifier

0 Medical and Surgical
D Gastrointestinal System
P Removal: Taking out or off a device from a body part

Body Part Character 4	Approach Character 5	Device Character 6	Qualifier Character 7
0 Upper Intestinal Tract **D** Lower Intestinal Tract	**0** Open **3** Percutaneous **4** Percutaneous Endoscopic **7** Via Natural or Artificial Opening **8** Via Natural or Artificial Opening Endoscopic	**0** Drainage Device **2** Monitoring Device **3** Infusion Device **7** Autologous Tissue Substitute **C** Extraluminal Device **D** Intraluminal Device **J** Synthetic Substitute **K** Nonautologous Tissue Substitute **U** Feeding Device **Y** Other Device	**Z** No Qualifier
0 Upper Intestinal Tract **D** Lower Intestinal Tract	**X** External	**0** Drainage Device **2** Monitoring Device **3** Infusion Device **D** Intraluminal Device **U** Feeding Device	**Z** No Qualifier
5 Esophagus	**0** Open **3** Percutaneous **4** Percutaneous Endoscopic	**1** Radioactive Element **2** Monitoring Device **3** Infusion Device **U** Feeding Device **Y** Other Device	**Z** No Qualifier
5 Esophagus	**7** Via Natural or Artificial Opening **8** Via Natural or Artificial Opening Endoscopic	**1** Radioactive Element **D** Intraluminal Device **Y** Other Device	**Z** No Qualifier
5 Esophagus	**X** External	**1** Radioactive Element **2** Monitoring Device **3** Infusion Device **D** Intraluminal Device **U** Feeding Device	**Z** No Qualifier
6 Stomach	**0** Open **3** Percutaneous **4** Percutaneous Endoscopic	**0** Drainage Device **2** Monitoring Device **3** Infusion Device **7** Autologous Tissue Substitute **C** Extraluminal Device **D** Intraluminal Device **J** Synthetic Substitute **K** Nonautologous Tissue Substitute **M** Stimulator Lead **U** Feeding Device **Y** Other Device	**Z** No Qualifier

0DP continued on next page

0DP continued from previous page

0 Medical and Surgical
D Gastrointestinal System
P Removal: Taking out or off a device from a body part

Body Part Character 4	Approach Character 5	Device Character 6	Qualifier Character 7
6 Stomach	**7** Via Natural or Artificial Opening **8** Via Natural or Artificial Opening Endoscopic	**0** Drainage Device **2** Monitoring Device **3** Infusion Device **7** Autologous Tissue Substitute **C** Extraluminal Device **D** Intraluminal Device **J** Synthetic Substitute **K** Nonautologous Tissue Substitute **U** Feeding Device **Y** Other Device	**Z** No Qualifier
6 Stomach	**X** External	**0** Drainage Device **2** Monitoring Device **3** Infusion Device **D** Intraluminal Device **U** Feeding Device	**Z** No Qualifier
P Rectum	**0** Open **3** Percutaneous **4** Percutaneous Endoscopic **7** Via Natural or Artificial Opening **8** Via Natural or Artificial Opening Endoscopic **X** External	**1** Radioactive Element	**Z** No Qualifier
Q Anus	**0** Open **3** Percutaneous **4** Percutaneous Endoscopic **7** Via Natural or Artificial Opening **8** Via Natural or Artificial Opening Endoscopic	**L** Artificial Sphincter	**Z** No Qualifier
R Anal Sphincter	**0** Open **3** Percutaneous **4** Percutaneous Endoscopic	**M** Stimulator Lead	**Z** No Qualifier
U Omentum **V** Mesentery **W** Peritoneum	**0** Open **3** Percutaneous **4** Percutaneous Endoscopic	**0** Drainage Device **1** Radioactive Element **7** Autologous Tissue Substitute **J** Synthetic Substitute **K** Nonautologous Tissue Substitute	**Z** No Qualifier

0 Medical and Surgical
D Gastrointestinal System
Q Repair: Restoring, to the extent possible, a body part to its normal anatomic structure and function

Body Part Character 4	Approach Character 5	Device Character 6	Qualifier Character 7
1 Esophagus, Upper **2** Esophagus, Middle **3** Esophagus, Lower **4** Esophagogastric Junction **5** Esophagus **6** Stomach **7** Stomach, Pylorus **8** Small Intestine CC **9** Duodenum CC **A** Jejunum CC **B** Ileum CC **C** Ileocecal Valve **E** Large Intestine CC **F** Large Intestine, Right CC **G** Large Intestine, Left CC **H** Cecum CC **J** Appendix **K** Ascending Colon CC **L** Transverse Colon CC **M** Descending Colon CC **N** Sigmoid Colon CC **P** Rectum	**0** Open **3** Percutaneous **4** Percutaneous Endoscopic **7** Via Natural or Artificial Opening **8** Via Natural or Artificial Opening Endoscopic	**Z** No Device	**Z** No Qualifier
Q Anus	**0** Open **3** Percutaneous **4** Percutaneous Endoscopic **7** Via Natural or Artificial Opening **8** Via Natural or Artificial Opening Endoscopic **X** External	**Z** No Device	**Z** No Qualifier
R Anal Sphincter **U** Omentum **V** Mesentery **W** Peritoneum	**0** Open **3** Percutaneous **4** Percutaneous Endoscopic	**Z** No Device	**Z** No Qualifier

CC 0DQ80ZZ 0DQ90ZZ 0DQA0ZZ 0DQB0ZZ 0DQE0ZZ 0DQF0ZZ 0DQG0ZZ 0DQH0ZZ 0DQK0ZZ 0DQL0ZZ 0DQM0ZZ 0DQN0ZZ

0 Medical and Surgical
D Gastrointestinal System
R Replacement: Putting in or on biological or synthetic material that physically takes the place and/or function of all or a portion of a body part

Body Part Character 4	Approach Character 5	Device Character 6	Qualifier Character 7
5 Esophagus	**0** Open **4** Percutaneous Endoscopic **7** Via Natural or Artificial Opening **8** Via Natural or Artificial Opening Endoscopic	**7** Autologous Tissue Substitute **J** Synthetic Substitute **K** Nonautologous Tissue Substitute	**Z** No Qualifier
R Anal Sphincter **U** Omentum **V** Mesentery **W** Peritoneum	**0** Open **4** Percutaneous Endoscopic	**7** Autologous Tissue Substitute **J** Synthetic Substitute **K** Nonautologous Tissue Substitute	**Z** No Qualifier

0 Medical and Surgical
D Gastrointestinal System
S Reposition: Moving to its normal location, or other suitable location, all or a portion of a body part

Body Part Character 4	Approach Character 5	Device Character 6	Qualifier Character 7
5 Esophagus **6** Stomach **9** Duodenum **A** Jejunum **B** Ileum **H** Cecum **K** Ascending Colon **L** Transverse Colon **M** Descending Colon **N** Sigmoid Colon **P** Rectum **Q** Anus	**0** Open **4** Percutaneous Endoscopic **7** Via Natural or Artificial Opening **8** Via Natural or Artificial Opening Endoscopic **X** External	**Z** No Device	**Z** No Qualifier
8 Small Intestine **E** Large Intestine	**0** Open **4** Percutaneous Endoscopic **7** Via Natural or Artificial Opening **8** Via Natural or Artificial Opening Endoscopic	**Z** No Device	**Z** No Qualifier

0 Medical and Surgical
D Gastrointestinal System
T Resection: Cutting out or off, without replacement, all of a body part

Body Part Character 4	Approach Character 5	Device Character 6	Qualifier Character 7
1 Esophagus, Upper **2** Esophagus, Middle **3** Esophagus, Lower **4** Esophagogastric Junction **5** Esophagus **6** Stomach **7** Stomach, Pylorus **8** Small Intestine **9** Duodenum CC **A** Jejunum **B** Ileum **C** Ileocecal Valve **E** Large Intestine **F** Large Intestine, Right **H** Cecum **J** Appendix **K** Ascending Colon **P** Rectum **Q** Anus	**0** Open **4** Percutaneous Endoscopic **7** Via Natural or Artificial Opening **8** Via Natural or Artificial Opening Endoscopic	**Z** No Device	**Z** No Qualifier
G Large Intestine, Left **L** Transverse Colon **M** Descending Colon **N** Sigmoid Colon	**0** Open **4** Percutaneous Endoscopic **7** Via Natural or Artificial Opening **8** Via Natural or Artificial Opening Endoscopic **F** Via Natural or Artificial Opening With Percutaneous Endoscopic Assistance	**Z** No Device	**Z** No Qualifier
R Anal Sphincter **U** Omentum	**0** Open **4** Percutaneous Endoscopic	**Z** No Device	**Z** No Qualifier

CC 0DT90ZZ

0 Medical and Surgical
D Gastrointestinal System
U Supplement: Putting in or on biological or synthetic material that physically reinforces and/or augments the function of a portion of a body part

Body Part Character 4	Approach Character 5	Device Character 6	Qualifier Character 7
1 Esophagus, Upper **2** Esophagus, Middle **3** Esophagus, Lower **4** Esophagogastric Junction **5** Esophagus **6** Stomach **7** Stomach, Pylorus **8** Small Intestine **9** Duodenum **A** Jejunum **B** Ileum **C** Ileocecal Valve **E** Large Intestine **F** Large Intestine, Right **G** Large Intestine, Left **H** Cecum **K** Ascending Colon **L** Transverse Colon **M** Descending Colon **N** Sigmoid Colon **P** Rectum	**0** Open **4** Percutaneous Endoscopic **7** Via Natural or Artificial Opening **8** Via Natural or Artificial Opening Endoscopic	**7** Autologous Tissue Substitute **J** Synthetic Substitute **K** Nonautologous Tissue Substitute	**Z** No Qualifier
Q Anus	**0** Open **4** Percutaneous Endoscopic **7** Via Natural or Artificial Opening **8** Via Natural or Artificial Opening Endoscopic **X** External	**7** Autologous Tissue Substitute **J** Synthetic Substitute **K** Nonautologous Tissue Substitute	**Z** No Qualifier
R Anal Sphincter **U** Omentum **V** Mesentery **W** Peritoneum	**0** Open **4** Percutaneous Endoscopic	**7** Autologous Tissue Substitute **J** Synthetic Substitute **K** Nonautologous Tissue Substitute	**Z** No Qualifier

0 Medical and Surgical
D Gastrointestinal System
V Restriction: Partially closing an orifice or the lumen of a tubular body part

Body Part Character 4	Approach Character 5	Device Character 6	Qualifier Character 7
1 Esophagus, Upper **2** Esophagus, Middle **3** Esophagus, Lower **4** Esophagogastric Junction **5** Esophagus **6** Stomach **7** Stomach, Pylorus **8** Small Intestine **9** Duodenum **A** Jejunum **B** Ileum **C** Ileocecal Valve **E** Large Intestine **F** Large Intestine, Right **G** Large Intestine, Left **H** Cecum **K** Ascending Colon **L** Transverse Colon **M** Descending Colon **N** Sigmoid Colon **P** Rectum	**0** Open **3** Percutaneous **4** Percutaneous Endoscopic	**C** Extraluminal Device **D** Intraluminal Device **Z** No Device	**Z** No Qualifier

0DV continued on next page

0DV continued from previous page

0 Medical and Surgical
D Gastrointestinal System
V Restriction: Partially closing an orifice or the lumen of a tubular body part

Body Part Character 4	Approach Character 5	Device Character 6	Qualifier Character 7
1 Esophagus, Upper **2** Esophagus, Middle **3** Esophagus, Lower **4** Esophagogastric Junction **5** Esophagus **6** Stomach NC HAC **7** Stomach, Pylorus **8** Small Intestine **9** Duodenum **A** Jejunum **B** Ileum **C** Ileocecal Valve **E** Large Intestine **F** Large Intestine, Right **G** Large Intestine, Left **H** Cecum **K** Ascending Colon **L** Transverse Colon **M** Descending Colon **N** Sigmoid Colon **P** Rectum	**7** Via Natural or Artificial Opening **8** Via Natural or Artificial Opening Endoscopic	**D** Intraluminal Device **Z** No Device	**Z** No Qualifier
Q Anus	**0** Open **3** Percutaneous **4** Percutaneous Endoscopic **X** External	**C** Extraluminal Device **D** Intraluminal Device **Z** No Device	**Z** No Qualifier
Q Anus	**7** Via Natural or Artificial Opening **8** Via Natural or Artificial Opening Endoscopic	**D** Intraluminal Device **Z** No Device	**Z** No Qualifier

NC 0DV67DZ 0DV68DZ
HAC 0DV64CZ
Surgical site infection following bariatric surgery procedures and principal diagnoses E66.01 and secondary diagnoses K68.11, K95.01, K95.81, T81.40XA, T81.41XA, T81.42XA, T81.43XA, T81.44XA, T81.49XA.

0 Medical and Surgical
D Gastrointestinal System
W Revision: Correcting, to the extent possible, a portion of a malfunctioning device or the position of a displaced device

Body Part Character 4	Approach Character 5	Device Character 6	Qualifier Character 7
0 Upper Intestinal Tract **D** Lower Intestinal Tract	**0** Open **3** Percutaneous **4** Percutaneous Endoscopic **7** Via Natural or Artificial Opening **8** Via Natural or Artificial Opening Endoscopic	**0** Drainage Device **2** Monitoring Device **3** Infusion Device **7** Autologous Tissue Substitute **C** Extraluminal Device **D** Intraluminal Device **J** Synthetic Substitute **K** Nonautologous Tissue Substitute **U** Feeding Device **Y** Other Device	**Z** No Qualifier
0 Upper Intestinal Tract **D** Lower Intestinal Tract	**X** External	**0** Drainage Device **2** Monitoring Device **3** Infusion Device **7** Autologous Tissue Substitute **C** Extraluminal Device **D** Intraluminal Device **J** Synthetic Substitute **K** Nonautologous Tissue Substitute **U** Feeding Device	**Z** No Qualifier

0DW continued on next page

0 Medical and Surgical
D Gastrointestinal System
W Revision: Correcting, to the extent possible, a portion of a malfunctioning device or the position of a displaced device

0DW continued from previous page

Body Part Character 4	Approach Character 5	Device Character 6	Qualifier Character 7
5 Esophagus	**0** Open **3** Percutaneous **4** Percutaneous Endoscopic	**Y** Other Device	**Z** No Qualifier
5 Esophagus	**7** Via Natural or Artificial Opening **8** Via Natural or Artificial Opening Endoscopic	**D** Intraluminal Device **Y** Other Device	**Z** No Qualifier
5 Esophagus	**X** External	**D** Intraluminal Device	**Z** No Qualifier
6 Stomach	**0** Open **3** Percutaneous **4** Percutaneous Endoscopic	**0** Drainage Device **2** Monitoring Device **3** Infusion Device **7** Autologous Tissue Substitute **C** Extraluminal Device **D** Intraluminal Device **J** Synthetic Substitute **K** Nonautologous Tissue Substitute **M** Stimulator Lead **U** Feeding Device **Y** Other Device	**Z** No Qualifier
6 Stomach	**7** Via Natural or Artificial Opening **8** Via Natural or Artificial Opening Endoscopic	**0** Drainage Device **2** Monitoring Device **3** Infusion Device **7** Autologous Tissue Substitute **C** Extraluminal Device **D** Intraluminal Device **J** Synthetic Substitute **K** Nonautologous Tissue Substitute **U** Feeding Device **Y** Other Device	**Z** No Qualifier
6 Stomach	**X** External	**0** Drainage Device **2** Monitoring Device **3** Infusion Device **7** Autologous Tissue Substitute **C** Extraluminal Device **D** Intraluminal Device **J** Synthetic Substitute **K** Nonautologous Tissue Substitute **U** Feeding Device	**Z** No Qualifier
8 Small Intestine **E** Large Intestine	**0** Open **4** Percutaneous Endoscopic **7** Via Natural or Artificial Opening **8** Via Natural or Artificial Opening Endoscopic	**7** Autologous Tissue Substitute **J** Synthetic Substitute **K** Nonautologous Tissue Substitute	**Z** No Qualifier
Q Anus	**0** Open **3** Percutaneous **4** Percutaneous Endoscopic **7** Via Natural or Artificial Opening **8** Via Natural or Artificial Opening Endoscopic	**L** Artificial Sphincter	**Z** No Qualifier
R Anal Sphincter	**0** Open **3** Percutaneous **4** Percutaneous Endoscopic	**M** Stimulator Lead	**Z** No Qualifier
U Omentum **V** Mesentery **W** Peritoneum	**0** Open **3** Percutaneous **4** Percutaneous Endoscopic	**0** Drainage Device **7** Autologous Tissue Substitute **J** Synthetic Substitute **K** Nonautologous Tissue Substitute	**Z** No Qualifier

0 Medical and Surgical
D Gastrointestinal System
X Transfer: Moving, without taking out, all or a portion of a body part to another location to take over the function of all or a portion of a body part

Body Part Character 4	Approach Character 5	Device Character 6	Qualifier Character 7
6 Stomach **8** Small Intestine	**0** Open **4** Percutaneous Endoscopic	**Z** No Device	**5** Esophagus
E Large Intestine ♀	**0** Open **4** Percutaneous Endoscopic	**Z** No Device	**5** Esophagus **7** Vagina

♀ 0DXE0Z7 0DXE4Z7

0 Medical and Surgical
D Gastrointestinal System
Y Transplantation: Putting in or on all or a portion of a living body part taken from another individual or animal to physically take the place and/or function of all or a portion of a similar body part

Body Part Character 4	Approach Character 5	Device Character 6	Qualifier Character 7
5 Esophagus **6** Stomach **8** Small Intestine LC **E** Large Intestine LC	**0** Open	**Z** No Device	**0** Allogeneic **1** Syngeneic **2** Zooplastic

LC 0DY80Z0 0DY80Z1 0DY80Z2 0DYE0Z0 0DYE0Z1 0DYE0Z2

NOTES

Hepatobiliary System and Pancreas 0F1-0FY

0 Medical and Surgical
F Hepatobiliary System and Pancreas
1 Bypass: Altering the route of passage of the contents of a tubular body part

Body Part Character 4	Approach Character 5	Device Character 6	Qualifier Character 7
4 Gallbladder **5** Hepatic Duct, Right **6** Hepatic Duct, Left **7** Hepatic Duct, Common **8** Cystic Duct **9** Common Bile Duct	**0** Open **4** Percutaneous Endoscopic	**D** Intraluminal Device **Z** No Device	**3** Duodenum **4** Stomach **5** Hepatic Duct, Right **6** Hepatic Duct, Left **7** Hepatic Duct, Caudate **8** Cystic Duct **9** Common Bile Duct **B** Small Intestine
D Pancreatic Duct **F** Pancreatic Duct, Accessory **G** Pancreas	**0** Open **4** Percutaneous Endoscopic	**D** Intraluminal Device **Z** No Device	**3** Duodenum **B** Small Intestine **C** Large Intestine

0 Medical and Surgical
F Hepatobiliary System and Pancreas
2 Change: Taking out or off a device from a body part and putting back an identical or similar device in or on the same body part without cutting or puncturing the skin or a mucous membrane

Body Part Character 4	Approach Character 5	Device Character 6	Qualifier Character 7
0 Liver **4** Gallbladder **B** Hepatobiliary Duct **D** Pancreatic Duct **G** Pancreas	**X** External	**0** Drainage Device **Y** Other Device	**Z** No Qualifier

0 Medical and Surgical
F Hepatobiliary System and Pancreas
5 Destruction: Physical eradication of all or a portion of a body part by the direct use of energy, force, or a destructive agent

Body Part Character 4	Approach Character 5	Device Character 6	Qualifier Character 7
0 Liver **1** Liver, Right Lobe **2** Liver, Left Lobe	**0** Open **3** Percutaneous **4** Percutaneous Endoscopic	**Z** No Device	**F** Irreversible Electroporation **Z** No Qualifier
4 Gallbladder	**0** Open **3** Percutaneous **4** Percutaneous Endoscopic **8** Via Natural or Artificial Opening Endoscopic	**Z** No Device	**Z** No Qualifier
5 Hepatic Duct, Right **6** Hepatic Duct, Left **7** Hepatic Duct, Common **8** Cystic Duct **9** Common Bile Duct **C** Ampulla of Vater **D** Pancreatic Duct **F** Pancreatic Duct, Accessory	**0** Open **3** Percutaneous **4** Percutaneous Endoscopic **7** Via Natural or Artificial Opening **8** Via Natural or Artificial Opening Endoscopic	**Z** No Device	**Z** No Qualifier
G Pancreas	**0** Open **3** Percutaneous **4** Percutaneous Endoscopic	**Z** No Device	**F** Irreversible Electroporation **Z** No Qualifier
G Pancreas	**8** Via Natural or Artificial Opening Endoscopic	**Z** No Device	**Z** No Qualifier

0 Medical and Surgical
F Hepatobiliary System and Pancreas
7 Dilation: Expanding an orifice or the lumen of a tubular body part

Body Part Character 4	Approach Character 5	Device Character 6	Qualifier Character 7
5 Hepatic Duct, Right **6** Hepatic Duct, Left **7** Hepatic Duct, Common **8** Cystic Duct **9** Common Bile Duct **C** Ampulla of Vater **D** Pancreatic Duct **F** Pancreatic Duct, Accessory	**0** Open **3** Percutaneous **4** Percutaneous Endoscopic **7** Via Natural or Artificial Opening **8** Via Natural or Artificial Opening Endoscopic	**D** Intraluminal Device **Z** No Device	**Z** No Qualifier

0 Medical and Surgical
F Hepatobiliary System and Pancreas
8 Division: Cutting into a body part, without draining fluids and/or gases from the body part, in order to separate or transect a body part

Body Part Character 4	Approach Character 5	Device Character 6	Qualifier Character 7
G Pancreas	**0** Open **3** Percutaneous **4** Percutaneous Endoscopic	**Z** No Device	**Z** No Qualifier

0 Medical and Surgical
F Hepatobiliary System and Pancreas
9 Drainage: Taking or letting out fluids and/or gases from a body part

Body Part Character 4	Approach Character 5	Device Character 6	Qualifier Character 7
0 Liver **1** Liver, Right Lobe **2** Liver, Left Lobe	**0** Open laparotomy **3** Percutaneous **4** Percutaneous Endoscopic	**0** Drainage Device	**Z** No Qualifier
0 Liver **1** Liver, Right Lobe **2** Liver, Left Lobe	**0** Open **3** Percutaneous **4** Percutaneous Endoscopic	**Z** No Device	**X** Diagnostic **Z** No Qualifier
4 Gallbladder **G** Pancreas	**0** Open **3** Percutaneous **4** Percutaneous Endoscopic **8** Via Natural or Artificial Opening Endoscopic	**0** Drainage Device	**Z** No Qualifier
4 Gallbladder **G** Pancreas	**0** Open **3** Percutaneous **4** Percutaneous Endoscopic **8** Via Natural or Artificial Opening Endoscopic	**Z** No Device	**X** Diagnostic **Z** No Qualifier
5 Hepatic Duct, Right **6** Hepatic Duct, Left **7** Hepatic Duct, Common **8** Cystic Duct **9** Common Bile Duct **C** Ampulla of Vater **D** Pancreatic Duct **F** Pancreatic Duct, Accessory	**0** Open **3** Percutaneous **4** Percutaneous Endoscopic **7** Via Natural or Artificial Opening **8** Via Natural or Artificial Opening Endoscopic	**0** Drainage Device	**Z** No Qualifier
5 Hepatic Duct, Right **6** Hepatic Duct, Left **7** Hepatic Duct, Common **8** Cystic Duct **9** Common Bile Duct **C** Ampulla of Vater **D** Pancreatic Duct **F** Pancreatic Duct, Accessory	**0** Open **3** Percutaneous **4** Percutaneous Endoscopic **7** Via Natural or Artificial Opening **8** Via Natural or Artificial Opening Endoscopic	**Z** No Device	**X** Diagnostic **Z** No Qualifier

0 Medical and Surgical
F Hepatobiliary System and Pancreas
B Excision: Cutting out or off, without replacement, a portion of a body part

Body Part Character 4	Approach Character 5	Device Character 6	Qualifier Character 7
0 Liver 1 Liver, Right Lobe 2 Liver, Left Lobe	0 Open 3 Percutaneous 4 Percutaneous Endoscopic	Z No Device	X Diagnostic Z No Qualifier
4 Gallbladder G Pancreas - maybe just tail	0 Open 3 Percutaneous 4 Percutaneous Endoscopic 8 Via Natural or Artificial Opening Endoscopic	Z No Device	X Diagnostic Z No Qualifier
5 Hepatic Duct, Right 6 Hepatic Duct, Left 7 Hepatic Duct, Common 8 Cystic Duct 9 Common Bile Duct C Ampulla of Vater D Pancreatic Duct F Pancreatic Duct, Accessory	0 Open pancreas 3 Percutaneous 4 Percutaneous Endoscopic 7 Via Natural or Artificial Opening 8 Via Natural or Artificial Opening Endoscopic	Z No Device	X Diagnostic Z No Qualifier

0 Medical and Surgical
F Hepatobiliary System and Pancreas
C Extirpation: Taking or cutting out solid matter from a body part

Body Part Character 4	Approach Character 5	Device Character 6	Qualifier Character 7
0 Liver 1 Liver, Right Lobe 2 Liver, Left Lobe	0 Open 3 Percutaneous 4 Percutaneous Endoscopic	Z No Device	Z No Qualifier
4 Gallbladder G Pancreas	0 Open 3 Percutaneous 4 Percutaneous Endoscopic 8 Via Natural or Artificial Opening Endoscopic	Z No Device	Z No Qualifier
5 Hepatic Duct, Right 6 Hepatic Duct, Left 7 Hepatic Duct, Common 8 Cystic Duct 9 Common Bile Duct C Ampulla of Vater D Pancreatic Duct F Pancreatic Duct, Accessory	0 Open 3 Percutaneous 4 Percutaneous Endoscopic 7 Via Natural or Artificial Opening 8 Via Natural or Artificial Opening Endoscopic	Z No Device	Z No Qualifier

0 Medical and Surgical
F Hepatobiliary System and Pancreas
D Extraction: Pulling or stripping out or off all or a portion of a body part by the use of force

Body Part Character 4	Approach Character 5	Device Character 6	Qualifier Character 7
0 Liver 1 Liver, Right Lobe 2 Liver, Left Lobe	3 Percutaneous 4 Percutaneous Endoscopic	Z No Device	X Diagnostic
4 Gallbladder 5 Hepatic Duct, Right 6 Hepatic Duct, Left 7 Hepatic Duct, Common 8 Cystic Duct 9 Common Bile Duct C Ampulla of Vater D Pancreatic Duct F Pancreatic Duct, Accessory G Pancreas	3 Percutaneous 4 Percutaneous Endoscopic 8 Via Natural or Artificial Opening Endoscopic	Z No Device	X Diagnostic

LC Limited Coverage NC Noncovered HAC HAC-associated Procedure CC Combination Cluster - See Appendix G for code lists
DRG Non-OR-Affecting MS-DRG Assignment New/Revised Text in **Orange** ♂ Male ♀ Female

0 Medical and Surgical
F Hepatobiliary System and Pancreas
F Fragmentation: Breaking solid matter in a body part into pieces

Body Part Character 4	Approach Character 5	Device Character 6	Qualifier Character 7
4 Gallbladder NC 5 Hepatic Duct, Right NC 6 Hepatic Duct, Left NC 7 Hepatic Duct, Common 8 Cystic Duct NC 9 Common Bile Duct NC C Ampulla of Vater NC D Pancreatic Duct NC F Pancreatic Duct, Accessory NC	0 Open 3 Percutaneous 4 Percutaneous Endoscopic 7 Via Natural or Artificial Opening 8 Via Natural or Artificial Opening Endoscopic X External	Z No Device	Z No Qualifier

NC 0FF4XZZ 0FF5XZZ 0FF6XZZ 0FF8XZZ 0FF9XZZ 0FFCXZZ 0FFDXZZ 0FFFXZZ

0 Medical and Surgical
F Hepatobiliary System and Pancreas
H Insertion: Putting in a nonbiological appliance that monitors, assists, performs, or prevents a physiological function but does not physically take the place of a body part

Body Part Character 4	Approach Character 5	Device Character 6	Qualifier Character 7
0 Liver 4 Gallbladder G Pancreas	0 Open 3 Percutaneous 4 Percutaneous Endoscopic	2 Monitoring Device 3 Infusion Device Y Other Device	Z No Qualifier
1 Liver, Right Lobe 2 Liver, Left Lobe	0 Open 3 Percutaneous 4 Percutaneous Endoscopic	2 Monitoring Device 3 Infusion Device	Z No Qualifier
B Hepatobiliary Duct D Pancreatic Duct	0 Open 3 Percutaneous 4 Percutaneous Endoscopic 7 Via Natural or Artificial Opening 8 Via Natural or Artificial Opening Endoscopic	1 Radioactive Element 2 Monitoring Device 3 Infusion Device D Intraluminal Device Y Other Device	Z No Qualifier

0 Medical and Surgical
F Hepatobiliary System and Pancreas
J Inspection: Visually and/or manually exploring a body part

Body Part Character 4	Approach Character 5	Device Character 6	Qualifier Character 7
0 Liver	0 Open 3 Percutaneous 4 Percutaneous Endoscopic X External	Z No Device	Z No Qualifier
4 Gallbladder G Pancreas	0 Open 3 Percutaneous 4 Percutaneous Endoscopic 8 Via Natural or Artificial Opening Endoscopic X External	Z No Device	Z No Qualifier
B Hepatobiliary Duct D Pancreatic Duct	0 Open 3 Percutaneous 4 Percutaneous Endoscopic 7 Via Natural or Artificial Opening 8 Via Natural or Artificial Opening Endoscopic	Z No Device	Z No Qualifier

0 Medical and Surgical
F Hepatobiliary System and Pancreas
L Occlusion: Completely closing an orifice or the lumen of a tubular body part

Body Part Character 4	Approach Character 5	Device Character 6	Qualifier Character 7
5 Hepatic Duct, Right **6** Hepatic Duct, Left **7** Hepatic Duct, Common **8** Cystic Duct **9** Common Bile Duct **C** Ampulla of Vater **D** Pancreatic Duct **F** Pancreatic Duct, Accessory	**0** Open **3** Percutaneous **4** Percutaneous Endoscopic	**C** Extraluminal Device **D** Intraluminal Device **Z** No Device	**Z** No Qualifier
5 Hepatic Duct, Right **6** Hepatic Duct, Left **7** Hepatic Duct, Common **8** Cystic Duct **9** Common Bile Duct **C** Ampulla of Vater **D** Pancreatic Duct **F** Pancreatic Duct, Accessory	**7** Via Natural or Artificial Opening **8** Via Natural or Artificial Opening Endoscopic	**D** Intraluminal Device **Z** No Device	**Z** No Qualifier

0 Medical and Surgical
F Hepatobiliary System and Pancreas
M Reattachment: Putting back in or on all or a portion of a separated body part to its normal location or other suitable location

Body Part Character 4	Approach Character 5	Device Character 6	Qualifier Character 7
0 Liver **1** Liver, Right Lobe **2** Liver, Left Lobe **4** Gallbladder **5** Hepatic Duct, Right **6** Hepatic Duct, Left **7** Hepatic Duct, Common **8** Cystic Duct **9** Common Bile Duct **C** Ampulla of Vater **D** Pancreatic Duct **F** Pancreatic Duct, Accessory **G** Pancreas	**0** Open **4** Percutaneous Endoscopic	**Z** No Device	**Z** No Qualifier

0 Medical and Surgical
F Hepatobiliary System and Pancreas
N Release: Freeing a body part from an abnormal physical constraint by cutting or by the use of force

Body Part Character 4	Approach Character 5	Device Character 6	Qualifier Character 7
0 Liver **1** Liver, Right Lobe **2** Liver, Left Lobe	**0** Open **3** Percutaneous **4** Percutaneous Endoscopic	**Z** No Device	**Z** No Qualifier
4 Gallbladder **G** Pancreas	**0** Open **3** Percutaneous **4** Percutaneous Endoscopic **8** Via Natural or Artificial Opening Endoscopic	**Z** No Device	**Z** No Qualifier
5 Hepatic Duct, Right **6** Hepatic Duct, Left **7** Hepatic Duct, Common **8** Cystic Duct **9** Common Bile Duct **C** Ampulla of Vater **D** Pancreatic Duct **F** Pancreatic Duct, Accessory	**0** Open **3** Percutaneous **4** Percutaneous Endoscopic **7** Via Natural or Artificial Opening **8** Via Natural or Artificial Opening Endoscopic	**Z** No Device	**Z** No Qualifier

0 Medical and Surgical
F Hepatobiliary System and Pancreas
P Removal: Taking out or off a device from a body part

Body Part Character 4	Approach Character 5	Device Character 6	Qualifier Character 7
0 Liver	**0** Open **3** Percutaneous **4** Percutaneous Endoscopic	**0** Drainage Device **2** Monitoring Device **3** Infusion Device **Y** Other Device	**Z** No Qualifier
0 Liver	**X** External	**0** Drainage Device **2** Monitoring Device **3** Infusion Device	**Z** No Qualifier
4 Gallbladder **G** Pancreas	**0** Open **3** Percutaneous **4** Percutaneous Endoscopic	**0** Drainage Device **2** Monitoring Device **3** Infusion Device **D** Intraluminal Device **Y** Other Device	**Z** No Qualifier
4 Gallbladder **G** Pancreas	**X** External	**0** Drainage Device **2** Monitoring Device **3** Infusion Device **D** Intraluminal Device	**Z** No Qualifier
B Hepatobiliary Duct **D** Pancreatic Duct	**0** Open **3** Percutaneous **4** Percutaneous Endoscopic **7** Via Natural or Artificial Opening **8** Via Natural or Artificial Opening Endoscopic	**0** Drainage Device **1** Radioactive Element **2** Monitoring Device **3** Infusion Device **7** Autologous Tissue Substitute **C** Extraluminal Device **D** Intraluminal Device **J** Synthetic Substitute **K** Nonautologous Tissue Substitute **Y** Other Device	**Z** No Qualifier
B Hepatobiliary Duct **D** Pancreatic Duct	**X** External	**0** Drainage Device **1** Radioactive Element **2** Monitoring Device **3** Infusion Device **D** Intraluminal Device	**Z** No Qualifier

0 Medical and Surgical
F Hepatobiliary System and Pancreas
Q Repair: Restoring, to the extent possible, a body part to its normal anatomic structure and function

Body Part Character 4	Approach Character 5	Device Character 6	Qualifier Character 7
0 Liver **1** Liver, Right Lobe **2** Liver, Left Lobe	**0** Open **3** Percutaneous **4** Percutaneous Endoscopic	**Z** No Device	**Z** No Qualifier
4 Gallbladder **G** Pancreas	**0** Open **3** Percutaneous **4** Percutaneous Endoscopic **8** Via Natural or Artificial Opening Endoscopic	**Z** No Device	**Z** No Qualifier
5 Hepatic Duct, Right **6** Hepatic Duct, Left **7** Hepatic Duct, Common **8** Cystic Duct **9** Common Bile Duct **C** Ampulla of Vater **D** Pancreatic Duct **F** Pancreatic Duct, Accessory	**0** Open **3** Percutaneous **4** Percutaneous Endoscopic **7** Via Natural or Artificial Opening **8** Via Natural or Artificial Opening Endoscopic	**Z** No Device	**Z** No Qualifier

0 Medical and Surgical
F Hepatobiliary System and Pancreas
R Replacement: Putting in or on biological or synthetic material that physically takes the place and/or function of all or a portion of a body part

Body Part Character 4	Approach Character 5	Device Character 6	Qualifier Character 7
5 Hepatic Duct, Right **6** Hepatic Duct, Left **7** Hepatic Duct, Common **8** Cystic Duct **9** Common Bile Duct **C** Ampulla of Vater **D** Pancreatic Duct **F** Pancreatic Duct, Accessory	**0** Open **4** Percutaneous Endoscopic **8** Via Natural or Artificial Opening Endoscopic	**7** Autologous Tissue Substitute **J** Synthetic Substitute **K** Nonautologous Tissue Substitute	**Z** No Qualifier

0 Medical and Surgical
F Hepatobiliary System and Pancreas
S Reposition: Moving to its normal location, or other suitable location, all or a portion of a body part

Body Part Character 4	Approach Character 5	Device Character 6	Qualifier Character 7
0 Liver **4** Gallbladder **5** Hepatic Duct, Right **6** Hepatic Duct, Left **7** Hepatic Duct, Common **8** Cystic Duct **9** Common Bile Duct **C** Ampulla of Vater **D** Pancreatic Duct **F** Pancreatic Duct, Accessory **G** Pancreas	**0** Open **4** Percutaneous Endoscopic	**Z** No Device	**Z** No Qualifier

0 Medical and Surgical
F Hepatobiliary System and Pancreas
T Resection: Cutting out or off, without replacement, all of a body part

Body Part Character 4	Approach Character 5	Device Character 6	Qualifier Character 7
0 Liver **1** Liver, Right Lobe **2** Liver, Left Lobe **4** Gallbladder Cholecyst **G** Pancreas CC	**0** Open **4** Percutaneous Endoscopic Laparoscope	**Z** No Device	**Z** No Qualifier
5 Hepatic Duct, Right **6** Hepatic Duct, Left **7** Hepatic Duct, Common **8** Cystic Duct **9** Common Bile Duct **C** Ampulla of Vater **D** Pancreatic Duct **F** Pancreatic Duct, Accessory	**0** Open **4** Percutaneous Endoscopic **7** Via Natural or Artificial Opening **8** Via Natural or Artificial Opening Endoscopic	**Z** No Device	**Z** No Qualifier

CC 0FTG0ZZ

0 Medical and Surgical
F Hepatobiliary System and Pancreas
U Supplement: Putting in or on biological or synthetic material that physically reinforces and/or augments the function of a portion of a body part

Body Part Character 4	Approach Character 5	Device Character 6	Qualifier Character 7
5 Hepatic Duct, Right 6 Hepatic Duct, Left 7 Hepatic Duct, Common 8 Cystic Duct 9 Common Bile Duct C Ampulla of Vater D Pancreatic Duct F Pancreatic Duct, Accessory	0 Open 3 Percutaneous 4 Percutaneous Endoscopic 8 Via Natural or Artificial Opening Endoscopic	7 Autologous Tissue Substitute J Synthetic Substitute K Nonautologous Tissue Substitute	Z No Qualifier

0 Medical and Surgical
F Hepatobiliary System and Pancreas
V Restriction: Partially closing an orifice or the lumen of a tubular body part

Body Part Character 4	Approach Character 5	Device Character 6	Qualifier Character 7
5 Hepatic Duct, Right 6 Hepatic Duct, Left 7 Hepatic Duct, Common 8 Cystic Duct 9 Common Bile Duct C Ampulla of Vater D Pancreatic Duct F Pancreatic Duct, Accessory	0 Open 3 Percutaneous 4 Percutaneous Endoscopic	C Extraluminal Device D Intraluminal Device Z No Device	Z No Qualifier
5 Hepatic Duct, Right 6 Hepatic Duct, Left 7 Hepatic Duct, Common 8 Cystic Duct 9 Common Bile Duct C Ampulla of Vater D Pancreatic Duct F Pancreatic Duct, Accessory	7 Via Natural or Artificial Opening 8 Via Natural or Artificial Opening Endoscopic	D Intraluminal Device Z No Device	Z No Qualifier

0 Medical and Surgical
F Hepatobiliary System and Pancreas
W Revision: Correcting, to the extent possible, a portion of a malfunctioning device or the position of a displaced device

Body Part Character 4	Approach Character 5	Device Character 6	Qualifier Character 7
0 Liver	0 Open 3 Percutaneous 4 Percutaneous Endoscopic	0 Drainage Device 2 Monitoring Device 3 Infusion Device Y Other Device	Z No Qualifier
0 Liver	X External	0 Drainage Device 2 Monitoring Device 3 Infusion Device	Z No Qualifier
4 Gallbladder G Pancreas	0 Open 3 Percutaneous 4 Percutaneous Endoscopic	0 Drainage Device 2 Monitoring Device 3 Infusion Device D Intraluminal Device Y Other Device	Z No Qualifier
4 Gallbladder G Pancreas	X External	0 Drainage Device 2 Monitoring Device 3 Infusion Device D Intraluminal Device	Z No Qualifier

0FW continued on next page

0FW continued from previous page

0 Medical and Surgical
F Hepatobiliary System and Pancreas
W Revision: Correcting, to the extent possible, a portion of a malfunctioning device or the position of a displaced device

Body Part Character 4	Approach Character 5	Device Character 6	Qualifier Character 7
B Hepatobiliary Duct **D** Pancreatic Duct	**0** Open **3** Percutaneous **4** Percutaneous Endoscopic **7** Via Natural or Artificial Opening **8** Via Natural or Artificial Opening Endoscopic	**0** Drainage Device **2** Monitoring Device **3** Infusion Device **7** Autologous Tissue Substitute **C** Extraluminal Device **D** Intraluminal Device **J** Synthetic Substitute **K** Nonautologous Tissue Substitute **Y** Other Device	**Z** No Qualifier
B Hepatobiliary Duct **D** Pancreatic Duct	**X** External	**0** Drainage Device **2** Monitoring Device **3** Infusion Device **7** Autologous Tissue Substitute **C** Extraluminal Device **D** Intraluminal Device **J** Synthetic Substitute **K** Nonautologous Tissue Substitute	**Z** No Qualifier

0 Medical and Surgical
F Hepatobiliary System and Pancreas
Y Transplantation: Putting in or on all or a portion of a living body part taken from another individual or animal to physically take the place and/or function of all or a portion of a similar body part

Body Part Character 4	Approach Character 5	Device Character 6	Qualifier Character 7
0 Liver LC **G** Pancreas LC NC CC	**0** Open	**Z** No Device	**0** Allogeneic **1** Syngeneic **2** Zooplastic

LC 0FY00Z0 0FY00Z1 0FY00Z2 0FYG0Z0 0FYG0Z1
NC 0FYG0Z2
NC 0FYG0Z0 0FYG0Z1
Codes in this list are identified as noncovered procedures except when combined with procedure codes 0TY00Z0, 0TY00Z1, 0TY00Z2, 0TY10Z0, 0TY10Z1, 0TY10Z2 and with diagnosis codes. E10.10, E10.11, E10.21, E10.22, E10.29, E10.311, E10.319, E10.3211, E10.3212, E10.3213, E10.3219, E10.3291, E10.3292, E10.3293, E10.3299, E10.3311, E10.3312, E10.3313, E10.3319, E10.3391, E10.3392, E10.3393, E10.3399, E10.3411, E10.3412, E10.3413, E10.3419, E10.3491, E10.3492, E10.3493, E10.3499, E10.3511, E10.3512, E10.3513, E10.3519, E10.3521, E10.3522, E10.3523, E10.3529, E10.3531, E10.3532, E10.3533, E10.3539, E10.3541, E10.3542, E10.3543, E10.3549, E10.3551, E10.3552, E10.3553, E10.3559, E10.3591, E10.3592, E10.3593, E10.3599, E10.36, E10.37X1, E10.37X2, E10.37X3, E10.37X9, E10.39, E10.40, E10.41, E10.42, E10.43, E10.44, E10.49, E10.51, E10.52, E10.59, E10.610, E10.618, E10.620, E10.621, E10.622, E10.628, E10.630, E10.638, E10.641, E10.649, E10.65, E10.69, E10.8, E10.9, E89.1.
CC 0FYG0Z0 0FYG0Z1 0FYG0Z2

NOTES

Types of thyroidectomy:

- Hemithyroidectomy - remove 1 lobe of thyroid + entire isthmus
- Partial ~~thyroidectomy - remove 1 lobe of thyroid~~ - remove gland in front of trachea
- Isthmectomy - removal of band of tissue (isthmus) connecting 2 lobes
- near total thyroidectomy - both lobes except the lower pole, which is very close to recurrent laryngeal nerve & parathyroid is removed
- Total thyroidectomy - entire gland is removed
- ~~Hartley Dunhill Operation~~ - remove 1 entire lateral lobe w/isthmus + partial/subtotal removal of opposite

Endocrine System 0G2-0GW

0 Medical and Surgical
G Endocrine System
2 Change: Taking out or off a device from a body part and putting back an identical or similar device in or on the same body part without cutting or puncturing the skin or a mucous membrane

Body Part	Approach	Device	Qualifier
Character 4	**Character 5**	**Character 6**	**Character 7**
0 Pituitary Gland **1** Pineal Body **5** Adrenal Gland **K** Thyroid Gland **R** Parathyroid Gland **S** Endocrine Gland	**X** External	**0** Drainage Device **Y** Other Device	**Z** No Qualifier

0 Medical and Surgical
G Endocrine System
5 Destruction: Physical eradication of all or a portion of a body part by the direct use of energy, force, or a destructive agent

Body Part	Approach	Device	Qualifier
Character 4	**Character 5**	**Character 6**	**Character 7**
0 Pituitary Gland **1** Pineal Body **2** Adrenal Gland, Left **3** Adrenal Gland, Right **4** Adrenal Glands, Bilateral **6** Carotid Body, Left **7** Carotid Body, Right **8** Carotid Bodies, Bilateral **9** Para-aortic Body **B** Coccygeal Glomus **C** Glomus Jugulare **D** Aortic Body **F** Paraganglion Extremity **G** Thyroid Gland Lobe, Left **H** Thyroid Gland Lobe, Right **K** Thyroid Gland **L** Superior Parathyroid Gland, Right **M** Superior Parathyroid Gland, Left **N** Inferior Parathyroid Gland, Right **P** Inferior Parathyroid Gland, Left **Q** Parathyroid Glands, Multiple **R** Parathyroid Gland	**0** Open **3** Percutaneous **4** Percutaneous Endoscopic	**Z** No Device	**Z** No Qualifier

0 Medical and Surgical
G Endocrine System
8 Division: Cutting into a body part, without draining fluids and/or gases from the body part, in order to separate or transect a body part

Body Part	Approach	Device	Qualifier
Character 4	**Character 5**	**Character 6**	**Character 7**
0 Pituitary Gland **J** Thyroid Gland Isthmus	**0** Open **3** Percutaneous **4** Percutaneous Endoscopic	**Z** No Device	**Z** No Qualifier

0 Medical and Surgical
G Endocrine System
9 Drainage: Taking or letting out fluids and/or gases from a body part

Body Part Character 4	Approach Character 5	Device Character 6	Qualifier Character 7
0 Pituitary Gland **1** Pineal Body **2** Adrenal Gland, Left **3** Adrenal Gland, Right **4** Adrenal Glands, Bilateral **6** Carotid Body, Left **7** Carotid Body, Right **8** Carotid Bodies, Bilateral **9** Para-aortic Body **B** Coccygeal Glomus **C** Glomus Jugulare **D** Aortic Body **F** Paraganglion Extremity **G** Thyroid Gland Lobe, Left **H** Thyroid Gland Lobe, Right **K** Thyroid Gland **L** Superior Parathyroid Gland, Right **M** Superior Parathyroid Gland, Left **N** Inferior Parathyroid Gland, Right **P** Inferior Parathyroid Gland, Left **Q** Parathyroid Glands, Multiple **R** Parathyroid Gland	**0** Open **3** Percutaneous **4** Percutaneous Endoscopic	**0** Drainage Device	**Z** No Qualifier
0 Pituitary Gland **1** Pineal Body **2** Adrenal Gland, Left **3** Adrenal Gland, Right **4** Adrenal Glands, Bilateral **6** Carotid Body, Left **7** Carotid Body, Right **8** Carotid Bodies, Bilateral **9** Para-aortic Body **B** Coccygeal Glomus **C** Glomus Jugulare **D** Aortic Body **F** Paraganglion Extremity **G** Thyroid Gland Lobe, Left **H** Thyroid Gland Lobe, Right **K** Thyroid Gland **L** Superior Parathyroid Gland, Right **M** Superior Parathyroid Gland, Left **N** Inferior Parathyroid Gland, Right **P** Inferior Parathyroid Gland, Left **Q** Parathyroid Glands, Multiple **R** Parathyroid Gland	**0** Open **3** Percutaneous **4** Percutaneous Endoscopic	**Z** No Device	**X** Diagnostic **Z** No Qualifier

near total thyroidectomy - remove both lobes, except small quantity of thyroid tissue & parathyroid

0 Medical and Surgical
G Endocrine System
B Excision: Cutting out or off, without replacement, a portion of a body part

If fluid-filled cyst- use drainage for biopsy

Body Part	Approach	Device	Qualifier
Character 4	**Character 5**	**Character 6**	**Character 7**
0 Pituitary Gland	**0** Open	**Z** No Device	**X** Diagnostic
1 Pineal Body	**3** Percutaneous — FNA		**Z** No Qualifier
2 Adrenal Gland, Left	**4** Percutaneous Endoscopic		
3 Adrenal Gland, Right			
4 Adrenal Glands, Bilateral	FNA- Fine Needle Aspiration		
6 Carotid Body, Left			
7 Carotid Body, Right			
8 Carotid Bodies, Bilateral			
9 Para-aortic Body			
B Coccygeal Glomus			
C Glomus Jugulare			
D Aortic Body			
F Paraganglion Extremity			
G Thyroid Gland Lobe, Left			
H Thyroid Gland Lobe, Right → Biopsy			
J Thyroid Gland Isthmus			
L Superior Parathyroid Gland, Right			
M Superior Parathyroid Gland, Left			
N Inferior Parathyroid Gland, Right			
P Inferior Parathyroid Gland, Left			
Q Parathyroid Glands, Multiple			
R Parathyroid Gland			

Ultrasound guidance thyroid biopsy BG44ZZZ

0 Medical and Surgical
G Endocrine System
C Extirpation: Taking or cutting out solid matter from a body part

Body Part	Approach	Device	Qualifier
Character 4	**Character 5**	**Character 6**	**Character 7**
0 Pituitary Gland	**0** Open	**Z** No Device	**Z** No Qualifier
1 Pineal Body	**3** Percutaneous		
2 Adrenal Gland, Left	**4** Percutaneous Endoscopic		
3 Adrenal Gland, Right			
4 Adrenal Glands, Bilateral			
6 Carotid Body, Left			
7 Carotid Body, Right			
8 Carotid Bodies, Bilateral			
9 Para-aortic Body			
B Coccygeal Glomus			
C Glomus Jugulare			
D Aortic Body			
F Paraganglion Extremity			
G Thyroid Gland Lobe, Left			
H Thyroid Gland Lobe, Right			
K Thyroid Gland			
L Superior Parathyroid Gland, Right			
M Superior Parathyroid Gland, Left			
N Inferior Parathyroid Gland, Right			
P Inferior Parathyroid Gland, Left			
Q Parathyroid Glands, Multiple			
R Parathyroid Gland			

0 Medical and Surgical
G Endocrine System
H Insertion: Putting in a nonbiological appliance that monitors, assists, performs, or prevents a physiological function but does not physically take the place of a body part

Body Part	Approach	Device	Qualifier
Character 4	Character 5	Character 6	Character 7
S Endocrine Gland	0 Open 3 Percutaneous 4 Percutaneous Endoscopic	2 Monitoring Device 3 Infusion Device Y Other Device	Z No Qualifier

0 Medical and Surgical
G Endocrine System
J Inspection: Visually and/or manually exploring a body part

Body Part	Approach	Device	Qualifier
Character 4	Character 5	Character 6	Character 7
0 Pituitary Gland 1 Pineal Body 5 Adrenal Gland K Thyroid Gland R Parathyroid Gland S Endocrine Gland	0 Open 3 Percutaneous 4 Percutaneous Endoscopic	Z No Device	Z No Qualifier

0 Medical and Surgical
G Endocrine System
M Reattachment: Putting back in or on all or a portion of a separated body part to its normal location or other suitable location

Body Part	Approach	Device	Qualifier
Character 4	Character 5	Character 6	Character 7
2 Adrenal Gland, Left 3 Adrenal Gland, Right G Thyroid Gland Lobe, Left H Thyroid Gland Lobe, Right L Superior Parathyroid Gland, Right M Superior Parathyroid Gland, Left N Inferior Parathyroid Gland, Right P Inferior Parathyroid Gland, Left Q Parathyroid Glands, Multiple R Parathyroid Gland	0 Open 4 Percutaneous Endoscopic	Z No Device	Z No Qualifier

0 Medical and Surgical
G Endocrine System
N Release: Freeing a body part from an abnormal physical constraint by cutting or by the use of force

Body Part Character 4	Approach Character 5	Device Character 6	Qualifier Character 7
0 Pituitary Gland **1** Pineal Body **2** Adrenal Gland, Left **3** Adrenal Gland, Right **4** Adrenal Glands, Bilateral **6** Carotid Body, Left **7** Carotid Body, Right **8** Carotid Bodies, Bilateral **9** Para-aortic Body **B** Coccygeal Glomus **C** Glomus Jugulare **D** Aortic Body **F** Paraganglion Extremity **G** Thyroid Gland Lobe, Left **H** Thyroid Gland Lobe, Right **K** Thyroid Gland **L** Superior Parathyroid Gland, Right **M** Superior Parathyroid Gland, Left **N** Inferior Parathyroid Gland, Right **P** Inferior Parathyroid Gland, Left **Q** Parathyroid Glands, Multiple **R** Parathyroid Gland	**0** Open **3** Percutaneous **4** Percutaneous Endoscopic	**Z** No Device	**Z** No Qualifier

0 Medical and Surgical
G Endocrine System
P Removal: Taking out or off a device from a body part

Body Part Character 4	Approach Character 5	Device Character 6	Qualifier Character 7
0 Pituitary Gland **1** Pineal Body **5** Adrenal Gland **K** Thyroid Gland **R** Parathyroid Gland	**0** Open **3** Percutaneous **4** Percutaneous Endoscopic **X** External	**0** Drainage Device	**Z** No Qualifier
S Endocrine Gland	**0** Open **3** Percutaneous **4** Percutaneous Endoscopic	**0** Drainage Device **2** Monitoring Device **3** Infusion Device **Y** Other Device	**Z** No Qualifier
S Endocrine Gland	**X** External	**0** Drainage Device **2** Monitoring Device **3** Infusion Device	**Z** No Qualifier

0 **Medical and Surgical**
G **Endocrine System**
Q **Repair:** Restoring, to the extent possible, a body part to its normal anatomic structure and function

Body Part	Approach	Device	Qualifier
Character 4	**Character 5**	**Character 6**	**Character 7**
0 Pituitary Gland **1** Pineal Body **2** Adrenal Gland, Left **3** Adrenal Gland, Right **4** Adrenal Glands, Bilateral **6** Carotid Body, Left **7** Carotid Body, Right **8** Carotid Bodies, Bilateral **9** Para-aortic Body **B** Coccygeal Glomus **C** Glomus Jugulare **D** Aortic Body **F** Paraganglion Extremity **G** Thyroid Gland Lobe, Left **H** Thyroid Gland Lobe, Right **J** Thyroid Gland Isthmus **K** Thyroid Gland **L** Superior Parathyroid Gland, Right **M** Superior Parathyroid Gland, Left **N** Inferior Parathyroid Gland, Right **P** Inferior Parathyroid Gland, Left **Q** Parathyroid Glands, Multiple **R** Parathyroid Gland	**0** Open **3** Percutaneous **4** Percutaneous Endoscopic	**Z** No Device	**Z** No Qualifier

0 **Medical and Surgical**
G **Endocrine System**
S **Reposition:** Moving to its normal location, or other suitable location, all or a portion of a body part

Body Part	Approach	Device	Qualifier
Character 4	**Character 5**	**Character 6**	**Character 7**
2 Adrenal Gland, Left **3** Adrenal Gland, Right **G** Thyroid Gland Lobe, Left **H** Thyroid Gland Lobe, Right **L** Superior Parathyroid Gland, Right **M** Superior Parathyroid Gland, Left **N** Inferior Parathyroid Gland, Right **P** Inferior Parathyroid Gland, Left **Q** Parathyroid Glands, Multiple **R** Parathyroid Gland	**0** Open **4** Percutaneous Endoscopic	**Z** No Device	**Z** No Qualifier

0 **Medical and Surgical** - Section
G **Endocrine System** · body system
T **Resection:** Cutting out or off, without replacement, all of a body part

Body Part	Approach	Device	Qualifier
Character 4	Character 5	Character 6	Character 7
0 Pituitary Gland	0 Open	Z No Device	Z No Qualifier
1 Pineal Body	4 Percutaneous Endoscopic *laproscopic*		
2 Adrenal Gland, Left			
3 Adrenal Gland, Right			
4 Adrenal Glands, Bilateral			
6 Carotid Body, Left			
7 Carotid Body, Right			
8 Carotid Bodies, Bilateral			
9 Para-aortic Body			
B Coccygeal Glomus			
C Glomus Jugulare			
D Aortic Body			
F Paraganglion Extremity	*thyroid-ectomy*		
G Thyroid Gland Lobe, Left	*> hemithyroidectomy*		
H Thyroid Gland Lobe, Right			
J Thyroid Gland Isthmus			
K Thyroid Gland *entire*			
L Superior Parathyroid Gland, Right			
M Superior Parathyroid Gland, Left			
N Inferior Parathyroid Gland, Right			
P Inferior Parathyroid Gland, Left			
Q Parathyroid Glands, Multiple			
R Parathyroid Gland			

0 **Medical and Surgical**
G **Endocrine System**
W **Revision:** Correcting, to the extent possible, a portion of a malfunctioning device or the position of a displaced device

Body Part	Approach	Device	Qualifier
Character 4	Character 5	Character 6	Character 7
0 Pituitary Gland	0 Open	0 Drainage Device	Z No Qualifier
1 Pineal Body	3 Percutaneous		
5 Adrenal Gland	4 Percutaneous Endoscopic		
K Thyroid Gland	X External		
R Parathyroid Gland			
S Endocrine Gland	0 Open	0 Drainage Device	Z No Qualifier
	3 Percutaneous	2 Monitoring Device	
	4 Percutaneous Endoscopic	3 Infusion Device	
		Y Other Device	
S Endocrine Gland	X External	0 Drainage Device	Z No Qualifier
		2 Monitoring Device	
		3 Infusion Device	

There is no Resection For skin

NOTES

Skin lesion removal = excision (B)

skin Flap = transfer

Skin substitutes = replacement

Skin and Breast 0H0-0HX

0 Medical and Surgical reconstruction of breast is considered cosmetic
H Skin and Breast
0 Alteration: Modifying the anatomic structure of a body part without affecting the function of the body part

Body Part Character 4	Approach Character 5	Device Character 6	Qualifier Character 7
T Breast, Right U Breast, Left V Breast, Bilateral	0 Open incision for implant 3 Percutaneous	7 Autologous Tissue Substitute J Synthetic Substitute silicone K Nonautologous Tissue Substitute Z No Device	Z No Qualifier

0 Medical and Surgical
H Skin and Breast
2 Change: Taking out or off a device from a body part and putting back an identical or similar device in or on the same body part without cutting or puncturing the skin or a mucous membrane

Body Part Character 4	Approach Character 5	Device Character 6	Qualifier Character 7
P Skin T Breast, Right U Breast, Left	X External	0 Drainage Device Y Other Device	Z No Qualifier

0 Medical and Surgical
H Skin and Breast
5 Destruction: Physical eradication of all or a portion of a body part by the direct use of energy, force, or a destructive agent

Body Part Character 4	Approach Character 5	Device Character 6	Qualifier Character 7
0 Skin, Scalp DRG 1 Skin, Face DRG 2 Skin, Right Ear 3 Skin, Left Ear 4 Skin, Neck DRG 5 Skin, Chest DRG 6 Skin, Back DRG 7 Skin, Abdomen DRG 8 Skin, Buttock DRG 9 Skin, Perineum DRG A Skin, Inguinal DRG B Skin, Right Upper Arm DRG C Skin, Left Upper Arm DRG D Skin, Right Lower Arm DRG E Skin, Left Lower Arm DRG F Skin, Right Hand DRG G Skin, Left Hand DRG H Skin, Right Upper Leg DRG J Skin, Left Upper Leg DRG K Skin, Right Lower Leg DRG L Skin, Left Lower Leg DRG M Skin, Right Foot DRG N Skin, Left Foot DRG	X External	Z No Device	D Multiple Z No Qualifier
Q Finger Nail DRG R Toe Nail DRG	X External	Z No Device	Z No Qualifier
T Breast, Right U Breast, Left V Breast, Bilateral	0 Open 3 Percutaneous 7 Via Natural or Artificial Opening 8 Via Natural or Artificial Opening Endoscopic	Z No Device	Z No Qualifier

0H5 continued on next page

LC Limited Coverage NC Noncovered HAC HAC-associated Procedure CC Combination Cluster - See Appendix G for code lists
DRG Non-OR-Affecting MS-DRG Assignment New/Revised Text in **Orange** ♂ Male ♀ Female

0 Medical and Surgical
H Skin and Breast
5 Destruction: Physical eradication of all or a portion of a body part by the direct use of energy, force, or a destructive agent

0H5 continued from previous page

Body Part Character 4	Approach Character 5	Device Character 6	Qualifier Character 7
W Nipple, Right X Nipple, Left	0 Open 3 Percutaneous 7 Via Natural or Artificial Opening 8 Via Natural or Artificial Opening Endoscopic X External	Z No Device	Z No Qualifier

DRG 0H50XZD 0H50XZZ 0H51XZD 0H51XZZ 0H54XZD 0H54XZZ 0H55XZD 0H55XZZ 0H56XZD 0H56XZZ 0H57XZD 0H57XZZ 0H58XZD 0H58XZZ 0H59XZD 0H59XZZ 0H5AXZD 0H5AXZZ 0H5BXZD 0H5BXZZ 0H5CXZD 0H5CXZZ 0H5DXZD 0H5DXZZ 0H5EXZD 0H5EXZZ 0H5FXZD 0H5FXZZ 0H5GXZD 0H5GXZZ 0H5HXZD 0H5HXZZ 0H5JXZD 0H5JXZZ 0H5KXZD 0H5KXZZ 0H5LXZD 0H5LXZZ 0H5MXZD 0H5MXZZ 0H5NXZD 0H5NXZZ 0H5QXZZ 0H5RXZZ

0 Medical and Surgical
H Skin and Breast
8 Division: Cutting into a body part, without draining fluids and/or gases from the body part, in order to separate or transect a body part

Body Part Character 4	Approach Character 5	Device Character 6	Qualifier Character 7
0 Skin, Scalp 1 Skin, Face 2 Skin, Right Ear 3 Skin, Left Ear 4 Skin, Neck 5 Skin, Chest 6 Skin, Back 7 Skin, Abdomen 8 Skin, Buttock 9 Skin, Perineum A Skin, Inguinal B Skin, Right Upper Arm C Skin, Left Upper Arm D Skin, Right Lower Arm E Skin, Left Lower Arm F Skin, Right Hand G Skin, Left Hand H Skin, Right Upper Leg J Skin, Left Upper Leg K Skin, Right Lower Leg L Skin, Left Lower Leg M Skin, Right Foot N Skin, Left Foot	X External	Z No Device	Z No Qualifier

0 Medical and Surgical
H Skin and Breast
9 Drainage: Taking or letting out fluids and/or gases from a body part

Body Part Character 4	Approach Character 5	Device Character 6	Qualifier Character 7
0 Skin, Scalp **1** Skin, Face **2** Skin, Right Ear **3** Skin, Left Ear **4** Skin, Neck **5** Skin, Chest **6** Skin, Back **7** Skin, Abdomen **8** Skin, Buttock **9** Skin, Perineum **A** Skin, Inguinal **B** Skin, Right Upper Arm **C** Skin, Left Upper Arm **D** Skin, Right Lower Arm **E** Skin, Left Lower Arm **F** Skin, Right Hand **G** Skin, Left Hand **H** Skin, Right Upper Leg **J** Skin, Left Upper Leg **K** Skin, Right Lower Leg **L** Skin, Left Lower Leg **M** Skin, Right Foot **N** Skin, Left Foot **Q** Finger Nail **R** Toe Nail	**X** External	**0** Drainage Device	**Z** No Qualifier
0 Skin, Scalp **1** Skin, Face **2** Skin, Right Ear **3** Skin, Left Ear **4** Skin, Neck **5** Skin, Chest **6** Skin, Back **7** Skin, Abdomen **8** Skin, Buttock **9** Skin, Perineum **A** Skin, Inguinal **B** Skin, Right Upper Arm **C** Skin, Left Upper Arm **D** Skin, Right Lower Arm **E** Skin, Left Lower Arm **F** Skin, Right Hand **G** Skin, Left Hand **H** Skin, Right Upper Leg **J** Skin, Left Upper Leg **K** Skin, Right Lower Leg **L** Skin, Left Lower Leg **M** Skin, Right Foot **N** Skin, Left Foot **Q** Finger Nail **R** Toe Nail	**X** External	**Z** No Device	**X** Diagnostic **Z** No Qualifier
T Breast, Right **U** Breast, Left **V** Breast, Bilateral	**0** Open **3** Percutaneous **7** Via Natural or Artificial Opening **8** Via Natural or Artificial Opening Endoscopic	**0** Drainage Device	**Z** No Qualifier

0H9 continued on next page

0 Medical and Surgical
H Skin and Breast
9 Drainage: Taking or letting out fluids and/or gases from a body part

0H9 continued from previous page

Body Part Character 4	Approach Character 5	Device Character 6	Qualifier Character 7
T Breast, Right **U** Breast, Left **V** Breast, Bilateral	**0** Open **3** Percutaneous **7** Via Natural or Artificial Opening **8** Via Natural or Artificial Opening Endoscopic	**Z** No Device	**X** Diagnostic **Z** No Qualifier
W Nipple, Right **X** Nipple, Left	**0** Open **3** Percutaneous **7** Via Natural or Artificial Opening **8** Via Natural or Artificial Opening Endoscopic **X** External	**0** Drainage Device	**Z** No Qualifier
W Nipple, Right **X** Nipple, Left	**0** Open **3** Percutaneous **7** Via Natural or Artificial Opening **8** Via Natural or Artificial Opening Endoscopic **X** External	**Z** No Device	**X** Diagnostic **Z** No Qualifier

0 Medical and Surgical
H Skin and Breast
B Excision: Cutting out or off, without replacement, a portion of a body part biopsy

Body Part Character 4	Approach Character 5	Device Character 6	Qualifier Character 7
0 Skin, Scalp **1** Skin, Face **2** Skin, Right Ear **3** Skin, Left Ear **4** Skin, Neck **5** Skin, Chest **6** Skin, Back **7** Skin, Abdomen **8** Skin, Buttock **9** Skin, Perineum DRG **A** Skin, Inguinal **B** Skin, Right Upper Arm **C** Skin, Left Upper Arm **D** Skin, Right Lower Arm **E** Skin, Left Lower Arm **F** Skin, Right Hand **G** Skin, Left Hand **H** Skin, Right Upper Leg **J** Skin, Left Upper Leg **K** Skin, Right Lower Leg **L** Skin, Left Lower Leg **M** Skin, Right Foot **N** Skin, Left Foot **Q** Finger Nail **R** Toe Nail	**X** External	**Z** No Device	**X** Diagnostic **Z** No Qualifier
T Breast, Right may be **U** Breast, Left needle biopsy **V** Breast, Bilateral **Y** Supernumerary Breast	**0** Open **3** Percutaneous 1/4" incision core **7** Via Natural or Artificial Opening **8** Via Natural or Artificial Opening Endoscopic	**Z** No Device	**X** Diagnostic **Z** No Qualifier
W Nipple, Right **X** Nipple, Left	**0** Open **3** Percutaneous **7** Via Natural or Artificial Opening **8** Via Natural or Artificial Opening Endoscopic **X** External	**Z** No Device	**X** Diagnostic **Z** No Qualifier

DRG 0HB9XZZ

If more than one biopsy done in same area - only code 1 time
ex: 2 biopsies of right breast = ØHBT3ZX

0 Medical and Surgical
H Skin and Breast
C Extirpation: Taking or cutting out solid matter from a body part

Body Part Character 4	Approach Character 5	Device Character 6	Qualifier Character 7
0 Skin, Scalp **1** Skin, Face **2** Skin, Right Ear **3** Skin, Left Ear **4** Skin, Neck **5** Skin, Chest **6** Skin, Back **7** Skin, Abdomen **8** Skin, Buttock **9** Skin, Perineum **A** Skin, Inguinal **B** Skin, Right Upper Arm **C** Skin, Left Upper Arm **D** Skin, Right Lower Arm **E** Skin, Left Lower Arm **F** Skin, Right Hand **G** Skin, Left Hand **H** Skin, Right Upper Leg **J** Skin, Left Upper Leg **K** Skin, Right Lower Leg **L** Skin, Left Lower Leg **M** Skin, Right Foot **N** Skin, Left Foot **Q** Finger Nail **R** Toe Nail	**X** External	**Z** No Device	**Z** No Qualifier
T Breast, Right **U** Breast, Left **V** Breast, Bilateral	**0** Open **3** Percutaneous **7** Via Natural or Artificial Opening **8** Via Natural or Artificial Opening Endoscopic	**Z** No Device	**Z** No Qualifier
W Nipple, Right **X** Nipple, Left	**0** Open **3** Percutaneous **7** Via Natural or Artificial Opening **8** Via Natural or Artificial Opening Endoscopic **X** External	**Z** No Device	**Z** No Qualifier

0HD6ZZ = L85.1

0 Medical and Surgical
H Skin and Breast
D Extraction: Pulling or stripping out or off all or a portion of a body part by the use of force

Body Part	Approach	Device	Qualifier
Character 4	Character 5	Character 6	Character 7
0 Skin, Scalp 1 Skin, Face 2 Skin, Right Ear 3 Skin, Left Ear 4 Skin, Neck 5 Skin, Chest 6 Skin, Back 7 Skin, Abdomen 8 Skin, Buttock 9 Skin, Perineum A Skin, Inguinal B Skin, Right Upper Arm C Skin, Left Upper Arm D Skin, Right Lower Arm E Skin, Left Lower Arm F Skin, Right Hand G Skin, Left Hand H Skin, Right Upper Leg J Skin, Left Upper Leg K Skin, Right Lower Leg L Skin, Left Lower Leg M Skin, Right Foot N Skin, Left Foot Q Finger Nail R Toe Nail S Hair	X External	Z No Device	Z No Qualifier
T Breast, Right U Breast, Left V Breast, Bilateral Y Supernumerary Breast	0 Open	Z No Device	Z No Qualifier

0 Medical and Surgical
H Skin and Breast
H Insertion: Putting in a nonbiological appliance that monitors, assists, performs, or prevents a physiological function but does not physically take the place of a body part

Body Part	Approach	Device	Qualifier
Character 4	Character 5	Character 6	Character 7
P Skin	X External	Y Other Device	Z No Qualifier
T Breast, Right U Breast, Left	0 Open 3 Percutaneous 7 Via Natural or Artificial Opening 8 Via Natural or Artificial Opening Endoscopic	1 Radioactive Element N Tissue Expander Y Other Device	Z No Qualifier
V Breast, Bilateral	0 Open 3 Percutaneous 7 Via Natural or Artificial Opening 8 Via Natural or Artificial Opening Endoscopic	1 Radioactive Element N Tissue	Z No Qualifier
W Nipple, Right X Nipple, Left	0 Open 3 Percutaneous 7 Via Natural or Artificial Opening 8 Via Natural or Artificial Opening Endoscopic	1 Radioactive Element N Tissue Expander	Z No Qualifier
W Nipple, Right X Nipple, Left	X External	1 Radioactive Element	Z No Qualifier

0 Medical and Surgical
H Skin and Breast
J Inspection: Visually and/or manually exploring a body part

Body Part Character 4	Approach Character 5	Device Character 6	Qualifier Character 7
P Skin **Q** Finger Nail **R** Toe Nail	**X** External	**Z** No Device	**Z** No Qualifier
T Breast, Right **U** Breast, Left	**0** Open **3** Percutaneous **7** Via Natural or Artificial Opening **8** Via Natural or Artificial Opening Endoscopic	**Z** No Device	**Z** No Qualifier

0 Medical and Surgical
H Skin and Breast
M Reattachment: Putting back in or on all or a portion of a separated body part to its normal location or other suitable location

Body Part Character 4	Approach Character 5	Device Character 6	Qualifier Character 7
0 Skin, Scalp **1** Skin, Face **2** Skin, Right Ear **3** Skin, Left Ear **4** Skin, Neck **5** Skin, Chest **6** Skin, Back **7** Skin, Abdomen **8** Skin, Buttock **9** Skin, Perineum **A** Skin, Inguinal **B** Skin, Right Upper Arm **C** Skin, Left Upper Arm **D** Skin, Right Lower Arm **E** Skin, Left Lower Arm **F** Skin, Right Hand **G** Skin, Left Hand **H** Skin, Right Upper Leg **J** Skin, Left Upper Leg **K** Skin, Right Lower Leg **L** Skin, Left Lower Leg **M** Skin, Right Foot **N** Skin, Left Foot **T** Breast, Right **U** Breast, Left **V** Breast, Bilateral **W** Nipple, Right **X** Nipple, Left	**X** External	**Z** No Device	**Z** No Qualifier

0 Medical and Surgical
H Skin and Breast
N Release: Freeing a body part from an abnormal physical constraint by cutting or by the use of force

Body Part Character 4	Approach Character 5	Device Character 6	Qualifier Character 7
0 Skin, Scalp **1** Skin, Face **2** Skin, Right Ear **3** Skin, Left Ear **4** Skin, Neck **5** Skin, Chest **6** Skin, Back **7** Skin, Abdomen **8** Skin, Buttock **9** Skin, Perineum **A** Skin, Inguinal **B** Skin, Right Upper Arm **C** Skin, Left Upper Arm **D** Skin, Right Lower Arm **E** Skin, Left Lower Arm **F** Skin, Right Hand **G** Skin, Left Hand **H** Skin, Right Upper Leg **J** Skin, Left Upper Leg **K** Skin, Right Lower Leg **L** Skin, Left Lower Leg **M** Skin, Right Foot **N** Skin, Left Foot **Q** Finger Nail **R** Toe Nail	**X** External	**Z** No Device	**Z** No Qualifier
T Breast, Right **U** Breast, Left **V** Breast, Bilateral	**0** Open **3** Percutaneous **7** Via Natural or Artificial Opening **8** Via Natural or Artificial Opening Endoscopic	**Z** No Device	**Z** No Qualifier
W Nipple, Right **X** Nipple, Left	**0** Open **3** Percutaneous **7** Via Natural or Artificial Opening **8** Via Natural or Artificial Opening Endoscopic **X** External	**Z** No Device	**Z** No Qualifier

0 Medical and Surgical
H Skin and Breast
P Removal: Taking out or off a device from a body part

Body Part Character 4	Approach Character 5	Device Character 6	Qualifier Character 7
P Skin	**X** External	**0** Drainage Device **7** Autologous Tissue Substitute **J** Synthetic Substitute **K** Nonautologous Tissue Substitute **Y** Other Device	**Z** No Qualifier
Q Finger Nail **R** Toe Nail	**X** External	**0** Drainage Device **7** Autologous Tissue Substitute **J** Synthetic Substitute **K** Nonautologous Tissue Substitute	**Z** No Qualifier
S Hair	**X** External	**7** Autologous Tissue Substitute **J** Synthetic Substitute **K** Nonautologous Tissue Substitute	**Z** No Qualifier

0HP continued on next page

0HP continued from previous page

0 Medical and Surgical
H Skin and Breast
P Removal: Taking out or off a device from a body part

Body Part Character 4	Approach Character 5	Device Character 6	Qualifier Character 7
T Breast, Right **U** Breast, Left	**0** Open **3** Percutaneous **7** Via Natural or Artificial Opening **8** Via Natural or Artificial Opening Endoscopic	**0** Drainage Device **1** Radioactive Element **7** Autologous Tissue Substitute **J** Synthetic Substitute **K** Nonautologous Tissue Substitute **N** Tissue Expander **Y** Other Device	**Z** No Qualifier

0 Medical and Surgical
H Skin and Breast
Q Repair: Restoring, to the extent possible, a body part to its normal anatomic structure and function

Body Part Character 4	Approach Character 5	Device Character 6	Qualifier Character 7
0 Skin, Scalp **1** Skin, Face **2** Skin, Right Ear **3** Skin, Left Ear **4** Skin, Neck **5** Skin, Chest **6** Skin, Back **7** Skin, Abdomen **8** Skin, Buttock **9** Skin, Perineum DRG delivery tear **A** Skin, Inguinal **B** Skin, Right Upper Arm **C** Skin, Left Upper Arm **D** Skin, Right Lower Arm **E** Skin, Left Lower Arm **F** Skin, Right Hand **G** Skin, Left Hand **H** Skin, Right Upper Leg **J** Skin, Left Upper Leg **K** Skin, Right Lower Leg **L** Skin, Left Lower Leg **M** Skin, Right Foot **N** Skin, Left Foot **Q** Finger Nail **R** Toe Nail	**X** External	**Z** No Device	**Z** No Qualifier
T Breast, Right **U** Breast, Left **V** Breast, Bilateral **Y** Supernumerary Breast	**0** Open **3** Percutaneous **7** Via Natural or Artificial Opening **8** Via Natural or Artificial Opening Endoscopic	**Z** No Device	**Z** No Qualifier
W Nipple, Right **X** Nipple, Left	**0** Open **3** Percutaneous **7** Via Natural or Artificial Opening **8** Via Natural or Artificial Opening Endoscopic **X** External	**Z** No Device	**Z** No Qualifier

DRG 0HQ9XZZ

LC Limited Coverage NC Noncovered HAC HAC-associated Procedure CC Combination Cluster - See Appendix G for code lists
DRG Non-OR-Affecting MS-DRG Assignment New/Revised Text in Orange ♂ Male ♀ Female
382 2020 ICD-10-PCS

0 Medical and Surgical
H Skin and Breast
R Replacement: Putting in or on biological or synthetic material that physically takes the place and/or function of all or a portion of a body part

Body Part	Approach	Device	Qualifier
Character 4	Character 5	Character 6	Character 7
0 Skin, Scalp **1** Skin, Face **2** Skin, Right Ear **3** Skin, Left Ear **4** Skin, Neck **5** Skin, Chest **6** Skin, Back **7** Skin, Abdomen **8** Skin, Buttock **9** Skin, Perineum **A** Skin, Inguinal **B** Skin, Right Upper Arm **C** Skin, Left Upper Arm **D** Skin, Right Lower Arm **E** Skin, Left Lower Arm **F** Skin, Right Hand **G** Skin, Left Hand **H** Skin, Right Upper Leg **J** Skin, Left Upper Leg **K** Skin, Right Lower Leg **L** Skin, Left Lower Leg **M** Skin, Right Foot **N** Skin, Left Foot	**X** External	**7** Autologous Tissue Substitute	**2** Cell Suspension Technique **3** Full Thickness **4** Partial Thickness
0 Skin, Scalp **1** Skin, Face **2** Skin, Right Ear **3** Skin, Left Ear **4** Skin, Neck **5** Skin, Chest **6** Skin, Back **7** Skin, Abdomen **8** Skin, Buttock **9** Skin, Perineum **A** Skin, Inguinal **B** Skin, Right Upper Arm **C** Skin, Left Upper Arm **D** Skin, Right Lower Arm **E** Skin, Left Lower Arm **F** Skin, Right Hand **G** Skin, Left Hand **H** Skin, Right Upper Leg **J** Skin, Left Upper Leg **K** Skin, Right Lower Leg **L** Skin, Left Lower Leg **M** Skin, Right Foot **N** Skin, Left Foot	**X** External	**J** Synthetic Substitute	**3** Full Thickness **4** Partial Thickness **Z** No Qualifier

0HR continued on next page

0 Medical and Surgical
H Skin and Breast
R Replacement: Putting in or on biological or synthetic material that physically takes the place and/or function of all or a portion of a body part

0HR continued from previous page

Body Part Character 4	Approach Character 5	Device Character 6	Qualifier Character 7
0 Skin, Scalp 1 Skin, Face 2 Skin, Right Ear 3 Skin, Left Ear 4 Skin, Neck 5 Skin, Chest 6 Skin, Back 7 Skin, Abdomen 8 Skin, Buttock 9 Skin, Perineum A Skin, Inguinal B Skin, Right Upper Arm C Skin, Left Upper Arm D Skin, Right Lower Arm E Skin, Left Lower Arm F Skin, Right Hand G Skin, Left Hand H Skin, Right Upper Leg J Skin, Left Upper Leg K Skin, Right Lower Leg L Skin, Left Lower Leg M Skin, Right Foot N Skin, Left Foot	X External	K Nonautologous Tissue Substitute	3 Full Thickness 4 Partial Thickness
Q Finger Nail R Toe Nail S Hair	X External	7 Autologous Tissue Substitute J Synthetic Substitute K Nonautologous Tissue Substitute	Z No Qualifier
T Breast, Right U Breast, Left V Breast, Bilateral	0 Open	7 Autologous Tissue Substitute	5 Latissimus Dorsi Myocutaneous Flap 6 Transverse Rectus Abdominis Myocutaneous Flap 7 Deep Inferior Epigastric Artery Perforator Flap 8 Superficial Inferior Epigastric Artery Flap 9 Gluteal Artery Perforator Flap Z No Qualifier
T Breast, Right U Breast, Left V Breast, Bilateral	0 Open	J Synthetic Substitute K Nonautologous Tissue Substitute	Z No Qualifier
T Breast, Right [CC] U Breast, Left [CC] V Breast, Bilateral [CC]	3 Percutaneous	7 Autologous Tissue Substitute J Synthetic Substitute K Nonautologous Tissue Substitute	Z No Qualifier
W Nipple, Right X Nipple, Left	0 Open 3 Percutaneous X External	7 Autologous Tissue Substitute J Synthetic Substitute K Nonautologous Tissue Substitute	Z No Qualifier

[CC] 0HRT37Z 0HRU37Z 0HRV37Z

0 Medical and Surgical
H Skin and Breast
S Reposition: Moving to its normal location, or other suitable location, all or a portion of a body part

Body Part Character 4	Approach Character 5	Device Character 6	Qualifier Character 7
S Hair **W** Nipple, Right **X** Nipple, Left	**X** External	**Z** No Device	**Z** No Qualifier
T Breast, Right **U** Breast, Left **V** Breast, Bilateral	**0** Open	**Z** No Device	**Z** No Qualifier

0 Medical and Surgical
H Skin and Breast
T Resection: Cutting out or off, without replacement, all of a body part

Body Part Character 4	Approach Character 5	Device Character 6	Qualifier Character 7
Q Finger Nail **R** Toe Nail **W** Nipple, Right **X** Nipple, Left	**X** External	**Z** No Device	**Z** No Qualifier
T Breast, Right CC **U** Breast, Left CC **V** Breast, Bilateral CC **Y** Supernumerary Breast	**0** Open	**Z** No Device	**Z** No Qualifier

CC 0HTT0ZZ 0HTU0ZZ 0HTV0ZZ

0 Medical and Surgical
H Skin and Breast
U Supplement: Putting in or on biological or synthetic material that physically reinforces and/or augments the function of a portion of a body part

Body Part Character 4	Approach Character 5	Device Character 6	Qualifier Character 7
T Breast, Right **U** Breast, Left **V** Breast, Bilateral	**0** Open **3** Percutaneous **7** Via Natural or Artificial Opening **8** Via Natural or Artificial Opening Endoscopic	**7** Autologous Tissue Substitute **J** Synthetic Substitute **K** Nonautologous Tissue Substitute	**Z** No Qualifier
W Nipple, Right **X** Nipple, Left	**0** Open **3** Percutaneous **7** Via Natural or Artificial Opening **8** Via Natural or Artificial Opening Endoscopic **X** External	**7** Autologous Tissue Substitute **J** Synthetic Substitute **K** Nonautologous Tissue Substitute	**Z** No Qualifier

0 Medical and Surgical
H Skin and Breast
W Revision: Correcting, to the extent possible, a portion of a malfunctioning device or the position of a displaced device

Body Part Character 4	Approach Character 5	Device Character 6	Qualifier Character 7
P Skin	**X** External	**0** Drainage Device **7** Autologous Tissue Substitute **J** Synthetic Substitute **K** Nonautologous Tissue Substitute **Y** Other Device	**Z** No Qualifier
Q Finger Nail **R** Toe Nail	**X** External	**0** Drainage Device **7** Autologous Tissue Substitute **J** Synthetic Substitute **K** Nonautologous Tissue Substitute	**Z** No Qualifier
S Hair	**X** External	**7** Autologous Tissue Substitute **J** Synthetic Substitute **K** Nonautologous Tissue Substitute	**Z** No Qualifier
T Breast, Right **U** Breast, Left	**0** Open **3** Percutaneous **7** Via Natural or Artificial Opening **8** Via Natural or Artificial Opening Endoscopic	**0** Drainage Device **7** Autologous Tissue Substitute **J** Synthetic Substitute **K** Nonautologous Tissue Substitute **N** Tissue Expander **Y** Other Device	**Z** No Qualifier

0 Medical and Surgical
H Skin and Breast
X Transfer: Moving, without taking out, all or a portion of a body part to another location to take over the function of all or a portion of a body part

Body Part Character 4	Approach Character 5	Device Character 6	Qualifier Character 7
0 Skin, Scalp **1** Skin, Face **2** Skin, Right Ear **3** Skin, Left Ear **4** Skin, Neck **5** Skin, Chest **6** Skin, Back **7** Skin, Abdomen **8** Skin, Buttock **9** Skin, Perineum **A** Skin, Inguinal **B** Skin, Right Upper Arm **C** Skin, Left Upper Arm **D** Skin, Right Lower Arm **E** Skin, Left Lower Arm **F** Skin, Right Hand **G** Skin, Left Hand **H** Skin, Right Upper Leg **J** Skin, Left Upper Leg **K** Skin, Right Lower Leg **L** Skin, Left Lower Leg **M** Skin, Right Foot **N** Skin, Left Foot	**X** External	**Z** No Device	**Z** No Qualifier

right scalp advancement Flap to R temple 0HX0XZZ

NOTES

NOTES

Subcutaneous Tissue and Fascia 0J0-0JX

0 Medical and Surgical
J Subcutaneous Tissue and Fascia
0 Alteration: Modifying the anatomic structure of a body part without affecting the function of the body part

Body Part Character 4	Approach Character 5	Device Character 6	Qualifier Character 7
1 Subcutaneous Tissue and Fascia, Face **4** Subcutaneous Tissue and Fascia, Right Neck **5** Subcutaneous Tissue and Fascia, Left Neck **6** Subcutaneous Tissue and Fascia, Chest **7** Subcutaneous Tissue and Fascia, Back **8** Subcutaneous Tissue and Fascia, Abdomen **9** Subcutaneous Tissue and Fascia, Buttock **D** Subcutaneous Tissue and Fascia, Right Upper Arm **F** Subcutaneous Tissue and Fascia, Left Upper Arm **G** Subcutaneous Tissue and Fascia, Right Lower Arm **H** Subcutaneous Tissue and Fascia, Left Lower Arm **L** Subcutaneous Tissue and Fascia, Right Upper Leg **M** Subcutaneous Tissue and Fascia, Left Upper Leg **N** Subcutaneous Tissue and Fascia, Right Lower Leg **P** Subcutaneous Tissue and Fascia, Left Lower Leg	**0** Open **3** Percutaneous	**Z** No Device	**Z** No Qualifier

0 Medical and Surgical
J Subcutaneous Tissue and Fascia
2 Change: Taking out or off a device from a body part and putting back an identical or similar device in or on the same body part without cutting or puncturing the skin or a mucous membrane

Body Part Character 4	Approach Character 5	Device Character 6	Qualifier Character 7
S Subcutaneous Tissue and Fascia, Head and Neck **T** Subcutaneous Tissue and Fascia, Trunk **V** Subcutaneous Tissue and Fascia, Upper Extremity **W** Subcutaneous Tissue and Fascia, Lower Extremity	**X** External	**0** Drainage Device **Y** Other Device	**Z** No Qualifier

LC Limited Coverage NC Noncovered HAC HAC-associated Procedure CC Combination Cluster - See Appendix G for code lists
DRG Non-OR-Affecting MS-DRG Assignment New/Revised Text in **Orange** ♂ Male ♀ Female

0 Medical and Surgical
J Subcutaneous Tissue and Fascia
5 Destruction: Physical eradication of all or a portion of a body part by the direct use of energy, force, or a destructive agent

Body Part Character 4	Approach Character 5	Device Character 6	Qualifier Character 7
0 Subcutaneous Tissue and Fascia, Scalp DRG **1** Subcutaneous Tissue and Fascia, Face DRG **4** Subcutaneous Tissue and Fascia, Right Neck DRG **5** Subcutaneous Tissue and Fascia, Left Neck DRG **6** Subcutaneous Tissue and Fascia, Chest DRG **7** Subcutaneous Tissue and Fascia, Back DRG **8** Subcutaneous Tissue and Fascia, Abdomen DRG **9** Subcutaneous Tissue and Fascia, Buttock DRG **B** Subcutaneous Tissue and Fascia, Perineum DRG **C** Subcutaneous Tissue and Fascia, Pelvic Region DRG **D** Subcutaneous Tissue and Fascia, Right Upper Arm DRG **F** Subcutaneous Tissue and Fascia, Left Upper Arm DRG **G** Subcutaneous Tissue and Fascia, Right Lower Arm DRG **H** Subcutaneous Tissue and Fascia, Left Lower Arm DRG **J** Subcutaneous Tissue and Fascia, Right Hand DRG **K** Subcutaneous Tissue and Fascia, Left Hand DRG **L** Subcutaneous Tissue and Fascia, Right Upper Leg DRG **M** Subcutaneous Tissue and Fascia, Left Upper Leg DRG **N** Subcutaneous Tissue and Fascia, Right Lower Leg DRG **P** Subcutaneous Tissue and Fascia, Left Lower Leg DRG **Q** Subcutaneous Tissue and Fascia, Right Foot DRG **R** Subcutaneous Tissue and Fascia, Left Foot DRG	**0** Open **3** Percutaneous	**Z** No Device	**Z** No Qualifier

DRG 0J500ZZ 0J503ZZ 0J510ZZ 0J513ZZ 0J540ZZ 0J543ZZ 0J550ZZ 0J553ZZ 0J560ZZ 0J563ZZ 0J570ZZ 0J573ZZ 0J580ZZ 0J583ZZ 0J590ZZ 0J593ZZ 0J5B0ZZ 0J5B3ZZ 0J5C0ZZ 0J5C3ZZ 0J5D0ZZ 0J5D3ZZ 0J5F0ZZ 0J5F3ZZ 0J5G0ZZ 0J5G3ZZ 0J5H0ZZ 0J5H3ZZ 0J5J0ZZ 0J5J3ZZ 0J5K0ZZ 0J5K3ZZ 0J5L0ZZ 0J5L3ZZ 0J5M0ZZ 0J5M3ZZ 0J5N0ZZ 0J5N3ZZ 0J5P0ZZ 0J5P3ZZ 0J5Q0ZZ 0J5Q3ZZ 0J5R0ZZ 0J5R3ZZ

0 Medical and Surgical
J Subcutaneous Tissue and Fascia
8 Division: Cutting into a body part, without draining fluids and/or gases from the body part, in order to separate or transect a body part

Body Part Character 4	Approach Character 5	Device Character 6	Qualifier Character 7
0 Subcutaneous Tissue and Fascia, Scalp **1** Subcutaneous Tissue and Fascia, Face **4** Subcutaneous Tissue and Fascia, Right Neck **5** Subcutaneous Tissue and Fascia, Left Neck **6** Subcutaneous Tissue and Fascia, Chest **7** Subcutaneous Tissue and Fascia, Back **8** Subcutaneous Tissue and Fascia, Abdomen **9** Subcutaneous Tissue and Fascia, Buttock **B** Subcutaneous Tissue and Fascia, Perineum **C** Subcutaneous Tissue and Fascia, Pelvic Region **D** Subcutaneous Tissue and Fascia, Right Upper Arm **F** Subcutaneous Tissue and Fascia, Left Upper Arm **G** Subcutaneous Tissue and Fascia, Right Lower Arm **H** Subcutaneous Tissue and Fascia, Left Lower Arm **J** Subcutaneous Tissue and Fascia, Right Hand **K** Subcutaneous Tissue and Fascia, Left Hand **L** Subcutaneous Tissue and Fascia, Right Upper Leg **M** Subcutaneous Tissue and Fascia, Left Upper Leg **N** Subcutaneous Tissue and Fascia, Right Lower Leg **P** Subcutaneous Tissue and Fascia, Left Lower Leg **Q** Subcutaneous Tissue and Fascia, Right Foot **R** Subcutaneous Tissue and Fascia, Left Foot **S** Subcutaneous Tissue and Fascia, Head and Neck **T** Subcutaneous Tissue and Fascia, Trunk **V** Subcutaneous Tissue and Fascia, Upper Extremity **W** Subcutaneous Tissue and Fascia, Lower Extremity	**0** Open **3** Percutaneous	**Z** No Device	**Z** No Qualifier

0 Medical and Surgical
J Subcutaneous Tissue and Fascia
9 Drainage: Taking or letting out fluids and/or gases from a body part

Body Part Character 4	Approach Character 5	Device Character 6	Qualifier Character 7
0 Subcutaneous Tissue and Fascia, Scalp **1** Subcutaneous Tissue and Fascia, Face **4** Subcutaneous Tissue and Fascia, Right Neck **5** Subcutaneous Tissue and Fascia, Left Neck **6** Subcutaneous Tissue and Fascia, Chest **7** Subcutaneous Tissue and Fascia, Back **8** Subcutaneous Tissue and Fascia, Abdomen **9** Subcutaneous Tissue and Fascia, Buttock **B** Subcutaneous Tissue and Fascia, Perineum **C** Subcutaneous Tissue and Fascia, Pelvic Region **D** Subcutaneous Tissue and Fascia, Right Upper Arm **F** Subcutaneous Tissue and Fascia, Left Upper Arm **G** Subcutaneous Tissue and Fascia, Right Lower Arm **H** Subcutaneous Tissue and Fascia, Left Lower Arm **J** Subcutaneous Tissue and Fascia, Right Hand **K** Subcutaneous Tissue and Fascia, Left Hand **L** Subcutaneous Tissue and Fascia, Right Upper Leg **M** Subcutaneous Tissue and Fascia, Left Upper Leg **N** Subcutaneous Tissue and Fascia, Right Lower Leg **P** Subcutaneous Tissue and Fascia, Left Lower Leg **Q** Subcutaneous Tissue and Fascia, Right Foot **R** Subcutaneous Tissue and Fascia, Left Foot	**0** Open **3** Percutaneous	**0** Drainage Device	**Z** No Qualifier

0J9 continued on next page

0J9 continued from previous page

0 Medical and Surgical
J Subcutaneous Tissue and Fascia
9 Drainage: Taking or letting out fluids and/or gases from a body part

Body Part Character 4	Approach Character 5	Device Character 6	Qualifier Character 7
0 Subcutaneous Tissue and Fascia, Scalp **1** Subcutaneous Tissue and Fascia, Face **4** Subcutaneous Tissue and Fascia, Right Neck **5** Subcutaneous Tissue and Fascia, Left Neck **6** Subcutaneous Tissue and Fascia, Chest **7** Subcutaneous Tissue and Fascia, Back **8** Subcutaneous Tissue and Fascia, Abdomen **9** Subcutaneous Tissue and Fascia, Buttock **B** Subcutaneous Tissue and Fascia, Perineum **C** Subcutaneous Tissue and Fascia, Pelvic Region **D** Subcutaneous Tissue and Fascia, Right Upper Arm **F** Subcutaneous Tissue and Fascia, Left Upper Arm **G** Subcutaneous Tissue and Fascia, Right Lower Arm **H** Subcutaneous Tissue and Fascia, Left Lower Arm **J** Subcutaneous Tissue and Fascia, Right Hand **K** Subcutaneous Tissue and Fascia, Left Hand **L** Subcutaneous Tissue and Fascia, Right Upper Leg **M** Subcutaneous Tissue and Fascia, Left Upper Leg **N** Subcutaneous Tissue and Fascia, Right Lower Leg **P** Subcutaneous Tissue and Fascia, Left Lower Leg **Q** Subcutaneous Tissue and Fascia, Right Foot **R** Subcutaneous Tissue and Fascia, Left Foot	**0** Open **3** Percutaneous	**Z** No Device	**X** Diagnostic **Z** No Qualifier

0 Medical and Surgical
J Subcutaneous Tissue and Fascia
B Excision: Cutting out or off, without replacement, a portion of a body part

Body Part Character 4	Approach Character 5	Device Character 6	Qualifier Character 7
0 Subcutaneous Tissue and Fascia, Scalp DRG **1** Subcutaneous Tissue and Fascia, Face **4** Subcutaneous Tissue and Fascia, Right Neck DRG **5** Subcutaneous Tissue and Fascia, Left Neck DRG **6** Subcutaneous Tissue and Fascia, Chest DRG **7** Subcutaneous Tissue and Fascia, Back DRG **8** Subcutaneous Tissue and Fascia, Abdomen DRG **9** Subcutaneous Tissue and Fascia, Buttock DRG **B** Subcutaneous Tissue and Fascia, Perineum DRG **C** Subcutaneous Tissue and Fascia, Pelvic Region DRG **D** Subcutaneous Tissue and Fascia, Right Upper Arm DRG **F** Subcutaneous Tissue and Fascia, Left Upper Arm DRG **G** Subcutaneous Tissue and Fascia, Right Lower Arm DRG **H** Subcutaneous Tissue and Fascia, Left Lower Arm DRG **J** Subcutaneous Tissue and Fascia, Right Hand **K** Subcutaneous Tissue and Fascia, Left Hand **L** Subcutaneous Tissue and Fascia, Right Upper Leg DRG **M** Subcutaneous Tissue and Fascia, Left Upper Leg DRG **N** Subcutaneous Tissue and Fascia, Right Lower Leg DRG **P** Subcutaneous Tissue and Fascia, Left Lower Leg DRG **Q** Subcutaneous Tissue and Fascia, Right Foot DRG **R** Subcutaneous Tissue and Fascia, Left Foot DRG	**0** Open **3** Percutaneous	**Z** No Device	**X** Diagnostic **Z** No Qualifier

DRG 0JB03ZZ 0JB43ZZ 0JB53ZZ 0JB63ZZ 0JB73ZZ 0JB83ZZ 0JB93ZZ 0JBB3ZZ 0JBC3ZZ 0JBD3ZZ 0JBF3ZZ 0JBG3ZZ 0JBH3ZZ 0JBL3ZZ 0JBM3ZZ 0JBN3ZZ 0JBP3ZZ 0JBQ3ZZ 0JBR3ZZ

0 Medical and Surgical
J Subcutaneous Tissue and Fascia
C Extirpation: Taking or cutting out solid matter from a body part

Body Part Character 4	Approach Character 5	Device Character 6	Qualifier Character 7
0 Subcutaneous Tissue and Fascia, Scalp **1** Subcutaneous Tissue and Fascia, Face **4** Subcutaneous Tissue and Fascia, Right Neck **5** Subcutaneous Tissue and Fascia, Left Neck **6** Subcutaneous Tissue and Fascia, Chest **7** Subcutaneous Tissue and Fascia, Back **8** Subcutaneous Tissue and Fascia, Abdomen **9** Subcutaneous Tissue and Fascia, Buttock **B** Subcutaneous Tissue and Fascia, Perineum **C** Subcutaneous Tissue and Fascia, Pelvic Region **D** Subcutaneous Tissue and Fascia, Right Upper Arm **F** Subcutaneous Tissue and Fascia, Left Upper Arm **G** Subcutaneous Tissue and Fascia, Right Lower Arm **H** Subcutaneous Tissue and Fascia, Left Lower Arm **J** Subcutaneous Tissue and Fascia, Right Hand **K** Subcutaneous Tissue and Fascia, Left Hand **L** Subcutaneous Tissue and Fascia, Right Upper Leg **M** Subcutaneous Tissue and Fascia, Left Upper Leg **N** Subcutaneous Tissue and Fascia, Right Lower Leg **P** Subcutaneous Tissue and Fascia, Left Lower Leg **Q** Subcutaneous Tissue and Fascia, Right Foot **R** Subcutaneous Tissue and Fascia, Left Foot	**0** Open **3** Percutaneous	**Z** No Device	**Z** No Qualifier

0 Medical and Surgical
J Subcutaneous Tissue and Fascia
D Extraction: Pulling or stripping out or off all or a portion of a body part by the use of force

Body Part Character 4	Approach Character 5	Device Character 6	Qualifier Character 7
0 Subcutaneous Tissue and Fascia, Scalp **1** Subcutaneous Tissue and Fascia, Face **4** Subcutaneous Tissue and Fascia, Right Neck **5** Subcutaneous Tissue and Fascia, Left Neck **6** Subcutaneous Tissue and Fascia, Chest DRG CC **7** Subcutaneous Tissue and Fascia, Back DRG CC **8** Subcutaneous Tissue and Fascia, Abdomen DRG CC **9** Subcutaneous Tissue and Fascia, Buttock DRG CC **B** Subcutaneous Tissue and Fascia, Perineum **C** Subcutaneous Tissue and Fascia, Pelvic Region **D** Subcutaneous Tissue and Fascia, Right Upper Arm **F** Subcutaneous Tissue and Fascia, Left Upper Arm **G** Subcutaneous Tissue and Fascia, Right Lower Arm **H** Subcutaneous Tissue and Fascia, Left Lower Arm **J** Subcutaneous Tissue and Fascia, Right Hand **K** Subcutaneous Tissue and Fascia, Left Hand **L** Subcutaneous Tissue and Fascia, Right Upper Leg DRG CC **M** Subcutaneous Tissue and Fascia, Left Upper Leg DRG CC **N** Subcutaneous Tissue and Fascia, Right Lower Leg **P** Subcutaneous Tissue and Fascia, Left Lower Leg **Q** Subcutaneous Tissue and Fascia, Right Foot **R** Subcutaneous Tissue and Fascia, Left Foot	**0** Open **3** Percutaneous	**Z** No Device	**Z** No Qualifier

DRG 0JD63ZZ 0JD73ZZ 0JD83ZZ 0JD93ZZ 0JDL3ZZ 0JDM3ZZ
CC 0JD63ZZ 0JD73ZZ 0JD83ZZ 0JD93ZZ 0JDL3ZZ 0JDM3ZZ

0 Medical and Surgical
J Subcutaneous Tissue and Fascia
H Insertion: Putting in a nonbiological appliance that monitors, assists, performs, or prevents a physiological function but does not physically take the place of a body part pacemaker - code leads seperate under 02H

Body Part Character 4	Approach Character 5	Device Character 6	Qualifier Character 7
0 Subcutaneous Tissue and Fascia, Scalp **1** Subcutaneous Tissue and Fascia, Face **4** Subcutaneous Tissue and Fascia, Right Neck **5** Subcutaneous Tissue and Fascia, Left Neck **9** Subcutaneous Tissue and Fascia, Buttock **B** Subcutaneous Tissue and Fascia, Perineum **C** Subcutaneous Tissue and Fascia, Pelvic Region **J** Subcutaneous Tissue and Fascia, Right Hand **K** Subcutaneous Tissue and Fascia, Left Hand **Q** Subcutaneous Tissue and Fascia, Right Foot **R** Subcutaneous Tissue and Fascia, Left Foot	**0** Open **3** Percutaneous	**N** Tissue Expander	**Z** No Qualifier
6 Subcutaneous Tissue and Fascia, Chest DRG HAC CC pocket for pacemaker	**0** Open **3** Percutaneous	**0** Monitoring Device, Hemodynamic **2** Monitoring Device **4** Pacemaker, Single Chamber **5** Pacemaker, Single Chamber Rate Responsive **6** Pacemaker, Dual Chamber **7** Cardiac Resynchronization Pacemaker Pulse Generator **8** Defibrillator Generator **9** Cardiac Resynchronization Defibrillator Pulse Generator **A** Contractility Modulation Device **B** Stimulator Generator, Single Array **C** Stimulator Generator, Single Array Rechargeable **D** Stimulator Generator, Multiple Array **E** Stimulator Generator, Multiple Array Rechargeable **F** Subcutaneous Defibrillator Lead **H** Contraceptive Device **M** Stimulator Generator **N** Tissue Expander **P** Cardiac Rhythm Related Device **V** Infusion Device, Pump **W** Vascular Access Device, Totally Implantable **X** Vascular Access Device, Tunneled	**Z** No Qualifier

0JH continued on next page

0JH continued from previous page

0 Medical and Surgical
J Subcutaneous Tissue and Fascia
H Insertion: Putting in a nonbiological appliance that monitors, assists, performs, or prevents a physiological function but does not physically take the place of a body part

Body Part Character 4	Approach Character 5	Device Character 6	Qualifier Character 7
7 Subcutaneous Tissue and Fascia, Back NC CC	**0** Open **3** Percutaneous	**B** Stimulator Generator, Single Array **C** Stimulator Generator, Single Array Rechargeable **D** Stimulator Generator, Multiple Array **E** Stimulator Generator, Multiple Array Rechargeable **M** Stimulator Generator **N** Tissue Expander **V** Infusion Device, Pump	**Z** No Qualifier
8 Subcutaneous Tissue and Fascia, Abdomen NC DRG HAC CC	**0** Open **3** Percutaneous	**0** Monitoring Device, Hemodynamic **2** Monitoring Device **4** Pacemaker, Single Chamber **5** Pacemaker, Single Chamber Rate Responsive **6** Pacemaker, Dual Chamber **7** Cardiac Resynchronization Pacemaker Pulse Generator **8** Defibrillator Generator **9** Cardiac Resynchronization Defibrillator Pulse Generator **A** Contractility Modulation Device **B** Stimulator Generator, Single Array **C** Stimulator Generator, Single Array Rechargeable **D** Stimulator Generator, Multiple Array **E** Stimulator Generator, Multiple Array Rechargeable **H** Contraceptive Device **M** Stimulator Generator **N** Tissue Expander **P** Cardiac Rhythm Related Device **V** Infusion Device, Pump **W** Vascular Access Device, Totally Implantable **X** Vascular Access Device, Tunneled	**Z** No Qualifier
D Subcutaneous Tissue and Fascia, Right Upper Arm DRG **F** Subcutaneous Tissue and Fascia, Left Upper Arm DRG **G** Subcutaneous Tissue and Fascia, Right Lower Arm DRG **H** Subcutaneous Tissue and Fascia, Left Lower Arm DRG **L** Subcutaneous Tissue and Fascia, Right Upper Leg DRG **M** Subcutaneous Tissue and Fascia, Left Upper Leg DRG **N** Subcutaneous Tissue and Fascia, Right Lower Leg DRG **P** Subcutaneous Tissue and Fascia, Left Lower Leg DRG	**0** Open **3** Percutaneous	**H** Contraceptive Device **N** Tissue Expander **V** Infusion Device, Pump **W** Vascular Access Device, Totally Implantable **X** Vascular Access Device, Tunneled	**Z** No Qualifier

0JH continued on next page

0JH continued from previous page

0 Medical and Surgical
J Subcutaneous Tissue and Fascia
H Insertion: Putting in a nonbiological appliance that monitors, assists, performs, or prevents a physiological function but does not physically take the place of a body part

Body Part Character 4	Approach Character 5	Device Character 6	Qualifier Character 7
S Subcutaneous Tissue and Fascia, Head and Neck **V** Subcutaneous Tissue and Fascia, Upper Extremity **W** Subcutaneous Tissue and Fascia, Lower Extremity	**0** Open **3** Percutaneous	**1** Radioactive Element **3** Infusion Device **Y** Other Device	**Z** No Qualifier
T Subcutaneous Tissue and Fascia, Trunk	**0** Open **3** Percutaneous	**1** Radioactive Element **3** Infusion Device **V** Infusion Device, Pump **Y** Other Device	**Z** No Qualifier

NC 0JH70MZ 0JH73MZ 0JH80MZ 0JH83MZ

DRG 0JH604Z 0JH605Z 0JH606Z 0JH607Z 0JH60HZ 0JH60PZ 0JH60XZ 0JH634Z 0JH635Z 0JH636Z 0JH637Z 0JH63HZ 0JH63PZ 0JH63WZ 0JH63XZ 0JH802Z 0JH804Z 0JH805Z 0JH806Z 0JH807Z 0JH80HZ 0JH80PZ 0JH80XZ 0JH832Z 0JH834Z 0JH835Z 0JH836Z 0JH837Z 0JH83HZ 0JH83PZ 0JH83WZ 0JH83XZ 0JHD0XZ 0JHD3WZ 0JHD3XZ 0JHF0XZ 0JHF3WZ 0JHF3XZ 0JHG0XZ 0JHG3WZ 0JHG3XZ 0JHH0XZ 0JHH3WZ 0JHH3XZ 0JHL0XZ 0JHL3WZ 0JHL3XZ 0JHM0XZ 0JHM3WZ 0JHM3XZ 0JHN0XZ 0JHN3HZ 0JHN3WZ 0JHN3XZ 0JHP0HZ 0JHP0XZ 0JHP3HZ 0JHP3WZ 0JHP3XZ

HAC 0JH604Z 0JH605Z 0JH606Z 0JH607Z 0JH608Z 0JH609Z 0JH60PZ 0JH634Z 0JH635Z 0JH636Z 0JH637Z 0JH638Z 0JH639Z 0JH63PZ 0JH804Z 0JH805Z 0JH806Z 0JH807Z 0JH808Z 0JH809Z 0JH80PZ 0JH834Z 0JH835Z 0JH836Z 0JH837Z 0JH838Z 0JH839Z 0JH83PZ

Surgical site infection (SSI) following cardiac implantable electronic device (CIED) procedures and secondary diagnosis K68.11, T81.40XA, T81.41XA, T81.42XA, T81.43XA, T81.44XA, T81.49XA, T82.6XXA, T82.7XXA.

HAC 0JH63XZ

Iatrogenic pneumothorax w/ venous catheterization procedures and secondary diagnosis J95.811.

CC 0JH604Z 0JH605Z 0JH606Z 0JH607Z 0JH608Z 0JH609Z 0JH60AZ 0JH60BZ 0JH60CZ 0JH60DZ 0JH60EZ 0JH60PZ 0JH634Z 0JH635Z 0JH636Z 0JH637Z 0JH638Z 0JH639Z 0JH63AZ 0JH63BZ 0JH63CZ 0JH63DZ 0JH63EZ 0JH63PZ 0JH70BZ 0JH70CZ 0JH70DZ 0JH70EZ 0JH73BZ 0JH73CZ 0JH73DZ 0JH73EZ 0JH804Z 0JH805Z 0JH806Z 0JH807Z 0JH808Z 0JH809Z 0JH80AZ 0JH80BZ 0JH80CZ 0JH80DZ 0JH80EZ 0JH80PZ 0JH834Z 0JH835Z 0JH836Z 0JH837Z 0JH838Z 0JH839Z 0JH83AZ 0JH83BZ 0JH83CZ 0JH83DZ 0JH83EZ 0JH83PZ

0 Medical and Surgical
J Subcutaneous Tissue and Fascia
J Inspection: Visually and/or manually exploring a body part

Body Part Character 4	Approach Character 5	Device Character 6	Qualifier Character 7
S Subcutaneous Tissue and Fascia, Head and Neck **T** Subcutaneous Tissue and Fascia, Trunk **V** Subcutaneous Tissue and Fascia, Upper Extremity **W** Subcutaneous Tissue and Fascia, Lower Extremity	**0** Open **3** Percutaneous **X** External	**Z** No Device	**Z** No Qualifier

0 Medical and Surgical
J Subcutaneous Tissue and Fascia
N Release: Freeing a body part from an abnormal physical constraint by cutting or by the use of force

Body Part Character 4	Approach Character 5	Device Character 6	Qualifier Character 7
0 Subcutaneous Tissue and Fascia, Scalp **1** Subcutaneous Tissue and Fascia, Face **4** Subcutaneous Tissue and Fascia, Right Neck **5** Subcutaneous Tissue and Fascia, Left Neck **6** Subcutaneous Tissue and Fascia, Chest **7** Subcutaneous Tissue and Fascia, Back **8** Subcutaneous Tissue and Fascia, Abdomen **9** Subcutaneous Tissue and Fascia, Buttock **B** Subcutaneous Tissue and Fascia, Perineum **C** Subcutaneous Tissue and Fascia, Pelvic Region **D** Subcutaneous Tissue and Fascia, Right Upper Arm **F** Subcutaneous Tissue and Fascia, Left Upper Arm **G** Subcutaneous Tissue and Fascia, Right Lower Arm **H** Subcutaneous Tissue and Fascia, Left Lower Arm **J** Subcutaneous Tissue and Fascia, Right Hand **K** Subcutaneous Tissue and Fascia, Left Hand **L** Subcutaneous Tissue and Fascia, Right Upper Leg **M** Subcutaneous Tissue and Fascia, Left Upper Leg **N** Subcutaneous Tissue and Fascia, Right Lower Leg **P** Subcutaneous Tissue and Fascia, Left Lower Leg **Q** Subcutaneous Tissue and Fascia, Right Foot **R** Subcutaneous Tissue and Fascia, Left Foot	**0** Open **3** Percutaneous **X** External	**Z** No Device	**Z** No Qualifier

0 Medical and Surgical
J Subcutaneous Tissue and Fascia
P Removal: Taking out or off a device from a body part

Body Part Character 4	Approach Character 5	Device Character 6	Qualifier Character 7
S Subcutaneous Tissue and Fascia, Head and Neck	**0** Open **3** Percutaneous	**0** Drainage Device **1** Radioactive Element **3** Infusion Device **7** Autologous Tissue Substitute **J** Synthetic Substitute **K** Nonautologous Tissue Substitute **N** Tissue Expander **Y** Other Device	**Z** No Qualifier
S Subcutaneous Tissue and Fascia, Head and Neck	**X** External	**0** Drainage Device **1** Radioactive Element **3** Infusion Device	**Z** No Qualifier
T Subcutaneous Tissue and Fascia, Trunk HAC	**0** Open **3** Percutaneous	**0** Drainage Device **1** Radioactive Element **2** Monitoring Device **3** Infusion Device **7** Autologous Tissue Substitute **F** Subcutaneous Defibrillator Lead **H** Contraceptive Device **J** Synthetic Substitute **K** Nonautologous Tissue Substitute **M** Stimulator Generator **N** Tissue Expander **P** Cardiac Rhythm Related Device **V** Infusion Device, Pump **W** Vascular Access Device, Totally Implantable **X** Vascular Access Device, Tunneled **Y** Other Device	**Z** No Qualifier
T Subcutaneous Tissue and Fascia, Trunk	**X** External	**0** Drainage Device **1** Radioactive Element **2** Monitoring Device **3** Infusion Device **H** Contraceptive Device **V** Infusion Device, Pump **X** Vascular Access Device, Tunneled	**Z** No Qualifier
V Subcutaneous Tissue and Fascia, Upper Extremity **W** Subcutaneous Tissue and Fascia, Lower Extremity	**0** Open **3** Percutaneous	**0** Drainage Device **1** Radioactive Element **3** Infusion Device **7** Autologous Tissue Substitute **H** Contraceptive Device **J** Synthetic Substitute **K** Nonautologous Tissue Substitute **N** Tissue Expander **V** Infusion Device, Pump **W** Vascular Access Device, Totally Implantable **X** Vascular Access Device, Tunneled **Y** Other Device	**Z** No Qualifier
V Subcutaneous Tissue and Fascia, Upper Extremity **W** Subcutaneous Tissue and Fascia, Lower Extremity	**X** External	**0** Drainage Device **1** Radioactive Element **3** Infusion Device **H** Contraceptive Device **V** Infusion Device, Pump **X** Vascular Access Device, Tunneled	**Z** No Qualifier

HAC 0JPT0PZ 0JPT3PZ
Surgical site infection (SSI) following cardiac implantable electronic device (CIED) procedures and secondary diagnosis K68.11, T81.40XA, T81.41XA, T81.42XA, T81.43XA, T81.44XA, T81.49XA, T82.6XXA, T82.7XXA.

0 Medical and Surgical
J Subcutaneous Tissue and Fascia
Q Repair: Restoring, to the extent possible, a body part to its normal anatomic structure and function

Body Part Character 4	Approach Character 5	Device Character 6	Qualifier Character 7
0 Subcutaneous Tissue and Fascia, Scalp **1** Subcutaneous Tissue and Fascia, Face **4** Subcutaneous Tissue and Fascia, Right Neck **5** Subcutaneous Tissue and Fascia, Left Neck **6** Subcutaneous Tissue and Fascia, Chest **7** Subcutaneous Tissue and Fascia, Back **8** Subcutaneous Tissue and Fascia, Abdomen **9** Subcutaneous Tissue and Fascia, Buttock **B** Subcutaneous Tissue and Fascia, Perineum **C** Subcutaneous Tissue and Fascia, Pelvic Region **D** Subcutaneous Tissue and Fascia, Right Upper Arm **F** Subcutaneous Tissue and Fascia, Left Upper Arm **G** Subcutaneous Tissue and Fascia, Right Lower Arm **H** Subcutaneous Tissue and Fascia, Left Lower Arm **J** Subcutaneous Tissue and Fascia, Right Hand **K** Subcutaneous Tissue and Fascia, Left Hand **L** Subcutaneous Tissue and Fascia, Right Upper Leg **M** Subcutaneous Tissue and Fascia, Left Upper Leg **N** Subcutaneous Tissue and Fascia, Right Lower Leg **P** Subcutaneous Tissue and Fascia, Left Lower Leg **Q** Subcutaneous Tissue and Fascia, Right Foot **R** Subcutaneous Tissue and Fascia, Left Foot	**0** Open **3** Percutaneous	**Z** No Device	**Z** No Qualifier

0 Medical and Surgical
J Subcutaneous Tissue and Fascia
R Replacement: Putting in or on biological or synthetic material that physically takes the place and/or function of all or a portion of a body part

Body Part Character 4	Approach Character 5	Device Character 6	Qualifier Character 7
0 Subcutaneous Tissue and Fascia, Scalp **1** Subcutaneous Tissue and Fascia, Face **4** Subcutaneous Tissue and Fascia, Right Neck **5** Subcutaneous Tissue and Fascia, Left Neck **6** Subcutaneous Tissue and Fascia, Chest **7** Subcutaneous Tissue and Fascia, Back **8** Subcutaneous Tissue and Fascia, Abdomen **9** Subcutaneous Tissue and Fascia, Buttock **B** Subcutaneous Tissue and Fascia, Perineum **C** Subcutaneous Tissue and Fascia, Pelvic Region **D** Subcutaneous Tissue and Fascia, Right Upper Arm **F** Subcutaneous Tissue and Fascia, Left Upper Arm **G** Subcutaneous Tissue and Fascia, Right Lower Arm **H** Subcutaneous Tissue and Fascia, Left Lower Arm **J** Subcutaneous Tissue and Fascia, Right Hand **K** Subcutaneous Tissue and Fascia, Left Hand **L** Subcutaneous Tissue and Fascia, Right Upper Leg **M** Subcutaneous Tissue and Fascia, Left Upper Leg **N** Subcutaneous Tissue and Fascia, Right Lower Leg **P** Subcutaneous Tissue and Fascia, Left Lower Leg **Q** Subcutaneous Tissue and Fascia, Right Foot **R** Subcutaneous Tissue and Fascia, Left Foot	**0** Open **3** Percutaneous	**7** Autologous Tissue Substitute **J** Synthetic Substitute **K** Nonautologous Tissue Substitute	**Z** No Qualifier

0 Medical and Surgical
J Subcutaneous Tissue and Fascia
U Supplement: Putting in or on biological or synthetic material that physically reinforces and/or augments the function of a portion of a body part

Body Part Character 4	Approach Character 5	Device Character 6	Qualifier Character 7
0 Subcutaneous Tissue and Fascia, Scalp	**0** Open	**7** Autologous Tissue Substitute	**Z** No Qualifier
1 Subcutaneous Tissue and Fascia, Face	**3** Percutaneous	**J** Synthetic Substitute mesh	
4 Subcutaneous Tissue and Fascia, Right Neck		**K** Nonautologous Tissue Substitute	
5 Subcutaneous Tissue and Fascia, Left Neck			
6 Subcutaneous Tissue and Fascia, Chest			
7 Subcutaneous Tissue and Fascia, Back			
8 Subcutaneous Tissue and Fascia, Abdomen			
9 Subcutaneous Tissue and Fascia, Buttock			
B Subcutaneous Tissue and Fascia, Perineum			
C Subcutaneous Tissue and Fascia, Pelvic Region cystocele			
D Subcutaneous Tissue and Fascia, Right Upper Arm			
F Subcutaneous Tissue and Fascia, Left Upper Arm			
G Subcutaneous Tissue and Fascia, Right Lower Arm			
H Subcutaneous Tissue and Fascia, Left Lower Arm			
J Subcutaneous Tissue and Fascia, Right Hand			
K Subcutaneous Tissue and Fascia, Left Hand			
L Subcutaneous Tissue and Fascia, Right Upper Leg			
M Subcutaneous Tissue and Fascia, Left Upper Leg			
N Subcutaneous Tissue and Fascia, Right Lower Leg			
P Subcutaneous Tissue and Fascia, Left Lower Leg			
Q Subcutaneous Tissue and Fascia, Right Foot			
R Subcutaneous Tissue and Fascia, Left Foot			

0 Medical and Surgical
J Subcutaneous Tissue and Fascia
W Revision: Correcting, to the extent possible, a portion of a malfunctioning device or the position of a displaced device

Body Part Character 4	Approach Character 5	Device Character 6	Qualifier Character 7
S Subcutaneous Tissue and Fascia, Head and Neck DRG	**0** Open **3** Percutaneous	**0** Drainage Device **3** Infusion Device **7** Autologous Tissue Substitute **J** Synthetic Substitute **K** Nonautologous Tissue Substitute **N** Tissue Expander **Y** Other Device	**Z** No Qualifier
S Subcutaneous Tissue and Fascia, Head and Neck	**X** External	**0** Drainage Device **3** Infusion Device **7** Autologous Tissue Substitute **J** Synthetic Substitute **K** Nonautologous Tissue Substitute **N** Tissue Expander	**Z** No Qualifier
T Subcutaneous Tissue and Fascia, Trunk DRG HAC	**0** Open **3** Percutaneous	**0** Drainage Device **2** Monitoring Device **3** Infusion Device **7** Autologous Tissue Substitute **F** Subcutaneous Defibrillator Lead **H** Contraceptive Device **J** Synthetic Substitute **K** Nonautologous Tissue Substitute **M** Stimulator Generator **N** Tissue Expander **P** Cardiac Rhythm Related Device **V** Infusion Device, Pump **W** Vascular Access Device, Totally Implantable **X** Vascular Access Device, Tunneled **Y** Other Device	**Z** No Qualifier
T Subcutaneous Tissue and Fascia, Trunk DRG	**X** External	**0** Drainage Device **2** Monitoring Device **3** Infusion Device **7** Autologous Tissue Substitute **F** Subcutaneous Defibrillator Lead **H** Contraceptive Device **J** Synthetic Substitute **K** Nonautologous Tissue Substitute **M** Stimulator Generator **N** Tissue Expander **P** Cardiac Rhythm Related Device **V** Infusion Device, Pump **W** Vascular Access Device, Totally Implantable **X** Vascular Access Device, Tunneled	**Z** No Qualifier

0JW continued on next page

LC Limited Coverage NC Noncovered HAC HAC-associated Procedure CC Combination Cluster - See Appendix G for code lists
DRG Non-OR-Affecting MS-DRG Assignment New/Revised Text in **Orange** ♂ Male ♀ Female

0 Medical and Surgical
J Subcutaneous Tissue and Fascia
W Revision: Correcting, to the extent possible, a portion of a malfunctioning device or the position of a displaced device

0JW continued from previous page

Body Part Character 4	Approach Character 5	Device Character 6	Qualifier Character 7
V Subcutaneous Tissue and Fascia, Upper Extremity DRG **W** Subcutaneous Tissue and Fascia, Lower Extremity DRG	**0** Open **3** Percutaneous	**0** Drainage Device **3** Infusion Device **7** Autologous Tissue Substitute **H** Contraceptive Device **J** Synthetic Substitute **K** Nonautologous Tissue Substitute **N** Tissue Expander **V** Infusion Device, Pump **W** Vascular Access Device, Totally Implantable **X** Vascular Access Device, Tunneled **Y** Other Device	**Z** No Qualifier
V Subcutaneous Tissue and Fascia, Upper Extremity **W** Subcutaneous Tissue and Fascia, Lower Extremity	**X** External	**0** Drainage Device **3** Infusion Device **7** Autologous Tissue Substitute **H** Contraceptive Device **J** Synthetic Substitute **K** Nonautologous Tissue Substitute **N** Tissue Expander **V** Infusion Device, Pump **W** Vascular Access Device, Totally Implantable **X** Vascular Access Device, Tunneled	**Z** No Qualifier

DRG 0JWS00Z 0JWS03Z 0JWS07Z 0JWS0JZ 0JWS0KZ 0JWS0NZ 0JWS0YZ 0JWS30Z 0JWS33Z 0JWS37Z 0JWS3JZ 0JWS3KZ 0JWS3NZ 0JWS3YZ 0JWT00Z 0JWT03Z 0JWT07Z 0JWT0HZ 0JWT0JZ 0JWT0KZ 0JWT0MZ 0JWT0NZ 0JWT0VZ 0JWT0WZ 0JWT0XZ 0JWT30Z 0JWT33Z 0JWT37Z 0JWT3HZ 0JWT3JZ 0JWT3KZ 0JWT3MZ 0JWT3NZ 0JWT3VZ 0JWT3WZ 0JWT3XZ 0JWTXMZ 0JWV00Z 0JWV03Z 0JWV07Z 0JWV0HZ 0JWV0JZ 0JWV0KZ 0JWV0NZ 0JWV0VZ 0JWV0WZ 0JWV0XZ 0JWV0YZ 0JWV30Z 0JWV33Z 0JWV37Z 0JWV3HZ 0JWV3JZ 0JWV3KZ 0JWV3NZ 0JWV3VZ 0JWV3WZ 0JWV3XZ 0JWV3YZ 0JWW00Z 0JWW03Z 0JWW07Z 0JWW0HZ 0JWW0JZ 0JWW0KZ 0JWW0NZ 0JWW0VZ 0JWW0WZ 0JWW0XZ 0JWW0YZ 0JWW30Z 0JWW33Z 0JWW37Z 0JWW3HZ 0JWW3JZ 0JWW3KZ 0JWW3NZ 0JWW3VZ 0JWW3WZ 0JWW3XZ 0JWW3YZ

HAC 0JWT0PZ 0JWT3PZ

0 Medical and Surgical
J Subcutaneous Tissue and Fascia
X Transfer: Moving, without taking out, all or a portion of a body part to another location to take over the function of all or a portion of a body part

Body Part Character 4	Approach Character 5	Device Character 6	Qualifier Character 7
0 Subcutaneous Tissue and Fascia, Scalp **1** Subcutaneous Tissue and Fascia, Face **4** Subcutaneous Tissue and Fascia, Right Neck may be anterior **5** Subcutaneous Tissue and Fascia, Left Neck **6** Subcutaneous Tissue and Fascia, Chest **7** Subcutaneous Tissue and Fascia, Back **8** Subcutaneous Tissue and Fascia, Abdomen **9** Subcutaneous Tissue and Fascia, Buttock **B** Subcutaneous Tissue and Fascia, Perineum **C** Subcutaneous Tissue and Fascia, Pelvic Region **D** Subcutaneous Tissue and Fascia, Right Upper Arm **F** Subcutaneous Tissue and Fascia, Left Upper Arm **G** Subcutaneous Tissue and Fascia, Right Lower Arm **H** Subcutaneous Tissue and Fascia, Left Lower Arm **J** Subcutaneous Tissue and Fascia, Right Hand **K** Subcutaneous Tissue and Fascia, Left Hand **L** Subcutaneous Tissue and Fascia, Right Upper Leg **M** Subcutaneous Tissue and Fascia, Left Upper Leg thigh **N** Subcutaneous Tissue and Fascia, Right Lower Leg **P** Subcutaneous Tissue and Fascia, Left Lower Leg **Q** Subcutaneous Tissue and Fascia, Right Foot **R** Subcutaneous Tissue and Fascia, Left Foot	**0** Open **3** Percutaneous	**Z** No Device	**B** Skin and Subcutaneous Tissue **C** Skin, Subcutaneous Tissue and Fascia fasciocutaneous **Z** No Qualifier

open fascio cutaneous flap closure of left thigh OJXMOZC

NOTES

Muscles 0K2-0KX

0 Medical and Surgical
K Muscles
2 Change: Taking out or off a device from a body part and putting back an identical or similar device in or on the same body part without cutting or puncturing the skin or a mucous membrane

Body Part	Approach	Device	Qualifier
Character 4	**Character 5**	**Character 6**	**Character 7**
X Upper Muscle **Y** Lower Muscle	**X** External	**0** Drainage Device **Y** Other Device	**Z** No Qualifier

0 Medical and Surgical
K Muscles
5 Destruction: Physical eradication of all or a portion of a body part by the direct use of energy, force, or a destructive agent

Body Part	Approach	Device	Qualifier
Character 4	**Character 5**	**Character 6**	**Character 7**
0 Head Muscle **1** Facial Muscle **2** Neck Muscle, Right **3** Neck Muscle, Left **4** Tongue, Palate, Pharynx Muscle **5** Shoulder Muscle, Right **6** Shoulder Muscle, Left **7** Upper Arm Muscle, Right **8** Upper Arm Muscle, Left **9** Lower Arm and Wrist Muscle, Right **B** Lower Arm and Wrist Muscle, Left **C** Hand Muscle, Right **D** Hand Muscle, Left **F** Trunk Muscle, Right **G** Trunk Muscle, Left **H** Thorax Muscle, Right **J** Thorax Muscle, Left **K** Abdomen Muscle, Right **L** Abdomen Muscle, Left **M** Perineum Muscle **N** Hip Muscle, Right **P** Hip Muscle, Left **Q** Upper Leg Muscle, Right **R** Upper Leg Muscle, Left **S** Lower Leg Muscle, Right **T** Lower Leg Muscle, Left **V** Foot Muscle, Right **W** Foot Muscle, Left	**0** Open **3** Percutaneous **4** Percutaneous Endoscopic	**Z** No Device	**Z** No Qualifier

0 Medical and Surgical
K Muscles
8 Division: Cutting into a body part, without draining fluids and/or gases from the body part, in order to separate or transect a body part

Body Part Character 4	Approach Character 5	Device Character 6	Qualifier Character 7
0 Head Muscle **1** Facial Muscle **2** Neck Muscle, Right **3** Neck Muscle, Left **4** Tongue, Palate, Pharynx Muscle **5** Shoulder Muscle, Right **6** Shoulder Muscle, Left **7** Upper Arm Muscle, Right **8** Upper Arm Muscle, Left **9** Lower Arm and Wrist Muscle, Right **B** Lower Arm and Wrist Muscle, Left **C** Hand Muscle, Right **D** Hand Muscle, Left **F** Trunk Muscle, Right **G** Trunk Muscle, Left **H** Thorax Muscle, Right **J** Thorax Muscle, Left **K** Abdomen Muscle, Right **L** Abdomen Muscle, Left **M** Perineum Muscle **N** Hip Muscle, Right **P** Hip Muscle, Left **Q** Upper Leg Muscle, Right **R** Upper Leg Muscle, Left **S** Lower Leg Muscle, Right **T** Lower Leg Muscle, Left **V** Foot Muscle, Right **W** Foot Muscle, Left	**0** Open **3** Percutaneous **4** Percutaneous Endoscopic	**Z** No Device	**Z** No Qualifier

0 Medical and Surgical
K Muscles
9 Drainage: Taking or letting out fluids and/or gases from a body part

Body Part Character 4	Approach Character 5	Device Character 6	Qualifier Character 7
0 Head Muscle **1** Facial Muscle **2** Neck Muscle, Right **3** Neck Muscle, Left **4** Tongue, Palate, Pharynx Muscle **5** Shoulder Muscle, Right **6** Shoulder Muscle, Left **7** Upper Arm Muscle, Right **8** Upper Arm Muscle, Left **9** Lower Arm and Wrist Muscle, Right **B** Lower Arm and Wrist Muscle, Left **C** Hand Muscle, Right **D** Hand Muscle, Left **F** Trunk Muscle, Right **G** Trunk Muscle, Left **H** Thorax Muscle, Right **J** Thorax Muscle, Left **K** Abdomen Muscle, Right **L** Abdomen Muscle, Left **M** Perineum Muscle **N** Hip Muscle, Right **P** Hip Muscle, Left **Q** Upper Leg Muscle, Right **R** Upper Leg Muscle, Left **S** Lower Leg Muscle, Right **T** Lower Leg Muscle, Left **V** Foot Muscle, Right **W** Foot Muscle, Left	**0** Open **3** Percutaneous **4** Percutaneous Endoscopic	**0** Drainage Device	**Z** No Qualifier
0 Head Muscle **1** Facial Muscle **2** Neck Muscle, Right **3** Neck Muscle, Left **4** Tongue, Palate, Pharynx Muscle **5** Shoulder Muscle, Right **6** Shoulder Muscle, Left **7** Upper Arm Muscle, Right **8** Upper Arm Muscle, Left **9** Lower Arm and Wrist Muscle, Right **B** Lower Arm and Wrist Muscle, Left **C** Hand Muscle, Right **D** Hand Muscle, Left **F** Trunk Muscle, Right **G** Trunk Muscle, Left **H** Thorax Muscle, Right **J** Thorax Muscle, Left **K** Abdomen Muscle, Right **L** Abdomen Muscle, Left **M** Perineum Muscle **N** Hip Muscle, Right **P** Hip Muscle, Left **Q** Upper Leg Muscle, Right **R** Upper Leg Muscle, Left **S** Lower Leg Muscle, Right **T** Lower Leg Muscle, Left **V** Foot Muscle, Right **W** Foot Muscle, Left	**0** Open **3** Percutaneous **4** Percutaneous Endoscopic	**Z** No Device	**X** Diagnostic **Z** No Qualifier

0 Medical and Surgical
K Muscles
B Excision: Cutting out or off, without replacement, a portion of a body part

Body Part Character 4	Approach Character 5	Device Character 6	Qualifier Character 7
0 Head Muscle **1** Facial Muscle **2** Neck Muscle, Right **3** Neck Muscle, Left **4** Tongue, Palate, Pharynx Muscle **5** Shoulder Muscle, Right **6** Shoulder Muscle, Left **7** Upper Arm Muscle, Right **8** Upper Arm Muscle, Left **9** Lower Arm and Wrist Muscle, Right **B** Lower Arm and Wrist Muscle, Left **C** Hand Muscle, Right **D** Hand Muscle, Left **F** Trunk Muscle, Right **G** Trunk Muscle, Left **H** Thorax Muscle, Right **J** Thorax Muscle, Left **K** Abdomen Muscle, Right **L** Abdomen Muscle, Left **M** Perineum Muscle **N** Hip Muscle, Right **P** Hip Muscle, Left **Q** Upper Leg Muscle, Right **R** Upper Leg Muscle, Left **S** Lower Leg Muscle, Right **T** Lower Leg Muscle, Left **V** Foot Muscle, Right **W** Foot Muscle, Left	**0** Open **3** Percutaneous **4** Percutaneous Endoscopic	**Z** No Device	**X** Diagnostic **Z** No Qualifier

0 Medical and Surgical
K Muscles
C Extirpation: Taking or cutting out solid matter from a body part

Body Part Character 4	Approach Character 5	Device Character 6	Qualifier Character 7
0 Head Muscle **1** Facial Muscle **2** Neck Muscle, Right **3** Neck Muscle, Left **4** Tongue, Palate, Pharynx Muscle **5** Shoulder Muscle, Right **6** Shoulder Muscle, Left **7** Upper Arm Muscle, Right **8** Upper Arm Muscle, Left **9** Lower Arm and Wrist Muscle, Right **B** Lower Arm and Wrist Muscle, Left **C** Hand Muscle, Right **D** Hand Muscle, Left **F** Trunk Muscle, Right **G** Trunk Muscle, Left **H** Thorax Muscle, Right **J** Thorax Muscle, Left **K** Abdomen Muscle, Right **L** Abdomen Muscle, Left **M** Perineum Muscle **N** Hip Muscle, Right **P** Hip Muscle, Left **Q** Upper Leg Muscle, Right **R** Upper Leg Muscle, Left **S** Lower Leg Muscle, Right **T** Lower Leg Muscle, Left **V** Foot Muscle, Right **W** Foot Muscle, Left	**0** Open **3** Percutaneous **4** Percutaneous Endoscopic	**Z** No Device	**Z** No Qualifier

LC Limited Coverage NC Noncovered HAC HAC-associated Procedure CC Combination Cluster - See Appendix G for code lists
DRG Non-OR-Affecting MS-DRG Assignment New/Revised Text in **Orange** ♂ Male ♀ Female
MUSCLES 0K2-0KX
412
2020 ICD-10-PCS

0 Medical and Surgical
K Muscles
D Extraction: Pulling or stripping out or off all or a portion of a body part by the use of force

Body Part	Approach	Device	Qualifier
Character 4	Character 5	Character 6	Character 7
0 Head Muscle **1** Facial Muscle **2** Neck Muscle, Right **3** Neck Muscle, Left **4** Tongue, Palate, Pharynx Muscle **5** Shoulder Muscle, Right **6** Shoulder Muscle, Left **7** Upper Arm Muscle, Right **8** Upper Arm Muscle, Left **9** Lower Arm and Wrist Muscle, Right **B** Lower Arm and Wrist Muscle, Left **C** Hand Muscle, Right **D** Hand Muscle, Left **F** Trunk Muscle, Right **G** Trunk Muscle, Left **H** Thorax Muscle, Right **J** Thorax Muscle, Left **K** Abdomen Muscle, Right **L** Abdomen Muscle, Left **M** Perineum Muscle **N** Hip Muscle, Right **P** Hip Muscle, Left **Q** Upper Leg Muscle, Right **R** Upper Leg Muscle, Left **S** Lower Leg Muscle, Right **T** Lower Leg Muscle, Left **V** Foot Muscle, Right **W** Foot Muscle, Left	**0** Open	**Z** No Device	**Z** No Qualifier

0 Medical and Surgical
K Muscles
H Insertion: Putting in a nonbiological appliance that monitors, assists, performs, or prevents a physiological function but does not physically take the place of a body part

Body Part	Approach	Device	Qualifier
Character 4	Character 5	Character 6	Character 7
X Upper Muscle **Y** Lower Muscle	**0** Open **3** Percutaneous **4** Percutaneous Endoscopic	**M** Stimulator Lead **Y** Other Device	**Z** No Qualifier

0 Medical and Surgical
K Muscles
J Inspection: Visually and/or manually exploring a body part

Body Part	Approach	Device	Qualifier
Character 4	Character 5	Character 6	Character 7
X Upper Muscle **Y** Lower Muscle	**0** Open **3** Percutaneous **4** Percutaneous Endoscopic **X** External	**Z** No Device	**Z** No Qualifier

0 Medical and Surgical
K Muscles
M Reattachment: Putting back in or on all or a portion of a separated body part to its normal location or other suitable location

Body Part Character 4	Approach Character 5	Device Character 6	Qualifier Character 7
0 Head Muscle **1** Facial Muscle **2** Neck Muscle, Right **3** Neck Muscle, Left **4** Tongue, Palate, Pharynx Muscle **5** Shoulder Muscle, Right **6** Shoulder Muscle, Left **7** Upper Arm Muscle, Right **8** Upper Arm Muscle, Left **9** Lower Arm and Wrist Muscle, Right **B** Lower Arm and Wrist Muscle, Left **C** Hand Muscle, Right **D** Hand Muscle, Left **F** Trunk Muscle, Right **G** Trunk Muscle, Left **H** Thorax Muscle, Right **J** Thorax Muscle, Left **K** Abdomen Muscle, Right **L** Abdomen Muscle, Left **M** Perineum Muscle **N** Hip Muscle, Right **P** Hip Muscle, Left **Q** Upper Leg Muscle, Right **R** Upper Leg Muscle, Left **S** Lower Leg Muscle, Right **T** Lower Leg Muscle, Left **V** Foot Muscle, Right **W** Foot Muscle, Left	**0** Open **4** Percutaneous Endoscopic	**Z** No Device	**Z** No Qualifier

0 Medical and Surgical
K Muscles
N Release: Freeing a body part from an abnormal physical constraint by cutting or by the use of force

Body Part Character 4	Approach Character 5	Device Character 6	Qualifier Character 7
0 Head Muscle **1** Facial Muscle **2** Neck Muscle, Right **3** Neck Muscle, Left **4** Tongue, Palate, Pharynx Muscle **5** Shoulder Muscle, Right **6** Shoulder Muscle, Left **7** Upper Arm Muscle, Right **8** Upper Arm Muscle, Left **9** Lower Arm and Wrist Muscle, Right **B** Lower Arm and Wrist Muscle, Left **C** Hand Muscle, Right **D** Hand Muscle, Left **F** Trunk Muscle, Right **G** Trunk Muscle, Left **H** Thorax Muscle, Right **J** Thorax Muscle, Left **K** Abdomen Muscle, Right **L** Abdomen Muscle, Left **M** Perineum Muscle **N** Hip Muscle, Right **P** Hip Muscle, Left **Q** Upper Leg Muscle, Right **R** Upper Leg Muscle, Left **S** Lower Leg Muscle, Right **T** Lower Leg Muscle, Left **V** Foot Muscle, Right **W** Foot Muscle, Left	**0** Open **3** Percutaneous **4** Percutaneous Endoscopic **X** External	**Z** No Device	**Z** No Qualifier

0 Medical and Surgical
K Muscles
P Removal: Taking out or off a device from a body part

Body Part Character 4	Approach Character 5	Device Character 6	Qualifier Character 7
X Upper Muscle **Y** Lower Muscle	**0** Open **3** Percutaneous **4** Percutaneous Endoscopic	**0** Drainage Device **7** Autologous Tissue Substitute **J** Synthetic Substitute **K** Nonautologous Tissue Substitute **M** Stimulator Lead **Y** Other Device	**Z** No Qualifier
X Upper Muscle **Y** Lower Muscle	**X** External	**0** Drainage Device **M** Stimulator Lead	**Z** No Qualifier

0 Medical and Surgical
K Muscles
Q Repair: Restoring, to the extent possible, a body part to its normal anatomic structure and function

Body Part Character 4	Approach Character 5	Device Character 6	Qualifier Character 7
0 Head Muscle **1** Facial Muscle **2** Neck Muscle, Right **3** Neck Muscle, Left **4** Tongue, Palate, Pharynx Muscle **5** Shoulder Muscle, Right **6** Shoulder Muscle, Left **7** Upper Arm Muscle, Right **8** Upper Arm Muscle, Left **9** Lower Arm and Wrist Muscle, Right **B** Lower Arm and Wrist Muscle, Left **C** Hand Muscle, Right **D** Hand Muscle, Left **F** Trunk Muscle, Right **G** Trunk Muscle, Left **H** Thorax Muscle, Right **J** Thorax Muscle, Left **K** Abdomen Muscle, Right **L** Abdomen Muscle, Left **M** Perineum Muscle **N** Hip Muscle, Right **P** Hip Muscle, Left **Q** Upper Leg Muscle, Right **R** Upper Leg Muscle, Left **S** Lower Leg Muscle, Right **T** Lower Leg Muscle, Left **V** Foot Muscle, Right **W** Foot Muscle, Left	**0** Open **3** Percutaneous **4** Percutaneous Endoscopic	**Z** No Device	**Z** No Qualifier

0 Medical and Surgical
K Muscles
R Replacement: Putting in or on biological or synthetic material that physically takes the place and/or function of all or a portion of a body part

Body Part Character 4	Approach Character 5	Device Character 6	Qualifier Character 7
0 Head Muscle **1** Facial Muscle **2** Neck Muscle, Right **3** Neck Muscle, Left **4** Tongue, Palate, Pharynx Muscle **5** Shoulder Muscle, Right **6** Shoulder Muscle, Left **7** Upper Arm Muscle, Right **8** Upper Arm Muscle, Left **9** Lower Arm and Wrist Muscle, Right **B** Lower Arm and Wrist Muscle, Left **C** Hand Muscle, Right **D** Hand Muscle, Left **F** Trunk Muscle, Right **G** Trunk Muscle, Left **H** Thorax Muscle, Right **J** Thorax Muscle, Left **K** Abdomen Muscle, Right **L** Abdomen Muscle, Left **M** Perineum Muscle **N** Hip Muscle, Right **P** Hip Muscle, Left **Q** Upper Leg Muscle, Right **R** Upper Leg Muscle, Left **S** Lower Leg Muscle, Right **T** Lower Leg Muscle, Left **V** Foot Muscle, Right **W** Foot Muscle, Left	**0** Open **4** Percutaneous Endoscopic	**7** Autologous Tissue Substitute **J** Synthetic Substitute **K** Nonautologous Tissue Substitute	**Z** No Qualifier

0 **Medical and Surgical**
K **Muscles**
S **Reposition:** Moving to its normal location, or other suitable location, all or a portion of a body part

Body Part Character 4	Approach Character 5	Device Character 6	Qualifier Character 7
0 Head Muscle 1 Facial Muscle 2 Neck Muscle, Right 3 Neck Muscle, Left 4 Tongue, Palate, Pharynx Muscle 5 Shoulder Muscle, Right 6 Shoulder Muscle, Left 7 Upper Arm Muscle, Right 8 Upper Arm Muscle, Left 9 Lower Arm and Wrist Muscle, Right B Lower Arm and Wrist Muscle, Left C Hand Muscle, Right D Hand Muscle, Left F Trunk Muscle, Right G Trunk Muscle, Left H Thorax Muscle, Right J Thorax Muscle, Left K Abdomen Muscle, Right L Abdomen Muscle, Left M Perineum Muscle N Hip Muscle, Right P Hip Muscle, Left Q Upper Leg Muscle, Right R Upper Leg Muscle, Left S Lower Leg Muscle, Right T Lower Leg Muscle, Left V Foot Muscle, Right W Foot Muscle, Left	0 Open 4 Percutaneous Endoscopic	Z No Device	Z No Qualifier

0 **Medical and Surgical**
K **Muscles**
T **Resection:** Cutting out or off, without replacement, all of a body part

Body Part Character 4	Approach Character 5	Device Character 6	Qualifier Character 7
0 Head Muscle 1 Facial Muscle 2 Neck Muscle, Right 3 Neck Muscle, Left 4 Tongue, Palate, Pharynx Muscle 5 Shoulder Muscle, Right 6 Shoulder Muscle, Left 7 Upper Arm Muscle, Right 8 Upper Arm Muscle, Left 9 Lower Arm and Wrist Muscle, Right B Lower Arm and Wrist Muscle, Left C Hand Muscle, Right D Hand Muscle, Left F Trunk Muscle, Right G Trunk Muscle, Left H Thorax Muscle, Right CC J Thorax Muscle, Left CC K Abdomen Muscle, Right L Abdomen Muscle, Left M Perineum Muscle N Hip Muscle, Right P Hip Muscle, Left Q Upper Leg Muscle, Right R Upper Leg Muscle, Left S Lower Leg Muscle, Right T Lower Leg Muscle, Left V Foot Muscle, Right W Foot Muscle, Left	0 Open 4 Percutaneous Endoscopic	Z No Device	Z No Qualifier

CC 0KTH0ZZ 0KTJ0ZZ

LC Limited Coverage NC Noncovered HAC HAC-associated Procedure CC Combination Cluster - See Appendix G for code lists
Non-OR-Affecting MS-DRG Assignment New/Revised Text in **Orange** ♂ Male ♀ Female

0 Medical and Surgical
K Muscles
U Supplement: Putting in or on biological or synthetic material that physically reinforces and/or augments the function of a portion of a body part

Body Part Character 4	Approach Character 5	Device Character 6	Qualifier Character 7
0 Head Muscle **1** Facial Muscle **2** Neck Muscle, Right **3** Neck Muscle, Left **4** Tongue, Palate, Pharynx Muscle **5** Shoulder Muscle, Right **6** Shoulder Muscle, Left **7** Upper Arm Muscle, Right **8** Upper Arm Muscle, Left **9** Lower Arm and Wrist Muscle, Right **B** Lower Arm and Wrist Muscle, Left **C** Hand Muscle, Right **D** Hand Muscle, Left **F** Trunk Muscle, Right **G** Trunk Muscle, Left **H** Thorax Muscle, Right **J** Thorax Muscle, Left **K** Abdomen Muscle, Right **L** Abdomen Muscle, Left **M** Perineum Muscle **N** Hip Muscle, Right **P** Hip Muscle, Left **Q** Upper Leg Muscle, Right **R** Upper Leg Muscle, Left **S** Lower Leg Muscle, Right **T** Lower Leg Muscle, Left **V** Foot Muscle, Right **W** Foot Muscle, Left	**0** Open **4** Percutaneous Endoscopic	**7** Autologous Tissue Substitute **J** Synthetic Substitute **K** Nonautologous Tissue Substitute	**Z** No Qualifier

0 Medical and Surgical
K Muscles
W Revision: Correcting, to the extent possible, a portion of a malfunctioning device or the position of a displaced device

Body Part Character 4	Approach Character 5	Device Character 6	Qualifier Character 7
X Upper Muscle **Y** Lower Muscle	**0** Open **3** Percutaneous **4** Percutaneous Endoscopic	**0** Drainage Device **7** Autologous Tissue Substitute **J** Synthetic Substitute **K** Nonautologous Tissue Substitute **M** Stimulator Lead **Y** Other Device	**Z** No Qualifier
X Upper Muscle **Y** Lower Muscle	**X** External	**0** Drainage Device **7** Autologous Tissue Substitute **J** Synthetic Substitute **K** Nonautologous Tissue Substitute **M** Stimulator Lead	**Z** No Qualifier

0 Medical and Surgical
K Muscles
X Transfer: Moving, without taking out, all or a portion of a body part to another location to take over the function of all or a portion of a body part

Body Part Character 4	Approach Character 5	Device Character 6	Qualifier Character 7
0 Head Muscle **1** Facial Muscle **2** Neck Muscle, Right **3** Neck Muscle, Left **4** Tongue, Palate, Pharynx Muscle **5** Shoulder Muscle, Right **6** Shoulder Muscle, Left **7** Upper Arm Muscle, Right **8** Upper Arm Muscle, Left **9** Lower Arm and Wrist Muscle, Right **B** Lower Arm and Wrist Muscle, Left **C** Hand Muscle, Right **D** Hand Muscle, Left **H** Thorax Muscle, Right **J** Thorax Muscle, Left **M** Perineum Muscle **N** Hip Muscle, Right **P** Hip Muscle, Left **Q** Upper Leg Muscle, Right **R** Upper Leg Muscle, Left **S** Lower Leg Muscle, Right **T** Lower Leg Muscle, Left **V** Foot Muscle, Right **W** Foot Muscle, Left	**0** Open **4** Percutaneous Endoscopic	**Z** No Device	**0** Skin **1** Subcutaneous Tissue **2** Skin and Subcutaneous Tissue **Z** No Qualifier
F Trunk Muscle, Right **G** Trunk Muscle, Left	**0** Open **4** Percutaneous Endoscopic	**Z** No Device	**0** Skin **1** Subcutaneous Tissue **2** Skin and Subcutaneous Tissue **5** Latissimus Dorsi Myocutaneous Flap **7** Deep Inferior Epigastric Artery Perforator Flap **8** Superficial Inferior Epigastric Artery Flap **9** Gluteal Artery Perforator Flap **Z** No Qualifier
K Abdomen Muscle, Right **L** Abdomen Muscle, Left	**0** Open **4** Percutaneous Endoscopic	**Z** No Device	**0** Skin **1** Subcutaneous Tissue **2** Skin and Subcutaneous Tissue **6** Transverse Rectus Abdominis Myocutaneous Flap **Z** No Qualifier

NOTES

Tendons 0L2-0LX

0 Medical and Surgical
L Tendons
2 Change: Taking out or off a device from a body part and putting back an identical or similar device in or on the same body part without cutting or puncturing the skin or a mucous membrane

Body Part Character 4	Approach Character 5	Device Character 6	Qualifier Character 7
X Upper Tendon Y Lower Tendon	X External	0 Drainage Device Y Other Device	Z No Qualifier

0 Medical and Surgical
L Tendons
5 Destruction: Physical eradication of all or a portion of a body part by the direct use of energy, force, or a destructive agent

Body Part Character 4	Approach Character 5	Device Character 6	Qualifier Character 7
0 Head and Neck Tendon 1 Shoulder Tendon, Right 2 Shoulder Tendon, Left 3 Upper Arm Tendon, Right 4 Upper Arm Tendon, Left 5 Lower Arm and Wrist Tendon, Right 6 Lower Arm and Wrist Tendon, Left 7 Hand Tendon, Right 8 Hand Tendon, Left 9 Trunk Tendon, Right B Trunk Tendon, Left C Thorax Tendon, Right D Thorax Tendon, Left F Abdomen Tendon, Right G Abdomen Tendon, Left H Perineum Tendon J Hip Tendon, Right K Hip Tendon, Left L Upper Leg Tendon, Right M Upper Leg Tendon, Left N Lower Leg Tendon, Right P Lower Leg Tendon, Left Q Knee Tendon, Right R Knee Tendon, Left S Ankle Tendon, Right T Ankle Tendon, Left V Foot Tendon, Right W Foot Tendon, Left	0 Open 3 Percutaneous 4 Percutaneous Endoscopic	Z No Device	Z No Qualifier

0 Medical and Surgical
L Tendons
8 Division: Cutting into a body part, without draining fluids and/or gases from the body part, in order to separate or transect a body part

Body Part Character 4	Approach Character 5	Device Character 6	Qualifier Character 7
0 Head and Neck Tendon **1** Shoulder Tendon, Right **2** Shoulder Tendon, Left **3** Upper Arm Tendon, Right **4** Upper Arm Tendon, Left **5** Lower Arm and Wrist Tendon, Right **6** Lower Arm and Wrist Tendon, Left **7** Hand Tendon, Right **8** Hand Tendon, Left **9** Trunk Tendon, Right **B** Trunk Tendon, Left **C** Thorax Tendon, Right **D** Thorax Tendon, Left **F** Abdomen Tendon, Right **G** Abdomen Tendon, Left **H** Perineum Tendon **J** Hip Tendon, Right **K** Hip Tendon, Left **L** Upper Leg Tendon, Right **M** Upper Leg Tendon, Left **N** Lower Leg Tendon, Right **P** Lower Leg Tendon, Left **Q** Knee Tendon, Right **R** Knee Tendon, Left **S** Ankle Tendon, Right **T** Ankle Tendon, Left **V** Foot Tendon, Right **W** Foot Tendon, Left	**0** Open **3** Percutaneous **4** Percutaneous Endoscopic	**Z** No Device	**Z** No Qualifier

0 Medical and Surgical
L Tendons
9 Drainage: Taking or letting out fluids and/or gases from a body part

Body Part Character 4	Approach Character 5	Device Character 6	Qualifier Character 7
0 Head and Neck Tendon 1 Shoulder Tendon, Right 2 Shoulder Tendon, Left 3 Upper Arm Tendon, Right 4 Upper Arm Tendon, Left 5 Lower Arm and Wrist Tendon, Right 6 Lower Arm and Wrist Tendon, Left 7 Hand Tendon, Right 8 Hand Tendon, Left 9 Trunk Tendon, Right B Trunk Tendon, Left C Thorax Tendon, Right D Thorax Tendon, Left F Abdomen Tendon, Right G Abdomen Tendon, Left H Perineum Tendon J Hip Tendon, Right K Hip Tendon, Left L Upper Leg Tendon, Right M Upper Leg Tendon, Left N Lower Leg Tendon, Right P Lower Leg Tendon, Left Q Knee Tendon, Right R Knee Tendon, Left S Ankle Tendon, Right T Ankle Tendon, Left V Foot Tendon, Right W Foot Tendon, Left	0 Open 3 Percutaneous 4 Percutaneous Endoscopic	0 Drainage Device	Z No Qualifier
0 Head and Neck Tendon 1 Shoulder Tendon, Right 2 Shoulder Tendon, Left 3 Upper Arm Tendon, Right 4 Upper Arm Tendon, Left 5 Lower Arm and Wrist Tendon, Right 6 Lower Arm and Wrist Tendon, Left 7 Hand Tendon, Right 8 Hand Tendon, Left 9 Trunk Tendon, Right B Trunk Tendon, Left C Thorax Tendon, Right D Thorax Tendon, Left F Abdomen Tendon, Right G Abdomen Tendon, Left H Perineum Tendon J Hip Tendon, Right K Hip Tendon, Left L Upper Leg Tendon, Right M Upper Leg Tendon, Left N Lower Leg Tendon, Right P Lower Leg Tendon, Left Q Knee Tendon, Right R Knee Tendon, Left S Ankle Tendon, Right T Ankle Tendon, Left V Foot Tendon, Right W Foot Tendon, Left	0 Open 3 Percutaneous 4 Percutaneous Endoscopic	Z No Device	X Diagnostic Z No Qualifier

0 Medical and Surgical
L Tendons
B Excision: Cutting out or off, without replacement, a portion of a body part

Body Part Character 4	Approach Character 5	Device Character 6	Qualifier Character 7
0 Head and Neck Tendon **1** Shoulder Tendon, Right **2** Shoulder Tendon, Left **3** Upper Arm Tendon, Right **4** Upper Arm Tendon, Left **5** Lower Arm and Wrist Tendon, Right **6** Lower Arm and Wrist Tendon, Left **7** Hand Tendon, Right **8** Hand Tendon, Left **9** Trunk Tendon, Right **B** Trunk Tendon, Left **C** Thorax Tendon, Right **D** Thorax Tendon, Left **F** Abdomen Tendon, Right **G** Abdomen Tendon, Left **H** Perineum Tendon **J** Hip Tendon, Right **K** Hip Tendon, Left **L** Upper Leg Tendon, Right **M** Upper Leg Tendon, Left **N** Lower Leg Tendon, Right **P** Lower Leg Tendon, Left **Q** Knee Tendon, Right **R** Knee Tendon, Left **S** Ankle Tendon, Right **T** Ankle Tendon, Left **V** Foot Tendon, Right **W** Foot Tendon, Left	**0** Open **3** Percutaneous **4** Percutaneous Endoscopic	**Z** No Device	**X** Diagnostic **Z** No Qualifier

0LB50ZZ- Excision of R L arm & tendon, open approach

0 Medical and Surgical
L Tendons
C Extirpation: Taking or cutting out solid matter from a body part

Body Part Character 4	Approach Character 5	Device Character 6	Qualifier Character 7
0 Head and Neck Tendon **1** Shoulder Tendon, Right **2** Shoulder Tendon, Left **3** Upper Arm Tendon, Right **4** Upper Arm Tendon, Left **5** Lower Arm and Wrist Tendon, Right **6** Lower Arm and Wrist Tendon, Left **7** Hand Tendon, Right **8** Hand Tendon, Left **9** Trunk Tendon, Right **B** Trunk Tendon, Left **C** Thorax Tendon, Right **D** Thorax Tendon, Left **F** Abdomen Tendon, Right **G** Abdomen Tendon, Left **H** Perineum Tendon **J** Hip Tendon, Right **K** Hip Tendon, Left **L** Upper Leg Tendon, Right **M** Upper Leg Tendon, Left **N** Lower Leg Tendon, Right **P** Lower Leg Tendon, Left **Q** Knee Tendon, Right **R** Knee Tendon, Left **S** Ankle Tendon, Right **T** Ankle Tendon, Left **V** Foot Tendon, Right **W** Foot Tendon, Left	**0** Open **3** Percutaneous **4** Percutaneous Endoscopic	**Z** No Device	**Z** No Qualifier

0 Medical and Surgical
L Tendons
D Extraction: Pulling or stripping out or off all or a portion of a body part by the use of force

Body Part Character 4	Approach Character 5	Device Character 6	Qualifier Character 7
0 Head and Neck Tendon **1** Shoulder Tendon, Right **2** Shoulder Tendon, Left **3** Upper Arm Tendon, Right **4** Upper Arm Tendon, Left **5** Lower Arm and Wrist Tendon, Right **6** Lower Arm and Wrist Tendon, Left **7** Hand Tendon, Right **8** Hand Tendon, Left **9** Trunk Tendon, Right **B** Trunk Tendon, Left **C** Thorax Tendon, Right **D** Thorax Tendon, Left **F** Abdomen Tendon, Right **G** Abdomen Tendon, Left **H** Perineum Tendon **J** Hip Tendon, Right **K** Hip Tendon, Left **L** Upper Leg Tendon, Right **M** Upper Leg Tendon, Left **N** Lower Leg Tendon, Right **P** Lower Leg Tendon, Left **Q** Knee Tendon, Right **R** Knee Tendon, Left **S** Ankle Tendon, Right **T** Ankle Tendon, Left **V** Foot Tendon, Right **W** Foot Tendon, Left	**0** Open	**Z** No Device	**Z** No Qualifier

0 Medical and Surgical
L Tendons
H Insertion: Putting in a nonbiological appliance that monitors, assists, performs, or prevents a physiological function but does not physically take the place of a body part

Body Part Character 4	Approach Character 5	Device Character 6	Qualifier Character 7
X Upper Tendon **Y** Lower Tendon	**0** Open **3** Percutaneous **4** Percutaneous Endoscopic	**Y** Other Device	**Z** No Qualifier

0 Medical and Surgical
L Tendons
J Inspection: Visually and/or manually exploring a body part

Body Part Character 4	Approach Character 5	Device Character 6	Qualifier Character 7
X Upper Tendon **Y** Lower Tendon	**0** Open **3** Percutaneous **4** Percutaneous Endoscopic **X** External	**Z** No Device	**Z** No Qualifier

0 Medical and Surgical
L Tendons
M Reattachment: Putting back in or on all or a portion of a separated body part to its normal location or other suitable location

Body Part Character 4	Approach Character 5	Device Character 6	Qualifier Character 7
0 Head and Neck Tendon **1** Shoulder Tendon, Right **2** Shoulder Tendon, Left **3** Upper Arm Tendon, Right **4** Upper Arm Tendon, Left **5** Lower Arm and Wrist Tendon, Right **6** Lower Arm and Wrist Tendon, Left **7** Hand Tendon, Right **8** Hand Tendon, Left **9** Trunk Tendon, Right **B** Trunk Tendon, Left **C** Thorax Tendon, Right **D** Thorax Tendon, Left **F** Abdomen Tendon, Right **G** Abdomen Tendon, Left **H** Perineum Tendon **J** Hip Tendon, Right **K** Hip Tendon, Left **L** Upper Leg Tendon, Right **M** Upper Leg Tendon, Left **N** Lower Leg Tendon, Right **P** Lower Leg Tendon, Left **Q** Knee Tendon, Right **R** Knee Tendon, Left **S** Ankle Tendon, Right **T** Ankle Tendon, Left **V** Foot Tendon, Right **W** Foot Tendon, Left	**0** Open **4** Percutaneous Endoscopic	**Z** No Device	**Z** No Qualifier

0 Medical and Surgical
L Tendons
N Release: Freeing a body part from an abnormal physical constraint by cutting or by the use of force

Body Part Character 4	Approach Character 5	Device Character 6	Qualifier Character 7
0 Head and Neck Tendon **1** Shoulder Tendon, Right **2** Shoulder Tendon, Left **3** Upper Arm Tendon, Right **4** Upper Arm Tendon, Left **5** Lower Arm and Wrist Tendon, Right **6** Lower Arm and Wrist Tendon, Left **7** Hand Tendon, Right **8** Hand Tendon, Left **9** Trunk Tendon, Right **B** Trunk Tendon, Left **C** Thorax Tendon, Right **D** Thorax Tendon, Left **F** Abdomen Tendon, Right **G** Abdomen Tendon, Left **H** Perineum Tendon **J** Hip Tendon, Right **K** Hip Tendon, Left **L** Upper Leg Tendon, Right **M** Upper Leg Tendon, Left **N** Lower Leg Tendon, Right **P** Lower Leg Tendon, Left achilles AKA cal caneal tendon **Q** Knee Tendon, Right **R** Knee Tendon, Left **S** Ankle Tendon, Right **T** Ankle Tendon, Left **V** Foot Tendon, Right **W** Foot Tendon, Left	**0** Open **3** Percutaneous **4** Percutaneous Endoscopic **X** External	**Z** No Device	**Z** No Qualifier

0 Medical and Surgical
L Tendons
P Removal: Taking out or off a device from a body part

Body Part Character 4	Approach Character 5	Device Character 6	Qualifier Character 7
X Upper Tendon **Y** Lower Tendon	**0** Open **3** Percutaneous **4** Percutaneous Endoscopic	**0** Drainage Device **7** Autologous Tissue Substitute **J** Synthetic Substitute **K** Nonautologous Tissue Substitute **Y** Other Device	**Z** No Qualifier
X Upper Tendon **Y** Lower Tendon	**X** External	**0** Drainage Device	**Z** No Qualifier

0 Medical and Surgical
L Tendons
Q Repair: Restoring, to the extent possible, a body part to its normal anatomic structure and function

Body Part Character 4	Approach Character 5	Device Character 6	Qualifier Character 7
0 Head and Neck Tendon **1** Shoulder Tendon, Right **2** Shoulder Tendon, Left **3** Upper Arm Tendon, Right **4** Upper Arm Tendon, Left **5** Lower Arm and Wrist Tendon, Right **6** Lower Arm and Wrist Tendon, Left **7** Hand Tendon, Right **8** Hand Tendon, Left **9** Trunk Tendon, Right **B** Trunk Tendon, Left **C** Thorax Tendon, Right **D** Thorax Tendon, Left **F** Abdomen Tendon, Right **G** Abdomen Tendon, Left **H** Perineum Tendon **J** Hip Tendon, Right **K** Hip Tendon, Left **L** Upper Leg Tendon, Right **M** Upper Leg Tendon, Left **N** Lower Leg Tendon, Right **P** Lower Leg Tendon, Left **Q** Knee Tendon, Right **R** Knee Tendon, Left **S** Ankle Tendon, Right **T** Ankle Tendon, Left **V** Foot Tendon, Right **W** Foot Tendon, Left	**0** Open **3** Percutaneous **4** Percutaneous Endoscopic	**Z** No Device	**Z** No Qualifier

0 Medical and Surgical
L Tendons
R Replacement: Putting in or on biological or synthetic material that physically takes the place and/or function of all or a portion of a body part

Body Part Character 4	Approach Character 5	Device Character 6	Qualifier Character 7
0 Head and Neck Tendon **1** Shoulder Tendon, Right **2** Shoulder Tendon, Left **3** Upper Arm Tendon, Right **4** Upper Arm Tendon, Left **5** Lower Arm and Wrist Tendon, Right **6** Lower Arm and Wrist Tendon, Left **7** Hand Tendon, Right **8** Hand Tendon, Left **9** Trunk Tendon, Right **B** Trunk Tendon, Left **C** Thorax Tendon, Right **D** Thorax Tendon, Left **F** Abdomen Tendon, Right **G** Abdomen Tendon, Left **H** Perineum Tendon **J** Hip Tendon, Right **K** Hip Tendon, Left **L** Upper Leg Tendon, Right **M** Upper Leg Tendon, Left **N** Lower Leg Tendon, Right **P** Lower Leg Tendon, Left **Q** Knee Tendon, Right **R** Knee Tendon, Left **S** Ankle Tendon, Right **T** Ankle Tendon, Left **V** Foot Tendon, Right **W** Foot Tendon, Left	**0** Open **4** Percutaneous Endoscopic	**7** Autologous Tissue Substitute **J** Synthetic Substitute **K** Nonautologous Tissue Substitute	**Z** No Qualifier

0 Medical and Surgical
L Tendons
S Reposition: Moving to its normal location, or other suitable location, all or a portion of a body part

Body Part Character 4	Approach Character 5	Device Character 6	Qualifier Character 7
0 Head and Neck Tendon **1** Shoulder Tendon, Right **2** Shoulder Tendon, Left **3** Upper Arm Tendon, Right **4** Upper Arm Tendon, Left **5** Lower Arm and Wrist Tendon, Right **6** Lower Arm and Wrist Tendon, Left **7** Hand Tendon, Right **8** Hand Tendon, Left **9** Trunk Tendon, Right **B** Trunk Tendon, Left **C** Thorax Tendon, Right **D** Thorax Tendon, Left **F** Abdomen Tendon, Right **G** Abdomen Tendon, Left **H** Perineum Tendon **J** Hip Tendon, Right **K** Hip Tendon, Left **L** Upper Leg Tendon, Right **M** Upper Leg Tendon, Left **N** Lower Leg Tendon, Right **P** Lower Leg Tendon, Left **Q** Knee Tendon, Right **R** Knee Tendon, Left **S** Ankle Tendon, Right **T** Ankle Tendon, Left **V** Foot Tendon, Right **W** Foot Tendon, Left	**0** Open **4** Percutaneous Endoscopic	**Z** No Device	**Z** No Qualifier

0 Medical and Surgical
L Tendons
T Resection: Cutting out or off, without replacement, all of a body part

Body Part Character 4	Approach Character 5	Device Character 6	Qualifier Character 7
0 Head and Neck Tendon **1** Shoulder Tendon, Right **2** Shoulder Tendon, Left **3** Upper Arm Tendon, Right **4** Upper Arm Tendon, Left **5** Lower Arm and Wrist Tendon, Right **6** Lower Arm and Wrist Tendon, Left **7** Hand Tendon, Right **8** Hand Tendon, Left **9** Trunk Tendon, Right **B** Trunk Tendon, Left **C** Thorax Tendon, Right **D** Thorax Tendon, Left **F** Abdomen Tendon, Right **G** Abdomen Tendon, Left **H** Perineum Tendon **J** Hip Tendon, Right **K** Hip Tendon, Left **L** Upper Leg Tendon, Right **M** Upper Leg Tendon, Left **N** Lower Leg Tendon, Right **P** Lower Leg Tendon, Left **Q** Knee Tendon, Right **R** Knee Tendon, Left **S** Ankle Tendon, Right **T** Ankle Tendon, Left **V** Foot Tendon, Right **W** Foot Tendon, Left	**0** Open **4** Percutaneous Endoscopic	**Z** No Device	**Z** No Qualifier

0 Medical and Surgical
L Tendons
U Supplement: Putting in or on biological or synthetic material that physically reinforces and/or augments the function of a portion of a body part

Body Part Character 4	Approach Character 5	Device Character 6	Qualifier Character 7
0 Head and Neck Tendon **1** Shoulder Tendon, Right **2** Shoulder Tendon, Left **3** Upper Arm Tendon, Right **4** Upper Arm Tendon, Left **5** Lower Arm and Wrist Tendon, Right **6** Lower Arm and Wrist Tendon, Left **7** Hand Tendon, Right **8** Hand Tendon, Left **9** Trunk Tendon, Right **B** Trunk Tendon, Left **C** Thorax Tendon, Right **D** Thorax Tendon, Left **F** Abdomen Tendon, Right **G** Abdomen Tendon, Left **H** Perineum Tendon **J** Hip Tendon, Right **K** Hip Tendon, Left **L** Upper Leg Tendon, Right **M** Upper Leg Tendon, Left **N** Lower Leg Tendon, Right **P** Lower Leg Tendon, Left **Q** Knee Tendon, Right **R** Knee Tendon, Left **S** Ankle Tendon, Right **T** Ankle Tendon, Left **V** Foot Tendon, Right **W** Foot Tendon, Left	**0** Open **4** Percutaneous Endoscopic	**7** Autologous Tissue Substitute **J** Synthetic Substitute **K** Nonautologous Tissue Substitute	**Z** No Qualifier

0 Medical and Surgical
L Tendons
W Revision: Correcting, to the extent possible, a portion of a malfunctioning device or the position of a displaced device

Body Part Character 4	Approach Character 5	Device Character 6	Qualifier Character 7
X Upper Tendon **Y** Lower Tendon	**0** Open **3** Percutaneous **4** Percutaneous Endoscopic	**0** Drainage Device **7** Autologous Tissue Substitute **J** Synthetic Substitute **K** Nonautologous Tissue Substitute **Y** Other Device	**Z** No Qualifier
X Upper Tendon **Y** Lower Tendon	**X** External	**0** Drainage Device **7** Autologous Tissue Substitute **J** Synthetic Substitute **K** Nonautologous Tissue Substitute	**Z** No Qualifier

0 Medical and Surgical
L Tendons
X Transfer: Moving, without taking out, all or a portion of a body part to another location to take over the function of all or a portion of a body part

Body Part Character 4	Approach Character 5	Device Character 6	Qualifier Character 7
0 Head and Neck Tendon **1** Shoulder Tendon, Right **2** Shoulder Tendon, Left **3** Upper Arm Tendon, Right **4** Upper Arm Tendon, Left **5** Lower Arm and Wrist Tendon, Right **6** Lower Arm and Wrist Tendon, Left **7** Hand Tendon, Right **8** Hand Tendon, Left **9** Trunk Tendon, Right **B** Trunk Tendon, Left **C** Thorax Tendon, Right **D** Thorax Tendon, Left **F** Abdomen Tendon, Right **G** Abdomen Tendon, Left **H** Perineum Tendon **J** Hip Tendon, Right **K** Hip Tendon, Left **L** Upper Leg Tendon, Right **M** Upper Leg Tendon, Left **N** Lower Leg Tendon, Right **P** Lower Leg Tendon, Left **Q** Knee Tendon, Right **R** Knee Tendon, Left **S** Ankle Tendon, Right **T** Ankle Tendon, Left **V** Foot Tendon, Right **W** Foot Tendon, Left	**0** Open **4** Percutaneous Endoscopic	**Z** No Device	**Z** No Qualifier

LC Limited Coverage NC Noncovered HAC HAC-associated Procedure CC Combination Cluster - See Appendix G for code lists
DRG Non-OR-Affecting MS-DRG Assignment New/Revised Text in **Orange** ♂ Male ♀ Female

2020 ICD-10-PCS 431

TENDONS 0L2-0LX

NOTES

Bursae and Ligaments 0M2-0MX

0 Medical and Surgical
M Bursae and Ligaments
2 Change: Taking out or off a device from a body part and putting back an identical or similar device in or on the same body part without cutting or puncturing the skin or a mucous membrane

Body Part Character 4	Approach Character 5	Device Character 6	Qualifier Character 7
X Upper Bursa and Ligament **Y** Lower Bursa and Ligament	**X** External	**0** Drainage Device **Y** Other Device	**Z** No Qualifier

0 Medical and Surgical
M Bursae and Ligaments
5 Destruction: Physical eradication of all or a portion of a body part by the direct use of energy, force, or a destructive agent

Body Part Character 4	Approach Character 5	Device Character 6	Qualifier Character 7
0 Head and Neck Bursa and Ligament **1** Shoulder Bursa and Ligament, Right **2** Shoulder Bursa and Ligament, Left **3** Elbow Bursa and Ligament, Right **4** Elbow Bursa and Ligament, Left **5** Wrist Bursa and Ligament, Right **6** Wrist Bursa and Ligament, Left **7** Hand Bursa and Ligament, Right **8** Hand Bursa and Ligament, Left **9** Upper Extremity Bursa and Ligament, Right **B** Upper Extremity Bursa and Ligament, Left **C** Upper Spine Bursa and Ligament **D** Lower Spine Bursa and Ligament **F** Sternum Bursa and Ligament **G** Rib(s) Bursa and Ligament **H** Abdomen Bursa and Ligament, Right **J** Abdomen Bursa and Ligament, Left **K** Perineum Bursa and Ligament **L** Hip Bursa and Ligament, Right **M** Hip Bursa and Ligament, Left **N** Knee Bursa and Ligament, Right **P** Knee Bursa and Ligament, Left **Q** Ankle Bursa and Ligament, Right **R** Ankle Bursa and Ligament, Left **S** Foot Bursa and Ligament, Right **T** Foot Bursa and Ligament, Left **V** Lower Extremity Bursa and Ligament, Right **W** Lower Extremity Bursa and Ligament, Left	**0** Open **3** Percutaneous **4** Percutaneous Endoscopic	**Z** No Device	**Z** No Qualifier

0 Medical and Surgical
M Bursae and Ligaments
8 Division: Cutting into a body part, without draining fluids and/or gases from the body part, in order to separate or transect a body part

Body Part Character 4	Approach Character 5	Device Character 6	Qualifier Character 7
0 Head and Neck Bursa and Ligament **1** Shoulder Bursa and Ligament, Right **2** Shoulder Bursa and Ligament, Left **3** Elbow Bursa and Ligament, Right **4** Elbow Bursa and Ligament, Left **5** Wrist Bursa and Ligament, Right **6** Wrist Bursa and Ligament, Left **7** Hand Bursa and Ligament, Right **8** Hand Bursa and Ligament, Left **9** Upper Extremity Bursa and Ligament, Right **B** Upper Extremity Bursa and Ligament, Left **C** Upper Spine Bursa and Ligament **D** Lower Spine Bursa and Ligament **F** Sternum Bursa and Ligament **G** Rib(s) Bursa and Ligament **H** Abdomen Bursa and Ligament, Right **J** Abdomen Bursa and Ligament, Left **K** Perineum Bursa and Ligament **L** Hip Bursa and Ligament, Right **M** Hip Bursa and Ligament, Left **N** Knee Bursa and Ligament, Right **P** Knee Bursa and Ligament, Left **Q** Ankle Bursa and Ligament, Right **R** Ankle Bursa and Ligament, Left **S** Foot Bursa and Ligament, Right **T** Foot Bursa and Ligament, Left **V** Lower Extremity Bursa and Ligament, Right **W** Lower Extremity Bursa and Ligament, Left	**0** Open **3** Percutaneous **4** Percutaneous Endoscopic	**Z** No Device	**Z** No Qualifier

0 Medical and Surgical
M Bursae and Ligaments
9 Drainage: Taking or letting out fluids and/or gases from a body part

Body Part Character 4	Approach Character 5	Device Character 6	Qualifier Character 7
0 Head and Neck Bursa and Ligament **1** Shoulder Bursa and Ligament, Right **2** Shoulder Bursa and Ligament, Left **3** Elbow Bursa and Ligament, Right **4** Elbow Bursa and Ligament, Left **5** Wrist Bursa and Ligament, Right **6** Wrist Bursa and Ligament, Left **7** Hand Bursa and Ligament, Right **8** Hand Bursa and Ligament, Left **9** Upper Extremity Bursa and Ligament, Right **B** Upper Extremity Bursa and Ligament, Left **C** Upper Spine Bursa and Ligament **D** Lower Spine Bursa and Ligament **F** Sternum Bursa and Ligament **G** Rib(s) Bursa and Ligament **H** Abdomen Bursa and Ligament, Right **J** Abdomen Bursa and Ligament, Left **K** Perineum Bursa and Ligament **L** Hip Bursa and Ligament, Right **M** Hip Bursa and Ligament, Left **N** Knee Bursa and Ligament, Right **P** Knee Bursa and Ligament, Left **Q** Ankle Bursa and Ligament, Right **R** Ankle Bursa and Ligament, Left **S** Foot Bursa and Ligament, Right **T** Foot Bursa and Ligament, Left **V** Lower Extremity Bursa and Ligament, Right **W** Lower Extremity Bursa and Ligament, Left	**0** Open **3** Percutaneous **4** Percutaneous Endoscopic	**0** Drainage Device	**Z** No Qualifier

0M9 continued on next page

0 Medical and Surgical
M Bursae and Ligaments
9 Drainage: Taking or letting out fluids and/or gases from a body part

0M9 continued from previous page

Body Part Character 4	Approach Character 5	Device Character 6	Qualifier Character 7
0 Head and Neck Bursa and Ligament **1** Shoulder Bursa and Ligament, Right **2** Shoulder Bursa and Ligament, Left **3** Elbow Bursa and Ligament, Right **4** Elbow Bursa and Ligament, Left **5** Wrist Bursa and Ligament, Right **6** Wrist Bursa and Ligament, Left **7** Hand Bursa and Ligament, Right **8** Hand Bursa and Ligament, Left **9** Upper Extremity Bursa and Ligament, Right **B** Upper Extremity Bursa and Ligament, Left **C** Upper Spine Bursa and Ligament **D** Lower Spine Bursa and Ligament **F** Sternum Bursa and Ligament **G** Rib(s) Bursa and Ligament **H** Abdomen Bursa and Ligament, Right **J** Abdomen Bursa and Ligament, Left **K** Perineum Bursa and Ligament **L** Hip Bursa and Ligament, Right **M** Hip Bursa and Ligament, Left **N** Knee Bursa and Ligament, Right **P** Knee Bursa and Ligament, Left **Q** Ankle Bursa and Ligament, Right **R** Ankle Bursa and Ligament, Left **S** Foot Bursa and Ligament, Right **T** Foot Bursa and Ligament, Left **V** Lower Extremity Bursa and Ligament, Right **W** Lower Extremity Bursa and Ligament, Left	**0** Open **3** Percutaneous **4** Percutaneous Endoscopic	**Z** No Device	**X** Diagnostic **Z** No Qualifier

0 Medical and Surgical
M Bursae and Ligaments
B Excision: Cutting out or off, without replacement, a portion of a body part

Body Part Character 4	Approach Character 5	Device Character 6	Qualifier Character 7
0 Head and Neck Bursa and Ligament **1** Shoulder Bursa and Ligament, Right **2** Shoulder Bursa and Ligament, Left **3** Elbow Bursa and Ligament, Right **4** Elbow Bursa and Ligament, Left **5** Wrist Bursa and Ligament, Right **6** Wrist Bursa and Ligament, Left **7** Hand Bursa and Ligament, Right **8** Hand Bursa and Ligament, Left **9** Upper Extremity Bursa and Ligament, Right **B** Upper Extremity Bursa and Ligament, Left **C** Upper Spine Bursa and Ligament **D** Lower Spine Bursa and Ligament **F** Sternum Bursa and Ligament **G** Rib(s) Bursa and Ligament **H** Abdomen Bursa and Ligament, Right **J** Abdomen Bursa and Ligament, Left **K** Perineum Bursa and Ligament **L** Hip Bursa and Ligament, Right **M** Hip Bursa and Ligament, Left **N** Knee Bursa and Ligament, Right **P** Knee Bursa and Ligament, Left **Q** Ankle Bursa and Ligament, Right **R** Ankle Bursa and Ligament, Left **S** Foot Bursa and Ligament, Right **T** Foot Bursa and Ligament, Left **V** Lower Extremity Bursa and Ligament, Right **W** Lower Extremity Bursa and Ligament, Left	**0** Open **3** Percutaneous **4** Percutaneous Endoscopic	**Z** No Device	**X** Diagnostic **Z** No Qualifier

0 Medical and Surgical
M Bursae and Ligaments
C Extirpation: Taking or cutting out solid matter from a body part

Body Part Character 4	Approach Character 5	Device Character 6	Qualifier Character 7
0 Head and Neck Bursa and Ligament **1** Shoulder Bursa and Ligament, Right **2** Shoulder Bursa and Ligament, Left **3** Elbow Bursa and Ligament, Right **4** Elbow Bursa and Ligament, Left **5** Wrist Bursa and Ligament, Right **6** Wrist Bursa and Ligament, Left **7** Hand Bursa and Ligament, Right **8** Hand Bursa and Ligament, Left **9** Upper Extremity Bursa and Ligament, Right **B** Upper Extremity Bursa and Ligament, Left **C** Upper Spine Bursa and Ligament **D** Lower Spine Bursa and Ligament **F** Sternum Bursa and Ligament **G** Rib(s) Bursa and Ligament **H** Abdomen Bursa and Ligament, Right **J** Abdomen Bursa and Ligament, Left **K** Perineum Bursa and Ligament **L** Hip Bursa and Ligament, Right **M** Hip Bursa and Ligament, Left **N** Knee Bursa and Ligament, Right **P** Knee Bursa and Ligament, Left **Q** Ankle Bursa and Ligament, Right **R** Ankle Bursa and Ligament, Left **S** Foot Bursa and Ligament, Right **T** Foot Bursa and Ligament, Left **V** Lower Extremity Bursa and Ligament, Right **W** Lower Extremity Bursa and Ligament, Left	**0** Open **3** Percutaneous **4** Percutaneous Endoscopic	**Z** No Device	**Z** No Qualifier

0 Medical and Surgical
M Bursae and Ligaments
D Extraction: Pulling or stripping out or off all or a portion of a body part by the use of force

Body Part Character 4	Approach Character 5	Device Character 6	Qualifier Character 7
0 Head and Neck Bursa and Ligament **1** Shoulder Bursa and Ligament, Right **2** Shoulder Bursa and Ligament, Left **3** Elbow Bursa and Ligament, Right **4** Elbow Bursa and Ligament, Left **5** Wrist Bursa and Ligament, Right **6** Wrist Bursa and Ligament, Left **7** Hand Bursa and Ligament, Right **8** Hand Bursa and Ligament, Left **9** Upper Extremity Bursa and Ligament, Right **B** Upper Extremity Bursa and Ligament, Left **C** Upper Spine Bursa and Ligament **D** Lower Spine Bursa and Ligament **F** Sternum Bursa and Ligament **G** Rib(s) Bursa and Ligament **H** Abdomen Bursa and Ligament, Right **J** Abdomen Bursa and Ligament, Left **K** Perineum Bursa and Ligament **L** Hip Bursa and Ligament, Right **M** Hip Bursa and Ligament, Left **N** Knee Bursa and Ligament, Right **P** Knee Bursa and Ligament, Left **Q** Ankle Bursa and Ligament, Right **R** Ankle Bursa and Ligament, Left **S** Foot Bursa and Ligament, Right **T** Foot Bursa and Ligament, Left **V** Lower Extremity Bursa and Ligament, Right **W** Lower Extremity Bursa and Ligament, Left	**0** Open **3** Percutaneous **4** Percutaneous Endoscopic	**Z** No Device	**Z** No Qualifier

0 Medical and Surgical
M Bursae and Ligaments
H Insertion: Putting in a nonbiological appliance that monitors, assists, performs, or prevents a physiological function but does not physically take the place of a body part

Body Part Character 4	Approach Character 5	Device Character 6	Qualifier Character 7
X Upper Bursa and Ligament **Y** Lower Bursa and Ligament	**0** Open **3** Percutaneous **4** Percutaneous Endoscopic	**Y** Other Device	**Z** No Qualifier

LC Limited Coverage NC Noncovered HAC HAC-associated Procedure CC Combination Cluster - See Appendix G for code lists
DRG Non-OR-Affecting MS-DRG Assignment New/Revised Text in Orange ♂ Male ♀ Female
2020 ICD-10-PCS 439

0 Medical and Surgical
M Bursae and Ligaments
J Inspection: Visually and/or manually exploring a body part

Body Part Character 4	Approach Character 5	Device Character 6	Qualifier Character 7
X Upper Bursa and Ligament Y Lower Bursa and Ligament	0 Open 3 Percutaneous 4 Percutaneous Endoscopic X External	Z No Device	Z No Qualifier

0 Medical and Surgical
M Bursae and Ligaments
M Reattachment: Putting back in or on all or a portion of a separated body part to its normal location or other suitable location

Body Part Character 4	Approach Character 5	Device Character 6	Qualifier Character 7
0 Head and Neck Bursa and Ligament 1 Shoulder Bursa and Ligament, Right 2 Shoulder Bursa and Ligament, Left 3 Elbow Bursa and Ligament, Right 4 Elbow Bursa and Ligament, Left 5 Wrist Bursa and Ligament, Right 6 Wrist Bursa and Ligament, Left 7 Hand Bursa and Ligament, Right 8 Hand Bursa and Ligament, Left 9 Upper Extremity Bursa and Ligament, Right B Upper Extremity Bursa and Ligament, Left C Upper Spine Bursa and Ligament D Lower Spine Bursa and Ligament F Sternum Bursa and Ligament G Rib(s) Bursa and Ligament H Abdomen Bursa and Ligament, Right J Abdomen Bursa and Ligament, Left K Perineum Bursa and Ligament L Hip Bursa and Ligament, Right M Hip Bursa and Ligament, Left N Knee Bursa and Ligament, Right P Knee Bursa and Ligament, Left Q Ankle Bursa and Ligament, Right R Ankle Bursa and Ligament, Left S Foot Bursa and Ligament, Right T Foot Bursa and Ligament, Left V Lower Extremity Bursa and Ligament, Right W Lower Extremity Bursa and Ligament, Left	0 Open 4 Percutaneous Endoscopic	Z No Device	Z No Qualifier

0 Medical and Surgical
M Bursae and Ligaments
N Release: Freeing a body part from an abnormal physical constraint by cutting or by the use of force

Body Part Character 4	Approach Character 5	Device Character 6	Qualifier Character 7
0 Head and Neck Bursa and Ligament **1** Shoulder Bursa and Ligament, Right coracoacromial **2** Shoulder Bursa and Ligament, Left **3** Elbow Bursa and Ligament, Right **4** Elbow Bursa and Ligament, Left **5** Wrist Bursa and Ligament, Right **6** Wrist Bursa and Ligament, Left **7** Hand Bursa and Ligament, Right **8** Hand Bursa and Ligament, Left **9** Upper Extremity Bursa and Ligament, Right **B** Upper Extremity Bursa and Ligament, Left **C** Upper Spine Bursa and Ligament **D** Lower Spine Bursa and Ligament **F** Sternum Bursa and Ligament **G** Rib(s) Bursa and Ligament **H** Abdomen Bursa and Ligament, Right **J** Abdomen Bursa and Ligament, Left **K** Perineum Bursa and Ligament **L** Hip Bursa and Ligament, Right **M** Hip Bursa and Ligament, Left **N** Knee Bursa and Ligament, Right **P** Knee Bursa and Ligament, Left **Q** Ankle Bursa and Ligament, Right **R** Ankle Bursa and Ligament, Left **S** Foot Bursa and Ligament, Right **T** Foot Bursa and Ligament, Left **V** Lower Extremity Bursa and Ligament, Right **W** Lower Extremity Bursa and Ligament, Left	**0** Open **3** Percutaneous **4** Percutaneous Endoscopic arthroscopy **X** External	**Z** No Device	**Z** No Qualifier

0 Medical and Surgical
M Bursae and Ligaments
P Removal: Taking out or off a device from a body part

Body Part Character 4	Approach Character 5	Device Character 6	Qualifier Character 7
X Upper Bursa and Ligament **Y** Lower Bursa and Ligament	**0** Open **3** Percutaneous **4** Percutaneous Endoscopic	**0** Drainage Device **7** Autologous Tissue Substitute **J** Synthetic Substitute **K** Nonautologous Tissue Substitute **Y** Other Device	**Z** No Qualifier
X Upper Bursa and Ligament **Y** Lower Bursa and Ligament	**X** External	**0** Drainage Device	**Z** No Qualifier

0 Medical and Surgical
M Bursae and Ligaments
Q Repair: Restoring, to the extent possible, a body part to its normal anatomic structure and function

Body Part Character 4	Approach Character 5	Device Character 6	Qualifier Character 7
0 Head and Neck Bursa and Ligament **1** Shoulder Bursa and Ligament, Right **2** Shoulder Bursa and Ligament, Left **3** Elbow Bursa and Ligament, Right **4** Elbow Bursa and Ligament, Left **5** Wrist Bursa and Ligament, Right **6** Wrist Bursa and Ligament, Left **7** Hand Bursa and Ligament, Right **8** Hand Bursa and Ligament, Left **9** Upper Extremity Bursa and Ligament, Right **B** Upper Extremity Bursa and Ligament, Left **C** Upper Spine Bursa and Ligament **D** Lower Spine Bursa and Ligament **F** Sternum Bursa and Ligament **G** Rib(s) Bursa and Ligament **H** Abdomen Bursa and Ligament, Right **J** Abdomen Bursa and Ligament, Left **K** Perineum Bursa and Ligament **L** Hip Bursa and Ligament, Right **M** Hip Bursa and Ligament, Left **N** Knee Bursa and Ligament, Right **P** Knee Bursa and Ligament, Left **Q** Ankle Bursa and Ligament, Right **R** Ankle Bursa and Ligament, Left **S** Foot Bursa and Ligament, Right **T** Foot Bursa and Ligament, Left **V** Lower Extremity Bursa and Ligament, Right **W** Lower Extremity Bursa and Ligament, Left	**0** Open **3** Percutaneous **4** Percutaneous Endoscopic	**Z** No Device	**Z** No Qualifier

0 Medical and Surgical
M Bursae and Ligaments
R Replacement: Putting in or on biological or synthetic material that physically takes the place and/or function of all or a portion of a body part

Body Part Character 4	Approach Character 5	Device Character 6	Qualifier Character 7
0 Head and Neck Bursa and Ligament **1** Shoulder Bursa and Ligament, Right **2** Shoulder Bursa and Ligament, Left **3** Elbow Bursa and Ligament, Right **4** Elbow Bursa and Ligament, Left **5** Wrist Bursa and Ligament, Right **6** Wrist Bursa and Ligament, Left **7** Hand Bursa and Ligament, Right **8** Hand Bursa and Ligament, Left **9** Upper Extremity Bursa and Ligament, Right **B** Upper Extremity Bursa and Ligament, Left **C** Upper Spine Bursa and Ligament **D** Lower Spine Bursa and Ligament **F** Sternum Bursa and Ligament **G** Rib(s) Bursa and Ligament **H** Abdomen Bursa and Ligament, Right **J** Abdomen Bursa and Ligament, Left **K** Perineum Bursa and Ligament **L** Hip Bursa and Ligament, Right **M** Hip Bursa and Ligament, Left **N** Knee Bursa and Ligament, Right **P** Knee Bursa and Ligament, Left **Q** Ankle Bursa and Ligament, Right **R** Ankle Bursa and Ligament, Left **S** Foot Bursa and Ligament, Right **T** Foot Bursa and Ligament, Left **V** Lower Extremity Bursa and Ligament, Right **W** Lower Extremity Bursa and Ligament, Left	**0** Open **4** Percutaneous Endoscopic	**7** Autologous Tissue Substitute **J** Synthetic Substitute **K** Nonautologous Tissue Substitute	**Z** No Qualifier

0 Medical and Surgical
M Bursae and Ligaments
S Reposition: Moving to its normal location, or other suitable location, all or a portion of a body part

Body Part Character 4	Approach Character 5	Device Character 6	Qualifier Character 7
0 Head and Neck Bursa and Ligament **1** Shoulder Bursa and Ligament, Right **2** Shoulder Bursa and Ligament, Left **3** Elbow Bursa and Ligament, Right **4** Elbow Bursa and Ligament, Left **5** Wrist Bursa and Ligament, Right **6** Wrist Bursa and Ligament, Left **7** Hand Bursa and Ligament, Right **8** Hand Bursa and Ligament, Left **9** Upper Extremity Bursa and Ligament, Right **B** Upper Extremity Bursa and Ligament, Left **C** Upper Spine Bursa and Ligament **D** Lower Spine Bursa and Ligament **F** Sternum Bursa and Ligament **G** Rib(s) Bursa and Ligament **H** Abdomen Bursa and Ligament, Right **J** Abdomen Bursa and Ligament, Left **K** Perineum Bursa and Ligament **L** Hip Bursa and Ligament, Right **M** Hip Bursa and Ligament, Left **N** Knee Bursa and Ligament, Right **P** Knee Bursa and Ligament, Left **Q** Ankle Bursa and Ligament, Right **R** Ankle Bursa and Ligament, Left **S** Foot Bursa and Ligament, Right **T** Foot Bursa and Ligament, Left **V** Lower Extremity Bursa and Ligament, Right **W** Lower Extremity Bursa and Ligament, Left	**0** Open **4** Percutaneous Endoscopic	**Z** No Device	**Z** No Qualifier

0 Medical and Surgical
M Bursae and Ligaments
T Resection: Cutting out or off, without replacement, all of a body part

Body Part Character 4	Approach Character 5	Device Character 6	Qualifier Character 7
0 Head and Neck Bursa and Ligament **1** Shoulder Bursa and Ligament, Right **2** Shoulder Bursa and Ligament, Left **3** Elbow Bursa and Ligament, Right **4** Elbow Bursa and Ligament, Left **5** Wrist Bursa and Ligament, Right **6** Wrist Bursa and Ligament, Left **7** Hand Bursa and Ligament, Right **8** Hand Bursa and Ligament, Left **9** Upper Extremity Bursa and Ligament, Right **B** Upper Extremity Bursa and Ligament, Left **C** Upper Spine Bursa and Ligament **D** Lower Spine Bursa and Ligament **F** Sternum Bursa and Ligament **G** Rib(s) Bursa and Ligament **H** Abdomen Bursa and Ligament, Right **J** Abdomen Bursa and Ligament, Left **K** Perineum Bursa and Ligament **L** Hip Bursa and Ligament, Right **M** Hip Bursa and Ligament, Left **N** Knee Bursa and Ligament, Right **P** Knee Bursa and Ligament, Left **Q** Ankle Bursa and Ligament, Right **R** Ankle Bursa and Ligament, Left **S** Foot Bursa and Ligament, Right **T** Foot Bursa and Ligament, Left **V** Lower Extremity Bursa and Ligament, Right **W** Lower Extremity Bursa and Ligament, Left	**0** Open **4** Percutaneous Endoscopic	**Z** No Device	**Z** No Qualifier

0 Medical and Surgical
M Bursae and Ligaments
U Supplement: Putting in or on biological or synthetic material that physically reinforces and/or augments the function of a portion of a body part

Body Part Character 4	Approach Character 5	Device Character 6	Qualifier Character 7
0 Head and Neck Bursa and Ligament **1** Shoulder Bursa and Ligament, Right **2** Shoulder Bursa and Ligament, Left **3** Elbow Bursa and Ligament, Right **4** Elbow Bursa and Ligament, Left **5** Wrist Bursa and Ligament, Right **6** Wrist Bursa and Ligament, Left **7** Hand Bursa and Ligament, Right **8** Hand Bursa and Ligament, Left **9** Upper Extremity Bursa and Ligament, Right **B** Upper Extremity Bursa and Ligament, Left **C** Upper Spine Bursa and Ligament **D** Lower Spine Bursa and Ligament **F** Sternum Bursa and Ligament **G** Rib(s) Bursa and Ligament **H** Abdomen Bursa and Ligament, Right **J** Abdomen Bursa and Ligament, Left **K** Perineum Bursa and Ligament **L** Hip Bursa and Ligament, Right **M** Hip Bursa and Ligament, Left **N** Knee Bursa and Ligament, Right **P** Knee Bursa and Ligament, Left **Q** Ankle Bursa and Ligament, Right **R** Ankle Bursa and Ligament, Left **S** Foot Bursa and Ligament, Right **T** Foot Bursa and Ligament, Left **V** Lower Extremity Bursa and Ligament, Right **W** Lower Extremity Bursa and Ligament, Left	**0** Open **4** Percutaneous Endoscopic	**7** Autologous Tissue Substitute **J** Synthetic Substitute **K** Nonautologous Tissue Substitute	**Z** No Qualifier

0 Medical and Surgical
M Bursae and Ligaments
W Revision: Correcting, to the extent possible, a portion of a malfunctioning device or the position of a displaced device

Body Part Character 4	Approach Character 5	Device Character 6	Qualifier Character 7
X Upper Bursa and Ligament **Y** Lower Bursa and Ligament	**0** Open **3** Percutaneous **4** Percutaneous Endoscopic	**0** Drainage Device **7** Autologous Tissue Substitute **J** Synthetic Substitute **K** Nonautologous Tissue Substitute **Y** Other Device	**Z** No Qualifier
X Upper Bursa and Ligament **Y** Lower Bursa and Ligament	**X** External	**0** Drainage Device **7** Autologous Tissue Substitute **J** Synthetic Substitute **K** Nonautologous Tissue Substitute	**Z** No Qualifier

0 Medical and Surgical
M Bursae and Ligaments
X Transfer: Moving, without taking out, all or a portion of a body part to another location to take over the function of all or a portion of a body part

Body Part Character 4	Approach Character 5	Device Character 6	Qualifier Character 7
0 Head and Neck Bursa and Ligament **1** Shoulder Bursa and Ligament, Right **2** Shoulder Bursa and Ligament, Left **3** Elbow Bursa and Ligament, Right **4** Elbow Bursa and Ligament, Left **5** Wrist Bursa and Ligament, Right **6** Wrist Bursa and Ligament, Left **7** Hand Bursa and Ligament, Right **8** Hand Bursa and Ligament, Left **9** Upper Extremity Bursa and Ligament, Right **B** Upper Extremity Bursa and Ligament, Left **C** Upper Spine Bursa and Ligament **D** Lower Spine Bursa and Ligament **F** Sternum Bursa and Ligament **G** Rib(s) Bursa and Ligament **H** Abdomen Bursa and Ligament, Right **J** Abdomen Bursa and Ligament, Left **K** Perineum Bursa and Ligament **L** Hip Bursa and Ligament, Right **M** Hip Bursa and Ligament, Left **N** Knee Bursa and Ligament, Right **P** Knee Bursa and Ligament, Left **Q** Ankle Bursa and Ligament, Right **R** Ankle Bursa and Ligament, Left **S** Foot Bursa and Ligament, Right **T** Foot Bursa and Ligament, Left **V** Lower Extremity Bursa and Ligament, Right **W** Lower Extremity Bursa and Ligament, Left	**0** Open **4** Percutaneous Endoscopic	**Z** No Device	**Z** No Qualifier

NOTES

Bone Fractures

1) surgical
2) conservative - thus non surgical such as pain management, immobilization or non-surgical stabilization

Classification

1) open - surgically opened
2) closed - not cut

Reduction - surgical procedure that restores a fracture or dislocation to the correct alignment

Closed Reduction - manipulation of bone fragments back into place w/o surgery

Open Reduction - expose fracture by dissecting tissue layers

ORIF - Open Reduction Internal Fixation - bones reinforced using implants

Immobilization - done prior to surgical reduction - use splint or cast

Head and Facial Bones 0N2-0NW

0 Medical and Surgical
N Head and Facial Bones
2 Change: Taking out or off a device from a body part and putting back an identical or similar device in or on the same body part without cutting or puncturing the skin or a mucous membrane

Body Part Character 4	Approach Character 5	Device Character 6	Qualifier Character 7
0 Skull B Nasal Bone W Facial Bone	X External	0 Drainage Device Y Other Device	Z No Qualifier

0 Medical and Surgical
N Head and Facial Bones
5 Destruction: Physical eradication of all or a portion of a body part by the direct use of energy, force, or a destructive agent

Body Part Character 4	Approach Character 5	Device Character 6	Qualifier Character 7
0 Skull 1 Frontal Bone 3 Parietal Bone, Right 4 Parietal Bone, Left 5 Temporal Bone, Right 6 Temporal Bone, Left 7 Occipital Bone B Nasal Bone C Sphenoid Bone F Ethmoid Bone, Right G Ethmoid Bone, Left H Lacrimal Bone, Right J Lacrimal Bone, Left K Palatine Bone, Right L Palatine Bone, Left M Zygomatic Bone, Right N Zygomatic Bone, Left P Orbit, Right Q Orbit, Left R Maxilla T Mandible, Right V Mandible, Left X Hyoid Bone	0 Open 3 Percutaneous 4 Percutaneous Endoscopic	Z No Device	Z No Qualifier

0 Medical and Surgical
N Head and Facial Bones
8 Division: Cutting into a body part, without draining fluids and/or gases from the body part, in order to separate or transect a body part

Body Part	Approach	Device	Qualifier
Character 4	**Character 5**	**Character 6**	**Character 7**
0 Skull **1** Frontal Bone **3** Parietal Bone, Right **4** Parietal Bone, Left **5** Temporal Bone, Right **6** Temporal Bone, Left **7** Occipital Bone **B** Nasal Bone **C** Sphenoid Bone **F** Ethmoid Bone, Right **G** Ethmoid Bone, Left **H** Lacrimal Bone, Right **J** Lacrimal Bone, Left **K** Palatine Bone, Right **L** Palatine Bone, Left **M** Zygomatic Bone, Right **N** Zygomatic Bone, Left **P** Orbit, Right **Q** Orbit, Left **R** Maxilla **T** Mandible, Right **V** Mandible, Left **X** Hyoid Bone	**0** Open **3** Percutaneous **4** Percutaneous Endoscopic	**Z** No Device	**Z** No Qualifier

0 Medical and Surgical
N Head and Facial Bones
9 Drainage: Taking or letting out fluids and/or gases from a body part

Body Part Character 4	Approach Character 5	Device Character 6	Qualifier Character 7
0 Skull **1** Frontal Bone **3** Parietal Bone, Right **4** Parietal Bone, Left **5** Temporal Bone, Right **6** Temporal Bone, Left **7** Occipital Bone **B** Nasal Bone **C** Sphenoid Bone **F** Ethmoid Bone, Right **G** Ethmoid Bone, Left **H** Lacrimal Bone, Right **J** Lacrimal Bone, Left **K** Palatine Bone, Right **L** Palatine Bone, Left **M** Zygomatic Bone, Right **N** Zygomatic Bone, Left **P** Orbit, Right **Q** Orbit, Left **R** Maxilla **T** Mandible, Right **V** Mandible, Left **X** Hyoid Bone	**0** Open **3** Percutaneous **4** Percutaneous Endoscopic	**0** Drainage Device	**Z** No Qualifier
0 Skull **1** Frontal Bone **3** Parietal Bone, Right **4** Parietal Bone, Left **5** Temporal Bone, Right **6** Temporal Bone, Left **7** Occipital Bone **B** Nasal Bone **C** Sphenoid Bone **F** Ethmoid Bone, Right **G** Ethmoid Bone, Left **H** Lacrimal Bone, Right **J** Lacrimal Bone, Left **K** Palatine Bone, Right **L** Palatine Bone, Left **M** Zygomatic Bone, Right **N** Zygomatic Bone, Left **P** Orbit, Right **Q** Orbit, Left **R** Maxilla **T** Mandible, Right **V** Mandible, Left **X** Hyoid Bone	**0** Open **3** Percutaneous **4** Percutaneous Endoscopic	**Z** No Device	**X** Diagnostic **Z** No Qualifier

0 Medical and Surgical
N Head and Facial Bones
B Excision: Cutting out or off, without replacement, a portion of a body part

Body Part Character 4	Approach Character 5	Device Character 6	Qualifier Character 7
0 Skull **1** Frontal Bone **3** Parietal Bone, Right **4** Parietal Bone, Left **5** Temporal Bone, Right **6** Temporal Bone, Left **7** Occipital Bone **B** Nasal Bone **C** Sphenoid Bone **F** Ethmoid Bone, Right **G** Ethmoid Bone, Left **H** Lacrimal Bone, Right **J** Lacrimal Bone, Left **K** Palatine Bone, Right **L** Palatine Bone, Left **M** Zygomatic Bone, Right **N** Zygomatic Bone, Left **P** Orbit, Right **Q** Orbit, Left **R** Maxilla **T** Mandible, Right **V** Mandible, Left **X** Hyoid Bone	**0** Open **3** Percutaneous **4** Percutaneous Endoscopic	**Z** No Device	**X** Diagnostic **Z** No Qualifier

0 Medical and Surgical
N Head and Facial Bones
C Extirpation: Taking or cutting out solid matter from a body part

Body Part Character 4	Approach Character 5	Device Character 6	Qualifier Character 7
1 Frontal Bone **3** Parietal Bone, Right **4** Parietal Bone, Left **5** Temporal Bone, Right **6** Temporal Bone, Left **7** Occipital Bone **B** Nasal Bone **C** Sphenoid Bone **F** Ethmoid Bone, Right **G** Ethmoid Bone, Left **H** Lacrimal Bone, Right **J** Lacrimal Bone, Left **K** Palatine Bone, Right **L** Palatine Bone, Left **M** Zygomatic Bone, Right **N** Zygomatic Bone, Left **P** Orbit, Right **Q** Orbit, Left **R** Maxilla **T** Mandible, Right **V** Mandible, Left **X** Hyoid Bone	**0** Open **3** Percutaneous **4** Percutaneous Endoscopic	**Z** No Device	**Z** No Qualifier

0 Medical and Surgical
N Head and Facial Bones
D Extraction: Pulling or stripping out or off all or a portion of a body part by the use of force

Body Part Character 4	Approach Character 5	Device Character 6	Qualifier Character 7
0 Skull **1** Frontal Bone **3** Parietal Bone, Right **4** Parietal Bone, Left **5** Temporal Bone, Right **6** Temporal Bone, Left **7** Occipital Bone **B** Nasal Bone **C** Sphenoid Bone **F** Ethmoid Bone, Right **G** Ethmoid Bone, Left **H** Lacrimal Bone, Right **J** Lacrimal Bone, Left **K** Palatine Bone, Right **L** Palatine Bone, Left **M** Zygomatic Bone, Right **N** Zygomatic Bone, Left **P** Orbit, Right **Q** Orbit, Left **R** Maxilla **T** Mandible, Right **V** Mandible, Left **X** Hyoid Bone	**0** Open	**Z** No Device	**Z** No Qualifier

0 Medical and Surgical
N Head and Facial Bones
H Insertion: Putting in a nonbiological appliance that monitors, assists, performs, or prevents a physiological function but does not physically take the place of a body part

Body Part Character 4	Approach Character 5	Device Character 6	Qualifier Character 7
0 Skull CC	**0** Open	**4** Internal Fixation Device **5** External Fixation Device **M** Bone Growth Stimulator **N** Neurostimulator Generator	**Z** No Qualifier
0 Skull	**3** Percutaneous **4** Percutaneous Endoscopic	**4** Internal Fixation Device **5** External Fixation Device **M** Bone Growth Stimulator	**Z** No Qualifier
1 Frontal Bone **3** Parietal Bone, Right **4** Parietal Bone, Left **7** Occipital Bone **C** Sphenoid Bone **F** Ethmoid Bone, Right **G** Ethmoid Bone, Left **H** Lacrimal Bone, Right **J** Lacrimal Bone, Left **K** Palatine Bone, Right **L** Palatine Bone, Left **M** Zygomatic Bone, Right **N** Zygomatic Bone, Left **P** Orbit, Right **Q** Orbit, Left **X** Hyoid Bone	**0** Open **3** Percutaneous **4** Percutaneous Endoscopic	**4** Internal Fixation Device	**Z** No Qualifier
5 Temporal Bone, Right **6** Temporal Bone, Left	**0** Open **3** Percutaneous **4** Percutaneous Endoscopic	**4** Internal Fixation Device **S** Hearing Device	**Z** No Qualifier
B Nasal Bone	**0** Open **3** Percutaneous **4** Percutaneous Endoscopic	**4** Internal Fixation Device **M** Bone Growth Stimulator	**Z** No Qualifier
R Maxilla **T** Mandible, Right **V** Mandible, Left	**0** Open **3** Percutaneous **4** Percutaneous Endoscopic	**4** Internal Fixation Device **5** External Fixation Device	**Z** No Qualifier
W Facial Bone	**0** Open **3** Percutaneous **4** Percutaneous Endoscopic	**M** Bone Growth Stimulator	**Z** No Qualifier

CC 0NH00NZ

0 Medical and Surgical
N Head and Facial Bones
J Inspection: Visually and/or manually exploring a body part

Body Part Character 4	Approach Character 5	Device Character 6	Qualifier Character 7
0 Skull **B** Nasal Bone **W** Facial Bone	**0** Open **3** Percutaneous **4** Percutaneous Endoscopic **X** External	**Z** No Device	**Z** No Qualifier

0 Medical and Surgical
N Head and Facial Bones
N Release: Freeing a body part from an abnormal physical constraint by cutting or by the use of force

Body Part Character 4	Approach Character 5	Device Character 6	Qualifier Character 7
1 Frontal Bone **3** Parietal Bone, Right **4** Parietal Bone, Left **5** Temporal Bone, Right **6** Temporal Bone, Left **7** Occipital Bone **B** Nasal Bone **C** Sphenoid Bone **F** Ethmoid Bone, Right **G** Ethmoid Bone, Left **H** Lacrimal Bone, Right **J** Lacrimal Bone, Left **K** Palatine Bone, Right **L** Palatine Bone, Left **M** Zygomatic Bone, Right **N** Zygomatic Bone, Left **P** Orbit, Right **Q** Orbit, Left **R** Maxilla **T** Mandible, Right **V** Mandible, Left **X** Hyoid Bone	**0** Open **3** Percutaneous **4** Percutaneous Endoscopic	**Z** No Device	**Z** No Qualifier

0 Medical and Surgical
N Head and Facial Bones
P Removal: Taking out or off a device from a body part

Body Part Character 4	Approach Character 5	Device Character 6	Qualifier Character 7
0 Skull	**0** Open	**0** Drainage Device **4** Internal Fixation Device **5** External Fixation Device **7** Autologous Tissue Substitute **J** Synthetic Substitute **K** Nonautologous Tissue Substitute **M** Bone Growth Stimulator **N** Neurostimulator Generator **S** Hearing Device	**Z** No Qualifier
0 Skull	**3** Percutaneous **4** Percutaneous Endoscopic	**0** Drainage Device **4** Internal Fixation Device **5** External Fixation Device **7** Autologous Tissue Substitute **J** Synthetic Substitute **K** Nonautologous Tissue Substitute **M** Bone Growth Stimulator **S** Hearing Device	**Z** No Qualifier
0 Skull	**X** External	**0** Drainage Device **4** Internal Fixation Device **5** External Fixation Device **M** Bone Growth Stimulator **S** Hearing Device	**Z** No Qualifier
B Nasal Bone **W** Facial Bone	**0** Open **3** Percutaneous **4** Percutaneous Endoscopic	**0** Drainage Device **4** Internal Fixation Device **7** Autologous Tissue Substitute **J** Synthetic Substitute **K** Nonautologous Tissue Substitute **M** Bone Growth Stimulator	**Z** No Qualifier
B Nasal Bone **W** Facial Bone	**X** External	**0** Drainage Device **4** Internal Fixation Device **M** Bone Growth Stimulator	**Z** No Qualifier

LC Limited Coverage NC Noncovered HAC HAC-associated Procedure CC Combination Cluster - See Appendix G for code lists
DRG Non-OR-Affecting MS-DRG Assignment New/Revised Text in **Orange** ♂ Male ♀ Female

0 Medical and Surgical
N Head and Facial Bones
Q Repair: Restoring, to the extent possible, a body part to its normal anatomic structure and function

Body Part Character 4	Approach Character 5	Device Character 6	Qualifier Character 7
0 Skull **1** Frontal Bone **3** Parietal Bone, Right **4** Parietal Bone, Left **5** Temporal Bone, Right **6** Temporal Bone, Left **7** Occipital Bone **B** Nasal Bone **C** Sphenoid Bone **F** Ethmoid Bone, Right **G** Ethmoid Bone, Left **H** Lacrimal Bone, Right **J** Lacrimal Bone, Left **K** Palatine Bone, Right **L** Palatine Bone, Left **M** Zygomatic Bone, Right **N** Zygomatic Bone, Left **P** Orbit, Right **Q** Orbit, Left **R** Maxilla **T** Mandible, Right **V** Mandible, Left **X** Hyoid Bone	**0** Open **3** Percutaneous **4** Percutaneous Endoscopic **X** External	**Z** No Device	**Z** No Qualifier

0 Medical and Surgical
N Head and Facial Bones
R Replacement: Putting in or on biological or synthetic material that physically takes the place and/or function of all or a portion of a body part

Body Part Character 4	Approach Character 5	Device Character 6	Qualifier Character 7
0 Skull **1** Frontal Bone **3** Parietal Bone, Right **4** Parietal Bone, Left **5** Temporal Bone, Right **6** Temporal Bone, Left **7** Occipital Bone **B** Nasal Bone **C** Sphenoid Bone **F** Ethmoid Bone, Right **G** Ethmoid Bone, Left **H** Lacrimal Bone, Right **J** Lacrimal Bone, Left **K** Palatine Bone, Right **L** Palatine Bone, Left **M** Zygomatic Bone, Right **N** Zygomatic Bone, Left **P** Orbit, Right **Q** Orbit, Left **R** Maxilla **T** Mandible, Right **V** Mandible, Left **X** Hyoid Bone	**0** Open **3** Percutaneous **4** Percutaneous Endoscopic	**7** Autologous Tissue Substitute **J** Synthetic Substitute **K** Nonautologous Tissue Substitute	**Z** No Qualifier

0 Medical and Surgical
N Head and Facial Bones
S Reposition: Moving to its normal location, or other suitable location, all or a portion of a body part

Body Part Character 4	Approach Character 5	Device Character 6	Qualifier Character 7
0 Skull **R** Maxilla **T** Mandible, Right **V** Mandible, Left	**0** Open **3** Percutaneous **4** Percutaneous Endoscopic	**4** Internal Fixation Device **5** External Fixation Device **Z** No Device	**Z** No Qualifier
0 Skull **R** Maxilla **T** Mandible, Right **V** Mandible, Left	**X** External	**Z** No Device	**Z** No Qualifier
1 Frontal Bone **3** Parietal Bone, Right **4** Parietal Bone, Left **5** Temporal Bone, Right **6** Temporal Bone, Left **7** Occipital Bone **B** Nasal Bone **C** Sphenoid Bone **F** Ethmoid Bone, Right **G** Ethmoid Bone, Left **H** Lacrimal Bone, Right **J** Lacrimal Bone, Left **K** Palatine Bone, Right **L** Palatine Bone, Left **M** Zygomatic Bone, Right **N** Zygomatic Bone, Left **P** Orbit, Right **Q** Orbit, Left **X** Hyoid Bone	**0** Open **3** Percutaneous **4** Percutaneous Endoscopic	**4** Internal Fixation Device **Z** No Device	**Z** No Qualifier
1 Frontal Bone **3** Parietal Bone, Right **4** Parietal Bone, Left **5** Temporal Bone, Right **6** Temporal Bone, Left **7** Occipital Bone **B** Nasal Bone **C** Sphenoid Bone **F** Ethmoid Bone, Right **G** Ethmoid Bone, Left **H** Lacrimal Bone, Right **J** Lacrimal Bone, Left **K** Palatine Bone, Right **L** Palatine Bone, Left **M** Zygomatic Bone, Right **N** Zygomatic Bone, Left **P** Orbit, Right **Q** Orbit, Left **X** Hyoid Bone	**X** External	**Z** No Device	**Z** No Qualifier

0 Medical and Surgical
N Head and Facial Bones
T Resection: Cutting out or off, without replacement, all of a body part

Body Part Character 4	Approach Character 5	Device Character 6	Qualifier Character 7
1 Frontal Bone **3** Parietal Bone, Right **4** Parietal Bone, Left **5** Temporal Bone, Right **6** Temporal Bone, Left **7** Occipital Bone **B** Nasal Bone **C** Sphenoid Bone **F** Ethmoid Bone, Right **G** Ethmoid Bone, Left **H** Lacrimal Bone, Right **J** Lacrimal Bone, Left **K** Palatine Bone, Right **L** Palatine Bone, Left **M** Zygomatic Bone, Right **N** Zygomatic Bone, Left **P** Orbit, Right **Q** Orbit, Left **R** Maxilla **T** Mandible, Right **V** Mandible, Left **X** Hyoid Bone	**0** Open	**Z** No Device	**Z** No Qualifier

0 Medical and Surgical
N Head and Facial Bones
U Supplement: Putting in or on biological or synthetic material that physically reinforces and/or augments the function of a portion of a body part

Body Part Character 4	Approach Character 5	Device Character 6	Qualifier Character 7
0 Skull **1** Frontal Bone **3** Parietal Bone, Right **4** Parietal Bone, Left **5** Temporal Bone, Right **6** Temporal Bone, Left **7** Occipital Bone **B** Nasal Bone **C** Sphenoid Bone **F** Ethmoid Bone, Right **G** Ethmoid Bone, Left **H** Lacrimal Bone, Right **J** Lacrimal Bone, Left **K** Palatine Bone, Right **L** Palatine Bone, Left **M** Zygomatic Bone, Right **N** Zygomatic Bone, Left **P** Orbit, Right **Q** Orbit, Left **R** Maxilla **T** Mandible, Right **V** Mandible, Left **X** Hyoid Bone	**0** Open **3** Percutaneous **4** Percutaneous Endoscopic	**7** Autologous Tissue Substitute **J** Synthetic Substitute **K** Nonautologous Tissue Substitute	**Z** No Qualifier

0 Medical and Surgical
N Head and Facial Bones
W Revision: Correcting, to the extent possible, a portion of a malfunctioning device or the position of a displaced device

Body Part Character 4	Approach Character 5	Device Character 6	Qualifier Character 7
0 Skull	**0** Open	**0** Drainage Device **4** Internal Fixation Device **5** External Fixation Device **7** Autologous Tissue Substitute **J** Synthetic Substitute **K** Nonautologous Tissue Substitute **M** Bone Growth Stimulator **N** Neurostimulator Generator **S** Hearing Device	**Z** No Qualifier
0 Skull	**3** Percutaneous **4** Percutaneous Endoscopic **X** External	**0** Drainage Device **4** Internal Fixation Device **5** External Fixation Device **7** Autologous Tissue Substitute **J** Synthetic Substitute **K** Nonautologous Tissue Substitute **M** Bone Growth Stimulator **S** Hearing Device	**Z** No Qualifier
B Nasal Bone **W** Facial Bone	**0** Open **3** Percutaneous **4** Percutaneous Endoscopic **X** External	**0** Drainage Device **4** Internal Fixation Device **7** Autologous Tissue Substitute **J** Synthetic Substitute **K** Nonautologous Tissue Substitute **M** Bone Growth Stimulator	**Z** No Qualifier

NOTES

Upper Bones 0P2-0PW

0 Medical and Surgical
P Upper Bones
2 Change: Taking out or off a device from a body part and putting back an identical or similar device in or on the same body part without cutting or puncturing the skin or a mucous membrane

Body Part	Approach	Device	Qualifier
Character 4	**Character 5**	**Character 6**	**Character 7**
Y Upper Bone	**X** External	**0** Drainage Device **Y** Other Device	**Z** No Qualifier

0 Medical and Surgical
P Upper Bones
5 Destruction: Physical eradication of all or a portion of a body part by the direct use of energy, force, or a destructive agent

Body Part	Approach	Device	Qualifier
Character 4	**Character 5**	**Character 6**	**Character 7**
0 Sternum **1** Ribs, 1 to 2 **2** Ribs, 3 or More **3** Cervical Vertebra **4** Thoracic Vertebra **5** Scapula, Right **6** Scapula, Left **7** Glenoid Cavity, Right **8** Glenoid Cavity, Left **9** Clavicle, Right **B** Clavicle, Left **C** Humeral Head, Right **D** Humeral Head, Left **F** Humeral Shaft, Right **G** Humeral Shaft, Left **H** Radius, Right **J** Radius, Left **K** Ulna, Right **L** Ulna, Left **M** Carpal, Right **N** Carpal, Left **P** Metacarpal, Right **Q** Metacarpal, Left **R** Thumb Phalanx, Right **S** Thumb Phalanx, Left **T** Finger Phalanx, Right **V** Finger Phalanx, Left	**0** Open **3** Percutaneous **4** Percutaneous Endoscopic	**Z** No Device	**Z** No Qualifier

0 Medical and Surgical
P Upper Bones
8 Division: Cutting into a body part, without draining fluids and/or gases from the body part, in order to separate or transect a body part

Body Part Character 4	Approach Character 5	Device Character 6	Qualifier Character 7
0 Sternum	**0** Open	**Z** No Device	**Z** No Qualifier
1 Ribs, 1 to 2	**3** Percutaneous		
2 Ribs, 3 or More	**4** Percutaneous Endoscopic		
3 Cervical Vertebra			
4 Thoracic Vertebra			
5 Scapula, Right			
6 Scapula, Left			
7 Glenoid Cavity, Right			
8 Glenoid Cavity, Left			
9 Clavicle, Right			
B Clavicle, Left			
C Humeral Head, Right			
D Humeral Head, Left			
F Humeral Shaft, Right			
G Humeral Shaft, Left			
H Radius, Right			
J Radius, Left			
K Ulna, Right			
L Ulna, Left			
M Carpal, Right			
N Carpal, Left capitate			
P Metacarpal, Right			
Q Metacarpal, Left			
R Thumb Phalanx, Right			
S Thumb Phalanx, Left			
T Finger Phalanx, Right			
V Finger Phalanx, Left			

0 Medical and Surgical
P Upper Bones
9 Drainage: Taking or letting out fluids and/or gases from a body part

Body Part Character 4	Approach Character 5	Device Character 6	Qualifier Character 7
0 Sternum **1** Ribs, 1 to 2 **2** Ribs, 3 or More **3** Cervical Vertebra **4** Thoracic Vertebra **5** Scapula, Right **6** Scapula, Left **7** Glenoid Cavity, Right **8** Glenoid Cavity, Left **9** Clavicle, Right **B** Clavicle, Left **C** Humeral Head, Right **D** Humeral Head, Left **F** Humeral Shaft, Right **G** Humeral Shaft, Left **H** Radius, Right **J** Radius, Left **K** Ulna, Right **L** Ulna, Left **M** Carpal, Right **N** Carpal, Left **P** Metacarpal, Right **Q** Metacarpal, Left **R** Thumb Phalanx, Right **S** Thumb Phalanx, Left **T** Finger Phalanx, Right **V** Finger Phalanx, Left	**0** Open **3** Percutaneous **4** Percutaneous Endoscopic	**0** Drainage Device	**Z** No Qualifier
0 Sternum **1** Ribs, 1 to 2 **2** Ribs, 3 or More **3** Cervical Vertebra **4** Thoracic Vertebra **5** Scapula, Right **6** Scapula, Left **7** Glenoid Cavity, Right **8** Glenoid Cavity, Left **9** Clavicle, Right **B** Clavicle, Left **C** Humeral Head, Right **D** Humeral Head, Left **F** Humeral Shaft, Right **G** Humeral Shaft, Left **H** Radius, Right **J** Radius, Left **K** Ulna, Right **L** Ulna, Left **M** Carpal, Right **N** Carpal, Left **P** Metacarpal, Right **Q** Metacarpal, Left **R** Thumb Phalanx, Right **S** Thumb Phalanx, Left **T** Finger Phalanx, Right **V** Finger Phalanx, Left	**0** Open **3** Percutaneous **4** Percutaneous Endoscopic	**Z** No Device	**X** Diagnostic **Z** No Qualifier

0 Medical and Surgical
P Upper Bones
B Excision: Cutting out or off, without replacement, a portion of a body part

Body Part Character 4	Approach Character 5	Device Character 6	Qualifier Character 7
0 Sternum **1** Ribs, 1 to 2 **2** Ribs, 3 or More **3** Cervical Vertebra **4** Thoracic Vertebra **5** Scapula, Right **6** Scapula, Left **7** Glenoid Cavity, Right **8** Glenoid Cavity, Left **9** Clavicle, Right **B** Clavicle, Left **C** Humeral Head, Right **D** Humeral Head, Left **F** Humeral Shaft, Right **G** Humeral Shaft, Left **H** Radius, Right **J** Radius, Left **K** Ulna, Right **L** Ulna, Left **M** Carpal, Right **N** Carpal, Left **P** Metacarpal, Right **Q** Metacarpal, Left **R** Thumb Phalanx, Right **S** Thumb Phalanx, Left **T** Finger Phalanx, Right **V** Finger Phalanx, Left	**0** Open **3** Percutaneous **4** Percutaneous Endoscopic	**Z** No Device	**X** Diagnostic **Z** No Qualifier

0 Medical and Surgical
P Upper Bones
C Extirpation: Taking or cutting out solid matter from a body part

Body Part Character 4	Approach Character 5	Device Character 6	Qualifier Character 7
0 Sternum **1** Ribs, 1 to 2 **2** Ribs, 3 or More **3** Cervical Vertebra **4** Thoracic Vertebra **5** Scapula, Right **6** Scapula, Left **7** Glenoid Cavity, Right **8** Glenoid Cavity, Left **9** Clavicle, Right **B** Clavicle, Left **C** Humeral Head, Right **D** Humeral Head, Left **F** Humeral Shaft, Right **G** Humeral Shaft, Left **H** Radius, Right **J** Radius, Left **K** Ulna, Right **L** Ulna, Left **M** Carpal, Right **N** Carpal, Left **P** Metacarpal, Right **Q** Metacarpal, Left **R** Thumb Phalanx, Right **S** Thumb Phalanx, Left **T** Finger Phalanx, Right **V** Finger Phalanx, Left	**0** Open **3** Percutaneous **4** Percutaneous Endoscopic	**Z** No Device	**Z** No Qualifier

0 Medical and Surgical
P Upper Bones
D Extraction: Pulling or stripping out or off all or a portion of a body part by the use of force

Body Part Character 4	Approach Character 5	Device Character 6	Qualifier Character 7
0 Sternum **1** Ribs, 1 to 2 **2** Ribs, 3 or More **3** Cervical Vertebra **4** Thoracic Vertebra **5** Scapula, Right **6** Scapula, Left **7** Glenoid Cavity, Right **8** Glenoid Cavity, Left **9** Clavicle, Right **B** Clavicle, Left **C** Humeral Head, Right **D** Humeral Head, Left **F** Humeral Shaft, Right **G** Humeral Shaft, Left **H** Radius, Right **J** Radius, Left **K** Ulna, Right **L** Ulna, Left **M** Carpal, Right **N** Carpal, Left **P** Metacarpal, Right **Q** Metacarpal, Left **R** Thumb Phalanx, Right **S** Thumb Phalanx, Left **T** Finger Phalanx, Right **V** Finger Phalanx, Left	**0** Open	**Z** No Device	**Z** No Qualifier

0 Medical and Surgical
P Upper Bones
H Insertion: Putting in a nonbiological appliance that monitors, assists, performs, or prevents a physiological function but does not physically take the place of a body part

Body Part Character 4	Approach Character 5	Device Character 6	Qualifier Character 7
0 Sternum	**0** Open **3** Percutaneous **4** Percutaneous Endoscopic	**0** Internal Fixation Device, Rigid Plate **4** Internal Fixation Device	**Z** No Qualifier
1 Ribs, 1 to 2 **2** Ribs, 3 or More **3** Cervical Vertebra **4** Thoracic Vertebra **5** Scapula, Right **6** Scapula, Left **7** Glenoid Cavity, Right **8** Glenoid Cavity, Left **9** Clavicle, Right **B** Clavicle, Left	**0** Open **3** Percutaneous **4** Percutaneous Endoscopic	**4** Internal Fixation Device	**Z** No Qualifier
C Humeral Head, Right **D** Humeral Head, Left **H** Radius, Right **J** Radius, Left **K** Ulna, Right **L** Ulna, Left	**0** Open **3** Percutaneous **4** Percutaneous Endoscopic	**4** Internal Fixation Device **5** External Fixation Device **6** Internal Fixation Device, Intramedullary **8** External Fixation Device, Limb Lengthening **B** External Fixation Device, Monoplanar **C** External Fixation Device, Ring **D** External Fixation Device, Hybrid	**Z** No Qualifier
F Humeral Shaft, Right **G** Humeral Shaft, Left	**0** Open **3** Percutaneous **4** Percutaneous Endoscopic	**4** Internal Fixation Device **5** External Fixation Device **6** Internal Fixation Device, Intramedullary **7** Internal Fixation Device, Intramedullary Limb Lengthening **8** External Fixation Device, Limb Lengthening **B** External Fixation Device, Monoplanar **C** External Fixation Device, Ring **D** External Fixation Device, Hybrid	**Z** No Qualifier
M Carpal, Right **N** Carpal, Left **P** Metacarpal, Right **Q** Metacarpal, Left **R** Thumb Phalanx, Right **S** Thumb Phalanx, Left **T** Finger Phalanx, Right **V** Finger Phalanx, Left	**0** Open **3** Percutaneous **4** Percutaneous Endoscopic	**4** Internal Fixation Device **5** External Fixation Device	**Z** No Qualifier
Y Upper Bone	**0** Open **3** Percutaneous **4** Percutaneous Endoscopic	**M** Bone Growth Stimulator	**Z** No Qualifier

0 Medical and Surgical
P Upper Bones
J Inspection: Visually and/or manually exploring a body part

Body Part Character 4	Approach Character 5	Device Character 6	Qualifier Character 7
Y Upper Bone	**0** Open **3** Percutaneous **4** Percutaneous Endoscopic **X** External	**Z** No Device	**Z** No Qualifier

0 **Medical and Surgical**
P **Upper Bones**
N **Release:** Freeing a body part from an abnormal physical constraint by cutting or by the use of force

Body Part Character 4	Approach Character 5	Device Character 6	Qualifier Character 7
0 Sternum **1** Ribs, 1 to 2 **2** Ribs, 3 or More **3** Cervical Vertebra **4** Thoracic Vertebra **5** Scapula, Right **6** Scapula, Left **7** Glenoid Cavity, Right **8** Glenoid Cavity, Left **9** Clavicle, Right **B** Clavicle, Left **C** Humeral Head, Right **D** Humeral Head, Left **F** Humeral Shaft, Right **G** Humeral Shaft, Left **H** Radius, Right **J** Radius, Left **K** Ulna, Right **L** Ulna, Left **M** Carpal, Right **N** Carpal, Left **P** Metacarpal, Right **Q** Metacarpal, Left **R** Thumb Phalanx, Right **S** Thumb Phalanx, Left **T** Finger Phalanx, Right **V** Finger Phalanx, Left	**0** Open **3** Percutaneous **4** Percutaneous Endoscopic	**Z** No Device	**Z** No Qualifier

0 **Medical and Surgical**
P **Upper Bones**
P **Removal:** Taking out or off a device from a body part

Body Part Character 4	Approach Character 5	Device Character 6	Qualifier Character 7
0 Sternum **1** Ribs, 1 to 2 **2** Ribs, 3 or More **3** Cervical Vertebra **4** Thoracic Vertebra **5** Scapula, Right **6** Scapula, Left **7** Glenoid Cavity, Right **8** Glenoid Cavity, Left **9** Clavicle, Right **B** Clavicle, Left	**0** Open **3** Percutaneous **4** Percutaneous Endoscopic	**4** Internal Fixation Device **7** Autologous Tissue Substitute **J** Synthetic Substitute **K** Nonautologous Tissue Substitute	**Z** No Qualifier
0 Sternum **1** Ribs, 1 to 2 **2** Ribs, 3 or More **3** Cervical Vertebra **4** Thoracic Vertebra **5** Scapula, Right **6** Scapula, Left **7** Glenoid Cavity, Right **8** Glenoid Cavity, Left **9** Clavicle, Right **B** Clavicle, Left	**X** External	**4** Internal Fixation Device	**Z** No Qualifier

0PP continued on next page

0PP continued from previous page

0 Medical and Surgical
P Upper Bones
P Removal: Taking out or off a device from a body part

Body Part Character 4	Approach Character 5	Device Character 6	Qualifier Character 7
C Humeral Head, Right **D** Humeral Head, Left **F** Humeral Shaft, Right **G** Humeral Shaft, Left **H** Radius, Right **J** Radius, Left **K** Ulna, Right **L** Ulna, Left **M** Carpal, Right **N** Carpal, Left **P** Metacarpal, Right **Q** Metacarpal, Left **R** Thumb Phalanx, Right **S** Thumb Phalanx, Left **T** Finger Phalanx, Right **V** Finger Phalanx, Left	**0** Open **3** Percutaneous **4** Percutaneous Endoscopic	**4** Internal Fixation Device **5** External Fixation Device **7** Autologous Tissue Substitute **J** Synthetic Substitute **K** Nonautologous Tissue Substitute	**Z** No Qualifier
C Humeral Head, Right **D** Humeral Head, Left **F** Humeral Shaft, Right **G** Humeral Shaft, Left **H** Radius, Right **J** Radius, Left **K** Ulna, Right **L** Ulna, Left **M** Carpal, Right **N** Carpal, Left **P** Metacarpal, Right **Q** Metacarpal, Left **R** Thumb Phalanx, Right **S** Thumb Phalanx, Left **T** Finger Phalanx, Right **V** Finger Phalanx, Left	**X** External	**4** Internal Fixation Device **5** External Fixation Device	**Z** No Qualifier
Y Upper Bone	**0** Open **3** Percutaneous **4** Percutaneous Endoscopic **X** External	**0** Drainage Device **M** Bone Growth Stimulator	**Z** No Qualifier

0 Medical and Surgical
P Upper Bones
Q Repair: Restoring, to the extent possible, a body part to its normal anatomic structure and function

Body Part Character 4	Approach Character 5	Device Character 6	Qualifier Character 7
0 Sternum **1** Ribs, 1 to 2 **2** Ribs, 3 or More **3** Cervical Vertebra **4** Thoracic Vertebra **5** Scapula, Right **6** Scapula, Left **7** Glenoid Cavity, Right **8** Glenoid Cavity, Left **9** Clavicle, Right **B** Clavicle, Left **C** Humeral Head, Right **D** Humeral Head, Left **F** Humeral Shaft, Right **G** Humeral Shaft, Left **H** Radius, Right **J** Radius, Left **K** Ulna, Right **L** Ulna, Left **M** Carpal, Right **N** Carpal, Left **P** Metacarpal, Right **Q** Metacarpal, Left **R** Thumb Phalanx, Right **S** Thumb Phalanx, Left **T** Finger Phalanx, Right **V** Finger Phalanx, Left	**0** Open **3** Percutaneous **4** Percutaneous Endoscopic **X** External	**Z** No Device	**Z** No Qualifier

0 Medical and Surgical
P Upper Bones
R Replacement: Putting in or on biological or synthetic material that physically takes the place and/or function of all or a portion of a body part

Body Part Character 4	Approach Character 5	Device Character 6	Qualifier Character 7
0 Sternum **1** Ribs, 1 to 2 **2** Ribs, 3 or More **3** Cervical Vertebra **4** Thoracic Vertebra **5** Scapula, Right **6** Scapula, Left **7** Glenoid Cavity, Right **8** Glenoid Cavity, Left **9** Clavicle, Right **B** Clavicle, Left **C** Humeral Head, Right **D** Humeral Head, Left **F** Humeral Shaft, Right **G** Humeral Shaft, Left **H** Radius, Right **J** Radius, Left **K** Ulna, Right **L** Ulna, Left **M** Carpal, Right **N** Carpal, Left **P** Metacarpal, Right **Q** Metacarpal, Left **R** Thumb Phalanx, Right **S** Thumb Phalanx, Left **T** Finger Phalanx, Right **V** Finger Phalanx, Left	**0** Open **3** Percutaneous **4** Percutaneous Endoscopic	**7** Autologous Tissue Substitute **J** Synthetic Substitute **K** Nonautologous Tissue Substitute	**Z** No Qualifier

0 Medical and Surgical
P Upper Bones
S Reposition: Moving to its normal location, or other suitable location, all or a portion of a body part

Body Part Character 4	Approach Character 5	Device Character 6	Qualifier Character 7
0 Sternum	0 Open 3 Percutaneous 4 Percutaneous Endoscopic	0 Internal Fixation Device, Rigid Plate 4 Internal Fixation Device Z No Device	Z No Qualifier
0 Sternum	X External	Z No Device	Z No Qualifier
1 Ribs, 1 to 2 2 Ribs, 3 or More 3 Cervical Vertebra CC 4 Thoracic Vertebra CC 5 Scapula, Right 6 Scapula, Left 7 Glenoid Cavity, Right 8 Glenoid Cavity, Left 9 Clavicle, Right B Clavicle, Left	0 Open 3 Percutaneous 4 Percutaneous Endoscopic	4 Internal Fixation Device Z No Device	Z No Qualifier
1 Ribs, 1 to 2 2 Ribs, 3 or More 3 Cervical Vertebra 4 Thoracic Vertebra 5 Scapula, Right 6 Scapula, Left 7 Glenoid Cavity, Right 8 Glenoid Cavity, Left 9 Clavicle, Right B Clavicle, Left	X External	Z No Device	Z No Qualifier
C Humeral Head, Right D Humeral Head, Left F Humeral Shaft, Right G Humeral Shaft, Left H Radius, Right J Radius, Left K Ulna, Right L Ulna, Left	0 Open 3 Percutaneous 4 Percutaneous Endoscopic	4 Internal Fixation Device 5 External Fixation Device 6 Internal Fixation Device, Intramedullary B External Fixation Device, Monoplanar C External Fixation Device, Ring D External Fixation Device, Hybrid Z No Device	Z No Qualifier
C Humeral Head, Right D Humeral Head, Left F Humeral Shaft, Right G Humeral Shaft, Left H Radius, Right J Radius, Left K Ulna, Right L Ulna, Left	X External	Z No Device	Z No Qualifier
M Carpal, Right N Carpal, Left P Metacarpal, Right Q Metacarpal, Left R Thumb Phalanx, Right S Thumb Phalanx, Left T Finger Phalanx, Right V Finger Phalanx, Left	0 Open 3 Percutaneous 4 Percutaneous Endoscopic	4 Internal Fixation Device 5 External Fixation Device Z No Device	Z No Qualifier
M Carpal, Right N Carpal, Left P Metacarpal, Right Q Metacarpal, Left R Thumb Phalanx, Right S Thumb Phalanx, Left T Finger Phalanx, Right V Finger Phalanx, Left	X External	Z No Device	Z No Qualifier

CC 0PS33ZZ 0PS43ZZ

0 Medical and Surgical
P Upper Bones
T Resection: Cutting out or off, without replacement, all of a body part

Body Part Character 4	Approach Character 5	Device Character 6	Qualifier Character 7
0 Sternum **1** Ribs, 1 to 2 **2** Ribs, 3 or More **5** Scapula, Right **6** Scapula, Left **7** Glenoid Cavity, Right **8** Glenoid Cavity, Left **9** Clavicle, Right **B** Clavicle, Left **C** Humeral Head, Right **D** Humeral Head, Left **F** Humeral Shaft, Right **G** Humeral Shaft, Left **H** Radius, Right **J** Radius, Left **K** Ulna, Right **L** Ulna, Left **M** Carpal, Right **N** Carpal, Left **P** Metacarpal, Right **Q** Metacarpal, Left **R** Thumb Phalanx, Right **S** Thumb Phalanx, Left **T** Finger Phalanx, Right **V** Finger Phalanx, Left	**0** Open	**Z** No Device	**Z** No Qualifier

0 Medical and Surgical
P Upper Bones
U Supplement: Putting in or on biological or synthetic material that physically reinforces and/or augments the function of a portion of a body part

Body Part Character 4	Approach Character 5	Device Character 6	Qualifier Character 7
0 Sternum **1** Ribs, 1 to 2 **2** Ribs, 3 or More **3** Cervical Vertebra CC **4** Thoracic Vertebra CC **5** Scapula, Right **6** Scapula, Left **7** Glenoid Cavity, Right **8** Glenoid Cavity, Left **9** Clavicle, Right **B** Clavicle, Left **C** Humeral Head, Right **D** Humeral Head, Left **F** Humeral Shaft, Right **G** Humeral Shaft, Left **H** Radius, Right **J** Radius, Left **K** Ulna, Right **L** Ulna, Left **M** Carpal, Right **N** Carpal, Left **P** Metacarpal, Right **Q** Metacarpal, Left **R** Thumb Phalanx, Right **S** Thumb Phalanx, Left **T** Finger Phalanx, Right **V** Finger Phalanx, Left	**0** Open **3** Percutaneous **4** Percutaneous Endoscopic	**7** Autologous Tissue Substitute **J** Synthetic Substitute **K** Nonautologous Tissue Substitute	**Z** No Qualifier

CC 0PU33JZ 0PU43JZ

0 Medical and Surgical
P Upper Bones
W Revision: Correcting, to the extent possible, a portion of a malfunctioning device or the position of a displaced device

Body Part Character 4	Approach Character 5	Device Character 6	Qualifier Character 7
0 Sternum **1** Ribs, 1 to 2 **2** Ribs, 3 or More **3** Cervical Vertebra **4** Thoracic Vertebra **5** Scapula, Right **6** Scapula, Left **7** Glenoid Cavity, Right **8** Glenoid Cavity, Left **9** Clavicle, Right **B** Clavicle, Left	**0** Open **3** Percutaneous **4** Percutaneous Endoscopic **X** External	**4** Internal Fixation Device **7** Autologous Tissue Substitute **J** Synthetic Substitute **K** Nonautologous Tissue Substitute	**Z** No Qualifier
C Humeral Head, Right **D** Humeral Head, Left **F** Humeral Shaft, Right **G** Humeral Shaft, Left **H** Radius, Right **J** Radius, Left **K** Ulna, Right **L** Ulna, Left **M** Carpal, Right **N** Carpal, Left **P** Metacarpal, Right **Q** Metacarpal, Left **R** Thumb Phalanx, Right **S** Thumb Phalanx, Left **T** Finger Phalanx, Right **V** Finger Phalanx, Left	**0** Open **3** Percutaneous **4** Percutaneous Endoscopic **X** External	**4** Internal Fixation Device **5** External Fixation Device **7** Autologous Tissue Substitute **J** Synthetic Substitute **K** Nonautologous Tissue Substitute	**Z** No Qualifier
Y Upper Bone	**0** Open **3** Percutaneous **4** Percutaneous Endoscopic **X** External	**0** Drainage Device **M** Bone Growth Stimulator	**Z** No Qualifier

NOTES

NOTES

Lower Bones 0Q2-0QW

0 Medical and Surgical
Q Lower Bones
2 Change: Taking out or off a device from a body part and putting back an identical or similar device in or on the same body part without cutting or puncturing the skin or a mucous membrane

Body Part Character 4	Approach Character 5	Device Character 6	Qualifier Character 7
Y Lower Bone	**X** External	**0** Drainage Device **Y** Other Device	**Z** No Qualifier

0 Medical and Surgical
Q Lower Bones
5 Destruction: Physical eradication of all or a portion of a body part by the direct use of energy, force, or a destructive agent

Body Part Character 4	Approach Character 5	Device Character 6	Qualifier Character 7
0 Lumbar Vertebra **1** Sacrum **2** Pelvic Bone, Right **3** Pelvic Bone, Left **4** Acetabulum, Right **5** Acetabulum, Left **6** Upper Femur, Right **7** Upper Femur, Left **8** Femoral Shaft, Right **9** Femoral Shaft, Left **B** Lower Femur, Right **C** Lower Femur, Left **D** Patella, Right **F** Patella, Left **G** Tibia, Right **H** Tibia, Left **J** Fibula, Right **K** Fibula, Left **L** Tarsal, Right **M** Tarsal, Left **N** Metatarsal, Right **P** Metatarsal, Left **Q** Toe Phalanx, Right **R** Toe Phalanx, Left **S** Coccyx	**0** Open **3** Percutaneous **4** Percutaneous Endoscopic	**Z** No Device	**Z** No Qualifier

0 Medical and Surgical
Q Lower Bones
8 Division: Cutting into a body part, without draining fluids and/or gases from the body part, in order to separate or transect a body part

Body Part Character 4	Approach Character 5	Device Character 6	Qualifier Character 7
0 Lumbar Vertebra **1** Sacrum **2** Pelvic Bone, Right **3** Pelvic Bone, Left **4** Acetabulum, Right **5** Acetabulum, Left **6** Upper Femur, Right **7** Upper Femur, Left **8** Femoral Shaft, Right **9** Femoral Shaft, Left **B** Lower Femur, Right **C** Lower Femur, Left **D** Patella, Right **F** Patella, Left **G** Tibia, Right **H** Tibia, Left **J** Fibula, Right **K** Fibula, Left **L** Tarsal, Right **M** Tarsal, Left **N** Metatarsal, Right **P** Metatarsal, Left **Q** Toe Phalanx, Right **R** Toe Phalanx, Left **S** Coccyx	**0** Open **3** Percutaneous **4** Percutaneous Endoscopic	**Z** No Device	**Z** No Qualifier

0 Medical and Surgical
Q Lower Bones
9 Drainage: Taking or letting out fluids and/or gases from a body part

Body Part Character 4	Approach Character 5	Device Character 6	Qualifier Character 7
0 Lumbar Vertebra **1** Sacrum **2** Pelvic Bone, Right **3** Pelvic Bone, Left **4** Acetabulum, Right **5** Acetabulum, Left **6** Upper Femur, Right **7** Upper Femur, Left **8** Femoral Shaft, Right **9** Femoral Shaft, Left **B** Lower Femur, Right **C** Lower Femur, Left **D** Patella, Right **F** Patella, Left **G** Tibia, Right **H** Tibia, Left **J** Fibula, Right **K** Fibula, Left **L** Tarsal, Right **M** Tarsal, Left **N** Metatarsal, Right **P** Metatarsal, Left **Q** Toe Phalanx, Right **R** Toe Phalanx, Left **S** Coccyx	**0** Open **3** Percutaneous **4** Percutaneous Endoscopic	**0** Drainage Device	**Z** No Qualifier
0 Lumbar Vertebra **1** Sacrum **2** Pelvic Bone, Right **3** Pelvic Bone, Left **4** Acetabulum, Right **5** Acetabulum, Left **6** Upper Femur, Right **7** Upper Femur, Left **8** Femoral Shaft, Right **9** Femoral Shaft, Left **B** Lower Femur, Right **C** Lower Femur, Left **D** Patella, Right **F** Patella, Left **G** Tibia, Right **H** Tibia, Left **J** Fibula, Right **K** Fibula, Left **L** Tarsal, Right **M** Tarsal, Left **N** Metatarsal, Right **P** Metatarsal, Left **Q** Toe Phalanx, Right **R** Toe Phalanx, Left **S** Coccyx	**0** Open **3** Percutaneous **4** Percutaneous Endoscopic	**Z** No Device	**X** Diagnostic **Z** No Qualifier

0 Medical and Surgical
Q Lower Bones
B Excision: Cutting out or off, without replacement, a portion of a body part

Body Part Character 4	Approach Character 5	Device Character 6	Qualifier Character 7
0 Lumbar Vertebra **1** Sacrum **2** Pelvic Bone, Right **3** Pelvic Bone, Left **4** Acetabulum, Right **5** Acetabulum, Left **6** Upper Femur, Right **7** Upper Femur, Left **8** Femoral Shaft, Right **9** Femoral Shaft, Left **B** Lower Femur, Right **C** Lower Femur, Left **D** Patella, Right **F** Patella, Left **G** Tibia, Right **H** Tibia, Left **J** Fibula, Right **K** Fibula, Left **L** Tarsal, Right **M** Tarsal, Left **N** Metatarsal, Right **P** Metatarsal, Left **Q** Toe Phalanx, Right **R** Toe Phalanx, Left **S** Coccyx	**0** Open **3** Percutaneous **4** Percutaneous Endoscopic	**Z** No Device	**X** Diagnostic **Z** No Qualifier

0 Medical and Surgical
Q Lower Bones
C Extirpation: Taking or cutting out solid matter from a body part

Body Part Character 4	Approach Character 5	Device Character 6	Qualifier Character 7
0 Lumbar Vertebra **1** Sacrum **2** Pelvic Bone, Right **3** Pelvic Bone, Left **4** Acetabulum, Right **5** Acetabulum, Left **6** Upper Femur, Right **7** Upper Femur, Left **8** Femoral Shaft, Right **9** Femoral Shaft, Left **B** Lower Femur, Right **C** Lower Femur, Left **D** Patella, Right **F** Patella, Left **G** Tibia, Right **H** Tibia, Left **J** Fibula, Right **K** Fibula, Left **L** Tarsal, Right **M** Tarsal, Left **N** Metatarsal, Right **P** Metatarsal, Left **Q** Toe Phalanx, Right **R** Toe Phalanx, Left **S** Coccyx	**0** Open **3** Percutaneous **4** Percutaneous Endoscopic	**Z** No Device	**Z** No Qualifier

0 **Medical and Surgical**
Q **Lower Bones**
D **Extraction:** Pulling or stripping out or off all or a portion of a body part by the use of force

Body Part Character 4	Approach Character 5	Device Character 6	Qualifier Character 7
0 Lumbar Vertebra **1** Sacrum **2** Pelvic Bone, Right **3** Pelvic Bone, Left **4** Acetabulum, Right **5** Acetabulum, Left **6** Upper Femur, Right **7** Upper Femur, Left **8** Femoral Shaft, Right **9** Femoral Shaft, Left **B** Lower Femur, Right **C** Lower Femur, Left **D** Patella, Right **F** Patella, Left **G** Tibia, Right **H** Tibia, Left **J** Fibula, Right **K** Fibula, Left **L** Tarsal, Right **M** Tarsal, Left **N** Metatarsal, Right **P** Metatarsal, Left **Q** Toe Phalanx, Right **R** Toe Phalanx, Left **S** Coccyx	**0** Open	**Z** No Device	**Z** No Qualifier

0 **Medical and Surgical**
Q **Lower Bones**
H **Insertion:** Putting in a nonbiological appliance that monitors, assists, performs, or prevents a physiological function but does not physically take the place of a body part

Body Part Character 4	Approach Character 5	Device Character 6	Qualifier Character 7
0 Lumbar Vertebra **1** Sacrum **2** Pelvic Bone, Right **3** Pelvic Bone, Left **4** Acetabulum, Right **5** Acetabulum, Left **D** Patella, Right **F** Patella, Left **L** Tarsal, Right **M** Tarsal, Left **N** Metatarsal, Right **P** Metatarsal, Left **Q** Toe Phalanx, Right **R** Toe Phalanx, Left **S** Coccyx	**0** Open **3** Percutaneous **4** Percutaneous Endoscopic	**4** Internal Fixation Device **5** External Fixation Device	**Z** No Qualifier
6 Upper Femur, Right **7** Upper Femur, Left **B** Lower Femur, Right **C** Lower Femur, Left **J** Fibula, Right **K** Fibula, Left	**0** Open **3** Percutaneous **4** Percutaneous Endoscopic	**4** Internal Fixation Device **5** External Fixation Device **6** Internal Fixation Device, Intramedullary **8** External Fixation Device, Limb Lengthening **B** External Fixation Device, Monoplanar **C** External Fixation Device, Ring **D** External Fixation Device, Hybrid	**Z** No Qualifier

0QH continued on next page

0QH continued from previous page

0 Medical and Surgical
Q Lower Bones
H Insertion: Putting in a nonbiological appliance that monitors, assists, performs, or prevents a physiological function but does not physically take the place of a body part

Body Part Character 4	Approach Character 5	Device Character 6	Qualifier Character 7
8 Femoral Shaft, Right **9** Femoral Shaft, Left **G** Tibia, Right **H** Tibia, Left	**0** Open **3** Percutaneous **4** Percutaneous Endoscopic	**4** Internal Fixation Device **5** External Fixation Device **6** Internal Fixation Device, Intramedullary **7** Internal Fixation Device, Intramedullary Limb Lengthening **8** External Fixation Device, Limb Lengthening **B** External Fixation Device, Monoplanar **C** External Fixation Device, Ring **D** External Fixation Device, Hybrid	**Z** No Qualifier
Y Lower Bone	**0** Open **3** Percutaneous **4** Percutaneous Endoscopic	**M** Bone Growth Stimulator	**Z** No Qualifier

0 Medical and Surgical
Q Lower Bones
J Inspection: Visually and/or manually exploring a body part

Body Part Character 4	Approach Character 5	Device Character 6	Qualifier Character 7
Y Lower Bone	**0** Open **3** Percutaneous **4** Percutaneous Endoscopic **X** External	**Z** No Device	**Z** No Qualifier

0 Medical and Surgical
Q Lower Bones
N Release: Freeing a body part from an abnormal physical constraint by cutting or by the use of force

Body Part Character 4	Approach Character 5	Device Character 6	Qualifier Character 7
0 Lumbar Vertebra **1** Sacrum **2** Pelvic Bone, Right **3** Pelvic Bone, Left **4** Acetabulum, Right **5** Acetabulum, Left **6** Upper Femur, Right **7** Upper Femur, Left **8** Femoral Shaft, Right **9** Femoral Shaft, Left **B** Lower Femur, Right **C** Lower Femur, Left **D** Patella, Right **F** Patella, Left **G** Tibia, Right **H** Tibia, Left **J** Fibula, Right **K** Fibula, Left **L** Tarsal, Right **M** Tarsal, Left **N** Metatarsal, Right **P** Metatarsal, Left **Q** Toe Phalanx, Right **R** Toe Phalanx, Left **S** Coccyx	**0** Open **3** Percutaneous **4** Percutaneous Endoscopic	**Z** No Device	**Z** No Qualifier

0 Medical and Surgical
Q Lower Bones
P Removal: Taking out or off a device from a body part

Body Part Character 4	Approach Character 5	Device Character 6	Qualifier Character 7
0 Lumbar Vertebra **1** Sacrum **4** Acetabulum, Right **5** Acetabulum, Left **S** Coccyx	**0** Open **3** Percutaneous **4** Percutaneous Endoscopic	**4** Internal Fixation Device **7** Autologous Tissue Substitute **J** Synthetic Substitute **K** Nonautologous Tissue Substitute	**Z** No Qualifier
0 Lumbar Vertebra **1** Sacrum **4** Acetabulum, Right **5** Acetabulum, Left **S** Coccyx	**X** External	**4** Internal Fixation Device	**Z** No Qualifier
2 Pelvic Bone, Right **3** Pelvic Bone, Left **6** Upper Femur, Right **7** Upper Femur, Left **8** Femoral Shaft, Right **9** Femoral Shaft, Left **B** Lower Femur, Right **C** Lower Femur, Left **D** Patella, Right **F** Patella, Left **G** Tibia, Right **H** Tibia, Left **J** Fibula, Right **K** Fibula, Left **L** Tarsal, Right **M** Tarsal, Left **N** Metatarsal, Right **P** Metatarsal, Left **Q** Toe Phalanx, Right **R** Toe Phalanx, Left	**0** Open **3** Percutaneous **4** Percutaneous Endoscopic	**4** Internal Fixation Device **5** External Fixation Device **7** Autologous Tissue Substitute **J** Synthetic Substitute **K** Nonautologous Tissue Substitute	**Z** No Qualifier
2 Pelvic Bone, Right **3** Pelvic Bone, Left **6** Upper Femur, Right **7** Upper Femur, Left **8** Femoral Shaft, Right **9** Femoral Shaft, Left **B** Lower Femur, Right **C** Lower Femur, Left **D** Patella, Right **F** Patella, Left **G** Tibia, Right **H** Tibia, Left **J** Fibula, Right **K** Fibula, Left **L** Tarsal, Right **M** Tarsal, Left **N** Metatarsal, Right **P** Metatarsal, Left **Q** Toe Phalanx, Right **R** Toe Phalanx, Left	**X** External	**4** Internal Fixation Device **5** External Fixation Device	**Z** No Qualifier
Y Lower Bone	**0** Open **3** Percutaneous **4** Percutaneous Endoscopic **X** External	**0** Drainage Device **M** Bone Growth Stimulator	**Z** No Qualifier

0 Medical and Surgical
Q Lower Bones
Q Repair: Restoring, to the extent possible, a body part to its normal anatomic structure and function

Body Part Character 4	Approach Character 5	Device Character 6	Qualifier Character 7
0 Lumbar Vertebra **1** Sacrum **2** Pelvic Bone, Right **3** Pelvic Bone, Left **4** Acetabulum, Right **5** Acetabulum, Left **6** Upper Femur, Right **7** Upper Femur, Left **8** Femoral Shaft, Right **9** Femoral Shaft, Left **B** Lower Femur, Right **C** Lower Femur, Left **D** Patella, Right **F** Patella, Left **G** Tibia, Right **H** Tibia, Left **J** Fibula, Right **K** Fibula, Left **L** Tarsal, Right **M** Tarsal, Left **N** Metatarsal, Right **P** Metatarsal, Left **Q** Toe Phalanx, Right **R** Toe Phalanx, Left **S** Coccyx	**0** Open **3** Percutaneous **4** Percutaneous Endoscopic **X** External	**Z** No Device	**Z** No Qualifier

0 Medical and Surgical
Q Lower Bones
R Replacement: Putting in or on biological or synthetic material that physically takes the place and/or function of all or a portion of a body part

Body Part Character 4	Approach Character 5	Device Character 6	Qualifier Character 7
0 Lumbar Vertebra **1** Sacrum **2** Pelvic Bone, Right **3** Pelvic Bone, Left **4** Acetabulum, Right **5** Acetabulum, Left **6** Upper Femur, Right head **7** Upper Femur, Left **8** Femoral Shaft, Right **9** Femoral Shaft, Left **B** Lower Femur, Right **C** Lower Femur, Left **D** Patella, Right **F** Patella, Left **G** Tibia, Right **H** Tibia, Left **J** Fibula, Right **K** Fibula, Left **L** Tarsal, Right **M** Tarsal, Left **N** Metatarsal, Right **P** Metatarsal, Left **Q** Toe Phalanx, Right **R** Toe Phalanx, Left **S** Coccyx	**0** Open **3** Percutaneous **4** Percutaneous Endoscopic	**7** Autologous Tissue Substitute **J** Synthetic Substitute **K** Nonautologous Tissue Substitute - bone bank	**Z** No Qualifier

0 Medical and Surgical
Q Lower Bones
S Reposition: Moving to its normal location, or other suitable location, all or a portion of a body part

Body Part Character 4	Approach Character 5	Device Character 6	Qualifier Character 7
0 Lumbar Vertebra CC **1** Sacrum CC **4** Acetabulum, Right **5** Acetabulum, Left **S** Coccyx CC	**0** Open **3** Percutaneous **4** Percutaneous Endoscopic	**4** Internal Fixation Device **Z** No Device	**Z** No Qualifier
0 Lumbar Vertebra **1** Sacrum **4** Acetabulum, Right **5** Acetabulum, Left **S** Coccyx	**X** External	**Z** No Device	**Z** No Qualifier
2 Pelvic Bone, Right **3** Pelvic Bone, Left **D** Patella, Right **F** Patella, Left **L** Tarsal, Right **M** Tarsal, Left **Q** Toe Phalanx, Right **R** Toe Phalanx, Left	**0** Open **3** Percutaneous **4** Percutaneous Endoscopic	**4** Internal Fixation Device **5** External Fixation Device **Z** No Device	**Z** No Qualifier
2 Pelvic Bone, Right **3** Pelvic Bone, Left **D** Patella, Right **F** Patella, Left **L** Tarsal, Right **M** Tarsal, Left **Q** Toe Phalanx, Right **R** Toe Phalanx, Left	**X** External	**Z** No Device	**Z** No Qualifier
6 Upper Femur, Right **7** Upper Femur, Left **8** Femoral Shaft, Right **9** Femoral Shaft, Left **B** Lower Femur, Right **C** Lower Femur, Left **G** Tibia, Right **H** Tibia, Left **J** Fibula, Right **K** Fibula, Left	**0** Open **3** Percutaneous **4** Percutaneous Endoscopic	**4** Internal Fixation Device **5** External Fixation Device **6** Internal Fixation Device, Intramedullary **B** External Fixation Device, Monoplanar **C** External Fixation Device, Ring **D** External Fixation Device, Hybrid **Z** No Device	**Z** No Qualifier
6 Upper Femur, Right **7** Upper Femur, Left **8** Femoral Shaft, Right **9** Femoral Shaft, Left **B** Lower Femur, Right **C** Lower Femur, Left **G** Tibia, Right **H** Tibia, Left **J** Fibula, Right **K** Fibula, Left	**X** External	**Z** No Device	**Z** No Qualifier
N Metatarsal, Right **P** Metatarsal, Left	**0** Open **3** Percutaneous **4** Percutaneous Endoscopic	**4** Internal Fixation Device **5** External Fixation Device **Z** No Device	**2** Sesamoid Bone(s) 1st Toe **Z** No Qualifier
N Metatarsal, Right **P** Metatarsal, Left	**X** External	**Z** No Device	**2** Sesamoid Bone(s) 1st Toe **Z** No Qualifier

CC 0QS03ZZ 0QS13ZZ 0QSS3ZZ

0 Medical and Surgical
Q Lower Bones
T Resection: Cutting out or off, without replacement, all of a body part

Body Part Character 4	Approach Character 5	Device Character 6	Qualifier Character 7
2 Pelvic Bone, Right **3** Pelvic Bone, Left **4** Acetabulum, Right **5** Acetabulum, Left **6** Upper Femur, Right **7** Upper Femur, Left **8** Femoral Shaft, Right **9** Femoral Shaft, Left **B** Lower Femur, Right **C** Lower Femur, Left **D** Patella, Right **F** Patella, Left **G** Tibia, Right **H** Tibia, Left **J** Fibula, Right **K** Fibula, Left **L** Tarsal, Right **M** Tarsal, Left **N** Metatarsal, Right **P** Metatarsal, Left **Q** Toe Phalanx, Right **R** Toe Phalanx, Left **S** Coccyx	**0** Open	**Z** No Device	**Z** No Qualifier

0 Medical and Surgical
Q Lower Bones
U Supplement: Putting in or on biological or synthetic material that physically reinforces and/or augments the function of a portion of a body part

Body Part Character 4	Approach Character 5	Device Character 6	Qualifier Character 7
0 Lumbar Vertebra CC **1** Sacrum CC **2** Pelvic Bone, Right **3** Pelvic Bone, Left **4** Acetabulum, Right **5** Acetabulum, Left **6** Upper Femur, Right **7** Upper Femur, Left **8** Femoral Shaft, Right **9** Femoral Shaft, Left **B** Lower Femur, Right **C** Lower Femur, Left **D** Patella, Right **F** Patella, Left **G** Tibia, Right **H** Tibia, Left **J** Fibula, Right **K** Fibula, Left **L** Tarsal, Right **M** Tarsal, Left **N** Metatarsal, Right **P** Metatarsal, Left **Q** Toe Phalanx, Right **R** Toe Phalanx, Left **S** Coccyx CC	**0** Open **3** Percutaneous **4** Percutaneous Endoscopic	**7** Autologous Tissue Substitute **J** Synthetic Substitute **K** Nonautologous Tissue Substitute	**Z** No Qualifier

CC 0QU03JZ 0QU13JZ 0QUS3JZ

0 Medical and Surgical
Q Lower Bones
W Revision: Correcting, to the extent possible, a portion of a malfunctioning device or the position of a displaced device

Body Part Character 4	Approach Character 5	Device Character 6	Qualifier Character 7
0 Lumbar Vertebra **1** Sacrum **4** Acetabulum, Right **5** Acetabulum, Left **S** Coccyx	**0** Open **3** Percutaneous **4** Percutaneous Endoscopic **X** External	**4** Internal Fixation Device **7** Autologous Tissue Substitute **J** Synthetic Substitute **K** Nonautologous Tissue Substitute	**Z** No Qualifier
2 Pelvic Bone, Right **3** Pelvic Bone, Left **6** Upper Femur, Right **7** Upper Femur, Left **8** Femoral Shaft, Right **9** Femoral Shaft, Left **B** Lower Femur, Right **C** Lower Femur, Left **D** Patella, Right **F** Patella, Left **G** Tibia, Right **H** Tibia, Left **J** Fibula, Right **K** Fibula, Left **L** Tarsal, Right **M** Tarsal, Left **N** Metatarsal, Right **P** Metatarsal, Left **Q** Toe Phalanx, Right **R** Toe Phalanx, Left	**0** Open **3** Percutaneous **4** Percutaneous Endoscopic **X** External	**4** Internal Fixation Device **5** External Fixation Device **7** Autologous Tissue Substitute **J** Synthetic Substitute **K** Nonautologous Tissue Substitute	**Z** No Qualifier
Y Lower Bone	**0** Open **3** Percutaneous **4** Percutaneous Endoscopic **X** External	**0** Drainage Device **M** Bone Growth Stimulator	**Z** No Qualifier

NOTES

Arthrodesis - Fusion of 2 joints in the body to eliminate bone-on-bone Friction and/or nerve compression
Treatment For: degenerative disc disease, spinal stenosis, Facet arthropathy. Done mainly on spine, hand, ankle & Foot, done w/ bone grafts - autograft or allograft, synthetic bone substitutes or metal implants

PLIF - Posterior Lumbar Interbody Fusion
a bone allograft using synthetic cages to stabilize the Fusion

Upper Joints 0R2-0RW

0 Medical and Surgical
R Upper Joints
2 Change: Taking out or off a device from a body part and putting back an identical or similar device in or on the same body part without cutting or puncturing the skin or a mucous membrane

Body Part Character 4	Approach Character 5	Device Character 6	Qualifier Character 7
Y Upper Joint	**X** External	**0** Drainage Device **Y** Other Device	**Z** No Qualifier

0 Medical and Surgical
R Upper Joints
5 Destruction: Physical eradication of all or a portion of a body part by the direct use of energy, force, or a destructive agent

Body Part Character 4	Approach Character 5	Device Character 6	Qualifier Character 7
0 Occipital-cervical Joint **1** Cervical Vertebral Joint **3** Cervical Vertebral Disc **4** Cervicothoracic Vertebral Joint **5** Cervicothoracic Vertebral Disc **6** Thoracic Vertebral Joint **9** Thoracic Vertebral Disc **A** Thoracolumbar Vertebral Joint **B** Thoracolumbar Vertebral Disc **C** Temporomandibular Joint, Right **D** Temporomandibular Joint, Left **E** Sternoclavicular Joint, Right **F** Sternoclavicular Joint, Left **G** Acromioclavicular Joint, Right **H** Acromioclavicular Joint, Left **J** Shoulder Joint, Right **K** Shoulder Joint, Left **L** Elbow Joint, Right **M** Elbow Joint, Left **N** Wrist Joint, Right **P** Wrist Joint, Left **Q** Carpal Joint, Right **R** Carpal Joint, Left **S** Carpometacarpal Joint, Right **T** Carpometacarpal Joint, Left **U** Metacarpophalangeal Joint, Right **V** Metacarpophalangeal Joint, Left **W** Finger Phalangeal Joint, Right **X** Finger Phalangeal Joint, Left	**0** Open **3** Percutaneous **4** Percutaneous Endoscopic	**Z** No Device	**Z** No Qualifier

0 Medical and Surgical
R Upper Joints
9 Drainage: Taking or letting out fluids and/or gases from a body part

Body Part Character 4	Approach Character 5	Device Character 6	Qualifier Character 7
0 Occipital-cervical Joint **1** Cervical Vertebral Joint **3** Cervical Vertebral Disc **4** Cervicothoracic Vertebral Joint **5** Cervicothoracic Vertebral Disc **6** Thoracic Vertebral Joint **9** Thoracic Vertebral Disc **A** Thoracolumbar Vertebral Joint **B** Thoracolumbar Vertebral Disc **C** Temporomandibular Joint, Right **D** Temporomandibular Joint, Left **E** Sternoclavicular Joint, Right **F** Sternoclavicular Joint, Left **G** Acromioclavicular Joint, Right **H** Acromioclavicular Joint, Left **J** Shoulder Joint, Right **K** Shoulder Joint, Left **L** Elbow Joint, Right **M** Elbow Joint, Left **N** Wrist Joint, Right **P** Wrist Joint, Left **Q** Carpal Joint, Right **R** Carpal Joint, Left **S** Carpometacarpal Joint, Right **T** Carpometacarpal Joint, Left **U** Metacarpophalangeal Joint, Right **V** Metacarpophalangeal Joint, Left **W** Finger Phalangeal Joint, Right **X** Finger Phalangeal Joint, Left	**0** Open **3** Percutaneous **4** Percutaneous Endoscopic	**0** Drainage Device	**Z** No Qualifier
0 Occipital-cervical Joint **1** Cervical Vertebral Joint **3** Cervical Vertebral Disc **4** Cervicothoracic Vertebral Joint **5** Cervicothoracic Vertebral Disc **6** Thoracic Vertebral Joint **9** Thoracic Vertebral Disc **A** Thoracolumbar Vertebral Joint **B** Thoracolumbar Vertebral Disc **C** Temporomandibular Joint, Right **D** Temporomandibular Joint, Left **E** Sternoclavicular Joint, Right **F** Sternoclavicular Joint, Left **G** Acromioclavicular Joint, Right **H** Acromioclavicular Joint, Left **J** Shoulder Joint, Right **K** Shoulder Joint, Left **L** Elbow Joint, Right **M** Elbow Joint, Left **N** Wrist Joint, Right **P** Wrist Joint, Left **Q** Carpal Joint, Right **R** Carpal Joint, Left **S** Carpometacarpal Joint, Right **T** Carpometacarpal Joint, Left **U** Metacarpophalangeal Joint, Right **V** Metacarpophalangeal Joint, Left **W** Finger Phalangeal Joint, Right **X** Finger Phalangeal Joint, Left	**0** Open **3** Percutaneous **4** Percutaneous Endoscopic	**Z** No Device	**X** Diagnostic **Z** No Qualifier

0 Medical and Surgical
R Upper Joints
B Excision: Cutting out or off, without replacement, a portion of a body part

Body Part Character 4	Approach Character 5	Device Character 6	Qualifier Character 7
0 Occipital-cervical Joint **1** Cervical Vertebral Joint **3** Cervical Vertebral Disc **4** Cervicothoracic Vertebral Joint **5** Cervicothoracic Vertebral Disc **6** Thoracic Vertebral Joint **9** Thoracic Vertebral Disc **A** Thoracolumbar Vertebral Joint **B** Thoracolumbar Vertebral Disc **C** Temporomandibular Joint, Right **D** Temporomandibular Joint, Left **E** Sternoclavicular Joint, Right **F** Sternoclavicular Joint, Left **G** Acromioclavicular Joint, Right **H** Acromioclavicular Joint, Left **J** Shoulder Joint, Right **K** Shoulder Joint, Left **L** Elbow Joint, Right **M** Elbow Joint, Left **N** Wrist Joint, Right **P** Wrist Joint, Left **Q** Carpal Joint, Right **R** Carpal Joint, Left **S** Carpometacarpal Joint, Right **T** Carpometacarpal Joint, Left **U** Metacarpophalangeal Joint, Right **V** Metacarpophalangeal Joint, Left **W** Finger Phalangeal Joint, Right **X** Finger Phalangeal Joint, Left	**0** Open **3** Percutaneous **4** Percutaneous Endoscopic	**Z** No Device	**X** Diagnostic **Z** No Qualifier

0 Medical and Surgical
R Upper Joints
C Extirpation: Taking or cutting out solid matter from a body part

Body Part Character 4	Approach Character 5	Device Character 6	Qualifier Character 7
0 Occipital-cervical Joint 1 Cervical Vertebral Joint 3 Cervical Vertebral Disc 4 Cervicothoracic Vertebral Joint 5 Cervicothoracic Vertebral Disc 6 Thoracic Vertebral Joint 9 Thoracic Vertebral Disc A Thoracolumbar Vertebral Joint B Thoracolumbar Vertebral Disc C Temporomandibular Joint, Right D Temporomandibular Joint, Left E Sternoclavicular Joint, Right F Sternoclavicular Joint, Left G Acromioclavicular Joint, Right H Acromioclavicular Joint, Left J Shoulder Joint, Right K Shoulder Joint, Left L Elbow Joint, Right M Elbow Joint, Left N Wrist Joint, Right P Wrist Joint, Left Q Carpal Joint, Right R Carpal Joint, Left S Carpometacarpal Joint, Right T Carpometacarpal Joint, Left U Metacarpophalangeal Joint, Right V Metacarpophalangeal Joint, Left W Finger Phalangeal Joint, Right X Finger Phalangeal Joint, Left	0 Open 3 Percutaneous 4 Percutaneous Endoscopic	Z No Device	Z No Qualifier

0 Medical and Surgical
R Upper Joints
G Fusion: Joining together portions of an articular body part rendering the articular body part immobile

Body Part Character 4	Approach Character 5	Device Character 6	Qualifier Character 7
0 Occipital-cervical Joint HAC 1 Cervical Vertebral Joint HAC 2 Cervical Vertebral Joints, 2 or more HAC 4 Cervicothoracic Vertebral Joint HAC 6 Thoracic Vertebral Joint HAC 7 Thoracic Vertebral Joints, 2 to 7 HAC CC 8 Thoracic Vertebral Joints, 8 or more HAC A Thoracolumbar Vertebral Joint HAC	0 Open 3 Percutaneous 4 Percutaneous Endoscopic	7 Autologous Tissue Substitute J Synthetic Substitute K Nonautologous Tissue Substitute	0 Anterior Approach, Anterior Column 1 Posterior Approach, Posterior Column J Posterior Approach, Anterior Column
0 Occipital-cervical Joint HAC 1 Cervical Vertebral Joint HAC 2 Cervical Vertebral Joints, 2 or more HAC 4 Cervicothoracic Vertebral Joint HAC 6 Thoracic Vertebral Joint HAC 7 Thoracic Vertebral Joints, 2 to 7 HAC CC 8 Thoracic Vertebral Joints, 8 or more HAC A Thoracolumbar Vertebral Joint HAC	0 Open 3 Percutaneous 4 Percutaneous Endoscopic	A Interbody Fusion Device Peek cages DynaTan Styker Plate & autoplus bone w/putty	0 Anterior Approach, Anterior Column J Posterior Approach, Anterior Column

0RG continued on next page

0 Medical and Surgical
R Upper Joints
G Fusion: Joining together portions of an articular body part rendering the articular body part immobile

0RG continued from previous page

Body Part Character 4	Approach Character 5	Device Character 6	Qualifier Character 7
C Temporomandibular Joint, Right **D** Temporomandibular Joint, Left **E** Sternoclavicular Joint, Right HAC **F** Sternoclavicular Joint, Left HAC **G** Acromioclavicular Joint, Right HAC **H** Acromioclavicular Joint, Left HAC **J** Shoulder Joint, Right HAC **K** Shoulder Joint, Left HAC	**0** Open **3** Percutaneous **4** Percutaneous Endoscopic	**4** Internal Fixation Device **7** Autologous Tissue Substitute **J** Synthetic Substitute **K** Nonautologous Tissue Substitute	**Z** No Qualifier
L Elbow Joint, Right HAC **M** Elbow Joint, Left HAC **N** Wrist Joint, Right **P** Wrist Joint, Left **Q** Carpal Joint, Right **R** Carpal Joint, Left **S** Carpometacarpal Joint, Right **T** Carpometacarpal Joint, Left **U** Metacarpophalangeal Joint, Right **V** Metacarpophalangeal Joint, Left **W** Finger Phalangeal Joint, Right **X** Finger Phalangeal Joint, Left	**0** Open **3** Percutaneous **4** Percutaneous Endoscopic	**4** Internal Fixation Device **5** External Fixation Device **7** Autologous Tissue Substitute **J** Synthetic Substitute **K** Nonautologous Tissue Substitute	**Z** No Qualifier

HAC 0RG0070 0RG0071 0RG007J 0RG00A0 0RG00AJ 0RG00J0 0RG00J1 0RG00JJ 0RG00K0 0RG00K1 0RG00KJ 0RG0370 0RG0371
0RG037J 0RG03A0 0RG03AJ 0RG03J0 0RG03J1 0RG03JJ 0RG03K0 0RG03K1 0RG03KJ 0RG0470 0RG0471 0RG047J 0RG04A0
0RG04AJ 0RG04J0 0RG04J1 0RG04JJ 0RG04K0 0RG04K1 0RG04KJ 0RG1070 0RG1071 0RG107J 0RG10A0 0RG10AJ 0RG10J0
0RG10J1 0RG10JJ 0RG10K0 0RG10K1 0RG10KJ 0RG1370 0RG1371 0RG137J 0RG13A0 0RG13AJ 0RG13J0 0RG13J1 0RG13JJ
0RG13K0 0RG13K1 0RG13KJ 0RG1470 0RG1471 0RG147J 0RG14A0 0RG14AJ 0RG14J0 0RG14J1 0RG14JJ 0RG14K0 0RG14K1
0RG14KJ 0RG2070 0RG2071 0RG207J 0RG20A0 0RG20AJ 0RG20J0 0RG20J1 0RG20JJ 0RG20K0 0RG20K1 0RG20KJ 0RG2370
0RG2371 0RG237J 0RG23A0 0RG23AJ 0RG23J0 0RG23J1 0RG23JJ 0RG23K0 0RG23K1 0RG23KJ 0RG2470 0RG2471 0RG247J
0RG24A0 0RG24AJ 0RG24J0 0RG24J1 0RG24JJ 0RG24K0 0RG24K1 0RG24KJ 0RG4070 0RG4071 0RG407J 0RG40A0 0RG40AJ
0RG40J0 0RG40J1 0RG40JJ 0RG40K0 0RG40K1 0RG40KJ 0RG4370 0RG4371 0RG437J 0RG43A0 0RG43AJ 0RG43J0 0RG43J1
0RG43JJ 0RG43K0 0RG43K1 0RG43KJ 0RG4470 0RG4471 0RG447J 0RG44A0 0RG44AJ 0RG44J0 0RG44J1 0RG44JJ 0RG44K0
0RG44K1 0RG44KJ 0RG6070 0RG6071 0RG607J 0RG60A0 0RG60AJ 0RG60J0 0RG60J1 0RG60JJ 0RG60K0 0RG60K1 0RG60KJ
0RG6370 0RG6371 0RG637J 0RG63A0 0RG63AJ 0RG63J0 0RG63J1 0RG63JJ 0RG63K0 0RG63K1 0RG63KJ 0RG6470 0RG6471
0RG647J 0RG64A0 0RG64AJ 0RG64J0 0RG64J1 0RG64JJ 0RG64K0 0RG64K1 0RG64KJ 0RG7070 0RG7071 0RG707J 0RG70A0
0RG70AJ 0RG70J0 0RG70J1 0RG70JJ 0RG70K0 0RG70K1 0RG70KJ 0RG7370 0RG7371 0RG737J 0RG73A0 0RG73AJ 0RG73J0
0RG73J1 0RG73JJ 0RG73K0 0RG73K1 0RG73KJ 0RG7470 0RG7471 0RG747J 0RG74A0 0RG74AJ 0RG74J0 0RG74J1 0RG74JJ
0RG74K0 0RG74K1 0RG74KJ 0RG8070 0RG8071 0RG807J 0RG80A0 0RG80AJ 0RG80J0 0RG80J1 0RG80JJ 0RG80K0 0RG80K1
0RG80KJ 0RG8370 0RG8371 0RG837J 0RG83A0 0RG83AJ 0RG83J0 0RG83J1 0RG83JJ 0RG83K0 0RG83K1 0RG83KJ 0RG8470
0RG8471 0RG847J 0RG84A0 0RG84AJ 0RG84J0 0RG84J1 0RG84JJ 0RG84K0 0RG84K1 0RG84KJ 0RGA070 0RGA071 0RGA07J
0RGA0A0 0RGA0AJ 0RGA0J0 0RGA0J1 0RGA0JJ 0RGA0K0 0RGA0K1 0RGA0KJ 0RGA370 0RGA371 0RGA37J 0RGA3A0 0RGA3AJ
0RGA3J0 0RGA3J1 0RGA3JJ 0RGA3K0 0RGA3K1 0RGA3KJ 0RGA470 0RGA471 0RGA47J 0RGA4A0 0RGA4AJ 0RGA4J0 0RGA4J1
0RGA4JJ 0RGA4K0 0RGA4K1 0RGA4KJ 0RGE04Z 0RGE07Z 0RGE0JZ 0RGE0KZ 0RGE34Z 0RGE37Z 0RGE3JZ 0RGE3KZ 0RGE44Z
0RGE47Z 0RGE4JZ 0RGE4KZ 0RGF04Z 0RGF07Z 0RGF0JZ 0RGF0KZ 0RGF34Z 0RGF37Z 0RGF3JZ 0RGF3KZ 0RGF44Z 0RGF47Z
0RGF4JZ 0RGF4KZ 0RGG04Z 0RGG07Z 0RGG0JZ 0RGG0KZ 0RGG34Z 0RGG37Z 0RGG3JZ 0RGG3KZ 0RGG44Z 0RGG47Z 0RGG4JZ
0RGG4KZ 0RGH04Z 0RGH07Z 0RGH0JZ 0RGH0KZ 0RGH34Z 0RGH37Z 0RGH3JZ 0RGH3KZ 0RGH44Z 0RGH47Z 0RGH4JZ 0RGH4KZ
0RGJ04Z 0RGJ07Z 0RGJ0JZ 0RGJ0KZ 0RGJ34Z 0RGJ37Z 0RGJ3JZ 0RGJ3KZ 0RGJ44Z 0RGJ47Z 0RGJ4JZ 0RGJ4KZ 0RGK04Z
0RGK07Z 0RGK0JZ 0RGK0KZ 0RGK34Z 0RGK37Z 0RGK3JZ 0RGK3KZ 0RGK44Z 0RGK47Z 0RGK4JZ 0RGK4KZ 0RGL04Z 0RGL05Z
0RGL07Z 0RGL0JZ 0RGL0KZ 0RGL34Z 0RGL35Z 0RGL37Z 0RGL3JZ 0RGL3KZ 0RGL44Z 0RGL45Z 0RGL47Z 0RGL4JZ 0RGL4KZ
0RGM04Z 0RGM05Z 0RGM07Z 0RGM0JZ 0RGM0KZ 0RGM34Z 0RGM35Z 0RGM37Z 0RGM3JZ 0RGM3KZ 0RGM44Z 0RGM45Z 0RGM47Z
0RGM4JZ 0RGM4KZ

Surgical site infection following certain orthopedic procedures of spine, shoulder or elbow procedures and secondary diagnosis K68.11, T81.40XA, T81.41XA, T81.42XA, T81.43XA, T81.44XA, T81.49XA, T84.60XA, T84.610A, T84.611A, T84.612A, T84.613A, T84.614A, T84.615A, T84.619A, T84.63XA, T84.69XA, T84.7XXA.

CC 0RG7070 0RG7071 0RG707J 0RG70A0 0RG70AJ 0RG70J0 0RG70J1 0RG70JJ 0RG70K0 0RG70K1 0RG70KJ 0RG7370 0RG7371
0RG737J 0RG73A0 0RG73AJ 0RG73J0 0RG73J1 0RG73JJ 0RG73K0 0RG73K1 0RG73KJ 0RG7470 0RG7471 0RG747J 0RG74A0
0RG74AJ 0RG74J0 0RG74J1 0RG74JJ 0RG74K0 0RG74K1 0RG74KJ

LC Limited Coverage NC Noncovered HAC HAC-associated Procedure CC Combination Cluster - See Appendix G for code lists
DRG Non-OR-Affecting MS-DRG Assignment New/Revised Text in **Orange** ♂ Male ♀ Female

0 Medical and Surgical
R Upper Joints
H Insertion: Putting in a nonbiological appliance that monitors, assists, performs, or prevents a physiological function but does not physically take the place of a body part

Body Part Character 4	Approach Character 5	Device Character 6	Qualifier Character 7
0 Occipital-cervical Joint **1** Cervical Vertebral Joint **4** Cervicothoracic Vertebral Joint **6** Thoracic Vertebral Joint **A** Thoracolumbar Vertebral Joint	**0** Open **3** Percutaneous **4** Percutaneous Endoscopic	**3** Infusion Device **4** Internal Fixation Device **8** Spacer **B** Spinal Stabilization Device, Interspinous Process **C** Spinal Stabilization Device, Pedicle-Based **D** Spinal Stabilization Device, Facet Replacement	**Z** No Qualifier
3 Cervical Vertebral Disc **5** Cervicothoracic Vertebral Disc **9** Thoracic Vertebral Disc **B** Thoracolumbar Vertebral Disc	**0** Open **3** Percutaneous **4** Percutaneous Endoscopic	**3** Infusion Device	**Z** No Qualifier
C Temporomandibular Joint, Right **D** Temporomandibular Joint, Left **E** Sternoclavicular Joint, Right **F** Sternoclavicular Joint, Left **G** Acromioclavicular Joint, Right **H** Acromioclavicular Joint, Left **J** Shoulder Joint, Right **K** Shoulder Joint, Left	**0** Open **3** Percutaneous **4** Percutaneous Endoscopic	**3** Infusion Device **4** Internal Fixation Device **8** Spacer	**Z** No Qualifier
L Elbow Joint, Right **M** Elbow Joint, Left **N** Wrist Joint, Right **P** Wrist Joint, Left **Q** Carpal Joint, Right **R** Carpal Joint, Left **S** Carpometacarpal Joint, Right **T** Carpometacarpal Joint, Left **U** Metacarpophalangeal Joint, Right **V** Metacarpophalangeal Joint, Left **W** Finger Phalangeal Joint, Right **X** Finger Phalangeal Joint, Left	**0** Open **3** Percutaneous **4** Percutaneous Endoscopic	**3** Infusion Device **4** Internal Fixation Device **5** External Fixation Device **8** Spacer	**Z** No Qualifier

0 Medical and Surgical
R Upper Joints
J Inspection: Visually and/or manually exploring a body part

Body Part Character 4	Approach Character 5	Device Character 6	Qualifier Character 7
0 Occipital-cervical Joint **1** Cervical Vertebral Joint **3** Cervical Vertebral Disc **4** Cervicothoracic Vertebral Joint **5** Cervicothoracic Vertebral Disc **6** Thoracic Vertebral Joint **9** Thoracic Vertebral Disc **A** Thoracolumbar Vertebral Joint **B** Thoracolumbar Vertebral Disc **C** Temporomandibular Joint, Right **D** Temporomandibular Joint, Left **E** Sternoclavicular Joint, Right **F** Sternoclavicular Joint, Left **G** Acromioclavicular Joint, Right **H** Acromioclavicular Joint, Left **J** Shoulder Joint, Right **K** Shoulder Joint, Left **L** Elbow Joint, Right **M** Elbow Joint, Left **N** Wrist Joint, Right **P** Wrist Joint, Left **Q** Carpal Joint, Right **R** Carpal Joint, Left **S** Carpometacarpal Joint, Right **T** Carpometacarpal Joint, Left **U** Metacarpophalangeal Joint, Right **V** Metacarpophalangeal Joint, Left **W** Finger Phalangeal Joint, Right **X** Finger Phalangeal Joint, Left	**0** Open **3** Percutaneous **4** Percutaneous Endoscopic **X** External	**Z** No Device	**Z** No Qualifier

0 Medical and Surgical
R Upper Joints
N Release: Freeing a body part from an abnormal physical constraint by cutting or by the use of force

Body Part Character 4	Approach Character 5	Device Character 6	Qualifier Character 7
0 Occipital-cervical Joint **1** Cervical Vertebral Joint **3** Cervical Vertebral Disc **4** Cervicothoracic Vertebral Joint **5** Cervicothoracic Vertebral Disc **6** Thoracic Vertebral Joint **9** Thoracic Vertebral Disc **A** Thoracolumbar Vertebral Joint **B** Thoracolumbar Vertebral Disc **C** Temporomandibular Joint, Right **D** Temporomandibular Joint, Left **E** Sternoclavicular Joint, Right **F** Sternoclavicular Joint, Left **G** Acromioclavicular Joint, Right **H** Acromioclavicular Joint, Left **J** Shoulder Joint, Right **K** Shoulder Joint, Left **L** Elbow Joint, Right **M** Elbow Joint, Left **N** Wrist Joint, Right **P** Wrist Joint, Left **Q** Carpal Joint, Right **R** Carpal Joint, Left **S** Carpometacarpal Joint, Right **T** Carpometacarpal Joint, Left **U** Metacarpophalangeal Joint, Right **V** Metacarpophalangeal Joint, Left **W** Finger Phalangeal Joint, Right **X** Finger Phalangeal Joint, Left	**0** Open **3** Percutaneous **4** Percutaneous Endoscopic **X** External	**Z** No Device	**Z** No Qualifier

0 Medical and Surgical
R Upper Joints
P Removal: Taking out or off a device from a body part

Body Part Character 4	Approach Character 5	Device Character 6	Qualifier Character 7
0 Occipital-cervical Joint **1** Cervical Vertebral Joint **4** Cervicothoracic Vertebral Joint **6** Thoracic Vertebral Joint **A** Thoracolumbar Vertebral Joint	**0** Open **3** Percutaneous **4** Percutaneous Endoscopic	**0** Drainage Device **3** Infusion Device **4** Internal Fixation Device **7** Autologous Tissue Substitute **8** Spacer **A** Interbody Fusion Device **J** Synthetic Substitute **K** Nonautologous Tissue Substitute	**Z** No Qualifier
0 Occipital-cervical Joint **1** Cervical Vertebral Joint **4** Cervicothoracic Vertebral Joint **6** Thoracic Vertebral Joint **A** Thoracolumbar Vertebral Joint	**X** External	**0** Drainage Device **3** Infusion Device **4** Internal Fixation Device	**Z** No Qualifier
3 Cervical Vertebral Disc **5** Cervicothoracic Vertebral Disc **9** Thoracic Vertebral Disc **B** Thoracolumbar Vertebral Disc	**0** Open **3** Percutaneous **4** Percutaneous Endoscopic	**0** Drainage Device **3** Infusion Device **7** Autologous Tissue Substitute **J** Synthetic Substitute **K** Nonautologous Tissue Substitute	**Z** No Qualifier

0RP continued on next page

0 Medical and Surgical
R Upper Joints
P Removal: Taking out or off a device from a body part

0RP continued from previous page

Body Part Character 4	Approach Character 5	Device Character 6	Qualifier Character 7
3 Cervical Vertebral Disc **5** Cervicothoracic Vertebral Disc **9** Thoracic Vertebral Disc **B** Thoracolumbar Vertebral Disc	**X** External	**0** Drainage Device **3** Infusion Device	**Z** No Qualifier
C Temporomandibular Joint, Right **D** Temporomandibular Joint, Left **E** Sternoclavicular Joint, Right **F** Sternoclavicular Joint, Left **G** Acromioclavicular Joint, Right **H** Acromioclavicular Joint, Left **J** Shoulder Joint, Right **K** Shoulder Joint, Left	**0** Open **3** Percutaneous **4** Percutaneous Endoscopic	**0** Drainage Device **3** Infusion Device **4** Internal Fixation Device **7** Autologous Tissue Substitute **8** Spacer **J** Synthetic Substitute **K** Nonautologous Tissue Substitute	**Z** No Qualifier
C Temporomandibular Joint, Right **D** Temporomandibular Joint, Left **E** Sternoclavicular Joint, Right **F** Sternoclavicular Joint, Left **G** Acromioclavicular Joint, Right **H** Acromioclavicular Joint, Left **J** Shoulder Joint, Right **K** Shoulder Joint, Left	**X** External	**0** Drainage Device **3** Infusion Device **4** Internal Fixation Device	**Z** No Qualifier
L Elbow Joint, Right **M** Elbow Joint, Left **N** Wrist Joint, Right **P** Wrist Joint, Left **Q** Carpal Joint, Right **R** Carpal Joint, Left **S** Carpometacarpal Joint, Right **T** Carpometacarpal Joint, Left **U** Metacarpophalangeal Joint, Right **V** Metacarpophalangeal Joint, Left **W** Finger Phalangeal Joint, Right **X** Finger Phalangeal Joint, Left	**0** Open **3** Percutaneous **4** Percutaneous Endoscopic	**0** Drainage Device **3** Infusion Device **4** Internal Fixation Device **5** External Fixation Device **7** Autologous Tissue Substitute **8** Spacer **J** Synthetic Substitute **K** Nonautologous Tissue Substitute	**Z** No Qualifier
L Elbow Joint, Right **M** Elbow Joint, Left **N** Wrist Joint, Right **P** Wrist Joint, Left **Q** Carpal Joint, Right **R** Carpal Joint, Left **S** Carpometacarpal Joint, Right **T** Carpometacarpal Joint, Left **U** Metacarpophalangeal Joint, Right **V** Metacarpophalangeal Joint, Left **W** Finger Phalangeal Joint, Right **X** Finger Phalangeal Joint, Left	**X** External	**0** Drainage Device **3** Infusion Device **4** Internal Fixation Device **5** External Fixation Device	**Z** No Qualifier

0 Medical and Surgical
R Upper Joints
Q Repair: Restoring, to the extent possible, a body part to its normal anatomic structure and function

Body Part Character 4	Approach Character 5	Device Character 6	Qualifier Character 7
0 Occipital-cervical Joint **1** Cervical Vertebral Joint **3** Cervical Vertebral Disc **4** Cervicothoracic Vertebral Joint **5** Cervicothoracic Vertebral Disc **6** Thoracic Vertebral Joint **9** Thoracic Vertebral Disc **A** Thoracolumbar Vertebral Joint **B** Thoracolumbar Vertebral Disc **C** Temporomandibular Joint, Right **D** Temporomandibular Joint, Left **E** Sternoclavicular Joint, Right HAC **F** Sternoclavicular Joint, Left HAC **G** Acromioclavicular Joint, Right HAC **H** Acromioclavicular Joint, Left HAC **J** Shoulder Joint, Right HAC **K** Shoulder Joint, Left HAC **L** Elbow Joint, Right HAC **M** Elbow Joint, Left HAC **N** Wrist Joint, Right **P** Wrist Joint, Left **Q** Carpal Joint, Right **R** Carpal Joint, Left **S** Carpometacarpal Joint, Right **T** Carpometacarpal Joint, Left **U** Metacarpophalangeal Joint, Right **V** Metacarpophalangeal Joint, Left **W** Finger Phalangeal Joint, Right **X** Finger Phalangeal Joint, Left	**0** Open **3** Percutaneous **4** Percutaneous Endoscopic **X** External	**Z** No Device	**Z** No Qualifier

HAC 0RQE0ZZ 0RQE3ZZ 0RQE4ZZ 0RQEXZZ 0RQF0ZZ 0RQF3ZZ 0RQF4ZZ 0RQFXZZ 0RQG0ZZ 0RQG3ZZ 0RQG4ZZ 0RQGXZZ 0RQH0ZZ 0RQH3ZZ 0RQH4ZZ 0RQHXZZ 0RQJ0ZZ 0RQJ3ZZ 0RQJ4ZZ 0RQJXZZ 0RQK0ZZ 0RQK3ZZ 0RQK4ZZ 0RQKXZZ 0RQL0ZZ 0RQL3ZZ 0RQL4ZZ 0RQLXZZ 0RQM0ZZ 0RQM3ZZ 0RQM4ZZ 0RQMXZZ
Surgical site infection following certain orthopedic procedures of spine, shoulder or elbow procedures and secondary diagnosis K68.11, T81.40XA, T81.41XA, T81.42XA, T81.43XA, T81.44XA, T81.49XA, T84.60XA, T84.610A, T84.611A, T84.612A, T84.613A, T84.614A, T84.615A, T84.619A, T84.63XA, T84.69XA, T84.7XXA.

0 Medical and Surgical
R Upper Joints
R Replacement: Putting in or on biological or synthetic material that physically takes the place and/or function of all or a portion of a body part

Body Part Character 4	Approach Character 5	Device Character 6	Qualifier Character 7
0 Occipital-cervical Joint **1** Cervical Vertebral Joint **3** Cervical Vertebral Disc **4** Cervicothoracic Vertebral Joint **5** Cervicothoracic Vertebral Disc **6** Thoracic Vertebral Joint **9** Thoracic Vertebral Disc **A** Thoracolumbar Vertebral Joint **B** Thoracolumbar Vertebral Disc **C** Temporomandibular Joint, Right **D** Temporomandibular Joint, Left **E** Sternoclavicular Joint, Right **F** Sternoclavicular Joint, Left **G** Acromioclavicular Joint, Right **H** Acromioclavicular Joint, Left **L** Elbow Joint, Right **M** Elbow Joint, Left **N** Wrist Joint, Right **P** Wrist Joint, Left **Q** Carpal Joint, Right **R** Carpal Joint, Left **S** Carpometacarpal Joint, Right **T** Carpometacarpal Joint, Left **U** Metacarpophalangeal Joint, Right **V** Metacarpophalangeal Joint, Left **W** Finger Phalangeal Joint, Right **X** Finger Phalangeal Joint, Left	**0** Open	**7** Autologous Tissue Substitute **J** Synthetic Substitute **K** Nonautologous Tissue Substitute	**Z** No Qualifier
J Shoulder Joint, Right **K** Shoulder Joint, Left	**0** Open	**0** Synthetic Substitute, Reverse Ball and Socket **7** Autologous Tissue Substitute **K** Nonautologous Tissue Substitute	**Z** No Qualifier
J Shoulder Joint, Right **K** Shoulder Joint, Left	**0** Open	**J** Synthetic Substitute	**6** Humeral Surface **7** Glenoid Surface **Z** No Qualifier

0 Medical and Surgical
R Upper Joints
S Reposition: Moving to its normal location, or other suitable location, all or a portion of a body part

Body Part Character 4	Approach Character 5	Device Character 6	Qualifier Character 7
0 Occipital-cervical Joint **1** Cervical Vertebral Joint **4** Cervicothoracic Vertebral Joint **6** Thoracic Vertebral Joint **A** Thoracolumbar Vertebral Joint **C** Temporomandibular Joint, Right **D** Temporomandibular Joint, Left **E** Sternoclavicular Joint, Right **F** Sternoclavicular Joint, Left **G** Acromioclavicular Joint, Right **H** Acromioclavicular Joint, Left **J** Shoulder Joint, Right **K** Shoulder Joint, Left	**0** Open **3** Percutaneous **4** Percutaneous Endoscopic **X** External	**4** Internal Fixation Device **Z** No Device	**Z** No Qualifier
L Elbow Joint, Right **M** Elbow Joint, Left **N** Wrist Joint, Right **P** Wrist Joint, Left **Q** Carpal Joint, Right **R** Carpal Joint, Left **S** Carpometacarpal Joint, Right **T** Carpometacarpal Joint, Left **U** Metacarpophalangeal Joint, Right **V** Metacarpophalangeal Joint, Left **W** Finger Phalangeal Joint, Right **X** Finger Phalangeal Joint, Left	**0** Open **3** Percutaneous **4** Percutaneous Endoscopic **X** External	**4** Internal Fixation Device **5** External Fixation Device **Z** No Device	**Z** No Qualifier

0 Medical and Surgical
R Upper Joints
T Resection: Cutting out or off, without replacement, all of a body part

Body Part Character 4	Approach Character 5	Device Character 6	Qualifier Character 7
3 Cervical Vertebral Disc **4** Cervicothoracic Vertebral Joint **5** Cervicothoracic Vertebral Disc **9** Thoracic Vertebral Disc **B** Thoracolumbar Vertebral Disc **C** Temporomandibular Joint, Right **D** Temporomandibular Joint, Left **E** Sternoclavicular Joint, Right **F** Sternoclavicular Joint, Left **G** Acromioclavicular Joint, Right **H** Acromioclavicular Joint, Left **J** Shoulder Joint, Right **K** Shoulder Joint, Left **L** Elbow Joint, Right **M** Elbow Joint, Left **N** Wrist Joint, Right **P** Wrist Joint, Left **Q** Carpal Joint, Right **R** Carpal Joint, Left **S** Carpometacarpal Joint, Right **T** Carpometacarpal Joint, Left **U** Metacarpophalangeal Joint, Right **V** Metacarpophalangeal Joint, Left **W** Finger Phalangeal Joint, Right **X** Finger Phalangeal Joint, Left	**0** Open	**Z** No Device	**Z** No Qualifier

0 Medical and Surgical
R Upper Joints
U Supplement: Putting in or on biological or synthetic material that physically reinforces and/or augments the function of a portion of a body part

Body Part	Approach	Device	Qualifier
Character 4	**Character 5**	**Character 6**	**Character 7**
0 Occipital-cervical Joint	**0** Open	**7** Autologous Tissue Substitute	**Z** No Qualifier
1 Cervical Vertebral Joint	**3** Percutaneous	**J** Synthetic Substitute	
3 Cervical Vertebral Disc	**4** Percutaneous Endoscopic	**K** Nonautologous Tissue Substitute	
4 Cervicothoracic Vertebral Joint			
5 Cervicothoracic Vertebral Disc			
6 Thoracic Vertebral Joint			
9 Thoracic Vertebral Disc			
A Thoracolumbar Vertebral Joint			
B Thoracolumbar Vertebral Disc			
C Temporomandibular Joint, Right			
D Temporomandibular Joint, Left			
E Sternoclavicular Joint, Right HAC			
F Sternoclavicular Joint, Left HAC			
G Acromioclavicular Joint, Right HAC			
H Acromioclavicular Joint, Left HAC			
J Shoulder Joint, Right HAC			
K Shoulder Joint, Left HAC			
L Elbow Joint, Right HAC			
M Elbow Joint, Left HAC			
N Wrist Joint, Right			
P Wrist Joint, Left			
Q Carpal Joint, Right			
R Carpal Joint, Left			
S Carpometacarpal Joint, Right			
T Carpometacarpal Joint, Left			
U Metacarpophalangeal Joint, Right			
V Metacarpophalangeal Joint, Left			
W Finger Phalangeal Joint, Right			
X Finger Phalangeal Joint, Left			

HAC 0RUE07Z 0RUE0JZ 0RUE0KZ 0RUE37Z 0RUE3JZ 0RUE3KZ 0RUE47Z 0RUE4JZ 0RUE4KZ 0RUF07Z 0RUF0JZ 0RUF0KZ 0RUF37Z 0RUF3JZ 0RUF3KZ 0RUF47Z 0RUF4JZ 0RUF4KZ 0RUG07Z 0RUG0JZ 0RUG0KZ 0RUG37Z 0RUG3JZ 0RUG3KZ 0RUG47Z 0RUG4JZ 0RUG4KZ 0RUH07Z 0RUH0JZ 0RUH0KZ 0RUH37Z 0RUH3JZ 0RUH3KZ 0RUH47Z 0RUH4JZ 0RUH4KZ 0RUJ07Z 0RUJ0JZ 0RUJ0KZ 0RUJ37Z 0RUJ3JZ 0RUJ3KZ 0RUJ47Z 0RUJ4JZ 0RUJ4KZ 0RUK07Z 0RUK0JZ 0RUK0KZ 0RUK37Z 0RUK3JZ 0RUK3KZ 0RUK47Z 0RUK4JZ 0RUK4KZ 0RUL07Z 0RUL0JZ 0RUL0KZ 0RUL37Z 0RUL3JZ 0RUL3KZ 0RUL47Z 0RUL4JZ 0RUL4KZ 0RUM07Z 0RUM0JZ 0RUM0KZ 0RUM37Z 0RUM3JZ 0RUM3KZ 0RUM47Z 0RUM4JZ 0RUM4KZ
Surgical site infection following certain orthopedic procedures of spine, shoulder or elbow procedures and secondary diagnosis K68.11, T81.40XA, T81.41XA, T81.42XA, T81.43XA, T81.44XA, T81.49XA, T84.60XA, T84.610A, T84.611A, T84.612A, T84.613A, T84.614A, T84.615A, T84.619A, T84.63XA, T84.69XA, T84.7XXA.

0 Medical and Surgical
R Upper Joints
W Revision: Correcting, to the extent possible, a portion of a malfunctioning device or the position of a displaced device

Body Part Character 4	Approach Character 5	Device Character 6	Qualifier Character 7
0 Occipital-cervical Joint **1** Cervical Vertebral Joint **4** Cervicothoracic Vertebral Joint **6** Thoracic Vertebral Joint **A** Thoracolumbar Vertebral Joint	**0** Open **3** Percutaneous **4** Percutaneous Endoscopic **X** External	**0** Drainage Device **3** Infusion Device **4** Internal Fixation Device **7** Autologous Tissue Substitute **8** Spacer **A** Interbody Fusion Device **J** Synthetic Substitute **K** Nonautologous Tissue Substitute	**Z** No Qualifier
3 Cervical Vertebral Disc **5** Cervicothoracic Vertebral Disc **9** Thoracic Vertebral Disc **B** Thoracolumbar Vertebral Disc	**0** Open **3** Percutaneous **4** Percutaneous Endoscopic **X** External	**0** Drainage Device **3** Infusion Device **7** Autologous Tissue Substitute **J** Synthetic Substitute **K** Nonautologous Tissue Substitute	**Z** No Qualifier
C Temporomandibular Joint, Right **D** Temporomandibular Joint, Left **E** Sternoclavicular Joint, Right **F** Sternoclavicular Joint, Left **G** Acromioclavicular Joint, Right **H** Acromioclavicular Joint, Left **J** Shoulder Joint, Right **K** Shoulder Joint, Left	**0** Open **3** Percutaneous **4** Percutaneous Endoscopic **X** External	**0** Drainage Device **3** Infusion Device **4** Internal Fixation Device **7** Autologous Tissue Substitute **8** Spacer **J** Synthetic Substitute **K** Nonautologous Tissue Substitute	**Z** No Qualifier
L Elbow Joint, Right **M** Elbow Joint, Left **N** Wrist Joint, Right **P** Wrist Joint, Left **Q** Carpal Joint, Right **R** Carpal Joint, Left **S** Carpometacarpal Joint, Right **T** Carpometacarpal Joint, Left **U** Metacarpophalangeal Joint, Right **V** Metacarpophalangeal Joint, Left **W** Finger Phalangeal Joint, Right **X** Finger Phalangeal Joint, Left	**0** Open **3** Percutaneous **4** Percutaneous Endoscopic **X** External	**0** Drainage Device **3** Infusion Device **4** Internal Fixation Device **5** External Fixation Device **7** Autologous Tissue Substitute **8** Spacer **J** Synthetic Substitute **K** Nonautologous Tissue Substitute	**Z** No Qualifier

NOTES

Lower Joints 0S2-0SW

0 Medical and Surgical
S Lower Joints
2 Change: Taking out or off a device from a body part and putting back an identical or similar device in or on the same body part without cutting or puncturing the skin or a mucous membrane

Body Part Character 4	Approach Character 5	Device Character 6	Qualifier Character 7
Y Lower Joint	**X** External	**0** Drainage Device **Y** Other Device	**Z** No Qualifier

0 Medical and Surgical
S Lower Joints
5 Destruction: Physical eradication of all or a portion of a body part by the direct use of energy, force, or a destructive agent

Body Part Character 4	Approach Character 5	Device Character 6	Qualifier Character 7
0 Lumbar Vertebral Joint **2** Lumbar Vertebral Disc **3** Lumbosacral Joint **4** Lumbosacral Disc **5** Sacrococcygeal Joint **6** Coccygeal Joint **7** Sacroiliac Joint, Right **8** Sacroiliac Joint, Left **9** Hip Joint, Right **B** Hip Joint, Left **C** Knee Joint, Right **D** Knee Joint, Left **F** Ankle Joint, Right **G** Ankle Joint, Left **H** Tarsal Joint, Right **J** Tarsal Joint, Left **K** Tarsometatarsal Joint, Right **L** Tarsometatarsal Joint, Left **M** Metatarsal-Phalangeal Joint, Right **N** Metatarsal-Phalangeal Joint, Left **P** Toe Phalangeal Joint, Right **Q** Toe Phalangeal Joint, Left	**0** Open **3** Percutaneous **4** Percutaneous Endoscopic	**Z** No Device	**Z** No Qualifier

0 Medical and Surgical
S Lower Joints
9 Drainage: Taking or letting out fluids and/or gases from a body part

Body Part Character 4	Approach Character 5	Device Character 6	Qualifier Character 7
0 Lumbar Vertebral Joint **2** Lumbar Vertebral Disc **3** Lumbosacral Joint **4** Lumbosacral Disc **5** Sacrococcygeal Joint **6** Coccygeal Joint **7** Sacroiliac Joint, Right **8** Sacroiliac Joint, Left **9** Hip Joint, Right **B** Hip Joint, Left **C** Knee Joint, Right **D** Knee Joint, Left **F** Ankle Joint, Right **G** Ankle Joint, Left **H** Tarsal Joint, Right **J** Tarsal Joint, Left **K** Tarsometatarsal Joint, Right **L** Tarsometatarsal Joint, Left **M** Metatarsal-Phalangeal Joint, Right **N** Metatarsal-Phalangeal Joint, Left **P** Toe Phalangeal Joint, Right **Q** Toe Phalangeal Joint, Left	**0** Open **3** Percutaneous **4** Percutaneous Endoscopic	**0** Drainage Device	**Z** No Qualifier
0 Lumbar Vertebral Joint **2** Lumbar Vertebral Disc **3** Lumbosacral Joint **4** Lumbosacral Disc **5** Sacrococcygeal Joint **6** Coccygeal Joint **7** Sacroiliac Joint, Right **8** Sacroiliac Joint, Left **9** Hip Joint, Right **B** Hip Joint, Left **C** Knee Joint, Right **D** Knee Joint, Left **F** Ankle Joint, Right **G** Ankle Joint, Left **H** Tarsal Joint, Right **J** Tarsal Joint, Left **K** Tarsometatarsal Joint, Right **L** Tarsometatarsal Joint, Left **M** Metatarsal-Phalangeal Joint, Right **N** Metatarsal-Phalangeal Joint, Left **P** Toe Phalangeal Joint, Right **Q** Toe Phalangeal Joint, Left	**0** Open **3** Percutaneous **4** Percutaneous Endoscopic	**Z** No Device	**X** Diagnostic **Z** No Qualifier

tricompartmental articular debridement knee 0SB C?

0 Medical and Surgical
S Lower Joints
B Excision: Cutting out or off, without replacement, a portion of a body part

Body Part Character 4	Approach Character 5	Device Character 6	Qualifier Character 7
0 Lumbar Vertebral Joint **2** Lumbar Vertebral Disc **3** Lumbosacral Joint **4** Lumbosacral Disc **5** Sacrococcygeal Joint **6** Coccygeal Joint **7** Sacroiliac Joint, Right **8** Sacroiliac Joint, Left **9** Hip Joint, Right **B** Hip Joint, Left **C** Knee Joint, Right **D** Knee Joint, Left **F** Ankle Joint, Right **G** Ankle Joint, Left **H** Tarsal Joint, Right **J** Tarsal Joint, Left **K** Tarsometatarsal Joint, Right **L** Tarsometatarsal Joint, Left **M** Metatarsal-Phalangeal Joint, Right **N** Metatarsal-Phalangeal Joint, Left **P** Toe Phalangeal Joint, Right **Q** Toe Phalangeal Joint, Left	**0** Open **3** Percutaneous **4** Percutaneous Endoscopic	**Z** No Device	**X** Diagnostic **Z** No Qualifier

0 Medical and Surgical
S Lower Joints
C Extirpation: Taking or cutting out solid matter from a body part

Body Part Character 4	Approach Character 5	Device Character 6	Qualifier Character 7
0 Lumbar Vertebral Joint **2** Lumbar Vertebral Disc **3** Lumbosacral Joint **4** Lumbosacral Disc **5** Sacrococcygeal Joint **6** Coccygeal Joint **7** Sacroiliac Joint, Right **8** Sacroiliac Joint, Left **9** Hip Joint, Right **B** Hip Joint, Left **C** Knee Joint, Right **D** Knee Joint, Left **F** Ankle Joint, Right **G** Ankle Joint, Left **H** Tarsal Joint, Right **J** Tarsal Joint, Left **K** Tarsometatarsal Joint, Right **L** Tarsometatarsal Joint, Left **M** Metatarsal-Phalangeal Joint, Right **N** Metatarsal-Phalangeal Joint, Left **P** Toe Phalangeal Joint, Right **Q** Toe Phalangeal Joint, Left	**0** Open **3** Percutaneous **4** Percutaneous Endoscopic	**Z** No Device	**Z** No Qualifier

0 Medical and Surgical
S Lower Joints
G Fusion: Joining together portions of an articular body part rendering the articular body part immobile

Body Part Character 4	Approach Character 5	Device Character 6	Qualifier Character 7
0 Lumbar Vertebral Joint HAC **1** Lumbar Vertebral Joints, 2 or more HAC CC **3** Lumbosacral Joint HAC	**0** Open **3** Percutaneous **4** Percutaneous Endoscopic	**7** Autologous Tissue Substitute **J** Synthetic Substitute **K** Nonautologous Tissue Substitute	**0** Anterior Approach, Anterior Column **1** Posterior Approach, Posterior Column **J** Posterior Approach, Anterior Column
0 Lumbar Vertebral Joint HAC **1** Lumbar Vertebral Joints, 2 or more HAC CC **3** Lumbosacral Joint HAC	**0** Open **3** Percutaneous **4** Percutaneous Endoscopic	**A** Interbody Fusion Device	**0** Anterior Approach, Anterior Column **J** Posterior Approach, Anterior Column
5 Sacrococcygeal Joint **6** Coccygeal Joint **7** Sacroiliac Joint, Right HAC **8** Sacroiliac Joint, Left HAC	**0** Open **3** Percutaneous **4** Percutaneous Endoscopic	**4** Internal Fixation Device **7** Autologous Tissue Substitute **J** Synthetic Substitute **K** Nonautologous Tissue Substitute	**Z** No Qualifier
9 Hip Joint, Right **B** Hip Joint, Left **C** Knee Joint, Right **D** Knee Joint, Left **F** Ankle Joint, Right **G** Ankle Joint, Left **H** Tarsal Joint, Right **J** Tarsal Joint, Left **K** Tarsometatarsal Joint, Right **L** Tarsometatarsal Joint, Left **M** Metatarsal-Phalangeal Joint, Right **N** Metatarsal-Phalangeal Joint, Left **P** Toe Phalangeal Joint, Right **Q** Toe Phalangeal Joint, Left	**0** Open **3** Percutaneous **4** Percutaneous Endoscopic	**4** Internal Fixation Device **5** External Fixation Device **7** Autologous Tissue Substitute **J** Synthetic Substitute **K** Nonautologous Tissue Substitute	**Z** No Qualifier

HAC 0SG0070 0SG0071 0SG007J 0SG00A0 0SG00AJ 0SG00J0 0SG00J1 0SG00JJ 0SG00K0 0SG00K1 0SG00KJ 0SG0370 0SG0371 0SG037J 0SG03A0 0SG03AJ 0SG03J0 0SG03J1 0SG03JJ 0SG03K0 0SG03K1 0SG03KJ 0SG0470 0SG0471 0SG047J 0SG04A0 0SG04AJ 0SG04J0 0SG04J1 0SG04JJ 0SG04K0 0SG04K1 0SG04KJ 0SG1070 0SG1071 0SG107J 0SG10A0 0SG10AJ 0SG10J0 0SG10J1 0SG10JJ 0SG10K0 0SG10K1 0SG10KJ 0SG1370 0SG1371 0SG137J 0SG13A0 0SG13AJ 0SG13J0 0SG13J1 0SG13JJ 0SG13K0 0SG13K1 0SG13KJ 0SG1470 0SG1471 0SG147J 0SG14A0 0SG14AJ 0SG14J0 0SG14J1 0SG14JJ 0SG14K0 0SG14K1 0SG14KJ 0SG3070 0SG3071 0SG307J 0SG30A0 0SG30AJ 0SG30J0 0SG30J1 0SG30JJ 0SG30K0 0SG30K1 0SG30KJ 0SG3370 0SG3371 0SG337J 0SG33A0 0SG33AJ 0SG33J0 0SG33J1 0SG33JJ 0SG33K0 0SG33K1 0SG33KJ 0SG3470 0SG3471 0SG347J 0SG34A0 0SG34AJ 0SG34J0 0SG34J1 0SG34JJ 0SG34K0 0SG34K1 0SG34KJ 0SG704Z 0SG707Z 0SG70JZ 0SG70KZ 0SG734Z 0SG737Z 0SG73JZ 0SG73KZ 0SG744Z 0SG747Z 0SG74JZ 0SG74KZ 0SG804Z 0SG807Z 0SG80JZ 0SG80KZ 0SG834Z 0SG837Z 0SG83JZ 0SG83KZ 0SG844Z 0SG847Z 0SG84JZ 0SG84KZ

Surgical site infection following certain orthopedic procedures of spine, shoulder or elbow procedures and secondary diagnosis K68.11, T81.40XA, T81.41XA, T81.42XA, T81.43XA, T81.44XA, T81.49XA, T84.60XA, T84.610A, T84.611A, T84.612A, T84.613A, T84.614A, T84.615A, T84.619A, T84.63XA, T84.69XA, T84.7XXA.

CC 0SG1070 0SG1071 0SG107J 0SG10A0 0SG10AJ 0SG10J0 0SG10J1 0SG10JJ 0SG10K0 0SG10K1 0SG10KJ 0SG1370 0SG1371 0SG137J 0SG13A0 0SG13AJ 0SG13J0 0SG13J1 0SG13JJ 0SG13K0 0SG13K1 0SG13KJ 0SG1470 0SG1471 0SG147J 0SG14A0 0SG14AJ 0SG14J0 0SG14J1 0SG14JJ 0SG14K0 0SG14K1 0SG14KJ

0 Medical and Surgical
S Lower Joints
H Insertion: Putting in a nonbiological appliance that monitors, assists, performs, or prevents a physiological function but does not physically take the place of a body part

Body Part Character 4	Approach Character 5	Device Character 6	Qualifier Character 7
0 Lumbar Vertebral Joint **3** Lumbosacral Joint	**0** Open **3** Percutaneous **4** Percutaneous Endoscopic	**3** Infusion Device **4** Internal Fixation Device **8** Spacer **B** Spinal Stabilization Device, Interspinous Process **C** Spinal Stabilization Device, Pedicle-Based **D** Spinal Stabilization Device, Facet Replacement	**Z** No Qualifier
2 Lumbar Vertebral Disc **4** Lumbosacral Disc	**0** Open **3** Percutaneous **4** Percutaneous Endoscopic	**3** Infusion Device **8** Spacer	**Z** No Qualifier
5 Sacrococcygeal Joint **6** Coccygeal Joint **7** Sacroiliac Joint, Right **8** Sacroiliac Joint, Left	**0** Open **3** Percutaneous **4** Percutaneous Endoscopic	**3** Infusion Device **4** Internal Fixation Device **8** Spacer	**Z** No Qualifier
9 Hip Joint, Right **B** Hip Joint, Left **C** Knee Joint, Right **D** Knee Joint, Left **F** Ankle Joint, Right **G** Ankle Joint, Left **H** Tarsal Joint, Right **J** Tarsal Joint, Left **K** Tarsometatarsal Joint, Right **L** Tarsometatarsal Joint, Left **M** Metatarsal-Phalangeal Joint, Right **N** Metatarsal-Phalangeal Joint, Left **P** Toe Phalangeal Joint, Right **Q** Toe Phalangeal Joint, Left	**0** Open **3** Percutaneous **4** Percutaneous Endoscopic	**3** Infusion Device **4** Internal Fixation Device **5** External Fixation Device **8** Spacer	**Z** No Qualifier

0 Medical and Surgical
S Lower Joints
J Inspection: Visually and/or manually exploring a body part

Body Part Character 4	Approach Character 5	Device Character 6	Qualifier Character 7
0 Lumbar Vertebral Joint	0 Open	Z No Device	Z No Qualifier
2 Lumbar Vertebral Disc	3 Percutaneous		
3 Lumbosacral Joint	4 Percutaneous Endoscopic =arthroscope		
4 Lumbosacral Disc	X External		
5 Sacrococcygeal Joint			
6 Coccygeal Joint			
7 Sacroiliac Joint, Right			
8 Sacroiliac Joint, Left			
9 Hip Joint, Right			
B Hip Joint, Left			
C Knee Joint, Right			
D Knee Joint, Left			
F Ankle Joint, Right			
G Ankle Joint, Left			
H Tarsal Joint, Right			
J Tarsal Joint, Left			
K Tarsometatarsal Joint, Right			
L Tarsometatarsal Joint, Left			
M Metatarsal-Phalangeal Joint, Right			
N Metatarsal-Phalangeal Joint, Left			
P Toe Phalangeal Joint, Right			
Q Toe Phalangeal Joint, Left			

0 Medical and Surgical
S Lower Joints
N Release: Freeing a body part from an abnormal physical constraint by cutting or by the use of force

Body Part Character 4	Approach Character 5	Device Character 6	Qualifier Character 7
0 Lumbar Vertebral Joint	0 Open	Z No Device	Z No Qualifier
2 Lumbar Vertebral Disc	3 Percutaneous		
3 Lumbosacral Joint	4 Percutaneous Endoscopic		
4 Lumbosacral Disc	X External		
5 Sacrococcygeal Joint			
6 Coccygeal Joint			
7 Sacroiliac Joint, Right			
8 Sacroiliac Joint, Left			
9 Hip Joint, Right			
B Hip Joint, Left			
C Knee Joint, Right			
D Knee Joint, Left			
F Ankle Joint, Right			
G Ankle Joint, Left			
H Tarsal Joint, Right			
J Tarsal Joint, Left			
K Tarsometatarsal Joint, Right			
L Tarsometatarsal Joint, Left			
M Metatarsal-Phalangeal Joint, Right			
N Metatarsal-Phalangeal Joint, Left			
P Toe Phalangeal Joint, Right			
Q Toe Phalangeal Joint, Left			

0 Medical and Surgical
S Lower Joints
P Removal: Taking out or off a device from a body part

Body Part Character 4	Approach Character 5	Device Character 6	Qualifier Character 7
0 Lumbar Vertebral Joint 3 Lumbosacral Joint	0 Open 3 Percutaneous 4 Percutaneous Endoscopic	0 Drainage Device 3 Infusion Device 4 Internal Fixation Device 7 Autologous Tissue Substitute 8 Spacer A Interbody Fusion Device J Synthetic Substitute K Nonautologous Tissue Substitute	Z No Qualifier
0 Lumbar Vertebral Joint 3 Lumbosacral Joint	X External	0 Drainage Device 3 Infusion Device 4 Internal Fixation Device	Z No Qualifier
2 Lumbar Vertebral Disc 4 Lumbosacral Disc	0 Open 3 Percutaneous 4 Percutaneous Endoscopic	0 Drainage Device 3 Infusion Device 7 Autologous Tissue Substitute J Synthetic Substitute K Nonautologous Tissue Substitute	Z No Qualifier
2 Lumbar Vertebral Disc 4 Lumbosacral Disc	X External	0 Drainage Device 3 Infusion Device	Z No Qualifier
5 Sacrococcygeal Joint 6 Coccygeal Joint 7 Sacroiliac Joint, Right 8 Sacroiliac Joint, Left	0 Open 3 Percutaneous 4 Percutaneous Endoscopic	0 Drainage Device 3 Infusion Device 4 Internal Fixation Device 7 Autologous Tissue Substitute 8 Spacer J Synthetic Substitute K Nonautologous Tissue Substitute	Z No Qualifier
5 Sacrococcygeal Joint 6 Coccygeal Joint 7 Sacroiliac Joint, Right 8 Sacroiliac Joint, Left	X External	0 Drainage Device 3 Infusion Device 4 Internal Fixation Device	Z No Qualifier
9 Hip Joint, Right CC B Hip Joint, Left CC	0 Open	0 Drainage Device 3 Infusion Device 4 Internal Fixation Device 5 External Fixation Device 7 Autologous Tissue Substitute 8 Spacer 9 Liner B Resurfacing Device E Articulating Spacer J Synthetic Substitute K Nonautologous Tissue Substitute	Z No Qualifier
9 Hip Joint, Right DRG CC B Hip Joint, Left CC	3 Percutaneous 4 Percutaneous Endoscopic	0 Drainage Device 3 Infusion Device 4 Internal Fixation Device 5 External Fixation Device 7 Autologous Tissue Substitute 8 Spacer J Synthetic Substitute K Nonautologous Tissue Substitute	Z No Qualifier
9 Hip Joint, Right B Hip Joint, Left	X External	0 Drainage Device 3 Infusion Device 4 Internal Fixation Device 5 External Fixation Device	Z No Qualifier

0SP continued on next page

0SP continued from previous page

0 Medical and Surgical
S Lower Joints
P Removal: Taking out or off a device from a body part

Body Part Character 4	Approach Character 5	Device Character 6	Qualifier Character 7
A Hip Joint, Acetabular Surface, Right CC E Hip Joint, Acetabular Surface, Left CC R Hip Joint, Femoral Surface, Right CC S Hip Joint, Femoral Surface, Left CC T Knee Joint, Femoral Surface, Right CC U Knee Joint, Femoral Surface, Left CC V Knee Joint, Tibial Surface, Right CC W Knee Joint, Tibial Surface, Left CC	0 Open 3 Percutaneous 4 Percutaneous Endoscopic	J Synthetic Substitute	Z No Qualifier
C Knee Joint, Right CC D Knee Joint, Left CC	0 Open	0 Drainage Device 3 Infusion Device 4 Internal Fixation Device 5 External Fixation Device 7 Autologous Tissue Substitute 8 Spacer 9 Liner E Articulating Spacer K Nonautologous Tissue Substitute L Synthetic Substitute, Unicondylar Medial M Synthetic Substitute, Unicondylar Lateral N Synthetic Substitute, Patellofemoral	Z No Qualifier
C Knee Joint, Right CC D Knee Joint, Left CC	0 Open	J Synthetic Substitute	C Patellar Surface Z No Qualifier
C Knee Joint, Right DRG CC D Knee Joint, Left DRG CC	3 Percutaneous 4 Percutaneous Endoscopic	0 Drainage Device 3 Infusion Device 4 Internal Fixation Device 5 External Fixation Device 7 Autologous Tissue Substitute 8 Spacer K Nonautologous Tissue Substitute L Synthetic Substitute, Unicondylar Medial M Synthetic Substitute, Unicondylar Lateral N Synthetic Substitute, Patellofemoral	Z No Qualifier
C Knee Joint, Right CC D Knee Joint, Left CC	3 Percutaneous 4 Percutaneous Endoscopic	J Synthetic Substitute	C Patellar Surface Z No Qualifier
C Knee Joint, Right D Knee Joint, Left	X External	0 Drainage Device 3 Infusion Device 4 Internal Fixation Device 5 External Fixation Device	Z No Qualifier

0SP continued on next page

0 Medical and Surgical
S Lower Joints
P Removal: Taking out or off a device from a body part

0SP continued from previous page

Body Part Character 4	Approach Character 5	Device Character 6	Qualifier Character 7
F Ankle Joint, Right **G** Ankle Joint, Left **H** Tarsal Joint, Right **J** Tarsal Joint, Left **K** Tarsometatarsal Joint, Right **L** Tarsometatarsal Joint, Left **M** Metatarsal-Phalangeal Joint, Right **N** Metatarsal-Phalangeal Joint, Left **P** Toe Phalangeal Joint, Right **Q** Toe Phalangeal Joint, Left	**0** Open **3** Percutaneous **4** Percutaneous Endoscopic	**0** Drainage Device **3** Infusion Device **4** Internal Fixation Device **5** External Fixation Device **7** Autologous Tissue Substitute **8** Spacer **J** Synthetic Substitute **K** Nonautologous Tissue Substitute	**Z** No Qualifier
F Ankle Joint, Right **G** Ankle Joint, Left **H** Tarsal Joint, Right **J** Tarsal Joint, Left **K** Tarsometatarsal Joint, Right **L** Tarsometatarsal Joint, Left **M** Metatarsal-Phalangeal Joint, Right **N** Metatarsal-Phalangeal Joint, Left **P** Toe Phalangeal Joint, Right **Q** Toe Phalangeal Joint, Left	**X** External	**0** Drainage Device **3** Infusion Device **4** Internal Fixation Device **5** External Fixation Device	**Z** No Qualifier

DRG 0SP948Z 0SPB48Z 0SPC38Z 0SPC48Z 0SPD38Z 0SPD48Z

CC 0SP908Z 0SP909Z 0SP90BZ 0SP90EZ 0SP90JZ 0SP948Z 0SP94JZ 0SPA0JZ 0SPA4JZ 0SPB08Z 0SPB09Z 0SPB0BZ 0SPB0EZ 0SPB0JZ 0SPB48Z 0SPB4JZ 0SPC08Z 0SPC09Z 0SPC0EZ 0SPC0JC 0SPC0JZ 0SPC0LZ 0SPC0MZ 0SPC0NZ 0SPC38Z 0SPC48Z 0SPC4JC 0SPC4JZ 0SPC4LZ 0SPC4MZ 0SPC4NZ 0SPD08Z 0SPD09Z 0SPD0EZ 0SPD0JC 0SPD0JZ 0SPD0LZ 0SPD0MZ 0SPD0NZ 0SPD38Z 0SPD48Z 0SPD4JC 0SPD4JZ 0SPD4LZ 0SPD4MZ 0SPD4NZ 0SPE0JZ 0SPE4JZ 0SPR0JZ 0SPR4JZ 0SPS0JZ 0SPS4JZ 0SPT0JZ 0SPT4JZ 0SPU0JZ 0SPU4JZ 0SPV0JZ 0SPV4JZ 0SPW0JZ 0SPW4JZ

0 Medical and Surgical
S Lower Joints
Q Repair: Restoring, to the extent possible, a body part to its normal anatomic structure and function

Body Part Character 4	Approach Character 5	Device Character 6	Qualifier Character 7
0 Lumbar Vertebral Joint **2** Lumbar Vertebral Disc **3** Lumbosacral Joint **4** Lumbosacral Disc **5** Sacrococcygeal Joint **6** Coccygeal Joint **7** Sacroiliac Joint, Right **8** Sacroiliac Joint, Left **9** Hip Joint, Right **B** Hip Joint, Left **C** Knee Joint, Right - medial femoral condyle **D** Knee Joint, Left **F** Ankle Joint, Right **G** Ankle Joint, Left **H** Tarsal Joint, Right **J** Tarsal Joint, Left **K** Tarsometatarsal Joint, Right **L** Tarsometatarsal Joint, Left **M** Metatarsal-Phalangeal Joint, Right **N** Metatarsal-Phalangeal Joint, Left **P** Toe Phalangeal Joint, Right **Q** Toe Phalangeal Joint, Left	**0** Open **3** Percutaneous **4** Percutaneous Endoscopic - arthroscopy **X** External	**Z** No Device	**Z** No Qualifier

0 **Medical and Surgical**
S **Lower Joints**
R **Replacement:** Putting in or on biological or synthetic material that physically takes the place and/or function of all or a portion of a body part

Body Part Character 4	Approach Character 5	Device Character 6	Qualifier Character 7
0 Lumbar Vertebral Joint 2 Lumbar Vertebral Disc NC 3 Lumbosacral Joint 4 Lumbosacral Disc NC 5 Sacrococcygeal Joint 6 Coccygeal Joint 7 Sacroiliac Joint, Right 8 Sacroiliac Joint, Left H Tarsal Joint, Right J Tarsal Joint, Left K Tarsometatarsal Joint, Right L Tarsometatarsal Joint, Left M Metatarsal-Phalangeal Joint, Right N Metatarsal-Phalangeal Joint, Left P Toe Phalangeal Joint, Right Q Toe Phalangeal Joint, Left	0 Open	7 Autologous Tissue Substitute J Synthetic Substitute K Nonautologous Tissue Substitute	Z No Qualifier
9 Hip Joint, Right HAC CC B Hip Joint, Left HAC CC	0 Open	1 Synthetic Substitute, Metal 2 Synthetic Substitute, Metal on Polyethylene 3 Synthetic Substitute, Ceramic 4 Synthetic Substitute, Ceramic on Polyethylene 6 Synthetic Substitute, Oxidized Zirconium on Polyethylene J Synthetic Substitute	9 Cemented A Uncemented Z No Qualifier
9 Hip Joint, Right HAC CC B Hip Joint, Left HAC CC	0 Open	7 Autologous Tissue Substitute E Articulating Spacer K Nonautologous Tissue Substitute	Z No Qualifier
A Hip Joint, Acetabular Surface, Right HAC CC E Hip Joint, Acetabular Surface, Left HAC CC	0 Open	0 Synthetic Substitute, Polyethylene 1 Synthetic Substitute, Metal 3 Synthetic Substitute, Ceramic J Synthetic Substitute	9 Cemented A Uncemented Z No Qualifier
A Hip Joint, Acetabular Surface, Right HAC E Hip Joint, Acetabular Surface, Left HAC	0 Open	7 Autologous Tissue Substitute K Nonautologous Tissue Substitute	Z No Qualifier
C Knee Joint, Right HAC CC D Knee Joint, Left HAC CC	0 Open	6 Synthetic Substitute, Oxidized Zirconium on Polyethylene J Synthetic Substitute L Synthetic Substitute, Unicondylar Medial M Synthetic Substitute, Unicondylar Lateral N Synthetic Substitute, Patellofemoral	9 Cemented A Uncemented Z No Qualifier
C Knee Joint, Right HAC CC D Knee Joint, Left HAC CC	0 Open	7 Autologous Tissue Substitute E Articulating Spacer K Nonautologous Tissue Substitute	Z No Qualifier

0SR continued on next page

0 Medical and Surgical
S Lower Joints
R Replacement: Putting in or on biological or synthetic material that physically takes the place and/or function of all or a portion of a body part

0SR continued from previous page

Body Part Character 4	Approach Character 5	Device Character 6	Qualifier Character 7
F Ankle Joint, Right **G** Ankle Joint, Left **T** Knee Joint, Femoral Surface, Right HAC **U** Knee Joint, Femoral Surface, Left HAC **V** Knee Joint, Tibial Surface, Right HAC **W** Knee Joint, Tibial Surface, Left HAC	**0** Open	**7** Autologous Tissue Substitute **K** Nonautologous Tissue Substitute	**Z** No Qualifier
F Ankle Joint, Right **G** Ankle Joint, Left **T** Knee Joint, Femoral Surface, Right HAC CC **U** Knee Joint, Femoral Surface, Left HAC CC **V** Knee Joint, Tibial Surface, Right HAC CC **W** Knee Joint, Tibial Surface, Left HAC CC	**0** Open	**J** Synthetic Substitute	**9** Cemented **A** Uncemented **Z** No Qualifier
R Hip Joint, Femoral Surface, Right HAC CC **S** Hip Joint, Femoral Surface, Left HAC CC	**0** Open	**1** Synthetic Substitute, Metal **3** Synthetic Substitute, Ceramic **J** Synthetic Substitute	**9** Cemented **A** Uncemented **Z** No Qualifier
R Hip Joint, Femoral Surface, Right HAC **S** Hip Joint, Femoral Surface, Left HAC	**0** Open	**7** Autologous Tissue Substitute **K** Nonautologous Tissue Substitute	**Z** No Qualifier

NC 0SR20JZ 0SR40JZ
When the beneficiary is over age 60.

HAC 0SR9019 0SR901A 0SR901Z 0SR9029 0SR902A 0SR902Z 0SR9039 0SR903A 0SR903Z 0SR9049 0SR904A 0SR904Z 0SR9069 0SR906A 0SR906Z 0SR907Z 0SR90EZ 0SR90J9 0SR90JA 0SR90JZ 0SR90KZ 0SRA009 0SRA00A 0SRA00Z 0SRA019 0SRA01A 0SRA01Z 0SRA039 0SRA03A 0SRA03Z 0SRA07Z 0SRA0J9 0SRA0JA 0SRA0JZ 0SRA0KZ 0SRB019 0SRB01A 0SRB01Z 0SRB029 0SRB02A 0SRB02Z 0SRB039 0SRB03A 0SRB03Z 0SRB049 0SRB04A 0SRB04Z 0SRB069 0SRB06A 0SRB06Z 0SRB07Z 0SRB0EZ 0SRB0J9 0SRB0JA 0SRB0JZ 0SRB0KZ 0SRC069 0SRC06A 0SRC06Z 0SRC07Z 0SRC0EZ 0SRC0J9 0SRC0JA 0SRC0JZ 0SRC0KZ 0SRC0L9 0SRC0LA 0SRC0LZ 0SRC0M9 0SRC0MA 0SRC0MZ 0SRC0N9 0SRC0NA 0SRC0NZ 0SRD069 0SRD06A 0SRD06Z 0SRD07Z 0SRD0EZ 0SRD0J9 0SRD0JA 0SRD0JZ 0SRD0KZ 0SRD0L9 0SRD0LA 0SRD0LZ 0SRD0M9 0SRD0MA 0SRD0MZ 0SRD0N9 0SRD0NA 0SRD0NZ 0SRE009 0SRE00A 0SRE00Z 0SRE019 0SRE01A 0SRE01Z 0SRE039 0SRE03A 0SRE03Z 0SRE07Z 0SRE0J9 0SRE0JA 0SRE0JZ 0SRE0KZ 0SRR019 0SRR01A 0SRR01Z 0SRR039 0SRR03A 0SRR03Z 0SRR07Z 0SRR0J9 0SRR0JA 0SRR0JZ 0SRR0KZ 0SRS019 0SRS01A 0SRS01Z 0SRS039 0SRS03A 0SRS03Z 0SRS07Z 0SRS0J9 0SRS0JA 0SRS0JZ 0SRS0KZ 0SRT07Z 0SRT0J9 0SRT0JA 0SRT0JZ 0SRT0KZ 0SRU07Z 0SRU0J9 0SRU0JA 0SRU0JZ 0SRU0KZ 0SRV07Z 0SRV0J9 0SRV0JA 0SRV0JZ 0SRV0KZ 0SRW07Z 0SRW0J9 0SRW0JA 0SRW0JZ 0SRW0KZ
Surgical site infection, mediastinitis, following coronary artery bypass graft (CABG) and secondary diagnosis I26.02, I26.09, I26.92. I26.99, I82.401, I82.402, I82.403, I82.409, I82.411, I82.412, I82.413, I82.419, I82.421, I82.422, I82.423, I82.429, I82.431, I82.432, I82.433, I82.439 I82.441, I82.442, I82.443, I82.449, I82.491, I82.492, I82.493, I82.499, I82.4Y1, I82.4Y2, I82.4Y3, I82.4Y9, I82.4Z1, I82.4Z2, I82.4Z3, I82.4Z9.

CC 0SR9019 0SR901A 0SR901Z 0SR9029 0SR902A 0SR902Z 0SR9039 0SR903A 0SR903Z 0SR9049 0SR904A 0SR904Z 0SR9069 0SR906A 0SR906Z 0SR90EZ 0SR90J9 0SR90JA 0SR90JZ 0SRA009 0SRA00A 0SRA00Z 0SRA019 0SRA01A 0SRA01Z 0SRA039 0SRA03A 0SRA03Z 0SRA0J9 0SRA0JA 0SRA0JZ 0SRB019 0SRB01A 0SRB01Z 0SRB029 0SRB02A 0SRB02Z 0SRB039 0SRB03A 0SRB03Z 0SRB049 0SRB04A 0SRB04Z 0SRB069 0SRB06A 0SRB06Z 0SRB0EZ 0SRB0J9 0SRB0JA 0SRB0JZ 0SRC069 0SRC06A 0SRC06Z 0SRC0EZ 0SRC0J9 0SRC0JA 0SRC0JZ 0SRC0L9 0SRC0LA 0SRC0LZ 0SRC0M9 0SRC0MA 0SRC0MZ 0SRC0N9 0SRC0NA 0SRC0NZ 0SRD069 0SRD06A 0SRD06Z 0SRD0EZ 0SRD0J9 0SRD0JA 0SRD0JZ 0SRD0L9 0SRD0LA 0SRD0LZ 0SRD0M9 0SRD0MA 0SRD0MZ 0SRD0N9 0SRD0NA 0SRD0NZ 0SRE009 0SRE00A 0SRE00Z 0SRE019 0SRE01A 0SRE01Z 0SRE039 0SRE03A 0SRE03Z 0SRE0J9 0SRE0JA 0SRE0JZ 0SRR019 0SRR01A 0SRR01Z 0SRR039 0SRR03A 0SRR03Z 0SRR0J9 0SRR0JA 0SRR0JZ 0SRS019 0SRS01A 0SRS01Z 0SRS039 0SRS03A 0SRS03Z 0SRS0J9 0SRS0JA 0SRS0JZ 0SRT0J9 0SRT0JA 0SRT0JZ 0SRU0J9 0SRU0JA 0SRU0JZ 0SRV0J9 0SRV0JA 0SRV0JZ 0SRW0J9 0SRW0JA 0SRW0JZ

0 Medical and Surgical
S Lower Joints
S Reposition: Moving to its normal location, or other suitable location, all or a portion of a body part

Body Part Character 4	Approach Character 5	Device Character 6	Qualifier Character 7
0 Lumbar Vertebral Joint **3** Lumbosacral Joint **5** Sacrococcygeal Joint **6** Coccygeal Joint **7** Sacroiliac Joint, Right **8** Sacroiliac Joint, Left	**0** Open **3** Percutaneous **4** Percutaneous Endoscopic **X** External	**4** Internal Fixation Device **Z** No Device	**Z** No Qualifier
9 Hip Joint, Right **B** Hip Joint, Left **C** Knee Joint, Right **D** Knee Joint, Left **F** Ankle Joint, Right **G** Ankle Joint, Left **H** Tarsal Joint, Right **J** Tarsal Joint, Left **K** Tarsometatarsal Joint, Right **L** Tarsometatarsal Joint, Left **M** Metatarsal-Phalangeal Joint, Right **N** Metatarsal-Phalangeal Joint, Left **P** Toe Phalangeal Joint, Right **Q** Toe Phalangeal Joint, Left	**0** Open **3** Percutaneous **4** Percutaneous Endoscopic **X** External	**4** Internal Fixation Device **5** External Fixation Device **Z** No Device	**Z** No Qualifier

0 Medical and Surgical
S Lower Joints
T Resection: Cutting out or off, without replacement, all of a body part

Body Part Character 4	Approach Character 5	Device Character 6	Qualifier Character 7
2 Lumbar Vertebral Disc **4** Lumbosacral Disc **5** Sacrococcygeal Joint **6** Coccygeal Joint **7** Sacroiliac Joint, Right **8** Sacroiliac Joint, Left **9** Hip Joint, Right **B** Hip Joint, Left **C** Knee Joint, Right **D** Knee Joint, Left **F** Ankle Joint, Right **G** Ankle Joint, Left **H** Tarsal Joint, Right **J** Tarsal Joint, Left **K** Tarsometatarsal Joint, Right **L** Tarsometatarsal Joint, Left **M** Metatarsal-Phalangeal Joint, Right **N** Metatarsal-Phalangeal Joint, Left **P** Toe Phalangeal Joint, Right **Q** Toe Phalangeal Joint, Left	**0** Open	**Z** No Device	**Z** No Qualifier

0 Medical and Surgical
S Lower Joints
U Supplement: Putting in or on biological or synthetic material that physically reinforces and/or augments the function of a portion of a body part

Body Part Character 4	Approach Character 5	Device Character 6	Qualifier Character 7
0 Lumbar Vertebral Joint **2** Lumbar Vertebral Disc **3** Lumbosacral Joint **4** Lumbosacral Disc **5** Sacrococcygeal Joint **6** Coccygeal Joint **7** Sacroiliac Joint, Right **8** Sacroiliac Joint, Left **F** Ankle Joint, Right **G** Ankle Joint, Left **H** Tarsal Joint, Right **J** Tarsal Joint, Left **K** Tarsometatarsal Joint, Right **L** Tarsometatarsal Joint, Left **M** Metatarsal-Phalangeal Joint, Right **N** Metatarsal-Phalangeal Joint, Left **P** Toe Phalangeal Joint, Right **Q** Toe Phalangeal Joint, Left	**0** Open **3** Percutaneous **4** Percutaneous Endoscopic	**7** Autologous Tissue Substitute **J** Synthetic Substitute **K** Nonautologous Tissue Substitute	**Z** No Qualifier
9 Hip Joint, Right HAC CC **B** Hip Joint, Left HAC CC	**0** Open	**7** Autologous Tissue Substitute **9** Liner **B** Resurfacing Device **J** Synthetic Substitute **K** Nonautologous Tissue Substitute	**Z** No Qualifier
9 Hip Joint, Right **B** Hip Joint, Left	**3** Percutaneous **4** Percutaneous Endoscopic	**7** Autologous Tissue Substitute **J** Synthetic Substitute **K** Nonautologous Tissue Substitute	**Z** No Qualifier
A Hip Joint, Acetabular Surface, Right HAC CC **E** Hip Joint, Acetabular Surface, Left HAC CC **R** Hip Joint, Femoral Surface, Right HAC CC **S** Hip Joint, Femoral Surface, Left HAC CC	**0** Open	**9** Liner **B** Resurfacing Device	**Z** No Qualifier
C Knee Joint, Right **D** Knee Joint, Left	**0** Open	**7** Autologous Tissue Substitute **J** Synthetic Substitute **K** Nonautologous Tissue Substitute	**Z** No Qualifier
C Knee Joint, Right **D** Knee Joint, Left	**0** Open	**9** Liner	**C** Patellar Surface **Z** No Qualifier
C Knee Joint, Right **D** Knee Joint, Left	**3** Percutaneous **4** Percutaneous Endoscopic	**7** Autologous Tissue Substitute **J** Synthetic Substitute **K** Nonautologous Tissue Substitute	**Z** No Qualifier
T Knee Joint, Femoral Surface, Right **U** Knee Joint, Femoral Surface, Left **V** Knee Joint, Tibial Surface, Right CC **W** Knee Joint, Tibial Surface, Left CC	**0** Open	**9** Liner	**Z** No Qualifier

HAC 0SU90BZ 0SUA0BZ 0SUB0BZ 0SUE0BZ 0SUR0BZ 0SUS0BZ
Surgical site infection, mediastinitis, following coronary artery bypass graft (CABG) and secondary diagnosis I26.02, I26.09, I26.92, I26.99, I82.401, I82.402, I82.403, I82.409, I82.411, I82.412, I82.413, I82.419, I82.421, I82.422, I82.423, I82.429, I82.431, I82.432, I82.433, I82.439, I82.441, I82.442, I82.443, I82.449, I82.491, I82.492, I82.493, I82.499, I82.4Y1, I82.4Y2, I82.4Y3, I82.4Y9, I82.4Z1, I82.4Z2, I82.4Z3, I82.4Z9.

CC 0SU909Z 0SUA09Z 0SUB09Z 0SUE09Z 0SUR09Z 0SUS09Z 0SUV09Z 0SUW09Z

LC Limited Coverage NC Noncovered HAC HAC-associated Procedure CC Combination Cluster - See Appendix G for code lists
ORG Non-OR-Affecting MS-DRG Assignment New/Revised Text in **Orange** ♂ Male ♀ Female

0 Medical and Surgical
S Lower Joints
W Revision: Correcting, to the extent possible, a portion of a malfunctioning device or the position of a displaced device

Body Part Character 4	Approach Character 5	Device Character 6	Qualifier Character 7
0 Lumbar Vertebral Joint **3** Lumbosacral Joint	**0** Open **3** Percutaneous **4** Percutaneous Endoscopic **X** External	**0** Drainage Device **3** Infusion Device **4** Internal Fixation Device **7** Autologous Tissue Substitute **8** Spacer **A** Interbody Fusion Device **J** Synthetic Substitute **K** Nonautologous Tissue Substitute	**Z** No Qualifier
2 Lumbar Vertebral Disc **4** Lumbosacral Disc	**0** Open **3** Percutaneous **4** Percutaneous Endoscopic **X** External	**0** Drainage Device **3** Infusion Device **7** Autologous Tissue Substitute **J** Synthetic Substitute **K** Nonautologous Tissue Substitute	**Z** No Qualifier
5 Sacrococcygeal Joint **6** Coccygeal Joint **7** Sacroiliac Joint, Right **8** Sacroiliac Joint, Left	**0** Open **3** Percutaneous **4** Percutaneous Endoscopic **X** External	**0** Drainage Device **3** Infusion Device **4** Internal Fixation Device **7** Autologous Tissue Substitute **8** Spacer **J** Synthetic Substitute **K** Nonautologous Tissue Substitute	**Z** No Qualifier
9 Hip Joint, Right **B** Hip Joint, Left	**0** Open	**0** Drainage Device **3** Infusion Device **4** Internal Fixation Device **5** External Fixation Device **7** Autologous Tissue Substitute **8** Spacer **9** Liner **B** Resurfacing Device **J** Synthetic Substitute **K** Nonautologous Tissue Substitute	**Z** No Qualifier
9 Hip Joint, Right **B** Hip Joint, Left	**3** Percutaneous **4** Percutaneous Endoscopic **X** External	**0** Drainage Device **3** Infusion Device **4** Internal Fixation Device **5** External Fixation Device **7** Autologous Tissue Substitute **8** Spacer **J** Synthetic Substitute **K** Nonautologous Tissue Substitute	**Z** No Qualifier
A Hip Joint, Acetabular Surface, Right **E** Hip Joint, Acetabular Surface, Left **R** Hip Joint, Femoral Surface, Right **S** Hip Joint, Femoral Surface, Left **T** Knee Joint, Femoral Surface, Right **U** Knee Joint, Femoral Surface, Left **V** Knee Joint, Tibial Surface, Right **W** Knee Joint, Tibial Surface, Left	**0** Open **3** Percutaneous **4** Percutaneous Endoscopic **X** External	**J** Synthetic Substitute	**Z** No Qualifier

0SW continued on next page

0 Medical and Surgical
S Lower Joints
W Revision: Correcting, to the extent possible, a portion of a malfunctioning device or the position of a displaced device

0SW continued from previous page

Body Part Character 4	Approach Character 5	Device Character 6	Qualifier Character 7
C Knee Joint, Right **D** Knee Joint, Left	**0** Open	**0** Drainage Device **3** Infusion Device **4** Internal Fixation Device **5** External Fixation Device **7** Autologous Tissue Substitute **8** Spacer **9** Liner **K** Nonautologous Tissue Substitute	**Z** No Qualifier
C Knee Joint, Right **D** Knee Joint, Left	**0** Open	**J** Synthetic Substitute	**C** Patellar Surface **Z** No Qualifier
C Knee Joint, Right **D** Knee Joint, Left	**3** Percutaneous **4** Percutaneous Endoscopic **X** External	**0** Drainage Device **3** Infusion Device **4** Internal Fixation Device **5** External Fixation Device **7** Autologous Tissue Substitute **8** Spacer **K** Nonautologous Tissue Substitute	**Z** No Qualifier
C Knee Joint, Right **D** Knee Joint, Left	**3** Percutaneous **4** Percutaneous Endoscopic **X** External	**J** Synthetic Substitute	**C** Patellar Surface **Z** No Qualifier
F Ankle Joint, Right **G** Ankle Joint, Left **H** Tarsal Joint, Right **J** Tarsal Joint, Left **K** Tarsometatarsal Joint, Right **L** Tarsometatarsal Joint, Left **M** Metatarsal-Phalangeal Joint, Right **N** Metatarsal-Phalangeal Joint, Left **P** Toe Phalangeal Joint, Right **Q** Toe Phalangeal Joint, Left	**0** Open **3** Percutaneous **4** Percutaneous Endoscopic **X** External	**0** Drainage Device **3** Infusion Device **4** Internal Fixation Device **5** External Fixation Device **7** Autologous Tissue Substitute **8** Spacer **J** Synthetic Substitute **K** Nonautologous Tissue Substitute	**Z** No Qualifier

PCNL- Percutaneous Nephrolithotomy-
a retrograde pyelgram is performed to locate calculas.
a percutaneous nephrolithotomy needle
is passed into the pelvis of the kidney

NOTES

+ confirmed under Fluoroscopy. A guide wire is passed through the needle into the pelvis. the needle is w/drawn, Leaving the guide wire in place. Dilators are placed over the guide wire + a sheath is introduced. then a nephroscope is passed inside + small stones are removed. Larger stones may be crushed first + then removed

Lithotripsy - Calculi are crushed

- ESWL - Extracorporeal Shock Wave Lithrotripsy
  crush calculi by acoustic pulse
- Laser Lithotripsy - a scope in inserted into urinary tract to locate calculas, then a laser fiber is inserted through the scope + the laser is directed emitted to the stone, disintegrating it. the remaining pieces are washed out the urinary tract

Urinary System 0T1-0TY

0 Medical and Surgical
T Urinary System
1 Bypass: Altering the route of passage of the contents of a tubular body part

Body Part From	Approach	Device	Qualifier to
Character 4	**Character 5**	**Character 6**	**Character 7**
3 Kidney Pelvis, Right **4** Kidney Pelvis, Left	**0** Open **4** Percutaneous Endoscopic	**7** Autologous Tissue Substitute **J** Synthetic Substitute **K** Nonautologous Tissue Substitute **Z** No Device - ileal conduit	**3** Kidney Pelvis, Right **4** Kidney Pelvis, Left **6** Ureter, Right **7** Ureter, Left **8** Colon **9** Colocutaneous **A** Ileum **B** Bladder **C** Ileocutaneous ileal conduit of skin **D** Cutaneous
3 Kidney Pelvis, Right **4** Kidney Pelvis, Left	**3** Percutaneous	**J** Synthetic Substitute	**D** Cutaneous
6 Ureter, Right **7** Ureter, Left **8** Ureters, Bilateral	**0** Open **4** Percutaneous Endoscopic	**7** Autologous Tissue Substitute **J** Synthetic Substitute **K** Nonautologous Tissue Substitute **Z** No Device ileal conduit	**6** Ureter, Right **7** Ureter, Left **8** Colon **9** Colocutaneous **A** Ileum **B** Bladder **C** Ileocutaneous - ileal conduit of skin **D** Cutaneous
6 Ureter, Right **7** Ureter, Left **8** Ureters, Bilateral	**3** Percutaneous	**J** Synthetic Substitute	**D** Cutaneous
B Bladder	**0** Open **4** Percutaneous Endoscopic	**7** Autologous Tissue Substitute **J** Synthetic Substitute **K** Nonautologous Tissue Substitute **Z** No Device	**9** Colocutaneous **C** Ileocutaneous **D** Cutaneous
B Bladder	**3** Percutaneous	**J** Synthetic Substitute	**D** Cutaneous

0 Medical and Surgical
T Urinary System
2 Change: Taking out or off a device from a body part and putting back an identical or similar device in or on the same body part without cutting or puncturing the skin or a mucous membrane

Body Part	Approach	Device	Qualifier
Character 4	**Character 5**	**Character 6**	**Character 7**
5 Kidney **9** Ureter **B** Bladder **D** Urethra	**X** External	**0** Drainage Device **Y** Other Device	**Z** No Qualifier

0 Medical and Surgical
T Urinary System
5 Destruction: Physical eradication of all or a portion of a body part by the direct use of energy, force, or a destructive agent

Body Part Character 4	Approach Character 5	Device Character 6	Qualifier Character 7
0 Kidney, Right 1 Kidney, Left 3 Kidney Pelvis, Right 4 Kidney Pelvis, Left 6 Ureter, Right 7 Ureter, Left B Bladder C Bladder Neck	0 Open 3 Percutaneous 4 Percutaneous Endoscopic 7 Via Natural or Artificial Opening 8 Via Natural or Artificial Opening Endoscopic	Z No Device	Z No Qualifier
D Urethra	0 Open 3 Percutaneous 4 Percutaneous Endoscopic 7 Via Natural or Artificial Opening 8 Via Natural or Artificial Opening Endoscopic X External	Z No Device	Z No Qualifier

0 Medical and Surgical
T Urinary System
7 Dilation: Expanding an orifice or the lumen of a tubular body part

Body Part Character 4	Approach Character 5	Device Character 6	Qualifier Character 7
3 Kidney Pelvis, Right 4 Kidney Pelvis, Left 6 Ureter, Right 7 Ureter, Left 8 Ureters, Bilateral B Bladder C Bladder Neck D Urethra	0 Open 3 Percutaneous 4 Percutaneous Endoscopic 7 Via Natural or Artificial Opening 8 Via Natural or Artificial Opening Endoscopic	D Intraluminal Device Z No Device	Z No Qualifier

0 Medical and Surgical
T Urinary System
8 Division: Cutting into a body part, without draining fluids and/or gases from the body part, in order to separate or transect a body part

Body Part Character 4	Approach Character 5	Device Character 6	Qualifier Character 7
2 Kidneys, Bilateral C Bladder Neck	0 Open 3 Percutaneous 4 Percutaneous Endoscopic	Z No Device	Z No Qualifier

0 Medical and Surgical
T Urinary System
9 Drainage: Taking or letting out fluids and/or gases from a body part

Body Part Character 4	Approach Character 5	Device Character 6	Qualifier Character 7
0 Kidney, Right **1** Kidney, Left **3** Kidney Pelvis, Right **4** Kidney Pelvis, Left **6** Ureter, Right **7** Ureter, Left **8** Ureters, Bilateral **B** Bladder **C** Bladder Neck	**0** Open **3** Percutaneous **4** Percutaneous Endoscopic **7** Via Natural or Artificial Opening **8** Via Natural or Artificial Opening Endoscopic	**0** Drainage Device	**Z** No Qualifier
0 Kidney, Right **1** Kidney, Left **3** Kidney Pelvis, Right **4** Kidney Pelvis, Left **6** Ureter, Right **7** Ureter, Left **8** Ureters, Bilateral **B** Bladder **C** Bladder Neck	**0** Open **3** Percutaneous **4** Percutaneous Endoscopic **7** Via Natural or Artificial Opening **8** Via Natural or Artificial Opening Endoscopic	**Z** No Device	**X** Diagnostic **Z** No Qualifier
D Urethra	**0** Open **3** Percutaneous **4** Percutaneous Endoscopic **7** Via Natural or Artificial Opening **8** Via Natural or Artificial Opening Endoscopic **X** External	**0** Drainage Device	**Z** No Qualifier
D Urethra	**0** Open **3** Percutaneous **4** Percutaneous Endoscopic **7** Via Natural or Artificial Opening **8** Via Natural or Artificial Opening Endoscopic **X** External	**Z** No Device	**X** Diagnostic **Z** No Qualifier

0 Medical and Surgical
T Urinary System
B Excision: Cutting out or off, without replacement, a portion of a body part

Body Part Character 4	Approach Character 5	Device Character 6	Qualifier Character 7
0 Kidney, Right **1** Kidney, Left **3** Kidney Pelvis, Right **4** Kidney Pelvis, Left **6** Ureter, Right **7** Ureter, Left **B** Bladder **C** Bladder Neck	**0** Open **3** Percutaneous **4** Percutaneous Endoscopic **7** Via Natural or Artificial Opening **8** Via Natural or Artificial Opening Endoscopic	**Z** No Device	**X** Diagnostic **Z** No Qualifier
D Urethra	**0** Open **3** Percutaneous **4** Percutaneous Endoscopic **7** Via Natural or Artificial Opening **8** Via Natural or Artificial Opening Endoscopic **X** External	**Z** No Device	**X** Diagnostic **Z** No Qualifier

0 Medical and Surgical
T Urinary System
C Extirpation: Taking or cutting out solid matter from a body part . Fragments removed

Body Part	Approach	Device	Qualifier
Character 4	**Character 5**	**Character 6**	**Character 7**
0 Kidney, Right **1** Kidney, Left **3** Kidney Pelvis, Right **4** Kidney Pelvis, Left **6** Ureter, Right **7** Ureter, Left **B** Bladder **C** Bladder Neck	**0** Open **3** Percutaneous **4** Percutaneous Endoscopic **7** Via Natural or Artificial Opening **8** Via Natural or Artificial Opening Endoscopic	**Z** No Device	**Z** No Qualifier
D Urethra	**0** Open **3** Percutaneous **4** Percutaneous Endoscopic **7** Via Natural or Artificial Opening **8** Via Natural or Artificial Opening Endoscopic **X** External	**Z** No Device	**Z** No Qualifier

0 Medical and Surgical
T Urinary System
D Extraction: Pulling or stripping out or off all or a portion of a body part by the use of force

Body Part	Approach	Device	Qualifier
Character 4	**Character 5**	**Character 6**	**Character 7**
0 Kidney, Right **1** Kidney, Left	**0** Open **3** Percutaneous **4** Percutaneous Endoscopic	**Z** No Device	**Z** No Qualifier

0 Medical and Surgical
T Urinary System no Fragments removed
F Fragmentation: Breaking solid matter in a body part into pieces renal calculus

Body Part	Approach	Device	Qualifier
Character 4	**Character 5**	**Character 6**	**Character 7**
3 Kidney Pelvis, Right DRG **4** Kidney Pelvis, Left DRG **6** Ureter, Right DRG **7** Ureter, Left DRG **B** Bladder DRG **C** Bladder Neck DRG **D** Urethra NC	**0** Open **3** Percutaneous litho **4** Percutaneous Endoscopic **7** Via Natural or Artificial Opening **8** Via Natural or Artificial Opening Endoscopic transurethral cystoscopy **X** External lithotripsy	**Z** No Device	**Z** No Qualifier

NC 0TFDXZZ
DRG 0TF3XZZ 0TF4XZZ 0TF6XZZ 0TF7XZZ 0TFBXZZ 0TFCXZZ

If near ureteropelvic junction (UPJ), the body part is kidney pelvis

LC Limited Coverage NC Noncovered HAC HAC-associated Procedure CC Combination Cluster - See Appendix G for code lists
DRG Non-OR-Affecting MS-DRG Assignment New/Revised Text in **Orange** ♂ Male ♀ Female

0 Medical and Surgical
T Urinary System
H Insertion: Putting in a nonbiological appliance that monitors, assists, performs, or prevents a physiological function but does not physically take the place of a body part

Body Part Character 4	Approach Character 5	Device Character 6	Qualifier Character 7
5 Kidney	**0** Open **3** Percutaneous **4** Percutaneous Endoscopic **7** Via Natural or Artificial Opening **8** Via Natural or Artificial Opening Endoscopic	**2** Monitoring Device **3** Infusion Device **Y** Other Device	**Z** No Qualifier
9 Ureter	**0** Open **3** Percutaneous **4** Percutaneous Endoscopic **7** Via Natural or Artificial Opening **8** Via Natural or Artificial Opening Endoscopic	**2** Monitoring Device **3** Infusion Device **M** Stimulator Lead **Y** Other Device	**Z** No Qualifier
B Bladder NC	**0** Open **3** Percutaneous **4** Percutaneous Endoscopic **7** Via Natural or Artificial Opening **8** Via Natural or Artificial Opening Endoscopic	**2** Monitoring Device **3** Infusion Device **L** Artificial Sphincter **M** Stimulator Lead **Y** Other Device	**Z** No Qualifier
C Bladder Neck	**0** Open **3** Percutaneous **4** Percutaneous Endoscopic **7** Via Natural or Artificial Opening **8** Via Natural or Artificial Opening Endoscopic	**L** Artificial Sphincter	**Z** No Qualifier
D Urethra	**0** Open **3** Percutaneous **4** Percutaneous Endoscopic **7** Via Natural or Artificial Opening **8** Via Natural or Artificial Opening Endoscopic	**2** Monitoring Device **3** Infusion Device **L** Artificial Sphincter **Y** Other Device	**Z** No Qualifier
D Urethra	**X** External	**2** Monitoring Device **3** Infusion Device **L** Artificial Sphincter	**Z** No Qualifier

NC 0THB0MZ 0THB3MZ 0THB4MZ 0THB7MZ 0THB8MZ

0 Medical and Surgical cystoscopy - endoscopy of urinary bladder via the urethra
T Urinary System
J Inspection: Visually and/or manually exploring a body part

Body Part Character 4	Approach Character 5	Device Character 6	Qualifier Character 7
5 Kidney **9** Ureter **B** Bladder transurethral **D** Urethra transurethral	**0** Open **3** Percutaneous **4** Percutaneous Endoscopic **7** Via Natural or Artificial Opening **8** Via Natural or Artificial Opening Endoscopic cystoscopy **X** External	**Z** No Device	**Z** No Qualifier

LC Limited Coverage NC Noncovered HAC HAC-associated Procedure CC Combination Cluster - See Appendix G for code lists
DRG Non-OR-Affecting MS-DRG Assignment New/Revised Text in **Orange** ♂ Male ♀ Female

0 Medical and Surgical
T Urinary System
L Occlusion: Completely closing an orifice or the lumen of a tubular body part

Body Part Character 4	Approach Character 5	Device Character 6	Qualifier Character 7
3 Kidney Pelvis, Right **4** Kidney Pelvis, Left **6** Ureter, Right **7** Ureter, Left **B** Bladder **C** Bladder Neck	**0** Open **3** Percutaneous **4** Percutaneous Endoscopic	**C** Extraluminal Device **D** Intraluminal Device **Z** No Device	**Z** No Qualifier
3 Kidney Pelvis, Right **4** Kidney Pelvis, Left **6** Ureter, Right **7** Ureter, Left **B** Bladder **C** Bladder Neck	**7** Via Natural or Artificial Opening **8** Via Natural or Artificial Opening Endoscopic	**D** Intraluminal Device **Z** No Device	**Z** No Qualifier
D Urethra	**0** Open **3** Percutaneous **4** Percutaneous Endoscopic **X** External	**C** Extraluminal Device **D** Intraluminal Device **Z** No Device	**Z** No Qualifier
D Urethra	**7** Via Natural or Artificial Opening **8** Via Natural or Artificial Opening Endoscopic	**D** Intraluminal Device **Z** No Device	**Z** No Qualifier

0 Medical and Surgical
T Urinary System
M Reattachment: Putting back in or on all or a portion of a separated body part to its normal location or other suitable location

Body Part Character 4	Approach Character 5	Device Character 6	Qualifier Character 7
0 Kidney, Right **1** Kidney, Left **2** Kidneys, Bilateral **3** Kidney Pelvis, Right **4** Kidney Pelvis, Left **6** Ureter, Right **7** Ureter, Left **8** Ureters, Bilateral **B** Bladder **C** Bladder Neck **D** Urethra	**0** Open **4** Percutaneous Endoscopic	**Z** No Device	**Z** No Qualifier

0 Medical and Surgical
T Urinary System
N Release: Freeing a body part from an abnormal physical constraint by cutting or by the use of force adhesiolysis

Body Part Character 4	Approach Character 5	Device Character 6	Qualifier Character 7
0 Kidney, Right **1** Kidney, Left **3** Kidney Pelvis, Right **4** Kidney Pelvis, Left **6** Ureter, Right **7** Ureter, Left **B** Bladder **C** Bladder Neck	**0** Open laparotomy **3** Percutaneous **4** Percutaneous Endoscopic **7** Via Natural or Artificial Opening **8** Via Natural or Artificial Opening Endoscopic	**Z** No Device	**Z** No Qualifier
D Urethra	**0** Open **3** Percutaneous **4** Percutaneous Endoscopic **7** Via Natural or Artificial Opening **8** Via Natural or Artificial Opening Endoscopic **X** External	**Z** No Device	**Z** No Qualifier

0 Medical and Surgical
T Urinary System
P Removal: Taking out or off a device from a body part

Body Part Character 4	Approach Character 5	Device Character 6	Qualifier Character 7
5 Kidney	**0** Open **3** Percutaneous **4** Percutaneous Endoscopic **7** Via Natural or Artificial Opening **8** Via Natural or Artificial Opening Endoscopic	**0** Drainage Device **2** Monitoring Device **3** Infusion Device **7** Autologous Tissue Substitute **C** Extraluminal Device **D** Intraluminal Device **J** Synthetic Substitute **K** Nonautologous Tissue Substitute **Y** Other Device	**Z** No Qualifier
5 Kidney	**X** External	**0** Drainage Device **2** Monitoring Device **3** Infusion Device **D** Intraluminal Device	**Z** No Qualifier
9 Ureter ureteral stent	**0** Open **3** Percutaneous **4** Percutaneous Endoscopic **7** Via Natural or Artificial Opening **8** Via Natural or Artificial Opening Endoscopic cystoscope	**0** Drainage Device **2** Monitoring Device **3** Infusion Device **7** Autologous Tissue Substitute **C** Extraluminal Device **D** Intraluminal Device stent **J** Synthetic Substitute **K** Nonautologous Tissue Substitute **M** Stimulator Lead **Y** Other Device	**Z** No Qualifier
9 Ureter ureteral stent	**X** External	**0** Drainage Device **2** Monitoring Device **3** Infusion Device **D** Intraluminal Device stent **M** Stimulator Lead	**Z** No Qualifier
B Bladder NC	**0** Open **3** Percutaneous **4** Percutaneous Endoscopic **7** Via Natural or Artificial Opening **8** Via Natural or Artificial Opening Endoscopic	**0** Drainage Device **2** Monitoring Device **3** Infusion Device **7** Autologous Tissue Substitute **C** Extraluminal Device **D** Intraluminal Device **J** Synthetic Substitute **K** Nonautologous Tissue Substitute **L** Artificial Sphincter **M** Stimulator Lead **Y** Other Device	**Z** No Qualifier
B Bladder	**X** External	**0** Drainage Device **2** Monitoring Device **3** Infusion Device **D** Intraluminal Device **L** Artificial Sphincter **M** Stimulator Lead	**Z** No Qualifier
D Urethra	**0** Open **3** Percutaneous **4** Percutaneous Endoscopic **7** Via Natural or Artificial Opening **8** Via Natural or Artificial Opening Endoscopic cystoscope	**0** Drainage Device **2** Monitoring Device **3** Infusion Device **7** Autologous Tissue Substitute **C** Extraluminal Device **D** Intraluminal Device **J** Synthetic Substitute **K** Nonautologous Tissue Substitute **L** Artificial Sphincter **Y** Other Device	**Z** No Qualifier

0TP continued on next page

0TP continued from previous page

0 Medical and Surgical
T Urinary System
P Removal: Taking out or off a device from a body part

Body Part Character 4	Approach Character 5	Device Character 6	Qualifier Character 7
D Urethra	X External	0 Drainage Device 2 Monitoring Device 3 Infusion Device D Intraluminal Device L Artificial Sphincter	Z No Qualifier

NC 0TPB0MZ 0TPB3MZ 0TPB4MZ 0TPB7MZ 0TPB8MZ

0 Medical and Surgical
T Urinary System
Q Repair: Restoring, to the extent possible, a body part to its normal anatomic structure and function

Body Part Character 4	Approach Character 5	Device Character 6	Qualifier Character 7
0 Kidney, Right 1 Kidney, Left 3 Kidney Pelvis, Right 4 Kidney Pelvis, Left 6 Ureter, Right 7 Ureter, Left B Bladder CC C Bladder Neck	0 Open 3 Percutaneous 4 Percutaneous Endoscopic 7 Via Natural or Artificial Opening 8 Via Natural or Artificial Opening Endoscopic	Z No Device	Z No Qualifier
D Urethra	0 Open 3 Percutaneous 4 Percutaneous Endoscopic 7 Via Natural or Artificial Opening 8 Via Natural or Artificial Opening Endoscopic X External	Z No Device	Z No Qualifier

CC 0TQB0ZZ 0TQB3ZZ 0TQB4ZZ

0 Medical and Surgical
T Urinary System
R Replacement: Putting in or on biological or synthetic material that physically takes the place and/or function of all or a portion of a body part

Body Part Character 4	Approach Character 5	Device Character 6	Qualifier Character 7
3 Kidney Pelvis, Right 4 Kidney Pelvis, Left 6 Ureter, Right 7 Ureter, Left B Bladder C Bladder Neck	0 Open 4 Percutaneous Endoscopic 7 Via Natural or Artificial Opening 8 Via Natural or Artificial Opening Endoscopic	7 Autologous Tissue Substitute J Synthetic Substitute K Nonautologous Tissue Substitute	Z No Qualifier
D Urethra	0 Open 4 Percutaneous Endoscopic 7 Via Natural or Artificial Opening 8 Via Natural or Artificial Opening Endoscopic X External	7 Autologous Tissue Substitute J Synthetic Substitute K Nonautologous Tissue Substitute	Z No Qualifier

0 Medical and Surgical
T Urinary System
S Reposition: Moving to its normal location, or other suitable location, all or a portion of a body part

may use sling or hammock to lift bladder neck
may use mesh

Body Part Character 4	Approach Character 5	Device Character 6	Qualifier Character 7
0 Kidney, Right **1** Kidney, Left **2** Kidneys, Bilateral **3** Kidney Pelvis, Right **4** Kidney Pelvis, Left **6** Ureter, Right **7** Ureter, Left **8** Ureters, Bilateral **B** Bladder **C** Bladder Neck - reinforce urethra & bladder neck **D** Urethra	**0** Open **4** Percutaneous Endoscopic	**Z** No Device	**Z** No Qualifier

0 Medical and Surgical
T Urinary System
T Resection: Cutting out or off, without replacement, all of a body part

Body Part Character 4	Approach Character 5	Device Character 6	Qualifier Character 7
0 Kidney, Right **1** Kidney, Left **2** Kidneys, Bilateral	**0** Open **4** Percutaneous Endoscopic	**Z** No Device	**Z** No Qualifier
3 Kidney Pelvis, Right **4** Kidney Pelvis, Left **6** Ureter, Right **7** Ureter, Left **B** Bladder CC **C** Bladder Neck **D** Urethra DRG CC	**0** Open **4** Percutaneous Endoscopic **7** Via Natural or Artificial Opening **8** Via Natural or Artificial Opening Endoscopic	**Z** No Device	**Z** No Qualifier

DRG 0TTD0ZZ
CC 0TTB0ZZ 0TTD0ZZ

0 Medical and Surgical
T Urinary System
U Supplement: Putting in or on biological or synthetic material that physically reinforces and/or augments the function of a portion of a body part

Body Part Character 4	Approach Character 5	Device Character 6	Qualifier Character 7
3 Kidney Pelvis, Right **4** Kidney Pelvis, Left **6** Ureter, Right **7** Ureter, Left **B** Bladder **C** Bladder Neck	**0** Open **4** Percutaneous Endoscopic **7** Via Natural or Artificial Opening **8** Via Natural or Artificial Opening Endoscopic	**7** Autologous Tissue Substitute **J** Synthetic Substitute **K** Nonautologous Tissue Substitute	**Z** No Qualifier
D Urethra	**0** Open **4** Percutaneous Endoscopic **7** Via Natural or Artificial Opening **8** Via Natural or Artificial Opening Endoscopic **X** External	**7** Autologous Tissue Substitute **J** Synthetic Substitute **K** Nonautologous Tissue Substitute	**Z** No Qualifier

0 Medical and Surgical
T Urinary System
V Restriction: Partially closing an orifice or the lumen of a tubular body part

Body Part Character 4	Approach Character 5	Device Character 6	Qualifier Character 7
3 Kidney Pelvis, Right **4** Kidney Pelvis, Left **6** Ureter, Right **7** Ureter, Left **B** Bladder **C** Bladder Neck	**0** Open **3** Percutaneous **4** Percutaneous Endoscopic	**C** Extraluminal Device **D** Intraluminal Device **Z** No Device	**Z** No Qualifier
3 Kidney Pelvis, Right **4** Kidney Pelvis, Left **6** Ureter, Right **7** Ureter, Left **B** Bladder **C** Bladder Neck	**7** Via Natural or Artificial Opening **8** Via Natural or Artificial Opening Endoscopic	**D** Intraluminal Device **Z** No Device	**Z** No Qualifier
D Urethra	**0** Open **3** Percutaneous **4** Percutaneous Endoscopic	**C** Extraluminal Device **D** Intraluminal Device **Z** No Device	**Z** No Qualifier
D Urethra	**7** Via Natural or Artificial Opening **8** Via Natural or Artificial Opening Endoscopic	**D** Intraluminal Device **Z** No Device	**Z** No Qualifier
D Urethra	**X** External	**Z** No Device	**Z** No Qualifier

0 Medical and Surgical
T Urinary System
W Revision: Correcting, to the extent possible, a portion of a malfunctioning device or the position of a displaced device

Body Part Character 4	Approach Character 5	Device Character 6	Qualifier Character 7
5 Kidney	**0** Open **3** Percutaneous **4** Percutaneous Endoscopic **7** Via Natural or Artificial Opening **8** Via Natural or Artificial Opening Endoscopic	**0** Drainage Device **2** Monitoring Device **3** Infusion Device **7** Autologous Tissue Substitute **C** Extraluminal Device **D** Intraluminal Device **J** Synthetic Substitute **K** Nonautologous Tissue Substitute **Y** Other Device	**Z** No Qualifier
5 Kidney	**X** External	**0** Drainage Device **2** Monitoring Device **3** Infusion Device **7** Autologous Tissue Substitute **C** Extraluminal Device **D** Intraluminal Device **J** Synthetic Substitute **K** Nonautologous Tissue Substitute	**Z** No Qualifier
9 Ureter	**0** Open **3** Percutaneous **4** Percutaneous Endoscopic **7** Via Natural or Artificial Opening **8** Via Natural or Artificial Opening Endoscopic	**0** Drainage Device **2** Monitoring Device **3** Infusion Device **7** Autologous Tissue Substitute **C** Extraluminal Device **D** Intraluminal Device **J** Synthetic Substitute **K** Nonautologous Tissue Substitute **M** Stimulator Lead **Y** Other Device	**Z** No Qualifier
9 Ureter	**X** External	**0** Drainage Device **2** Monitoring Device **3** Infusion Device **7** Autologous Tissue Substitute **C** Extraluminal Device **D** Intraluminal Device **J** Synthetic Substitute **K** Nonautologous Tissue Substitute **M** Stimulator Lead	**Z** No Qualifier

0TW continued on next page

0TW continued from previous page

0 Medical and Surgical
T Urinary System
W Revision: Correcting, to the extent possible, a portion of a malfunctioning device or the position of a displaced device

Body Part	Approach	Device	Qualifier
Character 4	Character 5	Character 6	Character 7
B Bladder	**0** Open **3** Percutaneous **4** Percutaneous Endoscopic **7** Via Natural or Artificial Opening **8** Via Natural or Artificial Opening Endoscopic	**0** Drainage Device **2** Monitoring Device **3** Infusion Device **7** Autologous Tissue Substitute **C** Extraluminal Device **D** Intraluminal Device **J** Synthetic Substitute **K** Nonautologous Tissue Substitute **L** Artificial Sphincter **M** Stimulator Lead **Y** Other Device	**Z** No Qualifier
B Bladder	**X** External	**0** Drainage Device **2** Monitoring Device **3** Infusion Device **7** Autologous Tissue Substitute **C** Extraluminal Device **D** Intraluminal Device **J** Synthetic Substitute **K** Nonautologous Tissue Substitute **L** Artificial Sphincter **M** Stimulator Lead	**Z** No Qualifier
D Urethra	**0** Open **3** Percutaneous **4** Percutaneous Endoscopic **7** Via Natural or Artificial Opening **8** Via Natural or Artificial Opening Endoscopic	**0** Drainage Device **2** Monitoring Device **3** Infusion Device **7** Autologous Tissue Substitute **C** Extraluminal Device **D** Intraluminal Device **J** Synthetic Substitute **K** Nonautologous Tissue Substitute **L** Artificial Sphincter **Y** Other Device	**Z** No Qualifier
D Urethra	**X** External	**0** Drainage Device **2** Monitoring Device **3** Infusion Device **7** Autologous Tissue Substitute **C** Extraluminal Device **D** Intraluminal Device **J** Synthetic Substitute **K** Nonautologous Tissue Substitute **L** Artificial Sphincter	**Z** No Qualifier

0 Medical and Surgical
T Urinary System
Y Transplantation: Putting in or on all or a portion of a living body part taken from another individual or animal to physically take the place and/or function of all or a portion of a similar body part

Body Part	Approach	Device	Qualifier
Character 4	Character 5	Character 6	Character 7
0 Kidney, Right LC CC **1** Kidney, Left LC CC	**0** Open	**Z** No Device	**0** Allogeneic **1** Syngeneic **2** Zooplastic

LC 0TY00Z0 0TY00Z1 0TY00Z2 0TY10Z0 0TY10Z1 0TY10Z2
CC 0TY00Z0 0TY00Z1 0TY00Z2 0TY10Z0 0TY10Z1 0TY10Z2

remember - X for diagnostic - only to be used for biopsy - sent to pathology
do not confuse w/ diagnostic laproscopy or diagnostic endoscopy

NOTES

Laproscopic = percutaneous endoscopic

pelvic laproscopic - involves small incision in the belly or lower adbomen

may diagnose: appendicitis, ovarian cancer, ectopic pregnancy, endometriosis, cholecystitis, pelvic inflammatory disease (PID)

Laproscopic also used to repair/replace/remove organs:
cholecystectomy (gallbladder) oophorectomy, salpingectomy, herniorrhaphy

Cervical Cerclage - Restriction - 3 types

1) McDonald - most common, purse string stitch used to cinch cervix shut

2) Shirodkar - sutures pass through wall of cervix so they aren't exposed
OUVC less common, more difficult. May involve more permanent stitch around the cervix that is not removed + a C-section delivers baby

3) Abdominal Cerclage - least common, permanent, involves stitching at the very top of the cervix, inside the abdomen. Used only if cervix is too short to attempt standard cerclage or if vaginal cerclage is not possible

Female Reproductive System 0U1-0UY

0 Medical and Surgical
U Female Reproductive System
1 Bypass: Altering the route of passage of the contents of a tubular body part

Body Part	Approach	Device	Qualifier
Character 4	**Character 5**	**Character 6**	**Character 7**
5 Fallopian Tube, Right ♀ **6** Fallopian Tube, Left ♀	**0** Open **4** Percutaneous Endoscopic	**7** Autologous Tissue Substitute **J** Synthetic Substitute **K** Nonautologous Tissue Substitute **Z** No Device	**5** Fallopian Tube, Right **6** Fallopian Tube, Left **9** Uterus

♀ 0U15075 0U15076 0U15079 0U150J5 0U150J6 0U150J9 0U150K5 0U150K6 0U150K9 0U150Z5 0U150Z6 0U150Z9 0U15475 0U15476 0U15479 0U154J5 0U154J6 0U154J9 0U154K5 0U154K6 0U154K9 0U154Z5 0U154Z6 0U154Z9 0U16075 0U16076 0U16079 0U160J5 0U160J6 0U160J9 0U160K5 0U160K6 0U160K9 0U160Z5 0U160Z6 0U160Z9 0U16475 0U16476 0U16479 0U164J5 0U164J6 0U164J9 0U164K5 0U164K6 0U164K9 0U164Z5 0U164Z6 0U164Z9

0 Medical and Surgical
U Female Reproductive System
2 Change: Taking out or off a device from a body part and putting back an identical or similar device in or on the same body part without cutting or puncturing the skin or a mucous membrane

Body Part	Approach	Device	Qualifier
Character 4	**Character 5**	**Character 6**	**Character 7**
3 Ovary ♀ **8** Fallopian Tube ♀ **M** Vulva ♀	**X** External	**0** Drainage Device **Y** Other Device	**Z** No Qualifier
D Uterus and Cervix ♀	**X** External	**0** Drainage Device **H** Contraceptive Device **Y** Other Device	**Z** No Qualifier
H Vagina and Cul-de-sac ♀	**X** External	**0** Drainage Device **G** Intraluminal Device, Pessary **Y** Other Device	**Z** No Qualifier

♀ 0U23X0Z 0U23XYZ 0U28X0Z 0U28XYZ 0U2DX0Z 0U2DXHZ 0U2DXYZ 0U2HX0Z 0U2HXGZ 0U2HXYZ 0U2MX0Z 0U2MXYZ

0 Medical and Surgical
U Female Reproductive System
5 Destruction: Physical eradication of all or a portion of a body part by the direct use of energy, force, or a destructive agent

Body Part	Approach	Device	Qualifier
Character 4	**Character 5**	**Character 6**	**Character 7**
0 Ovary, Right ♀ **1** Ovary, Left ♀ **2** Ovaries, Bilateral ♀ **4** Uterine Supporting Structure ♀	**0** Open **3** Percutaneous **4** Percutaneous Endoscopic **8** Via Natural or Artificial Opening Endoscopic	**Z** No Device	**Z** No Qualifier
5 Fallopian Tube, Right ♀ **6** Fallopian Tube, Left ♀ **7** Fallopian Tubes, Bilateral ♀ NC **9** Uterus ♀ **B** Endometrium ♀ **C** Cervix ♀ **F** Cul-de-sac ♀	**0** Open **3** Percutaneous **4** Percutaneous Endoscopic **7** Via Natural or Artificial Opening **8** Via Natural or Artificial Opening Endoscopic	**Z** No Device	**Z** No Qualifier
G Vagina ♀ **K** Hymen ♀	**0** Open **3** Percutaneous **4** Percutaneous Endoscopic **7** Via Natural or Artificial Opening **8** Via Natural or Artificial Opening Endoscopic **X** External	**Z** No Device	**Z** No Qualifier

0U5 continued on next page

0 **Medical and Surgical**
U **Female Reproductive System**

0U5 continued from previous page

5 **Destruction:** Physical eradication of all or a portion of a body part by the direct use of energy, force, or a destructive agent

Body Part	Approach	Device	Qualifier
Character 4	Character 5	Character 6	Character 7
J Clitoris ♀ L Vestibular Gland ♀ M Vulva ♀	0 Open X External	Z No Device	Z No Qualifier

♀ 0U500ZZ 0U503ZZ 0U504ZZ 0U508ZZ 0U510ZZ 0U513ZZ 0U514ZZ 0U518ZZ 0U520ZZ 0U523ZZ 0U524ZZ 0U528ZZ 0U540ZZ
0U543ZZ 0U544ZZ 0U548ZZ 0U550ZZ 0U553ZZ 0U554ZZ 0U557ZZ 0U558ZZ 0U560ZZ 0U563ZZ 0U564ZZ 0U567ZZ 0U568ZZ
0U570ZZ 0U573ZZ 0U574ZZ 0U577ZZ 0U578ZZ 0U590ZZ 0U593ZZ 0U594ZZ 0U597ZZ 0U598ZZ 0U5B0ZZ 0U5B3ZZ 0U5B4ZZ
0U5B7ZZ 0U5B8ZZ 0U5C0ZZ 0U5C3ZZ 0U5C4ZZ 0U5C7ZZ 0U5C8ZZ 0U5F0ZZ 0U5F3ZZ 0U5F4ZZ 0U5F7ZZ 0U5F8ZZ 0U5G0ZZ
0U5G3ZZ 0U5G4ZZ 0U5G7ZZ 0U5G8ZZ 0U5GXZZ 0U5J0ZZ 0U5JXZZ 0U5K0ZZ 0U5K3ZZ 0U5K4ZZ 0U5K7ZZ 0U5K8ZZ 0U5KXZZ
0U5L0ZZ 0U5LXZZ 0U5M0ZZ 0U5MXZZ

NC 0U570ZZ 0U573ZZ 0U574ZZ 0U577ZZ 0U578ZZ

Codes in this list are noncovered procedures only when reported with Z30.2 as either a principal or secondary diagnosis.

0 **Medical and Surgical**
U **Female Reproductive System**

7 **Dilation:** Expanding an orifice or the lumen of a tubular body part

Body Part	Approach	Device	Qualifier
Character 4	Character 5	Character 6	Character 7
5 Fallopian Tube, Right ♀ 6 Fallopian Tube, Left ♀ _fallow_ 7 Fallopian Tubes, Bilateral ♀ 9 Uterus ♀ C Cervix ♀ G Vagina ♀	0 Open 3 Percutaneous 4 Percutaneous Endoscopic 7 Via Natural or Artificial Opening 8 Via Natural or Artificial Opening Endoscopic _hysper scupy_	D Intraluminal Device _- must stay in body_ Z No Device	Z No Qualifier
K Hymen ♀	0 Open 3 Percutaneous 4 Percutaneous Endoscopic 7 Via Natural or Artificial Opening 8 Via Natural or Artificial Opening Endoscopic X External	D Intraluminal Device Z No Device	Z No Qualifier

♀ 0U750DZ 0U750ZZ 0U753DZ 0U753ZZ 0U754DZ 0U754ZZ 0U757DZ 0U757ZZ 0U758DZ 0U758ZZ 0U760DZ 0U760ZZ 0U763DZ
0U763ZZ 0U764DZ 0U764ZZ 0U767DZ 0U767ZZ 0U768DZ 0U768ZZ 0U770DZ 0U770ZZ 0U773DZ 0U773ZZ 0U774DZ 0U774ZZ
0U777DZ 0U777ZZ 0U778DZ 0U778ZZ 0U790DZ 0U790ZZ 0U793DZ 0U793ZZ 0U794DZ 0U794ZZ 0U797DZ 0U797ZZ 0U798DZ
0U798ZZ 0U7C0DZ 0U7C0ZZ 0U7C3DZ 0U7C3ZZ 0U7C4DZ 0U7C4ZZ 0U7C7DZ 0U7C7ZZ 0U7C8DZ 0U7C8ZZ 0U7G0DZ 0U7G0ZZ
0U7G3DZ 0U7G3ZZ 0U7G4DZ 0U7G4ZZ 0U7G7DZ 0U7G7ZZ 0U7G8DZ 0U7G8ZZ 0U7K0DZ 0U7K0ZZ 0U7K3DZ 0U7K3ZZ 0U7K4DZ
0U7K4ZZ 0U7K7DZ 0U7K7ZZ 0U7K8DZ 0U7K8ZZ 0U7KXDZ 0U7KXZZ

0 **Medical and Surgical**
U **Female Reproductive System**

8 **Division:** Cutting into a body part, without draining fluids and/or gases from the body part, in order to separate or transect a body part

Body Part	Approach	Device	Qualifier
Character 4	Character 5	Character 6	Character 7
0 Ovary, Right ♀ 1 Ovary, Left ♀ 2 Ovaries, Bilateral ♀ 4 Uterine Supporting Structure ♀	0 Open 3 Percutaneous 4 Percutaneous Endoscopic	Z No Device	Z No Qualifier
K Hymen ♀	7 Via Natural or Artificial Opening 8 Via Natural or Artificial Opening Endoscopic X External	Z No Device	Z No Qualifier

♀ 0U800ZZ 0U803ZZ 0U804ZZ 0U810ZZ 0U813ZZ 0U814ZZ 0U820ZZ 0U823ZZ 0U824ZZ 0U840ZZ 0U843ZZ 0U844ZZ 0U8K7ZZ
0U8K8ZZ 0U8KXZZ

LC Limited Coverage   NC Noncovered   HAC HAC-associated Procedure   CC Combination Cluster - See Appendix G for code lists
DRG Non-OR-Affecting MS-DRG Assignment   New/Revised Text in **Orange**   ♂ Male   ♀ Female

0 Medical and Surgical
U Female Reproductive System
9 Drainage: Taking or letting out fluids and/or gases from a body part

Body Part Character 4	Approach Character 5	Device Character 6	Qualifier Character 7
0 Ovary, Right ♀ **1** Ovary, Left ♀ **2** Ovaries, Bilateral ♀	**0** Open **3** Percutaneous **4** Percutaneous Endoscopic **8** Via Natural or Artificial Opening Endoscopic	**0** Drainage Device	**Z** No Qualifier
0 Ovary, Right ♀ **1** Ovary, Left ♀ **2** Ovaries, Bilateral ♀	**0** Open **3** Percutaneous **4** Percutaneous Endoscopic **8** Via Natural or Artificial Opening Endoscopic	**Z** No Device	**X** Diagnostic **Z** No Qualifier
0 Ovary, Right ♀ **1** Ovary, Left ♀ **2** Ovaries, Bilateral ♀	**X** External	**Z** No Device	**Z** No Qualifier
4 Uterine Supporting Structure ♀	**0** Open **3** Percutaneous **4** Percutaneous Endoscopic **8** Via Natural or Artificial Opening Endoscopic	**0** Drainage Device	**Z** No Qualifier
4 Uterine Supporting Structure ♀	**0** Open **3** Percutaneous **4** Percutaneous Endoscopic **8** Via Natural or Artificial Opening Endoscopic	**Z** No Device	**X** Diagnostic **Z** No Qualifier
5 Fallopian Tube, Right ♀ **6** Fallopian Tube, Left ♀ **7** Fallopian Tubes, Bilateral ♀ **9** Uterus ♀ **C** Cervix ♀ **F** Cul-de-sac ♀	**0** Open **3** Percutaneous **4** Percutaneous Endoscopic **7** Via Natural or Artificial Opening **8** Via Natural or Artificial Opening Endoscopic	**0** Drainage Device	**Z** No Qualifier
5 Fallopian Tube, Right ♀ **6** Fallopian Tube, Left ♀ **7** Fallopian Tubes, Bilateral ♀ **9** Uterus ♀ **C** Cervix ♀ **F** Cul-de-sac ♀	**0** Open **3** Percutaneous **4** Percutaneous Endoscopic **7** Via Natural or Artificial Opening **8** Via Natural or Artificial Opening Endoscopic	**Z** No Device	**X** Diagnostic **Z** No Qualifier
G Vagina ♀ **K** Hymen ♀	**0** Open **3** Percutaneous **4** Percutaneous Endoscopic **7** Via Natural or Artificial Opening **8** Via Natural or Artificial Opening Endoscopic **X** External	**0** Drainage Device	**Z** No Qualifier
G Vagina ♀ **K** Hymen ♀	**0** Open **3** Percutaneous **4** Percutaneous Endoscopic **7** Via Natural or Artificial Opening **8** Via Natural or Artificial Opening Endoscopic **X** External	**Z** No Device	**X** Diagnostic **Z** No Qualifier
J Clitoris ♀ **L** Vestibular Gland ♀ **M** Vulva ♀	**0** Open **X** External	**0** Drainage Device	**Z** No Qualifier

0U9 continued on next page

LC Limited Coverage NC Noncovered HAC HAC-associated Procedure CC Combination Cluster - See Appendix G for code lists
DRG Non-OR-Affecting MS-DRG Assignment New/Revised Text in **Orange** ♂ Male ♀ Female

0U9 continued from previous page

0 Medical and Surgical
U Female Reproductive System
9 Drainage: Taking or letting out fluids and/or gases from a body part

Body Part Character 4	Approach Character 5	Device Character 6	Qualifier Character 7
J Clitoris ♀ **L** Vestibular Gland ♀ **M** Vulva ♀	**0** Open **X** External	**Z** No Device	**X** Diagnostic **Z** No Qualifier

♀ 0U9000Z 0U900ZX 0U900ZZ 0U9030Z 0U903ZX 0U903ZZ 0U9040Z 0U904ZX 0U904ZZ 0U9080Z 0U908ZX 0U908ZZ 0U90XZZ
0U9100Z 0U910ZX 0U910ZZ 0U9130Z 0U913ZX 0U913ZZ 0U9140Z 0U914ZX 0U914ZZ 0U9180Z 0U918ZX 0U918ZZ 0U91XZZ
0U9200Z 0U920ZX 0U920ZZ 0U9230Z 0U923ZX 0U923ZZ 0U9240Z 0U924ZX 0U924ZZ 0U9280Z 0U928ZX 0U928ZZ 0U92XZZ
0U9400Z 0U940ZX 0U940ZZ 0U9430Z 0U943ZX 0U943ZZ 0U9440Z 0U944ZX 0U944ZZ 0U9480Z 0U948ZX 0U948ZZ 0U9500Z
0U950ZX 0U950ZZ 0U9530Z 0U953ZX 0U953ZZ 0U9540Z 0U954ZX 0U954ZZ 0U9570Z 0U957ZX 0U957ZZ 0U9580Z 0U958ZX
0U958ZZ 0U9600Z 0U960ZX 0U960ZZ 0U9630Z 0U963ZX 0U963ZZ 0U9640Z 0U964ZX 0U964ZZ 0U9670Z 0U967ZX 0U967ZZ
0U9680Z 0U968ZX 0U968ZZ 0U9700Z 0U970ZX 0U970ZZ 0U9730Z 0U973ZX 0U973ZZ 0U9740Z 0U974ZX 0U974ZZ 0U9770Z
0U977ZX 0U977ZZ 0U9780Z 0U978ZX 0U978ZZ 0U9900Z 0U990ZX 0U990ZZ 0U9930Z 0U993ZX 0U993ZZ 0U9940Z 0U994ZX
0U994ZZ 0U9970Z 0U997ZX 0U997ZZ 0U9980Z 0U998ZX 0U998ZZ 0U9C00Z 0U9C0ZX 0U9C0ZZ 0U9C30Z 0U9C3ZX 0U9C3ZZ
0U9C40Z 0U9C4ZX 0U9C4ZZ 0U9C70Z 0U9C7ZX 0U9C7ZZ 0U9C80Z 0U9C8ZX 0U9C8ZZ 0U9F00Z 0U9F0ZX 0U9F0ZZ 0U9F30Z
0U9F3ZX 0U9F3ZZ 0U9F40Z 0U9F4ZX 0U9F4ZZ 0U9F70Z 0U9F7ZX 0U9F7ZZ 0U9F80Z 0U9F8ZX 0U9F8ZZ 0U9G00Z 0U9G0ZX
0U9G0ZZ 0U9G30Z 0U9G3ZX 0U9G3ZZ 0U9G40Z 0U9G4ZX 0U9G4ZZ 0U9G70Z 0U9G7ZX 0U9G7ZZ 0U9G80Z 0U9G8ZX 0U9G8ZZ
0U9GX0Z 0U9GXZX 0U9GXZZ 0U9J00Z 0U9J0ZX 0U9J0ZZ 0U9JX0Z 0U9JXZX 0U9JXZZ 0U9K00Z 0U9K0ZX 0U9K0ZZ 0U9K30Z
0U9K3ZX 0U9K3ZZ 0U9K40Z 0U9K4ZX 0U9K4ZZ 0U9K70Z 0U9K7ZX 0U9K7ZZ 0U9K80Z 0U9K8ZX 0U9K8ZZ 0U9KX0Z 0U9KXZX
0U9KXZZ 0U9L00Z 0U9L0ZX 0U9L0ZZ 0U9LX0Z 0U9LXZX 0U9LXZZ 0U9M00Z 0U9M0ZX 0U9M0ZZ 0U9MX0Z 0U9MXZX 0U9MXZZ

0 Medical and Surgical
U Female Reproductive System
B Excision: Cutting out or off, without replacement, a portion of a body part endometrial implant L ovary 0UB14ZZ

Body Part Character 4	Approach Character 5	Device Character 6	Qualifier Character 7
0 Ovary, Right ♀ **1** Ovary, Left ♀ **2** Ovaries, Bilateral ♀ **4** Uterine Supporting Structure ♀ **5** Fallopian Tube, Right ♀ **6** Fallopian Tube, Left ♀ **7** Fallopian Tubes, Bilateral ♀ **9** Uterus ♀ **C** Cervix ♀ **F** Cul-de-sac ♀	**0** Open **3** Percutaneous **4** Percutaneous Endoscopic **7** Via Natural or Artificial Opening **8** Via Natural or Artificial Opening Endoscopic	**Z** No Device	**X** Diagnostic **Z** No Qualifier
G Vagina ♀ **K** Hymen ♀	**0** Open **3** Percutaneous **4** Percutaneous Endoscopic **7** Via Natural or Artificial Opening **8** Via Natural or Artificial Opening Endoscopic **X** External	**Z** No Device	**X** Diagnostic **Z** No Qualifier
J Clitoris ♀ **L** Vestibular Gland ♀ **M** Vulva ♀	**0** Open **X** External	**Z** No Device	**X** Diagnostic **Z** No Qualifier

♀ 0UB00ZX 0UB00ZZ 0UB03ZX 0UB03ZZ 0UB04ZX 0UB04ZZ 0UB07ZX 0UB07ZZ 0UB08ZX 0UB08ZZ 0UB10ZX 0UB10ZZ 0UB13ZX
0UB13ZZ 0UB14ZX 0UB14ZZ 0UB17ZX 0UB17ZZ 0UB18ZX 0UB18ZZ 0UB20ZX 0UB20ZZ 0UB23ZX 0UB23ZZ 0UB24ZX 0UB24ZZ
0UB27ZX 0UB27ZZ 0UB28ZX 0UB28ZZ 0UB40ZX 0UB40ZZ 0UB43ZX 0UB43ZZ 0UB44ZX 0UB44ZZ 0UB47ZX 0UB47ZZ 0UB48ZX
0UB48ZZ 0UB50ZX 0UB50ZZ 0UB53ZX 0UB53ZZ 0UB54ZX 0UB54ZZ 0UB57ZX 0UB57ZZ 0UB58ZX 0UB58ZZ 0UB60ZX 0UB60ZZ
0UB63ZX 0UB63ZZ 0UB64ZX 0UB64ZZ 0UB67ZX 0UB67ZZ 0UB68ZX 0UB68ZZ 0UB70ZX 0UB70ZZ 0UB73ZX 0UB73ZZ 0UB74ZX
0UB74ZZ 0UB77ZX 0UB77ZZ 0UB78ZX 0UB78ZZ 0UB90ZX 0UB90ZZ 0UB93ZX 0UB93ZZ 0UB94ZX 0UB94ZZ 0UB97ZX 0UB97ZZ
0UB98ZX 0UB98ZZ 0UBC0ZX 0UBC0ZZ 0UBC3ZX 0UBC3ZZ 0UBC4ZX 0UBC4ZZ 0UBC7ZX 0UBC7ZZ 0UBC8ZX 0UBC8ZZ 0UBF0ZX
0UBF0ZZ 0UBF3ZX 0UBF3ZZ 0UBF4ZX 0UBF4ZZ 0UBF7ZX 0UBF7ZZ 0UBF8ZX 0UBF8ZZ 0UBG0ZX 0UBG0ZZ 0UBG3ZX 0UBG3ZZ
0UBG4ZX 0UBG4ZZ 0UBG7ZX 0UBG7ZZ 0UBG8ZX 0UBG8ZZ 0UBGXZX 0UBGXZZ 0UBJ0ZX 0UBJ0ZZ 0UBJXZX 0UBJXZZ 0UBK0ZX
0UBK0ZZ 0UBK3ZX 0UBK3ZZ 0UBK4ZX 0UBK4ZZ 0UBK7ZX 0UBK7ZZ 0UBK8ZX 0UBK8ZZ 0UBKXZX 0UBKXZZ 0UBL0ZX 0UBL0ZZ
0UBLXZX 0UBLXZZ 0UBM0ZX 0UBM0ZZ 0UBMXZX 0UBMXZZ

LC Limited Coverage NC Noncovered HAC HAC-associated Procedure CC Combination Cluster - See Appendix G for code lists
DRG Non-OR-Affecting MS-DRG Assignment New/Revised Text in **Orange** ♂ Male ♀ Female

0 Medical and Surgical
U Female Reproductive System
C Extirpation: Taking or cutting out solid matter from a body part

Body Part Character 4	Approach Character 5	Device Character 6	Qualifier Character 7
0 Ovary, Right ♀ **1** Ovary, Left ♀ **2** Ovaries, Bilateral ♀ **4** Uterine Supporting Structure ♀	**0** Open **3** Percutaneous **4** Percutaneous Endoscopic **8** Via Natural or Artificial Opening Endoscopic	**Z** No Device	**Z** No Qualifier
5 Fallopian Tube, Right ♀ **6** Fallopian Tube, Left ♀ **7** Fallopian Tubes, Bilateral ♀ **9** Uterus ♀ **B** Endometrium ♀ **C** Cervix ♀ **F** Cul-de-sac ♀	**0** Open **3** Percutaneous **4** Percutaneous Endoscopic **7** Via Natural or Artificial Opening **8** Via Natural or Artificial Opening Endoscopic	**Z** No Device	**Z** No Qualifier
G Vagina ♀ **K** Hymen ♀	**0** Open **3** Percutaneous **4** Percutaneous Endoscopic **7** Via Natural or Artificial Opening **8** Via Natural or Artificial Opening Endoscopic **X** External	**Z** No Device	**Z** No Qualifier
J Clitoris ♀ **L** Vestibular Gland ♀ **M** Vulva ♀	**0** Open **X** External	**Z** No Device	**Z** No Qualifier

♀ 0UC00ZZ 0UC03ZZ 0UC04ZZ 0UC08ZZ 0UC10ZZ 0UC13ZZ 0UC14ZZ 0UC18ZZ 0UC20ZZ 0UC23ZZ 0UC24ZZ 0UC28ZZ 0UC40ZZ 0UC43ZZ 0UC44ZZ 0UC48ZZ 0UC50ZZ 0UC53ZZ 0UC54ZZ 0UC57ZZ 0UC58ZZ 0UC60ZZ 0UC63ZZ 0UC64ZZ 0UC67ZZ 0UC68ZZ 0UC70ZZ 0UC73ZZ 0UC74ZZ 0UC77ZZ 0UC78ZZ 0UC90ZZ 0UC93ZZ 0UC94ZZ 0UC97ZZ 0UC98ZZ 0UCB0ZZ 0UCB3ZZ 0UCB4ZZ 0UCB7ZZ 0UCB8ZZ 0UCC0ZZ 0UCC3ZZ 0UCC4ZZ 0UCC7ZZ 0UCC8ZZ 0UCF0ZZ 0UCF3ZZ 0UCF4ZZ 0UCF7ZZ 0UCF8ZZ 0UCG0ZZ 0UCG3ZZ 0UCG4ZZ 0UCG7ZZ 0UCG8ZZ 0UCGXZZ 0UCJ0ZZ 0UCJXZZ 0UCK0ZZ 0UCK3ZZ 0UCK4ZZ 0UCK7ZZ 0UCK8ZZ 0UCKXZZ 0UCL0ZZ 0UCLXZZ 0UCM0ZZ 0UCMXZZ

0 Medical and Surgical
U Female Reproductive System
D Extraction: Pulling or stripping out or off all or a portion of a body part by the use of force

Body Part Character 4	Approach Character 5	Device Character 6	Qualifier Character 7
B Endometrium ♀ D + C	**7** Via Natural or Artificial Opening **8** Via Natural or Artificial Opening Endoscopic hysterscope	**Z** No Device	**X** Diagnostic - biopsy **Z** No Qualifier
N Ova ♀	**0** Open **3** Percutaneous **4** Percutaneous Endoscopic	**Z** No Device	**Z** No Qualifier

♀ 0UDB7ZX 0UDB7ZZ 0UDB8ZX 0UDB8ZZ 0UDN0ZZ 0UDN3ZZ 0UDN4ZZ

0 Medical and Surgical
U Female Reproductive System
F Fragmentation: Breaking solid matter in a body part into pieces

Body Part Character 4	Approach Character 5	Device Character 6	Qualifier Character 7
5 Fallopian Tube, Right ♀ NC **6** Fallopian Tube, Left ♀ NC **7** Fallopian Tubes, Bilateral ♀ NC **9** Uterus ♀ NC	**0** Open **3** Percutaneous **4** Percutaneous Endoscopic **7** Via Natural or Artificial Opening **8** Via Natural or Artificial Opening Endoscopic **X** External	**Z** No Device	**Z** No Qualifier

♀ 0UF50ZZ 0UF53ZZ 0UF54ZZ 0UF57ZZ 0UF58ZZ 0UF5XZZ 0UF60ZZ 0UF63ZZ 0UF64ZZ 0UF67ZZ 0UF68ZZ 0UF6XZZ 0UF70ZZ 0UF73ZZ 0UF74ZZ 0UF77ZZ 0UF78ZZ 0UF7XZZ 0UF90ZZ 0UF93ZZ 0UF94ZZ 0UF97ZZ 0UF98ZZ 0UF9XZZ

NC 0UF5XZZ 0UF6XZZ 0UF7XZZ 0UF9XZZ

LC Limited Coverage NC Noncovered HAC HAC-associated Procedure CC Combination Cluster - See Appendix G for code lists
DRG Non-OR-Affecting MS-DRG Assignment New/Revised Text in **Orange** ♂ Male ♀ Female

0 Medical and Surgical
U Female Reproductive System
H Insertion: Putting in a nonbiological appliance that monitors, assists, performs, or prevents a physiological function but does not physically take the place of a body part

Body Part	Approach	Device	Qualifier
Character 4	Character 5	Character 6	Character 7
3 Ovary ♀	0 Open 3 Percutaneous 4 Percutaneous Endoscopic	3 Infusion Device Y Other Device	Z No Qualifier
3 Ovary ♀	7 Via Natural or Artificial Opening 8 Via Natural or Artificial Opening Endoscopic	Y Other Device	Z No Qualifier
8 Fallopian Tube ♀ D Uterus and Cervix ♀ H Vagina and Cul-de-sac ♀	0 Open 3 Percutaneous 4 Percutaneous Endoscopic 7 Via Natural or Artificial Opening 8 Via Natural or Artificial Opening Endoscopic	3 Infusion Device Y Other Device	Z No Qualifier
9 Uterus ♀	0 Open 7 Via Natural or Artificial Opening 8 Via Natural or Artificial Opening Endoscopic	H Contraceptive Device	Z No Qualifier
C Cervix ♀	0 Open 3 Percutaneous 4 Percutaneous Endoscopic	1 Radioactive Element	Z No Qualifier
C Cervix ♀	7 Via Natural or Artificial Opening 8 Via Natural or Artificial Opening Endoscopic	1 Radioactive Element H Contraceptive Device	Z No Qualifier
F Cul-de-sac ♀	7 Via Natural or Artificial Opening 8 Via Natural or Artificial Opening Endoscopic	G Intraluminal Device, Pessary	Z No Qualifier
G Vagina ♀	0 Open 3 Percutaneous 4 Percutaneous Endoscopic X External	1 Radioactive Element	Z No Qualifier
G Vagina ♀	7 Via Natural or Artificial Opening 8 Via Natural or Artificial Opening Endoscopic	1 Radioactive Element G Intraluminal Device, Pessary	Z No Qualifier

♀ 0UH303Z 0UH30YZ 0UH333Z 0UH33YZ 0UH343Z 0UH34YZ 0UH37YZ 0UH38YZ 0UH803Z 0UH80YZ 0UH833Z 0UH83YZ 0UH843Z 0UH84YZ 0UH873Z 0UH87YZ 0UH883Z 0UH88YZ 0UH90HZ 0UH97HZ 0UH98HZ 0UHC01Z 0UHC31Z 0UHC41Z 0UHC71Z 0UHC7HZ 0UHC81Z 0UHC8HZ 0UHD03Z 0UHD0YZ 0UHD33Z 0UHD3YZ 0UHD43Z 0UHD4YZ 0UHD73Z 0UHD7YZ 0UHD83Z 0UHD8YZ 0UHF7GZ 0UHF8GZ 0UHG01Z 0UHG31Z 0UHG41Z 0UHG71Z 0UHG7GZ 0UHG81Z 0UHG8GZ 0UHGX1Z 0UHH03Z 0UHH0YZ 0UHH33Z 0UHH3YZ 0UHH43Z 0UHH4YZ 0UHH73Z 0UHH7YZ 0UHH83Z 0UHH8YZ

0 Medical and Surgical
U Female Reproductive System
J Inspection: Visually and/or manually exploring a body part

Body Part	Approach	Device	Qualifier
Character 4	Character 5	Character 6	Character 7
3 Ovary ♀	0 Open 3 Percutaneous 4 Percutaneous Endoscopic 8 Via Natural or Artificial Opening Endoscopic X External	Z No Device	Z No Qualifier

0UJ continued on next page

0UJ continued from previous page

0 Medical and Surgical
U Female Reproductive System
J Inspection: Visually and/or manually exploring a body part

Body Part	Approach	Device	Qualifier
Character 4	**Character 5**	**Character 6**	**Character 7**
8 Fallopian Tube ♀ **D** Uterus and Cervix ♀ **H** Vagina and Cul-de-sac ♀	**0** Open **3** Percutaneous **4** Percutaneous Endoscopic **7** Via Natural or Artificial Opening **8** Via Natural or Artificial Opening Endoscopic **X** External	**Z** No Device	**Z** No Qualifier
M Vulva ♀	**0** Open **X** External	**Z** No Device	**Z** No Qualifier

♀ 0UJ30ZZ 0UJ33ZZ 0UJ34ZZ 0UJ38ZZ 0UJ3XZZ 0UJ80ZZ 0UJ83ZZ 0UJ84ZZ 0UJ87ZZ 0UJ88ZZ 0UJ8XZZ 0UJD0ZZ 0UJD3ZZ 0UJD4ZZ 0UJD7ZZ 0UJD8ZZ 0UJDXZZ 0UJH0ZZ 0UJH3ZZ 0UJH4ZZ 0UJH7ZZ 0UJH8ZZ 0UJHXZZ 0UJM0ZZ 0UJMXZZ

0 Medical and Surgical
U Female Reproductive System
L Occlusion: Completely closing an orifice or the lumen of a tubular body part

Body Part	Approach	Device	Qualifier
Character 4	**Character 5**	**Character 6**	**Character 7**
5 Fallopian Tube, Right ♀ **6** Fallopian Tube, Left ♀ **7** Fallopian Tubes, Bilateral ♀ NC	**0** Open **3** Percutaneous **4** Percutaneous Endoscopic	**C** Extraluminal Device **D** Intraluminal Device **Z** No Device	**Z** No Qualifier
5 Fallopian Tube, Right ♀ **6** Fallopian Tube, Left ♀ **7** Fallopian Tubes, Bilateral ♀ NC	**7** Via Natural or Artificial Opening **8** Via Natural or Artificial Opening Endoscopic	**D** Intraluminal Device **Z** No Device	**Z** No Qualifier
F Cul-de-sac ♀ **G** Vagina ♀	**7** Via Natural or Artificial Opening **8** Via Natural or Artificial Opening Endoscopic	**D** Intraluminal Device **Z** No Device	**Z** No Qualifier

♀ 0UL50CZ 0UL50DZ 0UL50ZZ 0UL53CZ 0UL53DZ 0UL53ZZ 0UL54CZ 0UL54DZ 0UL54ZZ 0UL57DZ 0UL57ZZ 0UL58DZ 0UL58ZZ 0UL60CZ 0UL60DZ 0UL60ZZ 0UL63CZ 0UL63DZ 0UL63ZZ 0UL64CZ 0UL64DZ 0UL64ZZ 0UL67DZ 0UL67ZZ 0UL68DZ 0UL68ZZ 0UL70CZ 0UL70DZ 0UL70ZZ 0UL73CZ 0UL73DZ 0UL73ZZ 0UL74CZ 0UL74DZ 0UL74ZZ 0UL77DZ 0UL77ZZ 0UL78DZ 0UL78ZZ 0ULF7DZ 0ULF7ZZ 0ULF8DZ 0ULF8ZZ 0ULG7DZ 0ULG7ZZ 0ULG8DZ 0ULG8ZZ

NC 0UL70CZ 0UL70DZ 0UL70ZZ 0UL73CZ 0UL73DZ 0UL73ZZ 0UL74CZ 0UL74DZ 0UL74ZZ 0UL77DZ 0UL77ZZ 0UL78DZ 0UL78ZZ
Codes in this list are noncovered procedures only when reported with Z30.2 as either a principal or secondary diagnosis.

0 Medical and Surgical
U Female Reproductive System
M Reattachment: Putting back in or on all or a portion of a separated body part to its normal location or other suitable location

Body Part	Approach	Device	Qualifier
Character 4	**Character 5**	**Character 6**	**Character 7**
0 Ovary, Right ♀ **1** Ovary, Left ♀ **2** Ovaries, Bilateral ♀ **4** Uterine Supporting Structure ♀ **5** Fallopian Tube, Right ♀ **6** Fallopian Tube, Left ♀ **7** Fallopian Tubes, Bilateral ♀ **9** Uterus ♀ **C** Cervix ♀ **F** Cul-de-sac ♀ **G** Vagina ♀	**0** Open **4** Percutaneous Endoscopic	**Z** No Device	**Z** No Qualifier
J Clitoris ♀ **M** Vulva ♀	**X** External	**Z** No Device	**Z** No Qualifier
K Hymen ♀	**0** Open **4** Percutaneous Endoscopic **X** External	**Z** No Device	**Z** No Qualifier

♀ 0UM00ZZ 0UM04ZZ 0UM10ZZ 0UM14ZZ 0UM20ZZ 0UM24ZZ 0UM40ZZ 0UM44ZZ 0UM50ZZ 0UM54ZZ 0UM60ZZ 0UM64ZZ 0UM70ZZ 0UM74ZZ 0UM90ZZ 0UM94ZZ 0UMC0ZZ 0UMC4ZZ 0UMF0ZZ 0UMF4ZZ 0UMG0ZZ 0UMG4ZZ 0UMJXZZ 0UMK0ZZ 0UMK4ZZ 0UMKXZZ 0UMMXZZ laparoscopic = percutaneous endoscopic

0 Medical and Surgical
U Female Reproductive System
N Release: Freeing a body part from an abnormal physical constraint by cutting or by the use of force

Body Part Character 4	Approach Character 5	Device Character 6	Qualifier Character 7
0 Ovary, Right ♀ **1** Ovary, Left ♀ **2** Ovaries, Bilateral ♀ **4** Uterine Supporting Structure ♀	**0** Open **3** Percutaneous **4** Percutaneous Endoscopic **8** Via Natural or Artificial Opening Endoscopic	**Z** No Device	**Z** No Qualifier
5 Fallopian Tube, Right ♀ **6** Fallopian Tube, Left ♀ **7** Fallopian Tubes, Bilateral ♀ **9** Uterus ♀ **C** Cervix ♀ **F** Cul-de-sac ♀	**0** Open **3** Percutaneous **4** Percutaneous Endoscopic laparoscopic **7** Via Natural or Artificial Opening **8** Via Natural or Artificial Opening Endoscopic	**Z** No Device	**Z** No Qualifier
G Vagina ♀ **K** Hymen ♀	**0** Open **3** Percutaneous **4** Percutaneous Endoscopic **7** Via Natural or Artificial Opening **8** Via Natural or Artificial Opening Endoscopic **X** External	**Z** No Device	**Z** No Qualifier
J Clitoris ♀ **L** Vestibular Gland ♀ **M** Vulva ♀	**0** Open **X** External	**Z** No Device	**Z** No Qualifier

♀ 0UN00ZZ 0UN03ZZ 0UN04ZZ 0UN08ZZ 0UN10ZZ 0UN13ZZ 0UN14ZZ 0UN18ZZ 0UN20ZZ 0UN23ZZ 0UN24ZZ 0UN28ZZ 0UN40ZZ 0UN43ZZ 0UN44ZZ 0UN48ZZ 0UN50ZZ 0UN53ZZ 0UN54ZZ 0UN57ZZ 0UN58ZZ 0UN60ZZ 0UN63ZZ 0UN64ZZ 0UN67ZZ 0UN68ZZ 0UN70ZZ 0UN73ZZ 0UN74ZZ 0UN77ZZ 0UN78ZZ 0UN90ZZ 0UN93ZZ 0UN94ZZ 0UN97ZZ 0UN98ZZ 0UNC0ZZ 0UNC3ZZ 0UNC4ZZ 0UNC7ZZ 0UNC8ZZ 0UNF0ZZ 0UNF3ZZ 0UNF4ZZ 0UNF7ZZ 0UNF8ZZ 0UNG0ZZ 0UNG3ZZ 0UNG4ZZ 0UNG7ZZ 0UNG8ZZ 0UNGXZZ 0UNJ0ZZ 0UNJXZZ 0UNK0ZZ 0UNK3ZZ 0UNK4ZZ 0UNK7ZZ 0UNK8ZZ 0UNKXZZ 0UNL0ZZ 0UNLXZZ 0UNM0ZZ 0UNMXZZ

0 Medical and Surgical
U Female Reproductive System
P Removal: Taking out or off a device from a body part

Body Part Character 4	Approach Character 5	Device Character 6	Qualifier Character 7
3 Ovary ♀	**0** Open **3** Percutaneous **4** Percutaneous Endoscopic	**0** Drainage Device **3** Infusion Device **Y** Other Device	**Z** No Qualifier
3 Ovary ♀	**7** Via Natural or Artificial Opening **8** Via Natural or Artificial Opening Endoscopic	**Y** Other Device	**Z** No Qualifier
3 Ovary ♀	**X** External	**0** Drainage Device **3** Infusion Device	**Z** No Qualifier
8 Fallopian Tube ♀	**0** Open **3** Percutaneous **4** Percutaneous Endoscopic **7** Via Natural or Artificial Opening **8** Via Natural or Artificial Opening Endoscopic	**0** Drainage Device **3** Infusion Device **7** Autologous Tissue Substitute **C** Extraluminal Device **D** Intraluminal Device **J** Synthetic Substitute **K** Nonautologous Tissue Substitute **Y** Other Device	**Z** No Qualifier
8 Fallopian Tube ♀	**X** External	**0** Drainage Device **3** Infusion Device **D** Intraluminal Device	**Z** No Qualifier

0UP continued on next page

0UP continued from previous page

0 Medical and Surgical
U Female Reproductive System
P Removal: Taking out or off a device from a body part

Body Part Character 4	Approach Character 5	Device Character 6	Qualifier Character 7
D Uterus and Cervix ♀	**0** Open **3** Percutaneous **4** Percutaneous Endoscopic **7** Via Natural or Artificial Opening **8** Via Natural or Artificial Opening Endoscopic	**0** Drainage Device **1** Radioactive Element **3** Infusion Device **7** Autologous Tissue Substitute **C** Extraluminal Device **D** Intraluminal Device **H** Contraceptive Device **J** Synthetic Substitute **K** Nonautologous Tissue Substitute **Y** Other Device	**Z** No Qualifier
D Uterus and Cervix ♀	**X** External	**0** Drainage Device **3** Infusion Device **D** Intraluminal Device **H** Contraceptive Device	**Z** No Qualifier
H Vagina and Cul-de-sac ♀	**0** Open **3** Percutaneous **4** Percutaneous Endoscopic **7** Via Natural or Artificial Opening **8** Via Natural or Artificial Opening Endoscopic	**0** Drainage Device **1** Radioactive Element **3** Infusion Device **7** Autologous Tissue Substitute **D** Intraluminal Device **J** Synthetic Substitute **K** Nonautologous Tissue Substitute **Y** Other Device	**Z** No Qualifier
H Vagina and Cul-de-sac ♀	**X** External	**0** Drainage Device **1** Radioactive Element **3** Infusion Device **D** Intraluminal Device	**Z** No Qualifier
M Vulva ♀	**0** Open	**0** Drainage Device **7** Autologous Tissue Substitute **J** Synthetic Substitute **K** Nonautologous Tissue Substitute	**Z** No Qualifier
M Vulva ♀	**X** External	**0** Drainage Device	**Z** No Qualifier

♀ 0UP300Z 0UP303Z 0UP30YZ 0UP330Z 0UP333Z 0UP33YZ 0UP340Z 0UP343Z 0UP34YZ 0UP37YZ 0UP38YZ 0UP3X0Z 0UP3X3Z 0UP800Z 0UP803Z 0UP807Z 0UP80CZ 0UP80DZ 0UP80JZ 0UP80KZ 0UP80YZ 0UP830Z 0UP833Z 0UP837Z 0UP83CZ 0UP83DZ 0UP83JZ 0UP83KZ 0UP83YZ 0UP840Z 0UP843Z 0UP847Z 0UP84CZ 0UP84DZ 0UP84JZ 0UP84KZ 0UP84YZ 0UP870Z 0UP873Z 0UP877Z 0UP87CZ 0UP87DZ 0UP87JZ 0UP87KZ 0UP87YZ 0UP880Z 0UP883Z 0UP887Z 0UP88CZ 0UP88DZ 0UP88JZ 0UP88KZ 0UP88YZ 0UP8X0Z 0UP8X3Z 0UP8XDZ 0UPD00Z 0UPD01Z 0UPD03Z 0UPD07Z 0UPD0CZ 0UPD0DZ 0UPD0HZ 0UPD0JZ 0UPD0KZ 0UPD0YZ 0UPD30Z 0UPD31Z 0UPD33Z 0UPD37Z 0UPD3CZ 0UPD3DZ 0UPD3HZ 0UPD3JZ 0UPD3KZ 0UPD3YZ 0UPD40Z 0UPD41Z 0UPD43Z 0UPD47Z 0UPD4CZ 0UPD4DZ 0UPD4HZ 0UPD4JZ 0UPD4KZ 0UPD4YZ 0UPD70Z 0UPD71Z 0UPD73Z 0UPD77Z 0UPD7CZ 0UPD7DZ 0UPD7HZ 0UPD7JZ 0UPD7KZ 0UPD7YZ 0UPD80Z 0UPD81Z 0UPD83Z 0UPD87Z 0UPD8CZ 0UPD8DZ 0UPD8HZ 0UPD8JZ 0UPD8KZ 0UPD8YZ 0UPDX0Z 0UPDX3Z 0UPDXDZ 0UPDXHZ 0UPH00Z 0UPH01Z 0UPH03Z 0UPH07Z 0UPH0DZ 0UPH0JZ 0UPH0KZ 0UPH0YZ 0UPH30Z 0UPH31Z 0UPH33Z 0UPH37Z 0UPH3DZ 0UPH3JZ 0UPH3KZ 0UPH3YZ 0UPH40Z 0UPH41Z 0UPH43Z 0UPH47Z 0UPH4DZ 0UPH4JZ 0UPH4KZ 0UPH4YZ 0UPH70Z 0UPH71Z 0UPH73Z 0UPH77Z 0UPH7DZ 0UPH7JZ 0UPH7KZ 0UPH7YZ 0UPH80Z 0UPH81Z 0UPH83Z 0UPH87Z 0UPH8DZ 0UPH8JZ 0UPH8KZ 0UPH8YZ 0UPHX0Z 0UPHX1Z 0UPHX3Z 0UPHXDZ 0UPM00Z 0UPM07Z 0UPM0JZ 0UPM0KZ 0UPMX0Z

0 Medical and Surgical
U Female Reproductive System
Q Repair: Restoring, to the extent possible, a body part to its normal anatomic structure and function

Body Part Character 4	Approach Character 5	Device Character 6	Qualifier Character 7
0 Ovary, Right ♀ **1** Ovary, Left ♀ **2** Ovaries, Bilateral ♀ **4** Uterine Supporting Structure ♀	**0** Open **3** Percutaneous **4** Percutaneous Endoscopic **8** Via Natural or Artificial Opening Endoscopic	**Z** No Device	**Z** No Qualifier
5 Fallopian Tube, Right ♀ **6** Fallopian Tube, Left ♀ **7** Fallopian Tubes, Bilateral ♀ **9** Uterus ♀ **C** Cervix ♀ **F** Cul-de-sac ♀	**0** Open **3** Percutaneous **4** Percutaneous Endoscopic **7** Via Natural or Artificial Opening **8** Via Natural or Artificial Opening Endoscopic	**Z** No Device	**Z** No Qualifier
G Vagina ♀ **K** Hymen ♀	**0** Open **3** Percutaneous **4** Percutaneous Endoscopic **7** Via Natural or Artificial Opening **8** Via Natural or Artificial Opening Endoscopic **X** External	**Z** No Device	**Z** No Qualifier
J Clitoris ♀ **L** Vestibular Gland ♀ **M** Vulva ♀	**0** Open **X** External	**Z** No Device	**Z** No Qualifier

♀ 0UQ00ZZ 0UQ03ZZ 0UQ04ZZ 0UQ08ZZ 0UQ10ZZ 0UQ13ZZ 0UQ14ZZ 0UQ18ZZ 0UQ20ZZ 0UQ23ZZ 0UQ24ZZ 0UQ28ZZ 0UQ40ZZ 0UQ43ZZ 0UQ44ZZ 0UQ48ZZ 0UQ50ZZ 0UQ53ZZ 0UQ54ZZ 0UQ57ZZ 0UQ58ZZ 0UQ60ZZ 0UQ63ZZ 0UQ64ZZ 0UQ67ZZ 0UQ68ZZ 0UQ70ZZ 0UQ73ZZ 0UQ74ZZ 0UQ77ZZ 0UQ78ZZ 0UQ90ZZ 0UQ93ZZ 0UQ94ZZ 0UQ97ZZ 0UQ98ZZ 0UQC0ZZ 0UQC3ZZ 0UQC4ZZ 0UQC7ZZ 0UQC8ZZ 0UQF0ZZ 0UQF3ZZ 0UQF4ZZ 0UQF7ZZ 0UQF8ZZ 0UQG0ZZ 0UQG3ZZ 0UQG4ZZ 0UQG7ZZ 0UQG8ZZ 0UQGXZZ 0UQJ0ZZ 0UQJXZZ 0UQK0ZZ 0UQK3ZZ 0UQK4ZZ 0UQK7ZZ 0UQK8ZZ 0UQKXZZ 0UQL0ZZ 0UQLXZZ 0UQM0ZZ 0UQMXZZ

0 Medical and Surgical
U Female Reproductive System
S Reposition: Moving to its normal location, or other suitable location, all or a portion of a body part

Body Part Character 4	Approach Character 5	Device Character 6	Qualifier Character 7
0 Ovary, Right ♀ **1** Ovary, Left ♀ **2** Ovaries, Bilateral ♀ **4** Uterine Supporting Structure ♀ **5** Fallopian Tube, Right ♀ **6** Fallopian Tube, Left ♀ **7** Fallopian Tubes, Bilateral ♀ **C** Cervix ♀ **F** Cul-de-sac ♀	**0** Open **4** Percutaneous Endoscopic **8** Via Natural or Artificial Opening Endoscopic	**Z** No Device	**Z** No Qualifier
9 Uterus ♀ **G** Vagina ♀	**0** Open **4** Percutaneous Endoscopic **7** Via Natural or Artificial Opening **8** Via Natural or Artificial Opening Endoscopic **X** External	**Z** No Device	**Z** No Qualifier

♀ 0US00ZZ 0US04ZZ 0US08ZZ 0US10ZZ 0US14ZZ 0US18ZZ 0US20ZZ 0US24ZZ 0US28ZZ 0US40ZZ 0US44ZZ 0US48ZZ 0US50ZZ 0US54ZZ 0US58ZZ 0US60ZZ 0US64ZZ 0US68ZZ 0US70ZZ 0US74ZZ 0US78ZZ 0US90ZZ 0US94ZZ 0US97ZZ 0US98ZZ 0US9XZZ 0USC0ZZ 0USC4ZZ 0USC8ZZ 0USF0ZZ 0USF4ZZ 0USF8ZZ 0USG0ZZ 0USG4ZZ 0USG7ZZ 0USG8ZZ 0USGXZZ

Supracervical- cervix remains

0 Medical and Surgical
U Female Reproductive System
T Resection: Cutting out or off, without replacement, all of a body part

Body Part Character 4	Approach Character 5	Device Character 6	Qualifier Character 7
0 Ovary, Right ♀ (Oopho) **1** Ovary, Left ♀ **2** Ovaries, Bilateral ♀ CC **5** Fallopian Tube, Right ♀ (salp) **6** Fallopian Tube, Left ♀ **7** Fallopian Tubes, Bilateral ♀ CC salping= tubes	**0** Open **4** Percutaneous Endoscopic **7** Via Natural or Artificial Opening **8** Via Natural or Artificial Opening Endoscopic **F** Via Natural or Artificial Opening With Percutaneous Endoscopic Assistance	**Z** No Device	**Z** No Qualifier
4 Uterine Supporting Structure ♀ CC **C** Cervix ♀ CC **F** Cul-de-sac ♀ **G** Vagina ♀ CC	**0** Open **4** Percutaneous Endoscopic **7** Via Natural or Artificial Opening **8** Via Natural or Artificial Opening Endoscopic	**Z** No Device	**Z** No Qualifier
9 Uterus ♀ CC hysterectomy	**0** Open (abdominal) **4** Percutaneous Endoscopic **7** Via Natural or Artificial Opening **8** Via Natural or Artificial Opening Endoscopic **F** Via Natural or Artificial Opening With Percutaneous Endoscopic Assistance	**Z** No Device	**L** Supracervical **Z** No Qualifier
J Clitoris ♀ **L** Vestibular Gland ♀ **M** Vulva ♀ CC	**0** Open **X** External	**Z** No Device	**Z** No Qualifier
K Hymen ♀	**0** Open **4** Percutaneous Endoscopic **7** Via Natural or Artificial Opening **8** Via Natural or Artificial Opening Endoscopic **X** External	**Z** No Device	**Z** No Qualifier

♀ 0UT00ZZ 0UT04ZZ 0UT07ZZ 0UT08ZZ 0UT0FZZ 0UT10ZZ 0UT14ZZ 0UT17ZZ 0UT18ZZ 0UT1FZZ 0UT20ZZ 0UT24ZZ 0UT27ZZ 0UT28ZZ 0UT2FZZ 0UT40ZZ 0UT44ZZ 0UT47ZZ 0UT48ZZ 0UT50ZZ 0UT54ZZ 0UT57ZZ 0UT58ZZ 0UT5FZZ 0UT60ZZ 0UT64ZZ 0UT67ZZ 0UT68ZZ 0UT6FZZ 0UT70ZZ 0UT74ZZ 0UT77ZZ 0UT78ZZ 0UT7FZZ 0UT90ZL 0UT90ZZ 0UT94ZL 0UT94ZZ 0UT97ZL 0UT97ZZ 0UT98ZL 0UT98ZZ 0UT9FZL 0UT9FZZ 0UTC0ZZ 0UTC4ZZ 0UTC7ZZ 0UTC8ZZ 0UTF0ZZ 0UTF4ZZ 0UTF7ZZ 0UTF8ZZ 0UTG0ZZ 0UTG4ZZ 0UTG7ZZ 0UTG8ZZ 0UTJ0ZZ 0UTJXZZ 0UTK0ZZ 0UTK4ZZ 0UTK7ZZ 0UTK8ZZ 0UTKXZZ 0UTL0ZZ 0UTLXZZ 0UTM0ZZ 0UTMXZZ

CC 0UT20ZZ 0UT40ZZ 0UT44ZZ 0UT47ZZ 0UT48ZZ 0UT70ZZ 0UT90ZZ 0UT94ZZ 0UT97ZZ 0UT98ZZ 0UT9FZZ 0UTC0ZZ 0UTC4ZZ 0UTC7ZZ 0UTC8ZZ 0UTG0ZZ 0UTM0ZZ 0UTMXZZ

0 Medical and Surgical
U Female Reproductive System
U Supplement: Putting in or on biological or synthetic material that physically reinforces and/or augments the function of a portion of a body part

Body Part Character 4	Approach Character 5	Device Character 6	Qualifier Character 7
4 Uterine Supporting Structure ♀	**0** Open **4** Percutaneous Endoscopic	**7** Autologous Tissue Substitute **J** Synthetic Substitute **K** Nonautologous Tissue Substitute	**Z** No Qualifier
5 Fallopian Tube, Right ♀ **6** Fallopian Tube, Left ♀ **7** Fallopian Tubes, Bilateral ♀ **F** Cul-de-sac ♀	**0** Open **4** Percutaneous Endoscopic **7** Via Natural or Artificial Opening **8** Via Natural or Artificial Opening Endoscopic	**7** Autologous Tissue Substitute **J** Synthetic Substitute **K** Nonautologous Tissue Substitute	**Z** No Qualifier

0UU continued on next page

0 Medical and Surgical
U Female Reproductive System
U Supplement: Putting in or on biological or synthetic material that physically reinforces and/or augments the function of a portion of a body part

0UU continued from previous page

Body Part Character 4	Approach Character 5	Device Character 6	Qualifier Character 7
G Vagina ♀ **K** Hymen ♀	**0** Open **4** Percutaneous Endoscopic **7** Via Natural or Artificial Opening **8** Via Natural or Artificial Opening Endoscopic **X** External	**7** Autologous Tissue Substitute **J** Synthetic Substitute **K** Nonautologous Tissue Substitute	**Z** No Qualifier
J Clitoris ♀ **M** Vulva ♀	**0** Open **X** External	**7** Autologous Tissue Substitute **J** Synthetic Substitute **K** Nonautologous Tissue Substitute	**Z** No Qualifier

♀ 0UU407Z 0UU40JZ 0UU40KZ 0UU447Z 0UU44JZ 0UU44KZ 0UU507Z 0UU50JZ 0UU50KZ 0UU547Z 0UU54JZ 0UU54KZ 0UU577Z 0UU57JZ 0UU57KZ 0UU587Z 0UU58JZ 0UU58KZ 0UU607Z 0UU60JZ 0UU60KZ 0UU647Z 0UU64JZ 0UU64KZ 0UU677Z 0UU67JZ 0UU67KZ 0UU687Z 0UU68JZ 0UU68KZ 0UU707Z 0UU70JZ 0UU70KZ 0UU747Z 0UU74JZ 0UU74KZ 0UU777Z 0UU77JZ 0UU77KZ 0UU787Z 0UU78JZ 0UU78KZ 0UUF07Z 0UUF0JZ 0UUF0KZ 0UUF47Z 0UUF4JZ 0UUF4KZ 0UUF77Z 0UUF7JZ 0UUF7KZ 0UUF87Z 0UUF8JZ 0UUF8KZ 0UUG07Z 0UUG0JZ 0UUG0KZ 0UUG47Z 0UUG4JZ 0UUG4KZ 0UUG77Z 0UUG7JZ 0UUG7KZ 0UUG87Z 0UUG8JZ 0UUG8KZ 0UUGX7Z 0UUGXJZ 0UUGXKZ 0UUJ07Z 0UUJ0JZ 0UUJ0KZ 0UUJX7Z 0UUJXJZ 0UUJXKZ 0UUK07Z 0UUK0JZ 0UUK0KZ 0UUK47Z 0UUK4JZ 0UUK4KZ 0UUK77Z 0UUK7JZ 0UUK7KZ 0UUK87Z 0UUK8JZ 0UUK8KZ 0UUKX7Z 0UUKXJZ 0UUKXKZ 0UUM07Z 0UUM0JZ 0UUM0KZ 0UUMX7Z 0UUMXJZ 0UUMXKZ

0 Medical and Surgical
U Female Reproductive System
V Restriction: Partially closing an orifice or the lumen of a tubular body part

Body Part Character 4	Approach Character 5	Device Character 6	Qualifier Character 7
C Cervix ♀	**0** Open **3** Percutaneous **4** Percutaneous Endoscopic	**C** Extraluminal Device **D** Intraluminal Device **Z** No Device	**Z** No Qualifier
C Cervix ♀	**7** Via Natural or Artificial Opening **8** Via Natural or Artificial Opening Endoscopic	**D** Intraluminal Device **Z** No Device	**Z** No Qualifier

♀ 0UVC0CZ 0UVC0DZ 0UVC0ZZ 0UVC3CZ 0UVC3DZ 0UVC3ZZ 0UVC4CZ 0UVC4DZ 0UVC4ZZ 0UVC7DZ 0UVC7ZZ 0UVC8DZ 0UVC8ZZ

0 Medical and Surgical
U Female Reproductive System
W Revision: Correcting, to the extent possible, a portion of a malfunctioning device or the position of a displaced device

Body Part Character 4	Approach Character 5	Device Character 6	Qualifier Character 7
3 Ovary ♀	**0** Open **3** Percutaneous **4** Percutaneous Endoscopic	**0** Drainage Device **3** Infusion Device **Y** Other Device	**Z** No Qualifier
3 Ovary ♀	**7** Via Natural or Artificial Opening **8** Via Natural or Artificial Opening Endoscopic	**Y** Other Device	**Z** No Qualifier
3 Ovary ♀	**X** External	**0** Drainage Device **3** Infusion Device	**Z** No Qualifier
8 Fallopian Tube ♀	**0** Open **3** Percutaneous **4** Percutaneous Endoscopic **7** Via Natural or Artificial Opening **8** Via Natural or Artificial Opening Endoscopic	**0** Drainage Device **3** Infusion Device **7** Autologous Tissue Substitute **C** Extraluminal Device **D** Intraluminal Device **J** Synthetic Substitute **K** Nonautologous Tissue Substitute **Y** Other Device	**Z** No Qualifier

0UW continued on next page

0UW continued from previous page

0 Medical and Surgical
U Female Reproductive System
W Revision: Correcting, to the extent possible, a portion of a malfunctioning device or the position of a displaced device

Body Part Character 4	Approach Character 5	Device Character 6	Qualifier Character 7
8 Fallopian Tube ♀	**X** External	**0** Drainage Device **3** Infusion Device **7** Autologous Tissue Substitute **C** Extraluminal Device **D** Intraluminal Device **J** Synthetic Substitute **K** Nonautologous Tissue Substitute	**Z** No Qualifier
D Uterus and Cervix ♀	**0** Open **3** Percutaneous **4** Percutaneous Endoscopic **7** Via Natural or Artificial Opening **8** Via Natural or Artificial Opening Endoscopic	**0** Drainage Device **1** Radioactive Element **3** Infusion Device **7** Autologous Tissue Substitute **C** Extraluminal Device **D** Intraluminal Device **H** Contraceptive Device **J** Synthetic Substitute **K** Nonautologous Tissue Substitute **Y** Other Device	**Z** No Qualifier
D Uterus and Cervix ♀	**X** External	**0** Drainage Device **3** Infusion Device **7** Autologous Tissue Substitute **C** Extraluminal Device **D** Intraluminal Device **H** Contraceptive Device **J** Synthetic Substitute **K** Nonautologous Tissue Substitute	**Z** No Qualifier
H Vagina and Cul-de-sac ♀	**0** Open **3** Percutaneous **4** Percutaneous Endoscopic **7** Via Natural or Artificial Opening **8** Via Natural or Artificial Opening Endoscopic	**0** Drainage Device **1** Radioactive Element **3** Infusion Device **7** Autologous Tissue Substitute **D** Intraluminal Device **J** Synthetic Substitute **K** Nonautologous Tissue Substitute **Y** Other Device	**Z** No Qualifier
H Vagina and Cul-de-sac ♀	**X** External	**0** Drainage Device **3** Infusion Device **7** Autologous Tissue Substitute **D** Intraluminal Device **J** Synthetic Substitute **K** Nonautologous Tissue Substitute	**Z** No Qualifier
M Vulva ♀	**0** Open **X** External	**0** Drainage Device **7** Autologous Tissue Substitute **J** Synthetic Substitute **K** Nonautologous Tissue Substitute	**Z** No Qualifier

♀ 0UW300Z 0UW303Z 0UW30YZ 0UW330Z 0UW333Z 0UW33YZ 0UW340Z 0UW343Z 0UW34YZ 0UW37YZ 0UW38YZ 0UW3X0Z 0UW3X3Z 0UW800Z 0UW803Z 0UW807Z 0UW80CZ 0UW80DZ 0UW80JZ 0UW80KZ 0UW80YZ 0UW830Z 0UW833Z 0UW837Z 0UW83CZ 0UW83DZ 0UW83JZ 0UW83KZ 0UW83YZ 0UW840Z 0UW843Z 0UW847Z 0UW84CZ 0UW84DZ 0UW84JZ 0UW84KZ 0UW84YZ 0UW870Z 0UW873Z 0UW877Z 0UW87CZ 0UW87DZ 0UW87JZ 0UW87KZ 0UW87YZ 0UW880Z 0UW883Z 0UW887Z 0UW88CZ 0UW88DZ 0UW88JZ 0UW88KZ 0UW88YZ 0UW8X0Z 0UW8X3Z 0UW8X7Z 0UW8XCZ 0UW8XDZ 0UW8XJZ 0UW8XKZ 0UWD00Z 0UWD01Z 0UWD03Z 0UWD07Z 0UWD0CZ 0UWD0DZ 0UWD0HZ 0UWD0JZ 0UWD0KZ 0UWD0YZ 0UWD30Z 0UWD31Z 0UWD33Z 0UWD37Z 0UWD3CZ 0UWD3DZ 0UWD3HZ 0UWD3JZ 0UWD3KZ 0UWD3YZ 0UWD40Z 0UWD41Z 0UWD43Z 0UWD47Z 0UWD4CZ 0UWD4DZ 0UWD4HZ 0UWD4JZ 0UWD4KZ 0UWD4YZ 0UWD70Z 0UWD71Z 0UWD73Z 0UWD77Z 0UWD7CZ 0UWD7DZ 0UWD7HZ 0UWD7JZ 0UWD7KZ 0UWD7YZ 0UWD80Z 0UWD81Z 0UWD83Z 0UWD87Z 0UWD8CZ 0UWD8DZ 0UWD8HZ 0UWD8JZ 0UWD8KZ 0UWD8YZ 0UWDX0Z 0UWDX3Z 0UWDX7Z 0UWDXCZ 0UWDXDZ 0UWDXHZ 0UWDXJZ 0UWDXKZ 0UWH00Z 0UWH01Z 0UWH03Z 0UWH07Z 0UWH0DZ 0UWH0JZ 0UWH0KZ 0UWH0YZ 0UWH30Z 0UWH31Z 0UWH33Z 0UWH37Z 0UWH3DZ 0UWH3JZ 0UWH3KZ 0UWH3YZ 0UWH40Z 0UWH41Z 0UWH43Z 0UWH47Z 0UWH4DZ 0UWH4JZ 0UWH4KZ 0UWH4YZ 0UWH70Z 0UWH71Z 0UWH73Z 0UWH77Z 0UWH7DZ 0UWH7JZ 0UWH7KZ 0UWH7YZ 0UWH80Z 0UWH81Z 0UWH83Z 0UWH87Z 0UWH8DZ 0UWH8JZ 0UWH8KZ 0UWH8YZ 0UWHX0Z 0UWHX3Z 0UWHX7Z 0UWHXDZ 0UWHXJZ 0UWHXKZ 0UWM00Z 0UWM07Z 0UWM0JZ 0UWM0KZ 0UWMX0Z 0UWMX7Z 0UWMXJZ 0UWMXKZ

0 Medical and Surgical
U Female Reproductive System
Y Transplantation: Putting in or on all or a portion of a living body part taken from another individual or animal to physically take the place and/or function of all or a portion of a similar body part

Body Part Character 4	Approach Character 5	Device Character 6	Qualifier Character 7
0 Ovary, Right ♀ **1** Ovary, Left ♀ **9** Uterus ♀	**0** Open	**Z** No Device	**0** Allogeneic **1** Syngeneic **2** Zooplastic

♀ 0UY00Z0 0UY00Z1 0UY00Z2 0UY10Z0 0UY10Z1 0UY10Z2 0UY90Z0 0UY90Z1 0UY90Z2

NOTES

NOTES

Male Reproductive System 0V1-0VX

0 Medical and Surgical
V Male Reproductive System
1 Bypass: Altering the route of passage of the contents of a tubular body part

Body Part	Approach	Device	Qualifier
Character 4	**Character 5**	**Character 6**	**Character 7**
N Vas Deferens, Right ♂ **P** Vas Deferens, Left ♂ **Q** Vas Deferens, Bilateral ♂	**0** Open **4** Percutaneous Endoscopic	**7** Autologous Tissue Substitute **J** Synthetic Substitute **K** Nonautologous Tissue Substitute **Z** No Device	**J** Epididymis, Right **K** Epididymis, Left **N** Vas Deferens, Right **P** Vas Deferens, Left

♂ 0V1N07J 0V1N07K 0V1N07N 0V1N07P 0V1N0JJ 0V1N0JK 0V1N0JN 0V1N0JP 0V1N0KJ 0V1N0KK 0V1N0KN 0V1N0KP 0V1N0ZJ 0V1N0ZK 0V1N0ZN 0V1N0ZP 0V1N47J 0V1N47K 0V1N47N 0V1N47P 0V1N4JJ 0V1N4JK 0V1N4JN 0V1N4JP 0V1N4KJ 0V1N4KK 0V1N4KN 0V1N4KP 0V1N4ZJ 0V1N4ZK 0V1N4ZN 0V1N4ZP 0V1P07J 0V1P07K 0V1P07N 0V1P07P 0V1P0JJ 0V1P0JK 0V1P0JN 0V1P0JP 0V1P0KJ 0V1P0KK 0V1P0KN 0V1P0KP 0V1P0ZJ 0V1P0ZK 0V1P0ZN 0V1P0ZP 0V1P47J 0V1P47K 0V1P47N 0V1P47P 0V1P4JJ 0V1P4JK 0V1P4JN 0V1P4JP 0V1P4KJ 0V1P4KK 0V1P4KN 0V1P4KP 0V1P4ZJ 0V1P4ZK 0V1P4ZN 0V1P4ZP 0V1Q07J 0V1Q07K 0V1Q07N 0V1Q07P 0V1Q0JJ 0V1Q0JK 0V1Q0JN 0V1Q0JP 0V1Q0KJ 0V1Q0KK 0V1Q0KN 0V1Q0KP 0V1Q0ZJ 0V1Q0ZK 0V1Q0ZN 0V1Q0ZP 0V1Q47J 0V1Q47K 0V1Q47N 0V1Q47P 0V1Q4JJ 0V1Q4JK 0V1Q4JN 0V1Q4JP 0V1Q4KJ 0V1Q4KK 0V1Q4KN 0V1Q4KP 0V1Q4ZJ 0V1Q4ZK 0V1Q4ZN 0V1Q4ZP

0 Medical and Surgical
V Male Reproductive System
2 Change: Taking out or off a device from a body part and putting back an identical or similar device in or on the same body part without cutting or puncturing the skin or a mucous membrane

Body Part	Approach	Device	Qualifier
Character 4	**Character 5**	**Character 6**	**Character 7**
4 Prostate and Seminal Vesicles ♂ **8** Scrotum and Tunica Vaginalis ♂ **D** Testis ♂ **M** Epididymis and Spermatic Cord ♂ **R** Vas Deferens ♂ **S** Penis ♂	**X** External	**0** Drainage Device **Y** Other Device	**Z** No Qualifier

♂ 0V24X0Z 0V24XYZ 0V28X0Z 0V28XYZ 0V2DX0Z 0V2DXYZ 0V2MX0Z 0V2MXYZ 0V2RX0Z 0V2RXYZ 0V2SX0Z 0V2SXYZ

0 Medical and Surgical
V Male Reproductive System
5 Destruction: Physical eradication of all or a portion of a body part by the direct use of energy, force, or a destructive agent

Body Part	Approach	Device	Qualifier
Character 4	**Character 5**	**Character 6**	**Character 7**
0 Prostate ♂	**0** Open **3** Percutaneous **4** Percutaneous Endoscopic **7** Via Natural or Artificial Opening transurethral **8** Via Natural or Artificial Opening Endoscopic transurethral endoscopic	**Z** No Device	**Z** No Qualifier
1 Seminal Vesicle, Right ♂ **2** Seminal Vesicle, Left ♂ **3** Seminal Vesicles, Bilateral ♂ **6** Tunica Vaginalis, Right ♂ **7** Tunica Vaginalis, Left ♂ **9** Testis, Right ♂ **B** Testis, Left ♂ **C** Testes, Bilateral ♂	**0** Open **3** Percutaneous **4** Percutaneous Endoscopic	**Z** No Device	**Z** No Qualifier
5 Scrotum ♂ **S** Penis ♂ **T** Prepuce ♂	**0** Open **3** Percutaneous **4** Percutaneous Endoscopic **X** External	**Z** No Device	**Z** No Qualifier
F Spermatic Cord, Right ♂ **G** Spermatic Cord, Left ♂ **H** Spermatic Cords, Bilateral ♂ **J** Epididymis, Right ♂ **K** Epididymis, Left ♂ **L** Epididymis, Bilateral ♂ **N** Vas Deferens, Right ♂ NC **P** Vas Deferens, Left ♂ NC **Q** Vas Deferens, Bilateral ♂ NC	**0** Open **3** Percutaneous **4** Percutaneous Endoscopic **8** Via Natural or Artificial Opening Endoscopic	**Z** No Device	**Z** No Qualifier

♂ 0V500ZZ 0V503ZZ 0V504ZZ 0V507ZZ 0V508ZZ 0V510ZZ 0V513ZZ 0V514ZZ 0V520ZZ 0V523ZZ 0V524ZZ 0V530ZZ 0V533ZZ 0V534ZZ 0V550ZZ 0V553ZZ 0V554ZZ 0V55XZZ 0V560ZZ 0V563ZZ 0V564ZZ 0V570ZZ 0V573ZZ 0V574ZZ 0V590ZZ 0V593ZZ 0V594ZZ 0V5B0ZZ 0V5B3ZZ 0V5B4ZZ 0V5C0ZZ 0V5C3ZZ 0V5C4ZZ 0V5F0ZZ 0V5F3ZZ 0V5F4ZZ 0V5F8ZZ 0V5G0ZZ 0V5G3ZZ 0V5G4ZZ 0V5G8ZZ 0V5H0ZZ 0V5H3ZZ 0V5H4ZZ 0V5H8ZZ 0V5J0ZZ 0V5J3ZZ 0V5J4ZZ 0V5J8ZZ 0V5K0ZZ 0V5K3ZZ 0V5K4ZZ 0V5K8ZZ 0V5L0ZZ 0V5L3ZZ 0V5L4ZZ 0V5L8ZZ 0V5N0ZZ 0V5N3ZZ 0V5N4ZZ 0V5N8ZZ 0V5P0ZZ 0V5P3ZZ 0V5P4ZZ 0V5P8ZZ 0V5Q0ZZ 0V5Q3ZZ 0V5Q4ZZ 0V5Q8ZZ 0V5S0ZZ 0V5S3ZZ 0V5S4ZZ 0V5SXZZ 0V5T0ZZ 0V5T3ZZ 0V5T4ZZ 0V5TXZZ

NC 0V5N0ZZ 0V5N3ZZ 0V5N4ZZ 0V5P0ZZ 0V5P3ZZ 0V5P4ZZ 0V5Q0ZZ 0V5Q3ZZ 0V5Q4ZZ
Codes in this list are noncovered procedures only when reported with Z30.2 as either a principal or secondary diagnosis.

0 Medical and Surgical
V Male Reproductive System
7 Dilation: Expanding an orifice or the lumen of a tubular body part

Body Part	Approach	Device	Qualifier
Character 4	**Character 5**	**Character 6**	**Character 7**
N Vas Deferens, Right ♂ **P** Vas Deferens, Left ♂ **Q** Vas Deferens, Bilateral ♂	**0** Open **3** Percutaneous **4** Percutaneous Endoscopic	**D** Intraluminal Device **Z** No Device	**Z** No Qualifier

♂ 0V7N0DZ 0V7N0ZZ 0V7N3DZ 0V7N3ZZ 0V7N4DZ 0V7N4ZZ 0V7P0DZ 0V7P0ZZ 0V7P3DZ 0V7P3ZZ 0V7P4DZ 0V7P4ZZ 0V7Q0DZ 0V7Q0ZZ 0V7Q3DZ 0V7Q3ZZ 0V7Q4DZ 0V7Q4ZZ

0 Medical and Surgical
V Male Reproductive System
9 Drainage: Taking or letting out fluids and/or gases from a body part

Body Part Character 4	Approach Character 5	Device Character 6	Qualifier Character 7
0 Prostate ♂	**0** Open **3** Percutaneous **4** Percutaneous Endoscopic **7** Via Natural or Artificial Opening **8** Via Natural or Artificial Opening Endoscopic	**0** Drainage Device	**Z** No Qualifier
0 Prostate ♂	**0** Open **3** Percutaneous **4** Percutaneous Endoscopic **7** Via Natural or Artificial Opening **8** Via Natural or Artificial Opening Endoscopic	**Z** No Device	**X** Diagnostic **Z** No Qualifier
1 Seminal Vesicle, Right ♂ **2** Seminal Vesicle, Left ♂ **3** Seminal Vesicles, Bilateral ♂ **6** Tunica Vaginalis, Right ♂ **7** Tunica Vaginalis, Left ♂ **9** Testis, Right ♂ **B** Testis, Left ♂ **C** Testes, Bilateral ♂ **F** Spermatic Cord, Right ♂ **G** Spermatic Cord, Left ♂ **H** Spermatic Cords, Bilateral ♂ **J** Epididymis, Right ♂ **K** Epididymis, Left ♂ **L** Epididymis, Bilateral ♂ **N** Vas Deferens, Right ♂ **P** Vas Deferens, Left ♂ **Q** Vas Deferens, Bilateral ♂	**0** Open **3** Percutaneous **4** Percutaneous Endoscopic	**0** Drainage Device	**Z** No Qualifier
1 Seminal Vesicle, Right ♂ **2** Seminal Vesicle, Left ♂ **3** Seminal Vesicles, Bilateral ♂ **6** Tunica Vaginalis, Right ♂ **7** Tunica Vaginalis, Left ♂ **9** Testis, Right ♂ **B** Testis, Left ♂ **C** Testes, Bilateral ♂ **F** Spermatic Cord, Right ♂ **G** Spermatic Cord, Left ♂ **H** Spermatic Cords, Bilateral ♂ **J** Epididymis, Right ♂ **K** Epididymis, Left ♂ **L** Epididymis, Bilateral ♂ **N** Vas Deferens, Right ♂ **P** Vas Deferens, Left ♂ **Q** Vas Deferens, Bilateral ♂	**0** Open **3** Percutaneous **4** Percutaneous Endoscopic	**Z** No Device	**X** Diagnostic **Z** No Qualifier
5 Scrotum ♂ **S** Penis ♂ **T** Prepuce ♂	**0** Open **3** Percutaneous **4** Percutaneous Endoscopic **X** External	**0** Drainage Device	**Z** No Qualifier
5 Scrotum ♂ **S** Penis ♂ **T** Prepuce ♂	**0** Open **3** Percutaneous **4** Percutaneous Endoscopic **X** External	**Z** No Device	**X** Diagnostic **Z** No Qualifier

♂ 0V9000Z 0V900ZX 0V900ZZ 0V9030Z 0V903ZX 0V903ZZ 0V9040Z 0V904ZX 0V904ZZ 0V9070Z 0V907ZX 0V907ZZ 0V9080Z 0V908ZX 0V908ZZ 0V9100Z 0V910ZX 0V910ZZ 0V9130Z 0V913ZX 0V913ZZ 0V9140Z 0V914ZX 0V914ZZ 0V9200Z 0V920ZX 0V920ZZ 0V9230Z 0V923ZX 0V923ZZ 0V9240Z 0V924ZX 0V924ZZ 0V9300Z 0V930ZX 0V930ZZ 0V9330Z 0V933ZX 0V933ZZ 0V9340Z 0V934ZX 0V934ZZ 0V9500Z 0V950ZX 0V950ZZ 0V9530Z 0V953ZX 0V953ZZ 0V9540Z 0V954ZX 0V954ZZ 0V95X0Z

0V9 continued on next page

0V9 continued from previous page

0V95XZX 0V95XZZ 0V9600Z 0V960ZX 0V960ZZ 0V9630Z 0V963ZX 0V963ZZ 0V9640Z 0V964ZX 0V964ZZ 0V9700Z 0V970ZX
0V970ZZ 0V9730Z 0V973ZX 0V973ZZ 0V9740Z 0V974ZX 0V974ZZ 0V9900Z 0V990ZX 0V990ZZ 0V9930Z 0V993ZX 0V993ZZ
0V9940Z 0V994ZX 0V994ZZ 0V9B00Z 0V9B0ZX 0V9B0ZZ 0V9B30Z 0V9B3ZX 0V9B3ZZ 0V9B40Z 0V9B4ZX 0V9B4ZZ 0V9C00Z
0V9C0ZX 0V9C0ZZ 0V9C30Z 0V9C3ZX 0V9C3ZZ 0V9C40Z 0V9C4ZX 0V9C4ZZ 0V9F00Z 0V9F0ZX 0V9F0ZZ 0V9F30Z 0V9F3ZX
0V9F3ZZ 0V9F40Z 0V9F4ZX 0V9F4ZZ 0V9G00Z 0V9G0ZX 0V9G0ZZ 0V9G30Z 0V9G3ZX 0V9G3ZZ 0V9G40Z 0V9G4ZX 0V9G4ZZ
0V9H00Z 0V9H0ZX 0V9H0ZZ 0V9H30Z 0V9H3ZX 0V9H3ZZ 0V9H40Z 0V9H4ZX 0V9H4ZZ 0V9J00Z 0V9J0ZX 0V9J0ZZ 0V9J30Z
0V9J3ZX 0V9J3ZZ 0V9J40Z 0V9J4ZX 0V9J4ZZ 0V9K00Z 0V9K0ZX 0V9K0ZZ 0V9K30Z 0V9K3ZX 0V9K3ZZ 0V9K40Z 0V9K4ZX
0V9K4ZZ 0V9L00Z 0V9L0ZX 0V9L0ZZ 0V9L30Z 0V9L3ZX 0V9L3ZZ 0V9L40Z 0V9L4ZX 0V9L4ZZ 0V9N00Z 0V9N0ZX 0V9N0ZZ
0V9N30Z 0V9N3ZX 0V9N3ZZ 0V9N40Z 0V9N4ZX 0V9N4ZZ 0V9P00Z 0V9P0ZX 0V9P0ZZ 0V9P30Z 0V9P3ZX 0V9P3ZZ 0V9P40Z
0V9P4ZX 0V9P4ZZ 0V9Q00Z 0V9Q0ZX 0V9Q0ZZ 0V9Q30Z 0V9Q3ZX 0V9Q3ZZ 0V9Q40Z 0V9Q4ZX 0V9Q4ZZ 0V9S00Z 0V9S0ZX
0V9S0ZZ 0V9S30Z 0V9S3ZX 0V9S3ZZ 0V9S40Z 0V9S4ZX 0V9S4ZZ 0V9SX0Z 0V9SXZX 0V9SXZZ 0V9T00Z 0V9T0ZX 0V9T0ZZ
0V9T30Z 0V9T3ZX 0V9T3ZZ 0V9T40Z 0V9T4ZX 0V9T4ZZ 0V9TX0Z 0V9TXZX 0V9TXZZ

0 Medical and Surgical
V Male Reproductive System
B Excision: Cutting out or off, without replacement, a portion of a body part

Body Part Character 4	Approach Character 5	Device Character 6	Qualifier Character 7
0 Prostate ♂	**0** Open **3** Percutaneous **4** Percutaneous Endoscopic **7** Via Natural or Artificial Opening **8** Via Natural or Artificial Opening Endoscopic	**Z** No Device	**X** Diagnostic **Z** No Qualifier
1 Seminal Vesicle, Right ♂ **2** Seminal Vesicle, Left ♂ **3** Seminal Vesicles, Bilateral ♂ **6** Tunica Vaginalis, Right ♂ **7** Tunica Vaginalis, Left ♂ **9** Testis, Right ♂ **B** Testis, Left ♂ **C** Testes, Bilateral ♂	**0** Open **3** Percutaneous **4** Percutaneous Endoscopic	**Z** No Device	**X** Diagnostic **Z** No Qualifier
5 Scrotum ♂ **S** Penis ♂ **T** Prepuce ♂	**0** Open **3** Percutaneous **4** Percutaneous Endoscopic **X** External	**Z** No Device	**X** Diagnostic **Z** No Qualifier
F Spermatic Cord, Right ♂ **G** Spermatic Cord, Left ♂ **H** Spermatic Cords, Bilateral ♂ **J** Epididymis, Right ♂ **K** Epididymis, Left ♂ **L** Epididymis, Bilateral ♂ **N** Vas Deferens, Right ♂ NC **P** Vas Deferens, Left ♂ NC **Q** Vas Deferens, Bilateral ♂ NC Vasectomy	**0** Open **3** Percutaneous through scrotum, may be key-hole w/sharp hemostat **4** Percutaneous Endoscopic **8** Via Natural or Artificial Opening Endoscopic	**Z** No Device	**X** Diagnostic **Z** No Qualifier

♂ 0VB00ZX 0VB00ZZ 0VB03ZX 0VB03ZZ 0VB04ZX 0VB04ZZ 0VB07ZX 0VB07ZZ 0VB08ZX 0VB08ZZ 0VB10ZX 0VB10ZZ 0VB13ZX
0VB13ZZ 0VB14ZX 0VB14ZZ 0VB20ZX 0VB20ZZ 0VB23ZX 0VB23ZZ 0VB24ZX 0VB24ZZ 0VB30ZX 0VB30ZZ 0VB33ZX 0VB33ZZ
0VB34ZX 0VB34ZZ 0VB50ZX 0VB50ZZ 0VB53ZX 0VB53ZZ 0VB54ZX 0VB54ZZ 0VB5XZX 0VB5XZZ 0VB60ZX 0VB60ZZ 0VB63ZX
0VB63ZZ 0VB64ZX 0VB64ZZ 0VB70ZX 0VB70ZZ 0VB73ZX 0VB73ZZ 0VB74ZX 0VB74ZZ 0VB90ZX 0VB90ZZ 0VB93ZX 0VB93ZZ
0VB94ZX 0VB94ZZ 0VBB0ZX 0VBB0ZZ 0VBB3ZX 0VBB3ZZ 0VBB4ZX 0VBB4ZZ 0VBC0ZX 0VBC0ZZ 0VBC3ZX 0VBC3ZZ 0VBC4ZX
0VBC4ZZ 0VBF0ZX 0VBF0ZZ 0VBF3ZX 0VBF3ZZ 0VBF4ZX 0VBF4ZZ 0VBF8ZX 0VBF8ZZ 0VBG0ZX 0VBG0ZZ 0VBG3ZX 0VBG3ZZ
0VBG4ZX 0VBG4ZZ 0VBG8ZX 0VBG8ZZ 0VBH0ZX 0VBH0ZZ 0VBH3ZX 0VBH3ZZ 0VBH4ZX 0VBH4ZZ 0VBH8ZX 0VBH8ZZ 0VBJ0ZX
0VBJ0ZZ 0VBJ3ZX 0VBJ3ZZ 0VBJ4ZX 0VBJ4ZZ 0VBJ8ZX 0VBJ8ZZ 0VBK0ZX 0VBK0ZZ 0VBK3ZX 0VBK3ZZ 0VBK4ZX 0VBK4ZZ
0VBK8ZX 0VBK8ZZ 0VBL0ZX 0VBL0ZZ 0VBL3ZX 0VBL3ZZ 0VBL4ZX 0VBL4ZZ 0VBL8ZX 0VBL8ZZ 0VBN0ZX 0VBN0ZZ 0VBN3ZX
0VBN3ZZ 0VBN4ZX 0VBN4ZZ 0VBN8ZX 0VBN8ZZ 0VBP0ZX 0VBP0ZZ 0VBP3ZX 0VBP3ZZ 0VBP4ZX 0VBP4ZZ 0VBP8ZX 0VBP8ZZ
0VBQ0ZX 0VBQ0ZZ 0VBQ3ZX 0VBQ3ZZ 0VBQ4ZX 0VBQ4ZZ 0VBQ8ZX 0VBQ8ZZ 0VBS0ZX 0VBS0ZZ 0VBS3ZX 0VBS3ZZ 0VBS4ZX
0VBS4ZZ 0VBSXZX 0VBSXZZ 0VBT0ZX 0VBT0ZZ 0VBT3ZX 0VBT3ZZ 0VBT4ZX 0VBT4ZZ 0VBTXZX 0VBTXZZ

NC 0VBN0ZZ 0VBN3ZZ 0VBN4ZZ 0VBP0ZZ 0VBP3ZZ 0VBP4ZZ 0VBQ0ZZ 0VBQ3ZZ 0VBQ4ZZ
Codes in this list are noncovered procedures only when reported with Z30.2 as either a principal or secondary diagnosis.

LC Limited Coverage NC Noncovered HAC HAC-associated Procedure CC Combination Cluster - See Appendix G for code lists
DRG Non-OR-Affecting MS-DRG Assignment New/Revised Text in **Orange** ♂ Male ♀ Female

0 Medical and Surgical
V Male Reproductive System
C Extirpation: Taking or cutting out solid matter from a body part

Body Part Character 4	Approach Character 5	Device Character 6	Qualifier Character 7
0 Prostate ♂	**0** Open **3** Percutaneous **4** Percutaneous Endoscopic **7** Via Natural or Artificial Opening **8** Via Natural or Artificial Opening Endoscopic	**Z** No Device	**Z** No Qualifier
1 Seminal Vesicle, Right ♂ **2** Seminal Vesicle, Left ♂ **3** Seminal Vesicles, Bilateral ♂ **6** Tunica Vaginalis, Right ♂ **7** Tunica Vaginalis, Left ♂ **9** Testis, Right ♂ **B** Testis, Left ♂ **C** Testes, Bilateral ♂ **F** Spermatic Cord, Right ♂ **G** Spermatic Cord, Left ♂ **H** Spermatic Cords, Bilateral ♂ **J** Epididymis, Right ♂ **K** Epididymis, Left ♂ **L** Epididymis, Bilateral ♂ **N** Vas Deferens, Right ♂ **P** Vas Deferens, Left ♂ **Q** Vas Deferens, Bilateral ♂	**0** Open **3** Percutaneous **4** Percutaneous Endoscopic	**Z** No Device	**Z** No Qualifier
5 Scrotum ♂ **S** Penis ♂ **T** Prepuce ♂	**0** Open **3** Percutaneous **4** Percutaneous Endoscopic **X** External	**Z** No Device	**Z** No Qualifier

♂ 0VC00ZZ 0VC03ZZ 0VC04ZZ 0VC07ZZ 0VC08ZZ 0VC10ZZ 0VC13ZZ 0VC14ZZ 0VC20ZZ 0VC23ZZ 0VC24ZZ 0VC30ZZ 0VC33ZZ 0VC34ZZ 0VC50ZZ 0VC53ZZ 0VC54ZZ 0VC5XZZ 0VC60ZZ 0VC63ZZ 0VC64ZZ 0VC70ZZ 0VC73ZZ 0VC74ZZ 0VC90ZZ 0VC93ZZ 0VC94ZZ 0VCB0ZZ 0VCB3ZZ 0VCB4ZZ 0VCC0ZZ 0VCC3ZZ 0VCC4ZZ 0VCF0ZZ 0VCF3ZZ 0VCF4ZZ 0VCG0ZZ 0VCG3ZZ 0VCG4ZZ 0VCH0ZZ 0VCH3ZZ 0VCH4ZZ 0VCJ0ZZ 0VCJ3ZZ 0VCJ4ZZ 0VCK0ZZ 0VCK3ZZ 0VCK4ZZ 0VCL0ZZ 0VCL3ZZ 0VCL4ZZ 0VCN0ZZ 0VCN3ZZ 0VCN4ZZ 0VCP0ZZ 0VCP3ZZ 0VCP4ZZ 0VCQ0ZZ 0VCQ3ZZ 0VCQ4ZZ 0VCS0ZZ 0VCS3ZZ 0VCS4ZZ 0VCSXZZ 0VCT0ZZ 0VCT3ZZ 0VCT4ZZ 0VCTXZZ

0 Medical and Surgical
V Male Reproductive System
H Insertion: Putting in a nonbiological appliance that monitors, assists, performs, or prevents a physiological function but does not physically take the place of a body part

Body Part Character 4	Approach Character 5	Device Character 6	Qualifier Character 7
0 Prostate ♂	**0** Open **3** Percutaneous **4** Percutaneous Endoscopic **7** Via Natural or Artificial Opening **8** Via Natural or Artificial Opening Endoscopic	**1** Radioactive Element	**Z** No Qualifier
4 Prostate and Seminal Vesicles ♂ **8** Scrotum and Tunica Vaginalis ♂ **D** Testis ♂ **M** Epididymis and Spermatic Cord ♂ **R** Vas Deferens ♂	**0** Open **3** Percutaneous **4** Percutaneous Endoscopic **7** Via Natural or Artificial Opening **8** Via Natural or Artificial Opening Endoscopic	**3** Infusion Device **Y** Other Device	**Z** No Qualifier
S Penis ♂	**0** Open **3** Percutaneous **4** Percutaneous Endoscopic	**3** Infusion Device **Y** Other Device	**Z** No Qualifier
S Penis ♂	**7** Via Natural or Artificial Opening **8** Via Natural or Artificial Opening Endoscopic	**Y** Other Device	**Z** No Qualifier
S Penis ♂	**X** External	**3** Infusion Device	**Z** No Qualifier

♂ 0VH001Z 0VH031Z 0VH041Z 0VH071Z 0VH081Z 0VH403Z 0VH40YZ 0VH433Z 0VH43YZ 0VH443Z 0VH44YZ 0VH473Z 0VH47YZ 0VH483Z 0VH48YZ 0VH803Z 0VH80YZ 0VH833Z 0VH83YZ 0VH843Z 0VH84YZ 0VH873Z 0VH87YZ 0VH883Z 0VH88YZ 0VHD03Z 0VHD0YZ 0VHD33Z 0VHD3YZ 0VHD43Z 0VHD4YZ 0VHD73Z 0VHD7YZ 0VHD83Z 0VHD8YZ 0VHM03Z 0VHM0YZ 0VHM33Z 0VHM3YZ 0VHM43Z 0VHM4YZ 0VHM73Z 0VHM7YZ 0VHM83Z 0VHM8YZ 0VHR03Z 0VHR0YZ 0VHR33Z 0VHR3YZ 0VHR43Z 0VHR4YZ 0VHR73Z 0VHR7YZ 0VHR83Z 0VHR8YZ 0VHS03Z 0VHS0YZ 0VHS33Z 0VHS3YZ 0VHS43Z 0VHS4YZ 0VHS7YZ 0VHS8YZ 0VHSX3Z

0 Medical and Surgical
V Male Reproductive System
J Inspection: Visually and/or manually exploring a body part

Body Part Character 4	Approach Character 5	Device Character 6	Qualifier Character 7
4 Prostate and Seminal Vesicles ♂ **8** Scrotum and Tunica Vaginalis ♂ **D** Testis ♂ **M** Epididymis and Spermatic Cord ♂ **R** Vas Deferens ♂ **S** Penis ♂	**0** Open **3** Percutaneous **4** Percutaneous Endoscopic **X** External	**Z** No Device	**Z** No Qualifier

♂ 0VJ40ZZ 0VJ43ZZ 0VJ44ZZ 0VJ4XZZ 0VJ80ZZ 0VJ83ZZ 0VJ84ZZ 0VJ8XZZ 0VJD0ZZ 0VJD3ZZ 0VJD4ZZ 0VJDXZZ 0VJM0ZZ 0VJM3ZZ 0VJM4ZZ 0VJMXZZ 0VJR0ZZ 0VJR3ZZ 0VJR4ZZ 0VJRXZZ 0VJS0ZZ 0VJS3ZZ 0VJS4ZZ 0VJSXZZ

Pro-Vas - use clip to squeeze shut the flow of sperm
Intra-Vas - insert plug into vas deferens
Injected plugs (MPU) medical grade polyurethane or (MSR) medical grade silicone rubber into vas deferens

0 Medical and Surgical
V Male Reproductive System
L Occlusion: Completely closing an orifice or the lumen of a tubular body part

Body Part Character 4	Approach Character 5	Device Character 6	Qualifier Character 7
F Spermatic Cord, Right ♂ NC **G** Spermatic Cord, Left ♂ NC **H** Spermatic Cords, Bilateral ♂ NC **N** Vas Deferens, Right ♂ NC Vas **P** Vas Deferens, Left ♂ NC clip **Q** Vas Deferens, Bilateral ♂ NC	**0** Open vas clip procedure **3** Percutaneous **4** Percutaneous Endoscopic **8** Via Natural or Artificial Opening Endoscopic	**C** Extraluminal Device Vas Clip **D** Intraluminal Device - IVD or injection plugs **Z** No Device	**Z** No Qualifier

♂ 0VLF0CZ 0VLF0DZ 0VLF0ZZ 0VLF3CZ 0VLF3DZ 0VLF3ZZ 0VLF4CZ 0VLF4DZ 0VLF4ZZ 0VLF8CZ 0VLF8DZ 0VLF8ZZ 0VLG0CZ 0VLG0DZ 0VLG0ZZ 0VLG3CZ 0VLG3DZ 0VLG3ZZ 0VLG4CZ 0VLG4DZ 0VLG4ZZ 0VLG8CZ 0VLG8DZ 0VLG8ZZ 0VLH0CZ 0VLH0DZ 0VLH0ZZ 0VLH3CZ 0VLH3DZ 0VLH3ZZ 0VLH4CZ 0VLH4DZ 0VLH4ZZ 0VLH8CZ 0VLH8DZ 0VLH8ZZ 0VLN0CZ 0VLN0DZ 0VLN0ZZ 0VLN3CZ 0VLN3DZ 0VLN3ZZ 0VLN4CZ 0VLN4DZ 0VLN4ZZ 0VLN8CZ 0VLN8DZ 0VLN8ZZ 0VLP0CZ 0VLP0DZ 0VLP0ZZ 0VLP3CZ 0VLP3DZ 0VLP3ZZ 0VLP4CZ 0VLP4DZ 0VLP4ZZ 0VLP8CZ 0VLP8DZ 0VLP8ZZ 0VLQ0CZ 0VLQ0DZ 0VLQ0ZZ 0VLQ3CZ 0VLQ3DZ 0VLQ3ZZ 0VLQ4CZ 0VLQ4DZ 0VLQ4ZZ 0VLQ8CZ 0VLQ8DZ 0VLQ8ZZ

NC 0VLF0CZ 0VLF0DZ 0VLF0ZZ 0VLF3CZ 0VLF3DZ 0VLF3ZZ 0VLF4CZ 0VLF4DZ 0VLF4ZZ 0VLG0CZ 0VLG0DZ 0VLG0ZZ 0VLG3CZ 0VLG3DZ 0VLG3ZZ 0VLG4CZ 0VLG4DZ 0VLG4ZZ 0VLH0CZ 0VLH0DZ 0VLH0ZZ 0VLH3CZ 0VLH3DZ 0VLH3ZZ 0VLH4CZ 0VLH4DZ 0VLH4ZZ 0VLN0CZ 0VLN0ZZ 0VLN3CZ 0VLN3ZZ 0VLN4CZ 0VLN4ZZ 0VLP0CZ 0VLP0ZZ 0VLP3CZ 0VLP3ZZ 0VLP4CZ 0VLP4ZZ 0VLQ0CZ 0VLQ0ZZ 0VLQ3CZ 0VLQ3ZZ 0VLQ4CZ 0VLQ4ZZ
Codes in this list are noncovered procedures only when reported with Z30.2 as either a principal or secondary diagnosis.

0 Medical and Surgical
V Male Reproductive System
M Reattachment: Putting back in or on all or a portion of a separated body part to its normal location or other suitable location

Body Part Character 4	Approach Character 5	Device Character 6	Qualifier Character 7
5 Scrotum ♂ **S** Penis ♂	**X** External	**Z** No Device	**Z** No Qualifier
6 Tunica Vaginalis, Right ♂ **7** Tunica Vaginalis, Left ♂ **9** Testis, Right ♂ **B** Testis, Left ♂ **C** Testes, Bilateral ♂ **F** Spermatic Cord, Right ♂ **G** Spermatic Cord, Left ♂ **H** Spermatic Cords, Bilateral ♂	**0** Open **4** Percutaneous Endoscopic	**Z** No Device	**Z** No Qualifier

♂ 0VM5XZZ 0VM60ZZ 0VM64ZZ 0VM70ZZ 0VM74ZZ 0VM90ZZ 0VM94ZZ 0VMB0ZZ 0VMB4ZZ 0VMC0ZZ 0VMC4ZZ 0VMF0ZZ 0VMF4ZZ 0VMG0ZZ 0VMG4ZZ 0VMH0ZZ 0VMH4ZZ 0VMSXZZ

0 Medical and Surgical
V Male Reproductive System
N Release: Freeing a body part from an abnormal physical constraint by cutting or by the use of force

Body Part Character 4	Approach Character 5	Device Character 6	Qualifier Character 7
0 Prostate ♂	**0** Open **3** Percutaneous **4** Percutaneous Endoscopic **7** Via Natural or Artificial Opening **8** Via Natural or Artificial Opening Endoscopic	**Z** No Device	**Z** No Qualifier
1 Seminal Vesicle, Right ♂ **2** Seminal Vesicle, Left ♂ **3** Seminal Vesicles, Bilateral ♂ **6** Tunica Vaginalis, Right ♂ **7** Tunica Vaginalis, Left ♂ **9** Testis, Right ♂ **B** Testis, Left ♂ **C** Testes, Bilateral ♂	**0** Open **3** Percutaneous **4** Percutaneous Endoscopic	**Z** No Device	**Z** No Qualifier
5 Scrotum ♂ **S** Penis ♂ **T** Prepuce ♂	**0** Open **3** Percutaneous **4** Percutaneous Endoscopic **X** External	**Z** No Device	**Z** No Qualifier
F Spermatic Cord, Right ♂ **G** Spermatic Cord, Left ♂ **H** Spermatic Cords, Bilateral ♂ **J** Epididymis, Right ♂ **K** Epididymis, Left ♂ **L** Epididymis, Bilateral ♂ **N** Vas Deferens, Right ♂ **P** Vas Deferens, Left ♂ **Q** Vas Deferens, Bilateral ♂	**0** Open **3** Percutaneous **4** Percutaneous Endoscopic **8** Via Natural or Artificial Opening Endoscopic	**Z** No Device	**Z** No Qualifier

♂ 0VN00ZZ 0VN03ZZ 0VN04ZZ 0VN07ZZ 0VN08ZZ 0VN10ZZ 0VN13ZZ 0VN14ZZ 0VN20ZZ 0VN23ZZ 0VN24ZZ 0VN30ZZ 0VN33ZZ 0VN34ZZ 0VN50ZZ 0VN53ZZ 0VN54ZZ 0VN5XZZ 0VN60ZZ 0VN63ZZ 0VN64ZZ 0VN70ZZ 0VN73ZZ 0VN74ZZ 0VN90ZZ 0VN93ZZ 0VN94ZZ 0VNB0ZZ 0VNB3ZZ 0VNB4ZZ 0VNC0ZZ 0VNC3ZZ 0VNC4ZZ 0VNF0ZZ 0VNF3ZZ 0VNF4ZZ 0VNF8ZZ 0VNG0ZZ 0VNG3ZZ 0VNG4ZZ 0VNG8ZZ 0VNH0ZZ 0VNH3ZZ 0VNH4ZZ 0VNH8ZZ 0VNJ0ZZ 0VNJ3ZZ 0VNJ4ZZ 0VNJ8ZZ 0VNK0ZZ 0VNK3ZZ 0VNK4ZZ 0VNK8ZZ 0VNL0ZZ 0VNL3ZZ 0VNL4ZZ 0VNL8ZZ 0VNN0ZZ 0VNN3ZZ 0VNN4ZZ 0VNN8ZZ 0VNP0ZZ 0VNP3ZZ 0VNP4ZZ 0VNP8ZZ 0VNQ0ZZ 0VNQ3ZZ 0VNQ4ZZ 0VNQ8ZZ 0VNS0ZZ 0VNS3ZZ 0VNS4ZZ 0VNSXZZ 0VNT0ZZ 0VNT3ZZ 0VNT4ZZ 0VNTXZZ

0 Medical and Surgical
V Male Reproductive System
P Removal: Taking out or off a device from a body part

Body Part Character 4	Approach Character 5	Device Character 6	Qualifier Character 7
4 Prostate and Seminal Vesicles ♂	**0** Open **3** Percutaneous **4** Percutaneous Endoscopic **7** Via Natural or Artificial Opening **8** Via Natural or Artificial Opening Endoscopic	**0** Drainage Device **1** Radioactive Element **3** Infusion Device **7** Autologous Tissue Substitute **J** Synthetic Substitute **K** Nonautologous Tissue Substitute **Y** Other Device	**Z** No Qualifier
4 Prostate and Seminal Vesicles ♂	**X** External	**0** Drainage Device **1** Radioactive Element **3** Infusion Device	**Z** No Qualifier
8 Scrotum and Tunica Vaginalis ♂ **D** Testis ♂ **S** Penis ♂	**0** Open **3** Percutaneous **4** Percutaneous Endoscopic **7** Via Natural or Artificial Opening **8** Via Natural or Artificial Opening Endoscopic	**0** Drainage Device **3** Infusion Device **7** Autologous Tissue Substitute **J** Synthetic Substitute **K** Nonautologous Tissue Substitute **Y** Other Device	**Z** No Qualifier
8 Scrotum and Tunica Vaginalis ♂ **D** Testis ♂ **S** Penis ♂	**X** External	**0** Drainage Device **3** Infusion Device	**Z** No Qualifier
M Epididymis and Spermatic Cord ♂	**0** Open **3** Percutaneous **4** Percutaneous Endoscopic **7** Via Natural or Artificial Opening **8** Via Natural or Artificial Opening Endoscopic	**0** Drainage Device **3** Infusion Device **7** Autologous Tissue Substitute **C** Extraluminal Device **J** Synthetic Substitute **K** Nonautologous Tissue Substitute **Y** Other Device	**Z** No Qualifier
M Epididymis and Spermatic Cord ♂	**X** External	**0** Drainage Device **3** Infusion Device	**Z** No Qualifier
R Vas Deferens ♂	**0** Open **3** Percutaneous **4** Percutaneous Endoscopic **7** Via Natural or Artificial Opening **8** Via Natural or Artificial Opening Endoscopic	**0** Drainage Device **3** Infusion Device **7** Autologous Tissue Substitute **C** Extraluminal Device **D** Intraluminal Device **J** Synthetic Substitute **K** Nonautologous Tissue Substitute **Y** Other Device	**Z** No Qualifier
R Vas Deferens ♂	**X** External	**0** Drainage Device **3** Infusion Device **D** Intraluminal Device	**Z** No Qualifier

♂ 0VP400Z 0VP401Z 0VP403Z 0VP407Z 0VP40JZ 0VP40KZ 0VP40YZ 0VP430Z 0VP431Z 0VP433Z 0VP437Z 0VP43JZ 0VP43KZ 0VP43YZ 0VP440Z 0VP441Z 0VP443Z 0VP447Z 0VP44JZ 0VP44KZ 0VP44YZ 0VP470Z 0VP471Z 0VP473Z 0VP477Z 0VP47JZ 0VP47KZ 0VP47YZ 0VP480Z 0VP481Z 0VP483Z 0VP487Z 0VP48JZ 0VP48KZ 0VP48YZ 0VP4X0Z 0VP4X1Z 0VP4X3Z 0VP800Z 0VP803Z 0VP807Z 0VP80JZ 0VP80KZ 0VP80YZ 0VP830Z 0VP833Z 0VP837Z 0VP83JZ 0VP83KZ 0VP83YZ 0VP840Z 0VP843Z 0VP847Z 0VP84JZ 0VP84KZ 0VP84YZ 0VP870Z 0VP873Z 0VP877Z 0VP87JZ 0VP87KZ 0VP87YZ 0VP880Z 0VP883Z 0VP887Z 0VP88JZ 0VP88KZ 0VP88YZ 0VP8X0Z 0VP8X3Z 0VPD00Z 0VPD03Z 0VPD07Z 0VPD0JZ 0VPD0KZ 0VPD0YZ 0VPD30Z 0VPD33Z 0VPD37Z 0VPD3JZ 0VPD3KZ 0VPD3YZ 0VPD40Z 0VPD43Z 0VPD47Z 0VPD4JZ 0VPD4KZ 0VPD4YZ 0VPD70Z 0VPD73Z 0VPD77Z 0VPD7JZ 0VPD7KZ 0VPD7YZ 0VPD80Z 0VPD83Z 0VPD87Z 0VPD8JZ 0VPD8KZ 0VPD8YZ 0VPDX0Z 0VPDX3Z 0VPM00Z 0VPM03Z 0VPM07Z 0VPM0CZ 0VPM0JZ 0VPM0KZ 0VPM0YZ 0VPM30Z 0VPM33Z 0VPM37Z 0VPM3CZ 0VPM3JZ 0VPM3KZ 0VPM3YZ 0VPM40Z 0VPM43Z 0VPM47Z 0VPM4CZ 0VPM4JZ 0VPM4KZ 0VPM4YZ 0VPM70Z 0VPM73Z 0VPM77Z 0VPM7CZ 0VPM7JZ 0VPM7KZ 0VPM7YZ 0VPM80Z 0VPM83Z 0VPM87Z 0VPM8CZ 0VPM8JZ 0VPM8KZ 0VPM8YZ 0VPMX0Z 0VPMX3Z 0VPR00Z 0VPR03Z 0VPR07Z 0VPR0CZ 0VPR0DZ 0VPR0JZ 0VPR0KZ 0VPR0YZ 0VPR30Z 0VPR33Z 0VPR37Z 0VPR3CZ 0VPR3DZ 0VPR3JZ 0VPR3KZ 0VPR3YZ 0VPR40Z 0VPR43Z 0VPR47Z 0VPR4CZ 0VPR4DZ 0VPR4JZ 0VPR4KZ 0VPR4YZ 0VPR70Z 0VPR73Z 0VPR77Z 0VPR7CZ 0VPR7DZ 0VPR7JZ 0VPR7KZ 0VPR7YZ 0VPR80Z 0VPR83Z 0VPR87Z 0VPR8CZ 0VPR8DZ 0VPR8JZ 0VPR8KZ 0VPR8YZ 0VPRX0Z 0VPRX3Z 0VPRXDZ 0VPS00Z 0VPS03Z 0VPS07Z 0VPS0JZ 0VPS0KZ 0VPS0YZ 0VPS30Z 0VPS33Z 0VPS37Z 0VPS3JZ 0VPS3KZ 0VPS3YZ 0VPS40Z 0VPS43Z 0VPS47Z 0VPS4JZ 0VPS4KZ 0VPS4YZ 0VPS70Z 0VPS73Z 0VPS77Z 0VPS7JZ 0VPS7KZ 0VPS7YZ 0VPS80Z 0VPS83Z 0VPS87Z 0VPS8JZ 0VPS8KZ 0VPS8YZ 0VPSX0Z 0VPSX3Z

0 Medical and Surgical
V Male Reproductive System
Q Repair: Restoring, to the extent possible, a body part to its normal anatomic structure and function

Body Part	Approach	Device	Qualifier
Character 4	**Character 5**	**Character 6**	**Character 7**
0 Prostate ♂	**0** Open **3** Percutaneous **4** Percutaneous Endoscopic **7** Via Natural or Artificial Opening **8** Via Natural or Artificial Opening Endoscopic	**Z** No Device	**Z** No Qualifier
1 Seminal Vesicle, Right ♂ **2** Seminal Vesicle, Left ♂ **3** Seminal Vesicles, Bilateral ♂ **6** Tunica Vaginalis, Right ♂ **7** Tunica Vaginalis, Left ♂ **9** Testis, Right ♂ **B** Testis, Left ♂ **C** Testes, Bilateral ♂	**0** Open **3** Percutaneous **4** Percutaneous Endoscopic	**Z** No Device	**Z** No Qualifier
5 Scrotum ♂ **S** Penis ♂ **T** Prepuce ♂	**0** Open **3** Percutaneous **4** Percutaneous Endoscopic **X** External	**Z** No Device	**Z** No Qualifier
F Spermatic Cord, Right ♂ **G** Spermatic Cord, Left ♂ **H** Spermatic Cords, Bilateral ♂ **J** Epididymis, Right ♂ **K** Epididymis, Left ♂ **L** Epididymis, Bilateral ♂ **N** Vas Deferens, Right ♂ **P** Vas Deferens, Left ♂ **Q** Vas Deferens, Bilateral ♂	**0** Open **3** Percutaneous **4** Percutaneous Endoscopic **8** Via Natural or Artificial Opening Endoscopic	**Z** No Device	**Z** No Qualifier

♂ 0VQ00ZZ 0VQ03ZZ 0VQ04ZZ 0VQ07ZZ 0VQ08ZZ 0VQ10ZZ 0VQ13ZZ 0VQ14ZZ 0VQ20ZZ 0VQ23ZZ 0VQ24ZZ 0VQ30ZZ 0VQ33ZZ
0VQ34ZZ 0VQ50ZZ 0VQ53ZZ 0VQ54ZZ 0VQ5XZZ 0VQ60ZZ 0VQ63ZZ 0VQ64ZZ 0VQ70ZZ 0VQ73ZZ 0VQ74ZZ 0VQ90ZZ 0VQ93ZZ
0VQ94ZZ 0VQB0ZZ 0VQB3ZZ 0VQB4ZZ 0VQC0ZZ 0VQC3ZZ 0VQC4ZZ 0VQF0ZZ 0VQF3ZZ 0VQF4ZZ 0VQF8ZZ 0VQG0ZZ 0VQG3ZZ
0VQG4ZZ 0VQG8ZZ 0VQH0ZZ 0VQH3ZZ 0VQH4ZZ 0VQH8ZZ 0VQJ0ZZ 0VQJ3ZZ 0VQJ4ZZ 0VQJ8ZZ 0VQK0ZZ 0VQK3ZZ 0VQK4ZZ
0VQK8ZZ 0VQL0ZZ 0VQL3ZZ 0VQL4ZZ 0VQL8ZZ 0VQN0ZZ 0VQN3ZZ 0VQN4ZZ 0VQN8ZZ 0VQP0ZZ 0VQP3ZZ 0VQP4ZZ 0VQP8ZZ
0VQQ0ZZ 0VQQ3ZZ 0VQQ4ZZ 0VQQ8ZZ 0VQS0ZZ 0VQS3ZZ 0VQS4ZZ 0VQSXZZ 0VQT0ZZ 0VQT3ZZ 0VQT4ZZ 0VQTXZZ

0 Medical and Surgical
V Male Reproductive System
R Replacement: Putting in or on biological or synthetic material that physically takes the place and/or function of all or a portion of a body part

Body Part	Approach	Device	Qualifier
Character 4	**Character 5**	**Character 6**	**Character 7**
9 Testis, Right ♂ **B** Testis, Left ♂ **C** Testes, Bilateral ♂	**0** Open	**J** Synthetic Substitute	**Z** No Qualifier

♂ 0VR90JZ 0VRB0JZ 0VRC0JZ

0 Medical and Surgical
V Male Reproductive System
S Reposition: Moving to its normal location, or other suitable location, all or a portion of a body part

Body Part Character 4	Approach Character 5	Device Character 6	Qualifier Character 7
9 Testis, Right ♂ **B** Testis, Left ♂ **C** Testes, Bilateral ♂ **F** Spermatic Cord, Right ♂ **G** Spermatic Cord, Left ♂ **H** Spermatic Cords, Bilateral ♂	**0** Open **3** Percutaneous **4** Percutaneous Endoscopic **8** Via Natural or Artificial Opening Endoscopic	**Z** No Device	**Z** No Qualifier

♂ 0VS90ZZ 0VS93ZZ 0VS94ZZ 0VS98ZZ 0VSB0ZZ 0VSB3ZZ 0VSB4ZZ 0VSB8ZZ 0VSC0ZZ 0VSC3ZZ 0VSC4ZZ 0VSC8ZZ 0VSF0ZZ 0VSF3ZZ 0VSF4ZZ 0VSF8ZZ 0VSG0ZZ 0VSG3ZZ 0VSG4ZZ 0VSG8ZZ 0VSH0ZZ 0VSH3ZZ 0VSH4ZZ 0VSH8ZZ

0 Medical and Surgical
V Male Reproductive System
T Resection: Cutting out or off, without replacement, all of a body part

Body Part Character 4	Approach Character 5	Device Character 6	Qualifier Character 7
0 Prostate ♂ CC radical, retropubic	**0** Open **4** Percutaneous Endoscopic **7** Via Natural or Artificial Opening **8** Via Natural or Artificial Opening Endoscopic	**Z** No Device	**Z** No Qualifier
1 Seminal Vesicle, Right ♂ **2** Seminal Vesicle, Left ♂ **3** Seminal Vesicles, Bilateral ♂ CC **6** Tunica Vaginalis, Right ♂ **7** Tunica Vaginalis, Left ♂ **9** Testis, Right ♂ **B** Testis, Left ♂ **C** Testes, Bilateral ♂ **F** Spermatic Cord, Right ♂ **G** Spermatic Cord, Left ♂ **H** Spermatic Cords, Bilateral ♂ **J** Epididymis, Right ♂ **K** Epididymis, Left ♂ **L** Epididymis, Bilateral ♂ **N** Vas Deferens, Right ♂ NC **P** Vas Deferens, Left ♂ NC **Q** Vas Deferens, Bilateral ♂ NC	**0** Open **4** Percutaneous Endoscopic	**Z** No Device	**Z** No Qualifier
5 Scrotum ♂ **S** Penis ♂ **T** Prepuce ♂	**0** Open **4** Percutaneous Endoscopic **X** External	**Z** No Device	**Z** No Qualifier

♂ 0VT00ZZ 0VT04ZZ 0VT07ZZ 0VT08ZZ 0VT10ZZ 0VT14ZZ 0VT20ZZ 0VT24ZZ 0VT30ZZ 0VT34ZZ 0VT50ZZ 0VT54ZZ 0VT5XZZ 0VT60ZZ 0VT64ZZ 0VT70ZZ 0VT74ZZ 0VT90ZZ 0VT94ZZ 0VTB0ZZ 0VTB4ZZ 0VTC0ZZ 0VTC4ZZ 0VTF0ZZ 0VTF4ZZ 0VTG0ZZ 0VTG4ZZ 0VTH0ZZ 0VTH4ZZ 0VTJ0ZZ 0VTJ4ZZ 0VTK0ZZ 0VTK4ZZ 0VTL0ZZ 0VTL4ZZ 0VTN0ZZ 0VTN4ZZ 0VTP0ZZ 0VTP4ZZ 0VTQ0ZZ 0VTQ4ZZ 0VTS0ZZ 0VTS4ZZ 0VTSXZZ 0VTT0ZZ 0VTT4ZZ 0VTTXZZ

NC 0VTN0ZZ 0VTN4ZZ 0VTP0ZZ 0VTP4ZZ 0VTQ0ZZ 0VTQ4ZZ
Codes in this list are noncovered procedures only when reported with Z30.2 as either a principal or secondary diagnosis.

CC 0VT00ZZ 0VT04ZZ 0VT07ZZ 0VT08ZZ 0VT30ZZ 0VT34ZZ

LC Limited Coverage NC Noncovered HAC HAC-associated Procedure CC Combination Cluster - See Appendix G for code lists
DRG Non-OR-Affecting MS-DRG Assignment New/Revised Text in **Orange** ♂ Male ♀ Female

0 Medical and Surgical
V Male Reproductive System
U Supplement: Putting in or on biological or synthetic material that physically reinforces and/or augments the function of a portion of a body part

Body Part Character 4	Approach Character 5	Device Character 6	Qualifier Character 7
1 Seminal Vesicle, Right ♂ **2** Seminal Vesicle, Left ♂ **3** Seminal Vesicles, Bilateral ♂ **6** Tunica Vaginalis, Right ♂ **7** Tunica Vaginalis, Left ♂ **F** Spermatic Cord, Right ♂ **G** Spermatic Cord, Left ♂ **H** Spermatic Cords, Bilateral ♂ **J** Epididymis, Right ♂ **K** Epididymis, Left ♂ **L** Epididymis, Bilateral ♂ **N** Vas Deferens, Right ♂ **P** Vas Deferens, Left ♂ **Q** Vas Deferens, Bilateral ♂	**0** Open **4** Percutaneous Endoscopic **8** Via Natural or Artificial Opening Endoscopic	**7** Autologous Tissue Substitute **J** Synthetic Substitute **K** Nonautologous Tissue Substitute	**Z** No Qualifier
5 Scrotum ♂ **S** Penis ♂ **T** Prepuce ♂	**0** Open **4** Percutaneous Endoscopic **X** External	**7** Autologous Tissue Substitute **J** Synthetic Substitute **K** Nonautologous Tissue Substitute	**Z** No Qualifier
9 Testis, Right ♂ **B** Testis, Left ♂ **C** Testes, Bilateral ♂	**0** Open	**7** Autologous Tissue Substitute **J** Synthetic Substitute **K** Nonautologous Tissue Substitute	**Z** No Qualifier

♂ 0VU107Z 0VU10JZ 0VU10KZ 0VU147Z 0VU14JZ 0VU14KZ 0VU187Z 0VU18JZ 0VU18KZ 0VU207Z 0VU20JZ 0VU20KZ 0VU247Z 0VU24JZ 0VU24KZ 0VU287Z 0VU28JZ 0VU28KZ 0VU307Z 0VU30JZ 0VU30KZ 0VU347Z 0VU34JZ 0VU34KZ 0VU387Z 0VU38JZ 0VU38KZ 0VU507Z 0VU50JZ 0VU50KZ 0VU547Z 0VU54JZ 0VU54KZ 0VU5X7Z 0VU5XJZ 0VU5XKZ 0VU607Z 0VU60JZ 0VU60KZ 0VU647Z 0VU64JZ 0VU64KZ 0VU687Z 0VU68JZ 0VU68KZ 0VU707Z 0VU70JZ 0VU70KZ 0VU747Z 0VU74JZ 0VU74KZ 0VU787Z 0VU78JZ 0VU78KZ 0VU907Z 0VU90JZ 0VU90KZ 0VUB07Z 0VUB0JZ 0VUB0KZ 0VUC07Z 0VUC0JZ 0VUC0KZ 0VUF07Z 0VUF0JZ 0VUF0KZ 0VUF47Z 0VUF4JZ 0VUF4KZ 0VUF87Z 0VUF8JZ 0VUF8KZ 0VUG07Z 0VUG0JZ 0VUG0KZ 0VUG47Z 0VUG4JZ 0VUG4KZ 0VUG87Z 0VUG8JZ 0VUG8KZ 0VUH07Z 0VUH0JZ 0VUH0KZ 0VUH47Z 0VUH4JZ 0VUH4KZ 0VUH87Z 0VUH8JZ 0VUH8KZ 0VUJ07Z 0VUJ0JZ 0VUJ0KZ 0VUJ47Z 0VUJ4JZ 0VUJ4KZ 0VUJ87Z 0VUJ8JZ 0VUJ8KZ 0VUK07Z 0VUK0JZ 0VUK0KZ 0VUK47Z 0VUK4JZ 0VUK4KZ 0VUK87Z 0VUK8JZ 0VUK8KZ 0VUL07Z 0VUL0JZ 0VUL0KZ 0VUL47Z 0VUL4JZ 0VUL4KZ 0VUL87Z 0VUL8JZ 0VUL8KZ 0VUN07Z 0VUN0JZ 0VUN0KZ 0VUN47Z 0VUN4JZ 0VUN4KZ 0VUN87Z 0VUN8JZ 0VUN8KZ 0VUP07Z 0VUP0JZ 0VUP0KZ 0VUP47Z 0VUP4JZ 0VUP4KZ 0VUP87Z 0VUP8JZ 0VUP8KZ 0VUQ07Z 0VUQ0JZ 0VUQ0KZ 0VUQ47Z 0VUQ4JZ 0VUQ4KZ 0VUQ87Z 0VUQ8JZ 0VUQ8KZ 0VUS07Z 0VUS0JZ 0VUS0KZ 0VUS47Z 0VUS4JZ 0VUS4KZ 0VUSX7Z 0VUSXJZ 0VUSXKZ 0VUT07Z 0VUT0JZ 0VUT0KZ 0VUT47Z 0VUT4JZ 0VUT4KZ 0VUTX7Z 0VUTXJZ 0VUTXKZ

0 Medical and Surgical
V Male Reproductive System
W Revision: Correcting, to the extent possible, a portion of a malfunctioning device or the position of a displaced device

Body Part	Approach	Device	Qualifier
Character 4	**Character 5**	**Character 6**	**Character 7**
4 Prostate and Seminal Vesicles ♂ **8** Scrotum and Tunica Vaginalis ♂ **D** Testis ♂ **S** Penis ♂	**0** Open **3** Percutaneous **4** Percutaneous Endoscopic **7** Via Natural or Artificial Opening **8** Via Natural or Artificial Opening Endoscopic	**0** Drainage Device **3** Infusion Device **7** Autologous Tissue Substitute **J** Synthetic Substitute **K** Nonautologous Tissue Substitute **Y** Other Device	**Z** No Qualifier
4 Prostate and Seminal Vesicles ♂ **8** Scrotum and Tunica Vaginalis ♂ **D** Testis ♂ **S** Penis ♂	**X** External	**0** Drainage Device **3** Infusion Device **7** Autologous Tissue Substitute **J** Synthetic Substitute **K** Nonautologous Tissue Substitute	**Z** No Qualifier
M Epididymis and Spermatic Cord ♂	**0** Open **3** Percutaneous **4** Percutaneous Endoscopic **7** Via Natural or Artificial Opening **8** Via Natural or Artificial Opening Endoscopic	**0** Drainage Device **3** Infusion Device **7** Autologous Tissue Substitute **C** Extraluminal Device **J** Synthetic Substitute **K** Nonautologous Tissue Substitute **Y** Other Device	**Z** No Qualifier
M Epididymis and Spermatic Cord ♂	**X** External	**0** Drainage Device **3** Infusion Device **7** Autologous Tissue Substitute **C** Extraluminal Device **J** Synthetic Substitute **K** Nonautologous Tissue Substitute	**Z** No Qualifier
R Vas Deferens ♂	**0** Open **3** Percutaneous **4** Percutaneous Endoscopic **7** Via Natural or Artificial Opening **8** Via Natural or Artificial Opening Endoscopic	**0** Drainage Device **3** Infusion Device **7** Autologous Tissue Substitute **C** Extraluminal Device **D** Intraluminal Device **J** Synthetic Substitute **K** Nonautologous Tissue Substitute **Y** Other Device	**Z** No Qualifier
R Vas Deferens ♂	**X** External	**0** Drainage Device **3** Infusion Device **7** Autologous Tissue Substitute **C** Extraluminal Device **D** Intraluminal Device **J** Synthetic Substitute **K** Nonautologous Tissue Substitute	**Z** No Qualifier

♂ 0VW400Z 0VW403Z 0VW407Z 0VW40JZ 0VW40KZ 0VW40YZ 0VW430Z 0VW433Z 0VW437Z 0VW43JZ 0VW43KZ 0VW43YZ 0VW440Z 0VW443Z 0VW447Z 0VW44JZ 0VW44KZ 0VW44YZ 0VW470Z 0VW473Z 0VW477Z 0VW47JZ 0VW47KZ 0VW47YZ 0VW480Z 0VW483Z 0VW487Z 0VW48JZ 0VW48KZ 0VW48YZ 0VW4X0Z 0VW4X3Z 0VW4X7Z 0VW4XJZ 0VW4XKZ 0VW800Z 0VW803Z 0VW807Z 0VW80JZ 0VW80KZ 0VW80YZ 0VW830Z 0VW833Z 0VW837Z 0VW83JZ 0VW83KZ 0VW83YZ 0VW840Z 0VW843Z 0VW847Z 0VW84JZ 0VW84KZ 0VW84YZ 0VW870Z 0VW873Z 0VW877Z 0VW87JZ 0VW87KZ 0VW87YZ 0VW880Z 0VW883Z 0VW887Z 0VW88JZ 0VW88KZ 0VW88YZ 0VW8X0Z 0VW8X3Z 0VW8X7Z 0VW8XJZ 0VW8XKZ 0VWD00Z 0VWD03Z 0VWD07Z 0VWD0JZ 0VWD0KZ 0VWD0YZ 0VWD30Z 0VWD33Z 0VWD37Z 0VWD3JZ 0VWD3KZ 0VWD3YZ 0VWD40Z 0VWD43Z 0VWD47Z 0VWD4JZ 0VWD4KZ 0VWD4YZ 0VWD70Z 0VWD73Z 0VWD77Z 0VWD7JZ 0VWD7KZ 0VWD7YZ 0VWD80Z 0VWD83Z 0VWD87Z 0VWD8JZ 0VWD8KZ 0VWD8YZ 0VWDX0Z 0VWDX3Z 0VWDX7Z 0VWDXJZ 0VWDXKZ 0VWM00Z 0VWM03Z 0VWM07Z 0VWM0CZ 0VWM0JZ 0VWM0KZ 0VWM0YZ 0VWM30Z 0VWM33Z 0VWM37Z 0VWM3CZ 0VWM3JZ 0VWM3KZ 0VWM3YZ 0VWM40Z 0VWM43Z 0VWM47Z 0VWM4CZ 0VWM4JZ 0VWM4KZ 0VWM4YZ 0VWM70Z 0VWM73Z 0VWM77Z 0VWM7CZ 0VWM7JZ 0VWM7KZ 0VWM7YZ 0VWM80Z 0VWM83Z 0VWM87Z 0VWM8CZ 0VWM8JZ 0VWM8KZ 0VWM8YZ 0VWMX0Z 0VWMX3Z 0VWMX7Z 0VWMXCZ 0VWMXJZ 0VWMXKZ 0VWR00Z 0VWR03Z 0VWR07Z 0VWR0CZ 0VWR0DZ 0VWR0JZ 0VWR0KZ 0VWR0YZ 0VWR30Z 0VWR33Z 0VWR37Z 0VWR3CZ 0VWR3DZ 0VWR3JZ 0VWR3KZ 0VWR3YZ 0VWR40Z 0VWR43Z 0VWR47Z 0VWR4CZ 0VWR4DZ 0VWR4JZ 0VWR4KZ 0VWR4YZ 0VWR70Z 0VWR73Z 0VWR77Z 0VWR7CZ 0VWR7DZ 0VWR7JZ 0VWR7KZ 0VWR7YZ 0VWR80Z 0VWR83Z 0VWR87Z 0VWR8CZ 0VWR8DZ 0VWR8JZ 0VWR8KZ 0VWR8YZ 0VWRX0Z 0VWRX3Z 0VWRX7Z 0VWRXCZ 0VWRXDZ 0VWRXJZ 0VWRXKZ 0VWS00Z 0VWS03Z 0VWS07Z 0VWS0JZ 0VWS0KZ 0VWS0YZ 0VWS30Z 0VWS33Z 0VWS37Z 0VWS3JZ 0VWS3KZ 0VWS3YZ 0VWS40Z 0VWS43Z 0VWS47Z 0VWS4JZ 0VWS4KZ 0VWS4YZ 0VWS70Z 0VWS73Z 0VWS77Z 0VWS7JZ 0VWS7KZ 0VWS7YZ 0VWS80Z 0VWS83Z 0VWS87Z 0VWS8JZ 0VWS8KZ 0VWS8YZ 0VWSX0Z 0VWSX3Z 0VWSX7Z 0VWSXJZ 0VWSXKZ

0 Medical and Surgical
V Male Reproductive System
X Transfer: Moving, without taking out, all or a portion of a body part to another location to take over the function of all or a portion of a body part

Body Part Character 4	Approach Character 5	Device Character 6	Qualifier Character 7
T Prepuce	**0** Open **X** External	**Z** No Device	**D** Urethra **S** Penis

NOTES

NOTES

Use Official Guidelines B2.1A

Anatomical Regions, General 0W0-0WY

0 Medical and Surgical
W Anatomical Regions, General
0 Alteration: Modifying the anatomic structure of a body part without affecting the function of the body part

Body Part Character 4	Approach Character 5	Device Character 6	Qualifier Character 7
0 Head **2** Face **4** Upper Jaw **5** Lower Jaw **6** Neck **8** Chest Wall **F** Abdominal Wall **K** Upper Back **L** Lower Back **M** Perineum, Male ♂ **N** Perineum, Female ♀	**0** Open **3** Percutaneous **4** Percutaneous Endoscopic	**7** Autologous Tissue Substitute **J** Synthetic Substitute **K** Nonautologous Tissue Substitute **Z** No Device	**Z** No Qualifier

♂ 0W0M07Z 0W0M0JZ 0W0M0KZ 0W0M0ZZ 0W0M37Z 0W0M3JZ 0W0M3KZ 0W0M3ZZ 0W0M47Z 0W0M4JZ 0W0M4KZ 0W0M4ZZ
♀ 0W0N07Z 0W0N0JZ 0W0N0KZ 0W0N0ZZ 0W0N37Z 0W0N3JZ 0W0N3KZ 0W0N3ZZ 0W0N47Z 0W0N4JZ 0W0N4KZ 0W0N4ZZ

0 Medical and Surgical
W Anatomical Regions, General
1 Bypass: Altering the route of passage of the contents of a tubular body part

Body Part Character 4	Approach Character 5	Device Character 6	Qualifier Character 7
1 Cranial Cavity	**0** Open	**J** Synthetic Substitute	**9** Pleural Cavity, Right **B** Pleural Cavity, Left **G** Peritoneal Cavity **J** Pelvic Cavity
9 Pleural Cavity, Right **B** Pleural Cavity, Left **G** Peritoneal Cavity **J** Pelvic Cavity	**0** Open **3** Percutaneous **4** Percutaneous Endoscopic	**J** Synthetic Substitute	**4** Cutaneous **9** Pleural Cavity, Right **B** Pleural Cavity, Left **G** Peritoneal Cavity **J** Pelvic Cavity **W** Upper Vein **Y** Lower Vein

0 Medical and Surgical
W Anatomical Regions, General
2 Change: Taking out or off a device from a body part and putting back an identical or similar device in or on the same body part without cutting or puncturing the skin or a mucous membrane

Body Part Character 4	Approach Character 5	Device Character 6	Qualifier Character 7
0 Head **1** Cranial Cavity **2** Face **4** Upper Jaw **5** Lower Jaw **6** Neck **8** Chest Wall **9** Pleural Cavity, Right **B** Pleural Cavity, Left **C** Mediastinum **D** Pericardial Cavity **F** Abdominal Wall **G** Peritoneal Cavity **H** Retroperitoneum **J** Pelvic Cavity **K** Upper Back **L** Lower Back **M** Perineum, Male ♂ **N** Perineum, Female ♀	**X** External	**0** Drainage Device **Y** Other Device	**Z** No Qualifier

♂ 0W2MX0Z 0W2MXYZ
♀ 0W2NX0Z 0W2NXYZ

0 Medical and Surgical
W Anatomical Regions, General
3 Control: Stopping, or attempting to stop, postprocedural or other acute bleeding post op bleed

Body Part Character 4	Approach Character 5	Device Character 6	Qualifier Character 7
0 Head **1** Cranial Cavity **2** Face **4** Upper Jaw **5** Lower Jaw **6** Neck **8** Chest Wall **9** Pleural Cavity, Right **B** Pleural Cavity, Left **C** Mediastinum **D** Pericardial Cavity **F** Abdominal Wall **G** Peritoneal Cavity **H** Retroperitoneum **J** Pelvic Cavity **K** Upper Back **L** Lower Back **M** Perineum, Male ♂ **N** Perineum, Female ♀	**0** Open **3** Percutaneous **4** Percutaneous Endoscopic	**Z** No Device	**Z** No Qualifier
3 Oral Cavity and Throat	**0** Open **3** Percutaneous **4** Percutaneous Endoscopic **7** Via Natural or Artificial Opening **8** Via Natural or Artificial Opening Endoscopic **X** External	**Z** No Device	**Z** No Qualifier
P Gastrointestinal Tract **Q** Respiratory Tract **R** Genitourinary Tract	**0** Open **3** Percutaneous **4** Percutaneous Endoscopic **7** Via Natural or Artificial Opening **8** Via Natural or Artificial Opening Endoscopic	**Z** No Device	**Z** No Qualifier

♂ 0W3M0ZZ 0W3M3ZZ 0W3M4ZZ
♀ 0W3N0ZZ 0W3N3ZZ 0W3N4ZZ

0 Medical and Surgical
W Anatomical Regions, General
4 Creation: Putting in or on biological or synthetic material to form a new body part that to the extent possible replicates the anatomic structure or function of an absent body part

Body Part Character 4	Approach Character 5	Device Character 6	Qualifier Character 7
M Perineum, Male ♂	**0** Open	**7** Autologous Tissue Substitute **J** Synthetic Substitute **K** Nonautologous Tissue Substitute	**0** Vagina
N Perineum, Female ♀	**0** Open	**7** Autologous Tissue Substitute **J** Synthetic Substitute **K** Nonautologous Tissue Substitute	**1** Penis

♂ 0W4M070 0W4M0J0 0W4M0K0
♀ 0W4N071 0W4N0J1 0W4N0K1

0 Medical and Surgical
W Anatomical Regions, General
8 Division: Cutting into a body part, without draining fluids and/or gases from the body part, in order to separate or transect a body part

Body Part Character 4	Approach Character 5	Device Character 6	Qualifier Character 7
N Perineum, Female ♀	**X** External	**Z** No Device	**Z** No Qualifier

♀ 0W8NXZZ

0 Medical and Surgical
W Anatomical Regions, General
9 Drainage: Taking or letting out fluids and/or gases from a body part

Body Part Character 4	Approach Character 5	Device Character 6	Qualifier Character 7
0 Head **1** Cranial Cavity **2** Face **3** Oral Cavity and Throat **4** Upper Jaw **5** Lower Jaw **6** Neck **8** Chest Wall **9** Pleural Cavity, Right **B** Pleural Cavity, Left **C** Mediastinum **D** Pericardial Cavity **F** Abdominal Wall **G** Peritoneal Cavity – abscess includes washing **H** Retroperitoneum **J** Pelvic Cavity **K** Upper Back **L** Lower Back **M** Perineum, Male ♂ **N** Perineum, Female ♀	**0** Open **3** Percutaneous **4** Percutaneous Endoscopic	**0** Drainage Device Pneumothorax- drain fluid or air	**Z** No Qualifier - not diagnostic w/ biopsy

0W9 continued on next page

0 Medical and Surgical
W Anatomical Regions, General
9 Drainage: Taking or letting out fluids and/or gases from a body part

0W9 continued from previous page

Body Part Character 4	Approach Character 5	Device Character 6	Qualifier Character 7
0 Head **1** Cranial Cavity **2** Face **3** Oral Cavity and Throat **4** Upper Jaw **5** Lower Jaw **6** Neck **8** Chest Wall **9** Pleural Cavity, Right **B** Pleural Cavity, Left **C** Mediastinum **D** Pericardial Cavity **F** Abdominal Wall **G** Peritoneal Cavity **H** Retroperitoneum **J** Pelvic Cavity **K** Upper Back **L** Lower Back **M** Perineum, Male ♂ **N** Perineum, Female ♀	**0** Open **3** Percutaneous **4** Percutaneous Endoscopic	**Z** No Device	**X** Diagnostic **Z** No Qualifier

♂ 0W9M00Z 0W9M0ZX 0W9M0ZZ 0W9M30Z 0W9M3ZX 0W9M3ZZ 0W9M40Z 0W9M4ZX 0W9M4ZZ
♀ 0W9N00Z 0W9N0ZX 0W9N0ZZ 0W9N30Z 0W9N3ZX 0W9N3ZZ 0W9N40Z 0W9N4ZZ

0 Medical and Surgical
W Anatomical Regions, General
B Excision: Cutting out or off, without replacement, a portion of a body part

Body Part Character 4	Approach Character 5	Device Character 6	Qualifier Character 7
0 Head **2** Face **3** Oral Cavity and Throat **4** Upper Jaw **5** Lower Jaw **8** Chest Wall **K** Upper Back **L** Lower Back **M** Perineum, Male ♂ **N** Perineum, Female ♀	**0** Open **3** Percutaneous **4** Percutaneous Endoscopic **X** External	**Z** No Device	**X** Diagnostic **Z** No Qualifier
6 Neck **F** Abdominal Wall	**0** Open **3** Percutaneous **4** Percutaneous Endoscopic	**Z** No Device	**X** Diagnostic **Z** No Qualifier
6 Neck **F** Abdominal Wall	**X** External	**Z** No Device	**2** Stoma **X** Diagnostic **Z** No Qualifier
C Mediastinum **H** Retroperitoneum	**0** Open **3** Percutaneous **4** Percutaneous Endoscopic	**Z** No Device	**X** Diagnostic **Z** No Qualifier

♂ 0WBM0ZX 0WBM0ZZ 0WBM3ZX 0WBM3ZZ 0WBM4ZX 0WBM4ZZ 0WBMXZX 0WBMXZZ
♀ 0WBN0ZX 0WBN0ZZ 0WBN3ZX 0WBN3ZZ 0WBN4ZX 0WBN4ZZ 0WBNXZX 0WBNXZZ

0 Medical and Surgical
W Anatomical Regions, General
C Extirpation: Taking or cutting out solid matter from a body part

Body Part Character 4	Approach Character 5	Device Character 6	Qualifier Character 7
1 Cranial Cavity 3 Oral Cavity and Throat 9 Pleural Cavity, Right B Pleural Cavity, Left C Mediastinum D Pericardial Cavity G Peritoneal Cavity H Retroperitoneum J Pelvic Cavity	0 Open 3 Percutaneous 4 Percutaneous Endoscopic X External	Z No Device	Z No Qualifier
4 Upper Jaw 5 Lower Jaw	0 Open 3 Percutaneous 4 Percutaneous Endoscopic	Z No Device	Z No Qualifier
P Gastrointestinal Tract Q Respiratory Tract R Genitourinary Tract	0 Open 3 Percutaneous 4 Percutaneous Endoscopic 7 Via Natural or Artificial Opening 8 Via Natural or Artificial Opening Endoscopic X External	Z No Device	Z No Qualifier

0 Medical and Surgical
W Anatomical Regions, General
F Fragmentation: Breaking solid matter in a body part into pieces

Body Part Character 4	Approach Character 5	Device Character 6	Qualifier Character 7
1 Cranial Cavity NC 3 Oral Cavity and Throat NC 9 Pleural Cavity, Right NC B Pleural Cavity, Left NC C Mediastinum NC D Pericardial Cavity G Peritoneal Cavity NC J Pelvic Cavity NC	0 Open 3 Percutaneous 4 Percutaneous Endoscopic X External	Z No Device	Z No Qualifier
P Gastrointestinal Tract NC Q Respiratory Tract NC R Genitourinary Tract DRG	0 Open 3 Percutaneous 4 Percutaneous Endoscopic 7 Via Natural or Artificial Opening 8 Via Natural or Artificial Opening Endoscopic X External	Z No Device	Z No Qualifier

NC 0WF1XZZ 0WF3XZZ 0WF9XZZ 0WFBXZZ 0WFCXZZ 0WFGXZZ 0WFJXZZ 0WFPXZZ 0WFQXZZ
DRG 0WFRXZZ

0 Medical and Surgical
W Anatomical Regions, General
H Insertion: Putting in a nonbiological appliance that monitors, assists, performs, or prevents a physiological function but does not physically take the place of a body part

Body Part Character 4	Approach Character 5	Device Character 6	Qualifier Character 7
0 Head DRG **1** Cranial Cavity **2** Face DRG **3** Oral Cavity and Throat **4** Upper Jaw DRG **5** Lower Jaw DRG **6** Neck DRG **8** Chest Wall **9** Pleural Cavity, Right **B** Pleural Cavity, Left **C** Mediastinum **D** Pericardial Cavity **F** Abdominal Wall **G** Peritoneal Cavity **H** Retroperitoneum **J** Pelvic Cavity **K** Upper Back DRG **L** Lower Back DRG **M** Perineum, Male DRG **N** Perineum, Female ♀	**0** Open **3** Percutaneous **4** Percutaneous Endoscopic	**1** Radioactive Element **3** Infusion Device **Y** Other Device	**Z** No Qualifier
P Gastrointestinal Tract **Q** Respiratory Tract **R** Genitourinary Tract	**0** Open **3** Percutaneous **4** Percutaneous Endoscopic **7** Via Natural or Artificial Opening **8** Via Natural or Artificial Opening Endoscopic	**1** Radioactive Element **3** Infusion Device **Y** Other Device	**Z** No Qualifier

♀ 0WHN03Z 0WHN0YZ 0WHN33Z 0WHN3YZ 0WHN43Z 0WHN4YZ

DRG 0WH003Z 0WH00YZ 0WH033Z 0WH03YZ 0WH043Z 0WH04YZ 0WH203Z 0WH20YZ 0WH233Z 0WH23YZ 0WH243Z 0WH24YZ 0WH403Z 0WH40YZ 0WH433Z 0WH43YZ 0WH443Z 0WH44YZ 0WH503Z 0WH50YZ 0WH533Z 0WH53YZ 0WH543Z 0WH54YZ 0WH603Z 0WH60YZ 0WH633Z 0WH63YZ 0WH643Z 0WH64YZ 0WHK03Z 0WHK0YZ 0WHK33Z 0WHK3YZ 0WHK43Z 0WHK4YZ 0WHL03Z 0WHL0YZ 0WHL33Z 0WHL3YZ 0WHL43Z 0WHL4YZ 0WHM03Z 0WHM0YZ 0WHM33Z 0WHM3YZ 0WHM43Z 0WHM4YZ

0 Medical and Surgical
W Anatomical Regions, General
J Inspection: Visually and/or manually exploring a body part

Body Part Character 4	Approach Character 5	Device Character 6	Qualifier Character 7
0 Head DRG **2** Face DRG **3** Oral Cavity and Throat **4** Upper Jaw DRG **5** Lower Jaw DRG **6** Neck **8** Chest Wall **F** Abdominal Wall **K** Upper Back DRG **L** Lower Back DRG **M** Perineum, Male ♂ **N** Perineum, Female ♀	**0** Open **3** Percutaneous **4** Percutaneous Endoscopic **X** External	**Z** No Device	**Z** No Qualifier
1 Cranial Cavity **9** Pleural Cavity, Right **B** Pleural Cavity, Left **C** Mediastinum **D** Pericardial Cavity **G** Peritoneal Cavity **H** Retroperitoneum **J** Pelvic Cavity	**0** Open **3** Percutaneous **4** Percutaneous Endoscopic	**Z** No Device	**Z** No Qualifier
P Gastrointestinal Tract **Q** Respiratory Tract **R** Genitourinary Tract	**0** Open **3** Percutaneous **4** Percutaneous Endoscopic **7** Via Natural or Artificial Opening **8** Via Natural or Artificial Opening Endoscopic	**Z** No Device	**Z** No Qualifier

♂ 0WJM0ZZ 0WJM3ZZ 0WJM4ZZ 0WJMXZZ
♀ 0WJN0ZZ 0WJN3ZZ 0WJN4ZZ 0WJNXZZ
DRG 0WJ00ZZ 0WJ20ZZ 0WJ40ZZ 0WJ50ZZ 0WJK0ZZ 0WJL0ZZ 0WJM0ZZ 0WJM4ZZ

0 Medical and Surgical
W Anatomical Regions, General
M Reattachment: Putting back in or on all or a portion of a separated body part to its normal location or other suitable location

Body Part Character 4	Approach Character 5	Device Character 6	Qualifier Character 7
2 Face **4** Upper Jaw **5** Lower Jaw **6** Neck **8** Chest Wall **F** Abdominal Wall **K** Upper Back **L** Lower Back **M** Perineum, Male ♂ **N** Perineum, Female ♀	**0** Open	**Z** No Device	**Z** No Qualifier

♂ 0WMM0ZZ
♀ 0WMN0ZZ

0 Medical and Surgical
W Anatomical Regions, General
P Removal: Taking out or off a device from a body part

Body Part	Approach	Device	Qualifier
Character 4	**Character 5**	**Character 6**	**Character 7**
0 Head **2** Face **4** Upper Jaw **5** Lower Jaw **6** Neck **8** Chest Wall **C** Mediastinum **F** Abdominal Wall **K** Upper Back **L** Lower Back **M** Perineum, Male ♂ **N** Perineum, Female ♀	**0** Open **3** Percutaneous **4** Percutaneous Endoscopic **X** External	**0** Drainage Device **1** Radioactive Element **3** Infusion Device **7** Autologous Tissue Substitute **J** Synthetic Substitute **K** Nonautologous Tissue Substitute **Y** Other Device	**Z** No Qualifier
1 Cranial Cavity **9** Pleural Cavity, Right **B** Pleural Cavity, Left **G** Peritoneal Cavity **J** Pelvic Cavity	**0** Open **3** Percutaneous **4** Percutaneous Endoscopic	**0** Drainage Device **1** Radioactive Element **3** Infusion Device **J** Synthetic Substitute **Y** Other Device	**Z** No Qualifier
1 Cranial Cavity **9** Pleural Cavity, Right **B** Pleural Cavity, Left **G** Peritoneal Cavity **J** Pelvic Cavity	**X** External	**0** Drainage Device **1** Radioactive Element **3** Infusion Device	**Z** No Qualifier
D Pericardial Cavity **H** Retroperitoneum	**0** Open **3** Percutaneous **4** Percutaneous Endoscopic	**0** Drainage Device **1** Radioactive Element **3** Infusion Device **Y** Other Device	**Z** No Qualifier
D Pericardial Cavity **H** Retroperitoneum	**X** External	**0** Drainage Device **1** Radioactive Element **3** Infusion Device	**Z** No Qualifier
P Gastrointestinal Tract **Q** Respiratory Tract **R** Genitourinary Tract	**0** Open **3** Percutaneous **4** Percutaneous Endoscopic **7** Via Natural or Artificial Opening **8** Via Natural or Artificial Opening Endoscopic **X** External	**1** Radioactive Element **3** Infusion Device **Y** Other Device	**Z** No Qualifier

♂ 0WPM00Z 0WPM01Z 0WPM03Z 0WPM07Z 0WPM0JZ 0WPM0KZ 0WPM0YZ 0WPM30Z 0WPM31Z 0WPM33Z 0WPM37Z 0WPM3JZ 0WPM3KZ 0WPM3YZ 0WPM40Z 0WPM41Z 0WPM43Z 0WPM47Z 0WPM4JZ 0WPM4KZ 0WPM4YZ 0WPMX0Z 0WPMX1Z 0WPMX3Z 0WPMX7Z 0WPMXJZ 0WPMXKZ 0WPMXYZ

♀ 0WPN00Z 0WPN01Z 0WPN03Z 0WPN07Z 0WPN0JZ 0WPN0KZ 0WPN0YZ 0WPN30Z 0WPN31Z 0WPN33Z 0WPN37Z 0WPN3JZ 0WPN3KZ 0WPN3YZ 0WPN40Z 0WPN41Z 0WPN43Z 0WPN47Z 0WPN4JZ 0WPN4KZ 0WPN4YZ 0WPNX0Z 0WPNX1Z 0WPNX3Z 0WPNX7Z 0WPNXJZ 0WPNXKZ 0WPNXYZ

0 Medical and Surgical
W Anatomical Regions, General
Q Repair: Restoring, to the extent possible, a body part to its normal anatomic structure and function

Body Part Character 4	Approach Character 5	Device Character 6	Qualifier Character 7
0 Head 2 Face 3 Oral Cavity and Throat 4 Upper Jaw 5 Lower Jaw 8 Chest Wall K Upper Back L Lower Back M Perineum, Male ♂ N Perineum, Female ♀	0 Open 3 Percutaneous 4 Percutaneous Endoscopic X External	Z No Device	Z No Qualifier
6 Neck F Abdominal Wall	0 Open 3 Percutaneous 4 Percutaneous Endoscopic	Z No Device	Z No Qualifier
6 Neck F Abdominal Wall CC	X External	Z No Device	2 Stoma Z No Qualifier
C Mediastinum	0 Open 3 Percutaneous 4 Percutaneous Endoscopic	Z No Device	Z No Qualifier

♂ 0WQM0ZZ 0WQM3ZZ 0WQM4ZZ 0WQMXZZ
♀ 0WQN0ZZ 0WQN3ZZ 0WQN4ZZ 0WQNXZZ
CC 0WQFXZ2 0WQFXZZ

0 Medical and Surgical
W Anatomical Regions, General
U Supplement: Putting in or on biological or synthetic material that physically reinforces and/or augments the function of a portion of a body part

Body Part Character 4	Approach Character 5	Device Character 6	Qualifier Character 7
0 Head 2 Face 4 Upper Jaw 5 Lower Jaw 6 Neck 8 Chest Wall C Mediastinum F Abdominal Wall K Upper Back L Lower Back M Perineum, Male ♂ N Perineum, Female ♀	0 Open 4 Percutaneous Endoscopic	7 Autologous Tissue Substitute J Synthetic Substitute K Nonautologous Tissue Substitute	Z No Qualifier

♂ 0WUM07Z 0WUM0JZ 0WUM0KZ 0WUM47Z 0WUM4JZ 0WUM4KZ
♀ 0WUN07Z 0WUN0JZ 0WUN0KZ 0WUN47Z 0WUN4JZ 0WUN4KZ

trocar - 3 sided cutting point enclosed in a tube
Endoscope = laproscope

0 Medical and Surgical
W Anatomical Regions, General
W Revision: Correcting, to the extent possible, a portion of a malfunctioning device or the position of a displaced device

Body Part Character 4	Approach Character 5	Device Character 6	Qualifier Character 7
0 Head DRG **2** Face DRG **4** Upper Jaw DRG **5** Lower Jaw DRG **6** Neck DRG **8** Chest Wall **C** Mediastinum **F** Abdominal Wall **K** Upper Back DRG **L** Lower Back DRG **M** Perineum, Male ♂ DRG **N** Perineum, Female ♀	**0** Open **3** Percutaneous **4** Percutaneous Endoscopic **X** External	**0** Drainage Device – not shunt **1** Radioactive Element **3** Infusion Device **7** Autologous Tissue Substitute **J** Synthetic Substitute - Shunt **K** Nonautologous Tissue Substitute **Y** Other Device	**Z** No Qualifier
1 Cranial Cavity **9** Pleural Cavity, Right **B** Pleural Cavity, Left **G** Peritoneal Cavity **J** Pelvic Cavity	**0** Open **3** Percutaneous trocar **4** Percutaneous Endoscopic trocar **X** External	**0** Drainage Device **1** Radioactive Element **3** Infusion Device **J** Synthetic Substitute shunt **Y** Other Device	**Z** No Qualifier
D Pericardial Cavity **H** Retroperitoneum	**0** Open **3** Percutaneous **4** Percutaneous Endoscopic **X** External	**0** Drainage Device **1** Radioactive Element **3** Infusion Device **Y** Other Device	**Z** No Qualifier
P Gastrointestinal Tract **Q** Respiratory Tract **R** Genitourinary Tract	**0** Open **3** Percutaneous **4** Percutaneous Endoscopic **7** Via Natural or Artificial Opening **8** Via Natural or Artificial Opening Endoscopic **X** External	**1** Radioactive Element **3** Infusion Device **Y** Other Device	**Z** No Qualifier

♂ 0WWM00Z 0WWM01Z 0WWM03Z 0WWM07Z 0WWM0JZ 0WWM0KZ 0WWM0YZ 0WWM30Z 0WWM31Z 0WWM33Z 0WWM37Z 0WWM3JZ 0WWM3KZ 0WWM3YZ 0WWM40Z 0WWM41Z 0WWM43Z 0WWM47Z 0WWM4JZ 0WWM4KZ 0WWM4YZ 0WWMX0Z 0WWMX1Z 0WWMX3Z 0WWMX7Z 0WWMXJZ 0WWMXKZ 0WWMXYZ

♀ 0WWN00Z 0WWN01Z 0WWN03Z 0WWN07Z 0WWN0JZ 0WWN0KZ 0WWN0YZ 0WWN30Z 0WWN31Z 0WWN33Z 0WWN37Z 0WWN3JZ 0WWN3KZ 0WWN3YZ 0WWN40Z 0WWN41Z 0WWN43Z 0WWN47Z 0WWN4JZ 0WWN4KZ 0WWN4YZ 0WWNX0Z 0WWNX1Z 0WWNX3Z 0WWNX7Z 0WWNXJZ 0WWNXKZ 0WWNXYZ

DRG 0WW000Z 0WW001Z 0WW003Z 0WW007Z 0WW00JZ 0WW00KZ 0WW00YZ 0WW030Z 0WW031Z 0WW033Z 0WW037Z 0WW03JZ 0WW03KZ 0WW03YZ 0WW040Z 0WW041Z 0WW043Z 0WW047Z 0WW04JZ 0WW04KZ 0WW04YZ 0WW200Z 0WW201Z 0WW203Z 0WW207Z 0WW20JZ 0WW20KZ 0WW20YZ 0WW230Z 0WW231Z 0WW233Z 0WW237Z 0WW23JZ 0WW23KZ 0WW23YZ 0WW240Z 0WW241Z 0WW243Z 0WW247Z 0WW24JZ 0WW24KZ 0WW24YZ 0WW400Z 0WW401Z 0WW403Z 0WW407Z 0WW40JZ 0WW40KZ 0WW40YZ 0WW430Z 0WW431Z 0WW433Z 0WW437Z 0WW43JZ 0WW43KZ 0WW43YZ 0WW440Z 0WW441Z 0WW443Z 0WW447Z 0WW44JZ 0WW44KZ 0WW44YZ 0WW500Z 0WW501Z 0WW503Z 0WW507Z 0WW50JZ 0WW50KZ 0WW50YZ 0WW530Z 0WW531Z 0WW533Z 0WW537Z 0WW53JZ 0WW53KZ 0WW53YZ 0WW540Z 0WW541Z 0WW543Z 0WW547Z 0WW54JZ 0WW54KZ 0WW54YZ 0WW600Z 0WW601Z 0WW603Z 0WW607Z 0WW60JZ 0WW60KZ 0WW60YZ 0WW630Z 0WW631Z 0WW633Z 0WW637Z 0WW63JZ 0WW63KZ 0WW63YZ 0WW640Z 0WW641Z 0WW643Z 0WW647Z 0WW64JZ 0WW64KZ 0WW64YZ 0WWK00Z 0WWK01Z 0WWK03Z 0WWK07Z 0WWK0JZ 0WWK0KZ 0WWK0YZ 0WWK30Z 0WWK31Z 0WWK33Z 0WWK37Z 0WWK3JZ 0WWK3KZ 0WWK3YZ 0WWK40Z 0WWK41Z 0WWK43Z 0WWK47Z 0WWK4JZ 0WWK4KZ 0WWK4YZ 0WWL00Z 0WWL01Z 0WWL03Z 0WWL07Z 0WWL0JZ 0WWL0KZ 0WWL0YZ 0WWL30Z 0WWL31Z 0WWL33Z 0WWL37Z 0WWL3JZ 0WWL3KZ 0WWL3YZ 0WWL40Z 0WWL41Z 0WWL43Z 0WWL47Z 0WWL4JZ 0WWL4KZ 0WWL4YZ 0WWM00Z 0WWM01Z 0WWM03Z 0WWM0JZ 0WWM0YZ 0WWM30Z 0WWM31Z 0WWM33Z 0WWM3JZ 0WWM3YZ 0WWM40Z 0WWM41Z 0WWM43Z 0WWM4JZ 0WWM4YZ

0 Medical and Surgical
W Anatomical Regions, General
Y Transplantation: Putting in or on all or a portion of a living body part taken from another individual or animal to physically take the place and/or function of all or a portion of a similar body part

Body Part Character 4	Approach Character 5	Device Character 6	Qualifier Character 7
2 Face	**0** Open	**Z** No Device	**0** Allogeneic **1** Syngeneic

NOTES

NOTES

upper arm/leg 1 = high: amputation at the proximal portion of humerous or Femur
2 = mid: amputation at the middle portion of the shaft of humerous or Femur
3 = low: amputation at the distal portion of the shaft of humerous or Femur

hand & Foot 0 = Complete
4 = complete 1st ray
5 = Complete 2nd ray

Anatomical Regions, Upper Extremities 0X0-0XY

0 Medical and Surgical
X Anatomical Regions, Upper Extremities
0 Alteration: Modifying the anatomic structure of a body part without affecting the function of the body part

Body Part Character 4	Approach Character 5	Device Character 6	Qualifier Character 7
2 Shoulder Region, Right **3** Shoulder Region, Left **4** Axilla, Right **5** Axilla, Left **6** Upper Extremity, Right **7** Upper Extremity, Left **8** Upper Arm, Right **9** Upper Arm, Left **B** Elbow Region, Right **C** Elbow Region, Left **D** Lower Arm, Right **F** Lower Arm, Left **G** Wrist Region, Right **H** Wrist Region, Left	**0** Open **3** Percutaneous **4** Percutaneous Endoscopic	**7** Autologous Tissue Substitute **J** Synthetic Substitute **K** Nonautologous Tissue Substitute **Z** No Device	**Z** No Qualifier

0 Medical and Surgical
X Anatomical Regions, Upper Extremities
2 Change: Taking out or off a device from a body part and putting back an identical or similar device in or on the same body part without cutting or puncturing the skin or a mucous membrane

Body Part Character 4	Approach Character 5	Device Character 6	Qualifier Character 7
6 Upper Extremity, Right **7** Upper Extremity, Left	**X** External	**0** Drainage Device **Y** Other Device	**Z** No Qualifier

0 Medical and Surgical
X Anatomical Regions, Upper Extremities
3 Control: Stopping, or attempting to stop, postprocedural or other acute bleeding

Body Part Character 4	Approach Character 5	Device Character 6	Qualifier Character 7
2 Shoulder Region, Right **3** Shoulder Region, Left **4** Axilla, Right **5** Axilla, Left **6** Upper Extremity, Right **7** Upper Extremity, Left **8** Upper Arm, Right **9** Upper Arm, Left **B** Elbow Region, Right **C** Elbow Region, Left **D** Lower Arm, Right **F** Lower Arm, Left **G** Wrist Region, Right **H** Wrist Region, Left **J** Hand, Right **K** Hand, Left	**0** Open **3** Percutaneous **4** Percutaneous Endoscopic	**Z** No Device	**Z** No Qualifier

0 Medical and Surgical
X Anatomical Regions, Upper Extremities
6 Detachment: Cutting off all or a portion of the upper or lower extremities

Body Part Character 4	Approach Character 5	Device Character 6	Qualifier Character 7
0 Forequarter, Right **1** Forequarter, Left **2** Shoulder Region, Right **3** Shoulder Region, Left **B** Elbow Region, Right **C** Elbow Region, Left	**0** Open	**Z** No Device	**Z** No Qualifier
8 Upper Arm, Right **9** Upper Arm, Left **D** Lower Arm, Right **F** Lower Arm, Left	**0** Open	**Z** No Device	**1** High **2** Mid **3** Low
J Hand, Right **K** Hand, Left	**0** Open	**Z** No Device	**0** Complete **4** Complete 1st Ray **5** Complete 2nd Ray **6** Complete 3rd Ray **7** Complete 4th Ray **8** Complete 5th Ray **9** Partial 1st Ray **B** Partial 2nd Ray **C** Partial 3rd Ray **D** Partial 4th Ray **F** Partial 5th Ray
L Thumb, Right **M** Thumb, Left **N** Index Finger, Right **P** Index Finger, Left **Q** Middle Finger, Right **R** Middle Finger, Left **S** Ring Finger, Right **T** Ring Finger, Left **V** Little Finger, Right **W** Little Finger, Left	**0** Open	**Z** No Device	**0** Complete **1** High **2** Mid **3** Low

0 Medical and Surgical
X Anatomical Regions, Upper Extremities
9 Drainage: Taking or letting out fluids and/or gases from a body part

Body Part Character 4	Approach Character 5	Device Character 6	Qualifier Character 7
2 Shoulder Region, Right **3** Shoulder Region, Left **4** Axilla, Right **5** Axilla, Left **6** Upper Extremity, Right **7** Upper Extremity, Left **8** Upper Arm, Right **9** Upper Arm, Left **B** Elbow Region, Right **C** Elbow Region, Left **D** Lower Arm, Right **F** Lower Arm, Left **G** Wrist Region, Right **H** Wrist Region, Left **J** Hand, Right **K** Hand, Left	**0** Open **3** Percutaneous **4** Percutaneous Endoscopic	**0** Drainage Device	**Z** No Qualifier
2 Shoulder Region, Right **3** Shoulder Region, Left **4** Axilla, Right **5** Axilla, Left **6** Upper Extremity, Right **7** Upper Extremity, Left **8** Upper Arm, Right **9** Upper Arm, Left **B** Elbow Region, Right **C** Elbow Region, Left **D** Lower Arm, Right **F** Lower Arm, Left **G** Wrist Region, Right **H** Wrist Region, Left **J** Hand, Right **K** Hand, Left	**0** Open **3** Percutaneous **4** Percutaneous Endoscopic	**Z** No Device	**X** Diagnostic **Z** No Qualifier

0 Medical and Surgical
X Anatomical Regions, Upper Extremities
B Excision: Cutting out or off, without replacement, a portion of a body part

Body Part Character 4	Approach Character 5	Device Character 6	Qualifier Character 7
2 Shoulder Region, Right **3** Shoulder Region, Left **4** Axilla, Right **5** Axilla, Left **6** Upper Extremity, Right **7** Upper Extremity, Left **8** Upper Arm, Right **9** Upper Arm, Left **B** Elbow Region, Right **C** Elbow Region, Left **D** Lower Arm, Right **F** Lower Arm, Left **G** Wrist Region, Right **H** Wrist Region, Left **J** Hand, Right **K** Hand, Left	**0** Open **3** Percutaneous **4** Percutaneous Endoscopic	**Z** No Device	**X** Diagnostic **Z** No Qualifier

0 Medical and Surgical
X Anatomical Regions, Upper Extremities
H Insertion: Putting in a nonbiological appliance that monitors, assists, performs, or prevents a physiological function but does not physically take the place of a body part

Body Part Character 4	Approach Character 5	Device Character 6	Qualifier Character 7
2 Shoulder Region, Right DRG **3** Shoulder Region, Left DRG **4** Axilla, Right DRG **5** Axilla, Left DRG **6** Upper Extremity, Right DRG **7** Upper Extremity, Left DRG **8** Upper Arm, Right DRG **9** Upper Arm, Left DRG **B** Elbow Region, Right DRG **C** Elbow Region, Left DRG **D** Lower Arm, Right DRG **F** Lower Arm, Left DRG **G** Wrist Region, Right DRG **H** Wrist Region, Left DRG **J** Hand, Right DRG **K** Hand, Left DRG	**0** Open **3** Percutaneous **4** Percutaneous Endoscopic	**1** Radioactive Element **3** Infusion Device **Y** Other Device	**Z** No Qualifier

DRG 0XH203Z 0XH20YZ 0XH233Z 0XH23YZ 0XH243Z 0XH24YZ 0XH303Z 0XH30YZ 0XH333Z 0XH33YZ 0XH343Z 0XH34YZ 0XH403Z
0XH40YZ 0XH433Z 0XH43YZ 0XH443Z 0XH44YZ 0XH503Z 0XH50YZ 0XH533Z 0XH53YZ 0XH543Z 0XH54YZ 0XH603Z 0XH60YZ
0XH633Z 0XH63YZ 0XH643Z 0XH64YZ 0XH703Z 0XH70YZ 0XH733Z 0XH73YZ 0XH743Z 0XH74YZ 0XH803Z 0XH80YZ 0XH833Z
0XH83YZ 0XH843Z 0XH84YZ 0XH903Z 0XH90YZ 0XH933Z 0XH93YZ 0XH943Z 0XH94YZ 0XHB03Z 0XHB0YZ 0XHB33Z 0XHB3YZ
0XHB43Z 0XHB4YZ 0XHC03Z 0XHC0YZ 0XHC33Z 0XHC3YZ 0XHC43Z 0XHC4YZ 0XHD03Z 0XHD0YZ 0XHD33Z 0XHD3YZ 0XHD43Z
0XHD4YZ 0XHF03Z 0XHF0YZ 0XHF33Z 0XHF3YZ 0XHF43Z 0XHF4YZ 0XHG03Z 0XHG0YZ 0XHG33Z 0XHG3YZ 0XHG43Z 0XHG4YZ
0XHH03Z 0XHH0YZ 0XHH33Z 0XHH3YZ 0XHH43Z 0XHH4YZ 0XHJ03Z 0XHJ0YZ 0XHJ33Z 0XHJ3YZ 0XHJ43Z 0XHJ4YZ 0XHK03Z
0XHK0YZ 0XHK33Z 0XHK3YZ 0XHK43Z 0XHK4YZ

0 Medical and Surgical
X Anatomical Regions, Upper Extremities
J Inspection: Visually and/or manually exploring a body part

Body Part Character 4	Approach Character 5	Device Character 6	Qualifier Character 7
2 Shoulder Region, Right DRG 3 Shoulder Region, Left DRG 4 Axilla, Right DRG 5 Axilla, Left DRG 6 Upper Extremity, Right DRG 7 Upper Extremity, Left DRG 8 Upper Arm, Right DRG 9 Upper Arm, Left DRG B Elbow Region, Right DRG C Elbow Region, Left DRG D Lower Arm, Right DRG F Lower Arm, Left DRG G Wrist Region, Right DRG H Wrist Region, Left DRG J Hand, Right DRG K Hand, Left DRG	0 Open 3 Percutaneous 4 Percutaneous Endoscopic X External	Z No Device	Z No Qualifier

DRG 0XJ20ZZ 0XJ30ZZ 0XJ40ZZ 0XJ50ZZ 0XJ60ZZ 0XJ70ZZ 0XJ80ZZ 0XJ90ZZ 0XJB0ZZ 0XJC0ZZ 0XJD0ZZ 0XJF0ZZ 0XJG0ZZ 0XJH0ZZ 0XJJ0ZZ 0XJK0ZZ

0 Medical and Surgical
X Anatomical Regions, Upper Extremities
M Reattachment: Putting back in or on all or a portion of a separated body part to its normal location or other suitable location

Body Part Character 4	Approach Character 5	Device Character 6	Qualifier Character 7
0 Forequarter, Right 1 Forequarter, Left 2 Shoulder Region, Right 3 Shoulder Region, Left 4 Axilla, Right 5 Axilla, Left 6 Upper Extremity, Right 7 Upper Extremity, Left 8 Upper Arm, Right 9 Upper Arm, Left B Elbow Region, Right C Elbow Region, Left D Lower Arm, Right F Lower Arm, Left G Wrist Region, Right H Wrist Region, Left J Hand, Right K Hand, Left L Thumb, Right M Thumb, Left N Index Finger, Right P Index Finger, Left Q Middle Finger, Right R Middle Finger, Left S Ring Finger, Right T Ring Finger, Left V Little Finger, Right W Little Finger, Left	0 Open	Z No Device	Z No Qualifier

0 Medical and Surgical
X Anatomical Regions, Upper Extremities
P Removal: Taking out or off a device from a body part

Body Part Character 4	Approach Character 5	Device Character 6	Qualifier Character 7
6 Upper Extremity, Right **7** Upper Extremity, Left	**0** Open **3** Percutaneous **4** Percutaneous Endoscopic **X** External	**0** Drainage Device **1** Radioactive Element **3** Infusion Device **7** Autologous Tissue Substitute **J** Synthetic Substitute **K** Nonautologous Tissue Substitute **Y** Other Device	**Z** No Qualifier

0 Medical and Surgical
X Anatomical Regions, Upper Extremities
Q Repair: Restoring, to the extent possible, a body part to its normal anatomic structure and function

Body Part Character 4	Approach Character 5	Device Character 6	Qualifier Character 7
2 Shoulder Region, Right **3** Shoulder Region, Left **4** Axilla, Right **5** Axilla, Left **6** Upper Extremity, Right **7** Upper Extremity, Left **8** Upper Arm, Right **9** Upper Arm, Left **B** Elbow Region, Right **C** Elbow Region, Left **D** Lower Arm, Right **F** Lower Arm, Left **G** Wrist Region, Right **H** Wrist Region, Left **J** Hand, Right **K** Hand, Left **L** Thumb, Right **M** Thumb, Left **N** Index Finger, Right **P** Index Finger, Left **Q** Middle Finger, Right **R** Middle Finger, Left **S** Ring Finger, Right **T** Ring Finger, Left **V** Little Finger, Right **W** Little Finger, Left	**0** Open **3** Percutaneous **4** Percutaneous Endoscopic **X** External	**Z** No Device	**Z** No Qualifier

0 Medical and Surgical
X Anatomical Regions, Upper Extremities
R Replacement: Putting in or on biological or synthetic material that physically takes the place and/or function of all or a portion of a body part

Body Part Character 4	Approach Character 5	Device Character 6	Qualifier Character 7
L Thumb, Right **M** Thumb, Left	**0** Open **4** Percutaneous Endoscopic	**7** Autologous Tissue Substitute	**N** Toe, Right **P** Toe, Left

0 Medical and Surgical
X Anatomical Regions, Upper Extremities
U Supplement: Putting in or on biological or synthetic material that physically reinforces and/or augments the function of a portion of a body part

Body Part Character 4	Approach Character 5	Device Character 6	Qualifier Character 7
2 Shoulder Region, Right **3** Shoulder Region, Left **4** Axilla, Right **5** Axilla, Left **6** Upper Extremity, Right **7** Upper Extremity, Left **8** Upper Arm, Right **9** Upper Arm, Left **B** Elbow Region, Right **C** Elbow Region, Left **D** Lower Arm, Right **F** Lower Arm, Left **G** Wrist Region, Right **H** Wrist Region, Left **J** Hand, Right **K** Hand, Left **L** Thumb, Right **M** Thumb, Left **N** Index Finger, Right **P** Index Finger, Left **Q** Middle Finger, Right **R** Middle Finger, Left **S** Ring Finger, Right **T** Ring Finger, Left **V** Little Finger, Right **W** Little Finger, Left	**0** Open **4** Percutaneous Endoscopic	**7** Autologous Tissue Substitute **J** Synthetic Substitute **K** Nonautologous Tissue Substitute	**Z** No Qualifier

0 Medical and Surgical
X Anatomical Regions, Upper Extremities
W Revision: Correcting, to the extent possible, a portion of a malfunctioning device or the position of a displaced device

Body Part Character 4	Approach Character 5	Device Character 6	Qualifier Character 7
6 Upper Extremity, Right DRG **7** Upper Extremity, Left DRG	**0** Open **3** Percutaneous **4** Percutaneous Endoscopic **X** External	**0** Drainage Device **3** Infusion Device **7** Autologous Tissue Substitute **J** Synthetic Substitute **K** Nonautologous Tissue Substitute **Y** Other Device	**Z** No Qualifier

DRG 0XW600Z 0XW603Z 0XW607Z 0XW60JZ 0XW60KZ 0XW60YZ 0XW630Z 0XW633Z 0XW637Z 0XW63JZ 0XW63KZ 0XW63YZ 0XW640Z 0XW643Z 0XW647Z 0XW64JZ 0XW64KZ 0XW64YZ 0XW700Z 0XW703Z 0XW707Z 0XW70JZ 0XW70KZ 0XW70YZ 0XW730Z 0XW733Z 0XW737Z 0XW73JZ 0XW73KZ 0XW73YZ 0XW740Z 0XW743Z 0XW747Z 0XW74JZ 0XW74KZ 0XW74YZ

0 Medical and Surgical
X Anatomical Regions, Upper Extremities
X Transfer: Moving, without taking out, all or a portion of a body part to another location to take over the function of all or a portion of a body part

Body Part Character 4	Approach Character 5	Device Character 6	Qualifier Character 7
N Index Finger, Right	**0** Open	**Z** No Device	**L** Thumb, Right
P Index Finger, Left	**0** Open	**Z** No Device	**M** Thumb, Left

0 Medical and Surgical
X Anatomical Regions, Upper Extremities
Y Transplantation: Putting in or on all or a portion of a living body part taken from another individual or animal to physically take the place and/or function of all or a portion of a similar body part

Body Part Character 4	Approach Character 5	Device Character 6	Qualifier Character 7
J Hand, Right **K** Hand, Left	**0** Open	**Z** No Device	**0** Allogeneic **1** Syngeneic

NOTES

amputation

1 high - proximal portion of shaft of humerous or femur

2 mid - middle portion of shaft of humerous or femur

3 low - distal portion of shaft of humerous or femur

Anatomical Regions, Lower Extremities 0Y0-0YW

0 Medical and Surgical
Y Anatomical Regions, Lower Extremities
0 Alteration: Modifying the anatomic structure of a body part without affecting the function of the body part

Body Part Character 4	Approach Character 5	Device Character 6	Qualifier Character 7
0 Buttock, Right **1** Buttock, Left **9** Lower Extremity, Right **B** Lower Extremity, Left **C** Upper Leg, Right **D** Upper Leg, Left **F** Knee Region, Right **G** Knee Region, Left **H** Lower Leg, Right **J** Lower Leg, Left **K** Ankle Region, Right **L** Ankle Region, Left	**0** Open **3** Percutaneous **4** Percutaneous Endoscopic	**7** Autologous Tissue Substitute **J** Synthetic Substitute **K** Nonautologous Tissue Substitute **Z** No Device	**Z** No Qualifier

0 Medical and Surgical
Y Anatomical Regions, Lower Extremities
2 Change: Taking out or off a device from a body part and putting back an identical or similar device in or on the same body part without cutting or puncturing the skin or a mucous membrane

Body Part Character 4	Approach Character 5	Device Character 6	Qualifier Character 7
9 Lower Extremity, Right **B** Lower Extremity, Left	**X** External	**0** Drainage Device **Y** Other Device	**Z** No Qualifier

0 Medical and Surgical
Y Anatomical Regions, Lower Extremities
3 Control: Stopping, or attempting to stop, postprocedural or other acute bleeding

Body Part Character 4	Approach Character 5	Device Character 6	Qualifier Character 7
0 Buttock, Right **1** Buttock, Left **5** Inguinal Region, Right **6** Inguinal Region, Left **7** Femoral Region, Right **8** Femoral Region, Left **9** Lower Extremity, Right **B** Lower Extremity, Left **C** Upper Leg, Right **D** Upper Leg, Left **F** Knee Region, Right **G** Knee Region, Left **H** Lower Leg, Right **J** Lower Leg, Left **K** Ankle Region, Right **L** Ankle Region, Left **M** Foot, Right **N** Foot, Left	**0** Open **3** Percutaneous **4** Percutaneous Endoscopic	**Z** No Device	**Z** No Qualifier

BKA- Below knee amputation

0 Medical and Surgical
Y Anatomical Regions, Lower Extremities
6 Detachment: Cutting off all or a portion of the upper or lower extremities

Body Part Character 4	Approach Character 5	Device Character 6	Qualifier Character 7
2 Hindquarter, Right **3** Hindquarter, Left **4** Hindquarter, Bilateral **7** Femoral Region, Right **8** Femoral Region, Left **F** Knee Region, Right **G** Knee Region, Left	**0** Open	**Z** No Device	**Z** No Qualifier
C Upper Leg, Right above **D** Upper Leg, Left the knee **H** Lower Leg, Right **J** Lower Leg, Left	**0** Open	**Z** No Device	**1** High See page **2** Mid 582 **3** Low
M Foot, Right **N** Foot, Left	**0** Open	**Z** No Device	**0** Complete **4** Complete 1st Ray **5** Complete 2nd Ray **6** Complete 3rd Ray **7** Complete 4th Ray **8** Complete 5th Ray **9** Partial 1st Ray **B** Partial 2nd Ray **C** Partial 3rd Ray **D** Partial 4th Ray **F** Partial 5th Ray
P 1st Toe, Right **Q** 1st Toe, Left **R** 2nd Toe, Right **S** 2nd Toe, Left **T** 3rd Toe, Right **U** 3rd Toe, Left **V** 4th Toe, Right **W** 4th Toe, Left **X** 5th Toe, Right **Y** 5th Toe, Left	**0** Open	**Z** No Device	**0** Complete **1** High **2** Mid **3** Low

0 Medical and Surgical
Y Anatomical Regions, Lower Extremities
9 Drainage: Taking or letting out fluids and/or gases from a body part

Body Part Character 4	Approach Character 5	Device Character 6	Qualifier Character 7
0 Buttock, Right **1** Buttock, Left **5** Inguinal Region, Right **6** Inguinal Region, Left **7** Femoral Region, Right **8** Femoral Region, Left **9** Lower Extremity, Right **B** Lower Extremity, Left **C** Upper Leg, Right **D** Upper Leg, Left **F** Knee Region, Right **G** Knee Region, Left **H** Lower Leg, Right **J** Lower Leg, Left **K** Ankle Region, Right **L** Ankle Region, Left **M** Foot, Right **N** Foot, Left	**0** Open **3** Percutaneous **4** Percutaneous Endoscopic	**0** Drainage Device	**Z** No Qualifier
0 Buttock, Right **1** Buttock, Left **5** Inguinal Region, Right **6** Inguinal Region, Left **7** Femoral Region, Right **8** Femoral Region, Left **9** Lower Extremity, Right **B** Lower Extremity, Left **C** Upper Leg, Right **D** Upper Leg, Left **F** Knee Region, Right **G** Knee Region, Left **H** Lower Leg, Right **J** Lower Leg, Left **K** Ankle Region, Right **L** Ankle Region, Left **M** Foot, Right **N** Foot, Left	**0** Open **3** Percutaneous **4** Percutaneous Endoscopic	**Z** No Device	**X** Diagnostic **Z** No Qualifier

0 Medical and Surgical
Y Anatomical Regions, Lower Extremities
B Excision: Cutting out or off, without replacement, a portion of a body part

Body Part Character 4	Approach Character 5	Device Character 6	Qualifier Character 7
0 Buttock, Right **1** Buttock, Left **5** Inguinal Region, Right **6** Inguinal Region, Left **7** Femoral Region, Right **8** Femoral Region, Left **9** Lower Extremity, Right **B** Lower Extremity, Left **C** Upper Leg, Right **D** Upper Leg, Left **F** Knee Region, Right **G** Knee Region, Left **H** Lower Leg, Right **J** Lower Leg, Left **K** Ankle Region, Right **L** Ankle Region, Left **M** Foot, Right **N** Foot, Left	**0** Open **3** Percutaneous **4** Percutaneous Endoscopic	**Z** No Device	**X** Diagnostic **Z** No Qualifier

gravida - pregnant Female

NOTES

Body Part (4th character)

- Products of Conception (∅)
  embroyo or Fetus any gestational age
- Products of conception retained (1)
  after incomplete or missed abortion, Also
  placenta retained in uterus after birth
- Products of conception (2) ectopic
  Fetus or Fertilized egg outside uterus
  May be in Fallioperan tubes or peritoneal cavity

Bimanual - dr has one hand of womans abdomen + 2 fingers other hand to Feel cervix + Fetal position

Approach (5th character)

abortion w/laminaria or abortifacient
use 7 - natural/artifical opening
Laminaria - ripens cervix

Cesarean Section - depends on incision made on uterus

- Classic w/midline longitudinal incision = high (∅) high on abdomen
- Lower segment C-section w/low transverse cut just above the edge of the bladder = low (1) most common
- Extraperitoneal - avoids letting contaminants from infected uterus to enter peritoneal space. Report w/qualifier 2
- emergency C-Section - performed once labor has started
- repeat C-Section - usually performed through old scar
- Cesarean Hysterectomy - C-section Followed by removal of uterus & may be done for intractable bleeding or when the placenta cannot be separated from the uterus.

Fetal procedures - treat birth defects in Fetus while in pregnant uterus

- open - completely open uterus to operate on Fetus
- minimally invasive - Fetoscopic surgery (Fetendo), uses small incisions & is guided by Fetoscopy & sonography
- endoscopic - may be done w/o incision. Done in real time, cross-sectional view provided by sonogram

Fetus, amnion, umbilical cord & placenta
also - zygote, embryo, fetus, retained products of conception
- codes not for pregnant female
must be product (baby) of conception
No differentiation based on gestational age

Obstetrics 102-10Y

1 Obstetrics
0 Pregnancy
2 Change: Taking out or off a device from a body part and putting back an identical or similar device in or on the same body part without cutting or puncturing the skin or a mucous membrane

Body Part	Approach	Device	Qualifier
Character 4	**Character 5**	**Character 6**	**Character 7**
0 Products of Conception ♀	**7** Via Natural or Artificial Opening	**3** Monitoring Electrode **Y** Other Device	**Z** No Qualifier

♀ 102073Z 10207YZ

1 Obstetrics Percutaneous spiral tab 10903ZA
0 Pregnancy
9 Drainage: Taking or letting out fluids and/or gases from a body part

type of fluid drained

Body Part	Approach	Device	Qualifier
Character 4	**Character 5**	**Character 6**	**Character 7**
0 Products of Conception ♀	**0** Open **3** Percutaneous **4** Percutaneous Endoscopic **7** Via Natural or Artificial Opening **8** Via Natural or Artificial Opening Endoscopic	**Z** No Device	**9** Fetal Blood **A** Fetal Cerebrospinal Fluid tap **B** Fetal Fluid, Other **C** Amniotic Fluid, Therapeutic **D** Fluid, Other **U** Amniotic Fluid, Diagnostic

♀ 10900Z9 10900ZA 10900ZB 10900ZC 10900ZD 10900ZU 10903Z9 10903ZA 10903ZB 10903ZC 10903ZD 10903ZU 10904Z9 10904ZA 10904ZB 10904ZC 10904ZD 10904ZU 10907Z9 10907ZA 10907ZB 10907ZC 10907ZD 10907ZU 10908Z9 10908ZA 10908ZB 10908ZC 10908ZD 10908ZU

1 Obstetrics therapeutic - to preserve health of mother
0 Pregnancy elective - anything other than therapeutic
A Abortion: Artificially terminating a pregnancy induced. If manually assisted, use delivery

Body Part	Approach	Device	Qualifier
Character 4	**Character 5**	**Character 6**	**Character 7**
0 Products of Conception ♀	**0** Open **3** Percutaneous **4** Percutaneous Endoscopic **8** Via Natural or Artificial Opening Endoscopic	**Z** No Device	**Z** No Qualifier
0 Products of Conception ♀	**7** Via Natural or Artificial Opening	**Z** No Device	**6** Vacuum **W** Laminaria - inserted in vagina to ripen **X** Abortifacient **Z** No Qualifier

♀ 10A00ZZ 10A03ZZ 10A04ZZ 10A07Z6 10A07ZW 10A07ZX 10A07ZZ 10A08ZZ

Abortion w/ dilation & evacuation w/ laminaria 10A07ZW

Following delivery or abortion curettage of endometrium or evacuation or retained products of conception

extraperitoneal C-section 10D00Z2

1 Obstetrics includes: c-section, internal inversion from
0 Pregnancy breech, vacuum forceps & other forceps
D Extraction: Pulling or stripping out or off all or a portion of a body part by the use of force

Body Part Character 4	Approach Character 5	Device Character 6	Qualifier Character 7
0 Products of Conception ♀ DRG QOA	**0** Open	**Z** No Device	**0** High **1** Low **2** Extraperitoneal
0 Products of Conception ♀ QOA	**7** Via Natural or Artificial Opening	**Z** No Device	**3** Low Forceps **4** Mid Forceps **5** High Forceps **6** Vacuum **7** Internal Version **8** Other
1 Products of Conception, Retained ♀	**7** Via Natural or Artificial Opening **8** Via Natural or Artificial Opening Endoscopic	**Z** No Device	**9** Manual **Z** No Qualifier
2 Products of Conception, Ectopic ♀	**7** Via Natural or Artificial Opening **8** Via Natural or Artificial Opening Endoscopic	**Z** No Device	**Z** No Qualifier

type of extraction or C-section

♀ 10D00Z0 10D00Z1 10D00Z2 10D07Z3 10D07Z4 10D07Z5 10D07Z6 10D07Z7 10D07Z8 10D17Z9 10D17ZZ 10D18Z9 10D18ZZ 10D27ZZ 10D28ZZ
DRG 10D07Z3 10D07Z4 10D07Z5 10D07Z6 10D07Z7 10D07Z8
QOA 10D00Z0 10D00Z1 10D00Z2 10D07Z3 10D07Z4 10D07Z5 10D07Z7
The list of codes is a questionable admission except when reported with a corresponding secondary diagnosis Z37.0, Z37.1, Z37.2, Z37.3, Z37.4, Z37.50, Z37.51, Z37.52, Z37.53, Z37.54, Z37.59, Z37.60, Z37.61, Z37.62, Z37.63, Z37.64, Z37.69, Z37.7, Z37.9.

1 Obstetrics manually assisted spontaneously delivery as it was not artificially terminated
0 Pregnancy Can be manually assisted spontaneous abortion - thus - no extraction
E Delivery: Assisting the passage of the products of conception from the genital canal

Body Part Character 4	Approach Character 5	Device Character 6	Qualifier Character 7
0 Products of Conception ♀ DRG QOA	**X** External	**Z** No Device	**Z** No Qualifier

♀ 10E0XZZ
DRG 10E0XZZ
QOA 10E0XZZ
can also code 0HQ9XZZ to repair 1st degree perineal lacerations
Can also code external fetal monitoring 4A1HXCZ
The list of codes is a questionable admission except when reported with a corresponding secondary diagnosis Z37.0, Z37.1, Z37.2, Z37.3, Z37.4, Z37.50, Z37.51, Z37.52, Z37.53, Z37.54, Z37.59, Z37.60, Z37.61, Z37.62, Z37.63, Z37.64, Z37.69, Z37.7, Z37.9.

1 Obstetrics
0 Pregnancy
H Insertion: Putting in a nonbiological appliance that monitors, assists, performs, or prevents a physiological function but does not physically take the place of a body part

Body Part Character 4	Approach Character 5	Device Character 6	Qualifier Character 7
0 Products of Conception ♀	**0** Open **7** Via Natural or Artificial Opening	**3** Monitoring Electrode **Y** Other Device	**Z** No Qualifier

♀ 10H003Z 10H00YZ 10H073Z 10H07YZ

1 Obstetrics
0 Pregnancy
J Inspection: Visually and/or manually exploring a body part

Body Part Character 4	Approach Character 5	Device Character 6	Qualifier Character 7
0 Products of Conception ♀ Fetus **1** Products of Conception, Retained ♀ **2** Products of Conception, Ectopic ♀	**0** Open **3** Percutaneous **4** Percutaneous Endoscopic **7** Via Natural or Artificial Opening bimanual **8** Via Natural or Artificial Opening Endoscopic **X** External	**Z** No Device	**Z** No Qualifier

♀ 10J00ZZ 10J03ZZ 10J04ZZ 10J07ZZ 10J08ZZ 10J0XZZ 10J10ZZ 10J13ZZ 10J14ZZ 10J17ZZ 10J18ZZ 10J1XZZ 10J20ZZ 10J23ZZ 10J24ZZ 10J27ZZ 10J28ZZ 10J2XZZ

1 Obstetrics
0 Pregnancy
P Removal: Taking out or off a device from a body part, region, or orifice

Body Part Character 4	Approach Character 5	Device Character 6	Qualifier Character 7
0 Products of Conception ♀	**0** Open **7** Via Natural or Artificial Opening	**3** Monitoring Electrode **Y** Other Device	**Z** No Qualifier

♀ 10P003Z 10P00YZ 10P073Z 10P07YZ

1 Obstetrics code urethral laceration in med/surg, code episiotomy to med/surg.
0 Pregnancy
Q Repair: Restoring, to the extent possible, a body part to its normal anatomic structure and function

Body Part Character 4	Approach Character 5	Device Character 6	Qualifier Character 7
0 Products of Conception ♀	**0** Open **3** Percutaneous **4** Percutaneous Endoscopic **7** Via Natural or Artificial Opening **8** Via Natural or Artificial Opening Endoscopic	**Y** Other Device **Z** No Device	**E** Nervous System **F** Cardiovascular System **G** Lymphatics and Hemic **H** Eye **J** Ear, Nose and Sinus **K** Respiratory System **L** Mouth and Throat **M** Gastrointestinal System **N** Hepatobiliary and Pancreas **P** Endocrine System **Q** Skin **R** Musculoskeletal System **S** Urinary System **T** Female Reproductive System **V** Male Reproductive System **Y** Other Body System

♀ 10Q00YE 10Q00YF 10Q00YG 10Q00YH 10Q00YJ 10Q00YK 10Q00YL 10Q00YM 10Q00YN 10Q00YP 10Q00YQ 10Q00YR 10Q00YS 10Q00YT 10Q00YV 10Q00YY 10Q00ZE 10Q00ZF 10Q00ZG 10Q00ZH 10Q00ZJ 10Q00ZK 10Q00ZL 10Q00ZM 10Q00ZN 10Q00ZP 10Q00ZQ 10Q00ZR 10Q00ZS 10Q00ZT 10Q00ZV 10Q00ZY 10Q03YE 10Q03YF 10Q03YG 10Q03YH 10Q03YJ 10Q03YK 10Q03YL 10Q03YM 10Q03YN 10Q03YP 10Q03YQ 10Q03YR 10Q03YS 10Q03YT 10Q03YV 10Q03YY 10Q03ZE 10Q03ZF 10Q03ZG 10Q03ZH 10Q03ZJ 10Q03ZK 10Q03ZL 10Q03ZM 10Q03ZN 10Q03ZP 10Q03ZQ 10Q03ZR 10Q03ZS 10Q03ZT 10Q03ZV 10Q03ZY 10Q04YE 10Q04YF 10Q04YG 10Q04YH 10Q04YJ 10Q04YK 10Q04YL 10Q04YM 10Q04YN 10Q04YP 10Q04YQ 10Q04YR 10Q04YS 10Q04YT 10Q04YV 10Q04YY 10Q04ZE 10Q04ZF 10Q04ZG 10Q04ZH 10Q04ZJ 10Q04ZK 10Q04ZL 10Q04ZM 10Q04ZN 10Q04ZP 10Q04ZQ 10Q04ZR 10Q04ZS 10Q04ZT 10Q04ZV 10Q04ZY 10Q07YE 10Q07YF 10Q07YG 10Q07YH 10Q07YJ 10Q07YK 10Q07YL 10Q07YM 10Q07YN 10Q07YP 10Q07YQ 10Q07YR 10Q07YS 10Q07YT 10Q07YV 10Q07YY 10Q07ZE 10Q07ZF 10Q07ZG 10Q07ZH 10Q07ZJ 10Q07ZK 10Q07ZL 10Q07ZM 10Q07ZN 10Q07ZP 10Q07ZQ 10Q07ZR 10Q07ZS 10Q07ZT 10Q07ZV 10Q07ZY 10Q08YE 10Q08YF 10Q08YG 10Q08YH 10Q08YJ 10Q08YK 10Q08YL 10Q08YM 10Q08YN 10Q08YP 10Q08YQ 10Q08YR 10Q08YS 10Q08YT 10Q08YV 10Q08YY 10Q08ZE 10Q08ZF 10Q08ZG 10Q08ZH 10Q08ZJ 10Q08ZK 10Q08ZL 10Q08ZM 10Q08ZN 10Q08ZP 10Q08ZQ 10Q08ZR 10Q08ZS 10Q08ZT 10Q08ZV 10Q08ZY

1 Obstetrics
0 Pregnancy
S Reposition: Moving to its normal location, or other suitable location, all or a portion of a body part

Body Part Character 4	Approach Character 5	Device Character 6	Qualifier Character 7
0 Products of Conception ♀	**7** Via Natural or Artificial Opening **X** External	**Z** No Device	**Z** No Qualifier
2 Products of Conception, Ectopic ♀	**0** Open **3** Percutaneous **4** Percutaneous Endoscopic **7** Via Natural or Artificial Opening **8** Via Natural or Artificial Opening Endoscopic	**Z** No Device	**Z** No Qualifier

♀ 10S07ZZ 10S0XZZ 10S20ZZ 10S23ZZ 10S24ZZ 10S27ZZ 10S28ZZ

1 Obstetrics
0 Pregnancy
T Resection: Cutting out or off, without replacement, all of a body part

Body Part Character 4	Approach Character 5	Device Character 6	Qualifier Character 7
2 Products of Conception, Ectopic ♀	**0** Open **3** Percutaneous **4** Percutaneous Endoscopic **7** Via Natural or Artificial Opening **8** Via Natural or Artificial Opening Endoscopic	**Z** No Device	**Z** No Qualifier

♀ 10T20ZZ 10T23ZZ 10T24ZZ 10T27ZZ 10T28ZZ

1 Obstetrics
0 Pregnancy
Y Transplantation: Putting in or on all or a portion of a living body part taken from another individual or animal to physically take the place and/or function of all or a portion of a similar body part

Body Part Character 4	Approach Character 5	Device Character 6	Qualifier Character 7
0 Products of Conception ♀	**3** Percutaneous **4** Percutaneous Endoscopic **7** Via Natural or Artificial Opening	**Z** No Device	**E** Nervous System **F** Cardiovascular System **G** Lymphatics and Hemic **H** Eye **J** Ear, Nose and Sinus **K** Respiratory System **L** Mouth and Throat **M** Gastrointestinal System **N** Hepatobiliary and Pancreas **P** Endocrine System **Q** Skin **R** Musculoskeletal System **S** Urinary System **T** Female Reproductive System **V** Male Reproductive System **Y** Other Body System

♀ 10Y03ZE 10Y03ZF 10Y03ZG 10Y03ZH 10Y03ZJ 10Y03ZK 10Y03ZL 10Y03ZM 10Y03ZN 10Y03ZP 10Y03ZQ 10Y03ZR 10Y03ZS 10Y03ZT 10Y03ZV 10Y03ZY 10Y04ZE 10Y04ZF 10Y04ZG 10Y04ZH 10Y04ZJ 10Y04ZK 10Y04ZL 10Y04ZM 10Y04ZN 10Y04ZP 10Y04ZQ 10Y04ZR 10Y04ZS 10Y04ZT 10Y04ZV 10Y04ZY 10Y07ZE 10Y07ZF 10Y07ZG 10Y07ZH 10Y07ZJ 10Y07ZK 10Y07ZL 10Y07ZM 10Y07ZN 10Y07ZP 10Y07ZQ 10Y07ZR 10Y07ZS 10Y07ZT 10Y07ZV 10Y07ZY

NOTES

NOTES

Body Section - 2 values

W = anatomical regions ⇒ chest wall, hindquarter, upper leg

Y = anatomical orifices ⇒ ear, mouth, pharynx, male genital tract

Root Operation (3rd character) include change or removal

all performed w/o making an incision or puncture

Device - placed during the procedure

- off the shelf & do not require any extensive design, fabrication, or fitting - includes casts for fractures
- If extensive design, fabrication or fitting needed - code in rehabilitation section as device fitting

Procedures for putting a device in or on a body region for protection, immobilization, stretching, compression or packing

Placement-Anatomical Regions 2W0-2W6

2 Placement
W Anatomical Regions
0 Change: Taking out or off a device from a body part and putting back an identical or similar device in or on the same body part without cutting or puncturing the skin or a mucous membrane

Body Region Character 4	Approach Character 5	Device Character 6	Qualifier Character 7
0 Head **2** Neck **3** Abdominal Wall **4** Chest Wall **5** Back **6** Inguinal Region, Right **7** Inguinal Region, Left **8** Upper Extremity, Right **9** Upper Extremity, Left **A** Upper Arm, Right **B** Upper Arm, Left **C** Lower Arm, Right **D** Lower Arm, Left **E** Hand, Right **F** Hand, Left **G** Thumb, Right **H** Thumb, Left **J** Finger, Right **K** Finger, Left **L** Lower Extremity, Right **M** Lower Extremity, Left **N** Upper Leg, Right **P** Upper Leg, Left **Q** Lower Leg, Right **R** Lower Leg, Left **S** Foot, Right **T** Foot, Left **U** Toe, Right **V** Toe, Left	**X** External - directly on the skin - directly on the mucus membrane - indirectly by applying external force through skin - indirectly by applying external force through mucus membrane	**0** Traction Apparatus **1** Splint **2** Cast **3** Brace **4** Bandage **5** Packing Material **6** Pressure Dressing **7** Intermittent Pressure Device **Y** Other Device	**Z** No Qualifier
1 Face	**X** External	**0** Traction Apparatus **1** Splint **2** Cast **3** Brace **4** Bandage **5** Packing Material **6** Pressure Dressing **7** Intermittent Pressure Device **9** Wire **Y** Other Device	**Z** No Qualifier

2 Placement
W Anatomical Regions
1 Compression: Putting pressure on a body region

Body Region	Approach	Device	Qualifier
Character 4	Character 5	Character 6	Character 7
0 Head 1 Face 2 Neck 3 Abdominal Wall 4 Chest Wall 5 Back 6 Inguinal Region, Right 7 Inguinal Region, Left 8 Upper Extremity, Right 9 Upper Extremity, Left A Upper Arm, Right B Upper Arm, Left C Lower Arm, Right D Lower Arm, Left E Hand, Right F Hand, Left G Thumb, Right H Thumb, Left J Finger, Right K Finger, Left L Lower Extremity, Right M Lower Extremity, Left N Upper Leg, Right P Upper Leg, Left Q Lower Leg, Right R Lower Leg, Left S Foot, Right T Foot, Left U Toe, Right V Toe, Left	X External	6 Pressure Dressing 7 Intermittent Pressure Device	Z No Qualifier

2 **Placement**
W **Anatomical Regions**
2 **Dressing:** Putting material on a body region for protection

Body Region Character 4	Approach Character 5	Device Character 6	Qualifier Character 7
0 Head **1** Face **2** Neck **3** Abdominal Wall **4** Chest Wall **5** Back **6** Inguinal Region, Right **7** Inguinal Region, Left **8** Upper Extremity, Right **9** Upper Extremity, Left **A** Upper Arm, Right **B** Upper Arm, Left **C** Lower Arm, Right **D** Lower Arm, Left **E** Hand, Right **F** Hand, Left **G** Thumb, Right **H** Thumb, Left **J** Finger, Right **K** Finger, Left **L** Lower Extremity, Right **M** Lower Extremity, Left **N** Upper Leg, Right **P** Upper Leg, Left **Q** Lower Leg, Right **R** Lower Leg, Left **S** Foot, Right **T** Foot, Left **U** Toe, Right **V** Toe, Left	**X** External	**4** Bandage	**Z** No Qualifier

2 Placement
W Anatomical Regions
3 Immobilization: Limiting or preventing motion of a body region

Body Region Character 4	Approach Character 5	Device Character 6	Qualifier Character 7
0 Head **2** Neck **3** Abdominal Wall **4** Chest Wall **5** Back **6** Inguinal Region, Right **7** Inguinal Region, Left **8** Upper Extremity, Right **9** Upper Extremity, Left **A** Upper Arm, Right **B** Upper Arm, Left **C** Lower Arm, Right **D** Lower Arm, Left **E** Hand, Right **F** Hand, Left **G** Thumb, Right **H** Thumb, Left **J** Finger, Right **K** Finger, Left **L** Lower Extremity, Right **M** Lower Extremity, Left **N** Upper Leg, Right **P** Upper Leg, Left **Q** Lower Leg, Right **R** Lower Leg, Left **S** Foot, Right **T** Foot, Left **U** Toe, Right **V** Toe, Left	**X** External	**1** Splint **2** Cast **3** Brace **Y** Other Device	**Z** No Qualifier
1 Face	**X** External	**1** Splint **2** Cast **3** Brace **9** Wire **Y** Other Device	**Z** No Qualifier

2 Placement
W Anatomical Regions
4 Packing: Putting material in a body region or orifice

Body Region	Approach	Device	Qualifier
Character 4	Character 5	Character 6	Character 7
0 Head **1** Face **2** Neck **3** Abdominal Wall **4** Chest Wall **5** Back **6** Inguinal Region, Right **7** Inguinal Region, Left **8** Upper Extremity, Right **9** Upper Extremity, Left **A** Upper Arm, Right **B** Upper Arm, Left **C** Lower Arm, Right **D** Lower Arm, Left **E** Hand, Right **F** Hand, Left **G** Thumb, Right **H** Thumb, Left **J** Finger, Right **K** Finger, Left **L** Lower Extremity, Right **M** Lower Extremity, Left **N** Upper Leg, Right **P** Upper Leg, Left **Q** Lower Leg, Right **R** Lower Leg, Left **S** Foot, Right **T** Foot, Left **U** Toe, Right **V** Toe, Left	**X** External	**5** Packing Material	**Z** No Qualifier

2 Placement
W Anatomical Regions
5 Removal: Taking out or off a device from a body part

Body Region Character 4	Approach Character 5	Device Character 6	Qualifier Character 7
0 Head **2** Neck **3** Abdominal Wall **4** Chest Wall **5** Back **6** Inguinal Region, Right **7** Inguinal Region, Left **8** Upper Extremity, Right > If not more specified **9** Upper Extremity, Left **A** Upper Arm, Right > shoulder **B** Upper Arm, Left **C** Lower Arm, Right **D** Lower Arm, Left **E** Hand, Right **F** Hand, Left **G** Thumb, Right **H** Thumb, Left **J** Finger, Right **K** Finger, Left **L** Lower Extremity, Right **M** Lower Extremity, Left **N** Upper Leg, Right **P** Upper Leg, Left **Q** Lower Leg, Right **R** Lower Leg, Left **S** Foot, Right **T** Foot, Left **U** Toe, Right **V** Toe, Left	**X** External	**0** Traction Apparatus **1** Splint **2** Cast **3** Brace **4** Bandage **5** Packing Material **6** Pressure Dressing **7** Intermittent Pressure Device **Y** Other Device	**Z** No Qualifier
1 Face	**X** External	**0** Traction Apparatus **1** Splint **2** Cast **3** Brace **4** Bandage **5** Packing Material **6** Pressure Dressing **7** Intermittent Pressure Device **9** Wire **Y** Other Device	**Z** No Qualifier

2 Placement
W Anatomical Regions
6 Traction: Exerting a pulling force on a body region in a distal direction

Body Region	Approach	Device	Qualifier
Character 4	Character 5	Character 6	Character 7
0 Head 1 Face 2 Neck 3 Abdominal Wall 4 Chest Wall 5 Back 6 Inguinal Region, Right 7 Inguinal Region, Left 8 Upper Extremity, Right 9 Upper Extremity, Left A Upper Arm, Right B Upper Arm, Left C Lower Arm, Right D Lower Arm, Left E Hand, Right F Hand, Left G Thumb, Right H Thumb, Left J Finger, Right K Finger, Left L Lower Extremity, Right M Lower Extremity, Left N Upper Leg, Right P Upper Leg, Left Q Lower Leg, Right R Lower Leg, Left S Foot, Right T Foot, Left U Toe, Right V Toe, Left	X External	0 Traction Apparatus Z No Device	Z No Qualifier

NOTES

Placement-Anatomical Orifices 2Y0-2Y5

2 Placement
Y Anatomical Orifices
0 Change: Taking out or off a device from a body part and putting back an identical or similar device in or on the same body part without cutting or puncturing the skin or a mucous membrane

Body Region	Approach	Device	Qualifier
Character 4	**Character 5**	**Character 6**	**Character 7**
0 Mouth and Pharynx **1** Nasal **2** Ear **3** Anorectal **4** Female Genital Tract ♀ vaginal **5** Urethra	**X** External	**5** Packing Material	**Z** No Qualifier

♀ 2Y04X5Z

2 Placement
Y Anatomical Orifices
4 Packing: Putting material in a body region or orifice

Body Region	Approach	Device	Qualifier
Character 4	**Character 5**	**Character 6**	**Character 7**
0 Mouth and Pharynx **1** Nasal **2** Ear **3** Anorectal **4** Female Genital Tract ♀ **5** Urethra	**X** External	**5** Packing Material	**Z** No Qualifier

♀ 2Y44X5Z

2 Placement
Y Anatomical Orifices
5 Removal: Taking out or off a device from a body part

Body Region	Approach	Device	Qualifier
Character 4	**Character 5**	**Character 6**	**Character 7**
0 Mouth and Pharynx **1** Nasal **2** Ear **3** Anorectal **4** Female Genital Tract ♀ **5** Urethra	**X** External	**5** Packing Material	**Z** No Qualifier

♀ 2Y54X5Z

NOTES

Body System (2nd character) - only 3 options

- Circulatory - transfusion
- Indwelling Device - Irrigation
- Physiological Systems / Anatomical Regions - administering drugs & other substances

2 types of central lines
1) PICC
2) Port A Cath

Body System / Region (4th character)

- where substance is administered, NOT where it takes effect
- Peripheral Artery / Vein - typically used for Chemo, percutaneous approach
- Implanted device for chemo into central artery / vein, not peripheral
- PICC - Peripherally Inserted Central Catheter - catheter 1st inserted into peripheral vein & advanced to central vein, ex: superior vena cava
- Central Artery / Vein typically used when the site where the substance is introduced is distant from the point of entry.
  Ex: Clot - introduction of a thrombolytic substance into a central artery / vein, percutaneous - usually local effect

AKA - Port A-Cath

Approach (5th character)

percutaneous (through the skin) includes intradermal, Sub-Q, & intramuscular (IM). Also catheter placed into an internal site w/in circulatory system.
Ex: catheter for heart angiography as contrast is placed into heart

Sclerotherapy - treat blood vessels malformations. Ex: varicose veins
Insert chemical substance - sclerosant to cause damage to internal lining of vein, causing scarring & forces blood to reroute to a healthier vein, thus the vein collapses & absorbs into tissue
may use alcohol injection

pleural cavity — talc prevent adhesion of 2 pleurae

Pleurodesis - pleural space is artificially obliterated (destroy)
Done to prevent recurrence of pneumothorax or pleural effusion to prevent fluid buildup. DO NOT USE Destruction (5) or Destructive Agent (T) Use INTRODUCTION 0 & THERAPEUTIC AGENT (G)

Peritoneal Dialysis - use IRRIGATION - catheter is inserted into peritoneal cavity (left in place) & use cleaning solution called dialysate (has H_2O, dextrose, electrolytes) to clean blood.

Putting in/on therapeutic, prophylactic, protective, diagnostic, nutritional, or physiological substance Includes: transfusions, injections, infusions irrigations & tattooing

Administration 302-3E1

3 Administration
0 Circulatory
2 Transfusion: Putting in blood or blood products

Body System / Region	Approach	Substance	Qualifier
Character 4	**Character 5**	**Character 6**	**Character 7**
3 Peripheral Vein NC DRG **4** Central Vein NC DRG	**0** Open **3** Percutaneous	**A** Stem Cells, Embryonic	**Z** No Qualifier
3 Peripheral Vein NC DRG **4** Central Vein NC DRG	**0** Open **3** Percutaneous	**G** Bone Marrow **X** Stem Cells, Cord Blood **Y** Stem Cells, Hematopoietic	**0** Autologous **2** Allogeneic, Related **3** Allogeneic, Unrelated **4** Allogeneic, Unspecified
3 Peripheral Vein **4** Central Vein	**0** Open **3** Percutaneous	**H** Whole Blood **J** Serum Albumin **K** Frozen Plasma **L** Fresh Plasma **M** Plasma Cryoprecipitate **N** Red Blood Cells **P** Frozen Red Cells **Q** White Cells **R** Platelets **S** Globulin **T** Fibrinogen **V** Antihemophilic Factors **W** Factor IX	**0** Autologous **1** Nonautologous
3 Peripheral Vein **4** Central Vein	**0** Open **3** Percutaneous	**U** Stem Cells, T-cell Depleted Hematopoietic	**2** Allogeneic, Related **3** Allogeneic, Unrelated **4** Allogeneic, Unspecified
7 Products of Conception, Circulatory ♀	**3** Percutaneous **7** Via Natural or Artificial Opening	**H** Whole Blood **J** Serum Albumin **K** Frozen Plasma **L** Fresh Plasma **M** Plasma Cryoprecipitate **N** Red Blood Cells **P** Frozen Red Cells **Q** White Cells **R** Platelets **S** Globulin **T** Fibrinogen **V** Antihemophilic Factors **W** Factor IX	**1** Nonautologous
8 Vein	**0** Open **3** Percutaneous	**B** 4-Factor Prothrombin Complex Concentrate	**1** Nonautologous

♀ 30273H1 30273J1 30273K1 30273L1 30273M1 30273N1 30273P1 30273Q1 30273R1 30273S1 30273T1 30273V1 30273W1 30277H1 30277J1 30277K1 30277L1 30277M1 30277N1 30277P1 30277Q1 30277R1 30277S1 30277T1 30277V1 30277W1

NC 30230AZ 30230G0 30230Y0 30233AZ 30233G0 30233Y0 30240AZ 30240G0 30240Y0 30243AZ 30243G0 30243Y0
Codes in this list are noncovered procedures only when reported with C91.00, C92.00, C92.10, C92.11, C92.40, C92.50, C92.60, C92.A0, C93.00, C94.00, C95.00 as either a principal or secondary diagnosis.

DRG 30233AZ 30233G0 30233X0 30233Y0 30243AZ 30243G0 30243X0 30243Y0

3 Administration
C Indwelling Device
1 Irrigation: Putting in or on a cleansing substance

Body System / Region	Approach	Substance	Qualifier
Character 4	**Character 5**	**Character 6**	**Character 7**
Z None	**X** External	**8** Irrigating Substance	**Z** No Qualifier

3 Administration
E Physiological Systems and Anatomical Regions
0 Introduction: Putting in or on a therapeutic, diagnostic, nutritional, physiological, or prophylactic substance except blood or blood products

Body System / Region Character 4	Approach Character 5	Substance Character 6	Qualifier Character 7
0 Skin and Mucous Membranes	**X** External	**0** Antineoplastic	**5** Other Antineoplastic **M** Monoclonal Antibody
0 Skin and Mucous Membranes	**X** External	**2** Anti-infective	**8** Oxazolidinones **9** Other Anti-infective
0 Skin and Mucous Membranes	**X** External	**3** Anti-inflammatory **4** Serum, Toxoid and Vaccine **B** Anesthetic Agent **K** Other Diagnostic Substance **M** Pigment **N** Analgesics, Hypnotics, Sedatives **T** Destructive Agent	**Z** No Qualifier
0 Skin and Mucous Membranes	**X** External	**G** Other Therapeutic Substance	**C** Other Substance
1 Subcutaneous Tissue	**0** Open	**2** Anti-infective	**A** Anti-Infective Envelope
1 Subcutaneous Tissue	**3** Percutaneous	**0** Antineoplastic	**5** Other Antineoplastic **M** Monoclonal Antibody
1 Subcutaneous Tissue	**3** Percutaneous	**2** Anti-infective	**8** Oxazolidinones **9** Other Anti-infective **A** Anti-Infective Envelope
1 Subcutaneous Tissue	**3** Percutaneous	**3** Anti-inflammatory **6** Nutritional Substance **7** Electrolytic and Water Balance Substance **B** Anesthetic Agent **H** Radioactive Substance **K** Other Diagnostic Substance **N** Analgesics, Hypnotics, Sedatives **T** Destructive Agent	**Z** No Qualifier
1 Subcutaneous Tissue	**3** Percutaneous	**4** Serum, Toxoid and Vaccine	**0** Influenza Vaccine **Z** No Qualifier
1 Subcutaneous Tissue	**3** Percutaneous	**G** Other Therapeutic Substance	**C** Other Substance
1 Subcutaneous Tissue	**3** Percutaneous	**V** Hormone	**G** Insulin **J** Other Hormone
2 Muscle	**3** Percutaneous	**0** Antineoplastic	**5** Other Antineoplastic **M** Monoclonal Antibody
2 Muscle	**3** Percutaneous	**2** Anti-infective	**8** Oxazolidinones **9** Other Anti-infective
2 Muscle	**3** Percutaneous	**3** Anti-inflammatory **6** Nutritional Substance **7** Electrolytic and Water Balance Substance **B** Anesthetic Agent **H** Radioactive Substance **K** Other Diagnostic Substance **N** Analgesics, Hypnotics, Sedatives **T** Destructive Agent	**Z** No Qualifier
2 Muscle	**3** Percutaneous	**4** Serum, Toxoid and Vaccine	**0** Influenza Vaccine **Z** No Qualifier
2 Muscle	**3** Percutaneous	**G** Other Therapeutic Substance	**C** Other Substance
3 Peripheral Vein DRG	**0** Open	**0** Antineoplastic	**2** High-dose Interleukin-2 **3** Low-dose Interleukin-2 **5** Other Antineoplastic **M** Monoclonal Antibody **P** Clofarabine

3E0 continued on next page

3 Administration
E Physiological Systems and Anatomical Regions
0 Introduction: Putting in or on a therapeutic, diagnostic, nutritional, physiological, or prophylactic substance except blood or blood products

3E0 continued from previous page

Body System / Region	Approach	Substance	Qualifier
Character 4	Character 5	Character 6	Character 7
3 Peripheral Vein DRG	0 Open	1 Thrombolytic	6 Recombinant Human-activated Protein C 7 Other Thrombolytic
3 Peripheral Vein	0 Open	2 Anti-infective	8 Oxazolidinones 9 Other Anti-infective
3 Peripheral Vein	0 Open	3 Anti-inflammatory 4 Serum, Toxoid and Vaccine 6 Nutritional Substance 7 Electrolytic and Water Balance Substance F Intracirculatory Anesthetic H Radioactive Substance K Other Diagnostic Substance N Analgesics, Hypnotics, Sedatives P Platelet Inhibitor R Antiarrhythmic T Destructive Agent X Vasopressor	Z No Qualifier
3 Peripheral Vein	0 Open	G Other Therapeutic Substance	C Other Substance N Blood Brain Barrier Disruption
3 Peripheral Vein DRG	0 Open	U Pancreatic Islet Cells	0 Autologous 1 Nonautologous
3 Peripheral Vein	0 Open	V Hormone	G Insulin H Human B -type Natriuretic Peptide J Other Hormone
3 Peripheral Vein	0 Open	W Immunotherapeutic	K Immunostimulator L Immunosuppressive
3 Peripheral Vein DRG	3 Percutaneous	0 Antineoplastic	2 High-dose Interleukin-2 3 Low-dose Interleukin-2 5 Other Antineoplastic M Monoclonal Antibody P Clofarabine
3 Peripheral Vein DRG	3 Percutaneous	1 Thrombolytic	6 Recombinant Human-activated Protein C 7 Other Thrombolytic
3 Peripheral Vein	3 Percutaneous	2 Anti-infective	8 Oxazolidinones 9 Other Anti-infective
3 Peripheral Vein	3 Percutaneous	3 Anti-inflammatory 4 Serum, Toxoid and Vaccine 6 Nutritional Substance 7 Electrolytic and Water Balance Substance F Intracirculatory Anesthetic H Radioactive Substance K Other Diagnostic Substance N Analgesics, Hypnotics, Sedatives P Platelet Inhibitor R Antiarrhythmic T Destructive Agent X Vasopressor	Z No Qualifier
3 Peripheral Vein	3 Percutaneous	G Other Therapeutic Substance	C Other Substance N Blood Brain Barrier Disruption Q Glucarpidase

3E0 continued on next page

3E0 continued from previous page

3 Administration
E Physiological Systems and Anatomical Regions
0 Introduction: Putting in or on a therapeutic, diagnostic, nutritional, physiological, or prophylactic substance except blood or blood products

Body System / Region Character 4	Approach Character 5	Substance Character 6	Qualifier Character 7
3 Peripheral Vein DRG	**3** Percutaneous	**U** Pancreatic Islet Cells	**0** Autologous **1** Nonautologous
3 Peripheral Vein	**3** Percutaneous	**V** Hormone	**G** Insulin **H** Human B-type Natriuretic Peptide **J** Other Hormone
3 Peripheral Vein	**3** Percutaneous	**W** Immunotherapeutic	**K** Immunostimulator **L** Immunosuppressive
4 Central Vein DRG	**0** Open	**0** Antineoplastic	**2** High-dose Interleukin-2 **3** Low-dose Interleukin-2 **5** Other Antineoplastic **M** Monoclonal Antibody **P** Clofarabine
4 Central Vein DRG	**0** Open	**1** Thrombolytic	**6** Recombinant Human-activated Protein C **7** Other Thrombolytic
4 Central Vein	**0** Open	**2** Anti-infective	**8** Oxazolidinones **9** Other Anti-infective
4 Central Vein	**0** Open	**3** Anti-inflammatory **4** Serum, Toxoid and Vaccine **6** Nutritional Substance **7** Electrolytic and Water Balance Substance **F** Intracirculatory Anesthetic **H** Radioactive Substance **K** Other Diagnostic Substance **N** Analgesics, Hypnotics, Sedatives **P** Platelet Inhibitor **R** Antiarrhythmic **T** Destructive Agent **X** Vasopressor	**Z** No Qualifier
4 Central Vein	**0** Open	**G** Other Therapeutic Substance	**C** Other Substance **N** Blood Brain Barrier Disruption
4 Central Vein	**0** Open	**V** Hormone	**G** Insulin **H** Human B-type Natriuretic Peptide **J** Other Hormone
4 Central Vein	**0** Open	**W** Immunotherapeutic	**K** Immunostimulator **L** Immunosuppressive
4 Central Vein DRG	**3** Percutaneous	**0** Antineoplastic	**2** High-dose Interleukin-2 **3** Low-dose Interleukin-2 **5** Other Antineoplastic **M** Monoclonal Antibody **P** Clofarabine
4 Central Vein DRG	**3** Percutaneous	**1** Thrombolytic	**6** Recombinant Human-activated Protein C **7** Other Thrombolytic
4 Central Vein	**3** Percutaneous	**2** Anti-infective	**8** Oxazolidinones **9** Other Anti-infective

3E0 continued on next page

LC Limited Coverage NC Noncovered HAC HAC-associated Procedure CC Combination Cluster - See Appendix G for code lists
DRG Non-OR-Affecting MS-DRG Assignment New/Revised Text in **Orange** ♂ Male ♀ Female

3 **Administration**
E **Physiological Systems and Anatomical Regions**
0 **Introduction:** Putting in or on a therapeutic, diagnostic, nutritional, physiological, or prophylactic substance except blood or blood products

3E0 continued from previous page

Body System / Region Character 4	Approach Character 5	Substance Character 6	Qualifier Character 7
4 Central Vein	3 Percutaneous	3 Anti-inflammatory 4 Serum, Toxoid and Vaccine 6 Nutritional Substance 7 Electrolytic and Water Balance Substance F Intracirculatory Anesthetic H Radioactive Substance K Other Diagnostic Substance N Analgesics, Hypnotics, Sedatives P Platelet Inhibitor R Antiarrhythmic T Destructive Agent X Vasopressor	Z No Qualifier
4 Central Vein	3 Percutaneous	G Other Therapeutic Substance	C Other Substance N Blood Brain Barrier Disruption Q Glucarpidase
4 Central Vein	3 Percutaneous	V Hormone	G Insulin H Human B-type Natriuretic Peptide J Other Hormone
4 Central Vein	3 Percutaneous	W Immunotherapeutic	K Immunostimulator L Immunosuppressive
5 Peripheral Artery DRG 6 Central Artery DRG	0 Open 3 Percutaneous	0 Antineoplastic	2 High-dose Interleukin-2 3 Low-dose Interleukin-2 5 Other Antineoplastic M Monoclonal Antibody P Clofarabine
5 Peripheral Artery DRG 6 Central Artery DRG	0 Open 3 Percutaneous	1 Thrombolytic	6 Recombinant Human-activated Protein C 7 Other Thrombolytic
5 Peripheral Artery 6 Central Artery	0 Open 3 Percutaneous	2 Anti-infective	8 Oxazolidinones 9 Other Anti-infective
5 Peripheral Artery 6 Central Artery	0 Open 3 Percutaneous	3 Anti-inflammatory 4 Serum, Toxoid and Vaccine 6 Nutritional Substance 7 Electrolytic and Water Balance Substance F Intracirculatory Anesthetic H Radioactive Substance K Other Diagnostic Substance N Analgesics, Hypnotics, Sedatives P Platelet Inhibitor R Antiarrhythmic T Destructive Agent X Vasopressor	Z No Qualifier
5 Peripheral Artery 6 Central Artery	0 Open 3 Percutaneous	G Other Therapeutic Substance	C Other Substance N Blood Brain Barrier Disruption
5 Peripheral Artery 6 Central Artery	0 Open 3 Percutaneous	V Hormone	G Insulin H Human B-type Natriuretic Peptide J Other Hormone
5 Peripheral Artery 6 Central Artery	0 Open 3 Percutaneous	W Immunotherapeutic	K Immunostimulator L Immunosuppressive

3E0 continued on next page

3E0 continued from previous page

3 Administration
E Physiological Systems and Anatomical Regions
0 Introduction: Putting in or on a therapeutic, diagnostic, nutritional, physiological, or prophylactic substance except blood or blood products

Body System / Region Character 4	Approach Character 5	Substance Character 6	Qualifier Character 7
7 Coronary Artery 8 Heart DRG	0 Open 3 Percutaneous	1 Thrombolytic	6 Recombinant Human-activated Protein C 7 Other Thrombolytic
7 Coronary Artery 8 Heart	0 Open 3 Percutaneous	G Other Therapeutic Substance	C Other Substance
7 Coronary Artery 8 Heart	0 Open 3 Percutaneous	K Other Diagnostic Substance P Platelet Inhibitor	Z No Qualifier
7 Coronary Artery 8 Heart	4 Percutaneous Endoscopic	G Other Therapeutic Substance	C Other Substance
9 Nose	3 Percutaneous 7 Via Natural or Artificial Opening X External	0 Antineoplastic	5 Other Antineoplastic M Monoclonal Antibody
9 Nose	3 Percutaneous 7 Via Natural or Artificial Opening X External	2 Anti-infective	8 Oxazolidinones 9 Other Anti-infective
9 Nose	3 Percutaneous 7 Via Natural or Artificial Opening X External	3 Anti-inflammatory 4 Serum, Toxoid and Vaccine B Anesthetic Agent H Radioactive Substance K Other Diagnostic Substance N Analgesics, Hypnotics, Sedatives T Destructive Agent	Z No Qualifier
9 Nose	3 Percutaneous 7 Via Natural or Artificial Opening X External	G Other Therapeutic Substance	C Other Substance
A Bone Marrow	3 Percutaneous	0 Antineoplastic	5 Other Antineoplastic M Monoclonal Antibody
A Bone Marrow	3 Percutaneous	G Other Therapeutic Substance	C Other Substance
B Ear	3 Percutaneous 7 Via Natural or Artificial Opening X External	0 Antineoplastic	4 Liquid Brachytherapy Radioisotope 5 Other Antineoplastic M Monoclonal Antibody
B Ear	3 Percutaneous 7 Via Natural or Artificial Opening X External	2 Anti-infective	8 Oxazolidinones 9 Other Anti-infective
B Ear	3 Percutaneous 7 Via Natural or Artificial Opening X External	3 Anti-inflammatory B Anesthetic Agent H Radioactive Substance K Other Diagnostic Substance N Analgesics, Hypnotics, Sedatives T Destructive Agent	Z No Qualifier
B Ear	3 Percutaneous 7 Via Natural or Artificial Opening X External	G Other Therapeutic Substance	C Other Substance
C Eye	3 Percutaneous 7 Via Natural or Artificial Opening X External	0 Antineoplastic	4 Liquid Brachytherapy Radioisotope 5 Other Antineoplastic M Monoclonal Antibody
C Eye	3 Percutaneous 7 Via Natural or Artificial Opening X External	2 Anti-infective	8 Oxazolidinones 9 Other Anti-infective

3E0 continued on next page

3E0 continued from previous page

3 Administration
E Physiological Systems and Anatomical Regions
0 Introduction: Putting in or on a therapeutic, diagnostic, nutritional, physiological, or prophylactic substance except blood or blood products

Body System / Region Character 4	Approach Character 5	Substance Character 6	Qualifier Character 7
C Eye	**3** Percutaneous **7** Via Natural or Artificial Opening **X** External	**3** Anti-inflammatory **B** Anesthetic Agent **H** Radioactive Substance **K** Other Diagnostic Substance **M** Pigment **N** Analgesics, Hypnotics, Sedatives **T** Destructive Agent	**Z** No Qualifier
C Eye	**3** Percutaneous **7** Via Natural or Artificial Opening **X** External	**G** Other Therapeutic Substance	**C** Other Substance
C Eye	**3** Percutaneous **7** Via Natural or Artificial Opening **X** External	**S** Gas	**F** Other Gas
D Mouth and Pharynx	**3** Percutaneous **7** Via Natural or Artificial Opening **X** External	**0** Antineoplastic	**4** Liquid Brachytherapy Radioisotope **5** Other Antineoplastic **M** Monoclonal Antibody
D Mouth and Pharynx	**3** Percutaneous **7** Via Natural or Artificial Opening **X** External	**2** Anti-infective	**8** Oxazolidinones **9** Other Anti-infective
D Mouth and Pharynx	**3** Percutaneous **7** Via Natural or Artificial Opening **X** External	**3** Anti-inflammatory **4** Serum, Toxoid and Vaccine **6** Nutritional Substance **7** Electrolytic and Water Balance Substance **B** Anesthetic Agent **H** Radioactive Substance **K** Other Diagnostic Substance **N** Analgesics, Hypnotics, Sedatives **R** Antiarrhythmic **T** Destructive Agent	**Z** No Qualifier
D Mouth and Pharynx	**3** Percutaneous **7** Via Natural or Artificial Opening **X** External	**G** Other Therapeutic Substance	**C** Other Substance
E Products of Conception ♀ **G** Upper GI **H** Lower GI **K** Genitourinary Tract **N** Male Reproductive ♂	**3** Percutaneous **7** Via Natural or Artificial Opening **8** Via Natural or Artificial Opening Endoscopic	**0** Antineoplastic	**4** Liquid Brachytherapy Radioisotope **5** Other Antineoplastic **M** Monoclonal Antibody
E Products of Conception ♀ **G** Upper GI **H** Lower GI **K** Genitourinary Tract **N** Male Reproductive ♂	**3** Percutaneous **7** Via Natural or Artificial Opening **8** Via Natural or Artificial Opening Endoscopic	**2** Anti-infective	**8** Oxazolidinones **9** Other Anti-infective
E Products of Conception ♀ **G** Upper GI **H** Lower GI **K** Genitourinary Tract **N** Male Reproductive ♂	**3** Percutaneous **7** Via Natural or Artificial Opening **8** Via Natural or Artificial Opening Endoscopic	**3** Anti-inflammatory **6** Nutritional Substance **7** Electrolytic and Water Balance Substance **B** Anesthetic Agent **H** Radioactive Substance **K** Other Diagnostic Substance **N** Analgesics, Hypnotics, Sedatives **T** Destructive Agent	**Z** No Qualifier

3E0 continued on next page

3E0 continued from previous page

3 **Administration**
E **Physiological Systems and Anatomical Regions**
0 **Introduction:** Putting in or on a therapeutic, diagnostic, nutritional, physiological, or prophylactic substance except blood or blood products

Body System / Region Character 4	Approach Character 5	Substance Character 6	Qualifier Character 7
E Products of Conception ♀ **G** Upper GI **H** Lower GI **K** Genitourinary Tract **N** Male Reproductive ♂	**3** Percutaneous **7** Via Natural or Artificial Opening **8** Via Natural or Artificial Opening Endoscopic	**G** Other Therapeutic Substance	**C** Other Substance
E Products of Conception ♀ **G** Upper GI **H** Lower GI **K** Genitourinary Tract **N** Male Reproductive ♂	**3** Percutaneous **7** Via Natural or Artificial Opening **8** Via Natural or Artificial Opening Endoscopic	**S** Gas	**F** Other Gas
E Products of Conception ♀ **G** Upper GI **H** Lower GI **K** Genitourinary Tract **N** Male Reproductive ♂	**4** Percutaneous Endoscopic	**G** Other Therapeutic Substance	**C** Other Substance
F Respiratory Tract	**3** Percutaneous **7** Via Natural or Artificial Opening **8** Via Natural or Artificial Opening Endoscopic	**0** Antineoplastic	**4** Liquid Brachytherapy Radioisotope **5** Other Antineoplastic **M** Monoclonal Antibody
F Respiratory Tract	**3** Percutaneous **7** Via Natural or Artificial Opening **8** Via Natural or Artificial Opening Endoscopic	**2** Anti-infective	**8** Oxazolidinones **9** Other Anti-infective
F Respiratory Tract	**3** Percutaneous **7** Via Natural or Artificial Opening **8** Via Natural or Artificial Opening Endoscopic	**3** Anti-inflammatory **6** Nutritional Substance **7** Electrolytic and Water Balance Substance **B** Anesthetic Agent **H** Radioactive Substance **K** Other Diagnostic Substance **N** Analgesics, Hypnotics, Sedatives **T** Destructive Agent	**Z** No Qualifier
F Respiratory Tract	**3** Percutaneous **7** Via Natural or Artificial Opening **8** Via Natural or Artificial Opening Endoscopic	**G** Other Therapeutic Substance	**C** Other Substance
F Respiratory Tract	**3** Percutaneous **7** Via Natural or Artificial Opening **8** Via Natural or Artificial Opening Endoscopic	**S** Gas	**D** Nitric Oxide **F** Other Gas
F Respiratory Tract	**4** Percutaneous Endoscopic	**G** Other Therapeutic Substance	**C** Other Substance
J Biliary and Pancreatic Tract	**3** Percutaneous **7** Via Natural or Artificial Opening **8** Via Natural or Artificial Opening Endoscopic	**0** Antineoplastic	**4** Liquid Brachytherapy Radioisotope **5** Other Antineoplastic **M** Monoclonal Antibody
J Biliary and Pancreatic Tract	**3** Percutaneous **7** Via Natural or Artificial Opening **8** Via Natural or Artificial Opening Endoscopic	**2** Anti-infective	**8** Oxazolidinones **9** Other Anti-infective

3E0 continued on next page

Pleurodesis w/TALC + VATS = 3E0L4GC

3E0 continued from previous page

3 Administration
E Physiological Systems and Anatomical Regions
0 Introduction: Putting in or on a therapeutic, diagnostic, nutritional, physiological, or prophylactic substance except blood or blood products

Body System / Region Character 4	Approach Character 5	Substance Character 6	Qualifier Character 7
J Biliary and Pancreatic Tract	3 Percutaneous 7 Via Natural or Artificial Opening 8 Via Natural or Artificial Opening Endoscopic	3 Anti-inflammatory 6 Nutritional Substance 7 Electrolytic and Water Balance Substance B Anesthetic Agent H Radioactive Substance K Other Diagnostic Substance N Analgesics, Hypnotics, Sedatives T Destructive Agent	Z No Qualifier
J Biliary and Pancreatic Tract	3 Percutaneous 7 Via Natural or Artificial Opening 8 Via Natural or Artificial Opening Endoscopic	G Other Therapeutic Substance	C Other Substance
J Biliary and Pancreatic Tract	3 Percutaneous 7 Via Natural or Artificial Opening 8 Via Natural or Artificial Opening Endoscopic	S Gas	F Other Gas
J Biliary and Pancreatic Tract DRG	3 Percutaneous 7 Via Natural or Artificial Opening 8 Via Natural or Artificial Opening Endoscopic	U Pancreatic Islet Cells	0 Autologous 1 Nonautologous
J Biliary and Pancreatic Tract	4 Percutaneous Endoscopic	G Other Therapeutic Substance	C Other Substance
L Pleural Cavity	0 Open	5 Adhesion Barrier	Z No Qualifier
L Pleural Cavity	3 Percutaneous	0 Antineoplastic	4 Liquid Brachytherapy Radioisotope 5 Other Antineoplastic M Monoclonal Antibody
L Pleural Cavity R or L	3 Percutaneous	2 Anti-infective	8 Oxazolidinones 9 Other Anti-infective
L Pleural Cavity R or L	3 Percutaneous	3 Anti-inflammatory 5 Adhesion Barrier 6 Nutritional Substance 7 Electrolytic and Water Balance Substance B Anesthetic Agent H Radioactive Substance K Other Diagnostic Substance N Analgesics, Hypnotics, Sedatives T Destructive Agent	Z No Qualifier
L Pleural Cavity R or L	3 Percutaneous	G Other Therapeutic Substance TALC	C Other Substance
L Pleural Cavity	3 Percutaneous	S Gas	F Other Gas
L Pleural Cavity	4 Percutaneous Endoscopic	5 Adhesion Barrier	Z No Qualifier
L Pleural Cavity R or L	4 Percutaneous Endoscopic VATS	G Other Therapeutic Substance TALC	C Other Substance
L Pleural Cavity	7 Via Natural or Artificial Opening	0 Antineoplastic	4 Liquid Brachytherapy Radioisotope 5 Other Antineoplastic M Monoclonal Antibody
L Pleural Cavity	7 Via Natural or Artificial Opening	S Gas	F Other Gas
M Peritoneal Cavity	0 Open	5 Adhesion Barrier	Z No Qualifier

VATS - Video Assisted Thoracoscopic Surgery

3E0 continued on next page

OTHER THERAPEUTIC Substance: bleomycin, tetracycline, providone iodine, or slurry of Talc through chest drain

LC Limited Coverage NC Noncovered HAC HAC-associated Procedure CC Combination Cluster - See Appendix G for code lists
DRG Non-OR-Affecting MS-DRG Assignment New/Revised Text in **Orange** ♂ Male ♀ Female

3E0 continued from previous page

3 Administration
E Physiological Systems and Anatomical Regions
0 Introduction: Putting in or on a therapeutic, diagnostic, nutritional, physiological, or prophylactic substance except blood or blood products

Body System / Region Character 4	Approach Character 5	Substance Character 6	Qualifier Character 7
M Peritoneal Cavity	**3** Percutaneous	**0** Antineoplastic	**4** Liquid Brachytherapy Radioisotope **5** Other Antineoplastic **M** Monoclonal Antibody **Y** Hyperthermic
M Peritoneal Cavity	**3** Percutaneous	**2** Anti-infective	**8** Oxazolidinones **9** Other Anti-infective
M Peritoneal Cavity	**3** Percutaneous	**3** Anti-inflammatory **5** Adhesion Barrier **6** Nutritional Substance **7** Electrolytic and Water Balance Substance **B** Anesthetic Agent **H** Radioactive Substance **K** Other Diagnostic Substance **N** Analgesics, Hypnotics, Sedatives **T** Destructive Agent	**Z** No Qualifier
M Peritoneal Cavity	**3** Percutaneous	**G** Other Therapeutic Substance	**C** Other Substance
M Peritoneal Cavity	**3** Percutaneous	**S** Gas	**F** Other Gas
M Peritoneal Cavity	**4** Percutaneous Endoscopic	**5** Adhesion Barrier	**Z** No Qualifier
M Peritoneal Cavity	**4** Percutaneous Endoscopic	**G** Other Therapeutic Substance	**C** Other Substance
M Peritoneal Cavity	**7** Via Natural or Artificial Opening	**0** Antineoplastic	**4** Liquid Brachytherapy Radioisotope **5** Other Antineoplastic **M** Monoclonal Antibody
M Peritoneal Cavity	**7** Via Natural or Artificial Opening	**S** Gas	**F** Other Gas
P Female Reproductive ♀	**0** Open	**5** Adhesion Barrier	**Z** No Qualifier
P Female Reproductive ♀	**3** Percutaneous	**0** Antineoplastic	**4** Liquid Brachytherapy Radioisotope **5** Other Antineoplastic **M** Monoclonal Antibody
P Female Reproductive ♀	**3** Percutaneous	**2** Anti-infective	**8** Oxazolidinones **9** Other Anti-infective
P Female Reproductive ♀	**3** Percutaneous	**3** Anti-inflammatory **5** Adhesion Barrier **6** Nutritional Substance **7** Electrolytic and Water Balance Substance **B** Anesthetic Agent **H** Radioactive Substance **K** Other Diagnostic Substance **L** Sperm **N** Analgesics, Hypnotics, Sedatives **T** Destructive Agent **V** Hormone	**Z** No Qualifier
P Female Reproductive ♀	**3** Percutaneous	**G** Other Therapeutic Substance	**C** Other Substance
P Female Reproductive ♀	**3** Percutaneous	**Q** Fertilized Ovum	**0** Autologous **1** Nonautologous
P Female Reproductive ♀	**3** Percutaneous	**S** Gas	**F** Other Gas
P Female Reproductive ♀	**4** Percutaneous Endoscopic	**5** Adhesion Barrier	**Z** No Qualifier
P Female Reproductive ♀	**4** Percutaneous Endoscopic	**G** Other Therapeutic Substance	**C** Other Substance

3E0 continued on next page

3E0 continued from previous page

3 Administration
E Physiological Systems and Anatomical Regions
0 Introduction: Putting in or on a therapeutic, diagnostic, nutritional, physiological, or prophylactic substance except blood or blood products

Body System / Region	Approach	Substance	Qualifier
Character 4	**Character 5**	**Character 6**	**Character 7**
P Female Reproductive ♀	**7** Via Natural or Artificial Opening	**0** Antineoplastic	**4** Liquid Brachytherapy Radioisotope **5** Other Antineoplastic **M** Monoclonal Antibody
P Female Reproductive ♀	**7** Via Natural or Artificial Opening	**2** Anti-infective	**8** Oxazolidinones **9** Other Anti-infective
P Female Reproductive ♀	**7** Via Natural or Artificial Opening transvaginal	**3** Anti-inflammatory **6** Nutritional Substance **7** Electrolytic and Water Balance Substance **B** Anesthetic Agent **H** Radioactive Substance **K** Other Diagnostic Substance **L** Sperm artifical insemination **N** Analgesics, Hypnotics, Sedatives **T** Destructive Agent **V** Hormone	**Z** No Qualifier
P Female Reproductive ♀	**7** Via Natural or Artificial Opening	**G** Other Therapeutic Substance	**C** Other Substance
P Female Reproductive ♀	**7** Via Natural or Artificial Opening	**Q** Fertilized Ovum	**0** Autologous **1** Nonautologous
P Female Reproductive ♀	**7** Via Natural or Artificial Opening	**S** Gas	**F** Other Gas
P Female Reproductive ♀	**8** Via Natural or Artificial Opening Endoscopic	**0** Antineoplastic	**4** Liquid Brachytherapy Radioisotope **5** Other Antineoplastic **M** Monoclonal Antibody
P Female Reproductive ♀	**8** Via Natural or Artificial Opening Endoscopic	**2** Anti-infective	**8** Oxazolidinones **9** Other Anti-infective
P Female Reproductive ♀	**8** Via Natural or Artificial Opening Endoscopic	**3** Anti-inflammatory **6** Nutritional Substance **7** Electrolytic and Water Balance Substance **B** Anesthetic Agent **H** Radioactive Substance **K** Other Diagnostic Substance **N** Analgesics, Hypnotics, Sedatives **T** Destructive Agent	**Z** No Qualifier
P Female Reproductive ♀	**8** Via Natural or Artificial Opening Endoscopic	**G** Other Therapeutic Substance	**C** Other Substance
P Female Reproductive ♀	**8** Via Natural or Artificial Opening Endoscopic	**S** Gas	**F** Other Gas
Q Cranial Cavity and Brain DRG	**0** Open **3** Percutaneous	**0** Antineoplastic	**4** Liquid Brachytherapy Radioisotope **5** Other Antineoplastic **M** Monoclonal Antibody
Q Cranial Cavity and Brain	**0** Open **3** Percutaneous	**2** Anti-infective	**8** Oxazolidinones **9** Other Anti-infective
Q Cranial Cavity and Brain	**0** Open **3** Percutaneous	**3** Anti-inflammatory **6** Nutritional Substance **7** Electrolytic and Water Balance Substance **A** Stem Cells, Embryonic **B** Anesthetic Agent **H** Radioactive Substance **K** Other Diagnostic Substance **N** Analgesics, Hypnotics, Sedatives **T** Destructive Agent	**Z** No Qualifier

3E0 continued on next page

3 Administration
E Physiological Systems and Anatomical Regions
0 Introduction: Putting in or on a therapeutic, diagnostic, nutritional, physiological, or prophylactic substance except blood or blood products

3E0 continued from previous page

Body System / Region Character 4	Approach Character 5	Substance Character 6	Qualifier Character 7
Q Cranial Cavity and Brain	**0** Open **3** Percutaneous	**E** Stem Cells, Somatic	**0** Autologous **1** Nonautologous
Q Cranial Cavity and Brain	**0** Open **3** Percutaneous	**G** Other Therapeutic Substance	**C** Other Substance
Q Cranial Cavity and Brain	**0** Open **3** Percutaneous	**S** Gas	**F** Other Gas
Q Cranial Cavity and Brain DRG	**7** Via Natural or Artificial Opening	**0** Antineoplastic	**4** Liquid Brachytherapy Radioisotope **5** Other Antineoplastic **M** Monoclonal Antibody
Q Cranial Cavity and Brain	**7** Via Natural or Artificial Opening	**S** Gas	**F** Other Gas
R Spinal Canal	**0** Open	**A** Stem Cells, Embryonic	**Z** No Qualifier
R Spinal Canal	**0** Open	**E** Stem Cells, Somatic	**0** Autologous **1** Nonautologous
R Spinal Canal DRG	**3** Percutaneous	**0** Antineoplastic	**2** High-dose Interleukin-2 **3** Low-dose Interleukin-2 **4** Liquid Brachytherapy Radioisotope **5** Other Antineoplastic **M** Monoclonal Antibody
R Spinal Canal	**3** Percutaneous	**2** Anti-infective	**8** Oxazolidinones **9** Other Anti-infective
R Spinal Canal	**3** Percutaneous	**3** Anti-inflammatory **6** Nutritional Substance **7** Electrolytic and Water Balance Substance **A** Stem Cells, Embryonic **B** Anesthetic Agent **H** Radioactive Substance **K** Other Diagnostic Substance **N** Analgesics, Hypnotics, Sedatives **T** Destructive Agent	**Z** No Qualifier
R Spinal Canal	**3** Percutaneous	**E** Stem Cells, Somatic	**0** Autologous **1** Nonautologous
R Spinal Canal	**3** Percutaneous	**G** Other Therapeutic Substance	**C** Other Substance
R Spinal Canal	**3** Percutaneous	**S** Gas	**F** Other Gas
R Spinal Canal	**7** Via Natural or Artificial Opening	**S** Gas	**F** Other Gas
S Epidural Space DRG	**3** Percutaneous	**0** Antineoplastic	**2** High-dose Interleukin-2 **3** Low-dose Interleukin-2 **4** Liquid Brachytherapy Radioisotope **5** Other Antineoplastic **M** Monoclonal Antibody
S Epidural Space	**3** Percutaneous	**2** Anti-infective	**8** Oxazolidinones **9** Other Anti-infective
S Epidural Space epidural injection	**3** Percutaneous transforaminal	**3** Anti-inflammatory Kenalog **6** Nutritional Substance **7** Electrolytic and Water Balance Substance **B** Anesthetic Agent bupivacaine **H** Radioactive Substance **K** Other Diagnostic Substance **N** Analgesics, Hypnotics, Sedatives **T** Destructive Agent	**Z** No Qualifier
S Epidural Space	**3** Percutaneous	**G** Other Therapeutic Substance	**C** Other Substance

3E0 continued on next page

T= brachial plexus

3E0 continued from previous page

3 Administration
E Physiological Systems and Anatomical Regions
0 Introduction: Putting in or on a therapeutic, diagnostic, nutritional, physiological, or prophylactic substance except blood or blood products

Body System / Region Character 4	Approach Character 5	Substance Character 6	Qualifier Character 7
S Epidural Space	**3** Percutaneous	**S** Gas	**F** Other Gas
S Epidural Space	**7** Via Natural or Artificial Opening	**S** Gas	**F** Other Gas
T Peripheral Nerves and Plexi **X** Cranial Nerves	**3** Percutaneous	**3** Anti-inflammatory **B** Anesthetic Agent **T** Destructive Agent	**Z** No Qualifier
T Peripheral Nerves and Plexi **X** Cranial Nerves	**3** Percutaneous	**G** Other Therapeutic Substance	**C** Other Substance
U Joints	**0** Open	**2** Anti-infective	**8** Oxazolidinones **9** Other Anti-infective
U Joints	**0** Open	**G** Other Therapeutic Substance	**B** Recombinant Bone Morphogenetic Protein
U Joints	**3** Percutaneous	**0** Antineoplastic	**4** Liquid Brachytherapy Radioisotope **5** Other Antineoplastic **M** Monoclonal Antibody
U Joints	**3** Percutaneous	**2** Anti-infective	**8** Oxazolidinones **9** Other Anti-infective
U Joints	**3** Percutaneous	**3** Anti-inflammatory **6** Nutritional Substance **7** Electrolytic and Water Balance Substance **B** Anesthetic Agent **H** Radioactive Substance **K** Other Diagnostic Substance **N** Analgesics, Hypnotics, Sedatives **T** Destructive Agent	**Z** No Qualifier
U Joints	**3** Percutaneous	**G** Other Therapeutic Substance	**B** Recombinant Bone Morphogenetic Protein **C** Other Substance
U Joints	**3** Percutaneous	**S** Gas	**F** Other Gas
U Joints	**4** Percutaneous Endoscopic	**G** Other Therapeutic Substance	**C** Other Substance
V Bones	**0** Open	**G** Other Therapeutic Substance	**B** Recombinant Bone Morphogenetic Protein
V Bones	**3** Percutaneous	**0** Antineoplastic	**5** Other Antineoplastic **M** Monoclonal Antibody
V Bones	**3** Percutaneous	**2** Anti-infective	**8** Oxazolidinones **9** Other Anti-infective
V Bones	**3** Percutaneous	**3** Anti-inflammatory **6** Nutritional Substance **7** Electrolytic and Water Balance Substance **B** Anesthetic Agent **H** Radioactive Substance **K** Other Diagnostic Substance **N** Analgesics, Hypnotics, Sedatives **T** Destructive Agent	**Z** No Qualifier
V Bones	**3** Percutaneous	**G** Other Therapeutic Substance	**B** Recombinant Bone Morphogenetic Protein **C** Other Substance
W Lymphatics	**3** Percutaneous	**0** Antineoplastic	**5** Other Antineoplastic **M** Monoclonal Antibody
W Lymphatics	**3** Percutaneous	**2** Anti-infective	**8** Oxazolidinones **9** Other Anti-infective

3E0 continued on next page

3 Administration
E Physiological Systems and Anatomical Regions
0 Introduction: Putting in or on a therapeutic, diagnostic, nutritional, physiological, or prophylactic substance except blood or blood products

3E0 continued from previous page

Body System / Region	Approach	Substance	Qualifier
Character 4	Character 5	Character 6	Character 7
W Lymphatics	**3** Percutaneous	**3** Anti-inflammatory **6** Nutritional Substance **7** Electrolytic and Water Balance Substance **B** Anesthetic Agent **H** Radioactive Substance **K** Other Diagnostic Substance **N** Analgesics, Hypnotics, Sedatives **T** Destructive Agent	**Z** No Qualifier
W Lymphatics	**3** Percutaneous	**G** Other Therapeutic Substance	**C** Other Substance
Y Pericardial Cavity	**3** Percutaneous	**0** Antineoplastic	**4** Liquid Brachytherapy Radioisotope **5** Other Antineoplastic **M** Monoclonal Antibody
Y Pericardial Cavity	**3** Percutaneous	**2** Anti-infective	**8** Oxazolidinones **9** Other Anti-infective
Y Pericardial Cavity	**3** Percutaneous	**3** Anti-inflammatory **6** Nutritional Substance **7** Electrolytic and Water Balance Substance **B** Anesthetic Agent **H** Radioactive Substance **K** Other Diagnostic Substance **N** Analgesics, Hypnotics, Sedatives **T** Destructive Agent	**Z** No Qualifier
Y Pericardial Cavity	**3** Percutaneous	**G** Other Therapeutic Substance	**C** Other Substance
Y Pericardial Cavity	**3** Percutaneous	**S** Gas	**F** Other Gas
Y Pericardial Cavity	**4** Percutaneous Endoscopic	**G** Other Therapeutic Substance	**C** Other Substance
Y Pericardial Cavity	**7** Via Natural or Artificial Opening	**0** Antineoplastic	**4** Liquid Brachytherapy Radioisotope **5** Other Antineoplastic **M** Monoclonal Antibody
Y Pericardial Cavity	**7** Via Natural or Artificial Opening	**S** Gas	**F** Other Gas

♀ 3E0E304 3E0E305 3E0E30M 3E0E328 3E0E329 3E0E33Z 3E0E36Z 3E0E37Z 3E0E3BZ 3E0E3GC 3E0E3HZ 3E0E3KZ 3E0E3NZ 3E0E3SF 3E0E3TZ 3E0E4GC 3E0E704 3E0E705 3E0E70M 3E0E728 3E0E729 3E0E73Z 3E0E76Z 3E0E77Z 3E0E7BZ 3E0E7GC 3E0E7HZ 3E0E7KZ 3E0E7NZ 3E0E7SF 3E0E7TZ 3E0E804 3E0E805 3E0E80M 3E0E828 3E0E829 3E0E83Z 3E0E86Z 3E0E87Z 3E0E8BZ 3E0E8GC 3E0E8HZ 3E0E8KZ 3E0E8NZ 3E0E8SF 3E0E8TZ 3E0P05Z 3E0P304 3E0P305 3E0P30M 3E0P328 3E0P329 3E0P33Z 3E0P35Z 3E0P36Z 3E0P37Z 3E0P3BZ 3E0P3GC 3E0P3HZ 3E0P3KZ 3E0P3LZ 3E0P3NZ 3E0P3Q0 3E0P3Q1 3E0P3SF 3E0P3TZ 3E0P3VZ 3E0P45Z 3E0P4GC 3E0P704 3E0P705 3E0P70M 3E0P728 3E0P729 3E0P73Z 3E0P76Z 3E0P77Z 3E0P7BZ 3E0P7GC 3E0P7HZ 3E0P7KZ 3E0P7LZ 3E0P7NZ 3E0P7Q0 3E0P7Q1 3E0P7SF 3E0P7TZ 3E0P7VZ 3E0P804 3E0P805 3E0P80M 3E0P828 3E0P829 3E0P83Z 3E0P86Z 3E0P87Z 3E0P8BZ 3E0P8GC 3E0P8HZ 3E0P8KZ 3E0P8NZ 3E0P8SF 3E0P8TZ

♂ 3E0N304 3E0N305 3E0N30M 3E0N328 3E0N329 3E0N33Z 3E0N36Z 3E0N37Z 3E0N3BZ 3E0N3GC 3E0N3HZ 3E0N3KZ 3E0N3NZ 3E0N3SF 3E0N3TZ 3E0N4GC 3E0N704 3E0N705 3E0N70M 3E0N728 3E0N729 3E0N73Z 3E0N76Z 3E0N77Z 3E0N7BZ 3E0N7GC 3E0N7HZ 3E0N7KZ 3E0N7NZ 3E0N7SF 3E0N7TZ 3E0N804 3E0N805 3E0N80M 3E0N828 3E0N829 3E0N83Z 3E0N86Z 3E0N87Z 3E0N8BZ 3E0N8GC 3E0N8HZ 3E0N8KZ 3E0N8NZ 3E0N8SF 3E0N8TZ

DRG 3E03002 3E03017 3E030U0 3E030U1 3E03302 3E03317 3E033U0 3E033U1 3E04002 3E04017 3E04302 3E04317 3E05002 3E05017 3E05302 3E05317 3E06002 3E06017 3E06302 3E06317 3E08017 3E08317 3E0J3U0 3E0J3U1 3E0J7U0 3E0J7U1 3E0J8U0 3E0J8U1 3E0Q005 3E0Q305 3E0Q705 3E0R302 3E0S302

3 Administration
E Physiological Systems and Anatomical Regions
1 Irrigation: Putting in or on a cleansing substance

Body System / Region Character 4	Approach Character 5	Substance Character 6	Qualifier Character 7
0 Skin and Mucous Membranes **C** Eye	**3** Percutaneous **X** External	**8** Irrigating Substance	**X** Diagnostic **Z** No Qualifier
9 Nose **B** Ear **F** Respiratory Tract **G** Upper GI **H** Lower GI **J** Biliary and Pancreatic Tract **K** Genitourinary Tract **N** Male Reproductive ♂ **P** Female Reproductive ♀	**3** Percutaneous **7** Via Natural or Artificial Opening **8** Via Natural or Artificial Opening Endoscopic	**8** Irrigating Substance	**X** Diagnostic **Z** No Qualifier
L Pleural Cavity **Q** Cranial Cavity and Brain **R** Spinal Canal **S** Epidural Space **Y** Pericardial Cavity	**3** Percutaneous	**8** Irrigating Substance	**X** Diagnostic **Z** No Qualifier
M Peritoneal Cavity	**3** Percutaneous	**8** Irrigating Substance	**X** Diagnostic **Z** No Qualifier
M Peritoneal Cavity	**3** Percutaneous indwelling catheter	**9** Dialysate for dialysis	**Z** No Qualifier
U Joints	**3** Percutaneous **4** Percutaneous Endoscopic	**8** Irrigating Substance	**X** Diagnostic **Z** No Qualifier

♀ 3E1P38X 3E1P38Z 3E1P78X 3E1P78Z 3E1P88X 3E1P88Z
♂ 3E1N38X 3E1N38Z 3E1N78X 3E1N78Z 3E1N88X 3E1N88Z

Peritoneal dialysis w/indwelling catheter 3E1M39Z

NOTES

Body System (2nd character) - 2 options
- A = physiological systems: conductivity, metabolism, pulse, temp, volume
- B = physiological devices: stimulator, pacemaker, defibrillator

Rooot (3rd character) - 2 options
- Measurement - at a point in time Ex: pressure
- monitoring - over a period of time

IF DEVICE is inserted & left in, code insertion from med & surg section

Function/Device (6th character)
device that measures or monitors or physical function monitored. Ex: O_2

Cardiac cath
- measures pressures in the chambers of heart
- go into coronary arteries to measure occlusion from artherosclerosis
- code also fluoscopic imaging

ECG - measures cardiac electrical activity
EEG - measures electrical activity of CNS
Cardia cath - pressure of heart - percutaneous

Left-sided pressures: Aortic (AKA AO), Left ventricular & diastolic pressure LVEDP

Right-sided pressures: pulmonary artery, cardiac output, right atrium, right ventricle, pulmonary capillary wedge pressure PCWP

Code Also: anything other than hemodynamics AKA - heart pressures

Angiography - done during heart cath, contrast injected into coronary arteries looking for occlusion - code in imaging
done on coronary arteries & bypass grafts

Ventriculogram - contrast injected into left ventricle to describe structure and function. May also do ejection fraction - measures percentage of blood leaving the heart to go through out body each time the heart contract. Code in imaging Done for CHF
measures thickness of ventricle walls

Revascularization - for occlusions - may be angioplasty, atherectomy & stent insertion - code from med/surg section
used to restore blood flow

Left cardiac cath w/ low osmolar contrast LVEDP measured 4A023N7
also code imaging of ventriculum B215122 &
fluoroscopy arteries B211122
Cardiac stress test monitoring
cardiac catheterizations

Measurement and Monitoring 4A0-4B0

4 Measurement and Monitoring
A Physiological Systems
0 Measurement: Determining the level of a physiological or physical function at a point in time

Body System Character 4	Approach Character 5	Function/Device Character 6	Qualifier Character 7
0 Central Nervous	0 Open	2 Conductivity 4 Electrical Activity B Pressure	Z No Qualifier
0 Central Nervous	3 Percutaneous 7 Via Natural or Artificial Opening 8 Via Natural or Artificial Opening Endoscopic	4 Electrical Activity	Z No Qualifier
0 Central Nervous	3 Percutaneous 7 Via Natural or Artificial Opening 8 Via Natural or Artificial Opening Endoscopic	B Pressure K Temperature R Saturation	D Intracranial
0 Central Nervous	X External	2 Conductivity 4 Electrical Activity	Z No Qualifier
1 Peripheral Nervous	0 Open 3 Percutaneous 7 Via Natural or Artificial Opening 8 Via Natural or Artificial Opening Endoscopic X External	2 Conductivity	9 Sensory B Motor
1 Peripheral Nervous	0 Open 3 Percutaneous 7 Via Natural or Artificial Opening 8 Via Natural or Artificial Opening Endoscopic X External	4 Electrical Activity	Z No Qualifier
2 Cardiac DRG heart cath	0 Open 3 Percutaneous cath 7 Via Natural or Artificial Opening 8 Via Natural or Artificial Opening Endoscopic	4 Electrical Activity 9 Output C Rate F Rhythm H Sound P Action Currents	Z No Qualifier
2 Cardiac DRG may be heart cath	0 Open 3 Percutaneous cath 7 Via Natural or Artificial Opening 8 Via Natural or Artificial Opening Endoscopic	N Sampling and Pressure end diastolic pressure 8 mm mercury (HG)	6 Right Heart 7 Left Heart LVEDP 8 Bilateral L+R
2 Cardiac	X External	4 Electrical Activity	A Guidance Z No Qualifier
2 Cardiac	X External	9 Output C Rate F Rhythm H Sound P Action Currents	Z No Qualifier
2 Cardiac	X External ECG	M Total Activity	4 Stress
3 Arterial	0 Open 3 Percutaneous	5 Flow J Pulse	1 Peripheral 3 Pulmonary C Coronary
3 Arterial	0 Open 3 Percutaneous	B Pressure	1 Peripheral 3 Pulmonary C Coronary F Other Thoracic

4A0 continued on next page

4A0 continued from previous page

4 Measurement and Monitoring
A Physiological Systems
0 Measurement: Determining the level of a physiological or physical function at a point in time

Body System Character 4	Approach Character 5	Function/Device Character 6	Qualifier Character 7
3 Arterial	**0** Open **3** Percutaneous	**H** Sound **R** Saturation	**1** Peripheral
3 Arterial	**X** External	**5** Flow **B** Pressure **H** Sound **J** Pulse **R** Saturation	**1** Peripheral
4 Venous	**0** Open **3** Percutaneous	**5** Flow **B** Pressure **J** Pulse	**0** Central **1** Peripheral **2** Portal **3** Pulmonary
4 Venous	**0** Open **3** Percutaneous	**R** Saturation	**1** Peripheral
4 Venous	**X** External	**5** Flow **B** Pressure **J** Pulse **R** Saturation	**1** Peripheral
5 Circulatory	**X** External	**L** Volume	**Z** No Qualifier
6 Lymphatic	**0** Open **3** Percutaneous **7** Via Natural or Artificial Opening **8** Via Natural or Artificial Opening Endoscopic	**5** Flow **B** Pressure	**Z** No Qualifier
7 Visual	**X** External	**0** Acuity **7** Mobility **B** Pressure	**Z** No Qualifier
8 Olfactory	**X** External	**0** Acuity	**Z** No Qualifier
9 Respiratory	**7** Via Natural or Artificial Opening **8** Via Natural or Artificial Opening Endoscopic **X** External	**1** Capacity **5** Flow **C** Rate **D** Resistance **L** Volume **M** Total Activity	**Z** No Qualifier
B Gastrointestinal	**7** Via Natural or Artificial Opening **8** Via Natural or Artificial Opening Endoscopic	**8** Motility **B** Pressure **G** Secretion	**Z** No Qualifier
C Biliary	**3** Percutaneous **4** Percutaneous Endoscopic **7** Via Natural or Artificial Opening **8** Via Natural or Artificial Opening Endoscopic	**5** Flow **B** Pressure	**Z** No Qualifier
D Urinary	**7** Via Natural or Artificial Opening **8** Via Natural or Artificial Opening Endoscopic	**3** Contractility **5** Flow **B** Pressure **D** Resistance **L** Volume	**Z** No Qualifier
F Musculoskeletal EmG	**3** Percutaneous **X** External	**3** Contractility	**Z** No Qualifier
H Products of Conception, Cardiac ♀	**7** Via Natural or Artificial Opening **8** Via Natural or Artificial Opening Endoscopic **X** External	**4** Electrical Activity **C** Rate **F** Rhythm **H** Sound	**Z** No Qualifier

4A0 continued on next page

4 **Measurement and Monitoring**
A **Physiological Systems**
0 **Measurement:** Determining the level of a physiological or physical function at a point in time

4A0 continued from previous page

Body System Character 4	Approach Character 5	Function/Device Character 6	Qualifier Character 7
J Products of Conception, Nervous ♀	**7** Via Natural or Artificial Opening **8** Via Natural or Artificial Opening Endoscopic **X** External	**2** Conductivity **4** Electrical Activity **B** Pressure	**Z** No Qualifier
Z None	**7** Via Natural or Artificial Opening	**6** Metabolism **K** Temperature	**Z** No Qualifier
Z None	**X** External	**6** Metabolism **K** Temperature **Q** Sleep	**Z** No Qualifier

♀ 4A0H74Z 4A0H7CZ 4A0H7FZ 4A0H7HZ 4A0H84Z 4A0H8CZ 4A0H8FZ 4A0H8HZ 4A0HX4Z 4A0HXCZ 4A0HXFZ 4A0HXHZ 4A0J72Z 4A0J74Z 4A0J7BZ 4A0J82Z 4A0J84Z 4A0J8BZ 4A0JX2Z 4A0JX4Z 4A0JXBZ

DRG 4A020N6 4A020N7 4A020N8 4A023FZ 4A023N6 4A023N7 4A023N8 4A027FZ 4A027N6 4A027N7 4A027N8 4A028FZ 4A028N6 4A028N7 4A028N8

4 **Measurement and Monitoring**
A **Physiological Systems**
1 **Monitoring:** Determining the level of a physiological or physical function repetitively over a period of time

Body System Character 4	Approach Character 5	Function/Device Character 6	Qualifier Character 7
0 Central Nervous	**0** Open	**2** Conductivity **B** Pressure	**Z** No Qualifier
0 Central Nervous	**0** Open	**4** Electrical Activity	**G** Intraoperative **Z** No Qualifier
0 Central Nervous	**3** Percutaneous **7** Via Natural or Artificial Opening **8** Via Natural or Artificial Opening Endoscopic	**4** Electrical Activity	**G** Intraoperative **Z** No Qualifier
0 Central Nervous	**3** Percutaneous **7** Via Natural or Artificial Opening **8** Via Natural or Artificial Opening Endoscopic	**B** Pressure **K** Temperature **R** Saturation	**D** Intracranial
0 Central Nervous	**X** External	**2** Conductivity	**Z** No Qualifier
0 Central Nervous	**X** External	**4** Electrical Activity	**G** Intraoperative **Z** No Qualifier
1 Peripheral Nervous	**0** Open **3** Percutaneous **7** Via Natural or Artificial Opening **8** Via Natural or Artificial Opening Endoscopic **X** External	**2** Conductivity	**9** Sensory **B** Motor
1 Peripheral Nervous	**0** Open **3** Percutaneous **7** Via Natural or Artificial Opening **8** Via Natural or Artificial Opening Endoscopic **X** External	**4** Electrical Activity	**G** Intraoperative **Z** No Qualifier
2 Cardiac	**0** Open **3** Percutaneous **7** Via Natural or Artificial Opening **8** Via Natural or Artificial Opening Endoscopic	**4** Electrical Activity **9** Output **C** Rate **F** Rhythm **H** Sound	**Z** No Qualifier

4A1 continued on next page

4 Measurement and Monitoring
A Physiological Systems
1 Monitoring: Determining the level of a physiological or physical function repetitively over a period of time

4A1 continued from previous page

Body System	Approach	Function/Device	Qualifier
Character 4	**Character 5**	**Character 6**	**Character 7**
2 Cardiac	**X** External	**4** Electrical Activity	**5** Ambulatory **Z** No Qualifier
2 Cardiac	**X** External	**9** Output **C** Rate **F** Rhythm **H** Sound	**Z** No Qualifier
2 Cardiac	**X** External	**M** Total Activity	**4** Stress
2 Cardiac	**X** External	**S** Vascular Perfusion	**H** Indocyanine Green Dye
3 Arterial	**0** Open **3** Percutaneous	**5** Flow **B** Pressure **J** Pulse	**1** Peripheral **3** Pulmonary **C** Coronary
3 Arterial	**0** Open **3** Percutaneous	**H** Sound **R** Saturation	**1** Peripheral
3 Arterial	**X** External	**5** Flow **B** Pressure **H** Sound **J** Pulse **R** Saturation	**1** Peripheral
4 Venous	**0** Open **3** Percutaneous	**5** Flow **B** Pressure **J** Pulse	**0** Central **1** Peripheral **2** Portal **3** Pulmonary
4 Venous	**0** Open **3** Percutaneous	**R** Saturation	**0** Central **2** Portal **3** Pulmonary
4 Venous	**X** External	**5** Flow **B** Pressure **J** Pulse	**1** Peripheral
6 Lymphatic	**0** Open **3** Percutaneous **7** Via Natural or Artificial Opening **8** Via Natural or Artificial Opening Endoscopic	**5** Flow	**H** Indocyanine Green Dye **Z** No Qualifier
6 Lymphatic	**0** Open **3** Percutaneous **7** Via Natural or Artificial Opening **8** Via Natural or Artificial Opening Endoscopic	**B** Pressure	**Z** No Qualifier
9 Respiratory	**7** Via Natural or Artificial Opening **X** External	**1** Capacity **5** Flow **C** Rate **D** Resistance **L** Volume	**Z** No Qualifier
B Gastrointestinal	**7** Via Natural or Artificial Opening **8** Via Natural or Artificial Opening Endoscopic	**8** Motility **B** Pressure **G** Secretion	**Z** No Qualifier
B Gastrointestinal	**X** External	**S** Vascular Perfusion	**H** Indocyanine Green Dye
D Urinary	**7** Via Natural or Artificial Opening **8** Via Natural or Artificial Opening Endoscopic	**3** Contractility **5** Flow **B** Pressure **D** Resistance **L** Volume	**Z** No Qualifier

4A1 continued on next page

monitor fetal heart rate during delivery 4A1HXCZ

4 Measurement and Monitoring
A Physiological Systems
1 Monitoring: Determining the level of a physiological or physical function repetitively over a period of time

4A1 continued from previous page

Body System	Approach	Function/Device	Qualifier
Character 4	**Character 5**	**Character 6**	**Character 7**
G Skin and Breast	**X** External	**S** Vascular Perfusion	**H** Indocyanine Green Dye
H Products of Conception, Cardiac ♀ fetal monitor	**7** Via Natural or Artificial Opening **8** Via Natural or Artificial Opening Endoscopic **X** External	**4** Electrical Activity **C** Rate **F** Rhythm **H** Sound	**Z** No Qualifier
J Products of Conception, Nervous ♀	**7** Via Natural or Artificial Opening **8** Via Natural or Artificial Opening Endoscopic **X** External	**2** Conductivity **4** Electrical Activity **B** Pressure	**Z** No Qualifier
Z None	**7** Via Natural or Artificial Opening (mouth or rectum)	**K** Temperature	**Z** No Qualifier
Z None	**X** External (wand over skin)	**K** Temperature **Q** Sleep	**Z** No Qualifier

♀ 4A1H74Z 4A1H7CZ 4A1H7FZ 4A1H7HZ 4A1H84Z 4A1H8CZ 4A1H8FZ 4A1H8HZ 4A1HX4Z 4A1HXCZ 4A1HXFZ 4A1HXHZ 4A1J72Z 4A1J74Z 4A1J7BZ 4A1J82Z 4A1J84Z 4A1J8BZ 4A1JX2Z 4A1JX4Z 4A1JXBZ

4 Measurement and Monitoring
B Physiological Devices
0 Measurement: Determining the level of a physiological or physical function at a point in time

Body System	Approach	Function/Device	Qualifier
Character 4	**Character 5**	**Character 6**	**Character 7**
0 Central Nervous **1** Peripheral Nervous **F** Musculoskeletal	**X** External	**V** Stimulator	**Z** No Qualifier
2 Cardiac	**X** External	**S** Pacemaker **T** Defibrillator	**Z** No Qualifier
9 Respiratory	**X** External	**S** Pacemaker	**Z** No Qualifier

LC Limited Coverage NC Noncovered HAC HAC-associated Procedure CC Combination Cluster - See Appendix G for code lists
DRG Non-OR-Affecting MS-DRG Assignment New/Revised Text in **Orange** ♂ Male ♀ Female

NOTES

Hemodialysis - removing waste products such as creatinine + urea + H_2O From blood when kidneys are in renal Failure

3 primary methods to gain access

1. Intravenous Catheter! Central Venous Catheter (CVC) inserted into large vein (usually vena cava). Catheter tunneled or non-tunneled
2. Arteriovenous (AV) Fistula. Join artery + vein together through anastomosis, thus bypass capillaries. Fistulas are usually created in non-dominant arm + may be situated on the hand (snuff box fistula), the Forearm (Brescia-Cimino Fistula) or elbow. Fistula takes 4-6 weeks to mature
3. Synthetic Graft - a synthetic AV graft is made when an artificial vessel is used to join the artery + vein. Graft may be Polytetrafluoroethylene (PTEE). Veins From animals may be used. Used when pts artery/vein cannot support a Fistula

Patient may have multiple accesses until graft mature

All vascular accesses require surgery

3 Types of Hemodialysis

1) Conventional - For chronic pts, usually done 3 x week For 3/4 hrs
2) Daily - done at home, done 6 days a wk For 2 hrs.
3) nocturnal - Similar to conventional. Done 6 nights/week For 6-10 hrs while pt sleeps

ECMO - Extracorporeal Membrane Oxygenation

- Similar to heart/lung bypass machine. Pumps + oxygenates pts blood outside body as heart + lungs can no longer Function as they are severely diseased.
- Done by inserting cannulae in large blood vessels, pt given heparin + blood pumps through a membrane oxygenator
- Several Forms of ECMO

VA - Venoarterial - blood is returned to arterial system

VV - Veno-Venous - blood is returned to Venous system - no cardiac support

Mechanical Ventilation - may be short term For ICU or long term For chronic illness. may include PAP ventilators

- Positive Airway Pressure (AKA CPAP), transport ventilator using AC or DC power, ICU ventilator - all are mechanical method
- Hand-held include - bag valve mask or Continuous Flow or Anesthesia (T-piece) bag - use to provide positive pressure ventilation to a pt who is not breathing or breathing inadequently

Extracorporeal or Systemic Assistance and Performance 5A0-5A2

5 Extracorporeal or Systemic Assistance and Performance
A Physiological Systems
0 Assistance: Taking over a portion of a physiological function by extracorporeal means

Body System Character 4	Approach Character 5	Function/Device Character 6	Qualifier Character 7
2 Cardiac	1 Intermittent 2 Continuous	1 Output	0 Balloon Pump 5 Pulsatile Compression 6 Other Pump D Impeller Pump
5 Circulatory	1 Intermittent 2 Continuous	2 Oxygenation	1 Hyperbaric C Supersaturated
9 Respiratory	2 Continuous	0 Filtration	Z No Qualifier
9 Respiratory	3 Less than 24 Consecutive Hours 4 24-96 Consecutive Hours 5 Greater than 96 Consecutive Hours	5 Ventilation	7 Continuous Positive Airway Pressure 8 Intermittent Positive Airway Pressure 9 Continuous Negative Airway Pressure B Intermittent Negative Airway Pressure Z No Qualifier

5 Extracorporeal or Systemic Assistance and Performance
A Physiological Systems
1 Performance: Completely taking over a physiological function by extracorporeal means

Body System Character 4	Approach Character 5	Function/Device Character 6	Qualifier Character 7
2 Cardiac	0 Single	1 Output	2 Manual
2 Cardiac	1 Intermittent	3 Pacing	Z No Qualifier
2 Cardiac	2 Continuous	1 Output 3 Pacing	Z No Qualifier
5 Circulatory DRG	2 Continuous A Intraoperative	2 Oxygenation	F Membrane, Central G Membrane, Peripheral Veno-arterial H Membrane, Peripheral Veno-venous
9 Respiratory	0 Single	5 Ventilation	4 Nonmechanical
9 Respiratory DRG	3 Less than 24 Consecutive Hours 4 24-96 Consecutive Hours 5 Greater than 96 Consecutive Hours	5 Ventilation	Z No Qualifier
C Biliary	0 Single 6 Multiple	0 Filtration	Z No Qualifier
D Urinary	7 Intermittent, Less than 6 Hours Per Day 8 Prolonged Intermittent, 6-18 hours Per Day 9 Continuous, Greater than 18 hours Per Day	0 Filtration	Z No Qualifier

DRG 5A1522G 5A1522H 5A1935Z 5A1945Z 5A1955Z

5 Extracorporeal or Systemic Assistance and Performance
A Physiological Systems
2 Restoration: Returning, or attempting to return, a physiological function to its original state by extracorporeal means.

Body System Character 4	Approach Character 5	Function/Device Character 6	Qualifier Character 7
2 Cardiac	0 Single	4 Rhythm	Z No Qualifier

LC Limited Coverage NC Noncovered HAC HAC-associated Procedure CC Combination Cluster - See Appendix G for code lists
DRG Non-OR-Affecting MS-DRG Assignment New/Revised Text in **Orange** ♂ Male ♀ Female

NOTES

outside the body - performed in critical care settings

Extracorporeal or Systemic Therapies 6A0-6AB

- phototherapy

does not involve assistance/performance of a physiological function

6 Extracorporeal or Systemic Therapies
A Physiological Systems
0 Atmospheric Control: Extracorporeal control of atmospheric pressure and composition

Body System	Duration	Qualifier	Qualifier
Character 4	**Character 5**	**Character 6**	**Character 7**
Z None	**0** Single **1** Multiple	**Z** No Qualifier	**Z** No Qualifier

hyperbaric oxygen treatment
for decompression sickness - the bends in hyperbaric chamber

6 Extracorporeal or Systemic Therapies
A Physiological Systems
1 Decompression: Extracorporeal elimination of undissolved gas from body fluids

Body System	Duration	Qualifier	Qualifier
Character 4	**Character 5**	**Character 6**	**Character 7**
5 Circulatory	**0** Single **1** Multiple	**Z** No Qualifier	**Z** No Qualifier

6 Extracorporeal or Systemic Therapies
A Physiological Systems
2 Electromagnetic Therapy: Extracorporeal treatment by electromagnetic rays

Body System	Duration	Qualifier	Qualifier
Character 4	**Character 5**	**Character 6**	**Character 7**
1 Urinary **2** Central Nervous	**0** Single **1** Multiple	**Z** No Qualifier	**Z** No Qualifier

For temperature imbalance treatment + adjunct to radiation treatment for cancer. Code for radiation in Section D - other radiation + modality qual for - hyperth

6 Extracorporeal or Systemic Therapies
A Physiological Systems
3 Hyperthermia: Extracorporeal raising of body temperature

Body System	Duration	Qualifier	Qualifier
Character 4	**Character 5**	**Character 6**	**Character 7**
Z None	**0** Single **1** Multiple	**Z** No Qualifier	**Z** No Qualifier

6 Extracorporeal or Systemic Therapies
A Physiological Systems
4 Hypothermia: Extracorporeal lowering of body temperature

Body System	Duration	Qualifier	Qualifier
Character 4	**Character 5**	**Character 6**	**Character 7**
Z None	**0** Single **1** Multiple	**Z** No Qualifier	**Z** No Qualifier

Used to treat disease (leukemia) when too much blood is produced or to remove a blood product (platelets) from a donor for transfusion into another pt

6 Extracorporeal or Systemic Therapies
A Physiological Systems
5 Pheresis: Extracorporeal separation of blood products

Body System	Duration	Qualifier	Qualifier
Character 4	**Character 5**	**Character 6**	**Character 7**
5 Circulatory	**0** Single **1** Multiple	**Z** No Qualifier	**0** Erythrocytes **1** Leukocytes **2** Platelets **3** Plasma **T** Stem Cells, Cord Blood **V** Stem Cells, Hematopoietic

peresis performed on

Bili-light - expose skin to light rays. Ex: newborns for jaundice who have excess bilirubin in blood - use Isolette. Also treat adults for psoriasis

6 Extracorporeal or Systemic Therapies
A Physiological Systems
6 Phototherapy: Extracorporeal treatment by light rays

Body System Character 4	Duration Character 5	Qualifier Character 6	Qualifier Character 7
0 Skin jaundice, psoriasis **5** Circulatory blood	**0** Single **1** Multiple series	**Z** No Qualifier	**Z** No Qualifier

6 Extracorporeal or Systemic Therapies
A Physiological Systems
7 Ultrasound Therapy: Extracorporeal treatment by ultrasound

Body System Character 4	Duration Character 5	Qualifier Character 6	Qualifier Character 7
5 Circulatory	**0** Single **1** Multiple	**Z** No Qualifier	**4** Head and Neck Vessels **5** Heart site of **6** Peripheral Vessels treatment **7** Other Vessels **Z** No Qualifier

6 Extracorporeal or Systemic Therapies NOT for bili-light
A Physiological Systems
8 Ultraviolet Light Therapy: Extracorporeal treatment by ultraviolet light narrow section of visual light spectrum

Body System Character 4	Duration Character 5	Qualifier Character 6	Qualifier Character 7
0 Skin	**0** Single **1** Multiple	**Z** No Qualifier	**Z** No Qualifier

6 Extracorporeal or Systemic Therapies
A Physiological Systems
9 Shock Wave Therapy: Extracorporeal treatment by shock waves

Body System Character 4	Duration Character 5	Qualifier Character 6	Qualifier Character 7
3 Musculoskeletal	**0** Single **1** Multiple	**Z** No Qualifier	**Z** No Qualifier

6 Extracorporeal or Systemic Therapies
A Physiological Systems
B Perfusion: Extracorporeal treatment by diffusion of therapeutic fluid

Body System Character 4	Duration Character 5	Qualifier Character 6	Qualifier Character 7
5 Circulatory **B** Respiratory System **F** Hepatobiliary System and Pancreas **T** Urinary System	**0** Single	**B** Donor Organ	**Z** No Qualifier

NOTES

NOTES

OMT done by Osteopathic physician to improve physiologic function and/or support homeostasis that has been altered by somatic dysfunction.

Somatic Dysfunction - impaired or altered function of related components of the somatic (body framework) system: skeletal, arthrodial & myofascial structures & their related vascular, lymphatic & neural elements

treatment techniques (methods)

- Active - pt performs osteopathic practitioner directed function
- Passive - pt refrains from voluntary muscle contraction
- Direct - the restrictive barrier is engaged & a final activating force is applied to correct somatic dysfunction
- Indirect - the restrictive barrier is disengaged & the dysfunctional body is removed away from the restrictive barrier until tissue tension is equal in on or all planes & direction

Osteopathic Manipulative Treatment

Osteopathic 7W0 -OMT Procedures

7 Osteopathic
W Anatomical Regions
0 Treatment: Manual treatment to eliminate or alleviate somatic dysfunction and related disorders

Body Region Character 4	Approach Character 5	Method Character 6	Qualifier Character 7
0 Head 1 Cervical 2 Thoracic 3 Lumbar 4 Sacrum 5 Pelvis 6 Lower Extremities leg 7 Upper Extremities 8 Rib Cage 9 Abdomen	X External	0 Articulatory-Raising 1 Fascial Release myofascial 2 General Mobilization 3 High Velocity-Low Amplitude 4 Indirect 5 Low Velocity-High Amplitude LVHA 6 Lymphatic Pump 7 Muscle Energy-Isometric 8 Muscle Energy-Isotonic 9 Other Method	Z None

NOTES

Methods - 6th character

non-manual: excercise, rehabilitation, electrical modalities, back school

Long level specific contact: spinal manipulation to stretch or loosen several vertebra at a time

Short level specific contact: spinal manipulation on a vertebral process to move a single vetebra

L+R cath B211 + 4A02

Cardiac Caths Reporting

- the left heart pressures are reported from Section 4, Measurement & monitoring (mm/Hg)
- The coronary angiography & ventriculography is reported from table B21 for heart fluorscopy imaging
- Frequently, revusculation procedures are performed during a 2nd heart cath setting to cut down on the amount of contrast administed in one day
- At times, the revascularation procedure will be performed during the left heart catherization - In that case, the
- revascularization procedures will be reported using ~~pcs codes from med/surg~~

Chiropractic 9WB

non-surgical treatment of disorders of the nervous system and/or musculoskeletal system by spinal manipulation & treatment of surrounding structures

9 Chiropractic
W Anatomical Regions
B Manipulation: Manual procedure that involves a directed thrust to move a joint past the physiological range of motion, without exceeding the anatomical limit

Body Region	Approach	Method	Qualifier
Character 4	**Character 5**	**Character 6**	**Character 7**
0 Head **1** Cervical **2** Thoracic **3** Lumbar **4** Sacrum **5** Pelvis hip **6** Lower Extremities hip **7** Upper Extremities **8** Rib Cage **9** Abdomen	**X** External	**B** Non-Manual **C** Indirect Visceral **D** Extra-Articular **F** Direct Visceral **G** Long Lever Specific Contact **H** Short Lever Specific Contact **J** Long and Short Lever Specific Contact **K** Mechanically Assisted **L** Other Method	**Z** None

B4.6

If a procedure is performed on the skin, sub Q tissue or covering fascia overlying a joint - code to the body part, thus hip is coded to upper leg.

If manipulation is performed on the fascia overlying the hip joint - use lower extremity

Ancillary Services: B-D, F-H, X (7 Sections)

NOTES

Low Osmolar contrast: Omnipaque, Optiray, Isovue, Hexabrix, Visipaque

High Osmolar contrast: Conray, Cystografin, Gastrografin, Cholografin

Qualifier

Unenhanced & Enhanced - used for CT & magnetic resonance

- Use Φ if study is done with and without contrast.
- If study is done without contrast, use none for contrast & none for qualifier
- If study is done with contrast, contrast is reported as appropiate & none for qualifier

Full left heart cath includes:
- left heart pressures - hemodynamics
- coronary angiography
- ventriculum

*Use B21 table see page 640

Cardiac Catheterization Imaging - 2 types

1) Angiogram - xray of blood or lymph vessels, use fluorscopy

For coronary angiography - use contrast & use fluorscopy

- If artery is completely open = patent or degree of occlusion.
- Body parts pertaining to coronary angiography: coronary artery - single or multiple / coronary artery bypass graft - single or multiple / internal mammary bypass graft - left or right / Bypass graft - other

A. report 1 pcs code for native (non-bypass) coronary arteries imaged

CAB6
B. report 1 pcs code for any coronary artery bypass graft imaged, that DID NOT involve the internal mammary (IM) arteries. EX: one type of non IM bypass graft is a saphenous vein graft

C. Then report a PCS code for each Internal mammary (IM) bypass graft
Use LIMA - left Internal Mammary Artery
RIMA - right Interal Mammary Artery

D. Finally report a PCS code for any other type of bypass (non-artery & non-internal mammary artery) which is rare.

2.) ventriculography - contrast injected into ventricles of heart to evaluate main pumping chamber of heart - the left ventricle. Dr will describe the thickness (width) of ventricular walls, the wall motion (ejection factor EF) expressed as a percentage.

- report 1 pcs code for the ventriculogram using body part 5 - heart, left, if it is a left ventriculogram - they are not always performed. Only report this code if the dr mentions the ejection fraction or describes the left ventricle

Imaging B00-BY4

B Imaging
0 Central Nervous System
0 Plain Radiography: Planar display of an image developed from the capture of external ionizing radiation on photographic or photoconductive plate

Body Part	Contrast	Qualifier	Qualifier
Character 4	**Character 5**	**Character 6**	**Character 7**
B Spinal Cord	**0** High Osmolar **1** Low Osmolar **Y** Other Contrast **Z** None	**Z** None	**Z** None

B Imaging
0 Central Nervous System
1 Fluoroscopy: Single plane or bi-plane real time display of an image developed from the capture of external ionizing radiation on a fluorescent screen. The image may also be stored by either digital or analog means

Body Part	Contrast	Qualifier	Qualifier
Character 4	**Character 5**	**Character 6**	**Character 7**
B Spinal Cord	**0** High Osmolar **1** Low Osmolar **Y** Other Contrast **Z** None	**Z** None	**Z** None

B Imaging
0 Central Nervous System
2 Computerized Tomography (CT Scan): Computer reformatted digital display of multiplanar images developed from the capture of multiple exposures of external ionizing radiation

Body Part	Contrast	Qualifier	Qualifier
Character 4	**Character 5**	**Character 6**	**Character 7**
0 Brain **7** Cisterna **8** Cerebral Ventricle(s) **9** Sella Turcica/Pituitary Gland **B** Spinal Cord	**0** High Osmolar **1** Low Osmolar **Y** Other Contrast	**0** Unenhanced and Enhanced **Z** None	**Z** None
0 Brain **7** Cisterna **8** Cerebral Ventricle(s) **9** Sella Turcica/Pituitary Gland **B** Spinal Cord	**Z** None	**Z** None	**Z** None

B Imaging
0 Central Nervous System
3 Magnetic Resonance Imaging (MRI): Computer reformatted digital display of multiplanar images developed from the capture of radiofrequency signals emitted by nuclei in a body site excited within a magnetic field

Body Part	Contrast	Qualifier	Qualifier
Character 4	**Character 5**	**Character 6**	**Character 7**
0 Brain **9** Sella Turcica/Pituitary Gland **B** Spinal Cord **C** Acoustic Nerves	**Y** Other Contrast	**0** Unenhanced and Enhanced **Z** None	**Z** None
0 Brain **9** Sella Turcica/Pituitary Gland **B** Spinal Cord **C** Acoustic Nerves	**Z** None	**Z** None	**Z** None

B Imaging real-time tomographic images, may be referred to as obstetric sonography in pregnancy
0 Central Nervous System
4 Ultrasonography: Real time display of images of anatomy or flow information developed from the capture of reflected and attenuated high frequency sound waves For muscles, tendons, internal organs captures size, structure & pathological lesions

Body Part	Contrast	Qualifier	Qualifier
Character 4	**Character 5**	**Character 6**	**Character 7**
0 Brain **B** Spinal Cord	**Z** None	**Z** None	**Z** None

B Imaging
2 Heart
0 Plain Radiography: Planar display of an image developed from the capture of external ionizing radiation on photographic or photoconductive plate

Body Part	Contrast	Qualifier	Qualifier
Character 4	**Character 5**	**Character 6**	**Character 7**
0 Coronary Artery, Single DRG **1** Coronary Arteries, Multiple DRG **2** Coronary Artery Bypass Graft, Single DRG **3** Coronary Artery Bypass Grafts, Multiple DRG **4** Heart, Right DRG **5** Heart, Left DRG **6** Heart, Right and Left DRG **7** Internal Mammary Bypass Graft, Right DRG **8** Internal Mammary Bypass Graft, Left DRG **F** Bypass Graft, Other DRG	**0** High Osmolar **1** Low Osmolar **Y** Other Contrast	**Z** None	**Z** None

DRG B2000ZZ B2001ZZ B200YZZ B2010ZZ B2011ZZ B201YZZ B2020ZZ B2021ZZ B202YZZ B2030ZZ B2031ZZ B203YZZ B2040ZZ B2041ZZ B204YZZ B2050ZZ B2051ZZ B205YZZ B2060ZZ B2061ZZ B206YZZ B2070ZZ B2071ZZ B207YZZ B2080ZZ B2081ZZ B208YZZ B20F0ZZ B20F1ZZ B20FYZZ

See page 640 — done for heart caths

Main arteries of heart: left main, left circumflex, left anterior descending, Ramus intermediate & right coronary

B Imaging
2 Heart
1 Fluoroscopy: Single plane or bi-plane real time display of an image developed from the capture of external ionizing radiation on a fluorescent screen. The image may also be stored by either digital or analog means

Body Part	Contrast	Qualifier	Qualifier
Character 4	**Character 5**	**Character 6**	**Character 7**
0 Coronary Artery, Single **1** Coronary Arteries, Multiple **2** Coronary Artery Bypass Graft, Single saphenous **3** Coronary Artery Bypass Grafts, Multiple saphenous	**0** High Osmolar **1** Low Osmolar Isovue, omnipaque **Y** Other Contrast one body part represents multiple grafts	**1** Laser	**0** Intraoperative
0 Coronary Artery, Single DRG **1** Coronary Arteries, Multiple DRG **2** Coronary Artery Bypass Graft, Single DRG **3** Coronary Artery Bypass Grafts, Multiple DRG	**0** High Osmolar **1** Low Osmolar **Y** Other Contrast	**Z** None Note! whether it is a native coronary artery, a coronary artery bypass graft created from the internal mammary arteries - only 1 PCS code is reported	**Z** None
4 Heart, Right DRG **5** Heart, Left DRG ventriculum **6** Heart, Right and Left DRG **7** Internal Mammary Bypass Graft, Right DRG **8** Internal Mammary Bypass Graft, Left DRG **F** Bypass Graft, Other DRG	**0** High Osmolar **1** Low Osmolar **Y** Other Contrast	**Z** None	**Z** None

DRG B2100ZZ B2101ZZ B210YZZ B2110ZZ B2111ZZ B211YZZ B2120ZZ B2121ZZ B212YZZ B2130ZZ B2131ZZ B213YZZ B2140ZZ B2141ZZ B214YZZ B2150ZZ B2151ZZ B215YZZ B2160ZZ B2161ZZ B216YZZ B2170ZZ B2171ZZ B217YZZ B2180ZZ B2181ZZ B218YZZ B21F0ZZ B21F1ZZ B21FYZZ

L Heart cath showing patent RCA & LCA & 90% occlusion LAD use Isovue B2111ZZ
L Heart cath showing 30% occlusion of LIMA bypass graft B2181ZZ - do not report original LAD artery since it was bypassed

LC Limited Coverage NC Noncovered HAC HAC-associated Procedure CC Combination Cluster - See Appendix G for code lists
DRG Non-OR-Affecting MS-DRG Assignment New/Revised Text in **Orange** ♂ Male ♀ Female

L heart cath - ventriculum - mild hypertrophy of wall & EJ 48% - B215122

B Imaging
2 Heart
2 Computerized Tomography (CT Scan): Computer reformatted digital display of multiplanar images developed from the capture of multiple exposures of external ionizing radiation

Body Part Character 4	Contrast Character 5	Qualifier Character 6	Qualifier Character 7
1 Coronary Arteries, Multiple **3** Coronary Artery Bypass Grafts, Multiple **6** Heart, Right and Left	**0** High Osmolar **1** Low Osmolar **Y** Other Contrast	**0** Unenhanced and Enhanced **Z** None	**Z** None
1 Coronary Arteries, Multiple **3** Coronary Artery Bypass Grafts, Multiple **6** Heart, Right and Left	**Z** None	**2** Intravascular Optical Coherence **Z** None	**Z** None

B Imaging
2 Heart
3 Magnetic Resonance Imaging (MRI): Computer reformatted digital display of multiplanar images developed from the capture of radiofrequency signals emitted by nuclei in a body site excited within a magnetic field

Body Part Character 4	Contrast Character 5	Qualifier Character 6	Qualifier Character 7
1 Coronary Arteries, Multiple **3** Coronary Artery Bypass Grafts, Multiple **6** Heart, Right and Left	**Y** Other Contrast	**0** Unenhanced and Enhanced **Z** None	**Z** None
1 Coronary Arteries, Multiple **3** Coronary Artery Bypass Grafts, Multiple **6** Heart, Right and Left	**Z** None	**Z** None	**Z** None

B Imaging
2 Heart
4 Ultrasonography: Real time display of images of anatomy or flow information developed from the capture of reflected and attenuated high frequency sound waves

Body Part Character 4	Contrast Character 5	Qualifier Character 6	Qualifier Character 7
0 Coronary Artery, Single **1** Coronary Arteries, Multiple **4** Heart, Right **5** Heart, Left **6** Heart, Right and Left **B** Heart with Aorta **C** Pericardium **D** Pediatric Heart	**Y** Other Contrast	**Z** None	**Z** None
0 Coronary Artery, Single **1** Coronary Arteries, Multiple **4** Heart, Right **5** Heart, Left **6** Heart, Right and Left **B** Heart with Aorta **C** Pericardium **D** Pediatric Heart	**Z** None	**Z** None	**3** Intravascular **4** Transesophageal **Z** None

B Imaging
3 Upper Arteries
0 Plain Radiography: Planar display of an image developed from the capture of external ionizing radiation on photographic or photoconductive plate

Body Part	Contrast	Qualifier	Qualifier
Character 4	**Character 5**	**Character 6**	**Character 7**
0 Thoracic Aorta **1** Brachiocephalic-Subclavian Artery, Right **2** Subclavian Artery, Left **3** Common Carotid Artery, Right **4** Common Carotid Artery, Left **5** Common Carotid Arteries, Bilateral **6** Internal Carotid Artery, Right **7** Internal Carotid Artery, Left **8** Internal Carotid Arteries, Bilateral **9** External Carotid Artery, Right **B** External Carotid Artery, Left **C** External Carotid Arteries, Bilateral **D** Vertebral Artery, Right **F** Vertebral Artery, Left **G** Vertebral Arteries, Bilateral **H** Upper Extremity Arteries, Right **J** Upper Extremity Arteries, Left **K** Upper Extremity Arteries, Bilateral **L** Intercostal and Bronchial Arteries **M** Spinal Arteries **N** Upper Arteries, Other **P** Thoraco-Abdominal Aorta **Q** Cervico-Cerebral Arch **R** Intracranial Arteries **S** Pulmonary Artery, Right **T** Pulmonary Artery, Left	**0** High Osmolar **1** Low Osmolar **Y** Other Contrast **Z** None	**Z** None	**Z** None

B Imaging
3 Upper Arteries
1 Fluoroscopy: Single plane or bi-plane real time display of an image developed from the capture of external ionizing radiation on a fluorescent screen. The image may also be stored by either digital or analog means

Body Part Character 4	Contrast Character 5	Qualifier Character 6	Qualifier Character 7
0 Thoracic Aorta **1** Brachiocephalic-Subclavian Artery, Right **2** Subclavian Artery, Left **3** Common Carotid Artery, Right **4** Common Carotid Artery, Left **5** Common Carotid Arteries, Bilateral **6** Internal Carotid Artery, Right **7** Internal Carotid Artery, Left **8** Internal Carotid Arteries, Bilateral **9** External Carotid Artery, Right **B** External Carotid Artery, Left **C** External Carotid Arteries, Bilateral **D** Vertebral Artery, Right **F** Vertebral Artery, Left **G** Vertebral Arteries, Bilateral **H** Upper Extremity Arteries, Right **J** Upper Extremity Arteries, Left **K** Upper Extremity Arteries, Bilateral **L** Intercostal and Bronchial Arteries **M** Spinal Arteries **N** Upper Arteries, Other **P** Thoraco-Abdominal Aorta **Q** Cervico-Cerebral Arch **R** Intracranial Arteries **S** Pulmonary Artery, Right **T** Pulmonary Artery, Left **U** Pulmonary Trunk	**0** High Osmolar **1** Low Osmolar **Y** Other Contrast	**1** Laser	**0** Intraoperative

B31 continued on next page

B31 continued from previous page

B Imaging
3 Upper Arteries
1 Fluoroscopy: Single plane or bi-plane real time display of an image developed from the capture of external ionizing radiation on a fluorescent screen. The image may also be stored by either digital or analog means

Body Part Character 4	Contrast Character 5	Qualifier Character 6	Qualifier Character 7
0 Thoracic Aorta **1** Brachiocephalic-Subclavian Artery, Right **2** Subclavian Artery, Left **3** Common Carotid Artery, Right **4** Common Carotid Artery, Left **5** Common Carotid Arteries, Bilateral **6** Internal Carotid Artery, Right **7** Internal Carotid Artery, Left **8** Internal Carotid Arteries, Bilateral **9** External Carotid Artery, Right **B** External Carotid Artery, Left **C** External Carotid Arteries, Bilateral **D** Vertebral Artery, Right **F** Vertebral Artery, Left **G** Vertebral Arteries, Bilateral **H** Upper Extremity Arteries, Right **J** Upper Extremity Arteries, Left **K** Upper Extremity Arteries, Bilateral **L** Intercostal and Bronchial Arteries **M** Spinal Arteries **N** Upper Arteries, Other **P** Thoraco-Abdominal Aorta **Q** Cervico-Cerebral Arch **R** Intracranial Arteries **S** Pulmonary Artery, Right **T** Pulmonary Artery, Left **U** Pulmonary Trunk	**0** High Osmolar **1** Low Osmolar **Y** Other Contrast	**Z** None	**Z** None

B31 continued on next page

B31 continued from previous page

B Imaging
3 Upper Arteries
1 Fluoroscopy: Single plane or bi-plane real time display of an image developed from the capture of external ionizing radiation on a fluorescent screen. The image may also be stored by either digital or analog means

Body Part Character 4	Contrast Character 5	Qualifier Character 6	Qualifier Character 7
0 Thoracic Aorta **1** Brachiocephalic-Subclavian Artery, Right **2** Subclavian Artery, Left **3** Common Carotid Artery, Right **4** Common Carotid Artery, Left **5** Common Carotid Arteries, Bilateral **6** Internal Carotid Artery, Right **7** Internal Carotid Artery, Left **8** Internal Carotid Arteries, Bilateral **9** External Carotid Artery, Right **B** External Carotid Artery, Left **C** External Carotid Arteries, Bilateral **D** Vertebral Artery, Right **F** Vertebral Artery, Left **G** Vertebral Arteries, Bilateral **H** Upper Extremity Arteries, Right **J** Upper Extremity Arteries, Left **K** Upper Extremity Arteries, Bilateral **L** Intercostal and Bronchial Arteries **M** Spinal Arteries **N** Upper Arteries, Other **P** Thoraco-Abdominal Aorta **Q** Cervico-Cerebral Arch **R** Intracranial Arteries **S** Pulmonary Artery, Right **T** Pulmonary Artery, Left **U** Pulmonary Trunk	**Z** None	**Z** None	**Z** None

B Imaging
3 Upper Arteries
2 Computerized Tomography (CT Scan): Computer reformatted digital display of multiplanar images developed from the capture of multiple exposures of external ionizing radiation

Body Part Character 4	Contrast Character 5	Qualifier Character 6	Qualifier Character 7
0 Thoracic Aorta **5** Common Carotid Arteries, Bilateral **8** Internal Carotid Arteries, Bilateral **G** Vertebral Arteries, Bilateral **R** Intracranial Arteries **S** Pulmonary Artery, Right **T** Pulmonary Artery, Left	**0** High Osmolar **1** Low Osmolar **Y** Other Contrast	**Z** None	**Z** None
0 Thoracic Aorta **5** Common Carotid Arteries, Bilateral **8** Internal Carotid Arteries, Bilateral **G** Vertebral Arteries, Bilateral **R** Intracranial Arteries **S** Pulmonary Artery, Right **T** Pulmonary Artery, Left	**Z** None	**2** Intravascular Optical Coherence **Z** None	**Z** None

B Imaging
3 Upper Arteries
3 Magnetic Resonance Imaging (MRI): Computer reformatted digital display of multiplanar images developed from the capture of radiofrequency signals emitted by nuclei in a body site excited within a magnetic field

Body Part	Contrast	Qualifier	Qualifier
Character 4	Character 5	Character 6	Character 7
0 Thoracic Aorta 5 Common Carotid Arteries, Bilateral 8 Internal Carotid Arteries, Bilateral G Vertebral Arteries, Bilateral H Upper Extremity Arteries, Right J Upper Extremity Arteries, Left K Upper Extremity Arteries, Bilateral M Spinal Arteries Q Cervico-Cerebral Arch R Intracranial Arteries	Y Other Contrast	0 Unenhanced and Enhanced Z None	Z None
0 Thoracic Aorta 5 Common Carotid Arteries, Bilateral 8 Internal Carotid Arteries, Bilateral G Vertebral Arteries, Bilateral H Upper Extremity Arteries, Right J Upper Extremity Arteries, Left K Upper Extremity Arteries, Bilateral M Spinal Arteries Q Cervico-Cerebral Arch R Intracranial Arteries	Z None	Z None	Z None

B Imaging
3 Upper Arteries
4 Ultrasonography: Real time display of images of anatomy or flow information developed from the capture of reflected and attenuated high frequency sound waves

Body Part	Contrast	Qualifier	Qualifier
Character 4	Character 5	Character 6	Character 7
0 Thoracic Aorta 1 Brachiocephalic-Subclavian Artery, Right 2 Subclavian Artery, Left 3 Common Carotid Artery, Right 4 Common Carotid Artery, Left 5 Common Carotid Arteries, Bilateral 6 Internal Carotid Artery, Right 7 Internal Carotid Artery, Left 8 Internal Carotid Arteries, Bilateral H Upper Extremity Arteries, Right J Upper Extremity Arteries, Left K Upper Extremity Arteries, Bilateral R Intracranial Arteries S Pulmonary Artery, Right T Pulmonary Artery, Left V Ophthalmic Arteries	Z None	Z None	3 Intravascular Z None

LC Limited Coverage NC Noncovered HAC HAC-associated Procedure CC Combination Cluster - See Appendix G for code lists
DRG Non-OR-Affecting MS-DRG Assignment New/Revised Text in Orange ♂ Male ♀ Female

IMAGING B00-BY4

650 2020 ICD-10-PCS

B Imaging
4 Lower Arteries
0 Plain Radiography: Planar display of an image developed from the capture of external ionizing radiation on photographic or photoconductive plate

Body Part	Contrast	Qualifier	Qualifier
Character 4	**Character 5**	**Character 6**	**Character 7**
0 Abdominal Aorta **2** Hepatic Artery **3** Splenic Arteries **4** Superior Mesenteric Artery **5** Inferior Mesenteric Artery **6** Renal Artery, Right **7** Renal Artery, Left **8** Renal Arteries, Bilateral **9** Lumbar Arteries **B** Intra-Abdominal Arteries, Other **C** Pelvic Arteries **D** Aorta and Bilateral Lower Extremity Arteries **F** Lower Extremity Arteries, Right **G** Lower Extremity Arteries, Left **J** Lower Arteries, Other **M** Renal Artery Transplant	**0** High Osmolar **1** Low Osmolar **Y** Other Contrast	**Z** None	**Z** None

B Imaging
4 Lower Arteries
1 Fluoroscopy: Single plane or bi-plane real time display of an image developed from the capture of external ionizing radiation on a fluorescent screen. The image may also be stored by either digital or analog means

Body Part Character 4	Contrast Character 5	Qualifier Character 6	Qualifier Character 7
0 Abdominal Aorta **2** Hepatic Artery **3** Splenic Arteries **4** Superior Mesenteric Artery **5** Inferior Mesenteric Artery **6** Renal Artery, Right **7** Renal Artery, Left **8** Renal Arteries, Bilateral **9** Lumbar Arteries **B** Intra-Abdominal Arteries, Other **C** Pelvic Arteries **D** Aorta and Bilateral Lower Extremity Arteries **F** Lower Extremity Arteries, Right **G** Lower Extremity Arteries, Left **J** Lower Arteries, Other	**0** High Osmolar **1** Low Osmolar **Y** Other Contrast	**1** Laser	**0** Intraoperative
0 Abdominal Aorta **2** Hepatic Artery **3** Splenic Arteries **4** Superior Mesenteric Artery **5** Inferior Mesenteric Artery **6** Renal Artery, Right **7** Renal Artery, Left **8** Renal Arteries, Bilateral **9** Lumbar Arteries **B** Intra-Abdominal Arteries, Other **C** Pelvic Arteries **D** Aorta and Bilateral Lower Extremity Arteries **F** Lower Extremity Arteries, Right **G** Lower Extremity Arteries, Left **J** Lower Arteries, Other	**0** High Osmolar **1** Low Osmolar **Y** Other Contrast	**Z** None	**Z** None
0 Abdominal Aorta **2** Hepatic Artery **3** Splenic Arteries **4** Superior Mesenteric Artery **5** Inferior Mesenteric Artery **6** Renal Artery, Right **7** Renal Artery, Left **8** Renal Arteries, Bilateral **9** Lumbar Arteries **B** Intra-Abdominal Arteries, Other **C** Pelvic Arteries **D** Aorta and Bilateral Lower Extremity Arteries **F** Lower Extremity Arteries, Right **G** Lower Extremity Arteries, Left **J** Lower Arteries, Other	**Z** None	**Z** None	**Z** None

LC Limited Coverage NC Noncovered HAC HAC-associated Procedure CC Combination Cluster - See Appendix G for code lists
DRG Non-OR-Affecting MS-DRG Assignment New/Revised Text in **Orange** ♂ Male ♀ Female

652 2020 ICD-10-PCS

IMAGING B00-BY4

B Imaging
4 Lower Arteries
2 Computerized Tomography (CT Scan): Computer reformatted digital display of multiplanar images developed from the capture of multiple exposures of external ionizing radiation

Body Part	Contrast	Qualifier	Qualifier
Character 4	**Character 5**	**Character 6**	**Character 7**
0 Abdominal Aorta **1** Celiac Artery **4** Superior Mesenteric Artery **8** Renal Arteries, Bilateral **C** Pelvic Arteries **F** Lower Extremity Arteries, Right **G** Lower Extremity Arteries, Left **H** Lower Extremity Arteries, Bilateral **M** Renal Artery Transplant	**0** High Osmolar **1** Low Osmolar **Y** Other Contrast	**Z** None	**Z** None
0 Abdominal Aorta **1** Celiac Artery **4** Superior Mesenteric Artery **8** Renal Arteries, Bilateral **C** Pelvic Arteries **F** Lower Extremity Arteries, Right **G** Lower Extremity Arteries, Left **H** Lower Extremity Arteries, Bilateral **M** Renal Artery Transplant	**Z** None	**2** Intravascular Optical Coherence **Z** None	**Z** None

B Imaging
4 Lower Arteries
3 Magnetic Resonance Imaging (MRI): Computer reformatted digital display of multiplanar images developed from the capture of radiofrequency signals emitted by nuclei in a body site excited within a magnetic field

Body Part	Contrast	Qualifier	Qualifier
Character 4	**Character 5**	**Character 6**	**Character 7**
0 Abdominal Aorta **1** Celiac Artery **4** Superior Mesenteric Artery **8** Renal Arteries, Bilateral **C** Pelvic Arteries **F** Lower Extremity Arteries, Right **G** Lower Extremity Arteries, Left **H** Lower Extremity Arteries, Bilateral	**Y** Other Contrast	**0** Unenhanced and Enhanced **Z** None	**Z** None
0 Abdominal Aorta **1** Celiac Artery **4** Superior Mesenteric Artery **8** Renal Arteries, Bilateral **C** Pelvic Arteries **F** Lower Extremity Arteries, Right **G** Lower Extremity Arteries, Left **H** Lower Extremity Arteries, Bilateral	**Z** None	**Z** None	**Z** None

B Imaging
4 Lower Arteries
4 Ultrasonography: Real time display of images of anatomy or flow information developed from the capture of reflected and attenuated high frequency sound waves

Body Part Character 4	Contrast Character 5	Qualifier Character 6	Qualifier Character 7
0 Abdominal Aorta **4** Superior Mesenteric Artery **5** Inferior Mesenteric Artery **6** Renal Artery, Right **7** Renal Artery, Left **8** Renal Arteries, Bilateral **B** Intra-Abdominal Arteries, Other **F** Lower Extremity Arteries, Right **G** Lower Extremity Arteries, Left **H** Lower Extremity Arteries, Bilateral **K** Celiac and Mesenteric Arteries **L** Femoral Artery **N** Penile Arteries	**Z** None	**Z** None	**3** Intravascular **Z** None

B Imaging
5 Veins
0 Plain Radiography: Planar display of an image developed from the capture of external ionizing radiation on photographic or photoconductive plate

Body Part Character 4	Contrast Character 5	Qualifier Character 6	Qualifier Character 7
0 Epidural Veins **1** Cerebral and Cerebellar Veins **2** Intracranial Sinuses **3** Jugular Veins, Right **4** Jugular Veins, Left **5** Jugular Veins, Bilateral **6** Subclavian Vein, Right **7** Subclavian Vein, Left **8** Superior Vena Cava **9** Inferior Vena Cava **B** Lower Extremity Veins, Right **C** Lower Extremity Veins, Left **D** Lower Extremity Veins, Bilateral **F** Pelvic (Iliac) Veins, Right **G** Pelvic (Iliac) Veins, Left **H** Pelvic (Iliac) Veins, Bilateral **J** Renal Vein, Right **K** Renal Vein, Left **L** Renal Veins, Bilateral **M** Upper Extremity Veins, Right **N** Upper Extremity Veins, Left **P** Upper Extremity Veins, Bilateral **Q** Pulmonary Vein, Right **R** Pulmonary Vein, Left **S** Pulmonary Veins, Bilateral **T** Portal and Splanchnic Veins **V** Veins, Other **W** Dialysis Shunt/Fistula	**0** High Osmolar **1** Low Osmolar **Y** Other Contrast	**Z** None	**Z** None

B Imaging
5 Veins
1 Fluoroscopy: Single plane or bi-plane real time display of an image developed from the capture of external ionizing radiation on a fluorescent screen. The image may also be stored by either digital or analog means

Body Part	Contrast	Qualifier	Qualifier
Character 4	**Character 5**	**Character 6**	**Character 7**
0 Epidural Veins **1** Cerebral and Cerebellar Veins **2** Intracranial Sinuses **3** Jugular Veins, Right **4** Jugular Veins, Left **5** Jugular Veins, Bilateral **6** Subclavian Vein, Right **7** Subclavian Vein, Left **8** Superior Vena Cava **9** Inferior Vena Cava **B** Lower Extremity Veins, Right **C** Lower Extremity Veins, Left **D** Lower Extremity Veins, Bilateral **F** Pelvic (Iliac) Veins, Right **G** Pelvic (Iliac) Veins, Left **H** Pelvic (Iliac) Veins, Bilateral **J** Renal Vein, Right **K** Renal Vein, Left **L** Renal Veins, Bilateral **M** Upper Extremity Veins, Right **N** Upper Extremity Veins, Left **P** Upper Extremity Veins, Bilateral **Q** Pulmonary Vein, Right **R** Pulmonary Vein, Left **S** Pulmonary Veins, Bilateral **T** Portal and Splanchnic Veins **V** Veins, Other **W** Dialysis Shunt/Fistula	**0** High Osmolar **1** Low Osmolar **Y** Other Contrast **Z** None	**Z** None	**A** Guidance **Z** None

PICC Supervir vena cava B5182ZA

B Imaging
5 Veins
2 Computerized Tomography (CT Scan): Computer reformatted digital display of multiplanar images developed from the capture of multiple exposures of external ionizing radiation

Body Part	Contrast	Qualifier	Qualifier
Character 4	Character 5	Character 6	Character 7
2 Intracranial Sinuses **8** Superior Vena Cava **9** Inferior Vena Cava **F** Pelvic (Iliac) Veins, Right **G** Pelvic (Iliac) Veins, Left **H** Pelvic (Iliac) Veins, Bilateral **J** Renal Vein, Right **K** Renal Vein, Left **L** Renal Veins, Bilateral **Q** Pulmonary Vein, Right **R** Pulmonary Vein, Left **S** Pulmonary Veins, Bilateral **T** Portal and Splanchnic Veins	**0** High Osmolar **1** Low Osmolar **Y** Other Contrast	**0** Unenhanced and Enhanced **Z** None	**Z** None
2 Intracranial Sinuses **8** Superior Vena Cava **9** Inferior Vena Cava **F** Pelvic (Iliac) Veins, Right **G** Pelvic (Iliac) Veins, Left **H** Pelvic (Iliac) Veins, Bilateral **J** Renal Vein, Right **K** Renal Vein, Left **L** Renal Veins, Bilateral **Q** Pulmonary Vein, Right **R** Pulmonary Vein, Left **S** Pulmonary Veins, Bilateral **T** Portal and Splanchnic Veins	**Z** None	**2** Intravascular Optical Coherence **Z** None	**Z** None

B Imaging
5 Veins
3 Magnetic Resonance Imaging (MRI): Computer reformatted digital display of multiplanar images developed from the capture of radiofrequency signals emitted by nuclei in a body site excited within a magnetic field

Body Part Character 4	Contrast Character 5	Qualifier Character 6	Qualifier Character 7
1 Cerebral and Cerebellar Veins **2** Intracranial Sinuses **5** Jugular Veins, Bilateral **8** Superior Vena Cava **9** Inferior Vena Cava **B** Lower Extremity Veins, Right **C** Lower Extremity Veins, Left **D** Lower Extremity Veins, Bilateral **H** Pelvic (Iliac) Veins, Bilateral **L** Renal Veins, Bilateral **M** Upper Extremity Veins, Right **N** Upper Extremity Veins, Left **P** Upper Extremity Veins, Bilateral **S** Pulmonary Veins, Bilateral **T** Portal and Splanchnic Veins **V** Veins, Other	**Y** Other Contrast	**0** Unenhanced and Enhanced **Z** None	**Z** None
1 Cerebral and Cerebellar Veins **2** Intracranial Sinuses **5** Jugular Veins, Bilateral **8** Superior Vena Cava **9** Inferior Vena Cava **B** Lower Extremity Veins, Right **C** Lower Extremity Veins, Left **D** Lower Extremity Veins, Bilateral **H** Pelvic (Iliac) Veins, Bilateral **L** Renal Veins, Bilateral **M** Upper Extremity Veins, Right **N** Upper Extremity Veins, Left **P** Upper Extremity Veins, Bilateral **S** Pulmonary Veins, Bilateral **T** Portal and Splanchnic Veins **V** Veins, Other	**Z** None	**Z** None	**Z** None

B Imaging
5 Veins
4 Ultrasonography: Real time display of images of anatomy or flow information developed from the capture of reflected and attenuated high frequency sound waves

Body Part	Contrast	Qualifier	Qualifier
Character 4	**Character 5**	**Character 6**	**Character 7**
3 Jugular Veins, Right **4** Jugular Veins, Left **6** Subclavian Vein, Right **7** Subclavian Vein, Left **8** Superior Vena Cava **9** Inferior Vena Cava **B** Lower Extremity Veins, Right **C** Lower Extremity Veins, Left **D** Lower Extremity Veins, Bilateral **J** Renal Vein, Right **K** Renal Vein, Left **L** Renal Veins, Bilateral **M** Upper Extremity Veins, Right **N** Upper Extremity Veins, Left **P** Upper Extremity Veins, Bilateral **T** Portal and Splanchnic Veins	**Z** None	**Z** None	**3** Intravascular **A** Guidance **Z** None

B Imaging
7 Lymphatic System
0 Plain Radiography: Planar display of an image developed from the capture of external ionizing radiation on photographic or photoconductive plate

Body Part	Contrast	Qualifier	Qualifier
Character 4	**Character 5**	**Character 6**	**Character 7**
0 Abdominal/Retroperitoneal Lymphatics, Unilateral **1** Abdominal/Retroperitoneal Lymphatics, Bilateral **4** Lymphatics, Head and Neck **5** Upper Extremity Lymphatics, Right **6** Upper Extremity Lymphatics, Left **7** Upper Extremity Lymphatics, Bilateral **8** Lower Extremity Lymphatics, Right **9** Lower Extremity Lymphatics, Left **B** Lower Extremity Lymphatics, Bilateral **C** Lymphatics, Pelvic	**0** High Osmolar **1** Low Osmolar **Y** Other Contrast	**Z** None	**Z** None

B Imaging
8 Eye
0 Plain Radiography: Planar display of an image developed from the capture of external ionizing radiation on photographic or photoconductive plate

Body Part	Contrast	Qualifier	Qualifier
Character 4	**Character 5**	**Character 6**	**Character 7**
0 Lacrimal Duct, Right 1 Lacrimal Duct, Left 2 Lacrimal Ducts, Bilateral	0 High Osmolar 1 Low Osmolar Y Other Contrast	Z None	Z None
3 Optic Foramina, Right 4 Optic Foramina, Left 5 Eye, Right 6 Eye, Left 7 Eyes, Bilateral	Z None	Z None	Z None

B Imaging
8 Eye
2 Computerized Tomography (CT Scan): Computer reformatted digital display of multiplanar images developed from the capture of multiple exposures of external ionizing radiation

Body Part	Contrast	Qualifier	Qualifier
Character 4	**Character 5**	**Character 6**	**Character 7**
5 Eye, Right 6 Eye, Left 7 Eyes, Bilateral	0 High Osmolar 1 Low Osmolar Y Other Contrast	0 Unenhanced and Enhanced Z None	Z None
5 Eye, Right 6 Eye, Left 7 Eyes, Bilateral	Z None	Z None	Z None

B Imaging
8 Eye
3 Magnetic Resonance Imaging (MRI): Computer reformatted digital display of multiplanar images developed from the capture of radiofrequency signals emitted by nuclei in a body site excited within a magnetic field

Body Part	Contrast	Qualifier	Qualifier
Character 4	**Character 5**	**Character 6**	**Character 7**
5 Eye, Right 6 Eye, Left 7 Eyes, Bilateral	Y Other Contrast	0 Unenhanced and Enhanced Z None	Z None
5 Eye, Right 6 Eye, Left 7 Eyes, Bilateral	Z None	Z None	Z None

B Imaging
8 Eye
4 Ultrasonography: Real time display of images of anatomy or flow information developed from the capture of reflected and attenuated high frequency sound waves

Body Part	Contrast	Qualifier	Qualifier
Character 4	**Character 5**	**Character 6**	**Character 7**
5 Eye, Right 6 Eye, Left 7 Eyes, Bilateral	Z None	Z None	Z None

B Imaging
9 Ear, Nose, Mouth and Throat
0 Plain Radiography: Planar display of an image developed from the capture of external ionizing radiation on photographic or photoconductive plate

Body Part Character 4	Contrast Character 5	Qualifier Character 6	Qualifier Character 7
2 Paranasal Sinuses **F** Nasopharynx/Oropharynx **H** Mastoids	**Z** None	**Z** None	**Z** None
4 Parotid Gland, Right **5** Parotid Gland, Left **6** Parotid Glands, Bilateral **7** Submandibular Gland, Right **8** Submandibular Gland, Left **9** Submandibular Glands, Bilateral **B** Salivary Gland, Right **C** Salivary Gland, Left **D** Salivary Glands, Bilateral	**0** High Osmolar **1** Low Osmolar **Y** Other Contrast	**Z** None	**Z** None

B Imaging
9 Ear, Nose, Mouth and Throat
1 Fluoroscopy: Single plane or bi-plane real time display of an image developed from the capture of external ionizing radiation on a fluorescent screen. The image may also be stored by either digital or analog means

Body Part Character 4	Contrast Character 5	Qualifier Character 6	Qualifier Character 7
G Pharynx and Epiglottis **J** Larynx	**Y** Other Contrast **Z** None	**Z** None	**Z** None

B Imaging
9 Ear, Nose, Mouth and Throat
2 Computerized Tomography (CT Scan): Computer reformatted digital display of multiplanar images developed from the capture of multiple exposures of external ionizing radiation

Body Part Character 4	Contrast Character 5	Qualifier Character 6	Qualifier Character 7
0 Ear **2** Paranasal Sinuses **6** Parotid Glands, Bilateral **9** Submandibular Glands, Bilateral **D** Salivary Glands, Bilateral **F** Nasopharynx/Oropharynx **J** Larynx	**0** High Osmolar **1** Low Osmolar **Y** Other Contrast	**0** Unenhanced and Enhanced **Z** None	**Z** None
0 Ear **2** Paranasal Sinuses **6** Parotid Glands, Bilateral **9** Submandibular Glands, Bilateral **D** Salivary Glands, Bilateral **F** Nasopharynx/Oropharynx **J** Larynx	**Z** None	**Z** None	**Z** None

B Imaging
9 Ear, Nose, Mouth and Throat
3 Magnetic Resonance Imaging (MRI): Computer reformatted digital display of multiplanar images developed from the capture of radiofrequency signals emitted by nuclei in a body site excited within a magnetic field

Body Part Character 4	Contrast Character 5	Qualifier Character 6	Qualifier Character 7
0 Ear 2 Paranasal Sinuses 6 Parotid Glands, Bilateral 9 Submandibular Glands, Bilateral D Salivary Glands, Bilateral F Nasopharynx/Oropharynx J Larynx	Y Other Contrast	0 Unenhanced and Enhanced Z None	Z None
0 Ear 2 Paranasal Sinuses 6 Parotid Glands, Bilateral 9 Submandibular Glands, Bilateral D Salivary Glands, Bilateral F Nasopharynx/Oropharynx J Larynx	Z None	Z None	Z None

B Imaging
B Respiratory System
0 Plain Radiography: Planar display of an image developed from the capture of external ionizing radiation on photographic or photoconductive plate

Body Part Character 4	Contrast Character 5	Qualifier Character 6	Qualifier Character 7
7 Tracheobronchial Tree, Right 8 Tracheobronchial Tree, Left 9 Tracheobronchial Trees, Bilateral	Y Other Contrast	Z None	Z None
D Upper Airways	Z None	Z None	Z None

B Imaging
B Respiratory System
1 Fluoroscopy: Single plane or bi-plane real time display of an image developed from the capture of external ionizing radiation on a fluorescent screen. The image may also be stored by either digital or analog means

Body Part Character 4	Contrast Character 5	Qualifier Character 6	Qualifier Character 7
2 Lung, Right 3 Lung, Left 4 Lungs, Bilateral 6 Diaphragm C Mediastinum D Upper Airways	Z None	Z None	Z None
7 Tracheobronchial Tree, Right 8 Tracheobronchial Tree, Left 9 Tracheobronchial Trees, Bilateral	Y Other Contrast	Z None	Z None

B Imaging
B Respiratory System
2 Computerized Tomography (CT Scan): Computer reformatted digital display of multiplanar images developed from the capture of multiple exposures of external ionizing radiation

Body Part	Contrast	Qualifier	Qualifier
Character 4	**Character 5**	**Character 6**	**Character 7**
4 Lungs, Bilateral **7** Tracheobronchial Tree, Right **8** Tracheobronchial Tree, Left **9** Tracheobronchial Trees, Bilateral **F** Trachea/Airways	**0** High Osmolar **1** Low Osmolar **Y** Other Contrast	**0** Unenhanced and Enhanced **Z** None	**Z** None
4 Lungs, Bilateral **7** Tracheobronchial Tree, Right **8** Tracheobronchial Tree, Left **9** Tracheobronchial Trees, Bilateral **F** Trachea/Airways	**Z** None	**Z** None	**Z** None

B Imaging
B Respiratory System
3 Magnetic Resonance Imaging (MRI): Computer reformatted digital display of multiplanar images developed from the capture of radiofrequency signals emitted by nuclei in a body site excited within a magnetic field

Body Part	Contrast	Qualifier	Qualifier
Character 4	**Character 5**	**Character 6**	**Character 7**
G Lung Apices	**Y** Other Contrast	**0** Unenhanced and Enhanced **Z** None	**Z** None
G Lung Apices	**Z** None	**Z** None	**Z** None

B Imaging
B Respiratory System
4 Ultrasonography: Real time display of images of anatomy or flow information developed from the capture of reflected and attenuated high frequency sound waves

Body Part	Contrast	Qualifier	Qualifier
Character 4	**Character 5**	**Character 6**	**Character 7**
B Pleura **C** Mediastinum	**Z** None	**Z** None	**Z** None

B Imaging
D Gastrointestinal System
1 Fluoroscopy: Single plane or bi-plane real time display of an image developed from the capture of external ionizing radiation on a fluorescent screen. The image may also be stored by either digital or analog means

Body Part	Contrast	Qualifier	Qualifier
Character 4	**Character 5**	**Character 6**	**Character 7**
1 Esophagus **2** Stomach **3** Small Bowel **4** Colon **5** Upper GI **6** Upper GI and Small Bowel **9** Duodenum **B** Mouth/Oropharynx	**Y** Other Contrast **Z** None	**Z** None	**Z** None

LC Limited Coverage NC Noncovered HAC HAC-associated Procedure CC Combination Cluster - See Appendix G for code lists
DRG Non-OR-Affecting MS-DRG Assignment New/Revised Text in **Orange** ♂ Male ♀ Female

IMAGING B00-BY4

662 2020 ICD-10-PCS

B Imaging
D Gastrointestinal System
2 Computerized Tomography (CT Scan): Computer reformatted digital display of multiplanar images developed from the capture of multiple exposures of external ionizing radiation

Body Part Character 4	Contrast Character 5	Qualifier Character 6	Qualifier Character 7
4 Colon	**0** High Osmolar **1** Low Osmolar **Y** Other Contrast	**0** Unenhanced and Enhanced **Z** None	**Z** None
4 Colon	**Z** None	**Z** None	**Z** None

B Imaging
D Gastrointestinal System
4 Ultrasonography: Real time display of images of anatomy or flow information developed from the capture of reflected and attenuated high frequency sound waves

Body Part Character 4	Contrast Character 5	Qualifier Character 6	Qualifier Character 7
1 Esophagus **2** Stomach **7** Gastrointestinal Tract **8** Appendix **9** Duodenum **C** Rectum	**Z** None	**Z** None	**Z** None

B Imaging
F Hepatobiliary System and Pancreas
0 Plain Radiography: Planar display of an image developed from the capture of external ionizing radiation on photographic or photoconductive plate

Body Part Character 4	Contrast Character 5	Qualifier Character 6	Qualifier Character 7
0 Bile Ducts **3** Gallbladder and Bile Ducts **C** Hepatobiliary System, All	**0** High Osmolar **1** Low Osmolar **Y** Other Contrast	**Z** None	**Z** None

B Imaging
F Hepatobiliary System and Pancreas
1 Fluoroscopy: Single plane or bi-plane real time display of an image developed from the capture of external ionizing radiation on a fluorescent screen. The image may also be stored by either digital or analog means

Body Part Character 4	Contrast Character 5	Qualifier Character 6	Qualifier Character 7
0 Bile Ducts **1** Biliary and Pancreatic Ducts **2** Gallbladder **3** Gallbladder and Bile Ducts **4** Gallbladder, Bile Ducts and Pancreatic Ducts **8** Pancreatic Ducts	**0** High Osmolar **1** Low Osmolar **Y** Other Contrast	**Z** None	**Z** None

B Imaging
F Hepatobiliary System and Pancreas
2 Computerized Tomography (CT Scan): Computer reformatted digital display of multiplanar images developed from the capture of multiple exposures of external ionizing radiation

Body Part Character 4	Contrast Character 5	Qualifier Character 6	Qualifier Character 7
5 Liver 6 Liver and Spleen 7 Pancreas C Hepatobiliary System, All	0 High Osmolar 1 Low Osmolar Y Other Contrast	0 Unenhanced and Enhanced Z None	Z None
5 Liver 6 Liver and Spleen 7 Pancreas C Hepatobiliary System, All	Z None	Z None	Z None

B Imaging
F Hepatobiliary System and Pancreas
3 Magnetic Resonance Imaging (MRI): Computer reformatted digital display of multiplanar images developed from the capture of radiofrequency signals emitted by nuclei in a body site excited within a magnetic field

Body Part Character 4	Contrast Character 5	Qualifier Character 6	Qualifier Character 7
5 Liver 6 Liver and Spleen 7 Pancreas	Y Other Contrast – gadoteridol	0 Unenhanced and Enhanced Z None w/ contrast	Z None
5 Liver 6 Liver and Spleen 7 Pancreas	Z None	Z None	Z None

B Imaging
F Hepatobiliary System and Pancreas
4 Ultrasonography: Real time display of images of anatomy or flow information developed from the capture of reflected and attenuated high frequency sound waves

Body Part Character 4	Contrast Character 5	Qualifier Character 6	Qualifier Character 7
0 Bile Ducts 2 Gallbladder 3 Gallbladder and Bile Ducts 5 Liver 6 Liver and Spleen 7 Pancreas C Hepatobiliary System, All	Z None	Z None	Z None

B Imaging
G Endocrine System
2 Computerized Tomography (CT Scan): Computer reformatted digital display of multiplanar images developed from the capture of multiple exposures of external ionizing radiation

Body Part Character 4	Contrast Character 5	Qualifier Character 6	Qualifier Character 7
2 Adrenal Glands, Bilateral 3 Parathyroid Glands 4 Thyroid Gland	0 High Osmolar 1 Low Osmolar Y Other Contrast	0 Unenhanced and Enhanced Z None	Z None
2 Adrenal Glands, Bilateral 3 Parathyroid Glands 4 Thyroid Gland	Z None	Z None	Z None

B Imaging
G Endocrine System
3 Magnetic Resonance Imaging (MRI): Computer reformatted digital display of multiplanar images developed from the capture of radiofrequency signals emitted by nuclei in a body site excited within a magnetic field

Body Part	Contrast	Qualifier	Qualifier
Character 4	Character 5	Character 6	Character 7
2 Adrenal Glands, Bilateral 3 Parathyroid Glands 4 Thyroid Gland	Y Other Contrast	0 Unenhanced and Enhanced Z None	Z None
2 Adrenal Glands, Bilateral 3 Parathyroid Glands 4 Thyroid Gland	Z None	Z None	Z None

B Imaging
G Endocrine System
4 Ultrasonography: Real time display of images of anatomy or flow information developed from the capture of reflected and attenuated high frequency sound waves

Body Part	Contrast	Qualifier	Qualifier
Character 4	Character 5	Character 6	Character 7
0 Adrenal Gland, Right 1 Adrenal Gland, Left 2 Adrenal Glands, Bilateral 3 Parathyroid Glands 4 Thyroid Gland	Z None	Z None	Z None

thyroid biopsy ØGBH3ZX

B Imaging
H Skin, Subcutaneous Tissue and Breast
0 Plain Radiography: Planar display of an image developed from the capture of external ionizing radiation on photographic or photoconductive plate

Body Part	Contrast	Qualifier	Qualifier
Character 4	Character 5	Character 6	Character 7
0 Breast, Right 1 Breast, Left 2 Breasts, Bilateral	Z None	Z None	Z None
3 Single Mammary Duct, Right 4 Single Mammary Duct, Left 5 Multiple Mammary Ducts, Right 6 Multiple Mammary Ducts, Left	0 High Osmolar 1 Low Osmolar Y Other Contrast Z None	Z None	Z None

B Imaging
H Skin, Subcutaneous Tissue and Breast
3 Magnetic Resonance Imaging (MRI): Computer reformatted digital display of multiplanar images developed from the capture of radiofrequency signals emitted by nuclei in a body site excited within a magnetic field

Body Part Character 4	Contrast Character 5	Qualifier Character 6	Qualifier Character 7
0 Breast, Right **1** Breast, Left **2** Breasts, Bilateral **D** Subcutaneous Tissue, Head/Neck **F** Subcutaneous Tissue, Upper Extremity **G** Subcutaneous Tissue, Thorax **H** Subcutaneous Tissue, Abdomen and Pelvis **J** Subcutaneous Tissue, Lower Extremity	**Y** Other Contrast	**0** Unenhanced and Enhanced **Z** None	**Z** None
0 Breast, Right **1** Breast, Left **2** Breasts, Bilateral **D** Subcutaneous Tissue, Head/Neck **F** Subcutaneous Tissue, Upper Extremity **G** Subcutaneous Tissue, Thorax **H** Subcutaneous Tissue, Abdomen and Pelvis **J** Subcutaneous Tissue, Lower Extremity	**Z** None	**Z** None	**Z** None

B Imaging
H Skin, Subcutaneous Tissue and Breast
4 Ultrasonography: Real time display of images of anatomy or flow information developed from the capture of reflected and attenuated high frequency sound waves

Body Part Character 4	Contrast Character 5	Qualifier Character 6	Qualifier Character 7
0 Breast, Right **1** Breast, Left **2** Breasts, Bilateral **7** Extremity, Upper **8** Extremity, Lower **9** Abdominal Wall **B** Chest Wall **C** Head and Neck	**Z** None	**Z** None	**Z** None

B Imaging
L Connective Tissue
3 Magnetic Resonance Imaging (MRI): Computer reformatted digital display of multiplanar images developed from the capture of radiofrequency signals emitted by nuclei in a body site excited within a magnetic field

Body Part	Contrast	Qualifier	Qualifier
Character 4	Character 5	Character 6	Character 7
0 Connective Tissue, Upper Extremity 1 Connective Tissue, Lower Extremity 2 Tendons, Upper Extremity 3 Tendons, Lower Extremity	Y Other Contrast	0 Unenhanced and Enhanced Z None	Z None
0 Connective Tissue, Upper Extremity 1 Connective Tissue, Lower Extremity 2 Tendons, Upper Extremity 3 Tendons, Lower Extremity	Z None	Z None	Z None

B Imaging
L Connective Tissue
4 Ultrasonography: Real time display of images of anatomy or flow information developed from the capture of reflected and attenuated high frequency sound waves

Body Part	Contrast	Qualifier	Qualifier
Character 4	Character 5	Character 6	Character 7
0 Connective Tissue, Upper Extremity 1 Connective Tissue, Lower Extremity 2 Tendons, Upper Extremity 3 Tendons, Lower Extremity	Z None	Z None	Z None

B Imaging
N Skull and Facial Bones
0 Plain Radiography: Planar display of an image developed from the capture of external ionizing radiation on photographic or photoconductive plate

Body Part	Contrast	Qualifier	Qualifier
Character 4	Character 5	Character 6	Character 7
0 Skull 1 Orbit, Right 2 Orbit, Left 3 Orbits, Bilateral 4 Nasal Bones 5 Facial Bones 6 Mandible B Zygomatic Arch, Right C Zygomatic Arch, Left D Zygomatic Arches, Bilateral G Tooth, Single H Teeth, Multiple J Teeth, All	Z None	Z None	Z None
7 Temporomandibular Joint, Right 8 Temporomandibular Joint, Left 9 Temporomandibular Joints, Bilateral	0 High Osmolar 1 Low Osmolar Y Other Contrast Z None	Z None	Z None

B Imaging
N Skull and Facial Bones
1 Fluoroscopy: Single plane or bi-plane real time display of an image developed from the capture of external ionizing radiation on a fluorescent screen. The image may also be stored by either digital or analog means

Body Part	Contrast	Qualifier	Qualifier
Character 4	Character 5	Character 6	Character 7
7 Temporomandibular Joint, Right 8 Temporomandibular Joint, Left 9 Temporomandibular Joints, Bilateral	0 High Osmolar 1 Low Osmolar Y Other Contrast Z None	Z None	Z None

B Imaging
N Skull and Facial Bones
2 Computerized Tomography (CT Scan): Computer reformatted digital display of multiplanar images developed from the capture of multiple exposures of external ionizing radiation

Body Part	Contrast	Qualifier	Qualifier
Character 4	Character 5	Character 6	Character 7
0 Skull 3 Orbits, Bilateral 5 Facial Bones 6 Mandible 9 Temporomandibular Joints, Bilateral F Temporal Bones	0 High Osmolar 1 Low Osmolar Y Other Contrast Z None	Z None	Z None

B Imaging
N Skull and Facial Bones
3 Magnetic Resonance Imaging (MRI): Computer reformatted digital display of multiplanar images developed from the capture of radiofrequency signals emitted by nuclei in a body site excited within a magnetic field

Body Part	Contrast	Qualifier	Qualifier
Character 4	Character 5	Character 6	Character 7
9 Temporomandibular Joints, Bilateral	Y Other Contrast Z None	Z None	Z None

B Imaging
P Non-Axial Upper Bones
0 Plain Radiography: Planar display of an image developed from the capture of external ionizing radiation on photographic or photoconductive plate

Body Part	Contrast	Qualifier	Qualifier
Character 4	Character 5	Character 6	Character 7
0 Sternoclavicular Joint, Right 1 Sternoclavicular Joint, Left 2 Sternoclavicular Joints, Bilateral 3 Acromioclavicular Joints, Bilateral 4 Clavicle, Right 5 Clavicle, Left 6 Scapula, Right 7 Scapula, Left A Humerus, Right B Humerus, Left E Upper Arm, Right F Upper Arm, Left J Forearm, Right K Forearm, Left N Hand, Right P Hand, Left R Finger(s), Right S Finger(s), Left X Ribs, Right Y Ribs, Left	Z None	Z None	Z None

BP0 continued on next page

BP0 continued from previous page

B Imaging
P Non-Axial Upper Bones
0 Plain Radiography: Planar display of an image developed from the capture of external ionizing radiation on photographic or photoconductive plate

Body Part Character 4	Contrast Character 5	Qualifier Character 6	Qualifier Character 7
8 Shoulder, Right **9** Shoulder, Left **C** Hand/Finger Joint, Right **D** Hand/Finger Joint, Left **G** Elbow, Right **H** Elbow, Left **L** Wrist, Right **M** Wrist, Left	**0** High Osmolar **1** Low Osmolar **Y** Other Contrast **Z** None	**Z** None	**Z** None

B Imaging
P Non-Axial Upper Bones
1 Fluoroscopy: Single plane or bi-plane real time display of an image developed from the capture of external ionizing radiation on a fluorescent screen. The image may also be stored by either digital or analog means

Body Part Character 4	Contrast Character 5	Qualifier Character 6	Qualifier Character 7
0 Sternoclavicular Joint, Right **1** Sternoclavicular Joint, Left **2** Sternoclavicular Joints, Bilateral **3** Acromioclavicular Joints, Bilateral **4** Clavicle, Right **5** Clavicle, Left **6** Scapula, Right **7** Scapula, Left **A** Humerus, Right **B** Humerus, Left **E** Upper Arm, Right **F** Upper Arm, Left **J** Forearm, Right **K** Forearm, Left **N** Hand, Right **P** Hand, Left **R** Finger(s), Right **S** Finger(s), Left **X** Ribs, Right **Y** Ribs, Left	**Z** None	**Z** None	**Z** None
8 Shoulder, Right **9** Shoulder, Left **L** Wrist, Right **M** Wrist, Left	**0** High Osmolar **1** Low Osmolar **Y** Other Contrast **Z** None	**Z** None	**Z** None
C Hand/Finger Joint, Right **D** Hand/Finger Joint, Left **G** Elbow, Right **H** Elbow, Left	**0** High Osmolar **1** Low Osmolar **Y** Other Contrast	**Z** None	**Z** None

B Imaging
P Non-Axial Upper Bones
2 Computerized Tomography (CT Scan): Computer reformatted digital display of multiplanar images developed from the capture of multiple exposures of external ionizing radiation

Body Part Character 4	Contrast Character 5	Qualifier Character 6	Qualifier Character 7
0 Sternoclavicular Joint, Right **1** Sternoclavicular Joint, Left **W** Thorax	**0** High Osmolar **1** Low Osmolar **Y** Other Contrast	**Z** None	**Z** None
2 Sternoclavicular Joints, Bilateral **3** Acromioclavicular Joints, Bilateral **4** Clavicle, Right **5** Clavicle, Left **6** Scapula, Right **7** Scapula, Left **8** Shoulder, Right **9** Shoulder, Left **A** Humerus, Right **B** Humerus, Left **E** Upper Arm, Right **F** Upper Arm, Left **G** Elbow, Right **H** Elbow, Left **J** Forearm, Right **K** Forearm, Left **L** Wrist, Right **M** Wrist, Left **N** Hand, Right **P** Hand, Left **Q** Hands and Wrists, Bilateral **R** Finger(s), Right **S** Finger(s), Left **T** Upper Extremity, Right **U** Upper Extremity, Left **V** Upper Extremities, Bilateral **X** Ribs, Right **Y** Ribs, Left	**0** High Osmolar **1** Low Osmolar **Y** Other Contrast **Z** None	**Z** None	**Z** None
C Hand/Finger Joint, Right **D** Hand/Finger Joint, Left	**Z** None	**Z** None	**Z** None

B Imaging
P Non-Axial Upper Bones
3 Magnetic Resonance Imaging (MRI): Computer reformatted digital display of multiplanar images developed from the capture of radiofrequency signals emitted by nuclei in a body site excited within a magnetic field

Body Part Character 4	Contrast Character 5	Qualifier Character 6	Qualifier Character 7
8 Shoulder, Right **9** Shoulder, Left **C** Hand/Finger Joint, Right **D** Hand/Finger Joint, Left **E** Upper Arm, Right **F** Upper Arm, Left **G** Elbow, Right **H** Elbow, Left **J** Forearm, Right **K** Forearm, Left **L** Wrist, Right **M** Wrist, Left	**Y** Other Contrast	**0** Unenhanced and Enhanced **Z** None	**Z** None

BP3 continued on next page

BP3 continued from previous page

B Imaging
P Non-Axial Upper Bones
3 Magnetic Resonance Imaging (MRI): Computer reformatted digital display of multiplanar images developed from the capture of radiofrequency signals emitted by nuclei in a body site excited within a magnetic field

Body Part Character 4	Contrast Character 5	Qualifier Character 6	Qualifier Character 7
8 Shoulder, Right **9** Shoulder, Left **C** Hand/Finger Joint, Right **D** Hand/Finger Joint, Left **E** Upper Arm, Right **F** Upper Arm, Left **G** Elbow, Right **H** Elbow, Left **J** Forearm, Right **K** Forearm, Left **L** Wrist, Right **M** Wrist, Left	**Z** None	**Z** None	**Z** None

B Imaging
P Non-Axial Upper Bones
4 Ultrasonography: Real time display of images of anatomy or flow information developed from the capture of reflected and attenuated high frequency sound waves

Body Part Character 4	Contrast Character 5	Qualifier Character 6	Qualifier Character 7
8 Shoulder, Right **9** Shoulder, Left **G** Elbow, Right **H** Elbow, Left **L** Wrist, Right **M** Wrist, Left **N** Hand, Right **P** Hand, Left	**Z** None	**Z** None	**1** Densitometry **Z** None

B Imaging
Q Non-Axial Lower Bones
0 Plain Radiography: Planar display of an image developed from the capture of external ionizing radiation on photographic or photoconductive plate

Body Part Character 4	Contrast Character 5	Qualifier Character 6	Qualifier Character 7
0 Hip, Right **1** Hip, Left	**0** High Osmolar **1** Low Osmolar **Y** Other Contrast	**Z** None	**Z** None
0 Hip, Right **1** Hip, Left	**Z** None	**Z** None	**1** Densitometry **Z** None
3 Femur, Right **4** Femur, Left	**Z** None	**Z** None	**1** Densitometry **Z** None
7 Knee, Right **8** Knee, Left **G** Ankle, Right **H** Ankle, Left	**0** High Osmolar **1** Low Osmolar **Y** Other Contrast **Z** None	**Z** None	**Z** None
D Lower Leg, Right **F** Lower Leg, Left **J** Calcaneus, Right **K** Calcaneus, Left **L** Foot, Right **M** Foot, Left **P** Toe(s), Right **Q** Toe(s), Left **V** Patella, Right **W** Patella, Left	**Z** None	**Z** None	**Z** None
X Foot/Toe Joint, Right **Y** Foot/Toe Joint, Left	**0** High Osmolar **1** Low Osmolar **Y** Other Contrast	**Z** None	**Z** None

LC Limited Coverage NC Noncovered HAC HAC-associated Procedure CC Combination Cluster - See Appendix G for code lists
DRG Non-OR-Affecting MS-DRG Assignment New/Revised Text in **Orange** ♂ Male ♀ Female

B Imaging
Q Non-Axial Lower Bones
1 Fluoroscopy: Single plane or bi-plane real time display of an image developed from the capture of external ionizing radiation on a fluorescent screen. The image may also be stored by either digital or analog means

Body Part Character 4	Contrast Character 5	Qualifier Character 6	Qualifier Character 7
0 Hip, Right **1** Hip, Left **7** Knee, Right **8** Knee, Left **G** Ankle, Right **H** Ankle, Left **X** Foot/Toe Joint, Right **Y** Foot/Toe Joint, Left	**0** High Osmolar **1** Low Osmolar **Y** Other Contrast **Z** None	**Z** None	**Z** None
3 Femur, Right **4** Femur, Left **D** Lower Leg, Right **F** Lower Leg, Left **J** Calcaneus, Right **K** Calcaneus, Left **L** Foot, Right **M** Foot, Left **P** Toe(s), Right **Q** Toe(s), Left **V** Patella, Right **W** Patella, Left	**Z** None	**Z** None	**Z** None

B Imaging
Q Non-Axial Lower Bones
2 Computerized Tomography (CT Scan): Computer reformatted digital display of multiplanar images developed from the capture of multiple exposures of external ionizing radiation

Body Part Character 4	Contrast Character 5	Qualifier Character 6	Qualifier Character 7
0 Hip, Right **1** Hip, Left **3** Femur, Right **4** Femur, Left **7** Knee, Right **8** Knee, Left **D** Lower Leg, Right **F** Lower Leg, Left **G** Ankle, Right **H** Ankle, Left **J** Calcaneus, Right **K** Calcaneus, Left **L** Foot, Right **M** Foot, Left **P** Toe(s), Right **Q** Toe(s), Left **R** Lower Extremity, Right **S** Lower Extremity, Left **V** Patella, Right **W** Patella, Left **X** Foot/Toe Joint, Right **Y** Foot/Toe Joint, Left	**0** High Osmolar **1** Low Osmolar **Y** Other Contrast **Z** None	**Z** None	**Z** None
B Tibia/Fibula, Right **C** Tibia/Fibula, Left	**0** High Osmolar **1** Low Osmolar **Y** Other Contrast	**Z** None	**Z** None

B Imaging
Q Non-Axial Lower Bones
3 Magnetic Resonance Imaging (MRI): Computer reformatted digital display of multiplanar images developed from the capture of radiofrequency signals emitted by nuclei in a body site excited within a magnetic field

Body Part Character 4	Contrast Character 5	Qualifier Character 6	Qualifier Character 7
0 Hip, Right **1** Hip, Left **3** Femur, Right **4** Femur, Left **7** Knee, Right **8** Knee, Left **D** Lower Leg, Right **F** Lower Leg, Left **G** Ankle, Right **H** Ankle, Left **J** Calcaneus, Right **K** Calcaneus, Left **L** Foot, Right **M** Foot, Left **P** Toe(s), Right **Q** Toe(s), Left **V** Patella, Right **W** Patella, Left	**Y** Other Contrast	**0** Unenhanced and Enhanced **Z** None	**Z** None
0 Hip, Right **1** Hip, Left **3** Femur, Right **4** Femur, Left **7** Knee, Right **8** Knee, Left **D** Lower Leg, Right **F** Lower Leg, Left **G** Ankle, Right **H** Ankle, Left **J** Calcaneus, Right **K** Calcaneus, Left **L** Foot, Right **M** Foot, Left **P** Toe(s), Right **Q** Toe(s), Left **V** Patella, Right **W** Patella, Left	**Z** None	**Z** None	**Z** None

B Imaging
Q Non-Axial Lower Bones
4 Ultrasonography: Real time display of images of anatomy or flow information developed from the capture of reflected and attenuated high frequency sound waves

Body Part Character 4	Contrast Character 5	Qualifier Character 6	Qualifier Character 7
0 Hip, Right **1** Hip, Left **2** Hips, Bilateral **7** Knee, Right **8** Knee, Left **9** Knees, Bilateral	**Z** None	**Z** None	**Z** None

B Imaging
R Axial Skeleton, Except Skull and Facial Bones
0 Plain Radiography: Planar display of an image developed from the capture of external ionizing radiation on photographic or photoconductive plate

Body Part	Contrast	Qualifier	Qualifier
Character 4	Character 5	Character 6	Character 7
0 Cervical Spine 7 Thoracic Spine 9 Lumbar Spine G Whole Spine	Z None	Z None	1 Densitometry Z None
1 Cervical Disc(s) 2 Thoracic Disc(s) 3 Lumbar Disc(s) 4 Cervical Facet Joint(s) 5 Thoracic Facet Joint(s) 6 Lumbar Facet Joint(s) D Sacroiliac Joints	0 High Osmolar 1 Low Osmolar Y Other Contrast Z None	Z None	Z None
8 Thoracolumbar Joint B Lumbosacral Joint C Pelvis F Sacrum and Coccyx H Sternum	Z None	Z None	Z None

B Imaging
R Axial Skeleton, Except Skull and Facial Bones
1 Fluoroscopy: Single plane or bi-plane real time display of an image developed from the capture of external ionizing radiation on a fluorescent screen. The image may also be stored by either digital or analog means

Body Part	Contrast	Qualifier	Qualifier
Character 4	Character 5	Character 6	Character 7
0 Cervical Spine 1 Cervical Disc(s) 2 Thoracic Disc(s) 3 Lumbar Disc(s) 4 Cervical Facet Joint(s) 5 Thoracic Facet Joint(s) 6 Lumbar Facet Joint(s) 7 Thoracic Spine 8 Thoracolumbar Joint 9 Lumbar Spine B Lumbosacral Joint C Pelvis D Sacroiliac Joints F Sacrum and Coccyx G Whole Spine H Sternum	0 High Osmolar 1 Low Osmolar Y Other Contrast Z None	Z None	Z None

B Imaging
R Axial Skeleton, Except Skull and Facial Bones
2 Computerized Tomography (CT Scan): Computer reformatted digital display of multiplanar images developed from the capture of multiple exposures of external ionizing radiation

Body Part	Contrast	Qualifier	Qualifier
Character 4	Character 5	Character 6	Character 7
0 Cervical Spine 7 Thoracic Spine 9 Lumbar Spine C Pelvis D Sacroiliac Joints F Sacrum and Coccyx	0 High Osmolar 1 Low Osmolar Y Other Contrast Z None	Z None	Z None

B Imaging
R Axial Skeleton, Except Skull and Facial Bones
3 Magnetic Resonance Imaging (MRI): Computer reformatted digital display of multiplanar images developed from the capture of radiofrequency signals emitted by nuclei in a body site excited within a magnetic field

Body Part	Contrast	Qualifier	Qualifier
Character 4	Character 5	Character 6	Character 7
0 Cervical Spine **1** Cervical Disc(s) **2** Thoracic Disc(s) **3** Lumbar Disc(s) **7** Thoracic Spine **9** Lumbar Spine **C** Pelvis **F** Sacrum and Coccyx	**Y** Other Contrast	**0** Unenhanced and Enhanced **Z** None	**Z** None
0 Cervical Spine **1** Cervical Disc(s) **2** Thoracic Disc(s) **3** Lumbar Disc(s) **7** Thoracic Spine **9** Lumbar Spine **C** Pelvis **F** Sacrum and Coccyx	**Z** None	**Z** None	**Z** None

B Imaging
R Axial Skeleton, Except Skull and Facial Bones
4 Ultrasonography: Real time display of images of anatomy or flow information developed from the capture of reflected and attenuated high frequency sound waves

Body Part	Contrast	Qualifier	Qualifier
Character 4	Character 5	Character 6	Character 7
0 Cervical Spine **7** Thoracic Spine **9** Lumbar Spine **F** Sacrum and Coccyx	**Z** None	**Z** None	**Z** None

B Imaging
T Urinary System
0 Plain Radiography: Planar display of an image developed from the capture of external ionizing radiation on photographic or photoconductive plate

Body Part	Contrast	Qualifier	Qualifier
Character 4	Character 5	Character 6	Character 7
0 Bladder **1** Kidney, Right **2** Kidney, Left **3** Kidneys, Bilateral **4** Kidneys, Ureters and Bladder **5** Urethra **6** Ureter, Right **7** Ureter, Left **8** Ureters, Bilateral **B** Bladder and Urethra **C** Ileal Diversion Loop	**0** High Osmolar **1** Low Osmolar **Y** Other Contrast **Z** None	**Z** None	**Z** None

B Imaging
T Urinary System
1 Fluoroscopy: Single plane or bi-plane real time display of an image developed from the capture of external ionizing radiation on a fluorescent screen. The image may also be stored by either digital or analog means

Body Part Character 4	Contrast Character 5	Qualifier Character 6	Qualifier Character 7
0 Bladder 1 Kidney, Right 2 Kidney, Left 3 Kidneys, Bilateral 4 Kidneys, Ureters and Bladder 5 Urethra 6 Ureter, Right 7 Ureter, Left B Bladder and Urethra C Ileal Diversion Loop D Kidney, Ureter and Bladder, Right F Kidney, Ureter and Bladder, Left G Ileal Loop, Ureters and Kidneys	0 High Osmolar 1 Low Osmolar Y Other Contrast Z None	Z None	Z None

B Imaging
T Urinary System
2 Computerized Tomography (CT Scan): Computer reformatted digital display of multiplanar images developed from the capture of multiple exposures of external ionizing radiation

Body Part Character 4	Contrast Character 5	Qualifier Character 6	Qualifier Character 7
0 Bladder 1 Kidney, Right 2 Kidney, Left 3 Kidneys, Bilateral 9 Kidney Transplant	0 High Osmolar 1 Low Osmolar Y Other Contrast	0 Unenhanced and Enhanced Z None	Z None
0 Bladder 1 Kidney, Right 2 Kidney, Left 3 Kidneys, Bilateral 9 Kidney Transplant	Z None	Z None	Z None

B Imaging
T Urinary System
3 Magnetic Resonance Imaging (MRI): Computer reformatted digital display of multiplanar images developed from the capture of radiofrequency signals emitted by nuclei in a body site excited within a magnetic field

Body Part Character 4	Contrast Character 5	Qualifier Character 6	Qualifier Character 7
0 Bladder 1 Kidney, Right 2 Kidney, Left 3 Kidneys, Bilateral 9 Kidney Transplant	Y Other Contrast	0 Unenhanced and Enhanced Z None	Z None
0 Bladder 1 Kidney, Right 2 Kidney, Left 3 Kidneys, Bilateral 9 Kidney Transplant	Z None	Z None	Z None

B Imaging
T Urinary System
4 Ultrasonography: Real time display of images of anatomy or flow information developed from the capture of reflected and attenuated high frequency sound waves

Body Part	Contrast	Qualifier	Qualifier
Character 4	**Character 5**	**Character 6**	**Character 7**
0 Bladder **1** Kidney, Right **2** Kidney, Left **3** Kidneys, Bilateral **5** Urethra **6** Ureter, Right **7** Ureter, Left **8** Ureters, Bilateral **9** Kidney Transplant **J** Kidneys and Bladder	**Z** None	**Z** None	**Z** None

B Imaging
U Female Reproductive System
0 Plain Radiography: Planar display of an image developed from the capture of external ionizing radiation on photographic or photoconductive plate

Body Part	Contrast	Qualifier	Qualifier
Character 4	**Character 5**	**Character 6**	**Character 7**
0 Fallopian Tube, Right ♀ **1** Fallopian Tube, Left ♀ **2** Fallopian Tubes, Bilateral ♀ **6** Uterus ♀ **8** Uterus and Fallopian Tubes ♀ **9** Vagina ♀	**0** High Osmolar **1** Low Osmolar **Y** Other Contrast	**Z** None	**Z** None

♀ BU000ZZ BU001ZZ BU00YZZ BU010ZZ BU011ZZ BU01YZZ BU020ZZ BU021ZZ BU02YZZ BU060ZZ BU061ZZ BU06YZZ BU080ZZ BU081ZZ BU08YZZ BU090ZZ BU091ZZ BU09YZZ

B Imaging
U Female Reproductive System
1 Fluoroscopy: Single plane or bi-plane real time display of an image developed from the capture of external ionizing radiation on a fluorescent screen. The image may also be stored by either digital or analog means

Body Part	Contrast	Qualifier	Qualifier
Character 4	**Character 5**	**Character 6**	**Character 7**
0 Fallopian Tube, Right ♀ **1** Fallopian Tube, Left ♀ **2** Fallopian Tubes, Bilateral ♀ **6** Uterus ♀ **8** Uterus and Fallopian Tubes ♀ **9** Vagina ♀	**0** High Osmolar **1** Low Osmolar **Y** Other Contrast **Z** None	**Z** None	**Z** None

♀ BU100ZZ BU101ZZ BU10YZZ BU10ZZZ BU110ZZ BU111ZZ BU11YZZ BU11ZZZ BU120ZZ BU121ZZ BU12YZZ BU12ZZZ BU160ZZ BU161ZZ BU16YZZ BU16ZZZ BU180ZZ BU181ZZ BU18YZZ BU18ZZZ BU190ZZ BU191ZZ BU19YZZ BU19ZZZ

B Imaging
U Female Reproductive System
3 Magnetic Resonance Imaging (MRI): Computer reformatted digital display of multiplanar images developed from the capture of radiofrequency signals emitted by nuclei in a body site excited within a magnetic field

Body Part Character 4	Contrast Character 5	Qualifier Character 6	Qualifier Character 7
3 Ovary, Right ♀ 4 Ovary, Left ♀ 5 Ovaries, Bilateral ♀ 6 Uterus ♀ 9 Vagina ♀ B Pregnant Uterus ♀ C Uterus and Ovaries ♀	Y Other Contrast	0 Unenhanced and Enhanced Z None	Z None
3 Ovary, Right ♀ 4 Ovary, Left ♀ 5 Ovaries, Bilateral ♀ 6 Uterus ♀ 9 Vagina ♀ B Pregnant Uterus ♀ C Uterus and Ovaries ♀	Z None	Z None	Z None

♀ BU33Y0Z BU33YZZ BU33ZZZ BU34Y0Z BU34YZZ BU34ZZZ BU35Y0Z BU35YZZ BU35ZZZ BU36Y0Z BU36YZZ BU36ZZZ BU39Y0Z BU39YZZ BU39ZZZ BU3BY0Z BU3BYZZ BU3BZZZ BU3CY0Z BU3CYZZ BU3CZZZ

B Imaging
U Female Reproductive System
4 Ultrasonography: Real time display of images of anatomy or flow information developed from the capture of reflected and attenuated high frequency sound waves

Body Part Character 4	Contrast Character 5	Qualifier Character 6	Qualifier Character 7
0 Fallopian Tube, Right ♀ 1 Fallopian Tube, Left ♀ 2 Fallopian Tubes, Bilateral ♀ 3 Ovary, Right ♀ 4 Ovary, Left ♀ 5 Ovaries, Bilateral ♀ 6 Uterus ♀ C Uterus and Ovaries ♀	Y Other Contrast Z None	Z None	Z None

♀ BU40YZZ BU40ZZZ BU41YZZ BU41ZZZ BU42YZZ BU42ZZZ BU43YZZ BU43ZZZ BU44YZZ BU44ZZZ BU45YZZ BU45ZZZ BU46YZZ BU46ZZZ BU4CYZZ BU4CZZZ

B Imaging
V Male Reproductive System
0 Plain Radiography: Planar display of an image developed from the capture of external ionizing radiation on photographic or photoconductive plate

Body Part Character 4	Contrast Character 5	Qualifier Character 6	Qualifier Character 7
0 Corpora Cavernosa ♂ 1 Epididymis, Right ♂ 2 Epididymis, Left ♂ 3 Prostate ♂ 5 Testicle, Right ♂ 6 Testicle, Left ♂ 8 Vasa Vasorum ♂	0 High Osmolar 1 Low Osmolar Y Other Contrast	Z None	Z None

♂ BV000ZZ BV001ZZ BV00YZZ BV010ZZ BV011ZZ BV01YZZ BV020ZZ BV021ZZ BV02YZZ BV030ZZ BV031ZZ BV03YZZ BV050ZZ BV051ZZ BV05YZZ BV060ZZ BV061ZZ BV06YZZ BV080ZZ BV081ZZ BV08YZZ

LC Limited Coverage NC Noncovered HAC HAC-associated Procedure CC Combination Cluster - See Appendix G for code lists
DRG Non-OR-Affecting MS-DRG Assignment New/Revised Text in **Orange** ♂ Male ♀ Female

IMAGING B00-BY4

678 2020 ICD-10-PCS

B Imaging
V Male Reproductive System
1 Fluoroscopy: Single plane or bi-plane real time display of an image developed from the capture of external ionizing radiation on a fluorescent screen. The image may also be stored by either digital or analog means

Body Part Character 4	Contrast Character 5	Qualifier Character 6	Qualifier Character 7
0 Corpora Cavernosa ♂ **8** Vasa Vasorum ♂	**0** High Osmolar **1** Low Osmolar **Y** Other Contrast **Z** None	**Z** None	**Z** None

♂ BV100ZZ BV101ZZ BV10YZZ BV10ZZZ BV180ZZ BV181ZZ BV18YZZ BV18ZZZ

B Imaging
V Male Reproductive System
2 Computerized Tomography (CT Scan): Computer reformatted digital display of multiplanar images developed from the capture of multiple exposures of external ionizing radiation

Body Part Character 4	Contrast Character 5	Qualifier Character 6	Qualifier Character 7
3 Prostate ♂	**0** High Osmolar **1** Low Osmolar **Y** Other Contrast	**0** Unenhanced and Enhanced **Z** None	**Z** None
3 Prostate ♂	**Z** None	**Z** None	**Z** None

♂ BV2300Z BV230ZZ BV2310Z BV23Y0Z BV23YZZ BV23ZZZ

B Imaging
V Male Reproductive System
3 Magnetic Resonance Imaging (MRI): Computer reformatted digital display of multiplanar images developed from the capture of radiofrequency signals emitted by nuclei in a body site excited within a magnetic field

Body Part Character 4	Contrast Character 5	Qualifier Character 6	Qualifier Character 7
0 Corpora Cavernosa ♂ **3** Prostate ♂ **4** Scrotum ♂ **5** Testicle, Right ♂ **6** Testicle, Left ♂ **7** Testicles, Bilateral ♂	**Y** Other Contrast	**0** Unenhanced and Enhanced **Z** None	**Z** None
0 Corpora Cavernosa ♂ **3** Prostate ♂ **4** Scrotum ♂ **5** Testicle, Right ♂ **6** Testicle, Left ♂ **7** Testicles, Bilateral ♂	**Z** None	**Z** None	**Z** None

♂ BV30Y0Z BV30YZZ BV30ZZZ BV33Y0Z BV33YZZ BV33ZZZ BV34Y0Z BV34YZZ BV34ZZZ BV35Y0Z BV35YZZ BV35ZZZ BV36Y0Z BV36YZZ BV36ZZZ BV37Y0Z BV37YZZ BV37ZZZ

B Imaging
V Male Reproductive System
4 Ultrasonography: Real time display of images of anatomy or flow information developed from the capture of reflected and attenuated high frequency sound waves

Body Part Character 4	Contrast Character 5	Qualifier Character 6	Qualifier Character 7
4 Scrotum ♂ **9** Prostate and Seminal Vesicles ♂ **B** Penis ♂	**Z** None	**Z** None	**Z** None

♂ BV44ZZZ BV49ZZZ BV4BZZZ

B Imaging
W Anatomical Regions
0 Plain Radiography: Planar display of an image developed from the capture of external ionizing radiation on photographic or photoconductive plate

Body Part Character 4	Contrast Character 5	Qualifier Character 6	Qualifier Character 7
0 Abdomen **1** Abdomen and Pelvis **3** Chest **B** Long Bones, All **C** Lower Extremity **J** Upper Extremity **K** Whole Body **L** Whole Skeleton **M** Whole Body, Infant	**Z** None	**Z** None	**Z** None

B Imaging
W Anatomical Regions
1 Fluoroscopy: Single plane or bi-plane real time display of an image developed from the capture of external ionizing radiation on a fluorescent screen. The image may also be stored by either digital or analog means

Body Part Character 4	Contrast Character 5	Qualifier Character 6	Qualifier Character 7
1 Abdomen and Pelvis **9** Head and Neck **C** Lower Extremity **J** Upper Extremity	**0** High Osmolar **1** Low Osmolar **Y** Other Contrast **Z** None	**Z** None	**Z** None

B Imaging
W Anatomical Regions
2 Computerized Tomography (CT Scan): Computer reformatted digital display of multiplanar images developed from the capture of multiple exposures of external ionizing radiation

Body Part Character 4	Contrast Character 5	Qualifier Character 6	Qualifier Character 7
0 Abdomen **1** Abdomen and Pelvis **4** Chest and Abdomen **5** Chest, Abdomen and Pelvis **8** Head **9** Head and Neck **F** Neck **G** Pelvic Region	**0** High Osmolar **1** Low Osmolar **Y** Other Contrast	**0** Unenhanced and Enhanced **Z** None	**Z** None
0 Abdomen **1** Abdomen and Pelvis **4** Chest and Abdomen **5** Chest, Abdomen and Pelvis **8** Head **9** Head and Neck **F** Neck **G** Pelvic Region	**Z** None	**Z** None	**Z** None

B Imaging
W Anatomical Regions
3 Magnetic Resonance Imaging (MRI): Computer reformatted digital display of multiplanar images developed from the capture of radiofrequency signals emitted by nuclei in a body site excited within a magnetic field

Body Part	Contrast	Qualifier	Qualifier
Character 4	**Character 5**	**Character 6**	**Character 7**
0 Abdomen **8** Head **F** Neck **G** Pelvic Region **H** Retroperitoneum **P** Brachial Plexus	**Y** Other Contrast	**0** Unenhanced and Enhanced **Z** None	**Z** None
0 Abdomen **8** Head **F** Neck **G** Pelvic Region **H** Retroperitoneum **P** Brachial Plexus	**Z** None	**Z** None	**Z** None
3 Chest	**Y** Other Contrast	**0** Unenhanced and Enhanced **Z** None	**Z** None

B Imaging
W Anatomical Regions
4 Ultrasonography: Real time display of images of anatomy or flow information developed from the capture of reflected and attenuated high frequency sound waves

Body Part	Contrast	Qualifier	Qualifier
Character 4	**Character 5**	**Character 6**	**Character 7**
0 Abdomen **1** Abdomen and Pelvis **F** Neck **G** Pelvic Region	**Z** None	**Z** None	**Z** None

B Imaging
Y Fetus and Obstetrical
3 Magnetic Resonance Imaging (MRI): Computer reformatted digital display of multiplanar images developed from the capture of radiofrequency signals emitted by nuclei in a body site excited within a magnetic field

Body Part	Contrast	Qualifier	Qualifier
Character 4	**Character 5**	**Character 6**	**Character 7**
0 Fetal Head ♀ **1** Fetal Heart ♀ **2** Fetal Thorax ♀ **3** Fetal Abdomen ♀ **4** Fetal Spine ♀ **5** Fetal Extremities ♀ **6** Whole Fetus ♀	**Y** Other Contrast	**0** Unenhanced and Enhanced **Z** None	**Z** None
0 Fetal Head ♀ **1** Fetal Heart ♀ **2** Fetal Thorax ♀ **3** Fetal Abdomen ♀ **4** Fetal Spine ♀ **5** Fetal Extremities ♀ **6** Whole Fetus ♀	**Z** None	**Z** None	**Z** None

♀ BY30Y0Z BY30YZZ BY30ZZZ BY31Y0Z BY31YZZ BY31ZZZ BY32Y0Z BY32YZZ BY32ZZZ BY33Y0Z BY33YZZ BY33ZZZ BY34YZZ BY34ZZZ BY35Y0Z BY35YZZ BY35ZZZ BY36Y0Z BY36YZZ BY36ZZZ

B Imaging
Y Fetus and Obstetrical
4 Ultrasonography: Real time display of images of anatomy or flow information developed from the capture of reflected and attenuated high frequency sound waves

Body Part Character 4	Contrast Character 5	Qualifier Character 6	Qualifier Character 7
7 Fetal Umbilical Cord ♀ **8** Placenta ♀ **9** First Trimester, Single Fetus ♀ **B** First Trimester, Multiple Gestation ♀ **C** Second Trimester, Single Fetus ♀ **D** Second Trimester, Multiple Gestation ♀ **F** Third Trimester, Single Fetus ♀ **G** Third Trimester, Multiple Gestation ♀	**Z** None	**Z** None	**Z** None

♀ BY47ZZZ BY48ZZZ BY49ZZZ BY4BZZZ BY4CZZZ BY4DZZZ BY4FZZZ BY4GZZZ

LC Limited Coverage NC Noncovered HAC HAC-associated Procedure CC Combination Cluster - See Appendix G for code lists
DRG Non-OR-Affecting MS-DRG Assignment New/Revised Text in **Orange** ♂ Male ♀ Female

682 2020 ICD-10-PCS

IMAGING B00-BY4

NOTES

NOTES

- Use radionuclides & relies on the process of radioactive decay in the diagnosis & treatment of disease
- differes from most other imaging in that it primarily shows the physiological function of the system being investigated
- the property of radiopharmaceutical, once administed to pt can localize & image the extent of disease process in the body, istead of relying on physical changes in tissue anatomy
- external detectors - gamma cameras used

most commonly used IV radionuclides are: (What is injected)

- technetium - 99m
- Iodine 123 & 131
- thallium 201
- gallium 67
- Fluoride - 18 Fluorodeoxyglucose
- Indium - 111 labeled leukocytes

most commonly used gaseous / aerosol radionuclides are:

- Xenon - 133
- krypton 81m
- Technetium - 99m technegas
- Technetium - 99m DTPA

technetium - AKA adenosine Sestamibi

Treatment w/ radiopharmaceuticals

- Scinigraphy - "Scint" - create 2-D or planar images
- SPECT - 3D tomagraphic technique using gamma camera
- PET - Positron Emission Tomography - uses considence detection to image functional processes

mdp - methylene diphosphonate - taken up by bone

5th character - "other radionuclide" = newly approved

* if more than one radiopharmaceutical is given, use more than 1 code

!5 body systems recognized

Nuclear Medicine C01-CW7

C Nuclear Medicine
0 Central Nervous System
1 Planar Nuclear Medicine Imaging: Introduction of radioactive materials into the body for single plane display of images developed from the capture of radioactive emissions

radiation source

Body Part	Radionuclide *Used*	Qualifier	Qualifier
Character 4	Character 5	Character 6	Character 7
0 Brain	**1** Technetium 99m (Tc-99m) **Y** Other Radionuclide	**Z** None	**Z** None
5 Cerebrospinal Fluid	**D** Indium 111 (In-111) **Y** Other Radionuclide	**Z** None	**Z** None
Y Central Nervous System	**Y** Other Radionuclide *— newly*	**Z** None	**Z** None

approved

C Nuclear Medicine
0 Central Nervous System
2 Tomographic (Tomo) Nuclear Medicine Imaging: Introduction of radioactive materials into the body for three dimensional display of images developed from the capture of radioactive emissions

Body Part	Radionuclide	Qualifier	Qualifier
Character 4	Character 5	Character 6	Character 7
0 Brain	**1** Technetium 99m (Tc-99m) **F** Iodine 123 (I-123) **S** Thallium 201 (Tl-201) **Y** Other Radionuclide	**Z** None	**Z** None
5 Cerebrospinal Fluid	**D** Indium 111 (In-111) **Y** Other Radionuclide	**Z** None	**Z** None
Y Central Nervous System	**Y** Other Radionuclide	**Z** None	**Z** None

C Nuclear Medicine
0 Central Nervous System
3 Positron Emission Tomographic (PET) Imaging: Introduction of radioactive materials into the body for three dimensional display of images developed from the simultaneous capture, 180 degrees apart, of radioactive emissions

Body Part	Radionuclide	Qualifier	Qualifier
Character 4	Character 5	Character 6	Character 7
0 Brain	**B** Carbon 11 (C-11) **K** Fluorine 18 (F-18) **M** Oxygen 15 (O-15) **Y** Other Radionuclide	**Z** None	**Z** None
Y Central Nervous System	**Y** Other Radionuclide	**Z** None	**Z** None

C Nuclear Medicine
0 Central Nervous System
5 Nonimaging Nuclear Medicine Probe: Introduction of radioactive materials into the body for the study of distribution and fate of certain substances by the detection of radioactive emissions; or, alternatively, measurement of absorption of radioactive emissions from an external source

Body Part	Radionuclide	Qualifier	Qualifier
Character 4	Character 5	Character 6	Character 7
0 Brain	**V** Xenon 133 (Xe-133) **Y** Other Radionuclide	**Z** None	**Z** None
Y Central Nervous System	**Y** Other Radionuclide	**Z** None	**Z** None

technetium = adenosine sestamibi

C Nuclear Medicine
2 Heart
1 Planar Nuclear Medicine Imaging: Introduction of radioactive materials into the body for single plane display of images developed from the capture of radioactive emissions planar scan

Body Part Character 4	Radionuclide Character 5	Qualifier Character 6	Qualifier Character 7
6 Heart, Right and Left	**1** Technetium 99m (Tc-99m) **Y** Other Radionuclide	**Z** None	**Z** None
G Myocardium heart muscle	**1** Technetium 99m (Tc-99m) **D** Indium 111 (In-111) **S** Thallium 201 (Tl-201) **Y** Other Radionuclide **Z** None	**Z** None adensoine sestamibi	**Z** None
Y Heart	**Y** Other Radionuclide	**Z** None	**Z** None

C Nuclear Medicine
2 Heart
2 Tomographic (Tomo) Nuclear Medicine Imaging: Introduction of radioactive materials into the body for three dimensional display of images developed from the capture of radioactive emissions

Body Part Character 4	Radionuclide Character 5	Qualifier Character 6	Qualifier Character 7
6 Heart, Right and Left	**1** Technetium 99m (Tc-99m) **Y** Other Radionuclide	**Z** None adenosine sestamibi	**Z** None
G Myocardium	**1** Technetium 99m (Tc-99m) **D** Indium 111 (In-111) **K** Fluorine 18 (F-18) **S** Thallium 201 (Tl-201) **Y** Other Radionuclide **Z** None	**Z** None	**Z** None
Y Heart	**Y** Other Radionuclide	**Z** None	**Z** None

C Nuclear Medicine
2 Heart
3 Positron Emission Tomographic (PET) Imaging: Introduction of radioactive materials into the body for three dimensional display of images developed from the simultaneous capture, 180 degrees apart, of radioactive emissions

Body Part Character 4	Radionuclide Character 5	Qualifier Character 6	Qualifier Character 7
G Myocardium	**K** Fluorine 18 (F-18) **M** Oxygen 15 (O-15) **Q** Rubidium 82 (Rb-82) **R** Nitrogen 13 (N-13) **Y** Other Radionuclide	**Z** None	**Z** None
Y Heart	**Y** Other Radionuclide	**Z** None	**Z** None

C Nuclear Medicine
2 Heart
5 Nonimaging Nuclear Medicine Probe: Introduction of radioactive materials into the body for the study of distribution and fate of certain substances by the detection of radioactive emissions; or, alternatively, measurement of absorption of radioactive emissions from an external source

Body Part Character 4	Radionuclide Character 5	Qualifier Character 6	Qualifier Character 7
6 Heart, Right and Left	**1** Technetium 99m (Tc-99m) **Y** Other Radionuclide	**Z** None	**Z** None
Y Heart	**Y** Other Radionuclide	**Z** None	**Z** None

LC Limited Coverage NC Noncovered HAC HAC-associated Procedure CC Combination Cluster - See Appendix G for code lists
DRG Non-OR-Affecting MS-DRG Assignment New/Revised Text in **Orange** ♂ Male ♀ Female

C Nuclear Medicine
5 Veins
1 Planar Nuclear Medicine Imaging: Introduction of radioactive materials into the body for single plane display of images developed from the capture of radioactive emissions

Body Part Character 4	Radionuclide Character 5	Qualifier Character 6	Qualifier Character 7
B Lower Extremity Veins, Right **C** Lower Extremity Veins, Left **D** Lower Extremity Veins, Bilateral **N** Upper Extremity Veins, Right **P** Upper Extremity Veins, Left **Q** Upper Extremity Veins, Bilateral **R** Central Veins	**1** Technetium 99m (Tc-99m) **Y** Other Radionuclide	**Z** None	**Z** None
Y Veins	**Y** Other Radionuclide	**Z** None	**Z** None

C Nuclear Medicine
7 Lymphatic and Hematologic System
1 Planar Nuclear Medicine Imaging: Introduction of radioactive materials into the body for single plane display of images developed from the capture of radioactive emissions

Body Part Character 4	Radionuclide Character 5	Qualifier Character 6	Qualifier Character 7
0 Bone Marrow	**1** Technetium 99m (Tc-99m) **D** Indium 111 (In-111) **Y** Other Radionuclide	**Z** None	**Z** None
2 Spleen **5** Lymphatics, Head and Neck **D** Lymphatics, Pelvic **J** Lymphatics, Head **K** Lymphatics, Neck **L** Lymphatics, Upper Chest **M** Lymphatics, Trunk **N** Lymphatics, Upper Extremity **P** Lymphatics, Lower Extremity	**1** Technetium 99m (Tc-99m) **Y** Other Radionuclide	**Z** None	**Z** None
3 Blood	**D** Indium 111 (In-111) **Y** Other Radionuclide	**Z** None	**Z** None
Y Lymphatic and Hematologic System	**Y** Other Radionuclide	**Z** None	**Z** None

C Nuclear Medicine
7 Lymphatic and Hematologic System
2 Tomographic (Tomo) Nuclear Medicine Imaging: Introduction of radioactive materials into the body for three dimensional display of images developed from the capture of radioactive emissions

Body Part Character 4	Radionuclide Character 5	Qualifier Character 6	Qualifier Character 7
2 Spleen	**1** Technetium 99m (Tc-99m) **Y** Other Radionuclide	**Z** None	**Z** None
Y Lymphatic and Hematologic System	**Y** Other Radionuclide	**Z** None	**Z** None

C Nuclear Medicine
7 Lymphatic and Hematologic System
5 Nonimaging Nuclear Medicine Probe: Introduction of radioactive materials into the body for the study of distribution and fate of certain substances by the detection of radioactive emissions; or, alternatively, measurement of absorption of radioactive emissions from an external source

Body Part	Radionuclide	Qualifier	Qualifier
Character 4	**Character 5**	**Character 6**	**Character 7**
5 Lymphatics, Head and Neck **D** Lymphatics, Pelvic **J** Lymphatics, Head **K** Lymphatics, Neck **L** Lymphatics, Upper Chest **M** Lymphatics, Trunk **N** Lymphatics, Upper Extremity **P** Lymphatics, Lower Extremity	**1** Technetium 99m (Tc-99m) **Y** Other Radionuclide	**Z** None	**Z** None
Y Lymphatic and Hematologic System	**Y** Other Radionuclide	**Z** None	**Z** None

C Nuclear Medicine
7 Lymphatic and Hematologic System
6 Nonimaging Nuclear Medicine Assay: Introduction of radioactive materials into the body for the study of body fluids and blood elements, by the detection of radioactive emissions

Body Part	Radionuclide	Qualifier	Qualifier
Character 4	**Character 5**	**Character 6**	**Character 7**
3 Blood	**1** Technetium 99m (Tc-99m) **7** Cobalt 58 (Co-58) **C** Cobalt 57 (Co-57) **D** Indium 111 (In-111) **H** Iodine 125 (I-125) **W** Chromium (Cr-51) **Y** Other Radionuclide	**Z** None	**Z** None
Y Lymphatic and Hematologic System	**Y** Other Radionuclide	**Z** None	**Z** None

C Nuclear Medicine
8 Eye
1 Planar Nuclear Medicine Imaging: Introduction of radioactive materials into the body for single plane display of images developed from the capture of radioactive emissions

Body Part	Radionuclide	Qualifier	Qualifier
Character 4	**Character 5**	**Character 6**	**Character 7**
9 Lacrimal Ducts, Bilateral	**1** Technetium 99m (Tc-99m) **Y** Other Radionuclide	**Z** None	**Z** None
Y Eye	**Y** Other Radionuclide	**Z** None	**Z** None

C Nuclear Medicine
9 Ear, Nose, Mouth and Throat
1 Planar Nuclear Medicine Imaging: Introduction of radioactive materials into the body for single plane display of images developed from the capture of radioactive emissions

Body Part	Radionuclide	Qualifier	Qualifier
Character 4	**Character 5**	**Character 6**	**Character 7**
B Salivary Glands, Bilateral	**1** Technetium 99m (Tc-99m) **Y** Other Radionuclide	**Z** None	**Z** None
Y Ear, Nose, Mouth and Throat	**Y** Other Radionuclide	**Z** None	**Z** None

C Nuclear Medicine
B Respiratory System
1 Planar Nuclear Medicine Imaging: Introduction of radioactive materials into the body for single plane display of images developed from the capture of radioactive emissions

Body Part	Radionuclide	Qualifier	Qualifier
Character 4	**Character 5**	**Character 6**	**Character 7**
2 Lungs and Bronchi	1 Technetium 99m (Tc-99m) 9 Krypton (Kr-81m) T Xenon 127 (Xe-127) V Xenon 133 (Xe-133) Y Other Radionuclide	Z None	Z None
Y Respiratory System	Y Other Radionuclide	Z None	Z None

C Nuclear Medicine
B Respiratory System
2 Tomographic (Tomo) Nuclear Medicine Imaging: Introduction of radioactive materials into the body for three dimensional display of images developed from the capture of radioactive emissions

Body Part	Radionuclide	Qualifier	Qualifier
Character 4	**Character 5**	**Character 6**	**Character 7**
2 Lungs and Bronchi	1 Technetium 99m (Tc-99m) 9 Krypton (Kr-81m) Y Other Radionuclide	Z None	Z None
Y Respiratory System	Y Other Radionuclide	Z None	Z None

C Nuclear Medicine
B Respiratory System
3 Positron Emission Tomographic (PET) Imaging: Introduction of radioactive materials into the body for three dimensional display of images developed from the simultaneous capture, 180 degrees apart, of radioactive emissions

Body Part	Radionuclide	Qualifier	Qualifier
Character 4	**Character 5**	**Character 6**	**Character 7**
2 Lungs and Bronchi	K Fluorine 18 (F-18) Y Other Radionuclide	Z None	Z None
Y Respiratory System	Y Other Radionuclide	Z None	Z None

C Nuclear Medicine
D Gastrointestinal System
1 Planar Nuclear Medicine Imaging: Introduction of radioactive materials into the body for single plane display of images developed from the capture of radioactive emissions

Body Part	Radionuclide	Qualifier	Qualifier
Character 4	**Character 5**	**Character 6**	**Character 7**
5 Upper Gastrointestinal Tract 7 Gastrointestinal Tract	1 Technetium 99m (Tc-99m) D Indium 111 (In-111) Y Other Radionuclide	Z None	Z None
Y Digestive System	Y Other Radionuclide	Z None	Z None

C Nuclear Medicine
D Gastrointestinal System
2 Tomographic (Tomo) Nuclear Medicine Imaging: Introduction of radioactive materials into the body for three dimensional display of images developed from the capture of radioactive emissions

Body Part	Radionuclide	Qualifier	Qualifier
Character 4	**Character 5**	**Character 6**	**Character 7**
7 Gastrointestinal Tract	1 Technetium 99m (Tc-99m) D Indium 111 (In-111) Y Other Radionuclide	Z None	Z None
Y Digestive System	Y Other Radionuclide	Z None	Z None

C Nuclear Medicine
F Hepatobiliary System and Pancreas
1 Planar Nuclear Medicine Imaging: Introduction of radioactive materials into the body for single plane display of images developed from the capture of radioactive emissions

Body Part Character 4	Radionuclide Character 5	Qualifier Character 6	Qualifier Character 7
4 Gallbladder **5** Liver **6** Liver and Spleen **C** Hepatobiliary System, All	**1** Technetium 99m (Tc-99m) **Y** Other Radionuclide	**Z** None	**Z** None
Y Hepatobiliary System and Pancreas	**Y** Other Radionuclide	**Z** None	**Z** None

C Nuclear Medicine
F Hepatobiliary System and Pancreas
2 Tomographic (Tomo) Nuclear Medicine Imaging: Introduction of radioactive materials into the body for three dimensional display of images developed from the capture of radioactive emissions

Body Part Character 4	Radionuclide Character 5	Qualifier Character 6	Qualifier Character 7
4 Gallbladder **5** Liver **6** Liver and Spleen	**1** Technetium 99m (Tc-99m) **Y** Other Radionuclide	**Z** None	**Z** None
Y Hepatobiliary System and Pancreas	**Y** Other Radionuclide	**Z** None	**Z** None

C Nuclear Medicine
G Endocrine System
1 Planar Nuclear Medicine Imaging: Introduction of radioactive materials into the body for single plane display of images developed from the capture of radioactive emissions

Body Part Character 4	Radionuclide Character 5	Qualifier Character 6	Qualifier Character 7
1 Parathyroid Glands	**1** Technetium 99m (Tc-99m) **S** Thallium 201 (Tl-201) **Y** Other Radionuclide	**Z** None	**Z** None
2 Thyroid Gland	**1** Technetium 99m (Tc-99m) **F** Iodine 123 (I-123) **G** Iodine 131 (I-131) **Y** Other Radionuclide	**Z** None	**Z** None
4 Adrenal Glands, Bilateral	**G** Iodine 131 (I-131) **Y** Other Radionuclide	**Z** None	**Z** None
Y Endocrine System	**Y** Other Radionuclide	**Z** None	**Z** None

C Nuclear Medicine
G Endocrine System
2 Tomographic (Tomo) Nuclear Medicine Imaging: Introduction of radioactive materials into the body for three dimensional display of images developed from the capture of radioactive emissions

Body Part Character 4	Radionuclide Character 5	Qualifier Character 6	Qualifier Character 7
1 Parathyroid Glands	**1** Technetium 99m (Tc-99m) **S** Thallium 201 (Tl-201) **Y** Other Radionuclide	**Z** None	**Z** None
Y Endocrine System	**Y** Other Radionuclide	**Z** None	**Z** None

C Nuclear Medicine
G Endocrine System
4 Nonimaging Nuclear Medicine Uptake: Introduction of radioactive materials into the body for measurements of organ function, from the detection of radioactive emissions

Body Part	Radionuclide	Qualifier	Qualifier
Character 4	**Character 5**	**Character 6**	**Character 7**
2 Thyroid Gland	1 Technetium 99m (Tc-99m) F Iodine 123 (I-123) G Iodine 131 (I-131) Y Other Radionuclide	Z None	Z None
Y Endocrine System	Y Other Radionuclide	Z None	Z None

C Nuclear Medicine
H Skin, Subcutaneous Tissue and Breast
1 Planar Nuclear Medicine Imaging: Introduction of radioactive materials into the body for single plane display of images developed from the capture of radioactive emissions

Body Part	Radionuclide	Qualifier	Qualifier
Character 4	**Character 5**	**Character 6**	**Character 7**
0 Breast, Right 1 Breast, Left 2 Breasts, Bilateral	1 Technetium 99m (Tc-99m) S Thallium 201 (Tl-201) Y Other Radionuclide	Z None	Z None
Y Skin, Subcutaneous Tissue and Breast	Y Other Radionuclide	Z None	Z None

C Nuclear Medicine
H Skin, Subcutaneous Tissue and Breast
2 Tomographic (Tomo) Nuclear Medicine Imaging: Introduction of radioactive materials into the body for three dimensional display of images developed from the capture of radioactive emissions

Body Part	Radionuclide	Qualifier	Qualifier
Character 4	**Character 5**	**Character 6**	**Character 7**
0 Breast, Right 1 Breast, Left 2 Breasts, Bilateral	1 Technetium 99m (Tc-99m) S Thallium 201 (Tl-201) Y Other Radionuclide	Z None	Z None
Y Skin, Subcutaneous Tissue and Breast	Y Other Radionuclide	Z None	Z None

C Nuclear Medicine
P Musculoskeletal System
1 Planar Nuclear Medicine Imaging: Introduction of radioactive materials into the body for single plane display of images developed from the capture of radioactive emissions

Body Part	Radionuclide	Qualifier	Qualifier
Character 4	**Character 5**	**Character 6**	**Character 7**
1 Skull 4 Thorax 5 Spine 6 Pelvis 7 Spine and Pelvis 8 Upper Extremity, Right 9 Upper Extremity, Left B Upper Extremities, Bilateral C Lower Extremity, Right D Lower Extremity, Left F Lower Extremities, Bilateral Z Musculoskeletal System, All	1 Technetium 99m (Tc-99m) Y Other Radionuclide	Z None	Z None
Y Musculoskeletal System, Other	Y Other Radionuclide	Z None	Z None

CG4-CP1
NUCLEAR MEDICINE C01-CW7

C Nuclear Medicine
P Musculoskeletal System
2 Tomographic (Tomo) Nuclear Medicine Imaging: Introduction of radioactive materials into the body for three dimensional display of images developed from the capture of radioactive emissions

Body Part	Radionuclide	Qualifier	Qualifier
Character 4	**Character 5**	**Character 6**	**Character 7**
1 Skull **2** Cervical Spine **3** Skull and Cervical Spine **4** Thorax **6** Pelvis **7** Spine and Pelvis **8** Upper Extremity, Right **9** Upper Extremity, Left **B** Upper Extremities, Bilateral **C** Lower Extremity, Right **D** Lower Extremity, Left **F** Lower Extremities, Bilateral **G** Thoracic Spine **H** Lumbar Spine **J** Thoracolumbar Spine	**1** Technetium 99m (Tc-99m) **Y** Other Radionuclide	**Z** None	**Z** None
Y Musculoskeletal System, Other	**Y** Other Radionuclide	**Z** None	**Z** None

C Nuclear Medicine
P Musculoskeletal System
5 Nonimaging Nuclear Medicine Probe: Introduction of radioactive materials into the body for the study of distribution and fate of certain substances by the detection of radioactive emissions; or, alternatively, measurement of absorption of radioactive emissions from an external source

Body Part	Radionuclide	Qualifier	Qualifier
Character 4	**Character 5**	**Character 6**	**Character 7**
5 Spine **N** Upper Extremities **P** Lower Extremities	**Z** None	**Z** None	**Z** None
Y Musculoskeletal System, Other	**Y** Other Radionuclide	**Z** None	**Z** None

C Nuclear Medicine
T Urinary System
1 Planar Nuclear Medicine Imaging: Introduction of radioactive materials into the body for single plane display of images developed from the capture of radioactive emissions

Body Part	Radionuclide	Qualifier	Qualifier
Character 4	**Character 5**	**Character 6**	**Character 7**
3 Kidneys, Ureters and Bladder	**1** Technetium 99m (Tc-99m) **F** Iodine 123 (I-123) **G** Iodine 131 (I-131) **Y** Other Radionuclide	**Z** None	**Z** None
H Bladder and Ureters	**1** Technetium 99m (Tc-99m) **Y** Other Radionuclide	**Z** None	**Z** None
Y Urinary System	**Y** Other Radionuclide	**Z** None	**Z** None

C Nuclear Medicine
T Urinary System
2 Tomographic (Tomo) Nuclear Medicine Imaging: Introduction of radioactive materials into the body for three dimensional display of images developed from the capture of radioactive emissions

Body Part	Radionuclide	Qualifier	Qualifier
Character 4	**Character 5**	**Character 6**	**Character 7**
3 Kidneys, Ureters and Bladder	**1** Technetium 99m (Tc-99m) **Y** Other Radionuclide	**Z** None	**Z** None
Y Urinary System	**Y** Other Radionuclide	**Z** None	**Z** None

C Nuclear Medicine non-imaging
T Urinary System
6 Nonimaging Nuclear Medicine Assay: Introduction of radioactive materials into the body for the study of body fluids and blood elements, by the detection of radioactive emissions

Body Part	Radionuclide	Qualifier	Qualifier
Character 4	Character 5	Character 6	Character 7
3 Kidneys, Ureters and Bladder	1 Technetium 99m (Tc-99m) F Iodine 123 (I-123) G Iodine 131 (I-131) H Iodine 125 (I-125) Y Other Radionuclide	Z None	Z None
Y Urinary System	Y Other Radionuclide	Z None	Z None

C Nuclear Medicine
V Male Reproductive System
1 Planar Nuclear Medicine Imaging: Introduction of radioactive materials into the body for single plane display of images developed from the capture of radioactive emissions

Body Part	Radionuclide	Qualifier	Qualifier
Character 4	Character 5	Character 6	Character 7
9 Testicles, Bilateral ♂	1 Technetium 99m (Tc-99m) Y Other Radionuclide	Z None	Z None
Y Male Reproductive System ♂	Y Other Radionuclide	Z None	Z None

♂ CV191ZZ CV19YZZ CV1YYZZ

C Nuclear Medicine
W Anatomical Regions
1 Planar Nuclear Medicine Imaging: Introduction of radioactive materials into the body for single plane display of images developed from the capture of radioactive emissions

Body Part	Radionuclide	Qualifier	Qualifier
Character 4	Character 5	Character 6	Character 7
0 Abdomen 1 Abdomen and Pelvis 4 Chest and Abdomen 6 Chest and Neck B Head and Neck D Lower Extremity J Pelvic Region M Upper Extremity N Whole Body	1 Technetium 99m (Tc-99m) D Indium 111 (In-111) F Iodine 123 (I-123) G Iodine 131 (I-131) L Gallium 67 (Ga-67) S Thallium 201 (Tl-201) Y Other Radionuclide	Z None	Z None
3 Chest	1 Technetium 99m (Tc-99m) D Indium 111 (In-111) F Iodine 123 (I-123) G Iodine 131 (I-131) K Fluorine 18 (F-18) L Gallium 67 (Ga-67) S Thallium 201 (Tl-201) Y Other Radionuclide	Z None	Z None
Y Anatomical Regions, Multiple	Y Other Radionuclide	Z None	Z None
Z Anatomical Region, Other	Z None	Z None	Z None

C Nuclear Medicine
W Anatomical Regions
2 Tomographic (Tomo) Nuclear Medicine Imaging: Introduction of radioactive materials into the body for three dimensional display of images developed from the capture of radioactive emissions

Body Part	Radionuclide	Qualifier	Qualifier
Character 4	**Character 5**	**Character 6**	**Character 7**
0 Abdomen **1** Abdomen and Pelvis **3** Chest **4** Chest and Abdomen **6** Chest and Neck **B** Head and Neck **D** Lower Extremity **J** Pelvic Region **M** Upper Extremity	**1** Technetium 99m (Tc-99m) **D** Indium 111 (In-111) **F** Iodine 123 (I-123) **G** Iodine 131 (I-131) **K** Fluorine 18 (F-18) **L** Gallium 67 (Ga-67) **S** Thallium 201 (Tl-201) **Y** Other Radionuclide	**Z** None	**Z** None
Y Anatomical Regions, Multiple	**Y** Other Radionuclide	**Z** None	**Z** None

C Nuclear Medicine
W Anatomical Regions
3 Positron Emission Tomographic (PET) Imaging: Introduction of radioactive materials into the body for three dimensional display of images developed from the simultaneous capture, 180 degrees apart, of radioactive emissions

Body Part	Radionuclide	Qualifier	Qualifier
Character 4	**Character 5**	**Character 6**	**Character 7**
N Whole Body	**Y** Other Radionuclide	**Z** None	**Z** None

C Nuclear Medicine
W Anatomical Regions
5 Nonimaging Nuclear Medicine Probe: Introduction of radioactive materials into the body for the study of distribution and fate of certain substances by the detection of radioactive emissions; or, alternatively, measurement of absorption of radioactive emissions from an external source

Body Part	Radionuclide	Qualifier	Qualifier
Character 4	**Character 5**	**Character 6**	**Character 7**
0 Abdomen **1** Abdomen and Pelvis **3** Chest **4** Chest and Abdomen **6** Chest and Neck **B** Head and Neck **D** Lower Extremity **J** Pelvic Region **M** Upper Extremity	**1** Technetium 99m (Tc-99m) **D** Indium 111 (In-111) **Y** Other Radionuclide	**Z** None	**Z** None

C Nuclear Medicine
W Anatomical Regions
7 Systemic Nuclear Medicine Therapy: Introduction of unsealed radioactive materials into the body for treatment

Body Part	Radionuclide	Qualifier	Qualifier
Character 4	**Character 5**	**Character 6**	**Character 7**
0 Abdomen **3** Chest	**N** Phosphorus 32 (P-32) **Y** Other Radionuclide	**Z** None	**Z** None
G Thyroid	**G** Iodine 131 (I-131) **Y** Other Radionuclide	**Z** None	**Z** None
N Whole Body	**8** Samarium 153 (Sm-153) **G** Iodine 131 (I-131) **N** Phosphorus 32 (P-32) **P** Strontium 89 (Sr-89) **Y** Other Radionuclide	**Z** None	**Z** None
Y Anatomical Regions, Multiple	**Y** Other Radionuclide	**Z** None	**Z** None

NOTES

NOTES

Use ionizing radiation as part of cancer treatment to control malignant cell, may be curative or adjuvant treatment, used as palliative or therapeutic treatment

TBI - total Body Irradiation - used to prepare body to recive bone marrow transplant

3 main types of radiation therapy - For cancer treatment
(0) • Beam - conventional external beam radiotherapy (2DXRT)
(1) • Stereotactic Radiosurgery (SRS) - For small tumors + radiation treatments of brain & spine
(2) • Brachytherapy - AKA internal radiotherapy Seeds placed inside the body - used in local area, AKA external beam radiotherapy

radiation therapy may be combined w/ surgery, chemo, hormone therapy, immunotherapy - or some mixture of the four mentioned

15 body systems recognized

Radiation Therapy D00-DWY

D Radiation Therapy
0 Central and Peripheral Nervous System
0 Beam Radiation

conventional external beam radiotherapy (2DXRT) delivered via 2-dimensional beams using linear accelerator machines - stimulator

Treatment Site Character 4	Modality Qualifier Character 5	Isotope Character 6	Qualifier Character 7
0 Brain **1** Brain Stem **6** Spinal Cord **7** Peripheral Nerve	**0** Photons <1 MeV **1** Photons 1 - 10 MeV **2** Photons >10 MeV **4** Heavy Particles (Protons, Ions) **5** Neutrons **6** Neutron Capture	**Z** None	**Z** None
0 Brain **1** Brain Stem **6** Spinal Cord **7** Peripheral Nerve	**3** Electrons	**Z** None	**0** Intraoperative **Z** None

indicates if performed intraoperatively

D Radiation Therapy
0 Central and Peripheral Nervous System
1 Brachytherapy

internal radiotherapy delivered by placing radiation sources inside or next to the area requiring treatment

Treatment Site Character 4	Modality Qualifier Character 5	Isotope (radioactive) Character 6	Qualifier Character 7
0 Brain **1** Brain Stem **6** Spinal Cord **7** Peripheral Nerve	**9** High Dose Rate (HDR)	**7** Cesium 137 (Cs-137) **8** Iridium 192 (Ir-192) **9** Iodine 125 (I-125) **B** Palladium 103 (Pd-103) **C** Californium 252 (Cf-252) **Y** Other Isotope	**Z** None
0 Brain **1** Brain Stem **6** Spinal Cord **7** Peripheral Nerve	**B** Low Dose Rate (LDR)	**7** Cesium 137 (Cs-137) **8** Iridium 192 (Ir-192) **9** Iodine 125 (I-125) **C** Californium 252 (Cf-252) **Y** Other Isotope	**Z** None
0 Brain **1** Brain Stem **6** Spinal Cord **7** Peripheral Nerve	**B** Low Dose Rate (LDR)	**B** Palladium 103 (Pd-103)	**1** Unidirectional Source **Z** None

D Radiation Therapy
0 Central and Peripheral Nervous System
2 Stereotactic Radiosurgery

uses focused radiation beams targeting a well-defined tumor using extremely detailed imaging scans

Treatment Site Character 4	Modality Qualifier Character 5	Isotope Character 6	Qualifier Character 7
0 Brain DRG **1** Brain Stem DRG **6** Spinal Cord DRG **7** Peripheral Nerve DRG	**D** Stereotactic Other Photon Radiosurgery **H** Stereotactic Particulate Radiosurgery **J** Stereotactic Gamma Beam Radiosurgery	**Z** None	**Z** None

DRG D020DZZ D020HZZ D020JZZ D021DZZ D021HZZ D021JZZ D026DZZ D026HZZ D026JZZ D027DZZ D027HZZ D027JZZ

LC Limited Coverage NC Noncovered HAC HAC-associated Procedure CC Combination Cluster - See Appendix G for code lists
DRG Non-OR-Affecting MS-DRG Assignment New/Revised Text in **Orange** ♂ Male ♀ Female

D Radiation Therapy
0 Central and Peripheral Nervous System
Y Other Radiation new technology

Treatment Site	Modality Qualifier	Isotope	Qualifier
Character 4	**Character 5**	**Character 6**	**Character 7**
0 Brain **1** Brain Stem **6** Spinal Cord **7** Peripheral Nerve	**7** Contact Radiation **8** Hyperthermia **F** Plaque Radiation **K** Laser Interstitial Thermal Therapy	**Z** None	**Z** None

D Radiation Therapy
7 Lymphatic and Hematologic System
0 Beam Radiation

Treatment Site	Modality Qualifier	Isotope	Qualifier
Character 4	**Character 5**	**Character 6**	**Character 7**
0 Bone Marrow **1** Thymus **2** Spleen **3** Lymphatics, Neck **4** Lymphatics, Axillary **5** Lymphatics, Thorax **6** Lymphatics, Abdomen **7** Lymphatics, Pelvis **8** Lymphatics, Inguinal	**0** Photons <1 MeV **1** Photons 1 - 10 MeV **2** Photons >10 MeV **4** Heavy Particles (Protons, Ions) **5** Neutrons **6** Neutron Capture	**Z** None	**Z** None
0 Bone Marrow **1** Thymus **2** Spleen **3** Lymphatics, Neck **4** Lymphatics, Axillary **5** Lymphatics, Thorax **6** Lymphatics, Abdomen **7** Lymphatics, Pelvis **8** Lymphatics, Inguinal	**3** Electrons	**Z** None	**0** Intraoperative **Z** None

D Radiation Therapy
7 Lymphatic and Hematologic System
1 Brachytherapy

Treatment Site Character 4	Modality Qualifier Character 5	Isotope Character 6	Qualifier Character 7
0 Bone Marrow **1** Thymus **2** Spleen **3** Lymphatics, Neck **4** Lymphatics, Axillary **5** Lymphatics, Thorax **6** Lymphatics, Abdomen **7** Lymphatics, Pelvis **8** Lymphatics, Inguinal	**9** High Dose Rate (HDR)	**7** Cesium 137 (Cs-137) **8** Iridium 192 (Ir-192) **9** Iodine 125 (I-125) **B** Palladium 103 (Pd-103) **C** Californium 252 (Cf-252) **Y** Other Isotope	**Z** None
0 Bone Marrow **1** Thymus **2** Spleen **3** Lymphatics, Neck **4** Lymphatics, Axillary **5** Lymphatics, Thorax **6** Lymphatics, Abdomen **7** Lymphatics, Pelvis **8** Lymphatics, Inguinal	**B** Low Dose Rate (LDR)	**7** Cesium 137 (Cs-137) **8** Iridium 192 (Ir-192) **9** Iodine 125 (I-125) **C** Californium 252 (Cf-252) **Y** Other Isotope	**Z** None
0 Bone Marrow **1** Thymus **2** Spleen **3** Lymphatics, Neck **4** Lymphatics, Axillary **5** Lymphatics, Thorax **6** Lymphatics, Abdomen **7** Lymphatics, Pelvis **8** Lymphatics, Inguinal	**B** Low Dose Rate (LDR)	**B** Palladium 103 (Pd-103)	**1** Unidirectional Source **Z** None

D Radiation Therapy
7 Lymphatic and Hematologic System
2 Stereotactic Radiosurgery

Treatment Site Character 4	Modality Qualifier Character 5	Isotope Character 6	Qualifier Character 7
0 Bone Marrow DRG **1** Thymus DRG **2** Spleen DRG **3** Lymphatics, Neck DRG **4** Lymphatics, Axillary DRG **5** Lymphatics, Thorax DRG **6** Lymphatics, Abdomen DRG **7** Lymphatics, Pelvis DRG **8** Lymphatics, Inguinal DRG	**D** Stereotactic Other Photon Radiosurgery **H** Stereotactic Particulate Radiosurgery **J** Stereotactic Gamma Beam Radiosurgery	**Z** None	**Z** None

DRG D720DZZ D720HZZ D720JZZ D721DZZ D721HZZ D721JZZ D722DZZ D722HZZ D722JZZ D723DZZ D723HZZ D723JZZ D724DZZ D724HZZ D724JZZ D725DZZ D725HZZ D725JZZ D726DZZ D726HZZ D726JZZ D727DZZ D727HZZ D727JZZ D728DZZ D728HZZ D728JZZ

D Radiation Therapy
7 Lymphatic and Hematologic System
Y Other Radiation

Treatment Site	Modality Qualifier	Isotope	Qualifier
Character 4	**Character 5**	**Character 6**	**Character 7**
0 Bone Marrow **1** Thymus **2** Spleen **3** Lymphatics, Neck **4** Lymphatics, Axillary **5** Lymphatics, Thorax **6** Lymphatics, Abdomen **7** Lymphatics, Pelvis **8** Lymphatics, Inguinal	**8** Hyperthermia **F** Plaque Radiation	**Z** None	**Z** None

D Radiation Therapy
8 Eye
0 Beam Radiation

Treatment Site	Modality Qualifier	Isotope	Qualifier
Character 4	**Character 5**	**Character 6**	**Character 7**
0 Eye	**0** Photons <1 MeV **1** Photons 1 - 10 MeV **2** Photons >10 MeV **4** Heavy Particles (Protons, Ions) **5** Neutrons **6** Neutron Capture	**Z** None	**Z** None
0 Eye	**3** Electrons	**Z** None	**0** Intraoperative **Z** None

D Radiation Therapy
8 Eye
1 Brachytherapy

Treatment Site	Modality Qualifier	Isotope	Qualifier
Character 4	**Character 5**	**Character 6**	**Character 7**
0 Eye	**9** High Dose Rate (HDR)	**7** Cesium 137 (Cs-137) **8** Iridium 192 (Ir-192) **9** Iodine 125 (I-125) **B** Palladium 103 (Pd-103) **C** Californium 252 (Cf-252) **Y** Other Isotope	**Z** None
0 Eye	**B** Low Dose Rate (LDR)	**7** Cesium 137 (Cs-137) **8** Iridium 192 (Ir-192) **9** Iodine 125 (I-125) **C** Californium 252 (Cf-252) **Y** Other Isotope	**Z** None
0 Eye	**B** Low Dose Rate (LDR)	**B** Palladium 103 (Pd-103)	**1** Unidirectional Source **Z** None

D Radiation Therapy
8 Eye
2 Stereotactic Radiosurgery

Treatment Site	Modality Qualifier	Isotope	Qualifier
Character 4	**Character 5**	**Character 6**	**Character 7**
0 Eye DRG	**D** Stereotactic Other Photon Radiosurgery **H** Stereotactic Particulate Radiosurgery **J** Stereotactic Gamma Beam Radiosurgery	**Z** None	**Z** None

DRG D820DZZ D820HZZ D820JZZ

Plaque irradiation of left eye, single port D8Y0FZZ

D Radiation Therapy
8 Eye
Y Other Radiation

Treatment Site Character 4	Modality Qualifier Character 5	Isotope Character 6	Qualifier Character 7
0 Eye	7 Contact Radiation 8 Hyperthermia F Plaque Radiation irradiation	Z None	Z None

D Radiation Therapy
9 Ear, Nose, Mouth and Throat
0 Beam Radiation

Treatment Site Character 4	Modality Qualifier Character 5	Isotope Character 6	Qualifier Character 7
0 Ear 1 Nose 3 Hypopharynx 4 Mouth 5 Tongue 6 Salivary Glands 7 Sinuses 8 Hard Palate 9 Soft Palate B Larynx D Nasopharynx F Oropharynx	0 Photons <1 MeV 1 Photons 1 - 10 MeV 2 Photons >10 MeV 4 Heavy Particles (Protons, Ions) 5 Neutrons 6 Neutron Capture	Z None	Z None
0 Ear 1 Nose 3 Hypopharynx 4 Mouth 5 Tongue 6 Salivary Glands 7 Sinuses 8 Hard Palate 9 Soft Palate B Larynx D Nasopharynx F Oropharynx	3 Electrons	Z None	0 Intraoperative Z None

D Radiation Therapy
9 Ear, Nose, Mouth and Throat
1 Brachytherapy

Treatment Site Character 4	Modality Qualifier Character 5	Isotope Character 6	Qualifier Character 7
0 Ear **1** Nose **3** Hypopharynx **4** Mouth **5** Tongue **6** Salivary Glands **7** Sinuses **8** Hard Palate **9** Soft Palate **B** Larynx **D** Nasopharynx **F** Oropharynx	**9** High Dose Rate (HDR)	**7** Cesium 137 (Cs-137) **8** Iridium 192 (Ir-192) **9** Iodine 125 (I-125) **B** Palladium 103 (Pd-103) **C** Californium 252 (Cf-252) **Y** Other Isotope	**Z** None
0 Ear **1** Nose **3** Hypopharynx **4** Mouth **5** Tongue **6** Salivary Glands **7** Sinuses **8** Hard Palate **9** Soft Palate **B** Larynx **D** Nasopharynx **F** Oropharynx	**B** Low Dose Rate (LDR)	**7** Cesium 137 (Cs-137) **8** Iridium 192 (Ir-192) **9** Iodine 125 (I-125) **C** Californium 252 (Cf-252) **Y** Other Isotope	**Z** None
0 Ear **1** Nose **3** Hypopharynx **4** Mouth **5** Tongue **6** Salivary Glands **7** Sinuses **8** Hard Palate **9** Soft Palate **B** Larynx **D** Nasopharynx **F** Oropharynx	**B** Low Dose Rate (LDR)	**B** Palladium 103 (Pd-103)	**1** Unidirectional Source **Z** None

D Radiation Therapy
9 Ear, Nose, Mouth and Throat
2 Stereotactic Radiosurgery

Treatment Site Character 4	Modality Qualifier Character 5	Isotope Character 6	Qualifier Character 7
0 Ear DRG **1** Nose DRG **4** Mouth DRG **5** Tongue DRG **6** Salivary Glands DRG **7** Sinuses DRG **8** Hard Palate DRG **9** Soft Palate DRG **B** Larynx DRG **C** Pharynx DRG **D** Nasopharynx DRG	**D** Stereotactic Other Photon Radiosurgery **H** Stereotactic Particulate Radiosurgery **J** Stereotactic Gamma Beam Radiosurgery	**Z** None	**Z** None

DRG D920DZZ D920HZZ D920JZZ D921DZZ D921HZZ D921JZZ D924DZZ D924HZZ D924JZZ D925DZZ D925HZZ D925JZZ D926DZZ D926HZZ D926JZZ D927DZZ D927HZZ D927JZZ D928DZZ D928HZZ D928JZZ D929DZZ D929HZZ D929JZZ D92BDZZ D92BHZZ D92BJZZ D92CDZZ D92CHZZ D92CJZZ D92DDZZ D92DHZZ D92DJZZ

D Radiation Therapy
9 Ear, Nose, Mouth and Throat
Y Other Radiation

Treatment Site Character 4	Modality Qualifier Character 5	Isotope Character 6	Qualifier Character 7
0 Ear **1** Nose **5** Tongue **6** Salivary Glands **7** Sinuses **8** Hard Palate **9** Soft Palate	**7** Contact Radiation **8** Hyperthermia **F** Plaque Radiation	**Z** None	**Z** None
3 Hypopharynx **F** Oropharynx	**7** Contact Radiation **8** Hyperthermia	**Z** None	**Z** None
4 Mouth **B** Larynx **D** Nasopharynx	**7** Contact Radiation **8** Hyperthermia **C** Intraoperative Radiation Therapy (IORT) **F** Plaque Radiation	**Z** None	**Z** None
C Pharynx	**C** Intraoperative Radiation Therapy (IORT) **F** Plaque Radiation	**Z** None	**Z** None

D Radiation Therapy
B Respiratory System
0 Beam Radiation

Treatment Site Character 4	Modality Qualifier Character 5	Isotope Character 6	Qualifier Character 7
0 Trachea **1** Bronchus **2** Lung **5** Pleura **6** Mediastinum **7** Chest Wall **8** Diaphragm	**0** Photons <1 MeV **1** Photons 1 - 10 MeV **2** Photons >10 MeV **4** Heavy Particles (Protons, Ions) **5** Neutrons **6** Neutron Capture	**Z** None	**Z** None
0 Trachea **1** Bronchus **2** Lung **5** Pleura **6** Mediastinum **7** Chest Wall **8** Diaphragm	**3** Electrons	**Z** None	**0** Intraoperative **Z** None

D Radiation Therapy
B Respiratory System
1 Brachytherapy

Treatment Site Character 4	Modality Qualifier Character 5	Isotope Character 6	Qualifier Character 7
0 Trachea **1** Bronchus **2** Lung **5** Pleura **6** Mediastinum **7** Chest Wall **8** Diaphragm	**9** High Dose Rate (HDR)	**7** Cesium 137 (Cs-137) **8** Iridium 192 (Ir-192) **9** Iodine 125 (I-125) **B** Palladium 103 (Pd-103) **C** Californium 252 (Cf-252) **Y** Other Isotope	**Z** None
0 Trachea **1** Bronchus **2** Lung **5** Pleura **6** Mediastinum **7** Chest Wall **8** Diaphragm	**B** Low Dose Rate (LDR)	**7** Cesium 137 (Cs-137) **8** Iridium 192 (Ir-192) **9** Iodine 125 (I-125) **C** Californium 252 (Cf-252) **Y** Other Isotope	**Z** None
0 Trachea **1** Bronchus **2** Lung **5** Pleura **6** Mediastinum **7** Chest Wall **8** Diaphragm	**B** Low Dose Rate (LDR)	**B** Palladium 103 (Pd-103)	**1** Unidirectional Source **Z** None

D Radiation Therapy
B Respiratory System
2 Stereotactic Radiosurgery

Treatment Site Character 4	Modality Qualifier Character 5	Isotope Character 6	Qualifier Character 7
0 Trachea DRG **1** Bronchus DRG **2** Lung DRG **5** Pleura DRG **6** Mediastinum DRG **7** Chest Wall DRG **8** Diaphragm DRG	**D** Stereotactic Other Photon Radiosurgery **H** Stereotactic Particulate Radiosurgery **J** Stereotactic Gamma Beam Radiosurgery	**Z** None	**Z** None

DRG DB20DZZ DB20HZZ DB20JZZ DB21DZZ DB21HZZ DB21JZZ DB22DZZ DB22HZZ DB22JZZ DB25DZZ DB25HZZ DB25JZZ DB26DZZ DB26HZZ DB26JZZ DB27DZZ DB27HZZ DB27JZZ DB28DZZ DB28HZZ DB28JZZ

D Radiation Therapy
B Respiratory System
Y Other Radiation

Treatment Site Character 4	Modality Qualifier Character 5	Isotope Character 6	Qualifier Character 7
0 Trachea **1** Bronchus **2** Lung **5** Pleura **6** Mediastinum **7** Chest Wall **8** Diaphragm	**7** Contact Radiation **8** Hyperthermia **F** Plaque Radiation **K** Laser Interstitial Thermal Therapy	**Z** None	**Z** None

D Radiation Therapy
D Gastrointestinal System
0 Beam Radiation

Treatment Site Character 4	Modality Qualifier Character 5	Isotope Character 6	Qualifier Character 7
0 Esophagus 1 Stomach 2 Duodenum 3 Jejunum 4 Ileum 5 Colon 7 Rectum	0 Photons <1 MeV 1 Photons 1 - 10 MeV 2 Photons >10 MeV 4 Heavy Particles (Protons, Ions) 5 Neutrons 6 Neutron Capture	Z None	Z None
0 Esophagus 1 Stomach 2 Duodenum 3 Jejunum 4 Ileum 5 Colon 7 Rectum	3 Electrons	Z None	0 Intraoperative Z None

D Radiation Therapy
D Gastrointestinal System
1 Brachytherapy

Treatment Site Character 4	Modality Qualifier Character 5	Isotope Character 6	Qualifier Character 7
0 Esophagus 1 Stomach 2 Duodenum 3 Jejunum 4 Ileum 5 Colon 7 Rectum	9 High Dose Rate (HDR)	7 Cesium 137 (Cs-137) 8 Iridium 192 (Ir-192) 9 Iodine 125 (I-125) B Palladium 103 (Pd-103) C Californium 252 (Cf-252) Y Other Isotope	Z None
0 Esophagus 1 Stomach 2 Duodenum 3 Jejunum 4 Ileum 5 Colon 7 Rectum	B Low Dose Rate (LDR)	7 Cesium 137 (Cs-137) 8 Iridium 192 (Ir-192) 9 Iodine 125 (I-125) C Californium 252 (Cf-252) Y Other Isotope	Z None
0 Esophagus 1 Stomach 2 Duodenum 3 Jejunum 4 Ileum 5 Colon 7 Rectum	B Low Dose Rate (LDR)	B Palladium 103 (Pd-103)	1 Unidirectional Source Z None

D Radiation Therapy
D Gastrointestinal System
2 Stereotactic Radiosurgery

Treatment Site Character 4	Modality Qualifier Character 5	Isotope Character 6	Qualifier Character 7
0 Esophagus DRG 1 Stomach DRG 2 Duodenum DRG 3 Jejunum DRG 4 Ileum DRG 5 Colon DRG 7 Rectum DRG	D Stereotactic Other Photon Radiosurgery H Stereotactic Particulate Radiosurgery J Stereotactic Gamma Beam Radiosurgery	Z None	Z None

DRG DD20DZZ DD20HZZ DD20JZZ DD21DZZ DD21HZZ DD21JZZ DD22DZZ DD22HZZ DD22JZZ DD23DZZ DD23HZZ DD23JZZ DD24DZZ DD24HZZ DD24JZZ DD25DZZ DD25HZZ DD25JZZ DD27DZZ DD27HZZ DD27JZZ

D Radiation Therapy
D Gastrointestinal System
Y Other Radiation

Treatment Site Character 4	Modality Qualifier Character 5	Isotope Character 6	Qualifier Character 7
0 Esophagus	**7** Contact Radiation **8** Hyperthermia **F** Plaque Radiation **K** Laser Interstitial Thermal Therapy	**Z** None	**Z** None
1 Stomach **2** Duodenum **3** Jejunum **4** Ileum **5** Colon **7** Rectum	**7** Contact Radiation **8** Hyperthermia **C** Intraoperative Radiation Therapy (IORT) **F** Plaque Radiation **K** Laser Interstitial Thermal Therapy	**Z** None	**Z** None
8 Anus	**C** Intraoperative Radiation Therapy (IORT) **F** Plaque Radiation **K** Laser Interstitial Thermal Therapy	**Z** None	**Z** None

D Radiation Therapy
F Hepatobiliary System and Pancreas
0 Beam Radiation

Treatment Site Character 4	Modality Qualifier Character 5	Isotope Character 6	Qualifier Character 7
0 Liver **1** Gallbladder **2** Bile Ducts **3** Pancreas	**0** Photons <1 MeV **1** Photons 1 - 10 MeV **2** Photons >10 MeV **4** Heavy Particles (Protons, Ions) **5** Neutrons **6** Neutron Capture	**Z** None	**Z** None
0 Liver **1** Gallbladder **2** Bile Ducts **3** Pancreas	**3** Electrons	**Z** None	**0** Intraoperative **Z** None

D Radiation Therapy
F Hepatobiliary System and Pancreas
1 Brachytherapy

Treatment Site Character 4	Modality Qualifier Character 5	Isotope Character 6	Qualifier Character 7
0 Liver **1** Gallbladder **2** Bile Ducts **3** Pancreas	**9** High Dose Rate (HDR)	**7** Cesium 137 (Cs-137) **8** Iridium 192 (Ir-192) **9** Iodine 125 (I-125) **B** Palladium 103 (Pd-103) **C** Californium 252 (Cf-252) **Y** Other Isotope	**Z** None
0 Liver **1** Gallbladder **2** Bile Ducts **3** Pancreas	**B** Low Dose Rate (LDR)	**7** Cesium 137 (Cs-137) **8** Iridium 192 (Ir-192) **9** Iodine 125 (I-125) **C** Californium 252 (Cf-252) **Y** Other Isotope	**Z** None
0 Liver **1** Gallbladder **2** Bile Ducts **3** Pancreas	**B** Low Dose Rate (LDR)	**B** Palladium 103 (Pd-103)	**1** Unidirectional Source **Z** None

D Radiation Therapy
F Hepatobiliary System and Pancreas
2 Stereotactic Radiosurgery

Treatment Site Character 4	Modality Qualifier Character 5	Isotope Character 6	Qualifier Character 7
0 Liver DRG 1 Gallbladder DRG 2 Bile Ducts DRG 3 Pancreas DRG	D Stereotactic Other Photon Radiosurgery H Stereotactic Particulate Radiosurgery J Stereotactic Gamma Beam Radiosurgery	Z None	Z None

DRG DF20DZZ DF20HZZ DF20JZZ DF21DZZ DF21HZZ DF21JZZ DF22DZZ DF22HZZ DF22JZZ DF23DZZ DF23HZZ DF23JZZ

D Radiation Therapy
F Hepatobiliary System and Pancreas
Y Other Radiation

Treatment Site Character 4	Modality Qualifier Character 5	Isotope Character 6	Qualifier Character 7
0 Liver 1 Gallbladder 2 Bile Ducts 3 Pancreas	7 Contact Radiation 8 Hyperthermia C Intraoperative Radiation Therapy (IORT) F Plaque Radiation K Laser Interstitial Thermal Therapy	Z None	Z None

D Radiation Therapy
G Endocrine System
0 Beam Radiation

Treatment Site Character 4	Modality Qualifier Character 5	Isotope Character 6	Qualifier Character 7
0 Pituitary Gland 1 Pineal Body 2 Adrenal Glands 4 Parathyroid Glands 5 Thyroid	0 Photons <1 MeV 1 Photons 1 - 10 MeV 2 Photons >10 MeV 5 Neutrons 6 Neutron Capture	Z None	Z None
0 Pituitary Gland 1 Pineal Body 2 Adrenal Glands 4 Parathyroid Glands 5 Thyroid	3 Electrons	Z None	0 Intraoperative Z None

D Radiation Therapy
G Endocrine System
1 Brachytherapy

Treatment Site Character 4	Modality Qualifier Character 5	Isotope Character 6	Qualifier Character 7
0 Pituitary Gland 1 Pineal Body 2 Adrenal Glands 4 Parathyroid Glands 5 Thyroid	9 High Dose Rate (HDR)	7 Cesium 137 (Cs-137) 8 Iridium 192 (Ir-192) 9 Iodine 125 (I-125) B Palladium 103 (Pd-103) C Californium 252 (Cf-252) Y Other Isotope	Z None
0 Pituitary Gland 1 Pineal Body 2 Adrenal Glands 4 Parathyroid Glands 5 Thyroid	B Low Dose Rate (LDR)	7 Cesium 137 (Cs-137) 8 Iridium 192 (Ir-192) 9 Iodine 125 (I-125) C Californium 252 (Cf-252) Y Other Isotope	Z None
0 Pituitary Gland 1 Pineal Body 2 Adrenal Glands 4 Parathyroid Glands 5 Thyroid	B Low Dose Rate (LDR)	B Palladium 103 (Pd-103)	1 Unidirectional Source Z None

D Radiation Therapy
G Endocrine System
2 Stereotactic Radiosurgery

Treatment Site	Modality Qualifier	Isotope	Qualifier
Character 4	Character 5	Character 6	Character 7
0 Pituitary Gland DRG 1 Pineal Body DRG 2 Adrenal Glands DRG 4 Parathyroid Glands DRG 5 Thyroid DRG	D Stereotactic Other Photon Radiosurgery H Stereotactic Particulate Radiosurgery J Stereotactic Gamma Beam Radiosurgery	Z None	Z None

DRG DG20DZZ DG20HZZ DG20JZZ DG21DZZ DG21HZZ DG21JZZ DG22DZZ DG22HZZ DG22JZZ DG24DZZ DG24HZZ DG24JZZ DG25DZZ DG25HZZ DG25JZZ

D Radiation Therapy
G Endocrine System
Y Other Radiation

Treatment Site	Modality Qualifier	Isotope	Qualifier
Character 4	Character 5	Character 6	Character 7
0 Pituitary Gland 1 Pineal Body 2 Adrenal Glands 4 Parathyroid Glands 5 Thyroid	7 Contact Radiation 8 Hyperthermia F Plaque Radiation K Laser Interstitial Thermal Therapy	Z None	Z None

D Radiation Therapy
H Skin
0 Beam Radiation

Treatment Site	Modality Qualifier	Isotope	Qualifier
Character 4	Character 5	Character 6	Character 7
2 Skin, Face 3 Skin, Neck 4 Skin, Arm 6 Skin, Chest 7 Skin, Back 8 Skin, Abdomen 9 Skin, Buttock B Skin, Leg	0 Photons <1 MeV 1 Photons 1 - 10 MeV 2 Photons >10 MeV 4 Heavy Particles (Protons, Ions) 5 Neutrons 6 Neutron Capture	Z None	Z None
2 Skin, Face 3 Skin, Neck 4 Skin, Arm 6 Skin, Chest 7 Skin, Back 8 Skin, Abdomen 9 Skin, Buttock B Skin, Leg	3 Electrons	Z None	0 Intraoperative Z None

D Radiation Therapy
H Skin
Y Other Radiation

Treatment Site Character 4	Modality Qualifier Character 5	Isotope Character 6	Qualifier Character 7
2 Skin, Face **3** Skin, Neck **4** Skin, Arm **6** Skin, Chest **7** Skin, Back **8** Skin, Abdomen **9** Skin, Buttock **B** Skin, Leg	**7** Contact Radiation **8** Hyperthermia **F** Plaque Radiation	**Z** None	**Z** None
5 Skin, Hand **C** Skin, Foot	**F** Plaque Radiation	**Z** None	**Z** None

D Radiation Therapy
M Breast
0 Beam Radiation

Treatment Site Character 4	Modality Qualifier Character 5	Isotope Character 6	Qualifier Character 7
0 Breast, Left **1** Breast, Right	**0** Photons <1 MeV **1** Photons 1 - 10 MeV **2** Photons >10 MeV **4** Heavy Particles (Protons, Ions) **5** Neutrons **6** Neutron Capture	**Z** None	**Z** None
0 Breast, Left **1** Breast, Right	**3** Electrons	**Z** None	**C** Intraoperative **Z** None

D Radiation Therapy
M Breast
1 Brachytherapy

Treatment Site Character 4	Modality Qualifier Character 5	Isotope Character 6	Qualifier Character 7
0 Breast, Left **1** Breast, Right	**9** High Dose Rate (HDR)	**7** Cesium 137 (Cs-137) **8** Iridium 192 (Ir-192) **9** Iodine 125 (I-125) **B** Palladium 103 (Pd-103) **C** Californium 252 (Cf-252) **Y** Other Isotope	**Z** None
0 Breast, Left **1** Breast, Right	**B** Low Dose Rate (LDR)	**7** Cesium 137 (Cs-137) **8** Iridium 192 (Ir-192) **9** Iodine 125 (I-125) **C** Californium 252 (Cf-252) **Y** Other Isotope	**Z** None
0 Breast, Left **1** Breast, Right	**B** Low Dose Rate (LDR)	**B** Palladium 103 (Pd-103)	**1** Unidirectional Source **Z** None

D Radiation Therapy
M Breast
2 Stereotactic Radiosurgery

Treatment Site Character 4	Modality Qualifier Character 5	Isotope Character 6	Qualifier Character 7
0 Breast, Left DRG **1** Breast, Right DRG	**D** Stereotactic Other Photon Radiosurgery **H** Stereotactic Particulate Radiosurgery **J** Stereotactic Gamma Beam Radiosurgery	**Z** None	**Z** None

DRG DM20DZZ DM20HZZ DM20JZZ DM21DZZ DM21HZZ DM21JZZ

D Radiation Therapy
M Breast
Y Other Radiation

Treatment Site Character 4	Modality Qualifier Character 5	Isotope Character 6	Qualifier Character 7
0 Breast, Left **1** Breast, Right	**7** Contact Radiation **8** Hyperthermia **F** Plaque Radiation **K** Laser Interstitial Thermal Therapy	**Z** None	**Z** None

D Radiation Therapy
P Musculoskeletal System
0 Beam Radiation

Treatment Site Character 4	Modality Qualifier Character 5	Isotope Character 6	Qualifier Character 7
0 Skull **2** Maxilla **3** Mandible **4** Sternum **5** Rib(s) **6** Humerus **7** Radius/Ulna **8** Pelvic Bones **9** Femur **B** Tibia/Fibula **C** Other Bone	**0** Photons <1 MeV **1** Photons 1 - 10 MeV **2** Photons >10 MeV **4** Heavy Particles (Protons, Ions) **5** Neutrons **6** Neutron Capture	**Z** None	**Z** None
0 Skull **2** Maxilla **3** Mandible **4** Sternum **5** Rib(s) **6** Humerus **7** Radius/Ulna **8** Pelvic Bones **9** Femur **B** Tibia/Fibula **C** Other Bone	**3** Electrons	**Z** None	**0** Intraoperative **Z** None

D Radiation Therapy
P Musculoskeletal System
Y Other Radiation

Treatment Site Character 4	Modality Qualifier Character 5	Isotope Character 6	Qualifier Character 7
0 Skull 2 Maxilla 3 Mandible 4 Sternum 5 Rib(s) 6 Humerus 7 Radius/Ulna 8 Pelvic Bones 9 Femur B Tibia/Fibula C Other Bone	7 Contact Radiation 8 Hyperthermia F Plaque Radiation	Z None	Z None

D Radiation Therapy
T Urinary System
0 Beam Radiation

Treatment Site Character 4	Modality Qualifier Character 5	Isotope Character 6	Qualifier Character 7
0 Kidney 1 Ureter 2 Bladder 3 Urethra	0 Photons <1 MeV 1 Photons 1 - 10 MeV 2 Photons >10 MeV 4 Heavy Particles (Protons, Ions) 5 Neutrons 6 Neutron Capture	Z None	Z None
0 Kidney 1 Ureter 2 Bladder 3 Urethra	3 Electrons	Z None	0 Intraoperative Z None

D Radiation Therapy
T Urinary System
1 Brachytherapy

Treatment Site Character 4	Modality Qualifier Character 5	Isotope Character 6	Qualifier Character 7
0 Kidney 1 Ureter 2 Bladder 3 Urethra	9 High Dose Rate (HDR)	7 Cesium 137 (Cs-137) 8 Iridium 192 (Ir-192) 9 Iodine 125 (I-125) B Palladium 103 (Pd-103) C Californium 252 (Cf-252) Y Other Isotope	Z None
0 Kidney 1 Ureter 2 Bladder 3 Urethra	B Low Dose Rate (LDR)	7 Cesium 137 (Cs-137) 8 Iridium 192 (Ir-192) 9 Iodine 125 (I-125) C Californium 252 (Cf-252) Y Other Isotope	Z None
0 Kidney 1 Ureter 2 Bladder 3 Urethra	B Low Dose Rate (LDR)	B Palladium 103 (Pd-103)	1 Unidirectional Source Z None

D Radiation Therapy
T Urinary System
2 Stereotactic Radiosurgery

Treatment Site Character 4	Modality Qualifier Character 5	Isotope Character 6	Qualifier Character 7
0 Kidney DRG 1 Ureter DRG 2 Bladder DRG 3 Urethra DRG	D Stereotactic Other Photon Radiosurgery H Stereotactic Particulate Radiosurgery J Stereotactic Gamma Beam Radiosurgery	Z None	Z None

DRG DT20DZZ DT20HZZ DT20JZZ DT21DZZ DT21HZZ DT21JZZ DT22DZZ DT22HZZ DT22JZZ DT23DZZ DT23HZZ DT23JZZ

D Radiation Therapy
T Urinary System
Y Other Radiation

Treatment Site Character 4	Modality Qualifier Character 5	Isotope Character 6	Qualifier Character 7
0 Kidney 1 Ureter 2 Bladder 3 Urethra	7 Contact Radiation 8 Hyperthermia C Intraoperative Radiation Therapy (IORT) F Plaque Radiation	Z None	Z None

D Radiation Therapy
U Female Reproductive System
0 Beam Radiation

Treatment Site Character 4	Modality Qualifier Character 5	Isotope Character 6	Qualifier Character 7
0 Ovary ♀ 1 Cervix ♀ 2 Uterus ♀	0 Photons <1 MeV 1 Photons 1 - 10 MeV 2 Photons >10 MeV 4 Heavy Particles (Protons, Ions) 5 Neutrons 6 Neutron Capture	Z None	Z None
0 Ovary ♀ 1 Cervix ♀ 2 Uterus ♀	3 Electrons	Z None	0 Intraoperative Z None

♀ DU000ZZ DU001ZZ DU002ZZ DU003Z0 DU003ZZ DU004ZZ DU005ZZ DU006ZZ DU010ZZ DU011ZZ DU012ZZ DU013Z0 DU013ZZ DU014ZZ DU015ZZ DU016ZZ DU020ZZ DU021ZZ DU022ZZ DU023Z0 DU023ZZ DU024ZZ DU025ZZ DU026ZZ

D Radiation Therapy
U Female Reproductive System
1 Brachytherapy

Treatment Site Character 4	Modality Qualifier Character 5	Isotope Character 6	Qualifier Character 7
0 Ovary ♀ **1** Cervix ♀ **2** Uterus ♀	**9** High Dose Rate (HDR)	**7** Cesium 137 (Cs-137) **8** Iridium 192 (Ir-192) **9** Iodine 125 (I-125) **B** Palladium 103 (Pd-103) **C** Californium 252 (Cf-252) **Y** Other Isotope	**Z** None
0 Ovary ♀ **1** Cervix ♀ **2** Uterus ♀	**B** Low Dose Rate (LDR)	**7** Cesium 137 (Cs-137) **8** Iridium 192 (Ir-192) **9** Iodine 125 (I-125) **C** Californium 252 (Cf-252) **Y** Other Isotope	**Z** None
0 Ovary ♀ **1** Cervix ♀ **2** Uterus ♀	**B** Low Dose Rate (LDR)	**B** Palladium 103 (Pd-103)	**1** Unidirectional Source **Z** None

♀ DU1097Z DU1098Z DU1099Z DU109BZ DU109CZ DU109YZ DU10B7Z DU10B8Z DU10B9Z DU10BB1 DU10BBZ DU10BCZ DU10BYZ DU1197Z DU1198Z DU1199Z DU119BZ DU119CZ DU119YZ DU11B7Z DU11B8Z DU11B9Z DU11BB1 DU11BBZ DU11BCZ DU11BYZ DU1297Z DU1298Z DU1299Z DU129BZ DU129CZ DU129YZ DU12B7Z DU12B8Z DU12B9Z DU12BB1 DU12BBZ DU12BCZ DU12BYZ

D Radiation Therapy
U Female Reproductive System
2 Stereotactic Radiosurgery

Treatment Site Character 4	Modality Qualifier Character 5	Isotope Character 6	Qualifier Character 7
0 Ovary ♀ DRG **1** Cervix ♀ DRG **2** Uterus ♀ DRG	**D** Stereotactic Other Photon Radiosurgery **H** Stereotactic Particulate Radiosurgery **J** Stereotactic Gamma Beam Radiosurgery	**Z** None	**Z** None

♀ DU20DZZ DU20HZZ DU20JZZ DU21DZZ DU21HZZ DU21JZZ DU22DZZ DU22HZZ DU22JZZ
DRG DU20DZZ DU20HZZ DU20JZZ DU21DZZ DU21HZZ DU21JZZ DU22DZZ DU22HZZ DU22JZZ

D Radiation Therapy
U Female Reproductive System
Y Other Radiation

Treatment Site Character 4	Modality Qualifier Character 5	Isotope Character 6	Qualifier Character 7
0 Ovary ♀ **1** Cervix ♀ **2** Uterus ♀	**7** Contact Radiation **8** Hyperthermia **C** Intraoperative Radiation Therapy (IORT) **F** Plaque Radiation	**Z** None	**Z** None

♀ DUY07ZZ DUY08ZZ DUY0CZZ DUY0FZZ DUY17ZZ DUY18ZZ DUY1CZZ DUY1FZZ DUY27ZZ DUY28ZZ DUY2CZZ DUY2FZZ

D Radiation Therapy
V Male Reproductive System
0 Beam Radiation

Treatment Site Character 4	Modality Qualifier Character 5	Isotope Character 6	Qualifier Character 7
0 Prostate ♂ **1** Testis ♂	**0** Photons <1 MeV **1** Photons 1 - 10 MeV **2** Photons >10 MeV **4** Heavy Particles (Protons, Ions) **5** Neutrons **6** Neutron Capture	**Z** None	**Z** None
0 Prostate ♂ **1** Testis ♂	**3** Electrons	**Z** None	**0** Intraoperative **Z** None

♂ DV000ZZ DV001ZZ DV002ZZ DV003Z0 DV003ZZ DV004ZZ DV005ZZ DV006ZZ DV010ZZ DV011ZZ DV012ZZ DV013Z0 DV013ZZ DV014ZZ DV015ZZ DV016ZZ

D Radiation Therapy
V Male Reproductive System
1 Brachytherapy

Treatment Site Character 4	Modality Qualifier Character 5	Isotope Character 6	Qualifier Character 7
0 Prostate ♂ **1** Testis ♂	**9** High Dose Rate (HDR)	**7** Cesium 137 (Cs-137) **8** Iridium 192 (Ir-192) **9** Iodine 125 (I-125) **B** Palladium 103 (Pd-103) **C** Californium 252 (Cf-252) **Y** Other Isotope	**Z** None
0 Prostate ♂ **1** Testis ♂	**B** Low Dose Rate (LDR)	**7** Cesium 137 (Cs-137) **8** Iridium 192 (Ir-192) **9** Iodine 125 (I-125) **C** Californium 252 (Cf-252) **Y** Other Isotope	**Z** None
0 Prostate ♂ **1** Testis ♂	**B** Low Dose Rate (LDR)	**B** Palladium 103 (Pd-103)	**1** Unidirectional Source **Z** None

♂ DV1097Z DV1098Z DV1099Z DV109BZ DV109CZ DV109YZ DV10B7Z DV10B8Z DV10B9Z DV10BB1 DV10BBZ DV10BCZ DV10BYZ DV1197Z DV1198Z DV1199Z DV119BZ DV119CZ DV119YZ DV11B7Z DV11B8Z DV11B9Z DV11BB1 DV11BBZ DV11BCZ DV11BYZ

D Radiation Therapy
V Male Reproductive System
2 Stereotactic Radiosurgery

Treatment Site Character 4	Modality Qualifier Character 5	Isotope Character 6	Qualifier Character 7
0 Prostate ♂ DRG **1** Testis ♂ DRG	**D** Stereotactic Other Photon Radiosurgery **H** Stereotactic Particulate Radiosurgery **J** Stereotactic Gamma Beam Radiosurgery	**Z** None	**Z** None

♂ DV20DZZ DV20HZZ DV20JZZ DV21DZZ DV21HZZ DV21JZZ
DRG DV20DZZ DV20HZZ DV20JZZ DV21DZZ DV21HZZ DV21JZZ

LC Limited Coverage NC Noncovered HAC HAC-associated Procedure CC Combination Cluster - See Appendix G for code lists
DRG Non-OR-Affecting MS-DRG Assignment New/Revised Text in **Orange** ♂ Male ♀ Female

D Radiation Therapy
V Male Reproductive System
Y Other Radiation

Treatment Site Character 4	Modality Qualifier Character 5	Isotope Character 6	Qualifier Character 7
0 Prostate ♂	7 Contact Radiation 8 Hyperthermia C Intraoperative Radiation Therapy (IORT) F Plaque Radiation K Laser Interstitial Thermal Therapy	Z None	Z None
1 Testis ♂	7 Contact Radiation 8 Hyperthermia F Plaque Radiation	Z None	Z None

♂ DVY07ZZ DVY08ZZ DVY0CZZ DVY0FZZ DVY0KZZ DVY17ZZ DVY18ZZ DVY1FZZ

D Radiation Therapy
W Anatomical Regions
0 Beam Radiation

Treatment Site Character 4	Modality Qualifier Character 5	Isotope Character 6	Qualifier Character 7
1 Head and Neck 2 Chest 3 Abdomen 4 Hemibody 5 Whole Body 6 Pelvic Region	0 Photons <1 MeV 1 Photons 1 - 10 MeV 2 Photons >10 MeV 4 Heavy Particles (Protons, Ions) 5 Neutrons 6 Neutron Capture	Z None	Z None
1 Head and Neck 2 Chest 3 Abdomen 4 Hemibody 5 Whole Body 6 Pelvic Region	3 Electrons	Z None	0 Intraoperative Z None

D Radiation Therapy
W Anatomical Regions
1 Brachytherapy

Treatment Site Character 4	Modality Qualifier Character 5	Isotope Character 6	Qualifier Character 7
0 Cranial Cavity **K** Upper Back **L** Lower Back **P** Gastrointestinal Tract **Q** Respiratory Tract **R** Genitourinary Tract **X** Upper Extremity **Y** Lower Extremity	**B** Low Dose Rate (LDR)	**B** Palladium 103 (Pd-103)	**1** Unidirectional Source **Z** None
1 Head and Neck **2** Chest **3** Abdomen **6** Pelvic Region	**9** High Dose Rate (HDR)	**7** Cesium 137 (Cs-137) **8** Iridium 192 (Ir-192) **9** Iodine 125 (I-125) **B** Palladium 103 (Pd-103) **C** Californium 252 (Cf-252) **Y** Other Isotope	**Z** None
1 Head and Neck **2** Chest **3** Abdomen **6** Pelvic Region	**B** Low Dose Rate (LDR)	**7** Cesium 137 (Cs-137) **8** Iridium 192 (Ir-192) **9** Iodine 125 (I-125) **B** Palladium 103 (Pd-103) **C** Californium 252 (Cf-252) **Y** Other Isotope	**Z** None
1 Head and Neck **2** Chest **3** Abdomen **6** Pelvic Region	**B** Low Dose Rate (LDR)	**B** Palladium 103 (Pd-103)	**1** Unidirectional Source **Z** None

D Radiation Therapy
W Anatomical Regions
2 Stereotactic Radiosurgery

Treatment Site Character 4	Modality Qualifier Character 5	Isotope Character 6	Qualifier Character 7
1 Head and Neck DRG **2** Chest DRG **3** Abdomen DRG **6** Pelvic Region DRG	**D** Stereotactic Other Photon Radiosurgery **H** Stereotactic Particulate Radiosurgery **J** Stereotactic Gamma Beam Radiosurgery	**Z** None	**Z** None

DRG DW21DZZ DW21HZZ DW21JZZ DW22DZZ DW22HZZ DW22JZZ DW23DZZ DW23HZZ DW23JZZ DW26DZZ DW26HZZ DW26JZZ

D Radiation Therapy
W Anatomical Regions
Y Other Radiation

Treatment Site Character 4	Modality Qualifier Character 5	Isotope Character 6	Qualifier Character 7
1 Head and Neck **2** Chest **3** Abdomen **4** Hemibody **6** Pelvic Region	**7** Contact Radiation **8** Hyperthermia **F** Plaque Radiation	**Z** None	**Z** None
5 Whole Body	**7** Contact Radiation **8** Hyperthermia **F** Plaque Radiation	**Z** None	**Z** None
5 Whole Body	**G** Isotope Administration	**D** Iodine 131 (I-131) **F** Phosphorus 32 (P-32) **G** Strontium 89 (Sr-89) **H** Strontium 90 (Sr-90) **Y** Other Isotope	**Z** None

NOTES

NOTES

Section qualifier (2nd character) - 2 options
1) rehabilitation
2) diagnostic audiology

Value	type qualifier	type qualifier definition
0	range of motion/joint mobility	- Exercises/activities to increase muscle strength & joint mobility
1	muscle performance	Exercises/activities to increase the capacity of a muscle to do work in terms of strength, power, endurance
2	Coordination/Dexterity	exercises/activity to facilitate gross coordination & fine coordination
3	motor function	exercises/activity to facilitate crossing midline, laterality, bilateral integration, praxis, neuromuscular relaxation, inhibition, facilitation, motor function & motor learning
4	manual therapy techniques	techniques the therapist uses hands to administer skilled movements, includes; connective tissue massage, joint mobilization, manual traction & soft tissue mobilization

Swallowing dysfunction exercises + wound management

14 root types

Physical Rehabilitation and Diagnostic Audiology F00-F15

PM&R

AKA Physiatry or rehabilitation

F Physical Rehabilitation and Diagnostic Audiology
0 Rehabilitation
0 Speech Assessment: Measurement of speech and related functions

Body system/ Region Character 4	Type Qualifier Character 5	Equipment (Used) Character 6	Qualifier Character 7
3 Neurological System - Whole Body DRG	**G** Communicative/Cognitive Integration Skills	**K** Audiovisual **M** Augmentative / Alternative Communication **P** Computer **Y** Other Equipment **Z** None	**Z** None
Z None DRG	**0** Filtered Speech **3** Staggered Spondaic Word **Q** Performance Intensity Phonetically Balanced Speech Discrimination **R** Brief Tone Stimuli **S** Distorted Speech **T** Dichotic Stimuli **V** Temporal Ordering of Stimuli **W** Masking Patterns	**1** Audiometer **2** Sound Field / Booth **K** Audiovisual **Z** None	**Z** None
Z None DRG	**1** Speech Threshold **2** Speech/Word Recognition	**1** Audiometer **2** Sound Field / Booth **9** Cochlear Implant **K** Audiovisual **Z** None	**Z** None
Z None DRG	**4** Sensorineural Acuity Level	**1** Audiometer **2** Sound Field / Booth **Z** None	**Z** None
Z None DRG	**5** Synthetic Sentence Identification	**1** Audiometer **2** Sound Field / Booth **9** Cochlear Implant **K** Audiovisual	**Z** None
Z None DRG	**6** Speech and/or Language Screening **7** Nonspoken Language **8** Receptive/Expressive Language **C** Aphasia **G** Communicative/Cognitive Integration Skills **L** Augmentative/Alternative Communication System	**K** Audiovisual **M** Augmentative / Alternative Communication **P** Computer **Y** Other Equipment **Z** None	**Z** None
Z None DRG	**9** Articulation/Phonology	**K** Audiovisual **P** Computer **Q** Speech Analysis - Spectrograph **Y** Other Equipment **Z** None	**Z** None
Z None DRG	**B** Motor Speech	**K** Audiovisual **N** Biosensory Feedback **P** Computer **Q** Speech Analysis **T** Aerodynamic Function **Y** Other Equipment **Z** None	**Z** None

F00 continued on next page

F Physical Rehabilitation and Diagnostic Audiology
0 Rehabilitation
0 Speech Assessment: Measurement of speech and related functions

F00 continued from previous page

Body system/ Region Character 4	Type Qualifier Character 5	Equipment Character 6	Qualifier Character 7
Z None DRG	**D** Fluency	**K** Audiovisual **N** Biosensory Feedback **P** Computer **Q** Speech Analysis **S** Voice Analysis **T** Aerodynamic Function **Y** Other Equipment **Z** None	**Z** None
Z None DRG	**F** Voice	**K** Audiovisual **N** Biosensory Feedback **P** Computer **S** Voice Analysis **T** Aerodynamic Function **Y** Other Equipment **Z** None	**Z** None
Z None DRG	**H** Bedside Swallowing and Oral Function **P** Oral Peripheral Mechanism	**Y** Other Equipment **Z** None	**Z** None
Z None DRG	**J** Instrumental Swallowing and Oral Function	**T** Aerodynamic Function **W** Swallowing **Y** Other Equipment	**Z** None
Z None DRG	**K** Orofacial Myofunctional	**K** Audiovisual **P** Computer **Y** Other Equipment **Z** None	**Z** None
Z None DRG	**M** Voice Prosthetic	**K** Audiovisual **P** Computer **S** Voice Analysis **V** Speech Prosthesis **Y** Other Equipment **Z** None	**Z** None
Z None DRG	**N** Non-invasive Instrumental Status	**N** Biosensory Feedback **P** Computer **Q** Speech Analysis **S** Voice Analysis **T** Aerodynamic Function **Y** Other Equipment	**Z** None
Z None DRG	**X** Other Specified Central Auditory Processing	**Z** None	**Z** None

DRG F003GKZ F003GMZ F003GPZ F003GYZ F003GZZ F00Z01Z F00Z02Z F00Z0KZ F00Z0ZZ F00Z11Z F00Z12Z F00Z19Z F00Z1KZ F00Z1ZZ F00Z21Z F00Z22Z F00Z29Z F00Z2KZ F00Z2ZZ F00Z31Z F00Z32Z F00Z3KZ F00Z3ZZ F00Z41Z F00Z42Z F00Z4ZZ F00Z51Z F00Z52Z F00Z59Z F00Z5KZ F00Z6KZ F00Z6MZ F00Z6PZ F00Z6YZ F00Z6ZZ F00Z7KZ F00Z7MZ F00Z7PZ F00Z7YZ F00Z7ZZ F00Z8KZ F00Z8MZ F00Z8PZ F00Z8YZ F00Z8ZZ F00Z9KZ F00Z9PZ F00Z9QZ F00Z9YZ F00Z9ZZ F00ZBKZ F00ZBNZ F00ZBPZ F00ZBQZ F00ZBTZ F00ZBYZ F00ZBZZ F00ZCKZ F00ZCMZ F00ZCPZ F00ZCYZ F00ZCZZ F00ZDKZ F00ZDNZ F00ZDPZ F00ZDQZ F00ZDSZ F00ZDTZ F00ZDYZ F00ZDZZ F00ZFKZ F00ZFNZ F00ZFPZ F00ZFSZ F00ZFTZ F00ZFYZ F00ZFZZ F00ZGKZ F00ZGMZ F00ZGPZ F00ZGYZ F00ZGZZ F00ZHYZ F00ZHZZ F00ZJTZ F00ZJWZ F00ZJYZ F00ZKKZ F00ZKPZ F00ZKYZ F00ZKZZ F00ZLKZ F00ZLMZ F00ZLPZ F00ZLYZ F00ZLZZ F00ZMKZ F00ZMPZ F00ZMSZ F00ZMVZ F00ZMYZ F00ZMZZ F00ZNNZ F00ZNPZ F00ZNQZ F00ZNSZ F00ZNTZ F00ZNYZ F00ZPYZ F00ZPZZ F00ZQ1Z F00ZQ2Z F00ZQKZ F00ZQZZ F00ZR1Z F00ZR2Z F00ZRKZ F00ZRZZ F00ZS1Z F00ZS2Z F00ZSKZ F00ZSZZ F00ZT1Z F00ZT2Z F00ZTKZ F00ZTZZ F00ZV1Z F00ZV2Z F00ZVKZ F00ZVZZ F00ZW1Z F00ZW2Z F00ZWKZ F00ZWZZ F00ZXZZ

F Physical Rehabilitation and Diagnostic Audiology
0 Rehabilitation
1 Motor and/or Nerve Function Assessment: Measurement of motor, nerve, and related functions

Body system/ Region Character 4	Type Qualifier Character 5	Equipment Character 6	Qualifier Character 7
0 Neurological System - Head and Neck DRG 1 Neurological System - Upper Back / Upper Extremity DRG 2 Neurological System - Lower Back / Lower Extremity DRG 3 Neurological System - Whole Body DRG	0 Muscle Performance	E Orthosis F Assistive, Adaptive, Supportive or Protective U Prosthesis Y Other Equipment Z None	Z None
0 Neurological System - Head and Neck DRG 1 Neurological System - Upper Back / Upper Extremity DRG 2 Neurological System - Lower Back / Lower Extremity DRG 3 Neurological System - Whole Body DRG	1 Integumentary Integrity 3 Coordination/Dexterity 4 Motor Function G Reflex Integrity	Z None	Z None
0 Neurological System - Head and Neck DRG 1 Neurological System - Upper Back / Upper Extremity DRG 2 Neurological System - Lower Back / Lower Extremity DRG 3 Neurological System - Whole Body DRG	5 Range of Motion and Joint Integrity 6 Sensory Awareness/Processing/ Integrity	Y Other Equipment Z None	Z None
D Integumentary System - Head and Neck DRG F Integumentary System - Upper Back / Upper Extremity DRG G Integumentary System - Lower Back / Lower Extremity DRG H Integumentary System - Whole Body DRG J Musculoskeletal System - Head and Neck DRG K Musculoskeletal System - Upper Back / Upper Extremity DRG L Musculoskeletal System - Lower Back / Lower Extremity DRG M Musculoskeletal System - Whole Body DRG	0 Muscle Performance	E Orthosis F Assistive, Adaptive, Supportive or Protective U Prosthesis Y Other Equipment Z None	Z None
D Integumentary System - Head and Neck DRG F Integumentary System - Upper Back / Upper Extremity DRG G Integumentary System - Lower Back / Lower Extremity DRG H Integumentary System - Whole Body DRG J Musculoskeletal System - Head and Neck DRG K Musculoskeletal System - Upper Back / Upper Extremity DRG L Musculoskeletal System - Lower Back / Lower Extremity DRG M Musculoskeletal System - Whole Body DRG	1 Integumentary Integrity	Z None	Z None

F01 continued on next page

F Physical Rehabilitation and Diagnostic Audiology
0 Rehabilitation
1 Motor and/or Nerve Function Assessment: Measurement of motor, nerve, and related functions

F01 continued from previous page

Body system/ Region Character 4	Type Qualifier Character 5	Equipment Character 6	Qualifier Character 7
D Integumentary System - Head and Neck DRG **F** Integumentary System - Upper Back / Upper Extremity DRG **G** Integumentary System - Lower Back / Lower Extremity DRG **H** Integumentary System - Whole Body DRG **J** Musculoskeletal System - Head and Neck DRG **K** Musculoskeletal System - Upper Back / Upper Extremity DRG **L** Musculoskeletal System - Lower Back / Lower Extremity DRG **M** Musculoskeletal System - Whole Body DRG	**5** Range of Motion and Joint Integrity **6** Sensory Awareness/Processing/ Integrity	**Y** Other Equipment **Z** None	**Z** None
N Genitourinary System DRG	**0** Muscle Performance	**E** Orthosis **F** Assistive, Adaptive, Supportive or Protective **U** Prosthesis **Y** Other Equipment **Z** None	**Z** None
Z None DRG	**2** Visual Motor Integration	**K** Audiovisual **M** Augmentative / Alternative Communication **N** Biosensory Feedback **P** Computer **Q** Speech Analysis **S** Voice Analysis **Y** Other Equipment **Z** None	**Z** None
Z None DRG	**7** Facial Nerve Function	**7** Electrophysiologic	**Z** None
Z None DRG	**9** Somatosensory Evoked Potentials	**J** Somatosensory	**Z** None
Z None DRG	**B** Bed Mobility **C** Transfer **F** Wheelchair Mobility	**E** Orthosis **F** Assistive, Adaptive, Supportive or Protective **U** Prosthesis **Z** None	**Z** None
Z None	**D** Gait and/or Balance	**E** Orthosis **F** Assistive, Adaptive, Supportive or Protective **U** Prosthesis **Y** Other Equipment **Z** None	**Z** None

DRG F0100EZ F0100FZ F0100UZ F0100YZ F0100ZZ F0101ZZ F0103ZZ F0104ZZ F0105YZ F0105ZZ F0106YZ F0106ZZ F010GZZ F0110EZ F0110FZ F0110UZ F0110YZ F0110ZZ F0111ZZ F0113ZZ F0114ZZ F0115YZ F0115ZZ F0116YZ F0116ZZ F011GZZ F0120EZ F0120FZ F0120UZ F0120YZ F0120ZZ F0121ZZ F0123ZZ F0124ZZ F0125YZ F0125ZZ F0126YZ F0126ZZ F012GZZ F0130EZ F0130FZ F0130UZ F0130YZ F0130ZZ F0131ZZ F0133ZZ F0134ZZ F0135YZ F0135ZZ F0136YZ F0136ZZ F013GZZ F01D0EZ F01D0FZ F01D0UZ F01D0YZ F01D0ZZ F01D1ZZ F01D5YZ F01D5ZZ F01D6YZ F01D6ZZ F01F0EZ F01F0FZ F01F0UZ F01F0YZ F01F0ZZ F01F1ZZ F01F5YZ F01F5ZZ F01F6YZ F01F6ZZ F01G0EZ F01G0FZ F01G0UZ F01G0YZ F01G0ZZ F01G1ZZ F01G5YZ F01G5ZZ F01G6YZ F01G6ZZ F01H0EZ F01H0FZ F01H0UZ F01H0YZ F01H0ZZ F01H1ZZ F01H5YZ F01H5ZZ F01H6YZ F01H6ZZ F01J0EZ F01J0FZ F01J0UZ F01J0YZ F01J0ZZ F01J1ZZ F01J5YZ F01J5ZZ F01J6YZ F01J6ZZ F01K0EZ F01K0FZ F01K0UZ F01K0YZ F01K0ZZ F01K1ZZ F01K5YZ F01K5ZZ F01K6YZ F01K6ZZ F01L0EZ F01L0FZ F01L0UZ F01L0YZ F01L0ZZ F01L1ZZ F01L5YZ F01L5ZZ F01L6YZ F01L6ZZ F01M0EZ F01M0FZ F01M0UZ F01M0YZ F01M0ZZ F01M1ZZ F01M5YZ F01M5ZZ F01M6YZ F01M6ZZ F01N0EZ F01N0FZ F01N0UZ F01N0YZ F01N0ZZ F01Z2KZ F01Z2MZ F01Z2NZ F01Z2PZ F01Z2QZ F01Z2SZ F01Z2YZ F01Z2ZZ F01Z77Z F01Z9JZ F01ZBEZ F01ZBFZ F01ZBUZ F01ZBZZ F01ZCEZ F01ZCFZ F01ZCUZ F01ZCZZ F01ZDEZ F01ZDFZ F01ZDUZ F01ZDYZ F01ZDZZ F01ZFEZ F01ZFFZ F01ZFUZ F01ZFZZ

LC Limited Coverage NC Noncovered HAC HAC-associated Procedure CC Combination Cluster - See Appendix G for code lists
DRG Non-OR-Affecting MS-DRG Assignment New/Revised Text in **Orange** ♂ Male ♀ Female

F Physical Rehabilitation and Diagnostic Audiology
0 Rehabilitation
2 Activities of Daily Living Assessment: Measurement of functional level for activities of daily living

Body system/ Region Character 4	Type Qualifier Character 5	Equipment Character 6	Qualifier Character 7
0 Neurological System - Head and Neck DRG	**9** Cranial Nerve Integrity **D** Neuromotor Development	**Y** Other Equipment **Z** None	**Z** None
1 Neurological System - Upper Back / Upper Extremity DRG **2** Neurological System - Lower Back / Lower Extremity DRG **3** Neurological System - Whole Body DRG	**D** Neuromotor Development	**Y** Other Equipment **Z** None	**Z** None
4 Circulatory System - Head and Neck DRG **5** Circulatory System - Upper Back / Upper Extremity DRG **6** Circulatory System - Lower Back / Lower Extremity DRG **8** Respiratory System - Head and Neck DRG **9** Respiratory System - Upper Back / Upper Extremity DRG **B** Respiratory System - Lower Back / Lower Extremity DRG	**G** Ventilation, Respiration and Circulation	**C** Mechanical **G** Aerobic Endurance and Conditioning **Y** Other Equipment **Z** None	**Z** None
7 Circulatory System - Whole Body DRG **C** Respiratory System - Whole Body DRG	**7** Aerobic Capacity and Endurance	**E** Orthosis **G** Aerobic Endurance and Conditioning **U** Prosthesis **Y** Other Equipment **Z** None	**Z** None
7 Circulatory System - Whole Body DRG **C** Respiratory System - Whole Body DRG	**G** Ventilation, Respiration and Circulation	**C** Mechanical **G** Aerobic Endurance and Conditioning **Y** Other Equipment **Z** None	**Z** None
Z None DRG	**0** Bathing/Showering **1** Dressing **3** Grooming/Personal Hygiene **4** Home Management	**E** Orthosis **F** Assistive, Adaptive, Supportive or Protective **U** Prosthesis **Z** None	**Z** None
Z None DRG	**2** Feeding/Eating **8** Anthropometric Characteristics **F** Pain	**Y** Other Equipment **Z** None	**Z** None
Z None DRG	**5** Perceptual Processing	**K** Audiovisual **M** Augmentative / Alternative Communication **N** Biosensory Feedback **P** Computer **Q** Speech Analysis **S** Voice Analysis **Y** Other Equipment **Z** None	**Z** None
Z None DRG	**6** Psychosocial Skills	**Z** None	**Z** None
Z None DRG	**B** Environmental, Home and Work Barriers **C** Ergonomics and Body Mechanics	**E** Orthosis **F** Assistive, Adaptive, Supportive or Protective **U** Prosthesis **Y** Other Equipment **Z** None	**Z** None

F02 continued on next page

F02 continued from previous page

F Physical Rehabilitation and Diagnostic Audiology
0 Rehabilitation
2 Activities of Daily Living Assessment: Measurement of functional level for activities of daily living

Body system/ Region Character 4	Type Qualifier Character 5	Equipment Character 6	Qualifier Character 7
Z None DRG	**H** Vocational Activities and Functional Community or Work Reintegration Skills	**E** Orthosis **F** Assistive, Adaptive, Supportive or Protective **G** Aerobic Endurance and Conditioning **U** Prosthesis **Y** Other Equipment **Z** None	**Z** None

DRG F0209YZ F0209ZZ F020DYZ F020DZZ F021DYZ F021DZZ F022DYZ F022DZZ F023DYZ F023DZZ F024GCZ F024GGZ F024GYZ F024GZZ F025GCZ F025GGZ F025GYZ F025GZZ F026GCZ F026GGZ F026GYZ F026GZZ F0277EZ F0277GZ F0277UZ F0277YZ F0277ZZ F027GCZ F027GGZ F027GYZ F027GZZ F028GCZ F028GGZ F028GYZ F028GZZ F029GCZ F029GGZ F029GYZ F029GZZ F02BGCZ F02BGGZ F02BGYZ F02BGZZ F02C7EZ F02C7GZ F02C7UZ F02C7YZ F02C7ZZ F02CGCZ F02CGGZ F02CGYZ F02CGZZ F02Z0EZ F02Z0FZ F02Z0UZ F02Z0ZZ F02Z1EZ F02Z1FZ F02Z1UZ F02Z1ZZ F02Z2YZ F02Z2ZZ F02Z3EZ F02Z3FZ F02Z3UZ F02Z3ZZ F02Z4EZ F02Z4FZ F02Z4UZ F02Z4ZZ F02Z5KZ F02Z5MZ F02Z5NZ F02Z5PZ F02Z5QZ F02Z5SZ F02Z5YZ F02Z5ZZ F02Z6ZZ F02Z8YZ F02Z8ZZ F02ZBEZ F02ZBFZ F02ZBUZ F02ZBYZ F02ZBZZ F02ZCEZ F02ZCFZ F02ZCUZ F02ZCYZ F02ZCZZ F02ZFYZ F02ZFZZ F02ZHEZ F02ZHFZ F02ZHGZ F02ZHUZ F02ZHYZ F02ZHZZ

F Physical Rehabilitation and Diagnostic Audiology
0 Rehabilitation
6 Speech Treatment: Application of techniques to improve, augment, or compensate for speech and related functional impairment

Body system/ Region Character 4	Type Qualifier Character 5	Equipment Character 6	Qualifier Character 7
3 Neurological System - Whole Body DRG	**6** Communicative/Cognitive Integration Skills	**K** Audiovisual **M** Augmentative / Alternative Communication **P** Computer **Y** Other Equipment **Z** None	**Z** None
Z None DRG	**0** Nonspoken Language **3** Aphasia **6** Communicative/Cognitive Integration Skills	**K** Audiovisual **M** Augmentative / Alternative Communication **P** Computer **Y** Other Equipment **Z** None	**Z** None
Z None DRG	**1** Speech-Language Pathology and Related Disorders Counseling **2** Speech-Language Pathology and Related Disorders Prevention	**K** Audiovisual **Z** None	**Z** None
Z None DRG	**4** Articulation/Phonology	**K** Audiovisual **P** Computer **Q** Speech Analysis **T** Aerodynamic Function **Y** Other Equipment **Z** None	**Z** None
Z None DRG	**5** Aural Rehabilitation	**K** Audiovisual **L** Assistive Listening **M** Augmentative / Alternative Communication **N** Biosensory Feedback **P** Computer **Q** Speech Analysis **S** Voice Analysis **Y** Other Equipment **Z** None	**Z** None

F06 continued on next page

F06 continued from previous page

F Physical Rehabilitation and Diagnostic Audiology
0 Rehabilitation
6 Speech Treatment: Application of techniques to improve, augment, or compensate for speech and related functional impairment

Body system/ Region Character 4	Type Qualifier Character 5	Equipment Character 6	Qualifier Character 7
Z None DRG	7 Fluency	4 Electroacoustic Immittance / Acoustic Reflex K Audiovisual N Biosensory Feedback Q Speech Analysis S Voice Analysis T Aerodynamic Function Y Other Equipment Z None	Z None
Z None DRG	8 Motor Speech	K Audiovisual N Biosensory Feedback P Computer Q Speech Analysis S Voice Analysis T Aerodynamic Function Y Other Equipment Z None	Z None
Z None DRG	9 Orofacial Myofunctional	K Audiovisual P Computer Y Other Equipment Z None	Z None
Z None DRG	B Receptive/Expressive Language	K Audiovisual L Assistive Listening M Augmentative / Alternative Communication P Computer Y Other Equipment Z None	Z None
Z None DRG	C Voice	K Audiovisual N Biosensory Feedback P Computer S Voice Analysis T Aerodynamic Function V Speech Prosthesis Y Other Equipment Z None	Z None
Z None DRG	D Swallowing Dysfunction	M Augmentative / Alternative Communication T Aerodynamic Function V Speech Prosthesis Y Other Equipment Z None	Z None

DRG F0636KZ F0636MZ F0636PZ F0636YZ F0636ZZ F06Z0KZ F06Z0MZ F06Z0PZ F06Z0YZ F06Z0ZZ F06Z1KZ F06Z1ZZ F06Z2KZ F06Z2ZZ F06Z3KZ F06Z3MZ F06Z3PZ F06Z3YZ F06Z3ZZ F06Z4KZ F06Z4PZ F06Z4QZ F06Z4TZ F06Z4YZ F06Z4ZZ F06Z5KZ F06Z5LZ F06Z5MZ F06Z5NZ F06Z5PZ F06Z5QZ F06Z5SZ F06Z5YZ F06Z5ZZ F06Z6KZ F06Z6MZ F06Z6PZ F06Z6YZ F06Z6ZZ F06Z74Z F06Z7KZ F06Z7NZ F06Z7QZ F06Z7SZ F06Z7TZ F06Z7YZ F06Z7ZZ F06Z8KZ F06Z8NZ F06Z8PZ F06Z8QZ F06Z8SZ F06Z8TZ F06Z8YZ F06Z8ZZ F06Z9KZ F06Z9PZ F06Z9YZ F06Z9ZZ F06ZBKZ F06ZBLZ F06ZBMZ F06ZBPZ F06ZBYZ F06ZBZZ F06ZCKZ F06ZCNZ F06ZCPZ F06ZCSZ F06ZCTZ F06ZCVZ F06ZCYZ F06ZCZZ F06ZDMZ F06ZDTZ F06ZDVZ F06ZDYZ F06ZDZZ

F Physical Rehabilitation and Diagnostic Audiology
0 Rehabilitation
7 Motor Treatment: Exercise or activities to increase or facilitate motor function

Body system/ Region Character 4	Type Qualifier Character 5	Equipment Character 6	Qualifier Character 7
0 Neurological System - Head and Neck DRG **1** Neurological System - Upper Back / Upper Extremity DRG **2** Neurological System - Lower Back / Lower Extremity DRG **3** Neurological System - Whole Body DRG **D** Integumentary System - Head and Neck DRG **F** Integumentary System - Upper Back / Upper Extremity DRG **G** Integumentary System - Lower Back / Lower Extremity DRG **H** Integumentary System - Whole Body DRG **J** Musculoskeletal System - Head and Neck DRG **K** Musculoskeletal System - Upper Back / Upper Extremity DRG **L** Musculoskeletal System - Lower Back / Lower Extremity DRG prone hip lumbar or may be knee **M** Musculoskeletal System - Whole Body DRG	**0** Range of Motion and Joint Mobility extensions **1** Muscle Performance **2** Coordination/Dexterity **3** Motor Function may be general strengthing	**E** Orthosis **F** Assistive, Adaptive, Supportive or Protective **U** Prosthesis **Y** Other Equipment **Z** None - pillow or weight set may see lbs written	**Z** None
0 Neurological System - Head and Neck DRG **1** Neurological System - Upper Back / Upper Extremity DRG **2** Neurological System - Lower Back / Lower Extremity DRG **3** Neurological System - Whole Body DRG **D** Integumentary System - Head and Neck DRG **F** Integumentary System - Upper Back / Upper Extremity DRG **G** Integumentary System - Lower Back / Lower Extremity DRG **H** Integumentary System - Whole Body DRG **J** Musculoskeletal System - Head and Neck DRG **K** Musculoskeletal System - Upper Back / Upper Extremity DRG **L** Musculoskeletal System - Lower Back / Lower Extremity DRG **M** Musculoskeletal System - Whole Body DRG	**6** Therapeutic Exercise	**B** Physical Agents **C** Mechanical **D** Electrotherapeutic **E** Orthosis **F** Assistive, Adaptive, Supportive or Protective **G** Aerobic Endurance and Conditioning **H** Mechanical or Electromechanical **U** Prosthesis **Y** Other Equipment **Z** None	**Z** None

F07 continued on next page

F Physical Rehabilitation and Diagnostic Audiology
0 Rehabilitation
7 Motor Treatment: Exercise or activities to increase or facilitate motor function

F07 continued from previous page

rationale for performing exercise

Body system/ Region Character 4	Type Qualifier Character 5	Equipment Character 6	Qualifier Character 7
0 Neurological System - Head and Neck DRG **1** Neurological System - Upper Back / Upper Extremity DRG **2** Neurological System - Lower Back / Lower Extremity DRG **3** Neurological System - Whole Body DRG **D** Integumentary System - Head and Neck DRG **F** Integumentary System - Upper Back / Upper Extremity DRG **G** Integumentary System - Lower Back / Lower Extremity DRG **H** Integumentary System - Whole Body DRG **J** Musculoskeletal System - Head and Neck DRG **K** Musculoskeletal System - Upper Back / Upper Extremity DRG **L** Musculoskeletal System - Lower Back / Lower Extremity DRG lumbar, paraspinal **M** Musculoskeletal System - Whole Body DRG	**7** Manual Therapy Techniques deep kneading massage	**Z** None	**Z** None
4 Circulatory System - Head and Neck DRG **5** Circulatory System - Upper Back / Upper Extremity DRG **6** Circulatory System - Lower Back / Lower Extremity DRG **7** Circulatory System - Whole Body DRG **8** Respiratory System - Head and Neck DRG **9** Respiratory System - Upper Back / Upper Extremity DRG **B** Respiratory System - Lower Back / Lower Extremity DRG **C** Respiratory System - Whole Body DRG	**6** Therapeutic Exercise	**B** Physical Agents **C** Mechanical **D** Electrotherapeutic **E** Orthosis **F** Assistive, Adaptive, Supportive or Protective **G** Aerobic Endurance and Conditioning **H** Mechanical or Electromechanical **U** Prosthesis **Y** Other Equipment **Z** None	**Z** None
N Genitourinary System DRG	**1** Muscle Performance	**E** Orthosis **F** Assistive, Adaptive, Supportive or Protective **U** Prosthesis **Y** Other Equipment **Z** None	**Z** None
N Genitourinary System DRG	**6** Therapeutic Exercise	**B** Physical Agents **C** Mechanical **D** Electrotherapeutic **E** Orthosis **F** Assistive, Adaptive, Supportive or Protective **G** Aerobic Endurance and Conditioning **H** Mechanical or Electromechanical **U** Prosthesis **Y** Other Equipment **Z** None	**Z** None

F07 continued on next page

F Physical Rehabilitation and Diagnostic Audiology
0 Rehabilitation
7 Motor Treatment: Exercise or activities to increase or facilitate motor function

F07 continued from previous page

Body system/ Region Character 4	Type Qualifier Character 5	Equipment Character 6	Qualifier Character 7
Z None DRG	**4** Wheelchair Mobility	**D** Electrotherapeutic **E** Orthosis **F** Assistive, Adaptive, Supportive or Protective **U** Prosthesis **Y** Other Equipment **Z** None	**Z** None
Z None DRG	**5** Bed Mobility	**C** Mechanical **E** Orthosis **F** Assistive, Adaptive, Supportive or Protective **U** Prosthesis **Y** Other Equipment **Z** None	**Z** None
Z None DRG	**8** Transfer Training	**C** Mechanical **D** Electrotherapeutic **E** Orthosis **F** Assistive, Adaptive, Supportive or Protective **U** Prosthesis **Y** Other Equipment **Z** None	**Z** None
Z None DRG	**9** Gait Training/Functional Ambulation	**C** Mechanical **D** Electrotherapeutic **E** Orthosis **F** Assistive, Adaptive, Supportive or Protective Crutches **G** Aerobic Endurance and Conditioning **U** Prosthesis **Y** Other Equipment **Z** None	**Z** None

DRG F0700EZ F0700FZ F0700UZ F0700YZ F0700ZZ F0701EZ F0701FZ F0701UZ F0701YZ F0701ZZ F0702EZ F0702FZ F0702UZ
F0702YZ F0702ZZ F0703EZ F0703FZ F0703UZ F0703YZ F0703ZZ F0706BZ F0706CZ F0706DZ F0706EZ F0706FZ F0706GZ
F0706HZ F0706UZ F0706YZ F0706ZZ F0707ZZ F0710EZ F0710FZ F0710UZ F0710YZ F0710ZZ F0711EZ F0711FZ F0711UZ
F0711YZ F0711ZZ F0712EZ F0712FZ F0712UZ F0712YZ F0712ZZ F0713EZ F0713FZ F0713UZ F0713YZ F0713ZZ F0716BZ
F0716CZ F0716DZ F0716EZ F0716FZ F0716GZ F0716HZ F0716UZ F0716YZ F0716ZZ F0717ZZ F0720EZ F0720FZ F0720UZ
F0720YZ F0720ZZ F0721EZ F0721FZ F0721UZ F0721YZ F0721ZZ F0722EZ F0722FZ F0722UZ F0722YZ F0722ZZ F0723EZ
F0723FZ F0723UZ F0723YZ F0723ZZ F0726BZ F0726CZ F0726DZ F0726EZ F0726FZ F0726GZ F0726HZ F0726UZ F0726YZ
F0726ZZ F0727ZZ F0730EZ F0730FZ F0730UZ F0730YZ F0730ZZ F0731EZ F0731FZ F0731UZ F0731YZ F0731ZZ F0732EZ
F0732FZ F0732UZ F0732YZ F0732ZZ F0733EZ F0733FZ F0733UZ F0733YZ F0733ZZ F0736BZ F0736CZ F0736DZ F0736EZ
F0736FZ F0736GZ F0736HZ F0736UZ F0736YZ F0736ZZ F0737ZZ F0746BZ F0746CZ F0746DZ F0746EZ F0746FZ F0746GZ
F0746HZ F0746UZ F0746YZ F0746ZZ F0756BZ F0756CZ F0756DZ F0756EZ F0756FZ F0756GZ F0756HZ F0756UZ F0756YZ
F0756ZZ F0766BZ F0766CZ F0766DZ F0766EZ F0766FZ F0766GZ F0766HZ F0766UZ F0766YZ F0766ZZ F0776BZ F0776CZ
F0776DZ F0776EZ F0776FZ F0776GZ F0776HZ F0776UZ F0776YZ F0776ZZ F0786BZ F0786CZ F0786DZ F0786EZ F0786FZ
F0786GZ F0786HZ F0786UZ F0786YZ F0786ZZ F0796BZ F0796CZ F0796DZ F0796EZ F0796FZ F0796GZ F0796HZ F0796UZ
F0796YZ F0796ZZ F07B6BZ F07B6CZ F07B6DZ F07B6EZ F07B6FZ F07B6GZ F07B6HZ F07B6UZ F07B6YZ F07B6ZZ F07C6BZ
F07C6CZ F07C6DZ F07C6EZ F07C6FZ F07C6GZ F07C6HZ F07C6UZ F07C6YZ F07C6ZZ F07D0EZ F07D0FZ F07D0UZ F07D0YZ
F07D0ZZ F07D1EZ F07D1FZ F07D1UZ F07D1YZ F07D1ZZ F07D2EZ F07D2FZ F07D2UZ F07D2YZ F07D2ZZ F07D3EZ F07D3FZ
F07D3UZ F07D3YZ F07D3ZZ F07D6BZ F07D6CZ F07D6DZ F07D6EZ F07D6FZ F07D6GZ F07D6HZ F07D6UZ F07D6YZ F07D6ZZ
F07D7ZZ F07F0EZ F07F0FZ F07F0UZ F07F0YZ F07F0ZZ F07F1EZ F07F1FZ F07F1UZ F07F1YZ F07F1ZZ F07F2EZ F07F2FZ
F07F2UZ F07F2YZ F07F2ZZ F07F3EZ F07F3FZ F07F3UZ F07F3YZ F07F3ZZ F07F6BZ F07F6CZ F07F6DZ F07F6EZ F07F6FZ
F07F6GZ F07F6HZ F07F6UZ F07F6YZ F07F6ZZ F07F7ZZ F07G0EZ F07G0FZ F07G0UZ F07G0YZ F07G0ZZ F07G1EZ F07G1FZ
F07G1UZ F07G1YZ F07G1ZZ F07G2EZ F07G2FZ F07G2UZ F07G2YZ F07G2ZZ F07G3EZ F07G3FZ F07G3UZ F07G3YZ F07G3ZZ
F07G6BZ F07G6CZ F07G6DZ F07G6EZ F07G6FZ F07G6GZ F07G6HZ F07G6UZ F07G6YZ F07G6ZZ F07G7ZZ F07H0EZ F07H0FZ
F07H0UZ F07H0YZ F07H0ZZ F07H1EZ F07H1FZ F07H1UZ F07H1YZ F07H1ZZ F07H2EZ F07H2FZ F07H2UZ F07H2YZ F07H2ZZ
F07H3EZ F07H3FZ F07H3UZ F07H3YZ F07H3ZZ F07H6BZ F07H6CZ F07H6DZ F07H6EZ F07H6FZ F07H6GZ F07H6HZ F07H6UZ
F07H6YZ F07H6ZZ F07H7ZZ F07J0EZ F07J0FZ F07J0UZ F07J0YZ F07J0ZZ F07J1EZ F07J1FZ F07J1UZ F07J1YZ F07J1ZZ
F07J2EZ F07J2FZ F07J2UZ F07J2YZ F07J2ZZ F07J3EZ F07J3FZ F07J3UZ F07J3YZ F07J3ZZ F07J6BZ F07J6CZ F07J6DZ
F07J6EZ F07J6FZ F07J6GZ F07J6HZ F07J6UZ F07J6YZ F07J6ZZ F07J7ZZ F07K0EZ F07K0FZ F07K0UZ F07K0YZ F07K0ZZ
F07K1EZ F07K1FZ F07K1UZ F07K1YZ F07K1ZZ F07K2EZ F07K2FZ F07K2UZ F07K2YZ F07K2ZZ F07K3EZ F07K3FZ F07K3UZ

F07 continued on next page

F07 continued from previous page

F07K3YZ	F07K3ZZ	F07K6BZ	F07K6CZ	F07K6DZ	F07K6EZ	F07K6FZ	F07K6GZ	F07K6HZ	F07K6UZ	F07K6YZ	F07K6ZZ	F07K7ZZ
F07L0EZ	F07L0FZ	F07L0UZ	F07L0YZ	F07L0ZZ	F07L1EZ	F07L1FZ	F07L1UZ	F07L1YZ	F07L1ZZ	F07L2EZ	F07L2FZ	F07L2UZ
F07L2YZ	F07L2ZZ	F07L3EZ	F07L3FZ	F07L3UZ	F07L3YZ	F07L3ZZ	F07L6BZ	F07L6CZ	F07L6DZ	F07L6EZ	F07L6FZ	F07L6GZ
F07L6HZ	F07L6UZ	F07L6YZ	F07L6ZZ	F07L7ZZ	F07M0EZ	F07M0FZ	F07M0UZ	F07M0YZ	F07M0ZZ	F07M1EZ	F07M1FZ	F07M1UZ
F07M1YZ	F07M1ZZ	F07M2EZ	F07M2FZ	F07M2UZ	F07M2YZ	F07M2ZZ	F07M3EZ	F07M3FZ	F07M3UZ	F07M3YZ	F07M3ZZ	F07M6BZ
F07M6CZ	F07M6DZ	F07M6EZ	F07M6FZ	F07M6GZ	F07M6HZ	F07M6UZ	F07M6YZ	F07M6ZZ	F07M7ZZ	F07N1EZ	F07N1FZ	F07N1UZ
F07N1YZ	F07N1ZZ	F07N6BZ	F07N6CZ	F07N6DZ	F07N6EZ	F07N6FZ	F07N6GZ	F07N6HZ	F07N6UZ	F07N6YZ	F07N6ZZ	F07Z4DZ
F07Z4EZ	F07Z4FZ	F07Z4UZ	F07Z4YZ	F07Z4ZZ	F07Z5CZ	F07Z5EZ	F07Z5FZ	F07Z5UZ	F07Z5YZ	F07Z5ZZ	F07Z8CZ	F07Z8DZ
F07Z8EZ	F07Z8FZ	F07Z8UZ	F07Z8YZ	F07Z8ZZ	F07Z9CZ	F07Z9DZ	F07Z9EZ	F07Z9FZ	F07Z9GZ	F07Z9UZ	F07Z9YZ	F07Z9ZZ

F Physical Rehabilitation and Diagnostic Audiology *includes wound management*
0 Rehabilitation
8 Activities of Daily Living Treatment: Exercise or activities to facilitate functional competence for activities of daily living

Body system/ Region Character 4	Type Qualifier Character 5	Equipment Character 6	Qualifier Character 7
D Integumentary System - Head and Neck DRG **F** Integumentary System - Upper Back / Upper Extremity DRG **G** Integumentary System - Lower Back / Lower Extremity DRG **H** Integumentary System - Whole Body DRG **J** Musculoskeletal System - Head and Neck DRG **K** Musculoskeletal System - Upper Back / Upper Extremity DRG **L** Musculoskeletal System - Lower Back / Lower Extremity DRG *- left calf ulcer extends to muscle* **M** Musculoskeletal System - Whole Body DRG	**5** Wound Management	**B** Physical Agents *- pulsative lavage* **C** Mechanical **D** Electrotherapeutic **E** Orthosis **F** Assistive, Adaptive, Supportive or Protective **U** Prosthesis **Y** Other Equipment **Z** None	**Z** None
Z None DRG	**0** Bathing/Showering Techniques **1** Dressing Techniques **2** Grooming/Personal Hygiene	**E** Orthosis **F** Assistive, Adaptive, Supportive or Protective **U** Prosthesis **Y** Other Equipment **Z** None	**Z** None
Z None DRG	**3** Feeding/Eating	**C** Mechanical **D** Electrotherapeutic **E** Orthosis **F** Assistive, Adaptive, Supportive or Protective **U** Prosthesis **Y** Other Equipment **Z** None	**Z** None
Z None DRG	**4** Home Management	**D** Electrotherapeutic **E** Orthosis **F** Assistive, Adaptive, Supportive or Protective **U** Prosthesis **Y** Other Equipment **Z** None	**Z** None
Z None DRG	**6** Psychosocial Skills	**Z** None	**Z** None
Z None DRG	**7** Vocational Activities and Functional Community or Work Reintegration Skills	**B** Physical Agents **C** Mechanical **D** Electrotherapeutic **E** Orthosis **F** Assistive, Adaptive, Supportive or Protective **G** Aerobic Endurance and Conditioning **U** Prosthesis **Y** Other Equipment **Z** None	**Z** None

DRG F08D5BZ F08D5CZ F08D5DZ F08D5EZ F08D5FZ F08D5UZ F08D5YZ F08D5ZZ F08F5BZ F08F5CZ F08F5DZ F08F5EZ F08F5FZ F08F5UZ F08F5YZ F08F5ZZ F08G5BZ F08G5CZ F08G5DZ F08G5EZ F08G5FZ F08G5UZ F08G5YZ F08G5ZZ F08H5BZ F08H5CZ

F08 continued on next page

F08 continued from previous page

F08H5DZ F08H5EZ F08H5FZ F08H5UZ F08H5YZ F08H5ZZ F08J5BZ F08J5CZ F08J5DZ F08J5EZ F08J5FZ F08J5UZ F08J5YZ
F08J5ZZ F08K5BZ F08K5CZ F08K5DZ F08K5EZ F08K5FZ F08K5UZ F08K5YZ F08K5ZZ F08L5BZ F08L5CZ F08L5DZ F08L5EZ
F08L5FZ F08L5UZ F08L5YZ F08L5ZZ F08M5BZ F08M5CZ F08M5DZ F08M5EZ F08M5FZ F08M5UZ F08M5YZ F08M5ZZ F08Z0EZ
F08Z0FZ F08Z0UZ F08Z0YZ F08Z0ZZ F08Z1EZ F08Z1FZ F08Z1UZ F08Z1YZ F08Z1ZZ F08Z2EZ F08Z2FZ F08Z2UZ F08Z2YZ
F08Z2ZZ F08Z3CZ F08Z3DZ F08Z3EZ F08Z3FZ F08Z3UZ F08Z3YZ F08Z3ZZ F08Z4DZ F08Z4EZ F08Z4FZ F08Z4UZ F08Z4YZ
F08Z4ZZ F08Z6ZZ F08Z7BZ F08Z7CZ F08Z7DZ F08Z7EZ F08Z7FZ F08Z7GZ F08Z7UZ F08Z7YZ F08Z7ZZ

F Physical Rehabilitation and Diagnostic Audiology
0 Rehabilitation
9 Hearing Treatment: Application of techniques to improve, augment, or compensate for hearing and related functional impairment

Body system/ Region	Type Qualifier	Equipment	Qualifier
Character 4	**Character 5**	**Character 6**	**Character 7**
Z None DRG	**0** Hearing and Related Disorders Counseling **1** Hearing and Related Disorders Prevention	**K** Audiovisual **Z** None	**Z** None
Z None DRG	**2** Auditory Processing	**K** Audiovisual **L** Assistive Listening **P** Computer **Y** Other Equipment **Z** None	**Z** None
Z None DRG	**3** Cerumen Management	**X** Cerumen Management **Z** None	**Z** None

DRG F09Z0KZ F09Z0ZZ F09Z1KZ F09Z1ZZ F09Z2KZ F09Z2LZ F09Z2PZ F09Z2YZ F09Z2ZZ F09Z3XZ F09Z3ZZ

F Physical Rehabilitation and Diagnostic Audiology
0 Rehabilitation
B Cochlear Implant Treatment: Application of techniques to improve the communication abilities of individuals with cochlear implant

Body system/ Region	Type Qualifier	Equipment	Qualifier
Character 4	**Character 5**	**Character 6**	**Character 7**
Z None DRG	**0** Cochlear Implant Rehabilitation	**1** Audiometer **2** Sound Field / Booth **9** Cochlear Implant **K** Audiovisual **P** Computer **Y** Other Equipment	**Z** None

DRG F0BZ01Z F0BZ02Z F0BZ09Z F0BZ0KZ F0BZ0PZ F0BZ0YZ

F Physical Rehabilitation and Diagnostic Audiology
0 Rehabilitation
C Vestibular Treatment: Application of techniques to improve, augment, or compensate for vestibular and related functional impairment

Body system/ Region	Type Qualifier	Equipment	Qualifier
Character 4	**Character 5**	**Character 6**	**Character 7**
3 Neurological System - Whole Body DRG **H** Integumentary System - Whole Body DRG **M** Musculoskeletal System - Whole Body DRG	**3** Postural Control	**E** Orthosis **F** Assistive, Adaptive, Supportive or Protective **U** Prosthesis **Y** Other Equipment **Z** None	**Z** None
Z None DRG	**0** Vestibular	**8** Vestibular / Balance **Z** None	**Z** None
Z None DRG	**1** Perceptual Processing **2** Visual Motor Integration	**K** Audiovisual **L** Assistive Listening **N** Biosensory Feedback **P** Computer **Q** Speech Analysis **S** Voice Analysis **T** Aerodynamic Function **Y** Other Equipment **Z** None	**Z** None

DRG F0C33EZ F0C33FZ F0C33UZ F0C33YZ F0C33ZZ F0CH3EZ F0CH3FZ F0CH3UZ F0CH3YZ F0CH3ZZ F0CM3EZ F0CM3FZ F0CM3UZ
F0CM3YZ F0CM3ZZ F0CZ08Z F0CZ0ZZ F0CZ1KZ F0CZ1LZ F0CZ1NZ F0CZ1PZ F0CZ1QZ F0CZ1SZ F0CZ1TZ F0CZ1YZ F0CZ1ZZ
F0CZ2KZ F0CZ2LZ F0CZ2NZ F0CZ2PZ F0CZ2QZ F0CZ2SZ F0CZ2TZ F0CZ2YZ F0CZ2ZZ

LC Limited Coverage NC Noncovered HAC HAC-associated Procedure CC Combination Cluster - See Appendix G for code lists
DRG Non-OR-Affecting MS-DRG Assignment New/Revised Text in **Orange** ♂ Male ♀ Female

F Physical Rehabilitation and Diagnostic Audiology
0 Rehabilitation
D Device Fitting: Fitting of a device designed to facilitate or support achievement of a higher level of function

Body system/ Region	Type Qualifier	Equipment	Qualifier
Character 4	**Character 5**	**Character 6**	**Character 7**
Z None DRG	**0** Tinnitus Masker	**5** Hearing Aid Selection / Fitting / Test **Z** None	**Z** None
Z None DRG	**1** Monaural Hearing Aid **2** Binaural Hearing Aid **5** Assistive Listening Device	**1** Audiometer **2** Sound Field / Booth **5** Hearing Aid Selection / Fitting / Test **K** Audiovisual **L** Assistive Listening **Z** None	**Z** None
Z None DRG	**3** Augmentative/Alternative Communication System	**M** Augmentative / Alternative Communication	**Z** None
Z None DRG	**4** Voice Prosthetic	**S** Voice Analysis **V** Speech Prosthesis	**Z** None
Z None DRG	**6** Dynamic Orthosis **7** Static Orthosis **8** Prosthesis **9** Assistive, Adaptive, Supportive or Protective Devices	**E** Orthosis **F** Assistive, Adaptive, Supportive or Protective **U** Prosthesis **Z** None	**Z** None

DRG F0DZ05Z F0DZ0ZZ F0DZ11Z F0DZ12Z F0DZ15Z F0DZ1KZ F0DZ1LZ F0DZ1ZZ F0DZ21Z F0DZ22Z F0DZ25Z F0DZ2KZ F0DZ2LZ F0DZ2ZZ F0DZ3MZ F0DZ4SZ F0DZ4VZ F0DZ51Z F0DZ52Z F0DZ55Z F0DZ5KZ F0DZ5LZ F0DZ5ZZ F0DZ6EZ F0DZ6FZ F0DZ6UZ F0DZ6ZZ F0DZ7EZ F0DZ7FZ F0DZ7UZ F0DZ7ZZ F0DZ8EZ F0DZ8FZ F0DZ8UZ

F Physical Rehabilitation and Diagnostic Audiology
0 Rehabilitation
F Caregiver Training: Training in activities to support patient's optimal level of function

Body system/ Region	Type Qualifier	Equipment	Qualifier
Character 4	**Character 5**	**Character 6**	**Character 7**
Z None DRG	**0** Bathing/Showering Technique **1** Dressing **2** Feeding and Eating **3** Grooming/Personal Hygiene **4** Bed Mobility **5** Transfer **6** Wheelchair Mobility **7** Therapeutic Exercise **8** Airway Clearance Techniques **9** Wound Management **B** Vocational Activities and Functional Community or Work Reintegration Skills **C** Gait Training/Functional Ambulation **D** Application, Proper Use and Care of Devices **F** Application, Proper Use and Care of Orthoses **G** Application, Proper Use and Care of Prosthesis **H** Home Management	**E** Orthosis **F** Assistive, Adaptive, Supportive or Protective **U** Prosthesis **Z** None	**Z** None
Z None DRG	**J** Communication Skills	**K** Audiovisual **L** Assistive Listening **M** Augmentative / Alternative Communication **P** Computer **Z** None	**Z** None

DRG F0FZ0EZ F0FZ0FZ F0FZ0UZ F0FZ0ZZ F0FZ1EZ F0FZ1FZ F0FZ1UZ F0FZ1ZZ F0FZ2EZ F0FZ2FZ F0FZ2UZ F0FZ2ZZ F0FZ3EZ F0FZ3FZ F0FZ3UZ F0FZ3ZZ F0FZ4EZ F0FZ4FZ F0FZ4UZ F0FZ4ZZ F0FZ5EZ F0FZ5FZ F0FZ5UZ F0FZ5ZZ F0FZ6EZ F0FZ6FZ F0FZ6UZ F0FZ6ZZ F0FZ7EZ F0FZ7FZ F0FZ7UZ F0FZ7ZZ F0FZ8EZ F0FZ8FZ F0FZ8UZ F0FZ8ZZ F0FZ9EZ F0FZ9FZ F0FZ9UZ F0FZ9ZZ F0FZBEZ F0FZBFZ F0FZBUZ F0FZBZZ F0FZCEZ F0FZCFZ F0FZCUZ F0FZCZZ F0FZDEZ F0FZDFZ F0FZDUZ F0FZDZZ F0FZFEZ F0FZFFZ F0FZFUZ F0FZFZZ F0FZGEZ F0FZGFZ F0FZGUZ F0FZGZZ F0FZHEZ F0FZHFZ F0FZHUZ F0FZHZZ F0FZJKZ F0FZJLZ F0FZJMZ F0FZJPZ F0FZJZZ

LC Limited Coverage NC Noncovered HAC HAC-associated Procedure CC Combination Cluster - See Appendix G for code lists
DRG Non-OR-Affecting MS-DRG Assignment New/Revised Text in **Orange** ♂ Male ♀ Female

F Physical Rehabilitation and Diagnostic Audiology
1 Diagnostic Audiology
3 Hearing Assessment: Measurement of hearing and related functions

Body system/ Region Character 4	Type Qualifier Character 5	Equipment Character 6	Qualifier Character 7
Z None	0 Hearing Screening	0 Occupational Hearing 1 Audiometer 2 Sound Field / Booth 3 Tympanometer 8 Vestibular / Balance 9 Cochlear Implant Z None	Z None
Z None	1 Pure Tone Audiometry, Air 2 Pure Tone Audiometry, Air and Bone	0 Occupational Hearing 1 Audiometer 2 Sound Field / Booth Z None	Z None
Z None	3 Bekesy Audiometry 6 Visual Reinforcement Audiometry 9 Short Increment Sensitivity Index B Stenger C Pure Tone Stenger	1 Audiometer 2 Sound Field / Booth Z None	Z None
Z None	4 Conditioned Play Audiometry 5 Select Picture Audiometry	1 Audiometer 2 Sound Field / Booth K Audiovisual Z None	Z None
Z None	7 Alternate Binaural or Monaural Loudness Balance	1 Audiometer K Audiovisual Z None	Z None
Z None	8 Tone Decay D Tympanometry F Eustachian Tube Function G Acoustic Reflex Patterns H Acoustic Reflex Threshold J Acoustic Reflex Decay	3 Tympanometer 4 Electroacoustic Immittance / Acoustic Reflex Z None	Z None
Z None	K Electrocochleography L Auditory Evoked Potentials	7 Electrophysiologic Z None	Z None
Z None	M Evoked Otoacoustic Emissions, Screening N Evoked Otoacoustic Emissions, Diagnostic	6 Otoacoustic Emission (OAE) Z None	Z None
Z None	P Aural Rehabilitation Status	1 Audiometer 2 Sound Field / Booth 4 Electroacoustic Immittance / Acoustic Reflex 9 Cochlear Implant K Audiovisual L Assistive Listening P Computer Z None	Z None
Z None	Q Auditory Processing	K Audiovisual P Computer Y Other Equipment Z None	Z None

F Physical Rehabilitation and Diagnostic Audiology
1 Diagnostic Audiology
4 Hearing Aid Assessment: Measurement of the appropriateness and/or effectiveness of a hearing device

Body system/ Region Character 4	Type Qualifier Character 5	Equipment Character 6	Qualifier Character 7
Z None	**0** Cochlear Implant	**1** Audiometer **2** Sound Field / Booth **3** Tympanometer **4** Electroacoustic Immittance / Acoustic Reflex **5** Hearing Aid Selection / Fitting / Test **7** Electrophysiologic **9** Cochlear Implant **K** Audiovisual **L** Assistive Listening **P** Computer **Y** Other Equipment **Z** None	**Z** None
Z None	**1** Ear Canal Probe Microphone **6** Binaural Electroacoustic Hearing Aid Check **8** Monaural Electroacoustic Hearing Aid Check	**5** Hearing Aid Selection / Fitting / Test **Z** None	**Z** None
Z None	**2** Monaural Hearing Aid **3** Binaural Hearing Aid	**1** Audiometer **2** Sound Field / Booth **3** Tympanometer **4** Electroacoustic Immittance / Acoustic Reflex **5** Hearing Aid Selection / Fitting / Test **K** Audiovisual **L** Assistive Listening **P** Computer **Z** None	**Z** None
Z None	**4** Assistive Listening System/ Device Selection	**1** Audiometer **2** Sound Field / Booth **3** Tympanometer **4** Electroacoustic Immittance / Acoustic Reflex **K** Audiovisual **L** Assistive Listening **Z** None	**Z** None
Z None	**5** Sensory Aids	**1** Audiometer **2** Sound Field / Booth **3** Tympanometer **4** Electroacoustic Immittance / Acoustic Reflex **5** Hearing Aid Selection / Fitting / Test **K** Audiovisual **L** Assistive Listening **Z** None	**Z** None
Z None	**7** Ear Protector Attenuation	**0** Occupational Hearing **Z** None	**Z** None

F Physical Rehabilitation and Diagnostic Audiology
1 Diagnostic Audiology
5 Vestibular Assessment: Measurement of the vestibular system and related functions

Body system/ Region	Type Qualifier	Equipment	Qualifier
Character 4	**Character 5**	**Character 6**	**Character 7**
Z None	**0** Bithermal, Binaural Caloric Irrigation **1** Bithermal, Monaural Caloric Irrigation **2** Unithermal Binaural Screen **3** Oscillating Tracking **4** Sinusoidal Vertical Axis Rotational **5** Dix-Hallpike Dynamic **6** Computerized Dynamic Posturography	**8** Vestibular / Balance **Z** None	**Z** None
Z None	**7** Tinnitus Masker	**5** Hearing Aid Selection / Fitting / Test **Z** None	**Z** None

NOTES

NOTES

Psychological Tests:

- Developmental: age normed developmental status of cognitive, social, and adaptive behavior skills
- Intellectual & Psychoeducational: Intellectual abilities, academic achievement, + learning capabilities (including behavior + emotional factors affecting learning)
- Neurobehavioral & Cognitive Status: Includes neurobehavioral status exam, interview(s), + observations for the clinical assessment of thinking, reasoning, & judgment, acquired knowledge, attention, memory, visual spatial abilities, language functions + planning

Neuropsychological: thinking, reasoning & judgment, acquired knowledge, attention, memory, visual spatial abilities, language functions, planning

Personality + behavioral: mood, emotion, behavior, social functioning, psychopathological conditions, personality traits + characteristics

Crisis Intervention: includes defusing, debriefing, counseling, psychotherapy, and/or coordination of care w/other providers/agencies

Individual Psychotherapy

- Behavior - primarily to modify behavior. Includes modeling + role-playing, positive reinforcement of target behaviors, response cost + training of self management skills
- Cognitive/Behavior - combining cognitive + behavior treatment strategies to improve functioning. Maladaptive responses are examined to determine how cognitions relate to behavior patterns in response to an event. Uses learning principles + information processing models
- Cognitive: primarily to correct cognitive distortions + errors
- Interactive: uses primarily physical aids + other forms of non-oral interaction w/a patient who is physically, psychologically, or developmentally unable to use ordinary language or communication
- Interpersonal: helps an individual make changes in interpersonal behavior to reduce psychological dysfunction. Includes exploratory techniques, encouragement of affective expression, clarification of pt statements, analysis of communication patterns, use of therapy relationship & behavior change technique.
- Psychoanalysis - methods of obtaining a detailed account of past + present mental + emotional experiences to determine the source & eliminate or diminish the undesirable effects of unconscious conflicts by making the individual aware of their existance, origin + inappropriate expression in emotions + behavior
- Psychodynamic - Exploration of past + present emotional experiences to understand motives + drives using insight-orientated technique to reduce the undesirable effects of internal conflicts on emotions + behavior
- Psychophysiological - monitoring + alteration of physiological processes to help the individual associate physiological reactions combined w/ cognitive + behavorial strategies to gain improved control of these processes to help the individual cope more effectively
- Supportive - Formation of therapeutic relationship primarily for providing emotional support to prevent further deterioration in functioning during periods of particular stress. Often used in conjunction w/other therapeutic approaches

12 root types

Mental Health GZ1-GZJ

Counseling & psychotherapy

G Mental Health
Z None
1 Psychological Tests: The administration and interpretation of standardized psychological tests and measurement instruments for the assessment of psychological function

Qualifier	Qualifier	Qualifier	Qualifier
Character 4	**Character 5**	**Character 6**	**Character 7**
0 Developmental 1 Personality and Behavioral 2 Intellectual and Psychoeducational 3 Neuropsychological 4 Neurobehavioral and Cognitive Status	Z None	Z None	Z None

Treatment of a traumatized, acutely distrubed or distressed individual for short term stabilization

G Mental Health
Z None
2 Crisis Intervention: Treatment of a traumatized, acutely disturbed or distressed individual for the purpose of short-term stabilization

Qualifier	Qualifier	Qualifier	Qualifier
Character 4	**Character 5**	**Character 6**	**Character 7**
Z None	Z None	Z None	Z None

G Mental Health
Z None
3 Medication Management: Monitoring and adjusting the use of medications for the treatment of a mental health disorder

Qualifier	Qualifier	Qualifier	Qualifier
Character 4	**Character 5**	**Character 6**	**Character 7**
Z None	Z None	Z None	Z None

G Mental Health
Z None
5 Individual Psychotherapy: Treatment of an individual with a mental health disorder by behavioral, cognitive, psychoanalytic, psychodynamic or psychophysiological means to improve functioning or well-being

Qualifier	Qualifier	Qualifier	Qualifier
Character 4	**Character 5**	**Character 6**	**Character 7**
0 Interactive 1 Behavioral 2 Cognitive 3 Interpersonal 4 Psychoanalysis 5 Psychodynamic 6 Supportive 8 Cognitive-Behavioral 9 Psychophysiological	Z None	Z None	Z None

Vocational - exploration of vocational interest, aptitudes & required adaptive behavior skills to develop & carry out a plan for achieving a successful vocational placement, enhancing work related adjustment &/or pursuing viable options in training education or preparation

G Mental Health
Z None
6 Counseling: The application of psychological methods to treat an individual with normal developmental issues and psychological problems in order to increase function, improve well-being, alleviate distress, maladjustment or resolve crises

Qualifier	Qualifier	Qualifier	Qualifier
Character 4	**Character 5**	**Character 6**	**Character 7**
0 Educational 1 Vocational 3 Other Counseling	Z None	Z None	Z None

remediation of emotional or behavorial problems presented by 1 or more family members when psychotherapy w/more than 1 family member is indicated

G Mental Health
Z None
7 Family Psychotherapy: Treatment that includes one or more family members of an individual with a mental health disorder by behavioral, cognitive, psychoanalytic, psychodynamic or psychophysiological means to improve functioning or well-being

Qualifier Character 4	Qualifier Character 5	Qualifier Character 6	Qualifier Character 7
2 Other Family Psychotherapy	Z None	Z None	Z None

G Mental Health
Z None ECT
B Electroconvulsive Therapy: The application of controlled electrical voltages to treat a mental health disorder

Qualifier Character 4	Qualifier Character 5	Qualifier Character 6	Qualifier Character 7
0 Unilateral-Single Seizure 1 Unilateral-Multiple Seizure 2 Bilateral-Single Seizure 3 Bilateral-Multiple Seizure 4 Other Electroconvulsive Therapy	Z None	Z None	Z None

G Mental Health
Z None
C Biofeedback: Provision of information from the monitoring and regulating of physiological processes in conjunction with cognitive-behavioral techniques to improve patient functioning or well-being galvonic skin response GSR

Qualifier Character 4	Qualifier Character 5	Qualifier Character 6	Qualifier Character 7
9 Other Biofeedback	Z None	Z None	Z None

Induction of a state of heightened suggestibility by auditory, visual & tactile techniques to elicit an emotional or behavioral response

G Mental Health
Z None
F Hypnosis: Induction of a state of heightened suggestibility by auditory, visual and tactile techniques to elicit an emotional or behavioral response

Qualifier Character 4	Qualifier Character 5	Qualifier Character 6	Qualifier Character 7
Z None	Z None	Z None	Z None

done under light anesthesia, or sometimes barbiturates are used. It is used to treat trauma, such as pts w/combat trauma or childhood trauma

G Mental Health
Z None
G Narcosynthesis: Administration of intravenous barbiturates in order to release suppressed or repressed thoughts

Qualifier Character 4	Qualifier Character 5	Qualifier Character 6	Qualifier Character 7
Z None	Z None	Z None	Z None

G Mental Health
Z None
H Group Psychotherapy: Treatment of two or more individuals with a mental health disorder by behavioral, cognitive, psychoanalytic, psychodynamic or psychophysiological means to improve functioning or well-being

Qualifier Character 4	Qualifier Character 5	Qualifier Character 6	Qualifier Character 7
Z None	Z None	Z None	Z None

G Mental Health
Z None
J Light Therapy: Application of specialized light treatments to improve functioning or well-being

Qualifier Character 4	Qualifier Character 5	Qualifier Character 6	Qualifier Character 7
Z None	Z None	Z None	Z None

LC Limited Coverage NC Noncovered HAC HAC-associated Procedure CC Combination Cluster - See Appendix G for code lists
DRG Non-OR-Affecting MS-DRG Assignment New/Revised Text in **Orange** ♂ Male ♀ Female

NOTES

Electroconvulsive Therapy (ECT) includes appropriate sedation & other preparation of the individual. ECT done under general anesthesia in which small currents are passed through the brain, which intentionally causes a brief seizure. Sometimes used to treat severe depression

Biofeedback: Includes electroencephalogram (EEG), blood pressure, skin temperature or peripheral blood flow, electrocardiogram (ECG), electroculogram, electromyogram (EMG), respirometry or capnometry, galvinic skin response (GSC) or electrodermal response (EDR) perineometry to monitor & regulate bowel or bladder activity, & electrogastrogram to monitor & regulate gastric motility

Biofeedback therapy is a non-drug treatment in which pts learn to control bodily processes that are normally involuntary, such as muscle tension, BP, or heart rate. It is believed to help a range of conditions, from chronic pain to urinary incontinence, high BP & other disorders

NOTES

7 root types

Substance Abuse Treatment HZ2-HZ9

- detoxification

H Substance Abuse Treatment
Z None
2 Detoxification Services: Detoxification from alcohol and/or drugs

not a treatment modality! but helps the pt stabalize physically & psychologically until the body becomes free of drugs & the effects of alchohol

Qualifier Character 4	Qualifier Character 5	Qualifier Character 6	Qualifier Character 7
Z None	Z None	Z None	Z None

H Substance Abuse Treatment
Z None
3 Individual Counseling: The application of psychological methods to treat an individual with addictive behavior

Consisting of several techniques, which apply various strategies to address drug addiction

Qualifier Character 4	Qualifier Character 5	Qualifier Character 6	Qualifier Character 7
0 Cognitive DRG	Z None	Z None	Z None
1 Behavioral DRG			
2 Cognitive-Behavioral DRG			
3 12-Step DRG			
4 Interpersonal DRG			
5 Vocational DRG			
6 Psychoeducation DRG			
7 Motivational Enhancement DRG			
8 Confrontational DRG			
9 Continuing Care DRG			
B Spiritual DRG			
C Pre/Post-Test Infectious Disease			

DRG HZ30ZZZ HZ31ZZZ HZ32ZZZ HZ33ZZZ HZ34ZZZ HZ35ZZZ HZ36ZZZ HZ37ZZZ HZ38ZZZ HZ39ZZZ HZ3BZZZ

H Substance Abuse Treatment
Z None
4 Group Counseling: The application of psychological methods to treat two or more individuals with addictive behavior

Provides structed group counseling sessions & healing power through the connections w/others

Qualifier Character 4	Qualifier Character 5	Qualifier Character 6	Qualifier Character 7
0 Cognitive DRG	Z None	Z None	Z None
1 Behavioral DRG			
2 Cognitive-Behavioral DRG			
3 12-Step DRG			
4 Interpersonal DRG			
5 Vocational DRG			
6 Psychoeducation DRG			
7 Motivational Enhancement DRG			
8 Confrontational DRG			
9 Continuing Care DRG			
B Spiritual DRG			
C Pre/Post-Test Infectious Disease			

DRG HZ40ZZZ HZ41ZZZ HZ42ZZZ HZ43ZZZ HZ44ZZZ HZ45ZZZ HZ46ZZZ HZ47ZZZ HZ48ZZZ HZ49ZZZ HZ4BZZZ

H Substance Abuse Treatment
Z None
5 Individual Psychotherapy: Treatment of an individual with addictive behavior by behavioral, cognitive, psychoanalytic, psychodynamic or psychophysiological means

Qualifier Character 4	Qualifier Character 5	Qualifier Character 6	Qualifier Character 7
0 Cognitive DRG	Z None	Z None	Z None
1 Behavioral DRG			
2 Cognitive-Behavioral DRG			
3 12-Step DRG			
4 Interpersonal DRG			
5 Interactive DRG			
6 Psychoeducation DRG			
7 Motivational Enhancement DRG			
8 Confrontational DRG			
9 Supportive DRG			
B Psychoanalysis DRG			
C Psychodynamic DRG			
D Psychophysiological DRG			

DRG HZ50ZZZ HZ51ZZZ HZ52ZZZ HZ53ZZZ HZ54ZZZ HZ55ZZZ HZ56ZZZ HZ57ZZZ HZ58ZZZ HZ59ZZZ HZ5BZZZ HZ5CZZZ HZ5DZZZ

H Substance Abuse Treatment Provides support & education for family members of addicted individuals.
Z None Family member participation is critical to substance abuse treatment
6 Family Counseling: The application of psychological methods that includes one or more family members to treat an individual with addictive behavior

Qualifier Character 4	Qualifier Character 5	Qualifier Character 6	Qualifier Character 7
3 Other Family Counseling	Z None	Z None	Z None

H Substance Abuse Treatment
Z None
8 Medication Management: Monitoring and adjusting the use of replacement medications for the treatment of addiction

Qualifier Character 4	Qualifier Character 5	Qualifier Character 6	Qualifier Character 7
0 Nicotine Replacement	Z None	Z None	Z None
1 Methadone Maintenance			
2 Levo-alpha-acetyl-methadol (LAAM)			
3 Antabuse			
4 Naltrexone			
5 Naloxone			
6 Clonidine			
7 Bupropion			
8 Psychiatric Medication			
9 Other Replacement Medication			

LC Limited Coverage NC Noncovered HAC HAC-associated Procedure CC Combination Cluster - See Appendix G for code lists
DRG Non-OR-Affecting MS-DRG Assignment New/Revised Text in **Orange** ♂ Male ♀ Female

H Substance Abuse Treatment
Z None
9 Pharmacotherapy: The use of replacement medications for the treatment of addiction

Qualifier Character 4	Qualifier Character 5	Qualifier Character 6	Qualifier Character 7
0 Nicotine Replacement **1** Methadone Maintenance **2** Levo-alpha-acetyl-methadol (LAAM) **3** Antabuse alcohol addiction **4** Naltrexone **5** Naloxone **6** Clonidine **7** Bupropion **8** Psychiatric Medication **9** Other Replacement Medication	**Z** None	**Z** None	**Z** None

antabuse may be alcohol addiction

NOTES

See Section E of Guidelines

8 body system values
7 root operations

New Technology X27-XY0

& new drugs

Cardiovascular System X27-X2R

X New Technology Section
2 Cardiovascular System body system
7 Dilation: Expanding an orifice or the lumen of a tubular body part Operation

Body Part Character 4	Approach Character 5	Device/Substance/Technology Character 6	Qualifier Character 7
H Femoral Artery, Right **J** Femoral Artery, Left **K** Popliteal Artery, Proximal Right **L** Popliteal Artery, Proximal Left **M** Popliteal Artery, Distal Right **N** Popliteal Artery, Distal Left **P** Anterior Tibial Artery, Right **Q** Anterior Tibial Artery, Left **R** Posterior Tibial Artery, Right **S** Posterior Tibial Artery, Left **T** Peroneal Artery, Right **U** Peroneal Artery, Left	**3** Percutaneous	**8** Intraluminal Device, Sustained Release Drug-eluting **9** Intraluminal Device, Sustained Release Drug-eluting, Two **B** Intraluminal Device, Sustained Release Drug-eluting, Three **C** Intraluminal Device, Sustained Release Drug-eluting, Four or More	**5** New Technology Group 5

X New Technology
2 Cardiovascular System
A Assistance: Taking over a portion of a physiological function by extracorporeal means

Body Part Character 4	Approach Character 5	Device/Substance/Technology Character 6	Qualifier Character 7
5 Innominate Artery and Left Common Carotid Artery	**3** Percutaneous	**1** Cerebral Embolic Filtration, Dual Filter	**2** New Technology Group 2
6 Aortic Arch	**3** Percutaneous	**2** Cerebral Embolic Filtration, Single Deflection Filter	**5** New Technology Group 5

X New Technology
2 Cardiovascular System
C Extirpation: Taking or cutting out solid matter from a body part

Body Part Character 4	Approach Character 5	Device/Substance/Technology Character 6	Qualifier Character 7
0 Coronary Artery, One Artery **1** Coronary Artery, Two Arteries **2** Coronary Artery, Three Arteries **3** Coronary Artery, Four or More Arteries	**3** Percutaneous	**6** Orbital Atherectomy Technology	**1** New Technology Group 1

X New Technology
2 Cardiovascular System
R Replacement: Putting in or on biological or synthetic material that physically takes the place and/or function of all or a portion of a body part

Body Part Character 4	Approach Character 5	Device/Substance/Technology Character 6	Qualifier Character 7
F Aortic Valve	**0** Open **3** Percutaneous **4** Percutaneous Endoscopic	**3** Zooplastic Tissue, Rapid Deployment Technique	**2** New Technology Group 2

NOTES

Skin, Subcutaneous Tissue, Fascia, and Breast XHR

X New Technology
H Skin, Subcutaneous Tissue, Fascia and Breast
R Replacement: Putting in or on biological or synthetic material that physically takes the place and/or function of all or a portion of a body part

Body Part	Approach	Device/Substance/Technology	Qualifier
Character 4	Character 5	Character 6	Character 7
P Skin	**X** External	**L** Skin Substitute, Porcine Liver Derived	**2** New Technology Group 2

NOTES

Muscles, Tendons, Bursae, and Ligaments XK0

X New Technology
K Muscles, Tendons, Bursae and Ligaments
0 Introduction: Putting in or on a therapeutic, diagnostic, nutritional, physiological, or prophylactic substance except blood or blood products

Body Part	Approach	Device/Substance/Technology	Qualifier
Character 4	**Character 5**	**Character 6**	**Character 7**
2 Muscle	**3** Percutaneous	**0** Concentrated Bone Marrow Aspirate	**3** New Technology Group 3

NOTES

Bones XNS

X New Technology
N Bones
S Reposition: Moving to its normal location, or other suitable location, all or a portion of a body part

Body Part Character 4	Approach Character 5	Device/Substance/Technology Character 6	Qualifier Character 7
0 Lumbar Vertebra **3** Cervical Vertebra **4** Thoracic Vertebra	**0** Open **3** Percutaneous	**3** Magnetically Controlled Growth Rod(s)	**2** New Technology Group 2

NOTES

Joints XR2-XRG

X New Technology
R Joints
2 Monitoring: Determining the level of a physiological or physical function repetitively over a period of time

Body Part	Approach	Device/Substance/Technology	Qualifier
Character 4	**Character 5**	**Character 6**	**Character 7**
G Knee Joint, Right **H** Knee Joint, Left	**0** Open	**2** Intraoperative Knee Replacement Sensor	**1** New Technology Group 1

X New Technology
R Joints
G Fusion: Joining together portions of an articular body part rendering the articular body part immobile

Body Part	Approach	Device/Substance/Technology	Qualifier
Character 4	**Character 5**	**Character 6**	**Character 7**
0 Occipital-cervical Joint HAC	**0** Open	**9** Interbody Fusion Device, Nanotextured Surface	**2** New Technology Group 2
0 Occipital-cervical Joint HAC	**0** Open	**F** Interbody Fusion Device, Radiolucent Porous	**3** New Technology Group 3
1 Cervical Vertebral Joint HAC	**0** Open	**9** Interbody Fusion Device, Nanotextured Surface	**2** New Technology Group 2
1 Cervical Vertebral Joint HAC	**0** Open	**F** Interbody Fusion Device, Radiolucent Porous	**3** New Technology Group 3
2 Cervical Vertebral Joints, 2 or more HAC	**0** Open	**9** Interbody Fusion Device, Nanotextured Surface	**2** New Technology Group 2
2 Cervical Vertebral Joints, 2 or more HAC	**0** Open	**F** Interbody Fusion Device, Radiolucent Porous	**3** New Technology Group 3
4 Cervicothoracic Vertebral Joint HAC	**0** Open	**9** Interbody Fusion Device, Nanotextured Surface	**2** New Technology Group 2
4 Cervicothoracic Vertebral Joint HAC	**0** Open	**F** Interbody Fusion Device, Radiolucent Porous	**3** New Technology Group 3
6 Thoracic Vertebral Joint HAC	**0** Open	**9** Interbody Fusion Device, Nanotextured Surface	**2** New Technology Group 2
6 Thoracic Vertebral Joint HAC	**0** Open	**F** Interbody Fusion Device, Radiolucent Porous	**3** New Technology Group 3
7 Thoracic Vertebral Joints, 2 to 7 HAC CC	**0** Open	**9** Interbody Fusion Device, Nanotextured Surface	**2** New Technology Group 2
7 Thoracic Vertebral Joints, 2 to 7 HAC CC	**0** Open	**F** Interbody Fusion Device, Radiolucent Porous	**3** New Technology Group 3
8 Thoracic Vertebral Joints, 8 or more HAC	**0** Open	**9** Interbody Fusion Device, Nanotextured Surface	**2** New Technology Group 2
8 Thoracic Vertebral Joints, 8 or more HAC	**0** Open	**F** Interbody Fusion Device, Radiolucent Porous	**3** New Technology Group 3
A Thoracolumbar Vertebral Joint HAC	**0** Open	**9** Interbody Fusion Device, Nanotextured Surface	**2** New Technology Group 2
A Thoracolumbar Vertebral Joint HAC	**0** Open	**F** Interbody Fusion Device, Radiolucent Porous	**3** New Technology Group 3
B Lumbar Vertebral Joint HAC	**0** Open	**9** Interbody Fusion Device, Nanotextured Surface	**2** New Technology Group 2
B Lumbar Vertebral Joint HAC	**0** Open	**F** Interbody Fusion Device, Radiolucent Porous	**3** New Technology Group 3
C Lumbar Vertebral Joints, 2 or more HAC CC	**0** Open	**9** Interbody Fusion Device, Nanotextured Surface	**2** New Technology Group 2

XRG continued on next page

LC Limited Coverage NC Noncovered HAC HAC-associated Procedure CC Combination Cluster - See Appendix G for code lists
DRG Non-OR-Affecting MS-DRG Assignment New/Revised Text in **Orange** ♂ Male ♀ Female
2020 ICD-10-PCS **753**
JOINTS XR2-XRG

XRG continued from previous page

X New Technology
R Joints
G Fusion: Joining together portions of an articular body part rendering the articular body part immobile

Body Part	Approach	Device/Substance/Technology	Qualifier
Character 4	**Character 5**	**Character 6**	**Character 7**
C Lumbar Vertebral Joints, 2 or more HAC CC	**0** Open	**F** Interbody Fusion Device, Radiolucent Porous	**3** New Technology Group 3
D Lumbosacral Joint HAC	**0** Open	**9** Interbody Fusion Device, Nanotextured Surface	**2** New Technology Group 2
D Lumbosacral Joint HAC	**0** Open	**F** Interbody Fusion Device, Radiolucent Porous	**3** New Technology Group 3

HAC XRG0092 XRG00F3 XRG1092 XRG10F3 XRG2092 XRG20F3 XRG4092 XRG40F3 XRG6092 XRG60F3 XRG7092 XRG70F3 XRG8092 XRG80F3 XRGA092 XRGA0F3 XRGB092 XRGB0F3 XRGC092 XRGC0F3 XRGD092 XRGD0F3
Surgical site infection following certain orthopedic procedures of spine, shoulder or elbow procedures and secondary diagnosis K68.11, T81.40XA, T81.41XA, T81.42XA, T81.43XA, T81.44XA, T81.49XA, T84.60XA, T84.610A, T84.611A, T84.612A, T84.613A, T84.614A, T84.615A, T84.619A, T84.63XA, T84.69XA, T84.7XXA.

CC XRG7092 XRG70F3 XRGC092 XRGC0F3

NOTES

NOTES

Urinary System XT2

X New Technology
T Urinary System
2 Monitoring: Determining the level of a physiological or physical function repetitively over a period of time

Body Part	Approach	Device/Substance/Technology	Qualifier
Character 4	**Character 5**	**Character 6**	**Character 7**
5 Kidney	**X** External	**E** Fluorescent Pyrazine	**5** New Technology Group 5

NOTES

Male Reproductive System XV5

X New Technology
V Male Reproductive System
5 Destruction: Physical eradication of all or a portion of a body part by the direct use of energy, force, or a destructive agent

Body Part Character 4	Approach Character 5	Device/Substance/Technology Character 6	Qualifier Character 7
0 Prostate	**8** Via Natural or Artificial Opening Endoscopic	**A** Robotic Waterjet Ablation	**4** New Technology Group 4

NOTES

Anatomical Regions XW0

X New Technology
W Anatomical Regions
0 Introduction: Putting in or on a therapeutic, diagnostic, nutritional, physiological, or prophylactic substance except blood or blood products

Body Part Character 4	Approach Character 5	Device/Substance/Technology Character 6	Qualifier Character 7
1 Subcutaneous Tissue	3 Percutaneous	W Caplacizumab	5 New Technology Group 5
3 Peripheral Vein	3 Percutaneous may be peripheral venous catheter	2 Ceftazidime-Avibactam Anti-infective – may only say ceftazidime 3 Idarucizumab, Dabigatran Reversal Agent 4 Isavuconazole Anti-infective 5 Blinatumomab Antineoplastic Immunotherapy	1 New Technology Group 1
3 Peripheral Vein	3 Percutaneous	7 Coagulation Factor Xa Inactivated 9 Defibrotide Sodium Anticoagulant	2 New Technology Group 2
3 Peripheral Vein DRG	3 Percutaneous	A Bezlotoxumab Monoclonal Antibody B Cytarabine and Daunorubicin Liposome Antineoplastic C Engineered Autologous Chimeric Antigen Receptor T-cell Immunotherapy F Other New Technology Therapeutic Substance	3 New Technology Group 3
3 Peripheral Vein	3 Percutaneous	G Plazomicin Anti-infective H Synthetic Human Angiotensin II	4 New Technology Group 4
3 Peripheral Vein	3 Percutaneous	K Fosfomycin Anti-infective N Meropenem-vaborbactam Anti-infective Q Tagraxofusp-erzs Antineoplastic S Iobenguane I-131 Antineoplastic U Imipenem-cilastatin-relebactam Anti-infective W Caplacizumab	5 New Technology Group 5
4 Central Vein	3 Percutaneous	2 Ceftazidime-Avibactam Anti-infective 3 Idarucizumab, Dabigatran Reversal Agent 4 Isavuconazole Antiinfective 5 Blinatumomab Antineoplastic Immunotherapy	1 New Technology Group 1
4 Central Vein	3 Percutaneous	7 Coagulation Factor Xa, Inactivated 9 Defibrotide Sodium Anticoagulant	2 New Technology Group 2
4 Central Vein DRG	3 Percutaneous	A Bezlotoxumab Monoclonal Antibody B Cytarabine and Daunorubicin Liposome Antineoplastic C Engineered Autologous Chimeric Antigen Receptor T-cell Immunotherapy F Other New Technology Therapeutic Substance	3 New Technology Group 3

XW0 continued on next page

X New Technology
W Anatomical Regions
0 Introduction: Putting in or on a therapeutic, diagnostic, nutritional, physiological, or prophylactic substance except blood or blood products

XW0 continued from previous page

Body Part	Approach	Device/Substance/Technology	Qualifier
Character 4	**Character 5**	**Character 6**	**Character 7**
4 Central Vein	**3** Percutaneous	**G** Plazomicin Anti-infective **H** Synthetic Human Angiotensin II	**4** New Technology Group 4
4 Central Vein	**3** Percutaneous	**K** Fosfomycin Anti-infective **N** Meropenem-vaborbactam Anti-infective **Q** Tagraxofusp-erzs Antineoplastic **S** Iobenguane I-131 Antineoplastic **U** Imipenem-cilastatin-relebactam Anti-infective **W** Caplacizumab	**5** New Technology Group 5
D Mouth and Pharynx	**X** External	**8** Uridine Triacetate	**2** New Technology Group 2
D Mouth and Pharynx	**X** External	**J** Apalutamide Antineoplastic **L** Erdafitinib Antineoplastic **R** Venetoclax Antineoplastic **T** Ruxolitinib **V** Gilteritinib Antineoplastic	**5** New Technology Group 5

DRG XW033C3 XW043C3

NOTES

NOTES

Physiological Systems XXE

X **New Technology**
X **Physiological Systems**
E **Measurement:** Determining the level of a physiological or physical function at a point in time

Body Part	Approach	Device/Substance/Technology	Qualifier
Character 4	Character 5	Character 6	Character 7
5 Circulatory	X External	M Infection, Whole Blood Nucleic Acid-base Microbial Detection	5 New Technology Group 5

NOTES

Extracorporeal XY0

X New Technology
Y Extracorporeal
0 Introduction: Putting in or on a therapeutic, diagnostic, nutritional, physiological, or prophylactic substance except blood or blood products

Body Part	Approach	Device/Substance/Technology	Qualifier
Character 4	**Character 5**	**Character 6**	**Character 7**
V Vein Graft	**X** External	**8** Endothelial Damage Inhibitor	**3** New Technology Group 3

NOTES

Complete or partial redo of orginial procedure is coded to root operation that ID's the procedure performed, rather than revision

Ex: redo of hip replacement - use replacement

Correction of malfunctioning or displaced device - use revision

post procedure hemorrage - use control

Lumen - cavity/channel within a tubular structure

tubular body parts - include cardiovascular, gastrointestinal, genitourinary systems, bilary + respiratory tract

VP shunt - 3 pieces: ① ventricular catheter (brain), ② peritoneal catheter (peritoneal cavity) ③ valve

do not code as drainage - it will be bypass, code as bypass if completely replaced, if only partly replaced, code revision, can also code removal of entire shunt *root operation is based on actual procedure performed - may/may not be the intended procedure. IF desired result is not obtained after completing procedure, root operation performed is still used. Root operation is determined by the FINAL procedure performed*

Appendix A: Root Operations Definitions *31 root operations*

		0 - Medical and Surgical
Value	**Root Operation**	**Definition/Explanation**
0	Alteration	**Definition:** Modifying the anatomic structure of a body part without affecting the function of the body part **Explanation:** Principal purpose is to improve appearance *require diagnostic confirmation for medical purposes* **Includes/Examples:** Face lift, breast augmentation
1	Bypass *Code graft separate - see notes -*	**Definition:** Altering the route of passage of the contents of a tubular body part *Guideline B3.6a* **Explanation:** Rerouting contents of a body part to a downstream area of the normal route, to a similar route and body part, or to an abnormal route and dissimilar body part. Includes one or more anastomoses, with or without the use of a device. *7th character qualifier IDs destination site of bypass* **Includes/Examples:** Coronary artery bypass, colostomy formation, *CABG, CSF-VP shunt - code also removal if replacing*
2	Change *w/o making new incision*	**Definition:** Taking out or off a device from a body part and putting back an identical or similar device in or on the same body part without cutting or puncturing the skin or a mucous membrane **Explanation:** All CHANGE procedures are coded using the approach EXTERNAL **Includes/Examples:** Urinary catheter change, gastrostomy tube change, *drainage & feeding devices* *tracheostomy tube exchange*
3	Control *do not use w/ bypass detachment, excision, extraction, reposition replacement, resection is used to stop the bleeding*	**Definition:** Stopping, or attempting to stop, postprocedural or other acute bleeding **Explanation:** The site of the bleeding is coded as an anatomical region and not to a specific body part **Includes/Examples:** Control of post-prostatectomy hemorrhage, control of intracranial subdural hemorrhage, control of bleeding duodenal ulcer, control of retroperitoneal hemorrhage *includes irrigation & evacuation of hematoma done at operative site*
4	Creation *Sex change Like Clit*	**Definition:** Putting in or on biological or synthetic material to form a new body part that to the extent possible replicates the anatomic structure or function of an absent body part **Explanation:** Used for gender reassignment surgery and corrective procedures in individuals with congenital anomalies **Includes/Examples:** Creation of vagina in a male, creation of right and left atrioventricular valve from common atrioventricular valve *site of procedure: perineum, when harvesting autografts, it separate procedure is performed to harvest tissue its coded also*
5	Destruction *Ablution*	**Definition:** Physical eradication of all or a portion of a body part by the direct use of energy, force, or a destructive agent **Explanation:** None of the body part is physically taken out **Includes/Examples:** Fulguration of rectal polyp, cautery of skin lesion, *Fulguration of endometrium* *laser coagulation*
6	Detachment	**Definition:** Cutting off all or a portion of the upper or lower extremities *See p. 574* **Explanation:** The body part value is the site of the detachment, with a qualifier if applicable to further specify the level where the extremity was detached **Includes/Examples:** Below knee amputation, disarticulation of shoulder
7	Dilation *device is integral part of procedure can still use if body part does not remain open*	*If dilation of urethra includes putting in a stent, still use dilation not insertion* **Definition:** Expanding an orifice or the lumen of a tubular body part **Explanation:** The orifice can be a natural orifice or an artificially created orifice. Accomplished by stretching a tubular body part using intraluminal pressure or by cutting part of the orifice or wall of the tubular body part. **Includes/Examples:** Percutaneous transluminal angioplasty, internal urethrotomy, *PTCA, Stent insertion*
8	Division *within Cut into*	**Definition:** Cutting into a body part, without draining fluids and/or gases from the body part, in order to separate or transect a body part, *transect or separate - within a body part* **Explanation:** All or a portion of the body part is separated into two or more portions **Includes/Examples:** Spinal cordotomy, osteotomy, *neurotomy*
9	Drainage *not for shunt must drain out of body*	**Definition:** Taking or letting out fluids and/or gases from a body part *used for diagnostic & therapeutic drainage procedures* **Explanation:** The qualifier DIAGNOSTIC is used to identify drainage procedures that are biopsies **Includes/Examples:** Thoracentesis, incision and drainage, *put in catheter, device 6th character* *tympanotomy w/ myringotomy tube*
B	Excision *irradicate Single lymph node breast lump Partial sigmoidectomy AKA- debridement of tumor snare polypectomy*	**Definition:** Cutting out or off, without replacement, a portion of a body part *cut w/ sharp instrument, snare includes scapel, wire, scissors bone saw, electro cautery tip* **Explanation:** The qualifier DIAGNOSTIC is used to identify excision procedures that are biopsies *If all of part removed - use resection* **Includes/Examples:** Partial nephrectomy, liver biopsy, *skin tumor*

Bone marrow & endometrial biopsies are NOT coded to excision. They are coded to extraction w/ qualifier diagnostic

Excision ex: segmentectomy (lung), wedge excision, biopsy of lung

0 - Medical and Surgical continued on next page

0 - Medical and Surgical continued from previous page

0 - Medical and Surgical		
Value	**Root Operation**	**Definition/Explanation**
C	Extirpation	**Definition:** Taking or cutting out solid matter from a body part **Explanation:** The solid matter may be an abnormal byproduct of a biological function or a foreign body; it may be imbedded in a body part or in the lumen of a tubular body part. The solid matter may or may not have been previously broken into pieces. **Includes/Examples:** Thrombectomy, choledocholithotomy
D	Extraction	**Definition:** Pulling or stripping out or off all or a portion of a body part by the use of force **Explanation:** The qualifier DIAGNOSTIC is used to identify extraction procedures that are biopsies **Includes/Examples:** Dilation and curettage, vein stripping
F	Fragmentation	**Definition:** Breaking solid matter in a body part into pieces **Explanation:** Physical force (e.g., manual, ultrasonic) applied directly or indirectly is used to break the solid matter into pieces. The solid matter may be an abnormal byproduct of a biological function or a foreign body. The pieces of solid matter are not taken out. **Includes/Examples:** Extracorporeal shockwave lithotripsy, transurethral lithotripsy
G	Fusion	**Definition:** Joining together portions of an articular body part rendering the articular body part immobile **Explanation:** The body part is joined together by fixation device, bone graft, or other means **Includes/Examples:** Spinal fusion, ankle arthrodesis
H	Insertion	**Definition:** Putting in a nonbiological appliance that monitors, assists, performs, or prevents a physiological function but does not physically take the place of a body part **Includes/Examples:** Insertion of radioactive implant, insertion of central venous catheter
J	Inspection	**Definition:** Visually and/or manually exploring a body part **Explanation:** Visual exploration may be performed with or without optical instrumentation. Manual exploration may be performed directly or through intervening body layers. **Includes/Examples:** Diagnostic arthroscopy, exploratory laparotomy
K	Map	**Definition:** Locating the route of passage of electrical impulses and/or locating functional areas in a body part **Explanation:** Applicable only to the cardiac conduction mechanism and the central nervous system **Includes/Examples:** Cardiac mapping, cortical mapping
L	Occlusion	**Definition:** Completely closing an orifice or the lumen of a tubular body part **Explanation:** The orifice can be a natural orifice or an artificially created orifice **Includes/Examples:** Fallopian tube ligation, ligation of inferior vena cava
M	Reattachment	**Definition:** Putting back in or on all or a portion of a separated body part to its normal location or other suitable location **Explanation:** Vascular circulation and nervous pathways may or may not be reestablished **Includes/Examples:** Reattachment of hand, reattachment of avulsed kidney
N	Release	**Definition:** Freeing a body part from an abnormal physical constraint by cutting or by the use of force **Explanation:** Some of the restraining tissue may be taken out but none of the body part is taken out **Includes/Examples:** Adhesiolysis, carpal tunnel release
P	Removal	**Definition:** Taking out or off a device from a body part **Explanation:** If a device is taken out and a similar device put in without cutting or puncturing the skin or mucous membrane, the procedure is coded to the root operation CHANGE. Otherwise, the procedure for taking out a device is coded to the root operation REMOVAL. **Includes/Examples:** Drainage tube removal, cardiac pacemaker removal
Q	Repair	**Definition:** Restoring, to the extent possible, a body part to its normal anatomic structure and function **Explanation:** Used only when the method to accomplish the repair is not one of the other root operations **Includes/Examples:** Colostomy takedown, suture of laceration

0 - Medical and Surgical continued on next page

not - drainage - VP shunt = CSF Shunt - has 3 pieces, use revision if only replacing a piece & replace if replacing all

0 - Medical and Surgical

Value	Root Operation	Definition/Explanation
R	Replacement	**Definition:** Putting in or on biological or synthetic material that physically takes the place and/or function of all or a portion of a body part
	code VP shunt as bypass even if replacing	**Explanation:** The body part may have been taken out or replaced, or may be taken out, physically eradicated, or rendered nonfunctional during the Replacement procedure. A Removal procedure is coded for taking out the device used in a previous replacement procedure. *If pedicle graft stays attached at one end do not code separate*
		Includes/Examples: Total hip replacement, bone graft, free skin graft, *cornea & lens*
S	Reposition *AKA reduction*	*Body parts only - do not use for devices like pacemakers - use revision* **Definition:** Moving to its normal location, or other suitable location, all or a portion of a body part *improve function*
to new or normal location to enhance ability to function AKA - transposition		**Explanation:** The body part is moved to a new location from an abnormal location, or from a normal location where it is not functioning correctly. The body part may or may not be cut out or off to be moved to the new location. *includes cast - do not code separate or splint*
		Includes/Examples: Reposition of undescended testicle, fracture reduction *ocular muscle*
T	Resection *radical pneumonectomy*	**Definition:** Cutting out or off, without replacement, all of a body part *1 lymph node = excision lymph node chain = resection*
		Includes/Examples: Total nephrectomy, total lobectomy of lung, *total excision of pituitary gland, total breast, transverse colon*
V	Restriction	**Definition:** Partially closing an orifice or the lumen of a tubular body part, *narrow diameter*
		Explanation: The orifice can be a natural orifice or an artificially created orifice. *can be intraluminar or extraluminal*
		Includes/Examples: Esophagogastric fundoplication, cervical cerclage, *aneurysm*
W	Revision	*For devices only not body parts* **Definition:** Correcting, to the extent possible, a portion of a malfunctioning device or the position of a displaced device
done mainly on mechanical devices, so not use if device is replaced - Ex: hip or entire shunt		**Explanation:** Revision can include correcting a malfunctioning or displaced device by taking out or putting in components of the device such as a screw or pin *correction of malfunctioning knee prosthesis*
		Includes/Examples: Adjustment of position of pacemaker lead, recementing of hip prosthesis *, piece of shunt*
U	Supplement	**Definition:** Putting in or on biological or synthetic material that physically reinforces and/or augments the function of a portion of a body part *does not take the place of existing body part*
		Explanation: The biological material is non-living, or is living and from the same individual. The body part may have been previously replaced, and the Supplement procedure is performed to physically reinforce and/or augment the function of the replaced body part.
		Includes/Examples: Herniorrhaphy using mesh, free nerve graft, *heart* mitral valve ring annuloplasty, put a new acetabular liner in a previous hip replacement *, If pedicle graft stays attached at one end. do not code separate*
X	Transfer *qualifier used for composite tissue transfers*	**Definition:** Moving, without taking out, all or a portion of a body part to another location to take over the function of all or a portion of a body part *, Body part is nerve being moved & Qualifier is receiving nerve*
		Explanation: The body part transferred remains connected to its vascular and nervous supply *- not disrupted*
		Includes/Examples: Tendon transfer, skin pedicle flap transfer, *muscular subcutaneous flap transfer*
Y	Transplantation	**Definition:** Putting in or on all or a portion of a living body part taken from another individual or animal to physically take the place and/or function of all or a portion of a similar body part
		Explanation: The native body part may or may not be taken out, and the transplanted body part may take over all or a portion of its function. *Putting in cells - code to administration*
		Includes/Examples: Kidney transplant, heart transplant

1 - Obstetrics

Value	Root Operation	Definition/Explanation
A	Abortion	**Definition:** Artificially terminating a pregnancy
2	Change	**Definition:** Taking out or off a device from a body part and putting back an identical or similar device in or on the same body part without cutting or puncturing the skin or a mucous membrane
E	Delivery	**Definition:** Assisting the passage of the products of conception from the genital canal
9	Drainage	**Definition:** Taking or letting out fluids and/or gases from a body part
D	Extraction	**Definition:** Pulling or stripping out or off all or a portion of a body part by the use of force

1 - Obstetrics continued on next page

1 - Obstetrics continued from previous page

1 - Obstetrics

Value	Root Operation	Definition/Explanation
H	Insertion	**Definition:** Putting in a nonbiological appliance that monitors, assists, performs, or prevents a physiological function but does not physically take the place of a body part
J	Inspection	**Definition:** Visually and/or manually exploring a body part **Explanation:** Visual exploration may be performed with or without optical instrumentation. Manual exploration may be performed directly or through intervening body layers
P	Removal	**Definition:** Taking out or off a device from a body part, region or orifice **Explanation:** If a device is taken out and a similar device put in without cutting or puncturing the skin or mucous membrane, the procedure is coded to the root operation CHANGE. Otherwise, the procedure for taking out a device is coded to the root operation REMOVAL.
Q	Repair	**Definition:** Restoring, to the extent possible, a body part to its normal anatomic structure and function **Explanation:** Used only when the method to accomplish the repair is not one of the other root operations
S	Reposition	**Definition:** Moving to its normal location, or other suitable location, all or a portion of a body part **Explanation:** The body part is moved to a new location from an abnormal location, or from a normal location where it is not functioning correctly. The body part may or may not be cut out or off to be moved to the new location.
T	Resection	**Definition:** Cutting out or off, without replacement, all of a body part
Y	Transplantation	**Definition:** Putting in or on all or a portion of a living body part taken from another individual or animal to physically take the place and/or function of all or a portion of a similar body part **Explanation:** The native body part may or may not be taken out, and the transplanted body part may take over all or a portion of its function

2 - Placement

Value	Root Operation	Definition/Explanation
0	Change	**Definition:** Taking out or off a device from a body part and putting back an identical or similar device in or on the same body part without cutting or puncturing the skin or a mucous membrane
1	Compression	**Definition:** Putting pressure on a body region
2	Dressing	**Definition:** Putting material on a body region for protection
3	Immobilization	**Definition:** Limiting or preventing motion of a body region apply cast
4	Packing	**Definition:** Putting material in a body region or orifice
5	Removal	**Definition:** Taking out or off a device from a body part
6	Traction	**Definition:** Exerting a pulling force on a body region in a distal direction

3 - Administration

Value	Root Operation	Definition/Explanation
0	Introduction	**Definition:** Putting in or on a therapeutic, diagnostic, nutritional, physiological, or prophylactic substance except blood or blood products
1	Irrigation	**Definition:** Putting in or on a cleansing substance
2	Transfusion	**Definition:** Putting in blood or blood products

4 - Measurement and Monitoring

Value	Root Operation	Definition/Explanation
0	Measurement	**Definition:** Determining the level of a physiological or physical function at a point in time
1	Monitoring	**Definition:** Determining the level of a physiological or physical function repetitively over a period of time

5 - Extracorporeal or Systemic Assistance and Performance

Value	Root Operation	Definition/Explanation
0	Assistance	**Definition:** Taking over a portion of a physiological function by extracorporeal means
1	Performance	**Definition:** Completely taking over a physiological function by extracorporeal means mechanical ventilation
2	Restoration	**Definition:** Returning, or attempting to return, a physiological function to its original state by extracorporeal means.

6 - Extracorporeal or Systemic Therapies

Value	Root Operation	Definition/Explanation
0	Atmospheric Control	**Definition:** Extracorporeal control of atmospheric pressure and composition
1	Decompression	**Definition:** Extracorporeal elimination of undissolved gas from body fluids
2	Electromagnetic Therapy	**Definition:** Extracorporeal treatment by electromagnetic rays
3	Hyperthermia	**Definition:** Extracorporeal raising of body temperature
4	Hypothermia	**Definition:** Extracorporeal lowering of body temperature
B	Perfusion	**Definition:** Extracorporeal treatment by diffusion of therapeutic fluid
5	Pheresis	**Definition:** Extracorporeal separation of blood products
6	Phototherapy	**Definition:** Extracorporeal treatment by light rays
9	Shock Wave Therapy	**Definition:** Extracorporeal treatment by shock waves
7	Ultrasound Therapy	**Definition:** Extracorporeal treatment by ultrasound
8	Ultraviolet Light Therapy	**Definition:** Extracorporeal treatment by ultraviolet light

7 - Osteopathic

Value	Root Operation	Definition/Explanation
0	Treatment	**Definition:** Manual treatment to eliminate or alleviate somatic dysfunction and related disorders

8 - Other Procedures

Value	Root Operation	Definition/Explanation
0	Other Procedures	**Definition:** Methodologies which attempt to remediate or cure a disorder or disease

9 - Chiropractic		
Value	**Root Operation**	**Definition/Explanation**
B	Manipulation	**Definition:** Manual procedure that involves a directed thrust to move a joint past the physiological range of motion, without exceeding the anatomical limit

X - New Technology		
Value	**Root Operation**	**Definition/Explanation**
A	Assistance	**Definition:** Taking over a portion of a physiological function by extracorporeal means
5	Destruction	**Definition:** Physical eradication of all or a portion of a body part by the direct use of energy, force, or a destructive agent **Explanation:** None of the body part is physically taken out **Includes/Examples:** Fulguration of rectal polyp, cautery of skin lesion
7	Dilation	**Definition:** Expanding an orifice or the lumen of a tubular body part **Explanation:** The orifice can be a natural orifice or an artificially created orifice. Accomplished by stretching a tubular body part using intraluminal pressure or by cutting part of the orifice or wall of the tubular body part
C	Extirpation	**Definition:** Taking or cutting out solid matter from a body part **Explanation:** The solid matter may be an abnormal byproduct of a biological function or a foreign body; it may be imbedded in a body part or in the lumen of a tubular body part. The solid matter may or may not have been previously broken into pieces. **Includes/Examples:** Thrombectomy, choledocholithotomy
G	Fusion	**Definition:** Joining together portions of an articular body part rendering the articular body part immobile **Explanation:** The body part is joined together by fixation device, bone graft, or other means **Includes/Examples:** Spinal fusion, ankle arthrodesis
0	Introduction	**Definition:** Putting in or on a therapeutic, diagnostic, nutritional, physiological, or prophylactic substance except blood or blood products
E	Measurement	**Definition:** Determining the level of a physiological or physical function at a point in time
2	Monitoring	**Definition:** Determining the level of a physiological or physical function repetitively over a period of time
R	Replacement	**Definition:** Putting in or on biological or synthetic material that physically takes the place and/or function of all or a portion of a body part **Explanation:** The body part may have been taken out or replaced, or may be taken out, physically eradicated, or rendered nonfunctional during the Replacement procedure. A Removal procedure is coded for taking out the device used in a previous replacement procedure. **Includes/Examples:** Total hip replacement, bone graft, free skin graft
S	Reposition	**Definition:** Moving to its normal location, or other suitable location, all or a portion of a body part **Explanation:** The body part is moved to a new location from an abnormal location, or from a normal location where it is not functioning correctly. The body part may or may not be cut out or off to be moved to the new location. **Includes/Examples:** Reposition of undescended testicle, fracture reduction

Appendix B: Body Part Key

Anatomical Term	ICD-10-PCS Value
Abdominal aortic plexus	Abdominal Sympathetic Nerve
Abdominal esophagus	Esophagus, Lower
Abductor hallucis muscle	Foot Muscle, Right
	Foot Muscle, Left
Accessory cephalic vein	Cephalic Vein, Right
	Cephalic Vein, Left
Accessory obturator nerve	Lumbar Plexus
Accessory phrenic nerve	Phrenic Nerve
Accessory spleen	Spleen
Acetabulofemoral joint	Hip Joint, Right
	Hip Joint, Left
Achilles tendon	Lower Leg Tendon, Right
	Lower Leg Tendon, Left
Acromioclavicular ligament	Shoulder Bursa and Ligament, Right
	Shoulder Bursa and Ligament, Left
Acromion (process)	Scapula, Right
	Scapula, Left
Adductor brevis muscle	Upper Leg Muscle, Right
	Upper Leg Muscle, Left
Adductor hallucis muscle	Foot Muscle, Right
	Foot Muscle, Left
Adductor longus muscle	Upper Leg Muscle, Right
	Upper Leg Muscle, Left
Adductor magnus muscle	Upper Leg Muscle, Right
	Upper Leg Muscle, Left
Adenohypophysis	Pituitary Gland
Alar ligament of axis	Head and Neck Bursa and Ligament
Alveolar process of mandible	Mandible, Right
	Mandible, Left
Alveolar process of maxilla	Maxilla
Anal orifice	Anus
Anatomical snuffbox	Lower Arm and Wrist Muscle, Right
	Lower Arm and Wrist Muscle, Left
Angular artery	Face Artery
Angular vein	Face Vein, Right
	Face Vein, Left
Annular ligament	Elbow Bursa and Ligament, Right
	Elbow Bursa and Ligament, Left
Anorectal junction	Rectum
Ansa cervicalis	Cervical Plexus
Antebrachial fascia	Subcutaneous Tissue and Fascia, Right Lower Arm
	Subcutaneous Tissue and Fascia, Left Lower Arm

Anatomical Term	ICD-10-PCS Value
Anterior (pectoral) lymph node	Lymphatic, Right Axillary
	Lymphatic, Left Axillary
Anterior cerebral artery	Intracranial Artery
Anterior cerebral vein	Intracranial Vein
Anterior choroidal artery	Intracranial Artery
Anterior circumflex humeral artery	Axillary Artery, Right
	Axillary Artery, Left
Anterior communicating artery	Intracranial Artery
Anterior cruciate ligament (ACL)	Knee Bursa and Ligament, Right
	Knee Bursa and Ligament, Left
Anterior crural nerve	Femoral Nerve
Anterior facial vein	Face Vein, Right
	Face Vein, Left
Anterior intercostal artery	Internal Mammary Artery, Right
	Internal Mammary Artery, Left
Anterior interosseous nerve	Median Nerve
Anterior lateral malleolar artery	Anterior Tibial Artery, Right
	Anterior Tibial Artery, Left
Anterior lingual gland	Minor Salivary Gland
Anterior medial malleolar artery	Anterior Tibial Artery, Right
	Anterior Tibial Artery, Left
Anterior spinal artery	Vertebral Artery, Right
	Vertebral Artery, Left
Anterior tibial recurrent artery	Anterior Tibial Artery, Right
	Anterior Tibial Artery, Left
Anterior ulnar recurrent artery	Ulnar Artery, Right
	Ulnar Artery, Left
Anterior vagal trunk	Vagus Nerve
Anterior vertebral muscle	Neck Muscle, Right
	Neck Muscle, Left
Antihelix	External Ear, Right
	External Ear, Left
	External Ear, Bilateral
Antitragus	External Ear, Right
	External Ear, Left
	External Ear, Bilateral
Antrum of Highmore	Maxillary Sinus, Right
	Maxillary Sinus, Left
Aortic annulus	Aortic Valve
Aortic arch	Thoracic Aorta, Ascending/Arch
Aortic intercostal artery	Upper Artery
Apical (subclavicular) lymph node	Lymphatic, Right Axillary
	Lymphatic, Left Axillary
Apneustic center	Pons
Aqueduct of Sylvius	Cerebral Ventricle

Peripheral nerve = brachial plexus = nerve network of 4 lower cervical nerves & upper thoracic nerve. It is in the neck & underarm region

Anatomical Term	ICD-10-PCS Value
Aqueous humour	Anterior Chamber, Right
	Anterior Chamber, Left
Arachnoid mater, intracranial	Cerebral Meninges
Arachnoid mater, spinal	Spinal Meninges
Arcuate artery	Foot Artery, Right
	Foot Artery, Left
Areola	Nipple, Right
	Nipple, Left
Arterial canal (duct)	Pulmonary Artery, Left
Aryepiglottic fold	Larynx
Arytenoid cartilage	Larynx
Arytenoid muscle	Neck Muscle, Right
	Neck Muscle, Left
Ascending aorta	Thoracic Aorta, Ascending/Arch
Ascending palatine artery	Face Artery
Ascending pharyngeal artery	External Carotid Artery, Right
	External Carotid Artery, Left
Atlantoaxial joint	Cervical Vertebral Joint
Atrioventricular node	Conduction Mechanism
Atrium dextrum cordis	Atrium, Right
Atrium pulmonale	Atrium, Left
Auditory tube	Eustachian Tube, Right
	Eustachian Tube, Left
Auerbach's (myenteric) plexus	Abdominal Sympathetic Nerve
Auricle	External Ear, Right
	External Ear, Left
	External Ear, Bilateral
Auricularis muscle	Head Muscle
Axillary fascia	Subcutaneous Tissue and Fascia, Right Upper Arm
	Subcutaneous Tissue and Fascia, Left Upper Arm
Axillary nerve	Brachial Plexus
Bartholin's (greater vestibular) gland	Vestibular Gland
Basal (internal) cerebral vein	Intracranial Vein
Basal nuclei	Basal Ganglia
Base of tongue	Pharynx
Basilar artery	Intracranial Artery
Basis pontis	Pons
Biceps brachii muscle	Upper Arm Muscle, Right
	Upper Arm Muscle, Left
Biceps femoris muscle	Upper Leg Muscle, Right
	Upper Leg Muscle, Left
Bicipital aponeurosis	Subcutaneous Tissue and Fascia, Right Lower Arm
	Subcutaneous Tissue and Fascia, Left Lower Arm

Anatomical Term	ICD-10-PCS Value
Bicuspid valve	Mitral Valve
Body of femur	Femoral Shaft, Right
	Femoral Shaft, Left
Body of fibula	Fibula, Right
	Fibula, Left
Bony labyrinth	Inner Ear, Right
	Inner Ear, Left
Bony orbit	Orbit, Right
	Orbit, Left
Bony vestibule	Inner Ear, Right
	Inner Ear, Left
Botallo's duct	Pulmonary Artery, Left
Brachial (lateral) lymph node	Lymphatic, Right Axillary
	Lymphatic, Left Axillary
Brachialis muscle	Upper Arm Muscle, Right
	Upper Arm Muscle, Left
Brachiocephalic artery	Innominate Artery
Brachiocephalic trunk	Innominate Artery
Brachiocephalic vein	Innominate Vein, Right
	Innominate Vein, Left
Brachioradialis muscle	Lower Arm and Wrist Muscle, Right
	Lower Arm and Wrist Muscle, Left
Breast procedures, skin only	Skin, Chest
Broad ligament	Uterine Supporting Structure
Bronchial artery	Upper Artery
Bronchus intermedius	Main Bronchus, Right
Buccal gland	Buccal Mucosa
Buccinator lymph node	Lymphatic, Head
Buccinator muscle	Facial Muscle
Bulbospongiosus muscle	Perineum Muscle
Bulbourethral (Cowper's) gland	Urethra
Bundle of His	Conduction Mechanism
Bundle of Kent	Conduction Mechanism
Calcaneocuboid joint	Tarsal Joint, Right
	Tarsal Joint, Left
Calcaneocuboid ligament	Foot Bursa and Ligament, Right
	Foot Bursa and Ligament, Left
Calcaneofibular ligament	Ankle Bursa and Ligament, Right
	Ankle Bursa and Ligament, Left
Calcaneus	Tarsal, Right
	Tarsal, Left
Capitate bone	Carpal, Right
	Carpal, Left
Cardia	Esophagogastric Junction
Cardiac plexus	Thoracic Sympathetic Nerve
Cardioesophageal junction	Esophagogastric Junction
Caroticotympanic artery	Internal Carotid Artery, Right
	Internal Carotid Artery, Left

Anatomical Term	ICD-10-PCS Value
Carotid glomus	Carotid Body, Left
	Carotid Body, Right
	Carotid Bodies, Bilateral
Carotid sinus	Internal Carotid Artery, Right
	Internal Carotid Artery, Left
Carotid sinus nerve	Glossopharyngeal Nerve
Carpometacarpal ligament	Hand Bursa and Ligament, Right
	Hand Bursa and Ligament, Left
Cauda equina	Lumbar Spinal Cord
Cavernous plexus	Head and Neck Sympathetic Nerve
Celiac (solar) plexus	Abdominal Sympathetic Nerve
Celiac ganglion	Abdominal Sympathetic Nerve
Celiac lymph node	Lymphatic, Aortic
Celiac trunk	Celiac Artery
Central axillary lymph node	Lymphatic, Right Axillary
	Lymphatic, Left Axillary
Cerebral aqueduct (Sylvius)	Cerebral Ventricle
Cerebrum	Brain
Cervical esophagus	Esophagus, Upper
Cervical facet joint	Cervical Vertebral Joint
	Cervical Vertebral Joints, 2 or more
Cervical ganglion	Head and Neck Sympathetic Nerve
Cervical interspinous ligament	Head and Neck Bursa and Ligament
Cervical intertransverse ligament	Head and Neck Bursa and Ligament
Cervical ligamentum flavum	Head and Neck Bursa and Ligament
Cervical lymph node	Lymphatic, Right Neck
	Lymphatic, Left Neck
Cervicothoracic facet joint	Cervicothoracic Vertebral Joint
Choana	Nasopharynx
Chondroglossus muscle	Tongue, Palate, Pharynx Muscle
Chorda tympani	Facial Nerve
Choroid plexus	Cerebral Ventricle
Ciliary body	Eye, Right
	Eye, Left
Ciliary ganglion	Head and Neck Sympathetic Nerve
Circle of Willis	Intracranial Artery
Circumflex iliac artery	Femoral Artery, Right
	Femoral Artery, Left
Claustrum	Basal Ganglia
Coccygeal body	Coccygeal Glomus
Coccygeus muscle	Trunk Muscle, Right
	Trunk Muscle, Left
Cochlea	Inner Ear, Right
	Inner Ear, Left
Cochlear nerve	Acoustic Nerve

Anatomical Term	ICD-10-PCS Value
Columella	Nasal Mucosa and Soft Tissue
Common digital vein	Foot Vein, Right
	Foot Vein, Left
Common facial vein	Face Vein, Right
	Face Vein, Left
Common fibular nerve	Peroneal Nerve
Common hepatic artery	Hepatic Artery
Common iliac (subaortic) lymph node	Lymphatic, Pelvis
Common interosseous artery	Ulnar Artery, Right
	Ulnar Artery, Left
Common peroneal nerve	Peroneal Nerve
Condyloid process	Mandible, Right
	Mandible, Left
Conus arteriosus	Ventricle, Right
Conus medullaris	Lumbar Spinal Cord
Coracoacromial ligament	Shoulder Bursa and Ligament, Right
	Shoulder Bursa and Ligament, Left
Coracobrachialis muscle	Upper Arm Muscle, Right
	Upper Arm Muscle, Left
Coracoclavicular ligament	Shoulder Bursa and Ligament, Right
	Shoulder Bursa and Ligament, Left
Coracohumeral ligament	Shoulder Bursa and Ligament, Right
	Shoulder Bursa and Ligament, Left
Coracoid process	Scapula, Right
	Scapula, Left
Corniculate cartilage	Larynx
Corpus callosum	Brain
Corpus cavernosum	Penis
Corpus spongiosum	Penis
Corpus striatum	Basal Ganglia
Corrugator supercilii muscle	Facial Muscle
Costocervical trunk	Subclavian Artery, Right
	Subclavian Artery, Left
Costoclavicular ligament	Shoulder Bursa and Ligament, Right
	Shoulder Bursa and Ligament, Left
Costotransverse joint	Thoracic Vertebral Joint
Costotransverse ligament	Rib(s) Bursa and Ligament
Costovertebral joint	Thoracic Vertebral Joint
Costoxiphoid ligament	Sternum Bursa and Ligament
Cowper's (bulbourethral) gland	Urethra
Cremaster muscle	Perineum Muscle
Cribriform plate	Ethmoid Bone, Right
	Ethmoid Bone, Left

Anatomical Term	ICD-10-PCS Value
Cricoid cartilage	Trachea
Cricothyroid artery	Thyroid Artery, Right
	Thyroid Artery, Left
Cricothyroid muscle	Neck Muscle, Right
	Neck Muscle, Left
Crural fascia	Subcutaneous Tissue and Fascia, Right Upper Leg
	Subcutaneous Tissue and Fascia, Left Upper Leg
Cubital lymph node	Lymphatic, Right Upper Extremity
	Lymphatic, Left Upper Extremity
Cubital nerve	Ulnar Nerve
Cuboid bone	Tarsal, Right
	Tarsal, Left
Cuboideonavicular joint	Tarsal Joint, Right
	Tarsal Joint, Left
Culmen	Cerebellum
Cuneiform cartilage	Larynx
Cuneonavicular joint	Tarsal Joint, Right
	Tarsal Joint, Left
Cuneonavicular ligament	Foot Bursa and Ligament, Right
	Foot Bursa and Ligament, Left
Cutaneous (transverse) cervical nerve	Cervical Plexus
Deep cervical fascia	Subcutaneous Tissue and Fascia, Right Neck
	Subcutaneous Tissue and Fascia, Left Neck
Deep cervical vein	Vertebral Vein, Right
	Vertebral Vein, Left
Deep circumflex iliac artery	External Iliac Artery, Right
	External Iliac Artery, Left
Deep facial vein	Face Vein, Right
	Face Vein, Left
Deep femoral (profunda femoris) vein	Femoral Vein, Right
	Femoral Vein, Left
Deep femoral artery	Femoral Artery, Right
	Femoral Artery, Left
Deep palmar arch	Hand Artery, Right
	Hand Artery, Left
Deep transverse perineal muscle	Perineum Muscle
Deferential artery	Internal Iliac Artery, Right
	Internal Iliac Artery, Left
Deltoid fascia	Subcutaneous Tissue and Fascia, Right Upper Arm
	Subcutaneous Tissue and Fascia, Left Upper Arm
Deltoid ligament	Ankle Bursa and Ligament, Right
	Ankle Bursa and Ligament, Left

Anatomical Term	ICD-10-PCS Value
Deltoid muscle	Shoulder Muscle, Right
	Shoulder Muscle, Left
Deltopectoral (infraclavicular) lymph node	Lymphatic, Right Upper Extremity
	Lymphatic, Left Upper Extremity
Dens	Cervical Vertebra
Denticulate (dentate) ligament	Spinal Meninges
Depressor anguli oris muscle	Facial Muscle
Depressor labii inferioris muscle	Facial Muscle
Depressor septi nasi muscle	Facial Muscle
Depressor supercilii muscle	Facial Muscle
Dermis	Skin
Descending genicular artery	Femoral Artery, Right
	Femoral Artery, Left
Diaphragma sellae	Dura Mater
Distal humerus	Humeral Shaft, Right
	Humeral Shaft, Left
Distal humerus, involving joint	Elbow Joint, Right
	Elbow Joint, Left
Distal radioulnar joint	Wrist Joint, Right
	Wrist Joint, Left
Dorsal digital nerve	Radial Nerve
Dorsal metacarpal vein	Hand Vein, Right
	Hand Vein, Left
Dorsal metatarsal artery	Foot Artery, Right
	Foot Artery, Left
Dorsal metatarsal vein	Foot Vein, Right
	Foot Vein, Left
Dorsal scapular artery	Subclavian Artery, Right
	Subclavian Artery, Left
Dorsal scapular nerve	Brachial Plexus
Dorsal venous arch	Foot Vein, Right
	Foot Vein, Left
Dorsalis pedis artery	Anterior Tibial Artery, Right
	Anterior Tibial Artery, Left
Duct of Santorini	Pancreatic Duct, Accessory
Duct of Wirsung	Pancreatic Duct
Ductus deferens	Vas Deferens, Right
	Vas Deferens, Left
	Vas Deferens, Bilateral
	Vas Deferens
Duodenal ampulla	Ampulla of Vater
Duodenojejunal flexure	Jejunum
Dura mater, intracranial	Dura Mater
Dura mater, spinal	Spinal Meninges
Dural venous sinus	Intracranial Vein

Anatomical Term	ICD-10-PCS Value
Earlobe	External Ear, Right
	External Ear, Left
	External Ear, Bilateral
Eighth cranial nerve	Acoustic Nerve
Ejaculatory duct	Vas Deferens, Right
	Vas Deferens, Left
	Vas Deferens, Bilateral
	Vas Deferens
Eleventh cranial nerve	Accessory Nerve
Encephalon	Brain
Ependyma	Cerebral Ventricle
Epidermis	Skin
Epidural space, spinal	Spinal Canal
Epiploic foramen	Peritoneum
Epithalamus	Thalamus
Epitrochlear lymph node	Lymphatic, Right Upper Extremity
	Lymphatic, Left Upper Extremity
Erector spinae muscle	Trunk Muscle, Right
	Trunk Muscle, Left
Esophageal artery	Upper Artery
Esophageal plexus	Thoracic Sympathetic Nerve
Ethmoidal air cell	Ethmoid Sinus, Right
	Ethmoid Sinus, Left
Extensor carpi radialis muscle	Lower Arm and Wrist Muscle, Right
	Lower Arm and Wrist Muscle, Left
Extensor carpi ulnaris muscle	Lower Arm and Wrist Muscle, Right
	Lower Arm and Wrist Muscle, Left
Extensor digitorum brevis muscle	Foot Muscle, Right
	Foot Muscle, Left
Extensor digitorum longus muscle	Lower Leg Muscle, Right
	Lower Leg Muscle, Left
Extensor hallucis brevis muscle	Foot Muscle, Right
	Foot Muscle, Left
Extensor hallucis longus muscle	Lower Leg Muscle, Right
	Lower Leg Muscle, Left
External anal sphincter	Anal Sphincter
External auditory meatus	External Auditory Canal, Right
	External Auditory Canal, Left
External maxillary artery	Face Artery
External naris	Nasal Mucosa and Soft Tissue
External oblique aponeurosis	Subcutaneous Tissue and Fascia, Trunk
External oblique muscle	Abdomen Muscle, Right
	Abdomen Muscle, Left
External popliteal nerve	Peroneal Nerve
External pudendal artery	Femoral Artery, Right
	Femoral Artery, Left
External pudendal vein	Saphenous Vein, Right
	Saphenous Vein, Left
External urethral sphincter	Urethra
Extradural space, intracranial	Epidural Space, Intracranial
Extradural space, spinal	Spinal Canal
Facial artery	Face Artery
False vocal cord	Larynx
Falx cerebri	Dura Mater
Fascia lata	Subcutaneous Tissue and Fascia, Right Upper Leg
	Subcutaneous Tissue and Fascia, Left Upper Leg
Femoral head	Upper Femur, Right
	Upper Femur, Left
Femoral lymph node	Lymphatic, Right Lower Extremity
	Lymphatic, Left Lower Extremity
Femoropatellar joint	Knee Joint, Right
	Knee Joint, Left
	Knee Joint, Femoral Surface, Right
	Knee Joint, Femoral Surface, Left
Femorotibial joint	Knee Joint, Right
	Knee Joint, Left
	Knee Joint, Tibial Surface, Right
	Knee Joint, Tibial Surface, Left
Fibular artery	Peroneal Artery, Right
	Peroneal Artery, Left
Fibularis brevis muscle	Lower Leg Muscle, Right
	Lower Leg Muscle, Left
Fibularis longus muscle	Lower Leg Muscle, Right
	Lower Leg Muscle, Left
Fifth cranial nerve	Trigeminal Nerve
Filum terminale	Spinal Meninges
First cranial nerve	Olfactory Nerve
First intercostal nerve	Brachial Plexus
Flexor carpi radialis muscle	Lower Arm and Wrist Muscle, Right
	Lower Arm and Wrist Muscle, Left
Flexor carpi ulnaris muscle	Lower Arm and Wrist Muscle, Right
	Lower Arm and Wrist Muscle, Left
Flexor digitorum brevis muscle	Foot Muscle, Right
	Foot Muscle, Left
Flexor digitorum longus muscle	Lower Leg Muscle, Right
	Lower Leg Muscle, Left
Flexor hallucis brevis muscle	Foot Muscle, Right
	Foot Muscle, Left
Flexor hallucis longus muscle	Lower Leg Muscle, Right
	Lower Leg Muscle, Left
Flexor pollicis longus muscle	Lower Arm and Wrist Muscle, Right
	Lower Arm and Wrist Muscle, Left

Anatomical Term	ICD-10-PCS Value
Foramen magnum	Occipital Bone
Foramen of Monro (intraventricular)	Cerebral Ventricle
Foreskin	Prepuce
Fossa of Rosenmuller	Nasopharynx
Fourth cranial nerve	Trochlear Nerve
Fourth ventricle	Cerebral Ventricle
Fovea	Retina, Right
	Retina, Left
Frenulum labii inferioris	Lower Lip
Frenulum labii superioris	Upper Lip
Frenulum linguae	Tongue
Frontal lobe	Cerebral Hemisphere
Frontal vein	Face Vein, Right
	Face Vein, Left
Fundus uteri	Uterus
Galea aponeurotica	Subcutaneous Tissue and Fascia, Scalp
Ganglion impar (ganglion of Walther)	Sacral Sympathetic Nerve
Gasserian ganglion	Trigeminal Nerve
Gastric lymph node	Lymphatic, Aortic
Gastric plexus	Abdominal Sympathetic Nerve
Gastrocnemius muscle	Lower Leg Muscle, Right
	Lower Leg Muscle, Left
Gastrocolic ligament	Omentum
Gastrocolic omentum	Omentum
Gastroduodenal artery	Hepatic Artery
Gastroesophageal (GE) junction	Esophagogastric Junction
Gastrohepatic omentum	Omentum
Gastrophrenic ligament	Omentum
Gastrosplenic ligament	Omentum
Gemellus muscle	Hip Muscle, Right
	Hip Muscle, Left
Geniculate ganglion	Facial Nerve
Geniculate nucleus	Thalamus
Genioglossus muscle	Tongue, Palate, Pharynx Muscle
Genitofemoral nerve	Lumbar Plexus
Glans penis	Prepuce
Glenohumeral joint	Shoulder Joint, Right
	Shoulder Joint, Left
Glenohumeral ligament	Shoulder Bursa and Ligament, Right
	Shoulder Bursa and Ligament, Left
Glenoid fossa (of scapula)	Glenoid Cavity, Right
	Glenoid Cavity, Left
Glenoid ligament (labrum)	Shoulder Joint, Right
	Shoulder Joint, Left

Anatomical Term	ICD-10-PCS Value
Globus pallidus	Basal Ganglia
Glossoepiglottic fold	Epiglottis
Glottis	Larynx
Gluteal lymph node	Lymphatic, Pelvis
Gluteal vein	Hypogastric Vein, Right
	Hypogastric Vein, Left
Gluteus maximus muscle	Hip Muscle, Right
	Hip Muscle, Left
Gluteus medius muscle	Hip Muscle, Right
	Hip Muscle, Left
Gluteus minimus muscle	Hip Muscle, Right
	Hip Muscle, Left
Gracilis muscle	Upper Leg Muscle, Right
	Upper Leg Muscle, Left
Great auricular nerve	Cervical Plexus
Great cerebral vein	Intracranial Vein
Great(er) saphenous vein	Saphenous Vein, Right
	Saphenous Vein, Left
Greater alar cartilage	Nasal Mucosa and Soft Tissue
Greater occipital nerve	Cervical Nerve
Greater omentum	Omentum
Greater splanchnic nerve	Thoracic Sympathetic Nerve
Greater superficial petrosal nerve	Facial Nerve
Greater trochanter	Upper Femur, Right
	Upper Femur, Left
Greater tuberosity	Humeral Head, Right
	Humeral Head, Left
Greater vestibular (Bartholin's) gland	Vestibular Gland
Greater wing	Sphenoid Bone
Hallux	1st Toe, Right
	1st Toe, Left
Hamate bone	Carpal, Right
	Carpal, Left
Head of fibula	Fibula, Right
	Fibula, Left
Helix	External Ear, Right
	External Ear, Left
	External Ear, Bilateral
Hepatic artery proper	Hepatic Artery
Hepatic flexure	Transverse Colon
Hepatic lymph node	Lymphatic, Aortic
Hepatic plexus	Abdominal Sympathetic Nerve
Hepatic portal vein	Portal Vein
Hepatogastric ligament	Omentum
Hepatopancreatic ampulla	Ampulla of Vater

Anatomical Term	ICD-10-PCS Value
Humeroradial joint	Elbow Joint, Right
	Elbow Joint, Left
Humeroulnar joint	Elbow Joint, Right
	Elbow Joint, Left
Humerus, distal	Humeral Shaft, Right
	Humeral Shaft, Left
Hyoglossus muscle	Tongue, Palate, Pharynx Muscle
Hyoid artery	Thyroid Artery, Right
	Thyroid Artery, Left
Hypogastric artery	Internal Iliac Artery, Right
	Internal Iliac Artery, Left
Hypopharynx	Pharynx
Hypophysis	Pituitary Gland
Hypothenar muscle	Hand Muscle, Right
	Hand Muscle, Left
Ileal artery	Superior Mesenteric Artery
Ileocolic artery	Superior Mesenteric Artery
Ileocolic vein	Colic Vein
Iliac crest	Pelvic Bone, Right
	Pelvic Bone, Left
Iliac fascia	Subcutaneous Tissue and Fascia, Right Upper Leg
	Subcutaneous Tissue and Fascia, Left Upper Leg
Iliac lymph node	Lymphatic, Pelvis
Iliacus muscle	Hip Muscle, Right
	Hip Muscle, Left
Iliofemoral ligament	Hip Bursa and Ligament, Right
	Hip Bursa and Ligament, Left
Iliohypogastric nerve	Lumbar Plexus
Ilioinguinal nerve	Lumbar Plexus
Iliolumbar artery	Internal Iliac Artery, Right
	Internal Iliac Artery, Left
Iliolumbar ligament	Lower Spine Bursa and Ligament
Iliotibial tract (band)	Subcutaneous Tissue and Fascia, Right Upper Leg
	Subcutaneous Tissue and Fascia, Left Upper Leg
Ilium	Pelvic Bone, Right
	Pelvic Bone, Left
Incus	Auditory Ossicle, Right
	Auditory Ossicle, Left
Inferior cardiac nerve	Thoracic Sympathetic Nerve
Inferior cerebellar vein	Intracranial Vein
Inferior cerebral vein	Intracranial Vein
Inferior epigastric artery	External Iliac Artery, Right
	External Iliac Artery, Left
Inferior epigastric lymph node	Lymphatic, Pelvis

Anatomical Term	ICD-10-PCS Value
Inferior genicular artery	Popliteal Artery, Right
	Popliteal Artery, Left
Inferior gluteal artery	Internal Iliac Artery, Right
	Internal Iliac Artery, Left
Inferior gluteal nerve	Sacral Plexus
Inferior hypogastric plexus	Abdominal Sympathetic Nerve
Inferior labial artery	Face Artery
Inferior longitudinal muscle	Tongue, Palate, Pharynx Muscle
Inferior mesenteric ganglion	Abdominal Sympathetic Nerve
Inferior mesenteric lymph node	Lymphatic, Mesenteric
Inferior mesenteric plexus	Abdominal Sympathetic Nerve
Inferior oblique muscle	Extraocular Muscle, Right
	Extraocular Muscle, Left
Inferior pancreaticoduodenal artery	Superior Mesenteric Artery
Inferior phrenic artery	Abdominal Aorta
Inferior rectus muscle	Extraocular Muscle, Right
	Extraocular Muscle, Left
Inferior suprarenal artery	Renal Artery, Right
	Renal Artery, Left
Inferior tarsal plate	Lower Eyelid, Right
	Lower Eyelid, Left
Inferior thyroid vein	Innominate Vein, Right
	Innominate Vein, Left
Inferior tibiofibular joint	Ankle Joint, Right
	Ankle Joint, Left
Inferior turbinate	Nasal Turbinate
Inferior ulnar collateral artery	Brachial Artery, Right
	Brachial Artery, Left
Inferior vesical artery	Internal Iliac Artery, Right
	Internal Iliac Artery, Left
Infraauricular lymph node	Lymphatic, Head
Infraclavicular (deltopectoral) lymph node	Lymphatic, Right Upper Extremity
	Lymphatic, Left Upper Extremity
Infrahyoid muscle	Neck Muscle, Right
	Neck Muscle, Left
Infraparotid lymph node	Lymphatic, Head
Infraspinatus fascia	Subcutaneous Tissue and Fascia, Right Upper Arm
	Subcutaneous Tissue and Fascia, Left Upper Arm
Infraspinatus muscle	Shoulder Muscle, Right
	Shoulder Muscle, Left
Infundibulopelvic ligament	Uterine Supporting Structure
Inguinal canal	Inguinal Region, Right
	Inguinal Region, Left
	Inguinal Region, Bilateral

Anatomical Term	ICD-10-PCS Value
Inguinal triangle	Inguinal Region, Right
	Inguinal Region, Left
	Inguinal Region, Bilateral
Interatrial septum	Atrial Septum
Intercarpal joint	Carpal Joint, Right
	Carpal Joint, Left
Intercarpal ligament	Hand Bursa and Ligament, Right
	Hand Bursa and Ligament, Left
Interclavicular ligament	Shoulder Bursa and Ligament, Right
	Shoulder Bursa and Ligament, Left
Intercostal lymph node	Lymphatic, Thorax
Intercostal muscle	Thorax Muscle, Right
	Thorax Muscle, Left
Intercostal nerve	Thoracic Nerve
Intercostobrachial nerve	Thoracic Nerve
Intercuneiform joint	Tarsal Joint, Right
	Tarsal Joint, Left
Intercuneiform ligament	Foot Bursa and Ligament, Right
	Foot Bursa and Ligament, Left
Intermediate bronchus	Main Bronchus, Right
Intermediate cuneiform bone	Tarsal, Right
	Tarsal, Left
Internal (basal) cerebral vein	Intracranial Vein
Internal anal sphincter	Anal Sphincter
Internal carotid artery, intracranial portion	Intracranial Artery
Internal carotid plexus	Head and Neck Sympathetic Nerve
Internal iliac vein	Hypogastric Vein, Right
	Hypogastric Vein, Left
Internal maxillary artery	External Carotid Artery, Right
	External Carotid Artery, Left
Internal naris	Nasal Mucosa and Soft Tissue
Internal oblique muscle	Abdomen Muscle, Right
	Abdomen Muscle, Left
Internal pudendal artery	Internal Iliac Artery, Right
	Internal Iliac Artery, Left
Internal pudendal vein	Hypogastric Vein, Right
	Hypogastric Vein, Left
Internal thoracic artery	Internal Mammary Artery, Right
	Internal Mammary Artery, Left
	Subclavian Artery, Right
	Subclavian Artery, Left
Internal urethral sphincter	Urethra
Interphalangeal (IP) joint	Finger Phalangeal Joint, Right
	Finger Phalangeal Joint, Left
	Toe Phalangeal Joint, Right
	Toe Phalangeal Joint, Left

Anatomical Term	ICD-10-PCS Value
Interphalangeal ligament	Hand Bursa and Ligament, Right
	Hand Bursa and Ligament, Left
	Foot Bursa and Ligament, Right
	Foot Bursa and Ligament, Left
Interspinalis muscle	Trunk Muscle, Right
	Trunk Muscle, Left
Interspinous ligament, cervical	Head and Neck Bursa and Ligament
Interspinous ligament, lumbar	Lower Spine Bursa and Ligament
Interspinous ligament, thoracic	Upper Spine Bursa and Ligament
Intertransversarius muscle	Trunk Muscle, Right
	Trunk Muscle, Left
Intertransverse ligament, cervical	Head and Neck Bursa and Ligament
Intertransverse ligament, lumbar	Lower Spine Bursa and Ligament
Intertransverse ligament, thoracic	Upper Spine Bursa and Ligament
Interventricular foramen (Monro)	Cerebral Ventricle
Interventricular septum	Ventricular Septum
Intestinal lymphatic trunk	Cisterna Chyli
Ischiatic nerve	Sciatic Nerve
Ischiocavernosus muscle	Perineum Muscle
Ischiofemoral ligament	Hip Bursa and Ligament, Right
	Hip Bursa and Ligament, Left
Ischium	Pelvic Bone, Right
	Pelvic Bone, Left
Jejunal artery	Superior Mesenteric Artery
Jugular body	Glomus Jugulare
Jugular lymph node	Lymphatic, Right Neck
	Lymphatic, Left Neck
Labia majora	Vulva
Labia minora	Vulva
Labial gland	Upper Lip
	Lower Lip
Lacrimal canaliculus	Lacrimal Duct, Right
	Lacrimal Duct, Left
Lacrimal punctum	Lacrimal Duct, Right
	Lacrimal Duct, Left
Lacrimal sac	Lacrimal Duct, Right
	Lacrimal Duct, Left
Laryngopharynx	Pharynx
Lateral (brachial) lymph node	Lymphatic, Right Axillary
	Lymphatic, Left Axillary
Lateral canthus	Upper Eyelid, Right
	Upper Eyelid, Left

Anatomical Term	ICD-10-PCS Value
Lateral collateral ligament (LCL)	Knee Bursa and Ligament, Right
	Knee Bursa and Ligament, Left
Lateral condyle of femur	Lower Femur, Right
	Lower Femur, Left
Lateral condyle of tibia	Tibia, Right
	Tibia, Left
Lateral cuneiform bone	Tarsal, Right
	Tarsal, Left
Lateral epicondyle of femur	Lower Femur, Right
	Lower Femur, Left
Lateral epicondyle of humerus	Humeral Shaft, Right
	Humeral Shaft, Left
Lateral femoral cutaneous nerve	Lumbar Plexus
Lateral malleolus	Fibula, Right
	Fibula, Left
Lateral meniscus	Knee Joint, Right
	Knee Joint, Left
Lateral nasal cartilage	Nasal Mucosa and Soft Tissue
Lateral plantar artery	Foot Artery, Right
	Foot Artery, Left
Lateral plantar nerve	Tibial Nerve
Lateral rectus muscle	Extraocular Muscle, Right
	Extraocular Muscle, Left
Lateral sacral artery	Internal Iliac Artery, Right
	Internal Iliac Artery, Left
Lateral sacral vein	Hypogastric Vein, Right
	Hypogastric Vein, Left
Lateral sural cutaneous nerve	Peroneal Nerve
Lateral tarsal artery	Foot Artery, Right
	Foot Artery, Left
Lateral temporomandibular ligament	Head and Neck Bursa and Ligament
Lateral thoracic artery	Axillary Artery, Right
	Axillary Artery, Left
Latissimus dorsi muscle	Trunk Muscle, Right
	Trunk Muscle, Left
Least splanchnic nerve	Thoracic Sympathetic Nerve
Left ascending lumbar vein	Hemiazygos Vein
Left atrioventricular valve	Mitral Valve
Left auricular appendix	Atrium, Left
Left colic vein	Colic Vein
Left coronary sulcus	Heart, Left
Left gastric artery	Gastric Artery
Left gastroepiploic artery	Splenic Artery
Left gastroepiploic vein	Splenic Vein
Left inferior phrenic vein	Renal Vein, Left
Left inferior pulmonary vein	Pulmonary Vein, Left
Left jugular trunk	Thoracic Duct
Left lateral ventricle	Cerebral Ventricle
Left ovarian vein	Renal Vein, Left
Left second lumbar vein	Renal Vein, Left
Left subclavian trunk	Thoracic Duct
Left subcostal vein	Hemiazygos Vein
Left superior pulmonary vein	Pulmonary Vein, Left
Left suprarenal vein	Renal Vein, Left
Left testicular vein	Renal Vein, Left
Leptomeninges, intracranial	Cerebral Meninges
Leptomeninges, spinal	Spinal Meninges
Lesser alar cartilage	Nasal Mucosa and Soft Tissue
Lesser occipital nerve	Cervical Plexus
Lesser omentum	Omentum
Lesser saphenous vein	Saphenous Vein, Right
	Saphenous Vein, Left
Lesser splanchnic nerve	Thoracic Sympathetic Nerve
Lesser trochanter	Upper Femur, Right
	Upper Femur, Left
Lesser tuberosity	Humeral Head, Right
	Humeral Head, Left
Lesser wing	Sphenoid Bone
Levator anguli oris muscle	Facial Muscle
Levator ani muscle	Perineum Muscle
Levator labii superioris alaeque nasi muscle	Facial Muscle
Levator labii superioris muscle	Facial Muscle
Levator palpebrae superioris muscle	Upper Eyelid, Right
	Upper Eyelid, Left
Levator scapulae muscle	Neck Muscle, Right
	Neck Muscle, Left
Levator veli palatini muscle	Tongue, Palate, Pharynx Muscle
Levatores costarum muscle	Thorax Muscle, Right
	Thorax Muscle, Left
Ligament of head of fibula	Knee Bursa and Ligament, Right
	Knee Bursa and Ligament, Left
Ligament of the lateral malleolus	Ankle Bursa and Ligament, Right
	Ankle Bursa and Ligament, Left
Ligamentum flavum, cervical	Head and Neck Bursa and Ligament
Ligamentum flavum, lumbar	Lower Spine Bursa and Ligament
Ligamentum flavum, thoracic	Upper Spine Bursa and Ligament
Lingual artery	External Carotid Artery, Right
	External Carotid Artery, Left
Lingual tonsil	Pharynx
Locus ceruleus	Pons
Long thoracic nerve	Brachial Plexus

Anatomical Term	ICD-10-PCS Value
Lumbar artery	Abdominal Aorta
Lumbar facet joint	Lumbar Vertebral Joint
Lumbar ganglion	Lumbar Sympathetic Nerve
Lumbar lymph node	Lymphatic, Aortic
Lumbar lymphatic trunk	Cisterna Chyli
Lumbar splanchnic nerve	Lumbar Sympathetic Nerve
Lumbosacral facet joint	Lumbosacral Joint
Lumbosacral trunk	Lumbar Nerve
Lunate bone	Carpal, Right
	Carpal, Left
Lunotriquetral ligament	Hand Bursa and Ligament, Right
	Hand Bursa and Ligament, Left
Macula	Retina, Right
	Retina, Left
Malleus	Auditory Ossicle, Right
	Auditory Ossicle, Left
Mammary duct	Breast, Right
	Breast, Left
	Breast, Bilateral
Mammary gland	Breast, Right
	Breast, Left
	Breast, Bilateral
Mammillary body	Hypothalamus
Mandibular nerve	Trigeminal Nerve
Mandibular notch	Mandible, Right
	Mandible, Left
Manubrium	Sternum
Masseter muscle	Head Muscle
Masseteric fascia	Subcutaneous Tissue and Fascia, Face
Mastoid (postauricular) lymph node	Lymphatic, Right Neck
	Lymphatic, Left Neck
Mastoid air cells	Mastoid Sinus, Right
	Mastoid Sinus, Left
Mastoid process	Temporal Bone, Right
	Temporal Bone, Left
Maxillary artery	External Carotid Artery, Right
	External Carotid Artery, Left
Maxillary nerve	Trigeminal Nerve
Medial canthus	Lower Eyelid, Right
	Lower Eyelid, Left
Medial collateral ligament (MCL)	Knee Bursa and Ligament, Right
	Knee Bursa and Ligament, Left
Medial condyle of femur	Lower Femur, Right
	Lower Femur, Left
Medial condyle of tibia	Tibia, Right
	Tibia, Left

Anatomical Term	ICD-10-PCS Value
Medial cuneiform bone	Tarsal, Right
	Tarsal, Left
Medial epicondyle of femur	Lower Femur, Right
	Lower Femur, Left
Medial epicondyle of humerus	Humeral Shaft, Right
	Humeral Shaft, Left
Medial malleolus	Tibia, Right
	Tibia, Left
Medial meniscus	Knee Joint, Right
	Knee Joint, Left
Medial plantar artery	Foot Artery, Right
	Foot Artery, Left
Medial plantar nerve	Tibial Nerve
Medial popliteal nerve	Tibial Nerve
Medial rectus muscle	Extraocular Muscle, Right
	Extraocular Muscle, Left
Medial sural cutaneous nerve	Tibial Nerve
Median antebrachial vein	Basilic Vein, Right
	Basilic Vein, Left
Median cubital vein	Basilic Vein, Right
	Basilic Vein, Left
Median sacral artery	Abdominal Aorta
Mediastinal cavity	Mediastinum
Mediastinal lymph node	Lymphatic, Thorax
Mediastinal space	Mediastinum
Meissner's (submucous) plexus	Abdominal Sympathetic Nerve
Membranous urethra	Urethra
Mental foramen	Mandible, Right
	Mandible, Left
Mentalis muscle	Facial Muscle
Mesoappendix	Mesentery
Mesocolon	Mesentery
Metacarpal ligament	Hand Bursa and Ligament, Right
	Hand Bursa and Ligament, Left
Metacarpophalangeal ligament	Hand Bursa and Ligament, Right
	Hand Bursa and Ligament, Left
Metatarsal ligament	Foot Bursa and Ligament, Right
	Foot Bursa and Ligament, Left
Metatarsophalangeal (MTP) joint	Metatarsal-Phalangeal Joint, Right
	Metatarsal-Phalangeal Joint, Left
Metatarsophalangeal ligament	Foot Bursa and Ligament, Right
	Foot Bursa and Ligament, Left
Metathalamus	Thalamus
Midcarpal joint	Carpal Joint, Right
	Carpal Joint, Left
Middle cardiac nerve	Thoracic Sympathetic Nerve
Middle cerebral artery	Intracranial Artery

Anatomical Term	ICD-10-PCS Value
Middle cerebral vein	Intracranial Vein
Middle colic vein	Colic Vein
Middle genicular artery	Popliteal Artery, Right
	Popliteal Artery, Left
Middle hemorrhoidal vein	Hypogastric Vein, Right
	Hypogastric Vein, Left
Middle rectal artery	Internal Iliac Artery, Right
	Internal Iliac Artery, Left
Middle suprarenal artery	Abdominal Aorta
Middle temporal artery	Temporal Artery, Right
	Temporal Artery, Left
Middle turbinate	Nasal Turbinate
Mitral annulus	Mitral Valve
Molar gland	Buccal Mucosa
Musculocutaneous nerve	Brachial Plexus
Musculophrenic artery	Internal Mammary Artery, Right
	Internal Mammary Artery, Left
Musculospiral nerve	Radial Nerve
Myelencephalon	Medulla Oblongata
Myenteric (Auerbach's) plexus	Abdominal Sympathetic Nerve
Myometrium	Uterus
Nail bed	Finger Nail
	Toe Nail
Nail plate	Finger Nail
	Toe Nail
Nasal cavity	Nasal Mucosa and Soft Tissue
Nasal concha	Nasal Turbinate
Nasalis muscle	Facial Muscle
Nasolacrimal duct	Lacrimal Duct, Right
	Lacrimal Duct, Left
Navicular bone	Tarsal, Right
	Tarsal, Left
Neck of femur	Upper Femur, Right
	Upper Femur, Left
Neck of humerus (anatomical) (surgical)	Humeral Head, Right
	Humeral Head, Left
Nerve to the stapedius	Facial Nerve
Neurohypophysis	Pituitary Gland
Ninth cranial nerve	Glossopharyngeal Nerve
Nostril	Nasal Mucosa and Soft Tissue
Obturator artery	Internal Iliac Artery, Right
	Internal Iliac Artery, Left
Obturator lymph node	Lymphatic, Pelvis
Obturator muscle	Hip Muscle, Right
	Hip Muscle, Left
Obturator nerve	Lumbar Plexus

Anatomical Term	ICD-10-PCS Value
Obturator vein	Hypogastric Vein, Right
	Hypogastric Vein, Left
Obtuse margin	Heart, Left
Occipital artery	External Carotid Artery, Right
	External Carotid Artery, Left
Occipital lobe	Cerebral Hemisphere
Occipital lymph node	Lymphatic, Right Neck
	Lymphatic, Left Neck
Occipitofrontalis muscle	Facial Muscle
Odontoid process	Cervical Vertebra
Olecranon bursa	Elbow Bursa and Ligament, Right
	Elbow Bursa and Ligament, Left
Olecranon process	Ulna, Right
	Ulna, Left
Olfactory bulb	Olfactory Nerve
Ophthalmic artery	Intracranial Artery
Ophthalmic nerve	Trigeminal Nerve
Ophthalmic vein	Intracranial Vein
Optic chiasma	Optic Nerve
Optic disc	Retina, Right
	Retina, Left
Optic foramen	Sphenoid Bone
Orbicularis oculi muscle	Upper Eyelid, Right
	Upper Eyelid, Left
Orbicularis oris muscle	Facial Muscle
Orbital fascia	Subcutaneous Tissue and Fascia, Face
Orbital portion of ethmoid bone	Orbit, Right
	Orbit, Left
Orbital portion of frontal bone	Orbit, Right
	Orbit, Left
Orbital portion of lacrimal bone	Orbit, Right
	Orbit, Left
Orbital portion of maxilla	Orbit, Right
	Orbit, Left
Orbital portion of palatine bone	Orbit, Right
	Orbit, Left
Orbital portion of sphenoid bone	Orbit, Right
	Orbit, Left
Orbital portion of zygomatic bone	Orbit, Right
	Orbit, Left
Oropharynx	Pharynx
Otic ganglion	Head and Neck Sympathetic Nerve
Oval window	Middle Ear, Right
	Middle Ear, Left
Ovarian artery	Abdominal Aorta
Ovarian ligament	Uterine Supporting Structure

Anatomical Term	ICD-10-PCS Value
Oviduct	Fallopian Tube, Right
	Fallopian Tube, Left
Palatine gland	Buccal Mucosa
Palatine tonsil	Tonsils
Palatine uvula	Uvula
Palatoglossal muscle	Tongue, Palate, Pharynx Muscle
Palatopharyngeal muscle	Tongue, Palate, Pharynx Muscle
Palmar (volar) digital vein	Hand Vein, Right
	Hand Vein, Left
Palmar (volar) metacarpal vein	Hand Vein, Right
	Hand Vein, Left
Palmar cutaneous nerve	Median Nerve
	Radial Nerve
Palmar fascia (aponeurosis)	Subcutaneous Tissue and Fascia, Right Hand
	Subcutaneous Tissue and Fascia, Left Hand
Palmar interosseous muscle	Hand Muscle, Right
	Hand Muscle, Left
Palmar ulnocarpal ligament	Wrist Bursa and Ligament, Right
	Wrist Bursa and Ligament, Left
Palmaris longus muscle	Lower Arm and Wrist Muscle, Right
	Lower Arm and Wrist Muscle, Left
Pancreatic artery	Splenic Artery
Pancreatic plexus	Abdominal Sympathetic Nerve
Pancreatic vein	Splenic Vein
Pancreaticosplenic lymph node	Lymphatic, Aortic
Paraaortic lymph node	Lymphatic, Aortic
Pararectal lymph node	Lymphatic, Mesenteric
Parasternal lymph node	Lymphatic, Thorax
Paratracheal lymph node	Lymphatic, Thorax
Paraurethral (Skene's) gland	Vestibular Gland
Parietal lobe	Cerebral Hemisphere
Parotid lymph node	Lymphatic, Head
Parotid plexus	Facial Nerve
Pars flaccida	Tympanic Membrane, Right
	Tympanic Membrane, Left
Patellar ligament	Knee Bursa and Ligament, Right
	Knee Bursa and Ligament, Left
Patellar tendon	Knee Tendon, Right
	Knee Tendon, Left
Patellofemoral joint	Knee Joint, Right
	Knee Joint, Left
	Knee Joint, Femoral Surface, Right
	Knee Joint, Femoral Surface, Left
Pectineus muscle	Upper Leg Muscle, Right
	Upper Leg Muscle, Left

Anatomical Term	ICD-10-PCS Value
Pectoral (anterior) lymph node	Lymphatic, Right Axillary
	Lymphatic, Left Axillary
Pectoral fascia	Subcutaneous Tissue and Fascia, Chest
Pectoralis major muscle	Thorax Muscle, Right
	Thorax Muscle, Left
Pectoralis minor muscle	Thorax Muscle, Right
	Thorax Muscle, Left
Pelvic splanchnic nerve	Abdominal Sympathetic Nerve
	Sacral Sympathetic Nerve
Penile urethra	Urethra
Pericardiophrenic artery	Internal Mammary Artery, Right
	Internal Mammary Artery, Left
Perimetrium	Uterus
Peroneus brevis muscle	Lower Leg Muscle, Right
	Lower Leg Muscle, Left
Peroneus longus muscle	Lower Leg Muscle, Right
	Lower Leg Muscle, Left
Petrous part of temporal bone	Temporal Bone, Right
	Temporal Bone, Left
Pharyngeal constrictor muscle	Tongue, Palate, Pharynx Muscle
Pharyngeal plexus	Vagus Nerve
Pharyngeal recess	Nasopharynx
Pharyngeal tonsil	Adenoids
Pharyngotympanic tube	Eustachian Tube, Right
	Eustachian Tube, Left
Pia mater, intracranial	Cerebral Meninges
Pia mater, spinal	Spinal Meninges
Pinna	External Ear, Right
	External Ear, Left
	External Ear, Bilateral
Piriform recess (sinus)	Pharynx
Piriformis muscle	Hip Muscle, Right
	Hip Muscle, Left
Pisiform bone	Carpal, Right
	Carpal, Left
Pisohamate ligament	Hand Bursa and Ligament, Right
	Hand Bursa and Ligament, Left
Pisometacarpal ligament	Hand Bursa and Ligament, Right
	Hand Bursa and Ligament, Left
Plantar digital vein	Foot Vein, Right
	Foot Vein, Left
Plantar fascia (aponeurosis)	Subcutaneous Tissue and Fascia, Right Foot
	Subcutaneous Tissue and Fascia, Left Foot

Anatomical Term	ICD-10-PCS Value
Plantar metatarsal vein	Foot Vein, Right
	Foot Vein, Left
Plantar venous arch	Foot Vein, Right
	Foot Vein, Left
Platysma muscle	Neck Muscle, Right
	Neck Muscle, Left
Plica semilunaris	Conjunctiva, Right
	Conjunctiva, Left
Pneumogastric nerve	Vagus Nerve
Pneumotaxic center	Pons
Pontine tegmentum	Pons
Popliteal ligament	Knee Bursa and Ligament, Right
	Knee Bursa and Ligament, Left
Popliteal lymph node	Lymphatic, Right Lower Extremity
	Lymphatic, Left Lower Extremity
Popliteal vein	Femoral Vein, Right
	Femoral Vein, Left
Popliteus muscle	Lower Leg Muscle, Right
	Lower Leg Muscle, Left
Postauricular (mastoid) lymph node	Lymphatic, Right Neck
	Lymphatic, Left Neck
Postcava	Inferior Vena Cava
Posterior (subscapular) lymph node	Lymphatic, Right Axillary
	Lymphatic, Left Axillary
Posterior auricular artery	External Carotid Artery, Right
	External Carotid Artery, Left
Posterior auricular nerve	Facial Nerve
Posterior auricular vein	External Jugular Vein, Right
	External Jugular Vein, Left
Posterior cerebral artery	Intracranial Artery
Posterior chamber	Eye, Right
	Eye, Left
Posterior circumflex humeral artery	Axillary Artery, Right
	Axillary Artery, Left
Posterior communicating artery	Intracranial Artery
Posterior cruciate ligament (PCL)	Knee Bursa and Ligament, Right
	Knee Bursa and Ligament, Left
Posterior facial (retromandibular) vein	Face Vein, Right
	Face Vein, Left
Posterior femoral cutaneous nerve	Sacral Plexus
Posterior inferior cerebellar artery (PICA)	Intracranial Artery
Posterior interosseous nerve	Radial Nerve
Posterior labial nerve	Pudendal Nerve
Posterior scrotal nerve	Pudendal Nerve

Anatomical Term	ICD-10-PCS Value
Posterior spinal artery	Vertebral Artery, Right
	Vertebral Artery, Left
Posterior tibial recurrent artery	Anterior Tibial Artery, Right
	Anterior Tibial Artery, Left
Posterior ulnar recurrent artery	Ulnar Artery, Right
	Ulnar Artery, Left
Posterior vagal trunk	Vagus Nerve
Preauricular lymph node	Lymphatic, Head
Precava	Superior Vena Cava
Prepatellar bursa	Knee Bursa and Ligament, Right
	Knee Bursa and Ligament, Left
Pretracheal fascia	Subcutaneous Tissue and Fascia, Right Neck
	Subcutaneous Tissue and Fascia, Left Neck
Prevertebral fascia	Subcutaneous Tissue and Fascia, Right Neck
	Subcutaneous Tissue and Fascia, Left Neck
Princeps pollicis artery	Hand Artery, Right
	Hand Artery, Left
Procerus muscle	Facial Muscle
Profunda brachii	Brachial Artery, Right
	Brachial Artery, Left
Profunda femoris (deep femoral) vein	Femoral Vein, Right
	Femoral Vein, Left
Pronator quadratus muscle	Lower Arm and Wrist Muscle, Right
	Lower Arm and Wrist Muscle, Left
Pronator teres muscle	Lower Arm and Wrist Muscle, Right
	Lower Arm and Wrist Muscle, Left
Prostatic urethra	Urethra
Proximal radioulnar joint	Elbow Joint, Right
	Elbow Joint, Left
Psoas muscle	Hip Muscle, Right
	Hip Muscle, Left
Pterygoid muscle	Head Muscle
Pterygoid process	Sphenoid Bone
Pterygopalatine (sphenopalatine) ganglion	Head and Neck Sympathetic Nerve
Pubis	Pelvic Bone, Right
	Pelvic Bone, Left
Pubofemoral ligament	Hip Bursa and Ligament, Right
	Hip Bursa and Ligament, Left
Pudendal nerve	Sacral Plexus
Pulmoaortic canal	Pulmonary Artery, Left
Pulmonary annulus	Pulmonary Valve
Pulmonary plexus	Vagus Nerve
	Thoracic Sympathetic Nerve

Anatomical Term	ICD-10-PCS Value
Pulmonic valve	Pulmonary Valve
Pulvinar	Thalamus
Pyloric antrum	Stomach, Pylorus
Pyloric canal	Stomach, Pylorus
Pyloric sphincter	Stomach, Pylorus
Pyramidalis muscle	Abdomen Muscle, Right
	Abdomen Muscle, Left
Quadrangular cartilage	Nasal Septum
Quadrate lobe	Liver
Quadratus femoris muscle	Hip Muscle, Right
	Hip Muscle, Left
Quadratus lumborum muscle	Trunk Muscle, Right
	Trunk Muscle, Left
Quadratus plantae muscle	Foot Muscle, Right
	Foot Muscle, Left
Quadriceps (femoris)	Upper Leg Muscle, Right
	Upper Leg Muscle, Left
Radial collateral carpal ligament	Wrist Bursa and Ligament, Right
	Wrist Bursa and Ligament, Left
Radial collateral ligament	Elbow Bursa and Ligament, Right
	Elbow Bursa and Ligament, Left
Radial notch	Ulna, Right
	Ulna, Left
Radial recurrent artery	Radial Artery, Right
	Radial Artery, Left
Radial vein	Brachial Vein, Right
	Brachial Vein, Left
Radialis indicis	Hand Artery, Right
	Hand Artery, Left
Radiocarpal joint	Wrist Joint, Right
	Wrist Joint, Left
Radiocarpal ligament	Wrist Bursa and Ligament, Right
	Wrist Bursa and Ligament, Left
Radioulnar ligament	Wrist Bursa and Ligament, Right
	Wrist Bursa and Ligament, Left
Rectosigmoid junction	Sigmoid Colon
Rectus abdominis muscle	Abdomen Muscle, Right
	Abdomen Muscle, Left
Rectus femoris muscle	Upper Leg Muscle, Right
	Upper Leg Muscle, Left
Recurrent laryngeal nerve	Vagus Nerve
Renal calyx	Kidney, Right
	Kidney, Left
	Kidneys, Bilateral
	Kidney

Anatomical Term	ICD-10-PCS Value
Renal capsule	Kidney, Right
	Kidney, Left
	Kidneys, Bilateral
	Kidney
Renal cortex	Kidney, Right
	Kidney, Left
	Kidneys, Bilateral
	Kidney
Renal plexus	Abdominal Sympathetic Nerve
Renal segment	Kidney, Right
	Kidney, Left
	Kidneys, Bilateral
	Kidney
Renal segmental artery	Renal Artery, Right
	Renal Artery, Left
Retroperitoneal cavity	Retroperitoneum
Retroperitoneal lymph node	Lymphatic, Aortic
Retroperitoneal space	Retroperitoneum
Retropharyngeal lymph node	Lymphatic, Right Neck
	Lymphatic, Left Neck
Retropubic space	Pelvic Cavity
Rhinopharynx	Nasopharynx
Rhomboid major muscle	Trunk Muscle, Right
	Trunk Muscle, Left
Rhomboid minor muscle	Trunk Muscle, Right
	Trunk Muscle, Left
Right ascending lumbar vein	Azygos Vein
Right atrioventricular valve	Tricuspid Valve
Right auricular appendix	Atrium, Right
Right colic vein	Colic Vein
Right coronary sulcus	Heart, Right
Right gastric artery	Gastric Artery
Right gastroepiploic vein	Superior Mesenteric Vein
Right inferior phrenic vein	Inferior Vena Cava
Right inferior pulmonary vein	Pulmonary Vein, Right
Right jugular trunk	Lymphatic, Right Neck
Right lateral ventricle	Cerebral Ventricle
Right lymphatic duct	Lymphatic, Right Neck
Right ovarian vein	Inferior Vena Cava
Right second lumbar vein	Inferior Vena Cava
Right subclavian trunk	Lymphatic, Right Neck
Right subcostal vein	Azygos Vein
Right superior pulmonary vein	Pulmonary Vein, Right
Right suprarenal vein	Inferior Vena Cava
Right testicular vein	Inferior Vena Cava
Rima glottidis	Larynx
Risorius muscle	Facial Muscle

Anatomical Term	ICD-10-PCS Value
Round ligament of uterus	Uterine Supporting Structure
Round window	Inner Ear, Right
	Inner Ear, Left
Sacral ganglion	Sacral Sympathetic Nerve
Sacral lymph node	Lymphatic, Pelvis
Sacral splanchnic nerve	Sacral Sympathetic Nerve
Sacrococcygeal ligament	Lower Spine Bursa and Ligament
Sacrococcygeal symphysis	Sacrococcygeal Joint
Sacroiliac ligament	Lower Spine Bursa and Ligament
Sacrospinous ligament	Lower Spine Bursa and Ligament
Sacrotuberous ligament	Lower Spine Bursa and Ligament
Salpingopharyngeus muscle	Tongue, Palate, Pharynx Muscle
Salpinx	Fallopian Tube, Right
	Fallopian Tube, Left
Saphenous nerve	Femoral Nerve
Sartorius muscle	Upper Leg Muscle, Right
	Upper Leg Muscle, Left
Scalene muscle	Neck Muscle, Right
	Neck Muscle, Left
Scaphoid bone	Carpal, Right
	Carpal, Left
Scapholunate ligament	Hand Bursa and Ligament, Right
	Hand Bursa and Ligament, Left
Scaphotrapezium ligament	Hand Bursa and Ligament, Right
	Hand Bursa and Ligament, Left
Scarpa's (vestibular) ganglion	Acoustic Nerve
Sebaceous gland	Skin
Second cranial nerve	Optic Nerve
Sella turcica	Sphenoid Bone
Semicircular canal	Inner Ear, Right
	Inner Ear, Left
Semimembranosus muscle	Upper Leg Muscle, Right
	Upper Leg Muscle, Left
Semitendinosus muscle	Upper Leg Muscle, Right
	Upper Leg Muscle, Left
Septal cartilage	Nasal Septum
Serratus anterior muscle	Thorax Muscle, Right
	Thorax Muscle, Left
Serratus posterior muscle	Trunk Muscle, Right
	Trunk Muscle, Left
Seventh cranial nerve	Facial Nerve
Short gastric artery	Splenic Artery
Sigmoid artery	Inferior Mesenteric Artery
Sigmoid flexure	Sigmoid Colon
Sigmoid vein	Inferior Mesenteric Vein
Sinoatrial node	Conduction Mechanism
Sinus venosus	Atrium, Right
Sixth cranial nerve	Abducens Nerve

Anatomical Term	ICD-10-PCS Value
Skene's (paraurethral) gland	Vestibular Gland
Small saphenous vein	Saphenous Vein, Right
	Saphenous Vein, Left
Solar (celiac) plexus	Abdominal Sympathetic Nerve
Soleus muscle	Lower Leg Muscle, Right
	Lower Leg Muscle, Left
Sphenomandibular ligament	Head and Neck Bursa and Ligament
Sphenopalatine (pterygopalatine) ganglion	Head and Neck Sympathetic Nerve
Spinal nerve, cervical	Cervical Nerve
Spinal nerve, lumbar	Lumbar Nerve
Spinal nerve, sacral	Sacral Nerve
Spinal nerve, thoracic	Thoracic Nerve
Spinous process	Cervical Vertebra
	Thoracic Vertebra
	Lumbar Vertebra
Spiral ganglion	Acoustic Nerve
Splenic flexure	Transverse Colon
Splenic plexus	Abdominal Sympathetic Nerve
Splenius capitis muscle	Head Muscle
Splenius cervicis muscle	Neck Muscle, Right
	Neck Muscle, Left
Stapes	Auditory Ossicle, Right
	Auditory Ossicle, Left
Stellate ganglion	Head and Neck Sympathetic Nerve
Stensen's duct	Parotid Duct, Right
	Parotid Duct, Left
Sternoclavicular ligament	Shoulder Bursa and Ligament, Right
	Shoulder Bursa and Ligament, Left
Sternocleidomastoid artery	Thyroid Artery, Right
	Thyroid Artery, Left
Sternocleidomastoid muscle	Neck Muscle, Right
	Neck Muscle, Left
Sternocostal ligament	Sternum Bursa and Ligament
Styloglossus muscle	Tongue, Palate, Pharynx Muscle
Stylomandibular ligament	Head and Neck Bursa and Ligament
Stylopharyngeus muscle	Tongue, Palate, Pharynx Muscle
Subacromial bursa	Shoulder Bursa and Ligament, Right
	Shoulder Bursa and Ligament, Left
Subaortic (common iliac) lymph node	Lymphatic, Pelvis
Subarachnoid space, spinal	Spinal Canal
Subclavicular (apical) lymph node	Lymphatic, Right Axillary
	Lymphatic, Left Axillary
Subclavius muscle	Thorax Muscle, Right
	Thorax Muscle, Left

Anatomical Term	ICD-10-PCS Value
Subclavius nerve	Brachial Plexus
Subcostal artery	Upper Artery
Subcostal muscle	Thorax Muscle, Right
	Thorax Muscle, Left
Subcostal nerve	Thoracic Nerve
Subdural space, spinal	Spinal Canal
Submandibular ganglion	Facial Nerve
	Head and Neck Sympathetic Nerve
Submandibular gland	Submaxillary Gland, Right
	Submaxillary Gland, Left
Submandibular lymph node	Lymphatic, Head
Submandibular space	Subcutaneous Tissue and Fascia, Face
Submaxillary ganglion	Head and Neck Sympathetic Nerve
Submaxillary lymph node	Lymphatic, Head
Submental artery	Face Artery
Submental lymph node	Lymphatic, Head
Submucous (Meissner's) plexus	Abdominal Sympathetic Nerve
Suboccipital nerve	Cervical Nerve
Suboccipital venous plexus	Vertebral Vein, Right
	Vertebral Vein, Left
Subparotid lymph node	Lymphatic, Head
Subscapular (posterior) lymph node	Lymphatic, Right Axillary
	Lymphatic, Left Axillary
Subscapular aponeurosis	Subcutaneous Tissue and Fascia, Right Upper Arm
	Subcutaneous Tissue and Fascia, Left Upper Arm
Subscapular artery	Axillary Artery, Right
	Axillary Artery, Left
Subscapularis muscle	Shoulder Muscle, Right
	Shoulder Muscle, Left
Substantia nigra	Basal Ganglia
Subtalar (talocalcaneal) joint	Tarsal Joint, Right
	Tarsal Joint, Left
Subtalar ligament	Foot Bursa and Ligament, Right
	Foot Bursa and Ligament, Left
Subthalamic nucleus	Basal Ganglia
Superficial circumflex iliac vein	Saphenous Vein, Right
	Saphenous Vein, Left
Superficial epigastric artery	Femoral Artery, Right
	Femoral Artery, Left
Superficial epigastric vein	Saphenous Vein, Right
	Saphenous Vein, Left
Superficial palmar arch	Hand Artery, Right
	Hand Artery, Left

Anatomical Term	ICD-10-PCS Value
Superficial palmar venous arch	Hand Vein, Right
	Hand Vein, Left
Superficial temporal artery	Temporal Artery, Right
	Temporal Artery, Left
Superficial transverse perineal muscle	Perineum Muscle
Superior cardiac nerve	Thoracic Sympathetic Nerve
Superior cerebellar vein	Intracranial Vein
Superior cerebral vein	Intracranial Vein
Superior clunic (cluneal) nerve	Lumbar Nerve
Superior epigastric artery	Internal Mammary Artery, Right
	Internal Mammary Artery, Left
Superior genicular artery	Popliteal Artery, Right
	Popliteal Artery, Left
Superior gluteal artery	Internal Iliac Artery, Right
	Internal Iliac Artery, Left
Superior gluteal nerve	Lumbar Plexus
Superior hypogastric plexus	Abdominal Sympathetic Nerve
Superior labial artery	Face Artery
Superior laryngeal artery	Thyroid Artery, Right
	Thyroid Artery, Left
Superior laryngeal nerve	Vagus Nerve
Superior longitudinal muscle	Tongue, Palate, Pharynx Muscle
Superior mesenteric ganglion	Abdominal Sympathetic Nerve
Superior mesenteric lymph node	Lymphatic, Mesenteric
Superior mesenteric plexus	Abdominal Sympathetic Nerve
Superior oblique muscle	Extraocular Muscle, Right
	Extraocular Muscle, Left
Superior olivary nucleus	Pons
Superior rectal artery	Inferior Mesenteric Artery
Superior rectal vein	Inferior Mesenteric Vein
Superior rectus muscle	Extraocular Muscle, Right
	Extraocular Muscle, Left
Superior tarsal plate	Upper Eyelid, Right
	Upper Eyelid, Left
Superior thoracic artery	Axillary Artery, Right
	Axillary Artery, Left
Superior thyroid artery	External Carotid Artery, Right
	External Carotid Artery, Left
	Thyroid Artery, Right
	Thyroid Artery, Left
Superior turbinate	Nasal Turbinate
Superior ulnar collateral artery	Brachial Artery, Right
	Brachial Artery, Left
Supraclavicular (Virchow's) lymph node	Lymphatic, Right Neck
	Lymphatic, Left Neck

Anatomical Term	ICD-10-PCS Value
Supraclavicular nerve	Cervical Plexus
Suprahyoid lymph node	Lymphatic, Head
Suprahyoid muscle	Neck Muscle, Right
	Neck Muscle, Left
Suprainguinal lymph node	Lymphatic, Pelvis
Supraorbital vein	Face Vein, Right
	Face Vein, Left
Suprarenal gland	Adrenal Gland, Left
	Adrenal Gland, Right
	Adrenal Glands, Bilateral
	Adrenal Gland
Suprarenal plexus	Abdominal Sympathetic Nerve
Suprascapular nerve	Brachial Plexus
Supraspinatus fascia	Subcutaneous Tissue and Fascia, Right Upper Arm
	Subcutaneous Tissue and Fascia, Left Upper Arm
Supraspinatus muscle	Shoulder Muscle, Right
	Shoulder Muscle, Left
Supraspinous ligament	Upper Spine Bursa and Ligament
	Lower Spine Bursa and Ligament
Suprasternal notch	Sternum
Supratrochlear lymph node	Lymphatic, Right Upper Extremity
	Lymphatic, Left Upper Extremity
Sural artery	Popliteal Artery, Right
	Popliteal Artery, Left
Sweat gland	Skin
Talocalcaneal (subtalar) joint	Tarsal Joint, Right
	Tarsal Joint, Left
Talocalcaneal ligament	Foot Bursa and Ligament, Right
	Foot Bursa and Ligament, Left
Talocalcaneonavicular joint	Tarsal Joint, Right
	Tarsal Joint, Left
Talocalcaneonavicular ligament	Foot Bursa and Ligament, Right
	Foot Bursa and Ligament, Left
Talocrural joint	Ankle Joint, Right
	Ankle Joint, Left
Talofibular ligament	Ankle Bursa and Ligament, Right
	Ankle Bursa and Ligament, Left
Talus bone	Tarsal, Right
	Tarsal, Left
Tarsometatarsal ligament	Foot Bursa and Ligament, Right
	Foot Bursa and Ligament, Left
Temporal lobe	Cerebral Hemisphere
Temporalis muscle	Head Muscle
Temporoparietalis muscle	Head Muscle
Tensor fasciae latae muscle	Hip Muscle, Right
	Hip Muscle, Left
Tensor veli palatini muscle	Tongue, Palate, Pharynx Muscle
Tenth cranial nerve	Vagus Nerve
Tentorium cerebelli	Dura Mater
Teres major muscle	Shoulder Muscle, Right
	Shoulder Muscle, Left
Teres minor muscle	Shoulder Muscle, Right
	Shoulder Muscle, Left
Testicular artery	Abdominal Aorta
Thenar muscle	Hand Muscle, Right
	Hand Muscle, Left
Third cranial nerve	Oculomotor Nerve
Third occipital nerve	Cervical Nerve
Third ventricle	Cerebral Ventricle
Thoracic aortic plexus	Thoracic Sympathetic Nerve
Thoracic esophagus	Esophagus, Middle
Thoracic facet joint	Thoracic Vertebral Joint
Thoracic ganglion	Thoracic Sympathetic Nerve
Thoracoacromial artery	Axillary Artery, Right
	Axillary Artery, Left
Thoracolumbar facet joint	Thoracolumbar Vertebral Joint
Thymus gland	Thymus
Thyroarytenoid muscle	Neck Muscle, Right
	Neck Muscle, Left
Thyrocervical trunk	Thyroid Artery, Right
	Thyroid Artery, Left
Thyroid cartilage	Larynx
Tibialis anterior muscle	Lower Leg Muscle, Right
	Lower Leg Muscle, Left
Tibialis posterior muscle	Lower Leg Muscle, Right
	Lower Leg Muscle, Left
Tibiofemoral joint	Knee Joint, Right
	Knee Joint, Left
	Knee Joint, Tibial Surface, Right
	Knee Joint, Tibial Surface, Left
Tibioperoneal trunk	Popliteal Artery, Right
	Popliteal Artery, Left
Tongue, base of	Pharynx
Tracheobronchial lymph node	Lymphatic, Thorax
Tragus	External Ear, Right
	External Ear, Left
	External Ear, Bilateral
Transversalis fascia	Subcutaneous Tissue and Fascia, Trunk
Transverse (cutaneous) cervical nerve	Cervical Plexus

Anatomical Term	ICD-10-PCS Value
Transverse acetabular ligament	Hip Bursa and Ligament, Right
	Hip Bursa and Ligament, Left
Transverse facial artery	Temporal Artery, Right
	Temporal Artery, Left
Transverse foramen	Cervical Vertebra
Transverse humeral ligament	Shoulder Bursa and Ligament, Right
	Shoulder Bursa and Ligament, Left
Transverse ligament of atlas	Head and Neck Bursa and Ligament
Transverse process	Cervical Vertebra
	Thoracic Vertebra
	Lumbar Vertebra
Transverse scapular ligament	Shoulder Bursa and Ligament, Right
	Shoulder Bursa and Ligament, Left
Transverse thoracis muscle	Thorax Muscle, Right
	Thorax Muscle, Left
Transversospinalis muscle	Trunk Muscle, Right
	Trunk Muscle, Left
Transversus abdominis muscle	Abdomen Muscle, Right
	Abdomen Muscle, Left
Trapezium bone	Carpal, Right
	Carpal, Left
Trapezius muscle	Trunk Muscle, Right
	Trunk Muscle, Left
Trapezoid bone	Carpal, Right
	Carpal, Left
Triceps brachii muscle	Upper Arm Muscle, Right
	Upper Arm Muscle, Left
Tricuspid annulus	Tricuspid Valve
Trifacial nerve	Trigeminal Nerve
Trigone of bladder	Bladder
Triquetral bone	Carpal, Right
	Carpal, Left
Trochanteric bursa	Hip Bursa and Ligament, Right
	Hip Bursa and Ligament, Left
Twelfth cranial nerve	Hypoglossal Nerve
Tympanic cavity	Middle Ear, Right
	Middle Ear, Left
Tympanic nerve	Glossopharyngeal Nerve
Tympanic part of temporal bone	Temporal Bone, Right
	Temporal Bone, Left
Ulnar collateral carpal ligament	Wrist Bursa and Ligament, Right
	Wrist Bursa and Ligament, Left
Ulnar collateral ligament	Elbow Bursa and Ligament, Right
	Elbow Bursa and Ligament, Left
Ulnar notch	Radius, Right
	Radius, Left

Anatomical Term	ICD-10-PCS Value
Ulnar vein	Brachial Vein, Right
	Brachial Vein, Left
Umbilical artery	Internal Iliac Artery, Right
	Internal Iliac Artery, Left
	Lower Artery
Ureteral orifice	Ureter, Right
	Ureter, Left
	Ureters, Bilateral
	Ureter
Ureteropelvic junction (UPJ)	Kidney Pelvis, Right
	Kidney Pelvis, Left
Ureterovesical orifice	Ureter, Right
	Ureter, Left
	Ureters, Bilateral
	Ureter
Uterine artery	Internal Iliac Artery, Right
	Internal Iliac Artery, Left
Uterine cornu	Uterus
Uterine tube	Fallopian Tube, Right
	Fallopian Tube, Left
Uterine vein	Hypogastric Vein, Right
	Hypogastric Vein, Left
Vaginal artery	Internal Iliac Artery, Right
	Internal Iliac Artery, Left
Vaginal vein	Hypogastric Vein, Right
	Hypogastric Vein, Left
Vastus intermedius muscle	Upper Leg Muscle, Right
	Upper Leg Muscle, Left
Vastus lateralis muscle	Upper Leg Muscle, Right
	Upper Leg Muscle, Left
Vastus medialis muscle	Upper Leg Muscle, Right
	Upper Leg Muscle, Left
Ventricular fold	Larynx
Vermiform appendix	Appendix
Vermilion border	Upper Lip
	Lower Lip
Vertebral arch	Cervical Vertebra
	Thoracic Vertebra
	Lumbar Vertebra
Vertebral body	Cervical Vertebra
	Thoracic Vertebra
	Lumbar Vertebra
Vertebral canal	Spinal Canal
Vertebral foramen	Cervical Vertebra
	Thoracic Vertebra
	Lumbar Vertebra

Anatomical Term	ICD-10-PCS Value
Vertebral lamina	Cervical Vertebra
	Thoracic Vertebra
	Lumbar Vertebra
Vertebral pedicle	Cervical Vertebra
	Thoracic Vertebra
	Lumbar Vertebra
Vesical vein	Hypogastric Vein, Right
	Hypogastric Vein, Left
Vestibular (Scarpa's) ganglion	Acoustic Nerve
Vestibular nerve	Acoustic Nerve
Vestibulocochlear nerve	Acoustic Nerve
Virchow's (supraclavicular) lymph node	Lymphatic, Right Neck
	Lymphatic, Left Neck
Vitreous body	Vitreous, Right
	Vitreous, Left
Vocal fold	Vocal Cord, Right
	Vocal Cord, Left
Volar (palmar) digital vein	Hand Vein, Right
	Hand Vein, Left
Volar (palmar) metacarpal vein	Hand Vein, Right
	Hand Vein, Left
Vomer bone	Nasal Septum
Vomer of nasal septum	Nasal Bone
Xiphoid process	Sternum
Zonule of Zinn	Lens, Right
	Lens, Left
Zygomatic process of frontal bone	Frontal Bone
Zygomatic process of temporal bone	Temporal Bone, Right
	Temporal Bone, Left
Zygomaticus muscle	Facial Muscle

Device - 6th character - remain after procedure is completed

4 General types of devices

1. Biological or synthetic material - takes the place of all/portion of body part
   ex: joint prosthesis
2. Biological or synthetic material that assists or prevents a physiological function
   ex: intrauterine device (IUD)
3. therapeutic material that is not absorbed by, eliminated by, or incorporated into a body part. Ex: radioactive material
4. mechanical or electronic appliances used to assist, monitor, take the place of, or prevent a physiological function. Ex: cardiac pacemaker

Devices may use root operation: alteration, bypass, creation, dilation, drainage
Fusion, occlusion, reposition, restriction

Specific device values must use: change, insertion, removal, replacement, revision

instruments used are specified in the approach, not the device

if objective of procedure is to put in a device, use: insertion

if device is put in other than the objective of insertion, use root operation underlying the objective of the procedure used, w/ the device used in the device character.

ex: hip joint replacement - use replacement, specify device in device character

materials incidental to procedure are not specified in device character

ex: clips, ligatures, sutures

This page intentionally left blank

devices left in place after surgery is complete

Appendix C: Device Key

Device Term	ICD-10-PCS Value
3f® (Aortic) Bioprosthesis valve	Zooplastic Tissue in Heart and Great Vessels
AbioCor® Total Replacement Heart	Synthetic Substitute
Absolute Pro® Vascular (OTW) Self-Expanding Stent System	Intraluminal Device
Acculink™ (RX) Carotid Stent System	Intraluminal Device
Acellular Hydrated Dermis	Nonautologous Tissue Substitute
Acetabular cup	Liner in Lower Joints
Activa PC® neurostimulator	Stimulator Generator, Multiple Array for Insertion in Subcutaneous Tissue and Fascia
Activa RC® neurostimulator	Stimulator Generator, Multiple Array Rechargeable for Insertion in Subcutaneous Tissue and Fascia
Activa SC® neurostimulator	Stimulator Generator, Single Array for Insertion in Subcutaneous Tissue and Fascia
ACUITY™ Steerable Lead	Cardiac Lead, Pacemaker for Insertion in Heart and Great Vessels
	Cardiac Lead, Defibrillator for Insertion in Heart and Great Vessels
Advisa MRI™	Pacemaker, Dual Chamber for Insertion in Subcutaneous Tissue and Fascia
AFX® Endovascular AAA System	Intraluminal Device
AMPLATZER® Muscular VSD Occluder	Synthetic Substitute
AMS 800® Urinary Control System	Artificial Sphincter in Urinary System
AneuRx® AAA Advantage®	Intraluminal Device
Annuloplasty ring	Synthetic Substitute
Articulating Spacer (Antibiotic)	Articulating Spacer in Lower Joints
Artificial anal sphincter (AAS)	Artificial Sphincter in Gastrointestinal System
Artificial bowel sphincter (neosphincter)	Artificial Sphincter in Gastrointestinal System
Artificial urinary sphincter (AUS)	Artificial Sphincter in Urinary System
Ascenda® Intrathecal Catheter	Infusion Device
Assurant (Cobalt)® stent	Intraluminal Device
AtriClip® LAA Exclusion System	Extraluminal Device
Attain Ability® lead	Cardiac Lead, Pacemaker for Insertion in Heart and Great Vessels
	Cardiac Lead, Defibrillator for Insertion in Heart and Great Vessels
Attain StarFix® (OTW) lead	Cardiac Lead, Pacemaker for Insertion in Heart and Great Vessels
	Cardiac Lead, Defibrillator for Insertion in Heart and Great Vessels
Autograft	Autologous Tissue Substitute
Autologous artery graft	Autologous Arterial Tissue in Heart and Great Vessels
	Autologous Arterial Tissue in Upper Arteries
	Autologous Arterial Tissue in Lower Arteries
	Autologous Arterial Tissue in Upper Veins
	Autologous Arterial Tissue in Lower Veins
Autologous vein graft	Autologous Venous Tissue in Heart and Great Vessels
	Autologous Venous Tissue in Upper Arteries
	Autologous Venous Tissue in Lower Arteries
	Autologous Venous Tissue in Upper Veins
	Autologous Venous Tissue in Lower Veins
Axial Lumbar Interbody Fusion System	Interbody Fusion Device in Lower Joints
AxiaLIF® System	Interbody Fusion Device in Lower Joints
BAK/C® Interbody Cervical Fusion System	Interbody Fusion Device in Upper Joints
Bard® Composix® (E/X) (LP) mesh	Synthetic Substitute
Bard® Composix® Kugel® patch	Synthetic Substitute
Bard® Dulex™ mesh	Synthetic Substitute
Bard® Ventralex™ hernia patch	Synthetic Substitute
Baroreflex Activation Therapy®(BAT®)	Stimulator Lead in Upper Arteries
	Stimulator Generator in Subcutaneous Tissue and Fascia
Berlin Heart® Ventricular Assist Device	Implantable Heart Assist System in Heart and Great Vessels
Bioactive embolization coil(s)	Intraluminal Device, Bioactive in Upper Arteries
Biventricular external heart assist system	Short-term External Heart Assist System in Heart and Great Vessels
Blood glucose monitoring system	Monitoring Device
Bone anchored hearing device	Hearing Device, Bone Conduction for Insertion in Ear, Nose, Sinus
	Hearing Device in Head and Facial Bones
Bone bank bone graft	Nonautologous Tissue Substitute
Bone screw (interlocking) (lag) (pedicle) (recessed)	Internal Fixation Device in Head and Facial Bones
	Internal Fixation Device in Upper Bones
	Internal Fixation Device in Lower Bones
Bovine pericardial valve	Zooplastic Tissue in Heart and Great Vessels
Bovine pericardium graft	Zooplastic Tissue in Heart and Great Vessels

Device Term	ICD-10-PCS Value
Brachytherapy seeds	Radioactive Element
BRYAN® Cervical Disc System	Synthetic Substitute
BVS 5000® Ventricular Assist Device	Short-term External Heart Assist System in Heart and Great Vessels
Cardiac contractility modulation lead	Cardiac Lead in Heart and Great Vessels
Cardiac event recorder	Monitoring Device
Cardiac resynchronization therapy (CRT) lead	Cardiac Lead, Pacemaker for Insertion in Heart and Great Vessels
	Cardiac Lead, Defibrillator for Insertion in Heart and Great Vessels
CardioMEMS® pressure sensor	Monitoring Device, Pressure Sensor for Insertion in Heart and Great Vessels
Carotid (artery) sinus (baroreceptor) lead	Stimulator Lead in Upper Arteries
Carotid WALLSTENT® Monorail® Endoprosthesis	Intraluminal Device
Centrimag® Blood Pump	Short-term External Heart Assist System in Heart and Great Vessels
Ceramic on ceramic bearing surface	Synthetic Substitute, Ceramic for Replacement in Lower Joints
Cesium-131 Collagen Implant	Radioactive Element, Cesium-131 Collagen Implant for Insertion in Central Nervous System and Cranial Nerves
CivaSheet®	Radioactive Element
Clamp and rod internal fixation system (CRIF)	Internal Fixation Device in Upper Bones
	Internal Fixation Device in Lower Bones
COALESCE® radiolucent interbody fusion device	Interbody Fusion Device, Radiolucent Porous in New Technology
CoAxia NeuroFlo™ catheter	Intraluminal Device
Cobalt/chromium head and polyethylene socket	Synthetic Substitute, Metal on Polyethylene for Replacement in Lower Joints
Cobalt/chromium head and socket	Synthetic Substitute, Metal for Replacement in Lower Joints
Cochlear implant (CI), multiple channel (electrode)	Hearing Device, Multiple Channel Cochlear Prosthesis for Insertion in Ear, Nose, Sinus
Cochlear implant (CI), single channel (electrode)	Hearing Device, Single Channel Cochlear Prosthesis for Insertion in Ear, Nose, Sinus
COGNIS® CRT-D	Cardiac Resynchronization Defibrillator Pulse Generator for Insertion in Subcutaneous Tissue and Fascia
COHERE® radiolucent interbody fusion device	Interbody Fusion Device, Radiolucent Porous in New Technology
Colonic Z-Stent®	Intraluminal Device
Complete® (SE) stent	Intraluminal Device

Device Term	ICD-10-PCS Value
Concerto® II CRT-D	Cardiac Resynchronization Defibrillator Pulse Generator for Insertion in Subcutaneous Tissue and Fascia
CONSERVE® PLUS Total Resurfacing Hip System	Resurfacing Device in Lower Joints
Consulta® CRT-D	Cardiac Resynchronization Defibrillator Pulse Generator for Insertion in Subcutaneous Tissue and Fascia
Consulta® CRT-P	Cardiac Resynchronization Pacemaker Pulse Generator for Insertion in Subcutaneous Tissue and Fascia
CONTAK RENEWAL® 3 RF (HE) CRT-D	Cardiac Resynchronization Defibrillator Pulse Generator for Insertion in Subcutaneous Tissue and Fascia
Contegra® Pulmonary Valved Conduit	Zooplastic Tissue in Heart and Great Vessels
Continuous Glucose Monitoring (CGM) device	Monitoring Device
Cook Biodesign® Fistula Plug(s)	Nonautologous Tissue Substitute
Cook Biodesign® Hernia Graft(s)	Nonautologous Tissue Substitute
Cook Biodesign® Layered Graft(s)	Nonautologous Tissue Substitute
Cook Zenapro™ Layered Graft(s)	Nonautologous Tissue Substitute
Cook Zenith® AAA Endovascular Graft	Intraluminal Device, Branched or Fenestrated, One or Two Arteries for Restriction in Lower Arteries
	Intraluminal Device, Branched or Fenestrated, Three or More Arteries for Restriction in Lower Arteries
	Intraluminal Device
CoreValve™ transcatheter aortic valve	Zooplastic Tissue in Heart and Great Vessels
Cormet™ Hip Resurfacing System	Resurfacing Device in Lower Joints
CoRoent® XL	Interbody Fusion Device in Lower Joints
Corox® (OTW) Bipolar Lead	Cardiac Lead, Pacemaker for Insertion in Heart and Great Vessels
	Cardiac Lead, Defibrillator for Insertion in Heart and Great Vessels
Cortical strip neurostimulator lead	Neurostimulator Lead in Central Nervous System and Cranial Nerves
Cultured epidermal cell autograft	Autologous Tissue Substitute
CYPHER® Stent	Intraluminal Device, Drug-eluting in Heart and Great Vessels
Cystostomy tube	Drainage Device
DBS™ lead	Neurostimulator Lead in Central Nervous System and Cranial Nerves
DeBakey® Left Ventricular Assist Device	Implantable Heart Assist System in Heart and Great Vessels

Device Term	ICD-10-PCS Value
Deep brain neurostimulator lead	Neurostimulator Lead in Central Nervous System and Cranial Nerves
Delta frame external fixator	External Fixation Device, Hybrid for Insertion in Upper Bones
	External Fixation Device, Hybrid for Reposition in Upper Bones
	External Fixation Device, Hybrid for Insertion in Lower Bones
	External Fixation Device, Hybrid for Reposition in Lower Bones
Delta III™ Reverse shoulder prosthesis	Synthetic Substitute, Reverse Ball and Socket for Replacement in Upper Joints
Diaphragmatic pacemaker generator	Stimulator Generator in Subcutaneous Tissue and Fascia
Direct Lateral Interbody Fusion (DLIF) device	Interbody Fusion Device in Lower Joints
Driver® stent (RX) (OTW)	Intraluminal Device
DuraHeart® Left Ventricular Assist System	Implantable Heart Assist System in Heart and Great Vessels
Durata® Defibrillation Lead	Cardiac Lead, Defibrillator for Insertion in Heart and Great Vessels
Dynesys® Dynamic Stabilization System	Spinal Stabilization Device, Pedicle-Based for Insertion in Upper Joints
	Spinal Stabilization Device, Pedicle-Based for Insertion in Lower Joints
E-Luminexx™ (Biliary) (Vascular) Stent	Intraluminal Device
EDWARDS INTUITY Elite™ valve system	Zooplastic Tissue, Rapid Deployment Technique in New Technology
Electrical bone growth stimulator (EBGS)	Bone Growth Stimulator in Head and Facial Bones
	Bone Growth Stimulator in Upper Bones
	Bone Growth Stimulator in Lower Bones
Electrical muscle stimulation (EMS) lead	Stimulator Lead in Muscles
Electronic muscle stimulator lead	Stimulator Lead in Muscles
Eluvia™ Drug-Eluting Vascular Stent System	Intraluminal Device, Sustained Release Drug-eluting in New Technology
	Intraluminal Device, Sustained Release Drug-eluting, Two in New Technology
	Intraluminal Device, Sustained Release Drug-eluting, Three in New Technology
	Intraluminal Device, Sustained Release Drug-eluting, Four or More in New Technology
Embolization coil(s)	Intraluminal Device
Endeavor® (III) (IV) (Sprint) Zotarolimus-eluting Coronary Stent System	Intraluminal Device, Drug-eluting in Heart and Great Vessels
Endologix AFX® Endovascular AAA System	Intraluminal Device
EndoSure® sensor	Monitoring Device, Pressure Sensor for Insertion in Heart and Great Vessels
ENDOTAK RELIANCE® (G) Defibrillation Lead	Cardiac Lead, Defibrillator for Insertion in Heart and Great Vessels
Endotracheal tube (cuffed) (double-lumen)	Intraluminal Device, Endotracheal Airway in Respiratory System
Endurant® Endovascular Stent Graft	Intraluminal Device
Endurant® II AAA stent graft system	Intraluminal Device
EnRhythm®	Pacemaker, Dual Chamber for Insertion in Subcutaneous Tissue and Fascia
Enterra® gastric neurostimulator	Stimulator Generator, Multiple Array for Insertion in Subcutaneous Tissue and Fascia
Epic™ Stented Tissue Valve (aortic)	Zooplastic Tissue in Heart and Great Vessels
Epicel® cultured epidermal autograft	Autologous Tissue Substitute
Esophageal obturator airway (EOA)	Intraluminal Device, Airway in Gastrointestinal System
Esteem® implantable hearing system	Hearing Device in Ear, Nose, Sinus
Evera™ (XT) (S) (DR/VR)	Defibrillator Generator for Insertion in Subcutaneous Tissue and Fascia
Everolimus-eluting coronary stent	Intraluminal Device, Drug-eluting in Heart and Great Vessels
Ex-PRESS™ mini glaucoma shunt	Synthetic Substitute
EXCLUDER® AAA Endoprosthesis	Intraluminal Device, Branched or Fenestrated, One or Two Arteries for Restriction in Lower Arteries
	Intraluminal Device, Branched or Fenestrated, Three or More Arteries for Restriction in Lower Arteries
	Intraluminal Device
EXCLUDER® IBE Endoprosthesis	Intraluminal Device, Branched or Fenestrated, One or Two Arteries for Restriction in Lower Arteries
Express® (LD) Premounted Stent System	Intraluminal Device
Express® Biliary SD Monorail® Premounted Stent System	Intraluminal Device
Express® SD Renal Monorail® Premounted Stent System	Intraluminal Device
External fixator	External Fixation Device in Head and Facial Bones
	External Fixation Device in Upper Bones
	External Fixation Device in Lower Bones
	External Fixation Device in Upper Joints
	External Fixation Device in Lower Joints

Device Term	ICD-10-PCS Value
EXtreme Lateral Interbody Fusion(XLIF) device	Interbody Fusion Device in Lower Joints
Facet replacement spinal stabilization device	Spinal Stabilization Device, Facet Replacement for Insertion in Upper Joints
	Spinal Stabilization Device, Facet Replacement for Insertion in Lower Joints
FLAIR® Endovascular Stent Graft	Intraluminal Device
Flexible Composite Mesh	Synthetic Substitute
Flow Diverter embolization device	Intraluminal Device, Flow Diverter for Restriction in Upper Arteries
Foley catheter	Drainage Device
Formula™ Balloon-Expandable Renal Stent System	Intraluminal Device
Freestyle® (Stentless) Aortic Root Bioprosthesis	Zooplastic Tissue in Heart and Great Vessels
Fusion screw (compression) (lag) (locking)	Internal Fixation Device in Upper Joints
	Internal Fixation Device in Lower Joints
GammaTile™	Radioactive Element, Cesium-131 Collagen Implant for Insertion in Central Nervous System and Cranial Nerves
Gastric electrical stimulation (GES) lead	Stimulator Lead in Gastrointestinal System
Gastric pacemaker lead	Stimulator Lead in Gastrointestinal System
GORE EXCLUDER® AAA Endoprosthesis	Intraluminal Device, Branched or Fenestrated, One or Two Arteries for Restriction in Lower Arteries
	Intraluminal Device, Branched or Fenestrated, Three or More Arteries for Restriction in Lower Arteries
	Intraluminal Device
GORE EXCLUDER® IBE Endoprosthesis	Intraluminal Device, Branched or Fenestrated, One or Two Arteries for Restriction in Lower Arteries
GORE TAG® Thoracic Endoprosthesis	Intraluminal Device
GORE® DUALMESH®	Synthetic Substitute
Guedel airway	Intraluminal Device, Airway in Mouth and Throat
Hancock® Bioprosthesis (aortic) (mitral) valve	Zooplastic Tissue in Heart and Great Vessels
Hancock® Bioprosthetic Valved Conduit	Zooplastic Tissue in Heart and Great Vessels
HeartMate 3™ LVAS	Implantable Heart Assist System in Heart and Great Vessels
HeartMate II® Left Ventricular Assist Device (LVAD)	Implantable Heart Assist System in Heart and Great Vessels
HeartMate XVE® Left Ventricular Assist Device (LVAD)	Implantable Heart Assist System in Heart and Great Vessels
Herculink® (RX) Elite Renal Stent System	Intraluminal Device
Hip (joint) liner	Liner in Lower Joints
Holter valve ventricular shunt	Synthetic Substitute

Device Term	ICD-10-PCS Value
Ilizarov external fixator	External Fixation Device, Ring for Insertion in Upper Bones
	External Fixation Device, Ring for Reposition in Upper Bones
	External Fixation Device, Ring for Insertion in Lower Bones
	External Fixation Device, Ring for Reposition in Lower Bones
Ilizarov-Vecklich device	External Fixation Device, Limb Lengthening for Insertion in Upper Bones
	External Fixation Device, Limb Lengthening for Insertion in Lower Bones
Impella® heart pump	Short-term External Heart Assist System in Heart and Great Vessels
Implantable cardioverter-defibrillator (ICD)	Defibrillator Generator for Insertion in Subcutaneous Tissue and Fascia
Implantable drug infusion pump (anti-spasmodic) (chemotherapy) (pain)	Infusion Device, Pump in Subcutaneous Tissue and Fascia
Implantable glucose monitoring device	Monitoring Device
Implantable hemodynamic monitor (IHM)	Monitoring Device, Hemodynamic for Insertion in Subcutaneous Tissue and Fascia
Implantable hemodynamic monitoring system (IHMS)	Monitoring Device, Hemodynamic for Insertion in Subcutaneous Tissue and Fascia
Implantable Miniature Telescope™(IMT)	Synthetic Substitute, Intraocular Telescope for Replacement in Eye
Implanted (venous) (access) port	Vascular Access Device, Totally Implantable in Subcutaneous Tissue and Fascia
InDura®, intrathecal catheter (1P) (spinal)	Infusion Device
Injection reservoir, port	Vascular Access Device, Totally Implantable in Subcutaneous Tissue and Fascia
Injection reservoir, pump	Infusion Device, Pump in Subcutaneous Tissue and Fascia
Interbody fusion (spine) cage	Interbody Fusion Device in Upper Joints
	Interbody Fusion Device in Lower Joints
Interspinous process spinal stabilization device	Spinal Stabilization Device, Interspinous Process for Insertion in Upper Joints
	Spinal Stabilization Device, Interspinous Process for Insertion in Lower Joints
InterStim® Therapy lead	Neurostimulator Lead in Peripheral Nervous System
InterStim® Therapy neurostimulator	Stimulator Generator, Single Array for Insertion in Subcutaneous Tissue and Fascia

Device Term	ICD-10-PCS Value
Intramedullary (IM) rod (nail)	Internal Fixation Device, Intramedullary in Upper Bones
	Internal Fixation Device, Intramedullary in Lower Bones
Intramedullary skeletal kinetic distractor (ISKD)	Internal Fixation Device, Intramedullary in Upper Bones
	Internal Fixation Device, Intramedullary in Lower Bones
Intrauterine device (IUD)	Contraceptive Device in Female Reproductive System
INTUITY Elite® valve system, EDWARDS	Zooplastic Tissue, Rapid Deployment Technique in New Technology
Itrel® (3) (4) neurostimulator	Stimulator Generator, Single Array for Insertion in Subcutaneous Tissue and Fascia
Joint fixation plate	Internal Fixation Device in Upper Joints
	Internal Fixation Device in Lower Joints
Joint liner (insert)	Liner in Lower Joints
Joint spacer (antibiotic)	Spacer in Upper Joints
	Spacer in Lower Joints
Kappa®	Pacemaker, Dual Chamber for Insertion in Subcutaneous Tissue and Fascia
Kirschner wire (K-wire)	Internal Fixation Device in Head and Facial Bones
	Internal Fixation Device in Upper Bones
	Internal Fixation Device in Lower Bones
	Internal Fixation Device in Upper Joints
	Internal Fixation Device in Lower Joints
Knee (implant) insert	Liner in Lower Joints
Kuntscher nail	Internal Fixation Device, Intramedullary in Upper Bones
	Internal Fixation Device, Intramedullary in Lower Bones
LAP-BAND® adjustable gastric banding system	Extraluminal Device
LifeStent® (Flexstar) (XL) Vascular Stent System	Intraluminal Device
LIVIAN™ CRT-D	Cardiac Resynchronization Defibrillator Pulse Generator for Insertion in Subcutaneous Tissue and Fascia
Loop recorder, implantable	Monitoring Device
MAGEC® Spinal Bracing and Distraction System	Magnetically Controlled Growth Rod(s) in New Technology
Mark IV™ Breathing Pacemaker System	Stimulator Generator in Subcutaneous Tissue and Fascia
Maximo® II DR (VR)	Defibrillator Generator for Insertion in Subcutaneous Tissue and Fascia
Maximo® II DR CRT-D	Cardiac Resynchronization Defibrillator Pulse Generator for Insertion in Subcutaneous Tissue and Fascia
Medtronic Endurant® II AAA stent graft system	Intraluminal Device
Melody® transcatheter pulmonary valve	Zooplastic Tissue in Heart and Great Vessels
Metal on metal bearing surface	Synthetic Substitute, Metal for Replacement in Lower Joints
Micro-Driver® stent (RX) (OTW)	Intraluminal Device
MicroMed HeartAssist™	Implantable Heart Assist System in Heart and Great Vessels
Micrus CERECYTE® microcoil	Intraluminal Device, Bioactive in Upper Arteries
MIRODERM™ Biologic Wound Matrix	Skin Substitute, Porcine Liver Derived in New Technology
MitraClip® valve repair system	Synthetic Substitute
Mitroflow® Aortic Pericardial Heart Valve	Zooplastic Tissue in Heart and Great Vessels
Mosaic® Bioprosthesis (aortic) (mitral) valve	Zooplastic Tissue in Heart and Great Vessels
MULTI-LINK (VISION®) (MINI-VISION VISION®) (ULTRA™) Coronary Stent System	Intraluminal Device
nanoLOCK™ interbody fusion device	Interbody Fusion Device, Nanotextured Surface in New Technology
Nasopharyngeal airway (NPA)	Intraluminal Device, Airway in Ear, Nose, Sinus
Neuromuscular electrical stimulation (NEMS) lead	Stimulator Lead in Muscles
Neurostimulator generator, multiple channel	Stimulator Generator, Multiple Array for Insertion in Subcutaneous Tissue and Fascia
Neurostimulator generator, multiple channel rechargeable	Stimulator Generator, Multiple Array Rechargeable for Insertion in Subcutaneous Tissue and Fascia
Neurostimulator generator, single channel	Stimulator Generator, Single Array for Insertion in Subcutaneous Tissue and Fascia
Neurostimulator generator, single channel rechargeable	Stimulator Generator, Single Array Rechargeable for Insertion in Subcutaneous Tissue and Fascia
Neutralization plate	Internal Fixation Device in Head and Facial Bones
	Internal Fixation Device in Upper Bones
	Internal Fixation Device in Lower Bones
Nitinol framed polymer mesh	Synthetic Substitute
Non-tunneled central venous catheter	Infusion Device

Device Term	ICD-10-PCS Value
Novacor® Left Ventricular Assist Device	Implantable Heart Assist System in Heart and Great Vessels
Novation® Ceramic AHS® (Articulation Hip System)	Synthetic Substitute, Ceramic for Replacement in Lower Joints
Omnilink Elite® Vascular Balloon Expandable Stent System	Intraluminal Device
Open Pivot™ (mechanical) valve	Synthetic Substitute
Open Pivot™ Aortic Valve Graft (AVG)	Synthetic Substitute
Optimizer™ III implantable pulse generator	Contractility Modulation Device for Insertion in Subcutaneous Tissue and Fascia
Oropharyngeal airway (OPA)	Intraluminal Device, Airway in Mouth and Throat
Ovatio™ CRT-D	Cardiac Resynchronization Defibrillator Pulse Generator for Insertion in Subcutaneous Tissue and Fascia
OXINIUM™	Synthetic Substitute, Oxidized Zirconium on Polyethylene for Replacement in Lower Joints
Paclitaxel-eluting coronary stent	Intraluminal Device, Drug-eluting in Heart and Great Vessels
Paclitaxel-eluting peripheral stent	Intraluminal Device, Drug-eluting in Upper Arteries
	Intraluminal Device, Drug-eluting in Lower Arteries
Partially absorbable mesh	Synthetic Substitute
Pedicle-based dynamic stabilization device	Spinal Stabilization Device, Pedicle-Based for Insertion in Upper Joints
	Spinal Stabilization Device, Pedicle-Based for Insertion in Lower Joints
Perceval sutureless valve	Zooplastic Tissue, Rapid Deployment Technique in New Technology
Percutaneous endoscopic gastrojejunostomy (PEG/J) tube	Feeding Device in Gastrointestinal System
Percutaneous endoscopic gastrostomy (PEG) tube	Feeding Device in Gastrointestinal System
Percutaneous nephrostomy catheter	Drainage Device
Peripherally inserted central catheter (PICC)	Infusion Device
Pessary ring	Intraluminal Device, Pessary in Female Reproductive System
Phrenic nerve stimulator generator	Stimulator Generator in Subcutaneous Tissue and Fascia
Phrenic nerve stimulator lead	Diaphragmatic Pacemaker Lead in Respiratory System
PHYSIOMESH™ Flexible Composite Mesh	Synthetic Substitute
Pipeline™ (Flex) embolization device	Intraluminal Device, Flow Diverter for Restriction in Upper Arteries
Polyethylene socket	Synthetic Substitute, Polyethylene for Replacement in Lower Joints

Device Term	ICD-10-PCS Value
Polymethylmethacrylate (PMMA)	Synthetic Substitute
Polypropylene mesh	Synthetic Substitute
Porcine (bioprosthetic) valve	Zooplastic Tissue in Heart and Great Vessels
PRECICE intramedullary limb lengthening system	Internal Fixation Device, Intramedullary Limb Lengthening for Insertion in Lower Bones
	Internal Fixation Device, Intramedullary Limb Lengthening for Insertion in Upper Bones
PRESTIGE® Cervical Disc	Synthetic Substitute
PrimeAdvanced® neurostimulator (SureScan®) (MRI Safe)	Stimulator Generator, Multiple Array for Insertion in Subcutaneous Tissue and Fascia
PROCEED™ Ventral Patch	Synthetic Substitute
Prodisc-C™	Synthetic Substitute
Prodisc-L™	Synthetic Substitute
PROLENE® Polypropylene Hernia System (PHS)	Synthetic Substitute
Protecta™ XT CRT-D	Cardiac Resynchronization Defibrillator Pulse Generator for Insertion in Subcutaneous Tissue and Fascia
Protecta™ XT DR (XT VR)	Defibrillator Generator for Insertion in Subcutaneous Tissue and Fascia
Protege® RX Carotid Stent System	Intraluminal Device
Pump reservoir	Infusion Device, Pump in Subcutaneous Tissue and Fascia
REALIZE® Adjustable Gastric Band	Extraluminal Device
Rebound HRD® (Hernia Repair Device)	Synthetic Substitute
RestoreAdvanced® neurostimulator (SureScan®) (MRI Safe)	Stimulator Generator, Multiple Array Rechargeable for Insertion in Subcutaneous Tissue and Fascia
RestoreSensor® neurostimulator (SureScan®) (MRI Safe)	Stimulator Generator, Multiple Array Rechargeable for Insertion in Subcutaneous Tissue and Fascia
RestoreUltra® neurostimulator (SureScan®) (MRI Safe)	Stimulator Generator, Multiple Array Rechargeable for Insertion in Subcutaneous Tissue and Fascia
Reveal® (LINQ) (DX) (XT)	Monitoring Device
Reverse® Shoulder Prosthesis	Synthetic Substitute, Reverse Ball and Socket for Replacement in Upper Joints
Revo MRI™ SureScan® pacemaker	Pacemaker, Dual Chamber for Insertion in Subcutaneous Tissue and Fascia
Rheos® System device	Stimulator Generator in Subcutaneous Tissue and Fascia
Rheos® System lead	Stimulator Lead in Upper Arteries
RNS® System lead	Neurostimulator Lead in Central Nervous System and Cranial Nerves
RNS® system neurostimulator generator	Neurostimulator Generator in Head and Facial Bones

Device Term	ICD-10-PCS Value
Sacral nerve modulation (SNM) lead	Stimulator Lead in Urinary System
S-ICD™ lead	Subcutaneous Defibrillator Lead in Subcutaneous Tissue and Fascia
Sacral neuromodulation lead	Stimulator Lead in Urinary System
SAPIEN® transcatheter aortic valve	Zooplastic Tissue in Heart and Great Vessels
SAVAL below-the-knee (BTK) drug-eluting stent system	Intraluminal Device, Sustained Release Drug-eluting in New Technology
	Intraluminal Device, Sustained Release Drug-eluting, Two in New Technology
	Intraluminal Device, Sustained Release Drug-eluting, Three in New Technology
	Intraluminal Device, Sustained Release Drug-eluting, Four or More in New Technology
Secura™ (DR) (VR)	Defibrillator Generator for Insertion in Subcutaneous Tissue and Fascia
Sheffield hybrid external fixator	External Fixation Device, Hybrid for Insertion in Upper Bones
	External Fixation Device, Hybrid for Reposition in Upper Bones
	External Fixation Device, Hybrid for Insertion in Lower Bones
	External Fixation Device, Hybrid for Reposition in Lower Bones
Sheffield ring external fixator	External Fixation Device, Ring for Insertion in Upper Bones
	External Fixation Device, Ring for Reposition in Upper Bones
	External Fixation Device, Ring for Insertion in Lower Bones
	External Fixation Device, Ring for Reposition in Lower Bones
Single lead pacemaker (atrium) (ventricle)	Pacemaker, Single Chamber for Insertion in Subcutaneous Tissue and Fascia
Single lead rate responsive pacemaker (atrium) (ventricle)	Pacemaker, Single Chamber Rate Responsive for Insertion in Subcutaneous Tissue and Fascia
Sirolimus-eluting coronary stent	Intraluminal Device, Drug-eluting in Heart and Great Vessels
SJM Biocor® Stented Valve System	Zooplastic Tissue in Heart and Great Vessels
Spacer, Articulating (Antibiotic)	Articulating Spacer in Lower Joints
Spacer, Static (Antibiotic)	Spacer in Lower Joints
Spinal cord neurostimulator lead	Neurostimulator Lead in Central Nervous System and Cranial Nerves
Spinal growth rods, magnetically controlled	Magnetically Controlled Growth Rod(s) in New Technology

Device Term	ICD-10-PCS Value
Spiration IBV™ Valve System	Intraluminal Device, Endobronchial Valve in Respiratory System
Static Spacer (Antibiotic)	Spacer in Lower Joints
Stent, intraluminal (cardiovascular) (gastrointestinal) (hepatobiliary) (urinary)	Intraluminal Device
Stented tissue valve	Zooplastic Tissue in Heart and Great Vessels
Stratos LV®	Cardiac Resynchronization Pacemaker Pulse Generator for Insertion in Subcutaneous Tissue and Fascia
Subcutaneous injection reservoir port	Vascular Access Device, Totally Implantable in Subcutaneous Tissue and Fascia
Subcutaneous injection reservoir pump	Infusion Device, Pump in Subcutaneous Tissue and Fascia
Subdermal progesterone implant	Contraceptive Device in Subcutaneous Tissue and Fascia
Surpass Streamline™ Flow Diverter	Intraluminal Device, Flow Diverter for Restriction in Upper Arteries
Sutureless valve, Perceval™	Zooplastic Tissue, Rapid Deployment Technique in New Technology
SynCardia™ Total Artificial Heart	Synthetic Substitute
Synchra™ CRT-P	Cardiac Resynchronization Pacemaker Pulse Generator for Insertion in Subcutaneous Tissue and Fascia
SynchroMed® pump	Infusion Device, Pump in Subcutaneous Tissue and Fascia
Talent® Converter	Intraluminal Device
Talent® Occluder	Intraluminal Device
Talent® Stent Graft (abdominal) (thoracic)	Intraluminal Device
TandemHeart® System	Short-term External Heart Assist System in Heart and Great Vessels
TAXUS® Liberte® Paclitaxel-eluting Coronary Stent System	Intraluminal Device, Drug-eluting in Heart and Great Vessels
Therapeutic occlusion coil(s)	Intraluminal Device
Thoracostomy tube	Drainage Device
Thoratec® IVAD (Implantable Ventricular Assist Device)	Implantable Heart Assist System in Heart and Great Vessels
Thoratec Paracorporeal Ventricular Assist Device	Short-term External Heart Assist System in Heart and Great Vessels
Tibial insert	Liner in Lower Joints
Tissue bank graft	Nonautologous Tissue Substitute
Tissue expander (inflatable) (injectable)	Tissue Expander in Skin and Breast
	Tissue Expander in Subcutaneous Tissue and Fascia
Titanium Sternal Fixation System (TSFS)	Internal Fixation Device, Rigid Plate for Insertion in Upper Bones
	Internal Fixation Device, Rigid Plate for Reposition in Upper Bones

Device Term	ICD-10-PCS Value
Total artificial (replacement) heart	Synthetic Substitute
Tracheostomy tube	Tracheostomy Device in Respiratory System
Trifecta™ Valve (aortic)	Zooplastic Tissue in Heart and Great Vessels
Tunneled central venous catheter	Vascular Access Device, Tunneled in Subcutaneous Tissue and Fascia
Tunneled spinal (intrathecal) catheter	Infusion Device
Two lead pacemaker	Pacemaker, Dual Chamber for Insertion in Subcutaneous Tissue and Fascia
Ultraflex™ Precision Colonic Stent System	Intraluminal Device
ULTRAPRO® Hernia System (UHS)	Synthetic Substitute
ULTRAPRO® Partially Absorbable Lightweight Mesh	Synthetic Substitute
ULTRAPRO® Plug	Synthetic Substitute
Ultrasonic osteogenic stimulator	Bone Growth Stimulator in Head and Facial Bones
	Bone Growth Stimulator in Upper Bones
	Bone Growth Stimulator in Lower Bones
Ultrasound bone healing system	Bone Growth Stimulator in Head and Facial Bones
	Bone Growth Stimulator in Upper Bones
	Bone Growth Stimulator in Lower Bones
Uniplanar external fixator	External Fixation Device, Monoplanar for Insertion in Upper Bones
	External Fixation Device, Monoplanar for Reposition in Upper Bones
	External Fixation Device, Monoplanar for Insertion in Lower Bones
	External Fixation Device, Monoplanar for Reposition in Lower Bones
Urinary incontinence stimulator lead	Stimulator Lead in Urinary System
Vaginal pessary	Intraluminal Device, Pessary in Female Reproductive System
Valiant® Thoracic Stent Graft	Intraluminal Device
Vectra® Vascular Access Graft	Vascular Access Device, Tunneled in Subcutaneous Tissue and Fascia

Device Term	ICD-10-PCS Value
Ventrio™ Hernia Patch	Synthetic Substitute
Versa®	Pacemaker, Dual Chamber for Insertion in Subcutaneous Tissue and Fascia
Virtuoso® (II) (DR) (VR)	Defibrillator Generator for Insertion in Subcutaneous Tissue and Fascia
Viva™ (XT) (S)	Cardiac Resynchronization Defibrillator Pulse Generator for Insertion in Subcutaneous Tissue and Fascia
WALLSTENT® Endoprosthesis	Intraluminal Device
X-STOP® Spacer	Spinal Stabilization Device, Interspinous Process for Insertion in Upper Joints
	Spinal Stabilization Device, Interspinous Process for Insertion in Lower Joints
Xact® Carotid Stent System	Intraluminal Device
Xenograft	Zooplastic Tissue in Heart and Great Vessels
XIENCE™ Everolimus Eluting Coronary Stent System	Intraluminal Device, Drug-eluting in Heart and Great Vessels
XLIF® System	Interbody Fusion Device in Lower Joints
Zenith® AAA Endovascular Graft	Intraluminal Device, Branched or Fenestrated, One or Two Arteries for Restriction in Lower Arteries
	Intraluminal Device, Branched or Fenestrated, Three or More Arteries for Restriction in Lower Arteries
	Intraluminal Device
Zenith Flex® AAA Endovascular Graft	Intraluminal Device
Zenith TX2® TAA Endovascular Graft	Intraluminal Device
Zenith® Renu™ AAA Ancillary Graft	Intraluminal Device
Zilver® PTX® (paclitaxel) Drug-eluting Peripheral Stent	Intraluminal Device, Drug-eluting in Upper Arteries
	Intraluminal Device, Drug-eluting in Lower Arteries
Zimmer® NexGen® LPS Mobile Bearing Knee	Synthetic Substitute
Zimmer® NexGen® LPS-Flex Mobile Knee	Synthetic Substitute
Zotarolimus-eluting coronary stent	Intraluminal Device, Drug-eluting in Heart and Great Vessels

ID's the appropriate device character value for specific root operations & body systems/parts

Appendix D: Device Aggregation Table

Specific Device	For Operation	In Body System	General Device
Autologous Arterial Tissue	All applicable	Heart and Great Vessels Lower Arteries Lower Veins Upper Arteries Upper Veins	**7** Autologous Tissue Substitute
Autologous Venous Tissue	All applicable	Heart and Great Vessels Lower Arteries Lower Veins Upper Arteries Upper Veins	**7** Autologous Tissue Substitute
Cardiac Lead, Defibrillator	Insertion	Heart and Great Vessels	**M** Cardiac Lead
Cardiac Lead, Pacemaker	Insertion	Heart and Great Vessels	**M** Cardiac Lead
Cardiac Resynchronization Defibrillator Pulse Generator	Insertion	Subcutaneous Tissue and Fascia	**P** Cardiac Rhythm Related Device
Cardiac Resynchronization Pacemaker Pulse Generator	Insertion	Subcutaneous Tissue and Fascia	**P** Cardiac Rhythm Related Device
Contractility Modulation Device	Insertion	Subcutaneous Tissue and Fascia	**P** Cardiac Rhythm Related Device
Defibrillator Generator	Insertion	Subcutaneous Tissue and Fascia	**P** Cardiac Rhythm Related Device
Epiretinal Visual Prosthesis	All applicable	Eye	**J** Synthetic Substitute
External Fixation Device, Hybrid	Insertion	Lower Bones Upper Bones	**5** External Fixation Device
External Fixation Device, Hybrid	Reposition	Lower Bones Upper Bones	**5** External Fixation Device
External Fixation Device, Limb Lengthening	Insertion	Lower Bones Upper Bones	**5** External Fixation Device
External Fixation Device, Monoplanar	Insertion	Lower Bones Upper Bones	**5** External Fixation Device
External Fixation Device, Monoplanar	Reposition	Lower Bones Upper Bones	**5** External Fixation Device
External Fixation Device, Ring	Insertion	Lower Bones Upper Bones	**5** External Fixation Device
External Fixation Device, Ring	Reposition	Lower Bones Upper Bones	**5** External Fixation Device
Hearing Device, Bone Conduction	Insertion	Ear, Nose, Sinus	**S** Hearing Device
Hearing Device, Multiple Channel Cochlear Prosthesis	Insertion	Ear, Nose, Sinus	**S** Hearing Device
Hearing Device, Single Channel Cochlear Prosthesis	Insertion	Ear, Nose, Sinus	**S** Hearing Device
Internal Fixation Device, Intramedullary	All applicable	Lower Bones Upper Bones	**4** Internal Fixation Device
Internal Fixation Device, Intramedullary Limb Lengthening	Insertion	Lower Bones Upper Bones	**6** Internal Fixation Device, Intramedullary
Internal Fixation Device, Rigid Plate	Insertion	Upper Bones	**4** Internal Fixation Device
Internal Fixation Device, Rigid Plate	Reposition	Upper Bones	**4** Internal Fixation Device

Specific Device	For Operation	In Body System	General Device
Intraluminal Device, Airway	All applicable	Ear, Nose, Sinus Gastrointestinal System Mouth and Throat	**D** Intraluminal Device
Intraluminal Device, Bioactive	All applicable	Upper Arteries	**D** Intraluminal Device
Intraluminal Device, Branched or Fenestrated, One or Two Arteries	Restriction	Heart and Great Vessels	**D** Intraluminal Device
		Lower Arteries	
Intraluminal Device, Branched or Fenestrated, Three or More Arteries	Restriction	Heart and Great Vessels	**D** Intraluminal Device
		Lower Arteries	
Intraluminal Device, Drug-eluting	All applicable	Heart and Great Vessels	**D** Intraluminal Device
		Lower Arteries	
		Upper Arteries	
Intraluminal Device, Drug-eluting, Four or More	All applicable	Heart and Great Vessels	**D** Intraluminal Device
		Lower Arteries	
		Upper Arteries	
Intraluminal Device, Drug-eluting, Three	All applicable	Heart and Great Vessels	**D** Intraluminal Device
		Lower Arteries	
		Upper Arteries	
Intraluminal Device, Drug-eluting, Two	All applicable	Heart and Great Vessels	**D** Intraluminal Device
		Lower Arteries	
		Upper Arteries	
Intraluminal Device, Endobronchial Valve	All applicable	Respiratory System	**D** Intraluminal Device
Intraluminal Device, Endotracheal Airway	All applicable	Respiratory System	**D** Intraluminal Device
Intraluminal Device, Flow Diverter	Restriction	Upper Arteries	**D** Intraluminal Device
Intraluminal Device, Four or More	All applicable	Heart and Great Vessels	**D** Intraluminal Device
		Lower Arteries	
		Upper Arteries	
Intraluminal Device, Pessary	All applicable	Female Reproductive System	**D** Intraluminal Device
Intraluminal Device, Radioactive	All applicable	Heart and Great Vessels	**D** Intraluminal Device
Intraluminal Device, Three	All applicable	Heart and Great Vessels	**D** Intraluminal Device
		Lower Arteries	
		Upper Arteries	
Intraluminal Device, Two	All applicable	Heart and Great Vessels	**D** Intraluminal Device
		Lower Arteries	
		Upper Arteries	
Monitoring Device, Hemodynamic	Insertion	Subcutaneous Tissue and Fascia	**2** Monitoring Device
Monitoring Device, Pressure Sensor	Insertion	Heart and Great Vessels	**2** Monitoring Device
Pacemaker, Dual Chamber	Insertion	Subcutaneous Tissue and Fascia	**P** Cardiac Rhythm Related Device
Pacemaker, Single Chamber	Insertion	Subcutaneous Tissue and Fascia	**P** Cardiac Rhythm Related Device
Pacemaker, Single Chamber Rate Responsive	Insertion	Subcutaneous Tissue and Fascia	**P** Cardiac Rhythm Related Device
Spinal Stabilization Device, Facet Replacement	Insertion	Lower Joints	**4** Internal Fixation Device
		Upper Joints	
Spinal Stabilization Device, Interspinous Process	Insertion	Lower Joints	**4** Internal Fixation Device
		Upper Joints	
Spinal Stabilization Device, Pedicle-Based	Insertion	Lower Joints	**4** Internal Fixation Device
		Upper Joints	

Specific Device	For Operation	In Body System	General Device
Stimulator Generator, Multiple Array	Insertion	Subcutaneous Tissue and Fascia	**M** Stimulator Generator
Stimulator Generator, Multiple Array Rechargeable	Insertion	Subcutaneous Tissue and Fascia	**M** Stimulator Generator
Stimulator Generator, Single Array	Insertion	Subcutaneous Tissue and Fascia	**M** Stimulator Generator
Stimulator Generator, Single Array Rechargeable	Insertion	Subcutaneous Tissue and Fascia	**M** Stimulator Generator
Synthetic Substitute, Ceramic	Replacement	Lower Joints	**J** Synthetic Substitute
Synthetic Substitute, Ceramic on Polyethylene	Replacement	Lower Joints	**J** Synthetic Substitute
Synthetic Substitute, Intraocular Telescope	Replacement	Eye	**J** Synthetic Substitute
Synthetic Substitute, Metal	Replacement	Lower Joints	**J** Synthetic Substitute
Synthetic Substitute, Metal on Polyethylene	Replacement	Lower Joints	**J** Synthetic Substitute
Synthetic Substitute, Oxidized Zirconium on Polyethylene	Replacement	Lower Joints	**J** Synthetic Substitute
Synthetic Substitute, Polyethylene	Replacement	Lower Joints	**J** Synthetic Substitute
Synthetic Substitute, Reverse Ball and Socket	Replacement	Upper Joints	**J** Synthetic Substitute

This page intentionally left blank

ID code options rather than starting at index

Appendix E: Character Meaning

0: Medical and Surgical
0: Central Nervous System and Cranial Nerves

Operation-Character 3	Body Part-Character 4	Approach-Character 5	Device-Character 6	Qualifier-Character 7
1 Bypass	**0** Brain	**0** Open	**0** Drainage Device	**0** Nasopharynx
2 Change	**1** Cerebral Meninges	**3** Percutaneous	**2** Monitoring Device	**1** Mastoid Sinus
5 Destruction	**2** Dura Mater	**4** Percutaneous Endoscopic	**3** Infusion Device	**2** Atrium
7 Dilation	**3** Epidural Space, Intracranial	**X** External	**4** Radioactive Element, Cesium-131 Collagen Implant	**3** Blood Vessel
8 Division	**4** Subdural Space, Intracranial		**7** Autologous Tissue Substitute	**4** Pleural Cavity
9 Drainage	**5** Subarachnoid Space, Intracranial		**J** Synthetic Substitute	**5** Intestine
B Excision	**6** Cerebral Ventricle		**K** Nonautologous Tissue Substitute	**6** Peritoneal Cavity
C Extirpation	**7** Cerebral Hemisphere		**M** Neurostimulator Lead	**7** Urinary Tract
D Extraction	**8** Basal Ganglia		**Y** Other Device	**8** Bone Marrow
F Fragmentation	**9** Thalamus		**Z** No Device	**9** Fallopian Tube
H Insertion	**A** Hypothalamus			**A** Subgaleal Space
J Inspection	**B** Pons			**B** Cerebral Cisterns
K Map	**C** Cerebellum			**F** Olfactory Nerve
N Release	**D** Medulla Oblongata			**G** Optic Nerve
P Removal	**E** Cranial Nerve			**H** Oculomotor Nerve
Q Repair	**F** Olfactory Nerve			**J** Trochlear Nerve
R Replacement	**G** Optic Nerve			**K** Trigeminal Nerve
S Reposition	**H** Oculomotor Nerve			**L** Abducens Nerve
T Resection	**J** Trochlear Nerve			**M** Facial Nerve
U Supplement	**K** Trigeminal Nerve			**N** Acoustic Nerve
W Revision	**L** Abducens Nerve			**P** Glossopharyngeal Nerve
X Transfer	**M** Facial Nerve			**Q** Vagus Nerve
	N Acoustic Nerve			**R** Accessory Nerve
	P Glossopharyngeal Nerve			**S** Hypoglossal Nerve
	Q Vagus Nerve			**X** Diagnostic
	R Accessory Nerve			**Z** No Qualifier
	S Hypoglossal Nerve			
	T Spinal Meninges			
	U Spinal Canal			
	V Spinal Cord			
	W Cervical Spinal Cord			
	X Thoracic Spinal Cord			
	Y Lumbar Spinal Cord			

0: Medical and Surgical
1: Peripheral Nervous System

Operation-Character 3	Body Part-Character 4	Approach-Character 5	Device-Character 6	Qualifier-Character 7
2 Change	**0** Cervical Plexus	**0** Open	**0** Drainage Device	**1** Cervical Nerve
5 Destruction	**1** Cervical Nerve	**3** Percutaneous	**2** Monitoring Device	**2** Phrenic Nerve
8 Division	**2** Phrenic Nerve	**4** Percutaneous Endoscopic	**7** Autologous Tissue Substitute	**4** Ulnar Nerve
9 Drainage	**3** Brachial Plexus	**X** External	**J** Synthetic Substitute	**5** Median Nerve
B Excision	**4** Ulnar Nerve		**K** Nonautologous Tissue Substitute	**6** Radial Nerve
C Extirpation	**5** Median Nerve		**M** Neurostimulator Lead	**8** Thoracic Nerve
D Extraction	**6** Radial Nerve		**Y** Other Device	**B** Lumbar Nerve
H Insertion	**8** Thoracic Nerve		**Z** No Device	**C** Perineal Nerve
J Inspection	**9** Lumbar Plexus			**D** Femoral Nerve
N Release	**A** Lumbosacral Plexus			**F** Sciatic Nerve
P Removal	**B** Lumbar Nerve			**G** Tibial Nerve
Q Repair	**C** Pudendal Nerve			**H** Peroneal Nerve
R Replacement	**D** Femoral Nerve			**X** Diagnostic
S Reposition	**F** Sciatic Nerve			**Z** No Qualifier
U Supplement	**G** Tibial Nerve			
W Revision	**H** Peroneal Nerve			
X Transfer	**K** Head and Neck Sympathetic Nerve			
	L Thoracic Sympathetic Nerve			
	M Abdominal Sympathetic Nerve			
	N Lumbar Sympathetic Nerve			
	P Sacral Sympathetic Nerve			
	Q Sacral Plexus			
	R Sacral Nerve			
	Y Peripheral Nerve			

0: Medical and Surgical
2: Heart and Great Vessels

Operation-Character 3	Body Part-Character 4	Approach-Character 5	Device-Character 6	Qualifier-Character 7
1 Bypass	**0** Coronary Artery, One Artery	**0** Open	**0** Monitoring Device, Pressure Sensor	**0** Allogeneic
4 Creation	**1** Coronary Artery, Two Arteries	**3** Percutaneous	**2** Monitoring Device	**1** Syngeneic
5 Destruction	**2** Coronary Artery, Three Arteries	**4** Percutaneous Endoscopic	**3** Infusion Device	**2** Zooplastic
7 Dilation	**3** Coronary Artery, Four or More Arteries	**X** External	**4** Intraluminal Device, Drug-eluting	**2** Common Atrioventricular Valve
8 Division	**4** Coronary Vein		**5** Intraluminal Device, Drug-eluting, Two	**3** Coronary Artery
B Excision	**5** Atrial Septum		**6** Intraluminal Device, Drug-eluting, Three	**4** Coronary Vein
C Extirpation	**6** Atrium, Right		**7** Intraluminal Device, Drug-eluting, Four or More	**5** Coronary Circulation
F Fragmentation	**7** Atrium, Left		**7** Autologous Tissue Substitute	**6** Bifurcation
H Insertion	**8** Conduction Mechanism		**8** Zooplastic Tissue	**7** Atrium, Left
J Inspection	**9** Chordae Tendineae		**9** Autologous Venous Tissue	**8** Internal Mammary, Right
K Map	**A** Heart		**A** Autologous Arterial Tissue	**9** Internal Mammary, Left
L Occlusion	**B** Heart, Right		**C** Extraluminal Device	**A** Innominate Artery
N Release	**C** Heart, Left		**D** Intraluminal Device	**B** Subclavian
P Removal	**D** Papillary Muscle		**E** Intraluminal Device, Two	**C** Thoracic Artery
Q Repair	**F** Aortic Valve		**E** Intraluminal Device, Branched or Fenestrated, One or Two Arteries	**D** Carotid
R Replacement	**G** Mitral Valve		**F** Intraluminal Device, Three	**E** Atrioventricular Valve, Left
S Reposition	**H** Pulmonary Valve		**F** Intraluminal Device, Branched or Fenestrated, Three or More Arteries	**F** Abdominal Artery
T Resection	**J** Tricuspid Valve		**G** Intraluminal Device, Four or More	**G** Atrioventricular Valve, Right
U Supplement	**K** Ventricle, Right		**J** Cardiac Lead, Pacemaker	**G** Axillary Artery
V Restriction	**L** Ventricle, Left		**J** Synthetic Substitute	**H** Transapical
W Revision	**M** Ventricular Septum		**K** Cardiac Lead, Defibrillator	**H** Brachial Artery
Y Transplantation	**N** Pericardium		**K** Nonautologous Tissue Substitute	**J** Intraoperative
	P Pulmonary Trunk		**M** Cardiac Lead	**J** Temporary
	Q Pulmonary Artery, Right		**N** Intracardiac Pacemaker	**J** Truncal Valve
	R Pulmonary Artery, Left		**Q** Implantable Heart Assist System	**K** Left Atrial Appendage
	S Pulmonary Vein, Right		**R** Short-term External Heart Assist System	**P** Pulmonary Trunk
	T Pulmonary Vein, Left		**T** Intraluminal Device, Radioactive	**Q** Pulmonary Artery, Right
	V Superior Vena Cava		**Y** Other Device	**R** Pulmonary Artery, Left
	W Thoracic Aorta, Descending		**Z** No Device	**S** Biventricular
	X Thoracic Aorta, Ascending/Arch			**S** Pulmonary Vein, Right
	Y Great Vessel			**T** Pulmonary Vein, Left
				T Ductus Arteriosus
				U Pulmonary Vein, Confluence
				V Lower Extremity Artery
				W Aorta
				X Diagnostic
				Z No Qualifier

0: Medical and Surgical
3: Upper Arteries

Operation-Character 3	Body Part-Character 4	Approach-Character 5	Device-Character 6	Qualifier-Character 7
1 Bypass	**0** Internal Mammary Artery, Right	**0** Open	**0** Drainage Device	**0** Upper Arm Artery, Right
5 Destruction	**1** Internal Mammary Artery, Left	**3** Percutaneous	**2** Monitoring Device	**1** Drug-Coated Balloon
7 Dilation	**2** Innominate Artery	**4** Percutaneous Endoscopic	**3** Infusion Device	**1** Upper Arm Artery, Left
9 Drainage	**3** Subclavian Artery, Right	**X** External	**4** Intraluminal Device, Drug-eluting	**2** Upper Arm Artery, Bilateral
B Excision	**4** Subclavian Artery, Left		**5** Intraluminal Device, Drug-eluting, Two	**3** Lower Arm Artery, Right
C Extirpation	**5** Axillary Artery, Right		**6** Intraluminal Device, Drug-eluting, Three	**4** Lower Arm Artery, Left
H Insertion	**6** Axillary Artery, Left		**7** Autologous Tissue Substitute	**5** Lower Arm Artery, Bilateral
J Inspection	**7** Brachial Artery, Right		**7** Intraluminal Device, Drug-eluting, Four or More	**6** Bifurcation
L Occlusion	**8** Brachial Artery, Left		**9** Autologous Venous Tissue	**6** Upper Leg Artery, Right
N Release	**9** Ulnar Artery, Right		**A** Autologous Arterial Tissue	**7** Stent Retriever
P Removal	**A** Ulnar Artery, Left		**B** Intraluminal Device, Bioactive	**7** Upper Leg Artery, Left
Q Repair	**B** Radial Artery, Right		**C** Extraluminal Device	**8** Upper Leg Artery, Bilateral
R Replacement	**C** Radial Artery, Left		**D** Intraluminal Device	**9** Lower Leg Artery, Right
S Reposition	**D** Hand Artery, Right		**E** Intraluminal Device, Two	**B** Lower Leg Artery, Left
U Supplement	**F** Hand Artery, Left		**F** Intraluminal Device, Three	**C** Lower Leg Artery, Bilateral
V Restriction	**G** Intracranial Artery		**G** Intraluminal Device, Four or More	**D** Upper Arm Vein
W Revision	**H** Common Carotid Artery, Right		**J** Synthetic Substitute	**F** Lower Arm Vein
	J Common Carotid Artery, Left		**K** Nonautologous Tissue Substitute	**G** Intracranial Artery
	K Internal Carotid Artery, Right		**M** Stimulator Lead	**J** Extracranial Artery, Right
	L Internal Carotid Artery, Left		**Y** Other Device	**K** Extracranial Artery, Left
	M External Carotid Artery, Right		**Z** No Device	**M** Pulmonary Artery, Right
	N External Carotid Artery, Left			**N** Pulmonary Artery, Left
	P Vertebral Artery, Right			**T** Abdominal Artery
	Q Vertebral Artery, Left			**V** Superior Vena Cava
	R Face Artery			**W** Lower Extremity Vein
	S Temporal Artery, Right			**X** Diagnostic
	T Temporal Artery, Left			**Y** Upper Artery
	U Thyroid Artery, Right			**Z** No Qualifier
	V Thyroid Artery, Left			
	Y Upper Artery			

0: Medical and Surgical
4: Lower Arteries

Operation-Character 3	Body Part-Character 4	Approach-Character 5	Device-Character 6	Qualifier-Character 7
1 Bypass	**0** Abdominal Aorta	**0** Open	**0** Drainage Device	**0** Abdominal Aorta
5 Destruction	**1** Celiac Artery	**3** Percutaneous	**1** Radioactive Element	**1** Celiac Artery
7 Dilation	**2** Gastric Artery	**4** Percutaneous Endoscopic	**2** Monitoring Device	**1** Drug-Coated Balloon
9 Drainage	**3** Hepatic Artery	**X** External	**3** Infusion Device	**2** Mesenteric Artery
B Excision	**4** Splenic Artery		**4** Intraluminal Device, Drug-eluting	**3** Renal Artery, Right
C Extirpation	**5** Superior Mesenteric Artery		**5** Intraluminal Device, Drug-eluting, Two	**4** Renal Artery, Left
H Insertion	**6** Colic Artery, Right		**6** Intraluminal Device, Drug-eluting, Three	**5** Renal Artery, Bilateral
J Inspection	**7** Colic Artery, Left		**7** Autologous Tissue Substitute	**6** Bifurcation
L Occlusion	**8** Colic Artery, Middle		**7** Intraluminal Device, Drug-eluting, Four or More	**6** Common Iliac Artery, Right
N Release	**9** Renal Artery, Right		**9** Autologous Venous Tissue	**7** Common Iliac Artery, Left
P Removal	**A** Renal Artery, Left		**A** Autologous Arterial Tissue	**8** Common Iliac Arteries, Bilateral
Q Repair	**B** Inferior Mesenteric Artery		**C** Extraluminal Device	**9** Internal Iliac Artery, Right
R Replacement	**C** Common Iliac Artery, Right		**D** Intraluminal Device	**B** Internal Iliac Artery, Left
S Reposition	**D** Common Iliac Artery, Left		**E** Intraluminal Device, Branched or Fenestrated, One or Two Arteries	**C** Internal Iliac Arteries, Bilateral
U Supplement	**E** Internal Iliac Artery, Right		**E** Intraluminal Device, Two	**D** External Iliac Artery, Right
V Restriction	**F** Internal Iliac Artery, Left		**F** Intraluminal Device, Branched or Fenestrated, Three or More Arteries	**F** External Iliac Artery, Left
W Revision	**H** External Iliac Artery, Right		**F** Intraluminal Device, Three	**G** External Iliac Arteries, Bilateral
	J External Iliac Artery, Left		**G** Intraluminal Device, Four or More	**H** Femoral Artery, Right
	K Femoral Artery, Right		**J** Synthetic Substitute	**J** Femoral Artery, Left
	L Femoral Artery, Left		**K** Nonautologous Tissue Substitute	**J** Temporary
	M Popliteal Artery, Right		**Y** Other Device	**K** Femoral Arteries, Bilateral
	N Popliteal Artery, Left		**Z** No Device	**L** Popliteal Artery
	P Anterior Tibial Artery, Right			**M** Peroneal Artery
	Q Anterior Tibial Artery, Left			**N** Posterior Tibial Artery
	R Posterior Tibial Artery, Right			**P** Foot Artery
	S Posterior Tibial Artery, Left			**Q** Lower Extremity Artery
	T Peroneal Artery, Right			**R** Lower Artery
	U Peroneal Artery, Left			**S** Lower Extremity Vein
	V Foot Artery, Right			**T** Uterine Artery, Right
	W Foot Artery, Left			**U** Uterine Artery, Left
	Y Lower Artery			**X** Diagnostic
				Z No Qualifier

0: Medical and Surgical
5: Upper Veins

Operation-Character 3	Body Part-Character 4	Approach-Character 5	Device-Character 6	Qualifier-Character 7
1 Bypass	**0** Azygos Vein	**0** Open	**0** Drainage Device	**1** Drug-Coated Balloon
5 Destruction	**1** Hemiazygos Vein	**3** Percutaneous	**2** Monitoring Device	**X** Diagnostic
7 Dilation	**3** Innominate Vein, Right	**4** Percutaneous Endoscopic	**3** Infusion Device	**Y** Upper Vein
9 Drainage	**4** Innominate Vein, Left	**X** External	**7** Autologous Tissue Substitute	**Z** No Qualifier
B Excision	**5** Subclavian Vein, Right		**9** Autologous Venous Tissue	
C Extirpation	**6** Subclavian Vein, Left		**A** Autologous Arterial Tissue	
D Extraction	**7** Axillary Vein, Right		**C** Extraluminal Device	
H Insertion	**8** Axillary Vein, Left		**D** Intraluminal Device	
J Inspection	**9** Brachial Vein, Right		**J** Synthetic Substitute	
L Occlusion	**A** Brachial Vein, Left		**K** Nonautologous Tissue Substitute	
N Release	**B** Basilic Vein, Right		**M** Neurostimulator Lead	
P Removal	**C** Basilic Vein, Left		**Y** Other Device	
Q Repair	**D** Cephalic Vein, Right		**Z** No Device	
R Replacement	**F** Cephalic Vein, Left			
S Reposition	**G** Hand Vein, Right			
U Supplement	**H** Hand Vein, Left			
V Restriction	**L** Intracranial Vein			
W Revision	**M** Internal Jugular Vein, Right			
	N Internal Jugular Vein, Left			
	P External Jugular Vein, Right			
	Q External Jugular Vein, Left			
	R Vertebral Vein, Right			
	S Vertebral Vein, Left			
	T Face Vein, Right			
	V Face Vein, Left			
	Y Upper Vein			

0: Medical and Surgical
6: Lower Veins

Operation-Character 3	Body Part-Character 4	Approach-Character 5	Device-Character 6	Qualifier-Character 7
1 Bypass	**0** Inferior Vena Cava	**0** Open	**0** Drainage Device	**4** Hepatic Vein
5 Destruction	**1** Splenic Vein	**3** Percutaneous	**2** Monitoring Device	**5** Superior Mesenteric Vein
7 Dilation	**2** Gastric Vein	**4** Percutaneous Endoscopic	**3** Infusion Device	**6** Inferior Mesenteric Vein
9 Drainage	**3** Esophageal Vein	**7** Via Natural or Artificial Opening	**7** Autologous Tissue Substitute	**9** Renal Vein, Right
B Excision	**4** Hepatic Vein	**8** Via Natural or Artificial Opening Endoscopic	**9** Autologous Venous Tissue	**B** Renal Vein, Left
C Extirpation	**5** Superior Mesenteric Vein	**X** External	**A** Autologous Arterial Tissue	**C** Hemorrhoidal Plexus
D Extraction	**6** Inferior Mesenteric Vein		**C** Extraluminal Device	**P** Pulmonary Trunk
H Insertion	**7** Colic Vein		**D** Intraluminal Device	**Q** Pulmonary Artery, Right
J Inspection	**8** Portal Vein		**J** Synthetic Substitute	**R** Pulmonary Artery, Left
L Occlusion	**9** Renal Vein, Right		**K** Nonautologous Tissue Substitute	**T** Via Umbilical Vein
N Release	**B** Renal Vein, Left		**Y** Other Device	**X** Diagnostic
P Removal	**C** Common Iliac Vein, Right		**Z** No Device	**Y** Lower Vein
Q Repair	**D** Common Iliac Vein, Left			**Z** No Qualifier
R Replacement	**F** External Iliac Vein, Right			
S Reposition	**G** External Iliac Vein, Left			
U Supplement	**H** Hypogastric Vein, Right			
V Restriction	**J** Hypogastric Vein, Left			
W Revision	**M** Femoral Vein, Right			
	N Femoral Vein, Left			
	P Saphenous Vein, Right			
	Q Saphenous Vein, Left			
	T Foot Vein, Right			
	V Foot Vein, Left			
	Y Lower Vein			

0: Medical and Surgical
7: Lymphatic and Hemic Systems

Operation-Character 3	Body Part-Character 4	Approach-Character 5	Device-Character 6	Qualifier-Character 7
2 Change	**0** Lymphatic, Head	**0** Open	**0** Drainage Device	**0** Allogeneic
5 Destruction	**1** Lymphatic, Right Neck	**3** Percutaneous	**3** Infusion Device	**1** Syngeneic
9 Drainage	**2** Lymphatic, Left Neck	**4** Percutaneous Endoscopic	**7** Autologous Tissue Substitute	**2** Zooplastic
B Excision	**3** Lymphatic, Right Upper Extremity	**8** Via Natural or Artificial Opening Endoscopic	**C** Extraluminal Device	**X** Diagnostic
C Extirpation	**4** Lymphatic, Left Upper Extremity	**X** External	**D** Intraluminal Device	**Z** No Qualifier
D Extraction	**5** Lymphatic, Right Axillary		**J** Synthetic Substitute	
H Insertion	**6** Lymphatic, Left Axillary		**K** Nonautologous Tissue Substitute	
J Inspection	**7** Lymphatic, Thorax		**Y** Other Device	
L Occlusion	**8** Lymphatic, Internal Mammary, Right		**Z** No Device	
N Release	**9** Lymphatic, Internal Mammary, Left			
P Removal	**B** Lymphatic, Mesenteric			
Q Repair	**C** Lymphatic, Pelvis			
S Reposition	**D** Lymphatic, Aortic			
T Resection	**F** Lymphatic, Right Lower Extremity			
U Supplement	**G** Lymphatic, Left Lower Extremity			
V Restriction	**H** Lymphatic, Right Inguinal			
W Revision	**J** Lymphatic, Left Inguinal			
Y Transplantation	**K** Thoracic Duct			
	L Cisterna Chyli			
	M Thymus			
	N Lymphatic			
	P Spleen			
	Q Bone Marrow, Sternum			
	R Bone Marrow, Iliac			
	S Bone Marrow, Vertebral			
	T Bone Marrow			

0: Medical and Surgical
8: Eye

Operation-Character 3	Body Part-Character 4	Approach-Character 5	Device-Character 6	Qualifier-Character 7
0 Alteration	**0** Eye, Right	**0** Open	**0** Drainage Device	**3** Nasal Cavity
1 Bypass	**1** Eye, Left	**3** Percutaneous	**0** Synthetic Substitute, Intraocular Telescope	**4** Sclera
2 Change	**2** Anterior Chamber, Right	**7** Via Natural or Artificial Opening	**1** Radioactive Element	**X** Diagnostic
5 Destruction	**3** Anterior Chamber, Left	**8** Via Natural or Artificial Opening Endoscopic	**3** Infusion Device	**Z** No Qualifier
7 Dilation	**4** Vitreous, Right	**X** External	**5** Epiretinal Visual Prosthesis	
9 Drainage	**5** Vitreous, Left		**7** Autologous Tissue Substitute	
B Excision	**6** Sclera, Right		**C** Extraluminal Device	
C Extirpation	**7** Sclera, Left		**D** Intraluminal Device	
D Extraction	**8** Cornea, Right		**J** Synthetic Substitute	
F Fragmentation	**9** Cornea, Left		**K** Nonautologous Tissue Substitute	
H Insertion	**A** Choroid, Right		**Y** Other Device	
J Inspection	**B** Choroid, Left		**Z** No Device	
L Occlusion	**C** Iris, Right			
M Reattachment	**D** Iris, Left			
N Release	**E** Retina, Right			
P Removal	**F** Retina, Left			
Q Repair	**G** Retinal Vessel, Right			
R Replacement	**H** Retinal Vessel, Left			
S Reposition	**J** Lens, Right			
T Resection	**K** Lens, Left			
U Supplement	**L** Extraocular Muscle, Right			
V Restriction	**M** Extraocular Muscle, Left			
W Revision	**N** Upper Eyelid, Right			
X Transfer	**P** Upper Eyelid, Left			
	Q Lower Eyelid, Right			
	R Lower Eyelid, Left			
	S Conjunctiva, Right			
	T Conjunctiva, Left			
	V Lacrimal Gland, Right			
	W Lacrimal Gland, Left			
	X Lacrimal Duct, Right			
	Y Lacrimal Duct, Left			

0: Medical and Surgical
9: Ear, Nose, Sinus

Operation-Character 3	Body Part-Character 4	Approach-Character 5	Device-Character 6	Qualifier-Character 7
0 Alteration	**0** External Ear, Right	**0** Open	**0** Drainage Device	**0** Endolymphatic
1 Bypass	**1** External Ear, Left	**3** Percutaneous	**4** Hearing Device, Bone Conduction	**X** Diagnostic
2 Change	**2** External Ear, Bilateral	**4** Percutaneous Endoscopic	**5** Hearing Device, Single Channel Cochlear Prosthesis	**Z** No Qualifier
3 Control	**3** External Auditory Canal, Right	**7** Via Natural or Artificial Opening	**6** Hearing Device, Multiple Channel Cochlear Prosthesis	
5 Destruction	**4** External Auditory Canal, Left	**8** Via Natural or Artificial Opening Endoscopic	**7** Autologous Tissue Substitute	
7 Dilation	**5** Middle Ear, Right	**X** External	**B** Intraluminal Device, Airway	
8 Division	**6** Middle Ear, Left		**D** Intraluminal Device	
9 Drainage	**7** Tympanic Membrane, Right		**J** Synthetic Substitute	
B Excision	**8** Tympanic Membrane, Left		**K** Nonautologous Tissue Substitute	
C Extirpation	**9** Auditory Ossicle, Right		**S** Hearing Device	
D Extraction	**A** Auditory Ossicle, Left		**Y** Other Device	
H Insertion	**B** Mastoid Sinus, Right		**Z** No Device	
J Inspection	**C** Mastoid Sinus, Left			
M Reattachment	**D** Inner Ear, Right			
N Release	**E** Inner Ear, Left			
P Removal	**F** Eustachian Tube, Right			
Q Repair	**G** Eustachian Tube, Left			
R Replacement	**H** Ear, Right			
S Reposition	**J** Ear, Left			
T Resection	**K** Nasal Mucosa and Soft Tissue			
U Supplement	**L** Nasal Turbinate			
W Revision	**M** Nasal Septum			
	N Nasopharynx			
	P Accessory Sinus			
	Q Maxillary Sinus, Right			
	R Maxillary Sinus, Left			
	S Frontal Sinus, Right			
	T Frontal Sinus, Left			
	U Ethmoid Sinus, Right			
	V Ethmoid Sinus, Left			
	W Sphenoid Sinus, Right			
	X Sphenoid Sinus, Left			
	Y Sinus			

0: Medical and Surgical
B: Respiratory System

Operation-Character 3	Body Part-Character 4	Approach-Character 5	Device-Character 6	Qualifier-Character 7
1 Bypass	**0** Tracheobronchial Tree	**0** Open	**0** Drainage Device	**0** Allogeneic
2 Change	**1** Trachea	**3** Percutaneous	**1** Radioactive Element	**1** Syngeneic
5 Destruction	**2** Carina	**4** Percutaneous Endoscopic	**2** Monitoring Device	**2** Zooplastic
7 Dilation	**3** Main Bronchus, Right	**7** Via Natural or Artificial Opening	**3** Infusion Device	**4** Cutaneous
9 Drainage	**4** Upper Lobe Bronchus, Right	**8** Via Natural or Artificial Opening Endoscopic	**7** Autologous Tissue Substitute	**6** Esophagus
B Excision	**5** Middle Lobe Bronchus, Right	**X** External	**C** Extraluminal Device	**X** Diagnostic
C Extirpation	**6** Lower Lobe Bronchus, Right		**D** Intraluminal Device	**Z** No Qualifier
D Extraction	**7** Main Bronchus, Left		**E** Intraluminal Device, Endotracheal Airway	
F Fragmentation	**8** Upper Lobe Bronchus, Left		**F** Tracheostomy Device	
H Insertion	**9** Lingula Bronchus		**G** Intraluminal Device, Endobronchial Valve	
J Inspection	**B** Lower Lobe Bronchus, Left		**J** Synthetic Substitute	
L Occlusion	**C** Upper Lung Lobe, Right		**K** Nonautologous Tissue Substitute	
M Reattachment	**D** Middle Lung Lobe, Right		**M** Diaphragmatic Pacemaker Lead	
N Release	**F** Lower Lung Lobe, Right		**Y** Other Device	
P Removal	**G** Upper Lung Lobe, Left		**Z** No Device	
Q Repair	**H** Lung Lingula			
R Replacement	**J** Lower Lung Lobe, Left			
S Reposition	**K** Lung, Right			
T Resection	**L** Lung, Left			
U Supplement	**M** Lungs, Bilateral			
V Restriction	**N** Pleura, Right			
W Revision	**P** Pleura, Left			
Y Transplantation	**Q** Pleura			
	T Diaphragm			

0: Medical and Surgical
C: Mouth and Throat

Operation-Character 3	Body Part-Character 4	Approach-Character 5	Device-Character 6	Qualifier-Character 7
0 Alteration	**0** Upper Lip	**0** Open	**0** Drainage Device	**0** Single
2 Change	**1** Lower Lip	**3** Percutaneous	**1** Radioactive Element	**1** Multiple
5 Destruction	**2** Hard Palate	**4** Percutaneous Endoscopic	**5** External Fixation Device	**2** All
7 Dilation	**3** Soft Palate	**7** Via Natural or Artificial Opening	**7** Autologous Tissue Substitute	**X** Diagnostic
9 Drainage	**4** Buccal Mucosa	**8** Via Natural or Artificial Opening Endoscopic	**B** Intraluminal Device, Airway	**Z** No Qualifier
B Excision	**5** Upper Gingiva	**X** External	**C** Extraluminal Device	
C Extirpation	**6** Lower Gingiva		**D** Intraluminal Device	
D Extraction	**7** Tongue		**J** Synthetic Substitute	
F Fragmentation	**8** Parotid Gland, Right		**K** Nonautologous Tissue Substitute	
H Insertion	**9** Parotid Gland, Left		**Y** Other Device	
J Inspection	**A** Salivary Gland		**Z** No Device	
L Occlusion	**B** Parotid Duct, Right			
M Reattachment	**C** Parotid Duct, Left			
N Release	**D** Sublingual Gland, Right			
P Removal	**F** Sublingual Gland, Left			
Q Repair	**G** Submaxillary Gland, Right			
R Replacement	**H** Submaxillary Gland, Left			
S Reposition	**J** Minor Salivary Gland			
T Resection	**M** Pharynx			
U Supplement	**N** Uvula			
V Restriction	**P** Tonsils			
W Revision	**Q** Adenoids			
X Transfer	**R** Epiglottis			
	S Larynx			
	T Vocal Cord, Right			
	V Vocal Cord, Left			
	W Upper Tooth			
	X Lower Tooth			
	Y Mouth and Throat			

0: Medical and Surgical
D: Gastrointestinal System

Operation-Character 3	Body Part-Character 4	Approach-Character 5	Device-Character 6	Qualifier-Character 7
1 Bypass	**0** Upper Intestinal Tract	**0** Open	**0** Drainage Device	**0** Allogeneic
2 Change	**1** Esophagus, Upper	**3** Percutaneous	**1** Radioactive Element	**1** Syngeneic
5 Destruction	**2** Esophagus, Middle	**4** Percutaneous Endoscopic	**2** Monitoring Device	**2** Zooplastic
7 Dilation	**3** Esophagus, Lower	**7** Via Natural or Artificial Opening	**3** Infusion Device	**3** Vertical
8 Division	**4** Esophagogastric Junction	**8** Via Natural or Artificial Opening Endoscopic	**7** Autologous Tissue Substitute	**4** Cutaneous
9 Drainage	**5** Esophagus	**X** External	**B** Intraluminal Device, Airway	**5** Esophagus
B Excision	**6** Stomach		**C** Extraluminal Device	**6** Stomach
C Extirpation	**7** Stomach, Pylorus		**D** Intraluminal Device	**7** Vagina
D Extraction	**8** Small Intestine		**J** Synthetic Substitute	**8** Small Intestine
F Fragmentation	**9** Duodenum		**K** Nonautologous Tissue Substitute	**9** Duodenum
H Insertion	**A** Jejunum		**L** Artificial Sphincter	**A** Jejunum
J Inspection	**B** Ileum		**M** Stimulator Lead	**B** Ileum
L Occlusion	**C** Ileocecal Valve		**U** Feeding Device	**H** Cecum
M Reattachment	**D** Lower Intestinal Tract		**Y** Other Device	**K** Ascending Colon
N Release	**E** Large Intestine		**Z** No Device	**L** Transverse Colon
P Removal	**F** Large Intestine, Right			**M** Descending Colon
Q Repair	**G** Large Intestine, Left			**N** Sigmoid Colon
R Replacement	**H** Cecum			**P** Rectum
S Reposition	**J** Appendix			**Q** Anus
T Resection	**K** Ascending Colon			**X** Diagnostic
U Supplement	**L** Transverse Colon			**Z** No Qualifier
V Restriction	**M** Descending Colon			
W Revision	**N** Sigmoid Colon			
X Transfer	**P** Rectum			
Y Transplantation	**Q** Anus			
	R Anal Sphincter			
	U Omentum			
	V Mesentery			
	W Peritoneum			

0: Medical and Surgical
F: Hepatobiliary System and Pancreas

Operation-Character 3	Body Part-Character 4	Approach-Character 5	Device-Character 6	Qualifier-Character 7
1 Bypass	**0** Liver	**0** Open	**0** Drainage Device	**0** Allogeneic
2 Change	**1** Liver, Right Lobe	**3** Percutaneous	**1** Radioactive Element	**1** Syngeneic
5 Destruction	**2** Liver, Left Lobe	**4** Percutaneous Endoscopic	**2** Monitoring Device	**2** Zooplastic
7 Dilation	**4** Gallbladder	**7** Via Natural or Artificial Opening	**3** Infusion Device	**3** Duodenum
8 Division	**5** Hepatic Duct, Right	**8** Via Natural or Artificial Opening Endoscopic	**7** Autologous Tissue Substitute	**4** Stomach
9 Drainage	**6** Hepatic Duct, Left	**X** External	**C** Extraluminal Device	**5** Hepatic Duct, Right
B Excision	**7** Hepatic Duct, Common		**D** Intraluminal Device	**6** Hepatic Duct, Left
C Extirpation	**8** Cystic Duct		**J** Synthetic Substitute	**7** Hepatic Duct, Caudate
D Extraction	**9** Common Bile Duct		**K** Nonautologous Tissue Substitute	**8** Cystic Duct
F Fragmentation	**B** Hepatobiliary Duct		**Y** Other Device	**9** Common Bile Duct
H Insertion	**C** Ampulla of Vater		**Z** No Device	**B** Small Intestine
J Inspection	**D** Pancreatic Duct			**C** Large Intestine
L Occlusion	**F** Pancreatic Duct, Accessory			**F** Irreversible Electroporation
M Reattachment	**G** Pancreas			**X** Diagnostic
N Release				**Z** No Qualifier
P Removal				
Q Repair				
R Replacement				
S Reposition				
T Resection				
U Supplement				
V Restriction				
W Revision				
Y Transplantation				

0: Medical and Surgical
G: Endocrine System

Operation-Character 3	Body Part-Character 4	Approach-Character 5	Device-Character 6	Qualifier-Character 7
2 Change	**0** Pituitary Gland	**0** Open	**0** Drainage Device	**X** Diagnostic
5 Destruction	**1** Pineal Body	**3** Percutaneous	**2** Monitoring Device	**Z** No Qualifier
8 Division	**2** Adrenal Gland, Left	**4** Percutaneous Endoscopic	**3** Infusion Device	
9 Drainage	**3** Adrenal Gland, Right	**X** External	**Y** Other Device	
B Excision	**4** Adrenal Glands, Bilateral		**Z** No Device	
C Extirpation	**5** Adrenal Gland			
H Insertion	**6** Carotid Body, Left			
J Inspection	**7** Carotid Body, Right			
M Reattachment	**8** Carotid Bodies, Bilateral			
N Release	**9** Para-aortic Body			
P Removal	**B** Coccygeal Glomus			
Q Repair	**C** Glomus Jugulare			
S Reposition	**D** Aortic Body			
T Resection	**F** Paraganglion Extremity			
W Revision	**G** Thyroid Gland Lobe, Left			
	H Thyroid Gland Lobe, Right			
	J Thyroid Gland Isthmus			
	K Thyroid Gland			
	L Superior Parathyroid Gland, Right			
	M Superior Parathyroid Gland, Left			
	N Inferior Parathyroid Gland, Right			
	P Inferior Parathyroid Gland, Left			
	Q Parathyroid Glands, Multiple			
	R Parathyroid Gland			
	S Endocrine Gland			

0: Medical and Surgical
H: Skin and Breast

Operation-Character 3	Body Part-Character 4	Approach-Character 5	Device-Character 6	Qualifier-Character 7
0 Alteration	**0** Skin, Scalp	**0** Open	**0** Drainage Device	**2** Cell Suspension Technique
2 Change	**1** Skin, Face	**3** Percutaneous	**1** Radioactive Element	**3** Full Thickness
5 Destruction	**2** Skin, Right Ear	**7** Via Natural or Artificial Opening	**7** Autologous Tissue Substitute	**4** Partial Thickness
8 Division	**3** Skin, Left Ear	**8** Via Natural or Artificial Opening Endoscopic	**J** Synthetic Substitute	**5** Latissimus Dorsi Myocutaneous Flap
9 Drainage	**4** Skin, Neck	**X** External	**K** Nonautologous Tissue Substitute	**6** Transverse Rectus Abdominis Myocutaneous Flap
B Excision	**5** Skin, Chest		**N** Tissue Expander	**7** Deep Inferior Epigastric Artery Perforator Flap
C Extirpation	**6** Skin, Back		**Y** Other Device	**8** Superficial Inferior Epigastric Artery Flap
D Extraction	**7** Skin, Abdomen		**Z** No Device	**9** Gluteal Artery Perforator Flap
H Insertion	**8** Skin, Buttock			**D** Multiple
J Inspection	**9** Skin, Perineum			**X** Diagnostic
M Reattachment	**A** Skin, Inguinal			**Z** No Qualifier
N Release	**B** Skin, Right Upper Arm			
P Removal	**C** Skin, Left Upper Arm			
Q Repair	**D** Skin, Right Lower Arm			
R Replacement	**E** Skin, Left Lower Arm			
S Reposition	**F** Skin, Right Hand			
T Resection	**G** Skin, Left Hand			
U Supplement	**H** Skin, Right Upper Leg			
W Revision	**J** Skin, Left Upper Leg			
X Transfer	**K** Skin, Right Lower Leg			
	L Skin, Left Lower Leg			
	M Skin, Right Foot			
	N Skin, Left Foot			
	P Skin			
	Q Finger Nail			
	R Toe Nail			
	S Hair			
	T Breast, Right			
	U Breast, Left			
	V Breast, Bilateral			
	W Nipple, Right			
	X Nipple, Left			
	Y Supernumerary Breast			

0: Medical and Surgical
J: Subcutaneous Tissue and Fascia

Operation-Character 3	Body Part-Character 4	Approach-Character 5	Device-Character 6	Qualifier-Character 7
0 Alteration	**0** Subcutaneous Tissue and Fascia, Scalp	**0** Open	**0** Drainage Device	**B** Skin and Subcutaneous Tissue
2 Change	**1** Subcutaneous Tissue and Fascia, Face	**3** Percutaneous	**0** Monitoring Device, Hemodynamic	**C** Skin, Subcutaneous Tissue and Fascia
5 Destruction	**4** Subcutaneous Tissue and Fascia, Right Neck	**X** External	**1** Radioactive Element	**X** Diagnostic
8 Division	**5** Subcutaneous Tissue and Fascia, Left Neck		**2** Monitoring Device	**Z** No Qualifier
9 Drainage	**6** Subcutaneous Tissue and Fascia, Chest		**3** Infusion Device	
B Excision	**7** Subcutaneous Tissue and Fascia, Back		**4** Pacemaker, Single Chamber	
C Extirpation	**8** Subcutaneous Tissue and Fascia, Abdomen		**5** Pacemaker, Single Chamber Rate Responsive	
D Extraction	**9** Subcutaneous Tissue and Fascia, Buttock		**6** Pacemaker, Dual Chamber	
H Insertion	**B** Subcutaneous Tissue and Fascia, Perineum		**7** Autologous Tissue Substitute	
J Inspection	**C** Subcutaneous Tissue and Fascia, Pelvic Region		**7** Cardiac Resynchronization Pacemaker Pulse Generator	
N Release	**D** Subcutaneous Tissue and Fascia, Right Upper Arm		**8** Defibrillator Generator	
P Removal	**F** Subcutaneous Tissue and Fascia, Left Upper Arm		**9** Cardiac Resynchronization Defibrillator Pulse Generator	
Q Repair	**G** Subcutaneous Tissue and Fascia, Right Lower Arm		**A** Contractility Modulation Device	
R Replacement	**H** Subcutaneous Tissue and Fascia, Left Lower Arm		**B** Stimulator Generator, Single Array	
U Supplement	**J** Subcutaneous Tissue and Fascia, Right Hand		**C** Stimulator Generator, Single Array Rechargeable	
W Revision	**K** Subcutaneous Tissue and Fascia, Left Hand		**D** Stimulator Generator, Multiple Array	
X Transfer	**L** Subcutaneous Tissue and Fascia, Right Upper Leg		**E** Stimulator Generator, Multiple Array Rechargeable	
	M Subcutaneous Tissue and Fascia, Left Upper Leg		**F** Subcutaneous Defibrillator Lead	
	N Subcutaneous Tissue and Fascia, Right Lower Leg		**H** Contraceptive Device	
	P Subcutaneous Tissue and Fascia, Left Lower Leg		**J** Synthetic Substitute	
	Q Subcutaneous Tissue and Fascia, Right Foot		**K** Nonautologous Tissue Substitute	
	R Subcutaneous Tissue and Fascia, Left Foot		**M** Stimulator Generator	
	S Subcutaneous Tissue and Fascia, Head and Neck		**N** Tissue Expander	
	T Subcutaneous Tissue and Fascia, Trunk		**P** Cardiac Rhythm Related Device	
	V Subcutaneous Tissue and Fascia, Upper Extremity		**V** Infusion Device, Pump	
	W Subcutaneous Tissue and Fascia, Lower Extremity		**W** Vascular Access Device, Totally Implantable	
			X Vascular Access Device, Tunneled	
			Y Other Device	
			Z No Device	

0: Medical and Surgical
K: Muscles

Operation-Character 3	Body Part-Character 4	Approach-Character 5	Device-Character 6	Qualifier-Character 7
2 Change	**0** Head Muscle	**0** Open	**0** Drainage Device	**0** Skin
5 Destruction	**1** Facial Muscle	**3** Percutaneous	**7** Autologous Tissue Substitute	**1** Subcutaneous Tissue
8 Division	**2** Neck Muscle, Right	**4** Percutaneous Endoscopic	**J** Synthetic Substitute	**2** Skin and Subcutaneous Tissue
9 Drainage	**3** Neck Muscle, Left	**X** External	**K** Nonautologous Tissue Substitute	**5** Latissimus Dorsi Myocutaneous Flap
B Excision	**4** Tongue, Palate, Pharynx Muscle		**M** Stimulator Lead	**6** Transverse Rectus Abdominis Myocutaneous Flap
C Extirpation	**5** Shoulder Muscle, Right		**Y** Other Device	**7** Deep Inferior Epigastric Artery Perforator Flap
D Extraction	**6** Shoulder Muscle, Left		**Z** No Device	**8** Superficial Inferior Epigastric Artery Flap
H Insertion	**7** Upper Arm Muscle, Right			**9** Gluteal Artery Perforator Flap
J Inspection	**8** Upper Arm Muscle, Left			**X** Diagnostic
M Reattachment	**9** Lower Arm and Wrist Muscle, Right			**Z** No Qualifier
N Release	**B** Lower Arm and Wrist Muscle, Left			
P Removal	**C** Hand Muscle, Right			
Q Repair	**D** Hand Muscle, Left			
R Replacement	**F** Trunk Muscle, Right			
S Reposition	**G** Trunk Muscle, Left			
T Resection	**H** Thorax Muscle, Right			
U Supplement	**J** Thorax Muscle, Left			
W Revision	**K** Abdomen Muscle, Right			
X Transfer	**L** Abdomen Muscle, Left			
	M Perineum Muscle			
	N Hip Muscle, Right			
	P Hip Muscle, Left			
	Q Upper Leg Muscle, Right			
	R Upper Leg Muscle, Left			
	S Lower Leg Muscle, Right			
	T Lower Leg Muscle, Left			
	V Foot Muscle, Right			
	W Foot Muscle, Left			
	X Upper Muscle			
	Y Lower Muscle			

0: Medical and Surgical
L: Tendons

Operation-Character 3	Body Part-Character 4	Approach-Character 5	Device-Character 6	Qualifier-Character 7
2 Change	**0** Head and Neck Tendon	**0** Open	**0** Drainage Device	**X** Diagnostic
5 Destruction	**1** Shoulder Tendon, Right	**3** Percutaneous	**7** Autologous Tissue Substitute	**Z** No Qualifier
8 Division	**2** Shoulder Tendon, Left	**4** Percutaneous Endoscopic	**J** Synthetic Substitute	
9 Drainage	**3** Upper Arm Tendon, Right	**X** External	**K** Nonautologous Tissue Substitute	
B Excision	**4** Upper Arm Tendon, Left		**Y** Other Device	
C Extirpation	**5** Lower Arm and Wrist Tendon, Right		**Z** No Device	
D Extraction	**6** Lower Arm and Wrist Tendon, Left			
H Insertion	**7** Hand Tendon, Right			
J Inspection	**8** Hand Tendon, Left			
M Reattachment	**9** Trunk Tendon, Right			
N Release	**B** Trunk Tendon, Left			
P Removal	**C** Thorax Tendon, Right			
Q Repair	**D** Thorax Tendon, Left			
R Replacement	**F** Abdomen Tendon, Right			
S Reposition	**G** Abdomen Tendon, Left			
T Resection	**H** Perineum Tendon			
U Supplement	**J** Hip Tendon, Right			
W Revision	**K** Hip Tendon, Left			
X Transfer	**L** Upper Leg Tendon, Right			
	M Upper Leg Tendon, Left			
	N Lower Leg Tendon, Right			
	P Lower Leg Tendon, Left			
	Q Knee Tendon, Right			
	R Knee Tendon, Left			
	S Ankle Tendon, Right			
	T Ankle Tendon, Left			
	V Foot Tendon, Right			
	W Foot Tendon, Left			
	X Upper Tendon			
	Y Lower Tendon			

0: Medical and Surgical
M: Bursae and Ligaments

Operation-Character 3	Body Part-Character 4	Approach-Character 5	Device-Character 6	Qualifier-Character 7
2 Change	**0** Head and Neck Bursa and Ligament	**0** Open	**0** Drainage Device	**X** Diagnostic
5 Destruction	**1** Shoulder Bursa and Ligament, Right	**3** Percutaneous	**7** Autologous Tissue Substitute	**Z** No Qualifier
8 Division	**2** Shoulder Bursa and Ligament, Left	**4** Percutaneous Endoscopic	**J** Synthetic Substitute	
9 Drainage	**3** Elbow Bursa and Ligament, Right	**X** External	**K** Nonautologous Tissue Substitute	
B Excision	**4** Elbow Bursa and Ligament, Left		**Y** Other Device	
C Extirpation	**5** Wrist Bursa and Ligament, Right		**Z** No Device	
D Extraction	**6** Wrist Bursa and Ligament, Left			
H Insertion	**7** Hand Bursa and Ligament, Right			
J Inspection	**8** Hand Bursa and Ligament, Left			
M Reattachment	**9** Upper Extremity Bursa and Ligament, Right			
N Release	**B** Upper Extremity Bursa and Ligament, Left			
P Removal	**C** Upper Spine Bursa and Ligament			
Q Repair	**D** Lower Spine Bursa and Ligament			
R Replacement	**F** Sternum Bursa and Ligament			
S Reposition	**G** Rib(s) Bursa and Ligament			
T Resection	**H** Abdomen Bursa and Ligament, Right			
U Supplement	**J** Abdomen Bursa and Ligament, Left			
W Revision	**K** Perineum Bursa and Ligament			
X Transfer	**L** Hip Bursa and Ligament, Right			
	M Hip Bursa and Ligament, Left			
	N Knee Bursa and Ligament, Right			
	P Knee Bursa and Ligament, Left			
	Q Ankle Bursa and Ligament, Right			
	R Ankle Bursa and Ligament, Left			
	S Foot Bursa and Ligament, Right			
	T Foot Bursa and Ligament, Left			
	V Lower Extremity Bursa and Ligament, Right			
	W Lower Extremity Bursa and Ligament, Left			
	X Upper Bursa and Ligament			
	Y Lower Bursa and Ligament			

0: Medical and Surgical
N: Head and Facial Bones

Operation-Character 3	Body Part-Character 4	Approach-Character 5	Device-Character 6	Qualifier-Character 7
2 Change	**0** Skull	**0** Open	**0** Drainage Device	**X** Diagnostic
5 Destruction	**1** Frontal Bone	**3** Percutaneous	**4** Internal Fixation Device	**Z** No Qualifier
8 Division	**3** Parietal Bone, Right	**4** Percutaneous Endoscopic	**5** External Fixation Device	
9 Drainage	**4** Parietal Bone, Left	**X** External	**7** Autologous Tissue Substitute	
B Excision	**5** Temporal Bone, Right		**J** Synthetic Substitute	
C Extirpation	**6** Temporal Bone, Left		**K** Nonautologous Tissue Substitute	
D Extraction	**7** Occipital Bone		**M** Bone Growth Stimulator	
H Insertion	**B** Nasal Bone		**N** Neurostimulator Generator	
J Inspection	**C** Sphenoid Bone		**S** Hearing Device	
N Release	**F** Ethmoid Bone, Right		**Y** Other Device	
P Removal	**G** Ethmoid Bone, Left		**Z** No Device	
Q Repair	**H** Lacrimal Bone, Right			
R Replacement	**J** Lacrimal Bone, Left			
S Reposition	**K** Palatine Bone, Right			
T Resection	**L** Palatine Bone, Left			
U Supplement	**M** Zygomatic Bone, Right			
W Revision	**N** Zygomatic Bone, Left			
	P Orbit, Right			
	Q Orbit, Left			
	R Maxilla			
	T Mandible, Right			
	V Mandible, Left			
	W Facial Bone			
	X Hyoid Bone			

0: Medical and Surgical
P: Upper Bones

Operation-Character 3	Body Part-Character 4	Approach-Character 5	Device-Character 6	Qualifier-Character 7
2 Change	**0** Sternum	**0** Open	**0** Drainage Device	**X** Diagnostic
5 Destruction	**1** Ribs, 1 to 2	**3** Percutaneous	**0** Internal Fixation Device, Rigid Plate	**Z** No Qualifier
8 Division	**2** Ribs, 3 or More	**4** Percutaneous Endoscopic	**4** Internal Fixation Device	
9 Drainage	**3** Cervical Vertebra	**X** External	**5** External Fixation Device	
B Excision	**4** Thoracic Vertebra		**6** Internal Fixation Device, Intramedullary	
C Extirpation	**5** Scapula, Right		**7** Autologous Tissue Substitute	
D Extraction	**6** Scapula, Left		**8** External Fixation Device, Limb Lengthening	
H Insertion	**7** Glenoid Cavity, Right		**B** External Fixation Device, Monoplanar	
J Inspection	**8** Glenoid Cavity, Left		**C** External Fixation Device, Ring	
N Release	**9** Clavicle, Right		**D** External Fixation Device, Hybrid	
P Removal	**B** Clavicle, Left		**J** Synthetic Substitute	
Q Repair	**C** Humeral Head, Right		**K** Nonautologous Tissue Substitute	
R Replacement	**D** Humeral Head, Left		**M** Bone Growth Stimulator	
S Reposition	**F** Humeral Shaft, Right		**Y** Other Device	
T Resection	**G** Humeral Shaft, Left		**Z** No Device	
U Supplement	**H** Radius, Right			
W Revision	**J** Radius, Left			
	K Ulna, Right			
	L Ulna, Left			
	M Carpal, Right			
	N Carpal, Left			
	P Metacarpal, Right			
	Q Metacarpal, Left			
	R Thumb Phalanx, Right			
	S Thumb Phalanx, Left			
	T Finger Phalanx, Right			
	V Finger Phalanx, Left			
	Y Upper Bone			

0: Medical and Surgical
Q: Lower Bones

Operation-Character 3	Body Part-Character 4	Approach-Character 5	Device-Character 6	Qualifier-Character 7
2 Change	**0** Lumbar Vertebra	**0** Open	**0** Drainage Device	**2** Sesamoid Bone(s) 1st Toe
5 Destruction	**1** Sacrum	**3** Percutaneous	**4** Internal Fixation Device	**X** Diagnostic
8 Division	**2** Pelvic Bone, Right	**4** Percutaneous Endoscopic	**5** External Fixation Device	**Z** No Qualifier
9 Drainage	**3** Pelvic Bone, Left	**X** External	**6** Internal Fixation Device, Intramedullary	
B Excision	**4** Acetabulum, Right		**7** Autologous Tissue Substitute	
C Extirpation	**5** Acetabulum, Left		**8** External Fixation Device, Limb Lengthening	
D Extraction	**6** Upper Femur, Right		**B** External Fixation Device, Monoplanar	
H Insertion	**7** Upper Femur, Left		**C** External Fixation Device, Ring	
J Inspection	**8** Femoral Shaft, Right		**D** External Fixation Device, Hybrid	
N Release	**9** Femoral Shaft, Left		**J** Synthetic Substitute	
P Removal	**B** Lower Femur, Right		**K** Nonautologous Tissue Substitute	
Q Repair	**C** Lower Femur, Left		**M** Bone Growth Stimulator	
R Replacement	**D** Patella, Right		**Y** Other Device	
S Reposition	**F** Patella, Left		**Z** No Device	
T Resection	**G** Tibia, Right			
U Supplement	**H** Tibia, Left			
W Revision	**J** Fibula, Right			
	K Fibula, Left			
	L Tarsal, Right			
	M Tarsal, Left			
	N Metatarsal, Right			
	P Metatarsal, Left			
	Q Toe Phalanx, Right			
	R Toe Phalanx, Left			
	S Coccyx			
	Y Lower Bone			

0: Medical and Surgical
R: Upper Joints

Operation-Character 3	Body Part-Character 4	Approach-Character 5	Device-Character 6	Qualifier-Character 7
2 Change	**0** Occipital-cervical Joint	**0** Open	**0** Drainage Device	**0** Anterior Approach, Anterior Column
5 Destruction	**1** Cervical Vertebral Joint	**3** Percutaneous	**0** Synthetic Substitute, Reverse Ball and Socket	**1** Posterior Approach, Posterior Column
9 Drainage	**2** Cervical Vertebral Joints, 2 or more	**4** Percutaneous Endoscopic	**3** Infusion Device	**6** Humeral Surface
B Excision	**3** Cervical Vertebral Disc	**X** External	**4** Internal Fixation Device	**7** Glenoid Surface
C Extirpation	**4** Cervicothoracic Vertebral Joint		**5** External Fixation Device	**J** Posterior Approach, Anterior Column
G Fusion	**5** Cervicothoracic Vertebral Disc		**7** Autologous Tissue Substitute	**X** Diagnostic
H Insertion	**6** Thoracic Vertebral Joint		**8** Spacer	**Z** No Qualifier
J Inspection	**7** Thoracic Vertebral Joints, 2 to 7		**A** Interbody Fusion Device	
N Release	**8** Thoracic Vertebral Joints, 8 or more		**B** Spinal Stabilization Device, Interspinous Process	
P Removal	**9** Thoracic Vertebral Disc		**C** Spinal Stabilization Device, Pedicle-Based	
Q Repair	**A** Thoracolumbar Vertebral Joint		**D** Spinal Stabilization Device, Facet Replacement	
R Replacement	**B** Thoracolumbar Vertebral Disc		**J** Synthetic Substitute	
S Reposition	**C** Temporomandibular Joint, Right		**K** Nonautologous Tissue Substitute	
T Resection	**D** Temporomandibular Joint, Left		**Y** Other Device	
U Supplement	**E** Sternoclavicular Joint, Right		**Z** No Device	
W Revision	**F** Sternoclavicular Joint, Left			
	G Acromioclavicular Joint, Right			
	H Acromioclavicular Joint, Left			
	J Shoulder Joint, Right			
	K Shoulder Joint, Left			
	L Elbow Joint, Right			
	M Elbow Joint, Left			
	N Wrist Joint, Right			
	P Wrist Joint, Left			
	Q Carpal Joint, Right			
	R Carpal Joint, Left			
	S Carpometacarpal Joint, Right			
	T Carpometacarpal Joint, Left			
	U Metacarpophalangeal Joint, Right			
	V Metacarpophalangeal Joint, Left			
	W Finger Phalangeal Joint, Right			
	X Finger Phalangeal Joint, Left			
	Y Upper Joint			

0: Medical and Surgical
S: Lower Joints

Operation-Character 3	Body Part-Character 4	Approach-Character 5	Device-Character 6	Qualifier-Character 7
2 Change	**0** Lumbar Vertebral Joint	**0** Open	**0** Drainage Device	**0** Anterior Approach, Anterior Column
5 Destruction	**1** Lumbar Vertebral Joints, 2 or more	**3** Percutaneous	**0** Synthetic Substitute, Polyethylene	**1** Posterior Approach, Posterior Column
9 Drainage	**2** Lumbar Vertebral Disc	**4** Percutaneous Endoscopic	**1** Synthetic Substitute, Metal	**9** Cemented
B Excision	**3** Lumbosacral Joint	**X** External	**2** Synthetic Substitute, Metal on Polyethylene	**A** Uncemented
C Extirpation	**4** Lumbosacral Disc		**3** Infusion Device	**C** Patellar Surface
G Fusion	**5** Sacrococcygeal Joint		**3** Synthetic Substitute, Ceramic	**J** Posterior Approach, Anterior Column
H Insertion	**6** Coccygeal Joint		**4** Internal Fixation Device	**X** Diagnostic
J Inspection	**7** Sacroiliac Joint, Right		**4** Synthetic Substitute, Ceramic on Polyethylene	**Z** No Qualifier
N Release	**8** Sacroiliac Joint, Left		**5** External Fixation Device	
P Removal	**9** Hip Joint, Right		**6** Synthetic Substitute, Oxidized Zirconium on Polyethylene	
Q Repair	**A** Hip Joint, Acetabular Surface, Right		**7** Autologous Tissue Substitute	
R Replacement	**B** Hip Joint, Left		**8** Spacer	
S Reposition	**C** Knee Joint, Right		**9** Liner	
T Resection	**D** Knee Joint, Left		**A** Interbody Fusion Device	
U Supplement	**E** Hip Joint, Acetabular Surface, Left		**B** Resurfacing Device	
W Revision	**F** Ankle Joint, Right		**B** Spinal Stabilization Device, Interspinous Process	
	G Ankle Joint, Left		**C** Spinal Stabilization Device, Pedicle-Based	
	H Tarsal Joint, Right		**D** Spinal Stabilization Device, Facet Replacement	
	J Tarsal Joint, Left		**E** Articulating Spacer	
	K Tarsometatarsal Joint, Right		**J** Synthetic Substitute	
	L Tarsometatarsal Joint, Left		**K** Nonautologous Tissue Substitute	
	M Metatarsal-Phalangeal Joint, Right		**L** Synthetic Substitute, Unicondylar Medial	
	N Metatarsal-Phalangeal Joint, Left		**M** Synthetic Substitute, Unicondylar Lateral	
	P Toe Phalangeal Joint, Right		**N** Synthetic Substitute, Patellofemoral	
	Q Toe Phalangeal Joint, Left		**Y** Other Device	
	R Hip Joint, Femoral Surface, Right		**Z** No Device	
	S Hip Joint, Femoral Surface, Left			
	T Knee Joint, Femoral Surface, Right			
	U Knee Joint, Femoral Surface, Left			
	V Knee Joint, Tibial Surface, Right			
	W Knee Joint, Tibial Surface, Left			
	Y Lower Joint			

0: Medical and Surgical
T: Urinary System

Operation-Character 3	Body Part-Character 4	Approach-Character 5	Device-Character 6	Qualifier-Character 7
1 Bypass	**0** Kidney, Right	**0** Open	**0** Drainage Device	**0** Allogeneic
2 Change	**1** Kidney, Left	**3** Percutaneous	**2** Monitoring Device	**1** Syngeneic
5 Destruction	**2** Kidneys, Bilateral	**4** Percutaneous Endoscopic	**3** Infusion Device	**2** Zooplastic
7 Dilation	**3** Kidney Pelvis, Right	**7** Via Natural or Artificial Opening	**7** Autologous Tissue Substitute	**3** Kidney Pelvis, Right
8 Division	**4** Kidney Pelvis, Left	**8** Via Natural or Artificial Opening Endoscopic	**C** Extraluminal Device	**4** Kidney Pelvis, Left
9 Drainage	**5** Kidney	**X** External	**D** Intraluminal Device	**6** Ureter, Right
B Excision	**6** Ureter, Right		**J** Synthetic Substitute	**7** Ureter, Left
C Extirpation	**7** Ureter, Left		**K** Nonautologous Tissue Substitute	**8** Colon
D Extraction	**8** Ureters, Bilateral		**L** Artificial Sphincter	**9** Colocutaneous
F Fragmentation	**9** Ureter		**M** Stimulator Lead	**A** Ileum
H Insertion	**B** Bladder		**Y** Other Device	**B** Bladder
J Inspection	**C** Bladder Neck		**Z** No Device	**C** Ileocutaneous
L Occlusion	**D** Urethra			**D** Cutaneous
M Reattachment				**X** Diagnostic
N Release				**Z** No Qualifier
P Removal				
Q Repair				
R Replacement				
S Reposition				
T Resection				
U Supplement				
V Restriction				
W Revision				
Y Transplantation				

0: Medical and Surgical
U: Female Reproductive System

Operation-Character 3	Body Part-Character 4	Approach-Character 5	Device-Character 6	Qualifier-Character 7
1 Bypass	**0** Ovary, Right	**0** Open	**0** Drainage Device	**0** Allogeneic
2 Change	**1** Ovary, Left	**3** Percutaneous	**1** Radioactive Element	**1** Syngeneic
5 Destruction	**2** Ovaries, Bilateral	**4** Percutaneous Endoscopic	**3** Infusion Device	**2** Zooplastic
7 Dilation	**3** Ovary	**7** Via Natural or Artificial Opening	**7** Autologous Tissue Substitute	**5** Fallopian Tube, Right
8 Division	**4** Uterine Supporting Structure	**8** Via Natural or Artificial Opening Endoscopic	**C** Extraluminal Device	**6** Fallopian Tube, Left
9 Drainage	**5** Fallopian Tube, Right	**F** Via Natural or Artificial Opening With Percutaneous Endoscopic Assistance	**D** Intraluminal Device	**9** Uterus
B Excision	**6** Fallopian Tube, Left	**X** External	**G** Intraluminal Device, Pessary	**L** Supracervical
C Extirpation	**7** Fallopian Tubes, Bilateral		**H** Contraceptive Device	**X** Diagnostic
D Extraction	**8** Fallopian Tube		**J** Synthetic Substitute	**Z** No Qualifier
F Fragmentation	**9** Uterus		**K** Nonautologous Tissue Substitute	
H Insertion	**B** Endometrium		**Y** Other Device	
J Inspection	**C** Cervix		**Z** No Device	
L Occlusion	**D** Uterus and Cervix			
M Reattachment	**F** Cul-de-sac			
N Release	**G** Vagina			
P Removal	**H** Vagina and Cul-de-sac			
Q Repair	**J** Clitoris			
S Reposition	**K** Hymen			
T Resection	**L** Vestibular Gland			
U Supplement	**M** Vulva			
V Restriction	**N** Ova			
W Revision				
Y Transplantation				

0: Medical and Surgical
V: Male Reproductive System

Operation-Character 3	Body Part-Character 4	Approach-Character 5	Device-Character 6	Qualifier-Character 7
1 Bypass	**0** Prostate	**0** Open	**0** Drainage Device	**D** Urethra
2 Change	**1** Seminal Vesicle, Right	**3** Percutaneous	**1** Radioactive Element	**J** Epididymis, Right
5 Destruction	**2** Seminal Vesicle, Left	**4** Percutaneous Endoscopic	**3** Infusion Device	**K** Epididymis, Left
7 Dilation	**3** Seminal Vesicles, Bilateral	**7** Via Natural or Artificial Opening	**7** Autologous Tissue Substitute	**N** Vas Deferens, Right
9 Drainage	**4** Prostate and Seminal Vesicles	**8** Via Natural or Artificial Opening Endoscopic	**C** Extraluminal Device	**P** Vas Deferens, Left
B Excision	**5** Scrotum	**X** External	**D** Intraluminal Device	**S** Penis
C Extirpation	**6** Tunica Vaginalis, Right		**J** Synthetic Substitute	**X** Diagnostic
H Insertion	**7** Tunica Vaginalis, Left		**K** Nonautologous Tissue Substitute	**Z** No Qualifier
J Inspection	**8** Scrotum and Tunica Vaginalis		**Y** Other Device	
L Occlusion	**9** Testis, Right		**Z** No Device	
M Reattachment	**B** Testis, Left			
N Release	**C** Testes, Bilateral			
P Removal	**D** Testis			
Q Repair	**F** Spermatic Cord, Right			
R Replacement	**G** Spermatic Cord, Left			
S Reposition	**H** Spermatic Cords, Bilateral			
T Resection	**J** Epididymis, Right			
U Supplement	**K** Epididymis, Left			
W Revision	**L** Epididymis, Bilateral			
X Transfer	**M** Epididymis and Spermatic Cord			
	N Vas Deferens, Right			
	P Vas Deferens, Left			
	Q Vas Deferens, Bilateral			
	R Vas Deferens			
	S Penis			
	T Prepuce			

0: Medical and Surgical
W: Anatomical Regions, General

Operation-Character 3	Body Part-Character 4	Approach-Character 5	Device-Character 6	Qualifier-Character 7
0 Alteration	**0** Head	**0** Open	**0** Drainage Device	**0** Allogeneic
1 Bypass	**1** Cranial Cavity	**3** Percutaneous	**1** Radioactive Element	**0** Vagina
2 Change	**2** Face	**4** Percutaneous Endoscopic	**3** Infusion Device	**1** Penis
3 Control	**3** Oral Cavity and Throat	**7** Via Natural or Artificial Opening	**7** Autologous Tissue Substitute	**1** Syngeneic
4 Creation	**4** Upper Jaw	**8** Via Natural or Artificial Opening Endoscopic	**J** Synthetic Substitute	**2** Stoma
8 Division	**5** Lower Jaw	**X** External	**K** Nonautologous Tissue Substitute	**4** Cutaneous
9 Drainage	**6** Neck		**Y** Other Device	**9** Pleural Cavity, Right
B Excision	**8** Chest Wall		**Z** No Device	**B** Pleural Cavity, Left
C Extirpation	**9** Pleural Cavity, Right			**G** Peritoneal Cavity
F Fragmentation	**B** Pleural Cavity, Left			**J** Pelvic Cavity
H Insertion	**C** Mediastinum			**W** Upper Vein
J Inspection	**D** Pericardial Cavity			**X** Diagnostic
M Reattachment	**F** Abdominal Wall			**Y** Lower Vein
P Removal	**G** Peritoneal Cavity			**Z** No Qualifier
Q Repair	**H** Retroperitoneum			
U Supplement	**J** Pelvic Cavity			
W Revision	**K** Upper Back			
Y Transplantation	**L** Lower Back			
	M Perineum, Male			
	N Perineum, Female			
	P Gastrointestinal Tract			
	Q Respiratory Tract			
	R Genitourinary Tract			

0: Medical and Surgical
X: Anatomical Regions, Upper Extremities

Operation-Character 3	Body Part-Character 4	Approach-Character 5	Device-Character 6	Qualifier-Character 7
0 Alteration	**0** Forequarter, Right	**0** Open	**0** Drainage Device	**0** Allogeneic
2 Change	**1** Forequarter, Left	**3** Percutaneous	**1** Radioactive Element	**0** Complete
3 Control	**2** Shoulder Region, Right	**4** Percutaneous Endoscopic	**3** Infusion Device	**1** High
6 Detachment	**3** Shoulder Region, Left	**X** External	**7** Autologous Tissue Substitute	**1** Syngeneic
9 Drainage	**4** Axilla, Right		**J** Synthetic Substitute	**2** Mid
B Excision	**5** Axilla, Left		**K** Nonautologous Tissue Substitute	**3** Low
H Insertion	**6** Upper Extremity, Right		**Y** Other Device	**4** Complete 1st Ray
J Inspection	**7** Upper Extremity, Left		**Z** No Device	**5** Complete 2nd Ray
M Reattachment	**8** Upper Arm, Right			**6** Complete 3rd Ray
P Removal	**9** Upper Arm, Left			**7** Complete 4th Ray
Q Repair	**B** Elbow Region, Right			**8** Complete 5th Ray
R Replacement	**C** Elbow Region, Left			**9** Partial 1st Ray
U Supplement	**D** Lower Arm, Right			**B** Partial 2nd Ray
W Revision	**F** Lower Arm, Left			**C** Partial 3rd Ray
X Transfer	**G** Wrist Region, Right			**D** Partial 4th Ray
Y Transplantation	**H** Wrist Region, Left			**F** Partial 5th Ray
	J Hand, Right			**L** Thumb, Right
	K Hand, Left			**M** Thumb, Left
	L Thumb, Right			**N** Toe, Right
	M Thumb, Left			**P** Toe, Left
	N Index Finger, Right			**X** Diagnostic
	P Index Finger, Left			**Z** No Qualifier
	Q Middle Finger, Right			
	R Middle Finger, Left			
	S Ring Finger, Right			
	T Ring Finger, Left			
	V Little Finger, Right			
	W Little Finger, Left			

0: Medical and Surgical
Y: Anatomical Regions, Lower Extremities

Operation-Character 3	Body Part-Character 4	Approach-Character 5	Device-Character 6	Qualifier-Character 7
0 Alteration	**0** Buttock, Right	**0** Open	**0** Drainage Device	**0** Complete
2 Change	**1** Buttock, Left	**3** Percutaneous	**1** Radioactive Element	**1** High
3 Control	**2** Hindquarter, Right	**4** Percutaneous Endoscopic	**3** Infusion Device	**2** Mid
6 Detachment	**3** Hindquarter, Left	**X** External	**7** Autologous Tissue Substitute	**3** Low
9 Drainage	**4** Hindquarter, Bilateral		**J** Synthetic Substitute	**4** Complete 1st Ray
B Excision	**5** Inguinal Region, Right		**K** Nonautologous Tissue Substitute	**5** Complete 2nd Ray
H Insertion	**6** Inguinal Region, Left		**Y** Other Device	**6** Complete 3rd Ray
J Inspection	**7** Femoral Region, Right		**Z** No Device	**7** Complete 4th Ray
M Reattachment	**8** Femoral Region, Left			**8** Complete 5th Ray
P Removal	**9** Lower Extremity, Right			**9** Partial 1st Ray
Q Repair	**A** Inguinal Region, Bilateral			**B** Partial 2nd Ray
U Supplement	**B** Lower Extremity, Left			**C** Partial 3rd Ray
W Revision	**C** Upper Leg, Right			**D** Partial 4th Ray
	D Upper Leg, Left			**F** Partial 5th Ray
	E Femoral Region, Bilateral			**X** Diagnostic
	F Knee Region, Right			**Z** No Qualifier
	G Knee Region, Left			
	H Lower Leg, Right			
	J Lower Leg, Left			
	K Ankle Region, Right			
	L Ankle Region, Left			
	M Foot, Right			
	N Foot, Left			
	P 1st Toe, Right			
	Q 1st Toe, Left			
	R 2nd Toe, Right			
	S 2nd Toe, Left			
	T 3rd Toe, Right			
	U 3rd Toe, Left			
	V 4th Toe, Right			
	W 4th Toe, Left			
	X 5th Toe, Right			
	Y 5th Toe, Left			

1: Obstetrics
0: Pregnancy

Operation-Character 3	Body Part-Character 4	Approach-Character 5	Device-Character 6	Qualifier-Character 7
2 Change	**0** Products of Conception	**0** Open	**3** Monitoring Electrode	**0** High
9 Drainage	**1** Products of Conception, Retained	**3** Percutaneous	**Y** Other Device	**1** Low
A Abortion	**2** Products of Conception, Ectopic	**4** Percutaneous Endoscopic	**Z** No Device	**2** Extraperitoneal
D Extraction		**7** Via Natural or Artificial Opening		**3** Low Forceps
E Delivery		**8** Via Natural or Artificial Opening Endoscopic		**4** Mid Forceps
H Insertion		**X** External		**5** High Forceps
J Inspection				**6** Vacuum
P Removal				**7** Internal Version
Q Repair				**8** Other
S Reposition				**9** Fetal Blood
T Resection				**9** Manual
Y Transplantation				**A** Fetal Cerebrospinal Fluid
				B Fetal Fluid, Other
				C Amniotic Fluid, Therapeutic
				D Fluid, Other
				E Nervous System
				F Cardiovascular System
				G Lymphatics and Hemic
				H Eye
				J Ear, Nose and Sinus
				K Respiratory System
				L Mouth and Throat
				M Gastrointestinal System
				N Hepatobiliary and Pancreas
				P Endocrine System
				Q Skin
				R Musculoskeletal System
				S Urinary System
				T Female Reproductive System
				U Amniotic Fluid, Diagnostic
				V Male Reproductive System
				W Laminaria
				X Abortifacient
				Y Other Body System
				Z No Qualifier

2: Placement
W: Anatomical Regions

Operation-Character 3	Body Region-Character 4	Approach-Character 5	Device-Character 6	Qualifier-Character 7
0 Change	**0** Head	**X** External	**0** Traction Apparatus	**Z** No Qualifier
1 Compression	**1** Face		**1** Splint	
2 Dressing	**2** Neck		**2** Cast	
3 Immobilization	**3** Abdominal Wall		**3** Brace	
4 Packing	**4** Chest Wall		**4** Bandage	
5 Removal	**5** Back		**5** Packing Material	
6 Traction	**6** Inguinal Region, Right		**6** Pressure Dressing	
	7 Inguinal Region, Left		**7** Intermittent Pressure Device	
	8 Upper Extremity, Right		**9** Wire	
	9 Upper Extremity, Left		**Y** Other Device	
	A Upper Arm, Right		**Z** No Device	
	B Upper Arm, Left			
	C Lower Arm, Right			
	D Lower Arm, Left			
	E Hand, Right			
	F Hand, Left			
	G Thumb, Right			
	H Thumb, Left			
	J Finger, Right			
	K Finger, Left			
	L Lower Extremity, Right			
	M Lower Extremity, Left			
	N Upper Leg, Right			
	P Upper Leg, Left			
	Q Lower Leg, Right			
	R Lower Leg, Left			
	S Foot, Right			
	T Foot, Left			
	U Toe, Right			
	V Toe, Left			

2: Placement
Y: Anatomical Orifices

Operation-Character 3	Body Region-Character 4	Approach-Character 5	Device-Character 6	Qualifier-Character 7
0 Change	**0** Mouth and Pharynx	**X** External	**5** Packing Material	**Z** No Qualifier
4 Packing	**1** Nasal			
5 Removal	**2** Ear			
	3 Anorectal			
	4 Female Genital Tract			
	5 Urethra			

3: Administration
0: Circulatory

Operation-Character 3	Body System/Region-Character 4	Approach-Character 5	Substance-Character 6	Qualifier-Character 7
2 Transfusion	**3** Peripheral Vein	**0** Open	**A** Stem Cells, Embryonic	**0** Autologous
	4 Central Vein	**3** Percutaneous	**B** 4-Factor Prothrombin Complex Concentrate	**1** Nonautologous
	5 Peripheral Artery	**7** Via Natural or Artificial Opening	**G** Bone Marrow	**2** Allogeneic, Related
	6 Central Artery		**H** Whole Blood	**3** Allogeneic, Unrelated
	7 Products of Conception, Circulatory		**J** Serum Albumin	**4** Allogeneic, Unspecified
	8 Vein		**K** Frozen Plasma	**Z** No Qualifier
			L Fresh Plasma	
			M Plasma Cryoprecipitate	
			N Red Blood Cells	
			P Frozen Red Cells	
			Q White Cells	
			R Platelets	
			S Globulin	
			T Fibrinogen	
			U Stem Cells, T-cell Depleted Hematopoietic	
			V Antihemophilic Factors	
			W Factor IX	
			X Stem Cells, Cord Blood	
			Y Stem Cells, Hematopoietic	

3: Administration
C: Indwelling Device

Operation-Character 3	Body System/Region-Character 4	Approach-Character 5	Substance-Character 6	Qualifier-Character 7
1 Irrigation	**Z** None	**X** External	**8** Irrigating Substance	**Z** No Qualifier

3: Administration
E: Physiological Systems and Anatomical Regions

Operation-Character 3	Body System/Region-Character 4	Approach-Character 5	Substance-Character 6	Qualifier-Character 7
0 Introduction	**0** Skin and Mucous Membranes	**0** Open	**0** Antineoplastic	**0** Autologous
1 Irrigation	**1** Subcutaneous Tissue	**3** Percutaneous	**1** Thrombolytic	**0** Influenza Vaccine
	2 Muscle	**4** Percutaneous Endoscopic	**2** Anti-infective	**1** Nonautologous
	3 Peripheral Vein	**7** Via Natural or Artificial Opening	**3** Anti-inflammatory	**2** High-dose Interleukin-2
	4 Central Vein	**8** Via Natural or Artificial Opening Endoscopic	**4** Serum, Toxoid and Vaccine	**3** Low-dose Interleukin-2
	5 Peripheral Artery	**X** External	**5** Adhesion Barrier	**4** Liquid Brachytherapy Radioisotope
	6 Central Artery		**6** Nutritional Substance	**5** Other Antineoplastic
	7 Coronary Artery		**7** Electrolytic and Water Balance Substance	**6** Recombinant Human-activated Protein C
	8 Heart		**8** Irrigating Substance	**7** Other Thrombolytic
	9 Nose		**9** Dialysate	**8** Oxazolidinones
	A Bone Marrow		**A** Stem Cells, Embryonic	**9** Other Anti-infective
	B Ear		**B** Anesthetic Agent	**A** Anti-Infective Envelope
	C Eye		**E** Stem Cells, Somatic	**B** Recombinant Bone Morphogenetic Protein
	D Mouth and Pharynx		**F** Intracirculatory Anesthetic	**C** Other Substance
	E Products of Conception		**G** Other Therapeutic Substance	**D** Nitric Oxide
	F Respiratory Tract		**H** Radioactive Substance	**F** Other Gas
	G Upper GI		**K** Other Diagnostic Substance	**G** Insulin
	H Lower GI		**L** Sperm	**H** Human B-type Natriuretic Peptide
	J Biliary and Pancreatic Tract		**M** Pigment	**J** Other Hormone
	K Genitourinary Tract		**N** Analgesics, Hypnotics, Sedatives	**K** Immunostimulator
	L Pleural Cavity		**P** Platelet Inhibitor	**L** Immunosuppressive
	M Peritoneal Cavity		**Q** Fertilized Ovum	**M** Monoclonal Antibody
	N Male Reproductive		**R** Antiarrhythmic	**N** Blood Brain Barrier Disruption
	P Female Reproductive		**S** Gas	**P** Clofarabine
	Q Cranial Cavity and Brain		**T** Destructive Agent	**Q** Glucarpidase
	R Spinal Canal		**U** Pancreatic Islet Cells	**X** Diagnostic
	S Epidural Space		**V** Hormone	**Y** Hyperthermic
	T Peripheral Nerves and Plexi		**W** Immunotherapeutic	**Z** No Qualifier
	U Joints		**X** Vasopressor	
	V Bones			
	W Lymphatics			
	X Cranial Nerves			
	Y Pericardial Cavity			

4: Measurement and Monitoring
A: Physiological Systems

Operation-Character 3	Body System-Character 4	Approach-Character 5	Function/Device-Character 6	Qualifier-Character 7
0 Measurement	**0** Central Nervous	**0** Open	**0** Acuity	**0** Central
1 Monitoring	**1** Peripheral Nervous	**3** Percutaneous	**1** Capacity	**1** Peripheral
	2 Cardiac	**4** Percutaneous Endoscopic	**2** Conductivity	**2** Portal
	3 Arterial	**7** Via Natural or Artificial Opening	**3** Contractility	**3** Pulmonary
	4 Venous	**8** Via Natural or Artificial Opening Endoscopic	**4** Electrical Activity	**4** Stress
	5 Circulatory	**X** External	**5** Flow	**5** Ambulatory
	6 Lymphatic		**6** Metabolism	**6** Right Heart
	7 Visual		**7** Mobility	**7** Left Heart
	8 Olfactory		**8** Motility	**8** Bilateral
	9 Respiratory		**9** Output	**9** Sensory
	B Gastrointestinal		**B** Pressure	**A** Guidance
	C Biliary		**C** Rate	**B** Motor
	D Urinary		**D** Resistance	**C** Coronary
	F Musculoskeletal		**F** Rhythm	**D** Intracranial
	G Skin and Breast		**G** Secretion	**F** Other Thoracic
	H Products of Conception, Cardiac		**H** Sound	**G** Intraoperative
	J Products of Conception, Nervous		**J** Pulse	**H** Indocyanine Green Dye
	Z None		**K** Temperature	**Z** No Qualifier
			L Volume	
			M Total Activity	
			N Sampling and Pressure	
			P Action Currents	
			Q Sleep	
			R Saturation	
			S Vascular Perfusion	

4: Measurement and Monitoring
B: Physiological Devices

Operation-Character 3	Body System-Character 4	Approach-Character 5	Function/Device-Character 6	Qualifier-Character 7
0 Measurement	**0** Central Nervous	**X** External	**S** Pacemaker	**Z** No Qualifier
	1 Peripheral Nervous		**T** Defibrillator	
	2 Cardiac		**V** Stimulator	
	9 Respiratory			
	F Musculoskeletal			

5: Extracorporeal Assistance and Performance
A: Physiological Systems

Operation-Character 3	Body System-Character 4	Duration-Character 5	Function-Character 6	Qualifier-Character 7
0 Assistance	**2** Cardiac	**0** Single	**0** Filtration	**0** Balloon Pump
1 Performance	**5** Circulatory	**1** Intermittent	**1** Output	**1** Hyperbaric
2 Restoration	**9** Respiratory	**2** Continuous	**2** Oxygenation	**2** Manual
	C Biliary	**3** Less than 24 Consecutive Hours	**3** Pacing	**4** Nonmechanical
	D Urinary	**4** 24-96 Consecutive Hours	**4** Rhythm	**5** Pulsatile Compression
		5 Greater than 96 Consecutive Hours	**5** Ventilation	**6** Other Pump
		6 Multiple		**7** Continuous Positive Airway Pressure
		7 Intermittent, Less than 6 Hours Per Day		**8** Intermittent Positive Airway Pressure
		8 Prolonged Intermittent, 6-18 hours Per Day		**9** Continuous Negative Airway Pressure
		9 Continuous, Greater than18 hours Per Day		**B** Intermittent Negative Airway Pressure
		A Intraoperative		**C** Supersaturated
				D Impeller Pump
				F Membrane, Central
				G Membrane, Peripheral Veno-arterial
				H Membrane, Peripheral Veno-venous
				Z No Qualifier

6: Extracorporeal Therapies
A: Physiological Systems

Operation-Character 3	Body System-Character 4	Duration-Character 5	Qualifier-Character 6	Qualifier-Character 7
0 Atmospheric Control	**0** Skin	**0** Single	**B** Donor Organ	**0** Erythrocytes
1 Decompression	**1** Urinary	**1** Multiple	**Z** No Qualifier	**1** Leukocytes
2 Electromagnetic Therapy	**2** Central Nervous			**2** Platelets
3 Hyperthermia	**3** Musculoskeletal			**3** Plasma
4 Hypothermia	**5** Circulatory			**4** Head and Neck Vessels
5 Pheresis	**B** Respiratory System			**5** Heart
6 Phototherapy	**F** Hepatobiliary System and Pancreas			**6** Peripheral Vessels
7 Ultrasound Therapy	**T** Urinary System			**7** Other Vessels
8 Ultraviolet Light Therapy	**Z** None			**T** Stem Cells, Cord Blood
9 Shock Wave Therapy				**V** Stem Cells, Hematopoietic
B Perfusion				**Z** No Qualifier

7: Osteopathic
W: Anatomical Regions

Operation-Character 3	Body Region-Character 4	Approach-Character 5	Method-Character 6	Qualifier-Character 7
0 Treatment	**0** Head	**X** External	**0** Articulatory-Raising	**Z** None
	1 Cervical		**1** Fascial Release	
	2 Thoracic		**2** General Mobilization	
	3 Lumbar		**3** High Velocity-Low Amplitude	
	4 Sacrum		**4** Indirect	
	5 Pelvis		**5** Low Velocity-High Amplitude	
	6 Lower Extremities		**6** Lymphatic Pump	
	7 Upper Extremities		**7** Muscle Energy-Isometric	
	8 Rib Cage		**8** Muscle Energy-Isotonic	
	9 Abdomen		**9** Other Method	

8: Other Procedures
C: Indwelling Device

Operation-Character 3	Body Region-Character 4	Approach-Character 5	Method-Character 6	Qualifier-Character 7
0 Other Procedures	**1** Nervous System	**X** External	**6** Collection	**J** Cerebrospinal Fluid
	2 Circulatory System			**K** Blood
				L Other Fluid

8: Other Procedures
E: Physiological Systems and Anatomical Regions

Operation-Character 3	Body Region-Character 4	Approach-Character 5	Method-Character 6	Qualifier-Character 7
0 Other Procedures	**1** Nervous System	**0** Open	**0** Acupuncture	**0** Anesthesia
	2 Circulatory System	**3** Percutaneous	**1** Therapeutic Massage	**1** In Vitro Fertilization
	9 Head and Neck Region	**4** Percutaneous Endoscopic	**6** Collection	**2** Breast Milk
	H Integumentary System and Breast	**7** Via Natural or Artificial Opening	**B** Computer Assisted Procedure	**3** Sperm
	K Musculoskeletal System	**8** Via Natural or Artificial Opening Endoscopic	**C** Robotic Assisted Procedure	**4** Yoga Therapy
	U Female Reproductive System	**X** External	**D** Near Infrared Spectroscopy	**5** Meditation
	V Male Reproductive System		**E** Fluorescence Guided Procedure	**6** Isolation
	W Trunk Region		**Y** Other Method	**7** Examination
	X Upper Extremity			**8** Suture Removal
	Y Lower Extremity			**9** Piercing
	Z None			**C** Prostate
				D Rectum
				F With Fluoroscopy
				G With Computerized Tomography
				H With Magnetic Resonance Imaging
				M Aminolevulinic Acid
				Z No Qualifier

9: Chiropractic
W: Anatomical Regions

Operation-Character 3	Body Region-Character 4	Approach-Character 5	Method-Character 6	Qualifier-Character 7
B Manipulation	**0** Head	**X** External	**B** Non-Manual	**Z** None
	1 Cervical		**C** Indirect Visceral	
	2 Thoracic		**D** Extra-Articular	
	3 Lumbar		**F** Direct Visceral	
	4 Sacrum		**G** Long Lever Specific Contact	
	5 Pelvis		**H** Short Lever Specific Contact	
	6 Lower Extremities		**J** Long and Short Lever Specific Contact	
	7 Upper Extremities		**K** Mechanically Assisted	
	8 Rib Cage		**L** Other Method	
	9 Abdomen			

B: Imaging
0: Central Nervous System

Type-Character 3	Body Part-Character 4	Contrast-Character 5	Qualifier-Character 6	Qualifier-Character 7
0 Plain Radiography	**0** Brain	**0** High Osmolar	**0** Unenhanced and Enhanced	**Z** None
1 Fluoroscopy	**7** Cisterna	**1** Low Osmolar	**Z** None	
2 Computerized Tomography (CT Scan)	**8** Cerebral Ventricle(s)	**Y** Other Contrast		
3 Magnetic Resonance Imaging (MRI)	**9** Sella Turcica/Pituitary Gland	**Z** None		
4 Ultrasonography	**B** Spinal Cord			
	C Acoustic Nerves			

B: Imaging
2: Heart

Type-Character 3	Body Part-Character 4	Contrast-Character 5	Qualifier-Character 6	Qualifier-Character 7
0 Plain Radiography	**0** Coronary Artery, Single	**0** High Osmolar	**0** Unenhanced and Enhanced	**0** Intraoperative
1 Fluoroscopy	**1** Coronary Arteries, Multiple	**1** Low Osmolar	**1** Laser	**3** Intravascular
2 Computerized Tomography (CT Scan)	**2** Coronary Artery Bypass Graft, Single	**Y** Other Contrast	**2** Intravascular Optical Coherence	**4** Transesophageal
3 Magnetic Resonance Imaging (MRI)	**3** Coronary Artery Bypass Grafts, Multiple	**Z** None	**Z** None	**Z** None
4 Ultrasonography	**4** Heart, Right			
	5 Heart, Left			
	6 Heart, Right and Left			
	7 Internal Mammary Bypass Graft, Right			
	8 Internal Mammary Bypass Graft, Left			
	B Heart with Aorta			
	C Pericardium			
	D Pediatric Heart			
	F Bypass Graft, Other			

B: Imaging
3: Upper Arteries

Type-Character 3	Body Part-Character 4	Contrast-Character 5	Qualifier-Character 6	Qualifier-Character 7
0 Plain Radiography	**0** Thoracic Aorta	**0** High Osmolar	**0** Unenhanced and Enhanced	**0** Intraoperative
1 Fluoroscopy	**1** Brachiocephalic-Subclavian Artery, Right	**1** Low Osmolar	**1** Laser	**3** Intravascular
2 Computerized Tomography (CT Scan)	**2** Subclavian Artery, Left	**Y** Other Contrast	**2** Intravascular Optical Coherence	**Z** None
3 Magnetic Resonance Imaging (MRI)	**3** Common Carotid Artery, Right	**Z** None	**Z** None	
4 Ultrasonography	**4** Common Carotid Artery, Left			
	5 Common Carotid Arteries, Bilateral			
	6 Internal Carotid Artery, Right			
	7 Internal Carotid Artery, Left			
	8 Internal Carotid Arteries, Bilateral			
	9 External Carotid Artery, Right			
	B External Carotid Artery, Left			
	C External Carotid Arteries, Bilateral			
	D Vertebral Artery, Right			
	F Vertebral Artery, Left			
	G Vertebral Arteries, Bilateral			
	H Upper Extremity Arteries, Right			
	J Upper Extremity Arteries, Left			
	K Upper Extremity Arteries, Bilateral			
	L Intercostal and Bronchial Arteries			
	M Spinal Arteries			
	N Upper Arteries, Other			
	P Thoraco-Abdominal Aorta			
	Q Cervico-Cerebral Arch			
	R Intracranial Arteries			
	S Pulmonary Artery, Right			
	T Pulmonary Artery, Left			
	U Pulmonary Trunk			
	V Ophthalmic Arteries			

B: Imaging
4: Lower Arteries

Type-Character 3	Body Part-Character 4	Contrast-Character 5	Qualifier-Character 6	Qualifier-Character 7
0 Plain Radiography	**0** Abdominal Aorta	**0** High Osmolar	**0** Unenhanced and Enhanced	**0** Intraoperative
1 Fluoroscopy	**1** Celiac Artery	**1** Low Osmolar	**1** Laser	**3** Intravascular
2 Computerized Tomography (CT Scan)	**2** Hepatic Artery	**Y** Other Contrast	**2** Intravascular Optical Coherence	**Z** None
3 Magnetic Resonance Imaging (MRI)	**3** Splenic Arteries	**Z** None	**Z** None	
4 Ultrasonography	**4** Superior Mesenteric Artery			
	5 Inferior Mesenteric Artery			
	6 Renal Artery, Right			
	7 Renal Artery, Left			
	8 Renal Arteries, Bilateral			
	9 Lumbar Arteries			
	B Intra-Abdominal Arteries, Other			
	C Pelvic Arteries			
	D Aorta and Bilateral Lower Extremity Arteries			
	F Lower Extremity Arteries, Right			
	G Lower Extremity Arteries, Left			
	H Lower Extremity Arteries, Bilateral			
	J Lower Arteries, Other			
	K Celiac and Mesenteric Arteries			
	L Femoral Artery			
	M Renal Artery Transplant			
	N Penile Arteries			

B: Imaging
5: Veins

Type-Character 3	Body Part-Character 4	Contrast-Character 5	Qualifier-Character 6	Qualifier-Character 7
0 Plain Radiography	**0** Epidural Veins	**0** High Osmolar	**0** Unenhanced and Enhanced	**3** Intravascular
1 Fluoroscopy	**1** Cerebral and Cerebellar Veins	**1** Low Osmolar	**2** Intravascular Optical Coherence	**A** Guidance
2 Computerized Tomography (CT Scan)	**2** Intracranial Sinuses	**Y** Other Contrast	**Z** None	**Z** None
3 Magnetic Resonance Imaging (MRI)	**3** Jugular Veins, Right	**Z** None		
4 Ultrasonography	**4** Jugular Veins, Left			
	5 Jugular Veins, Bilateral			
	6 Subclavian Vein, Right			
	7 Subclavian Vein, Left			
	8 Superior Vena Cava			
	9 Inferior Vena Cava			
	B Lower Extremity Veins, Right			
	C Lower Extremity Veins, Left			
	D Lower Extremity Veins, Bilateral			
	F Pelvic (Iliac) Veins, Right			
	G Pelvic (Iliac) Veins, Left			
	H Pelvic (Iliac) Veins, Bilateral			
	J Renal Vein, Right			
	K Renal Vein, Left			
	L Renal Veins, Bilateral			
	M Upper Extremity Veins, Right			
	N Upper Extremity Veins, Left			
	P Upper Extremity Veins, Bilateral			
	Q Pulmonary Vein, Right			
	R Pulmonary Vein, Left			
	S Pulmonary Veins, Bilateral			
	T Portal and Splanchnic Veins			
	V Veins, Other			
	W Dialysis Shunt/Fistula			

B: Imaging
7: Lymphatic System

Type-Character 3	Body Part-Character 4	Contrast-Character 5	Qualifier-Character 6	Qualifier-Character 7
0 Plain Radiography	**0** Abdominal/Retroperitoneal Lymphatics, Unilateral	**0** High Osmolar	**Z** None	**Z** None
	1 Abdominal/Retroperitoneal Lymphatics, Bilateral	**1** Low Osmolar		
	4 Lymphatics, Head and Neck	**Y** Other Contrast		
	5 Upper Extremity Lymphatics, Right			
	6 Upper Extremity Lymphatics, Left			
	7 Upper Extremity Lymphatics, Bilateral			
	8 Lower Extremity Lymphatics, Right			
	9 Lower Extremity Lymphatics, Left			
	B Lower Extremity Lymphatics, Bilateral			
	C Lymphatics, Pelvic			

B: Imaging
8: Eye

Type-Character 3	Body Part-Character 4	Contrast-Character 5	Qualifier-Character 6	Qualifier-Character 7
0 Plain Radiography	**0** Lacrimal Duct, Right	**0** High Osmolar	**0** Unenhanced and Enhanced	**Z** None
2 Computerized Tomography (CT Scan)	**1** Lacrimal Duct, Left	**1** Low Osmolar	**Z** None	
3 Magnetic Resonance Imaging (MRI)	**2** Lacrimal Ducts, Bilateral	**Y** Other Contrast		
4 Ultrasonography	**3** Optic Foramina, Right	**Z** None		
	4 Optic Foramina, Left			
	5 Eye, Right			
	6 Eye, Left			
	7 Eyes, Bilateral			

B: Imaging
9: Ear, Nose, Mouth and Throat

Type-Character 3	Body Part-Character 4	Contrast-Character 5	Qualifier-Character 6	Qualifier-Character 7
0 Plain Radiography	**0** Ear	**0** High Osmolar	**0** Unenhanced and Enhanced	**Z** None
1 Fluoroscopy	**2** Paranasal Sinuses	**1** Low Osmolar	**Z** None	
2 Computerized Tomography (CT Scan)	**4** Parotid Gland, Right	**Y** Other Contrast		
3 Magnetic Resonance Imaging (MRI)	**5** Parotid Gland, Left	**Z** None		
	6 Parotid Glands, Bilateral			
	7 Submandibular Gland, Right			
	8 Submandibular Gland, Left			
	9 Submandibular Glands, Bilateral			
	B Salivary Gland, Right			
	C Salivary Gland, Left			
	D Salivary Glands, Bilateral			
	F Nasopharynx/Oropharynx			
	G Pharynx and Epiglottis			
	H Mastoids			
	J Larynx			

B: Imaging
B: Respiratory System

Type-Character 3	Body Part-Character 4	Contrast-Character 5	Qualifier-Character 6	Qualifier-Character 7
0 Plain Radiography	**2** Lung, Right	**0** High Osmolar	**0** Unenhanced and Enhanced	**Z** None
1 Fluoroscopy	**3** Lung, Left	**1** Low Osmolar	**Z** None	
2 Computerized Tomography (CT Scan)	**4** Lungs, Bilateral	**Y** Other Contrast		
3 Magnetic Resonance Imaging (MRI)	**6** Diaphragm	**Z** None		
4 Ultrasonography	**7** Tracheobronchial Tree, Right			
	8 Tracheobronchial Tree, Left			
	9 Tracheobronchial Trees, Bilateral			
	B Pleura			
	C Mediastinum			
	D Upper Airways			
	F Trachea/Airways			
	G Lung Apices			

B: Imaging
D: Gastrointestinal System

Type-Character 3	Body Part-Character 4	Contrast-Character 5	Qualifier-Character 6	Qualifier-Character 7
1 Fluoroscopy	**1** Esophagus	**0** High Osmolar	**0** Unenhanced and Enhanced	**Z** None
2 Computerized Tomography (CT Scan)	**2** Stomach	**1** Low Osmolar	**Z** None	
4 Ultrasonography	**3** Small Bowel	**Y** Other Contrast		
	4 Colon	**Z** None		
	5 Upper GI			
	6 Upper GI and Small Bowel			
	7 Gastrointestinal Tract			
	8 Appendix			
	9 Duodenum			
	B Mouth/Oropharynx			
	C Rectum			

B: Imaging
F: Hepatobiliary System and Pancreas

Type-Character 3	Body Part-Character 4	Contrast-Character 5	Qualifier-Character 6	Qualifier-Character 7
0 Plain Radiography	**0** Bile Ducts	**0** High Osmolar	**0** Unenhanced and Enhanced	**Z** None
1 Fluoroscopy	**1** Biliary and Pancreatic Ducts	**1** Low Osmolar	**Z** None	
2 Computerized Tomography (CT Scan)	**2** Gallbladder	**Y** Other Contrast		
3 Magnetic Resonance Imaging (MRI)	**3** Gallbladder and Bile Ducts	**Z** None		
4 Ultrasonography	**4** Gallbladder, Bile Ducts and Pancreatic Ducts			
	5 Liver			
	6 Liver and Spleen			
	7 Pancreas			
	8 Pancreatic Ducts			
	C Hepatobiliary System, All			

B: Imaging
G: Endocrine System

Type-Character 3	Body Part-Character 4	Contrast-Character 5	Qualifier-Character 6	Qualifier-Character 7
2 Computerized Tomography (CT Scan)	**0** Adrenal Gland, Right	**0** High Osmolar	**0** Unenhanced and Enhanced	**Z** None
3 Magnetic Resonance Imaging (MRI)	**1** Adrenal Gland, Left	**1** Low Osmolar	**Z** None	
4 Ultrasonography	**2** Adrenal Glands, Bilateral	**Y** Other Contrast		
	3 Parathyroid Glands	**Z** None		
	4 Thyroid Gland			

B: Imaging
H: Skin, Subcutaneous Tissue and Breast

Type-Character 3	Body Part-Character 4	Contrast-Character 5	Qualifier-Character 6	Qualifier-Character 7
0 Plain Radiography	**0** Breast, Right	**0** High Osmolar	**0** Unenhanced and Enhanced	**Z** None
3 Magnetic Resonance Imaging (MRI)	**1** Breast, Left	**1** Low Osmolar	**Z** None	
4 Ultrasonography	**2** Breasts, Bilateral	**Y** Other Contrast		
	3 Single Mammary Duct, Right	**Z** None		
	4 Single Mammary Duct, Left			
	5 Multiple Mammary Ducts, Right			
	6 Multiple Mammary Ducts, Left			
	7 Extremity, Upper			
	8 Extremity, Lower			
	9 Abdominal Wall			
	B Chest Wall			
	C Head and Neck			
	D Subcutaneous Tissue, Head/Neck			
	F Subcutaneous Tissue, Upper Extremity			
	G Subcutaneous Tissue, Thorax			
	H Subcutaneous Tissue, Abdomen and Pelvis			
	J Subcutaneous Tissue, Lower Extremity			

B: Imaging
L: Connective Tissue

Type-Character 3	Body Part-Character 4	Contrast-Character 5	Qualifier-Character 6	Qualifier-Character 7
3 Magnetic Resonance Imaging (MRI)	**0** Connective Tissue, Upper Extremity	**Y** Other Contrast	**0** Unenhanced and Enhanced	**Z** None
4 Ultrasonography	**1** Connective Tissue, Lower Extremity	**Z** None	**Z** None	
	2 Tendons, Upper Extremity			
	3 Tendons, Lower Extremity			

B: Imaging
N: Skull and Facial Bones

Type-Character 3	Body Part-Character 4	Contrast-Character 5	Qualifier-Character 6	Qualifier-Character 7
0 Plain Radiography	**0** Skull	**0** High Osmolar	**Z** None	**Z** None
1 Fluoroscopy	**1** Orbit, Right	**1** Low Osmolar		
2 Computerized Tomography (CT Scan)	**2** Orbit, Left	**Y** Other Contrast		
3 Magnetic Resonance Imaging (MRI)	**3** Orbits, Bilateral	**Z** None		
	4 Nasal Bones			
	5 Facial Bones			
	6 Mandible			
	7 Temporomandibular Joint, Right			
	8 Temporomandibular Joint, Left			
	9 Temporomandibular Joints, Bilateral			
	B Zygomatic Arch, Right			
	C Zygomatic Arch, Left			
	D Zygomatic Arches, Bilateral			
	F Temporal Bones			
	G Tooth, Single			
	H Teeth, Multiple			
	J Teeth, All			

B: Imaging
P: Non-Axial Upper Bones

Type-Character 3	Body Part-Character 4	Contrast-Character 5	Qualifier-Character 6	Qualifier-Character 7
0 Plain Radiography	**0** Sternoclavicular Joint, Right	**0** High Osmolar	**0** Unenhanced and Enhanced	**1** Densitometry
1 Fluoroscopy	**1** Sternoclavicular Joint, Left	**1** Low Osmolar	**Z** None	**Z** None
2 Computerized Tomography (CT Scan)	**2** Sternoclavicular Joints, Bilateral	**Y** Other Contrast		
3 Magnetic Resonance Imaging (MRI)	**3** Acromioclavicular Joints, Bilateral	**Z** None		
4 Ultrasonography	**4** Clavicle, Right			
	5 Clavicle, Left			
	6 Scapula, Right			
	7 Scapula, Left			
	8 Shoulder, Right			
	9 Shoulder, Left			
	A Humerus, Right			
	B Humerus, Left			
	C Hand/Finger Joint, Right			
	D Hand/Finger Joint, Left			
	E Upper Arm, Right			
	F Upper Arm, Left			
	G Elbow, Right			
	H Elbow, Left			
	J Forearm, Right			
	K Forearm, Left			
	L Wrist, Right			
	M Wrist, Left			
	N Hand, Right			
	P Hand, Left			
	Q Hands and Wrists, Bilateral			
	R Finger(s), Right			
	S Finger(s), Left			
	T Upper Extremity, Right			
	U Upper Extremity, Left			
	V Upper Extremities, Bilateral			
	W Thorax			
	X Ribs, Right			
	Y Ribs, Left			

B: Imaging
Q: Non-Axial Lower Bones

Type-Character 3	Body Part-Character 4	Contrast-Character 5	Qualifier-Character 6	Qualifier-Character 7
0 Plain Radiography	**0** Hip, Right	**0** High Osmolar	**0** Unenhanced and Enhanced	**1** Densitometry
1 Fluoroscopy	**1** Hip, Left	**1** Low Osmolar	**Z** None	**Z** None
2 Computerized Tomography (CT Scan)	**2** Hips, Bilateral	**Y** Other Contrast		
3 Magnetic Resonance Imaging (MRI)	**3** Femur, Right	**Z** None		
4 Ultrasonography	**4** Femur, Left			
	7 Knee, Right			
	8 Knee, Left			
	9 Knees, Bilateral			
	B Tibia/Fibula, Right			
	C Tibia/Fibula, Left			
	D Lower Leg, Right			
	F Lower Leg, Left			
	G Ankle, Right			
	H Ankle, Left			
	J Calcaneus, Right			
	K Calcaneus, Left			
	L Foot, Right			
	M Foot, Left			
	P Toe(s), Right			
	Q Toe(s), Left			
	R Lower Extremity, Right			
	S Lower Extremity, Left			
	V Patella, Right			
	W Patella, Left			
	X Foot/Toe Joint, Right			
	Y Foot/Toe Joint, Left			

B: Imaging
R: Axial Skeleton, Except Skull and Facial Bones

Type-Character 3	Body Part-Character 4	Contrast-Character 5	Qualifier-Character 6	Qualifier-Character 7
0 Plain Radiography	**0** Cervical Spine	**0** High Osmolar	**0** Unenhanced and Enhanced	**1** Densitometry
1 Fluoroscopy	**1** Cervical Disc(s)	**1** Low Osmolar	**Z** None	**Z** None
2 Computerized Tomography (CT Scan)	**2** Thoracic Disc(s)	**Y** Other Contrast		
3 Magnetic Resonance Imaging (MRI)	**3** Lumbar Disc(s)	**Z** None		
4 Ultrasonography	**4** Cervical Facet Joint(s)			
	5 Thoracic Facet Joint(s)			
	6 Lumbar Facet Joint(s)			
	7 Thoracic Spine			
	8 Thoracolumbar Joint			
	9 Lumbar Spine			
	B Lumbosacral Joint			
	C Pelvis			
	D Sacroiliac Joints			
	F Sacrum and Coccyx			
	G Whole Spine			
	H Sternum			

B: Imaging
T: Urinary System

Type-Character 3	Body Part-Character 4	Contrast-Character 5	Qualifier-Character 6	Qualifier-Character 7
0 Plain Radiography	**0** Bladder	**0** High Osmolar	**0** Unenhanced and Enhanced	**Z** None
1 Fluoroscopy	**1** Kidney, Right	**1** Low Osmolar	**Z** None	
2 Computerized Tomography (CT Scan)	**2** Kidney, Left	**Y** Other Contrast		
3 Magnetic Resonance Imaging (MRI)	**3** Kidneys, Bilateral	**Z** None		
4 Ultrasonography	**4** Kidneys, Ureters and Bladder			
	5 Urethra			
	6 Ureter, Right			
	7 Ureter, Left			
	8 Ureters, Bilateral			
	9 Kidney Transplant			
	B Bladder and Urethra			
	C Ileal Diversion Loop			
	D Kidney, Ureter and Bladder, Right			
	F Kidney, Ureter and Bladder, Left			
	G Ileal Loop, Ureters and Kidneys			
	J Kidneys and Bladder			

B: Imaging
U: Female Reproductive System

Type-Character 3	Body Part-Character 4	Contrast-Character 5	Qualifier-Character 6	Qualifier-Character 7
0 Plain Radiography	**0** Fallopian Tube, Right	**0** High Osmolar	**0** Unenhanced and Enhanced	**Z** None
1 Fluoroscopy	**1** Fallopian Tube, Left	**1** Low Osmolar	**Z** None	
3 Magnetic Resonance Imaging (MRI)	**2** Fallopian Tubes, Bilateral	**Y** Other Contrast		
4 Ultrasonography	**3** Ovary, Right	**Z** None		
	4 Ovary, Left			
	5 Ovaries, Bilateral			
	6 Uterus			
	8 Uterus and Fallopian Tubes			
	9 Vagina			
	B Pregnant Uterus			
	C Uterus and Ovaries			

B: Imaging
V: Male Reproductive System

Type-Character 3	Body Part-Character 4	Contrast-Character 5	Qualifier-Character 6	Qualifier-Character 7
0 Plain Radiography	**0** Corpora Cavernosa	**0** High Osmolar	**0** Unenhanced and Enhanced	**Z** None
1 Fluoroscopy	**1** Epididymis, Right	**1** Low Osmolar	**Z** None	
2 Computerized Tomography (CT Scan)	**2** Epididymis, Left	**Y** Other Contrast		
3 Magnetic Resonance Imaging (MRI)	**3** Prostate	**Z** None		
4 Ultrasonography	**4** Scrotum			
	5 Testicle, Right			
	6 Testicle, Left			
	7 Testicles, Bilateral			
	8 Vasa Vasorum			
	9 Prostate and Seminal Vesicles			
	B Penis			

B: Imaging
W: Anatomical Regions

Type-Character 3	Body Part-Character 4	Contrast-Character 5	Qualifier-Character 6	Qualifier-Character 7
0 Plain Radiography	**0** Abdomen	**0** High Osmolar	**0** Unenhanced and Enhanced	**Z** None
1 Fluoroscopy	**1** Abdomen and Pelvis	**1** Low Osmolar	**Z** None	
2 Computerized Tomography (CT Scan)	**3** Chest	**Y** Other Contrast		
3 Magnetic Resonance Imaging (MRI)	**4** Chest and Abdomen	**Z** None		
4 Ultrasonography	**5** Chest, Abdomen and Pelvis			
	8 Head			
	9 Head and Neck			
	B Long Bones, All			
	C Lower Extremity			
	F Neck			
	G Pelvic Region			
	H Retroperitoneum			
	J Upper Extremity			
	K Whole Body			
	L Whole Skeleton			
	M Whole Body, Infant			
	P Brachial Plexus			

B: Imaging
Y: Fetus and Obstetrical

Type-Character 3	Body Part-Character 4	Contrast-Character 5	Qualifier-Character 6	Qualifier-Character 7
3 Magnetic Resonance Imaging (MRI)	**0** Fetal Head	**Y** Other Contrast	**0** Unenhanced and Enhanced	**Z** None
4 Ultrasonography	**1** Fetal Heart	**Z** None	**Z** None	
	2 Fetal Thorax			
	3 Fetal Abdomen			
	4 Fetal Spine			
	5 Fetal Extremities			
	6 Whole Fetus			
	7 Fetal Umbilical Cord			
	8 Placenta			
	9 First Trimester, Single Fetus			
	B First Trimester, Multiple Gestation			
	C Second Trimester, Single Fetus			
	D Second Trimester, Multiple Gestation			
	F Third Trimester, Single Fetus			
	G Third Trimester, Multiple Gestation			

C: Nuclear Medicine
0: Central Nervous System

Type-Character 3	Body Part-Character 4	Radionuclide-Character 5	Qualifier-Character 6	Qualifier-Character 7
1 Planar Nuclear Medicine Imaging	**0** Brain	**1** Technetium 99m (Tc-99m)	**Z** None	**Z** None
2 Tomographic (Tomo) Nuclear Medicine Imaging	**5** Cerebrospinal Fluid	**B** Carbon 11 (C-11)		
3 Positron Emission Tomographic (PET) Imaging	**Y** Central Nervous System	**D** Indium 111 (In-111)		
5 Nonimaging Nuclear Medicine Probe		**F** Iodine 123 (I-123)		
		K Fluorine 18 (F-18)		
		M Oxygen 15 (O-15)		
		S Thallium 201 (Tl-201)		
		V Xenon 133 (Xe-133)		
		Y Other Radionuclide		

C: Nuclear Medicine
2: Heart

Type-Character 3	Body Part-Character 4	Radionuclide-Character 5	Qualifier-Character 6	Qualifier-Character 7
1 Planar Nuclear Medicine Imaging	**6** Heart, Right and Left	**1** Technetium 99m (Tc-99m)	**Z** None	**Z** None
2 Tomographic (Tomo) Nuclear Medicine Imaging	**G** Myocardium	**D** Indium 111 (In-111)		
3 Positron Emission Tomographic (PET) Imaging	**Y** Heart	**K** Fluorine 18 (F-18)		
5 Nonimaging Nuclear Medicine Probe		**M** Oxygen 15 (O-15)		
		Q Rubidium 82 (Rb-82)		
		R Nitrogen 13 (N-13)		
		S Thallium 201 (Tl-201)		
		Y Other Radionuclide		
		Z None		

C: Nuclear Medicine
5: Veins

Type-Character 3	Body Part-Character 4	Radionuclide-Character 5	Qualifier-Character 6	Qualifier-Character 7
1 Planar Nuclear Medicine Imaging	**B** Lower Extremity Veins, Right	**1** Technetium 99m (Tc-99m)	**Z** None	**Z** None
	C Lower Extremity Veins, Left	**Y** Other Radionuclide		
	D Lower Extremity Veins, Bilateral			
	N Upper Extremity Veins, Right			
	P Upper Extremity Veins, Left			
	Q Upper Extremity Veins, Bilateral			
	R Central Veins			
	Y Veins			

C: Nuclear Medicine
7: Lymphatic and Hematologic System

Type-Character 3	Body Part-Character 4	Radionuclide-Character 5	Qualifier-Character 6	Qualifier-Character 7
1 Planar Nuclear Medicine Imaging	**0** Bone Marrow	**1** Technetium 99m (Tc-99m)	**Z** None	**Z** None
2 Tomographic (Tomo) Nuclear Medicine Imaging	**2** Spleen	**7** Cobalt 58 (Co-58)		
5 Nonimaging Nuclear Medicine Probe	**3** Blood	**C** Cobalt 57 (Co-57)		
6 Nonimaging Nuclear Medicine Assay	**5** Lymphatics, Head and Neck	**D** Indium 111 (In-111)		
	D Lymphatics, Pelvic	**H** Iodine 125 (I-125)		
	J Lymphatics, Head	**W** Chromium (Cr-51)		
	K Lymphatics, Neck	**Y** Other Radionuclide		
	L Lymphatics, Upper Chest			
	M Lymphatics, Trunk			
	N Lymphatics, Upper Extremity			
	P Lymphatics, Lower Extremity			
	Y Lymphatic and Hematologic System			

C: Nuclear Medicine
8: Eye

Type-Character 3	Body Part-Character 4	Radionuclide-Character 5	Qualifier-Character 6	Qualifier-Character 7
1 Planar Nuclear Medicine Imaging	**9** Lacrimal Ducts, Bilateral	**1** Technetium 99m (Tc-99m)	**Z** None	**Z** None
	Y Eye	**Y** Other Radionuclide		

C: Nuclear Medicine
9: Ear, Nose, Mouth and Throat

Type-Character 3	Body Part-Character 4	Radionuclide-Character 5	Qualifier-Character 6	Qualifier-Character 7
1 Planar Nuclear Medicine Imaging	**B** Salivary Glands, Bilateral	**1** Technetium 99m (Tc-99m)	**Z** None	**Z** None
	Y Ear, Nose, Mouth and Throat	**Y** Other Radionuclide		

C: Nuclear Medicine
B: Respiratory System

Type-Character 3	Body Part-Character 4	Radionuclide-Character 5	Qualifier-Character 6	Qualifier-Character 7
1 Planar Nuclear Medicine Imaging	**2** Lungs and Bronchi	**1** Technetium 99m (Tc-99m)	**Z** None	**Z** None
2 Tomographic (Tomo) Nuclear Medicine Imaging	**Y** Respiratory System	**9** Krypton (Kr-81m)		
3 Positron Emission Tomographic (PET) Imaging		**K** Fluorine 18 (F-18)		
		T Xenon 127 (Xe-127)		
		V Xenon 133 (Xe-133)		
		Y Other Radionuclide		

C: Nuclear Medicine
D: Gastrointestinal System

Type-Character 3	Body Part-Character 4	Radionuclide-Character 5	Qualifier-Character 6	Qualifier-Character 7
1 Planar Nuclear Medicine Imaging	**5** Upper Gastrointestinal Tract	**1** Technetium 99m (Tc-99m)	**Z** None	**Z** None
2 Tomographic (Tomo) Nuclear Medicine Imaging	**7** Gastrointestinal Tract	**D** Indium 111 (In-111)		
	Y Digestive System	**Y** Other Radionuclide		

C: Nuclear Medicine
F: Hepatobiliary System and Pancreas

Type-Character 3	Body Part-Character 4	Radionuclide-Character 5	Qualifier-Character 6	Qualifier-Character 7
1 Planar Nuclear Medicine Imaging	**4** Gallbladder	**1** Technetium 99m (Tc-99m)	**Z** None	**Z** None
2 Tomographic (Tomo) Nuclear Medicine Imaging	**5** Liver	**Y** Other Radionuclide		
	6 Liver and Spleen			
	C Hepatobiliary System, All			
	Y Hepatobiliary System and Pancreas			

C: Nuclear Medicine
G: Endocrine System

Type-Character 3	Body Part-Character 4	Radionuclide-Character 5	Qualifier-Character 6	Qualifier-Character 7
1 Planar Nuclear Medicine Imaging	**1** Parathyroid Glands	**1** Technetium 99m (Tc-99m)	**Z** None	**Z** None
2 Tomographic (Tomo) Nuclear Medicine Imaging	**2** Thyroid Gland	**F** Iodine 123 (I-123)		
4 Nonimaging Nuclear Medicine Uptake	**4** Adrenal Glands, Bilateral	**G** Iodine 131 (I-131)		
	Y Endocrine System	**S** Thallium 201 (Tl-201)		
		Y Other Radionuclide		

C: Nuclear Medicine
H: Skin, Subcutaneous Tissue and Breast

Type-Character 3	Body Part-Character 4	Radionuclide-Character 5	Qualifier-Character 6	Qualifier-Character 7
1 Planar Nuclear Medicine Imaging	**0** Breast, Right	**1** Technetium 99m (Tc-99m)	**Z** None	**Z** None
2 Tomographic (Tomo) Nuclear Medicine Imaging	**1** Breast, Left	**S** Thallium 201 (Tl-201)		
	2 Breasts, Bilateral	**Y** Other Radionuclide		
	Y Skin, Subcutaneous Tissue and Breast			

C: Nuclear Medicine
P: Musculoskeletal System

Type-Character 3	Body Part-Character 4	Radionuclide-Character 5	Qualifier-Character 6	Qualifier-Character 7
1 Planar Nuclear Medicine Imaging	**1** Skull	**1** Technetium 99m (Tc-99m)	**Z** None	**Z** None
2 Tomographic (Tomo) Nuclear Medicine Imaging	**2** Cervical Spine	**Y** Other Radionuclide		
5 Nonimaging Nuclear Medicine Probe	**3** Skull and Cervical Spine	**Z** None		
	4 Thorax			
	5 Spine			
	6 Pelvis			
	7 Spine and Pelvis			
	8 Upper Extremity, Right			
	9 Upper Extremity, Left			
	B Upper Extremities, Bilateral			
	C Lower Extremity, Right			
	D Lower Extremity, Left			
	F Lower Extremities, Bilateral			
	G Thoracic Spine			
	H Lumbar Spine			
	J Thoracolumbar Spine			
	N Upper Extremities			
	P Lower Extremities			
	Y Musculoskeletal System, Other			
	Z Musculoskeletal System, All			

C: Nuclear Medicine
T: Urinary System

Type-Character 3	Body Part-Character 4	Radionuclide-Character 5	Qualifier-Character 6	Qualifier-Character 7
1 Planar Nuclear Medicine Imaging	**3** Kidneys, Ureters and Bladder	**1** Technetium 99m (Tc-99m)	**Z** None	**Z** None
2 Tomographic (Tomo) Nuclear Medicine Imaging	**H** Bladder and Ureters	**F** Iodine 123 (I-123)		
6 Nonimaging Nuclear Medicine Assay	**Y** Urinary System	**G** Iodine 131 (I-131)		
		H Iodine 125 (I-125)		
		Y Other Radionuclide		

C: Nuclear Medicine
V: Male Reproductive System

Type-Character 3	Body Part-Character 4	Radionuclide-Character 5	Qualifier-Character 6	Qualifier-Character 7
1 Planar Nuclear Medicine Imaging	**9** Testicles, Bilateral	**1** Technetium 99m (Tc-99m)	**Z** None	**Z** None
	Y Male Reproductive System	**Y** Other Radionuclide		

C: Nuclear Medicine
W: Anatomical Regions

Type-Character 3	Body Part-Character 4	Radionuclide-Character 5	Qualifier-Character 6	Qualifier-Character 7
1 Planar Nuclear Medicine Imaging	**0** Abdomen	**1** Technetium 99m (Tc-99m)	**Z** None	**Z** None
2 Tomographic (Tomo) Nuclear Medicine Imaging	**1** Abdomen and Pelvis	**8** Samarium 153 (Sm-153)		
3 Positron Emission Tomographic (PET) Imaging	**3** Chest	**D** Indium 111 (In-111)		
5 Nonimaging Nuclear Medicine Probe	**4** Chest and Abdomen	**F** Iodine 123 (I-123)		
7 Systemic Nuclear Medicine Therapy	**6** Chest and Neck	**G** Iodine 131 (I-131)		
	B Head and Neck	**K** Fluorine 18 (F-18)		
	D Lower Extremity	**L** Gallium 67 (Ga-67)		
	G Thyroid	**N** Phosphorus 32 (P-32)		
	J Pelvic Region	**P** Strontium 89 (Sr-89)		
	M Upper Extremity	**S** Thallium 201 (Tl-201)		
	N Whole Body	**Y** Other Radionuclide		
	Y Anatomical Regions, Multiple	**Z** None		
	Z Anatomical Region, Other			

D: Radiation Therapy
0: Central and Peripheral Nervous System

Modality-Character 3	Treatment Site -Character 4	Modality Qualifier-Character 5	Isotope -Character 6	Qualifier-Character 7
0 Beam Radiation	**0** Brain	**0** Photons <1 MeV	**7** Cesium 137 (Cs-137)	**0** Intraoperative
1 Brachytherapy	**1** Brain Stem	**1** Photons 1 - 10 MeV	**8** Iridium 192 (Ir-192)	**1** Unidirectional Source
2 Stereotactic Radiosurgery	**6** Spinal Cord	**2** Photons >10 MeV	**9** Iodine 125 (I-125)	**Z** None
Y Other Radiation	**7** Peripheral Nerve	**3** Electrons	**B** Palladium 103 (Pd-103)	
		4 Heavy Particles (Protons, Ions)	**C** Californium 252 (Cf-252)	
		5 Neutrons	**Y** Other Isotope	
		6 Neutron Capture	**Z** None	
		7 Contact Radiation		
		8 Hyperthermia		
		9 High Dose Rate (HDR)		
		B Low Dose Rate (LDR)		
		D Stereotactic Other Photon Radiosurgery		
		F Plaque Radiation		
		H Stereotactic Particulate Radiosurgery		
		J Stereotactic Gamma Beam Radiosurgery		
		K Laser Interstitial Thermal Therapy		

D: Radiation Therapy
7: Lymphatic and Hematologic System

Modality-Character 3	Treatment Site -Character 4	Modality Qualifier-Character 5	Isotope -Character 6	Qualifier-Character 7
0 Beam Radiation	**0** Bone Marrow	**0** Photons <1 MeV	**7** Cesium 137 (Cs-137)	**0** Intraoperative
1 Brachytherapy	**1** Thymus	**1** Photons 1 - 10 MeV	**8** Iridium 192 (Ir-192)	**1** Unidirectional Source
2 Stereotactic Radiosurgery	**2** Spleen	**2** Photons >10 MeV	**9** Iodine 125 (I-125)	**Z** None
Y Other Radiation	**3** Lymphatics, Neck	**3** Electrons	**B** Palladium 103 (Pd-103)	
	4 Lymphatics, Axillary	**4** Heavy Particles (Protons, Ions)	**C** Californium 252 (Cf-252)	
	5 Lymphatics, Thorax	**5** Neutrons	**Y** Other Isotope	
	6 Lymphatics, Abdomen	**6** Neutron Capture	**Z** None	
	7 Lymphatics, Pelvis	**8** Hyperthermia		
	8 Lymphatics, Inguinal	**9** High Dose Rate (HDR)		
		B Low Dose Rate (LDR)		
		D Stereotactic Other Photon Radiosurgery		
		F Plaque Radiation		
		H Stereotactic Particulate Radiosurgery		
		J Stereotactic Gamma Beam Radiosurgery		

D: Radiation Therapy
8: Eye

Modality-Character 3	Treatment Site -Character 4	Modality Qualifier-Character 5	Isotope -Character 6	Qualifier-Character 7
0 Beam Radiation	**0** Eye	**0** Photons <1 MeV	**7** Cesium 137 (Cs-137)	**0** Intraoperative
1 Brachytherapy		**1** Photons 1 - 10 MeV	**8** Iridium 192 (Ir-192)	**1** Unidirectional Source
2 Stereotactic Radiosurgery		**2** Photons >10 MeV	**9** Iodine 125 (I-125)	**Z** None
Y Other Radiation		**3** Electrons	**B** Palladium 103 (Pd-103)	
		4 Heavy Particles (Protons, Ions)	**C** Californium 252 (Cf-252)	
		5 Neutrons	**Y** Other Isotope	
		6 Neutron Capture	**Z** None	
		7 Contact Radiation		
		8 Hyperthermia		
		9 High Dose Rate (HDR)		
		B Low Dose Rate (LDR)		
		D Stereotactic Other Photon Radiosurgery		
		F Plaque Radiation		
		H Stereotactic Particulate Radiosurgery		
		J Stereotactic Gamma Beam Radiosurgery		

D: Radiation Therapy
9: Ear, Nose, Mouth and Throat

Modality-Character 3	Treatment Site -Character 4	Modality Qualifier-Character 5	Isotope -Character 6	Qualifier-Character 7
0 Beam Radiation	**0** Ear	**0** Photons <1 MeV	**7** Cesium 137 (Cs-137)	**0** Intraoperative
1 Brachytherapy	**1** Nose	**1** Photons 1 - 10 MeV	**8** Iridium 192 (Ir-192)	**1** Unidirectional Source
2 Stereotactic Radiosurgery	**3** Hypopharynx	**2** Photons >10 MeV	**9** Iodine 125 (I-125)	**Z** None
Y Other Radiation	**4** Mouth	**3** Electrons	**B** Palladium 103 (Pd-103)	
	5 Tongue	**4** Heavy Particles (Protons, Ions)	**C** Californium 252 (Cf-252)	
	6 Salivary Glands	**5** Neutrons	**Y** Other Isotope	
	7 Sinuses	**6** Neutron Capture	**Z** None	
	8 Hard Palate	**7** Contact Radiation		
	9 Soft Palate	**8** Hyperthermia		
	B Larynx	**9** High Dose Rate (HDR)		
	C Pharynx	**B** Low Dose Rate (LDR)		
	D Nasopharynx	**C** Intraoperative Radiation Therapy (IORT)		
	F Oropharynx	**D** Stereotactic Other Photon Radiosurgery		
		F Plaque Radiation		
		H Stereotactic Particulate Radiosurgery		
		J Stereotactic Gamma Beam Radiosurgery		

D: Radiation Therapy
B: Respiratory System

Modality-Character 3	Treatment Site -Character 4	Modality Qualifier-Character 5	Isotope -Character 6	Qualifier-Character 7
0 Beam Radiation	**0** Trachea	**0** Photons <1 MeV	**7** Cesium 137 (Cs-137)	**0** Intraoperative
1 Brachytherapy	**1** Bronchus	**1** Photons 1 - 10 MeV	**8** Iridium 192 (Ir-192)	**1** Unidirectional Source
2 Stereotactic Radiosurgery	**2** Lung	**2** Photons >10 MeV	**9** Iodine 125 (I-125)	**Z** None
Y Other Radiation	**5** Pleura	**3** Electrons	**B** Palladium 103 (Pd-103)	
	6 Mediastinum	**4** Heavy Particles (Protons, Ions)	**C** Californium 252 (Cf-252)	
	7 Chest Wall	**5** Neutrons	**Y** Other Isotope	
	8 Diaphragm	**6** Neutron Capture	**Z** None	
		7 Contact Radiation		
		8 Hyperthermia		
		9 High Dose Rate (HDR)		
		B Low Dose Rate (LDR)		
		D Stereotactic Other Photon Radiosurgery		
		F Plaque Radiation		
		H Stereotactic Particulate Radiosurgery		
		J Stereotactic Gamma Beam Radiosurgery		
		K Laser Interstitial Thermal Therapy		

D: Radiation Therapy
D: Gastrointestinal System

Modality-Character 3	Treatment Site -Character 4	Modality Qualifier-Character 5	Isotope -Character 6	Qualifier-Character 7
0 Beam Radiation	**0** Esophagus	**0** Photons <1 MeV	**7** Cesium 137 (Cs-137)	**0** Intraoperative
1 Brachytherapy	**1** Stomach	**1** Photons 1 - 10 MeV	**8** Iridium 192 (Ir-192)	**1** Unidirectional Source
2 Stereotactic Radiosurgery	**2** Duodenum	**2** Photons >10 MeV	**9** Iodine 125 (I-125)	**Z** None
Y Other Radiation	**3** Jejunum	**3** Electrons	**B** Palladium 103 (Pd-103)	
	4 Ileum	**4** Heavy Particles (Protons, Ions)	**C** Californium 252 (Cf-252)	
	5 Colon	**5** Neutrons	**Y** Other Isotope	
	7 Rectum	**6** Neutron Capture	**Z** None	
	8 Anus	**7** Contact Radiation		
		8 Hyperthermia		
		9 High Dose Rate (HDR)		
		B Low Dose Rate (LDR)		
		C Intraoperative Radiation Therapy (IORT)		
		D Stereotactic Other Photon Radiosurgery		
		F Plaque Radiation		
		H Stereotactic Particulate Radiosurgery		
		J Stereotactic Gamma Beam Radiosurgery		
		K Laser Interstitial Thermal Therapy		

D: Radiation Therapy
F: Hepatobiliary System and Pancreas

Modality-Character 3	Treatment Site -Character 4	Modality Qualifier-Character 5	Isotope -Character 6	Qualifier-Character 7
0 Beam Radiation	**0** Liver	**0** Photons <1 MeV	**7** Cesium 137 (Cs-137)	**0** Intraoperative
1 Brachytherapy	**1** Gallbladder	**1** Photons 1 - 10 MeV	**8** Iridium 192 (Ir-192)	**1** Unidirectional Source
2 Stereotactic Radiosurgery	**2** Bile Ducts	**2** Photons >10 MeV	**9** Iodine 125 (I-125)	**Z** None
Y Other Radiation	**3** Pancreas	**3** Electrons	**B** Palladium 103 (Pd-103)	
		4 Heavy Particles (Protons, Ions)	**C** Californium 252 (Cf-252)	
		5 Neutrons	**Y** Other Isotope	
		6 Neutron Capture	**Z** None	
		7 Contact Radiation		
		8 Hyperthermia		
		9 High Dose Rate (HDR)		
		B Low Dose Rate (LDR)		
		C Intraoperative Radiation Therapy (IORT)		
		D Stereotactic Other Photon Radiosurgery		
		F Plaque Radiation		
		H Stereotactic Particulate Radiosurgery		
		J Stereotactic Gamma Beam Radiosurgery		
		K Laser Interstitial Thermal Therapy		

D: Radiation Therapy
G: Endocrine System

Modality-Character 3	Treatment Site -Character 4	Modality Qualifier-Character 5	Isotope -Character 6	Qualifier-Character 7
0 Beam Radiation	**0** Pituitary Gland	**0** Photons <1 MeV	**7** Cesium 137 (Cs-137)	**0** Intraoperative
1 Brachytherapy	**1** Pineal Body	**1** Photons 1 - 10 MeV	**8** Iridium 192 (Ir-192)	**1** Unidirectional Source
2 Stereotactic Radiosurgery	**2** Adrenal Glands	**2** Photons >10 MeV	**9** Iodine 125 (I-125)	**Z** None
Y Other Radiation	**4** Parathyroid Glands	**3** Electrons	**B** Palladium 103 (Pd-103)	
	5 Thyroid	**5** Neutrons	**C** Californium 252 (Cf-252)	
		6 Neutron Capture	**Y** Other Isotope	
		7 Contact Radiation	**Z** None	
		8 Hyperthermia		
		9 High Dose Rate (HDR)		
		B Low Dose Rate (LDR)		
		D Stereotactic Other Photon Radiosurgery		
		F Plaque Radiation		
		H Stereotactic Particulate Radiosurgery		
		J Stereotactic Gamma Beam Radiosurgery		
		K Laser Interstitial Thermal Therapy		

D: Radiation Therapy
H: Skin

Modality-Character 3	Treatment Site -Character 4	Modality Qualifier-Character 5	Isotope -Character 6	Qualifier-Character 7
0 Beam Radiation	**2** Skin, Face	**0** Photons <1 MeV	**Z** None	**0** Intraoperative
Y Other Radiation	**3** Skin, Neck	**1** Photons 1 - 10 MeV		**Z** None
	4 Skin, Arm	**2** Photons >10 MeV		
	5 Skin, Hand	**3** Electrons		
	6 Skin, Chest	**4** Heavy Particles (Protons, Ions)		
	7 Skin, Back	**5** Neutrons		
	8 Skin, Abdomen	**6** Neutron Capture		
	9 Skin, Buttock	**7** Contact Radiation		
	B Skin, Leg	**8** Hyperthermia		
	C Skin, Foot	**F** Plaque Radiation		

D: Radiation Therapy
M: Breast

Modality-Character 3	Treatment Site -Character 4	Modality Qualifier-Character 5	Isotope -Character 6	Qualifier-Character 7
0 Beam Radiation	**0** Breast, Left	**0** Photons <1 MeV	**7** Cesium 137 (Cs-137)	**0** Intraoperative
1 Brachytherapy	**1** Breast, Right	**1** Photons 1 - 10 MeV	**8** Iridium 192 (Ir-192)	**1** Unidirectional Source
2 Stereotactic Radiosurgery		**2** Photons >10 MeV	**9** Iodine 125 (I-125)	**Z** None
Y Other Radiation		**3** Electrons	**B** Palladium 103 (Pd-103)	
		4 Heavy Particles (Protons, Ions)	**C** Californium 252 (Cf-252)	
		5 Neutrons	**Y** Other Isotope	
		6 Neutron Capture	**Z** None	
		7 Contact Radiation		
		8 Hyperthermia		
		9 High Dose Rate (HDR)		
		B Low Dose Rate (LDR)		
		D Stereotactic Other Photon Radiosurgery		
		F Plaque Radiation		
		H Stereotactic Particulate Radiosurgery		
		J Stereotactic Gamma Beam Radiosurgery		
		K Laser Interstitial Thermal Therapy		

D: Radiation Therapy
P: Musculoskeletal System

Modality-Character 3	Treatment Site -Character 4	Modality Qualifier-Character 5	Isotope -Character 6	Qualifier-Character 7
0 Beam Radiation	**0** Skull	**0** Photons <1 MeV	**Z** None	**0** Intraoperative
Y Other Radiation	**2** Maxilla	**1** Photons 1 - 10 MeV		**Z** None
	3 Mandible	**2** Photons >10 MeV		
	4 Sternum	**3** Electrons		
	5 Rib(s)	**4** Heavy Particles (Protons, Ions)		
	6 Humerus	**5** Neutrons		
	7 Radius/Ulna	**6** Neutron Capture		
	8 Pelvic Bones	**7** Contact Radiation		
	9 Femur	**8** Hyperthermia		
	B Tibia/Fibula	**F** Plaque Radiation		
	C Other Bone			

D: Radiation Therapy
T: Urinary System

Modality-Character 3	Treatment Site -Character 4	Modality Qualifier-Character 5	Isotope -Character 6	Qualifier-Character 7
0 Beam Radiation	**0** Kidney	**0** Photons <1 MeV	**7** Cesium 137 (Cs-137)	**0** Intraoperative
1 Brachytherapy	**1** Ureter	**1** Photons 1 - 10 MeV	**8** Iridium 192 (Ir-192)	**1** Unidirectional Source
2 Stereotactic Radiosurgery	**2** Bladder	**2** Photons >10 MeV	**9** Iodine 125 (I-125)	**Z** None
Y Other Radiation	**3** Urethra	**3** Electrons	**B** Palladium 103 (Pd-103)	
		4 Heavy Particles (Protons, Ions)	**C** Californium 252 (Cf-252)	
		5 Neutrons	**Y** Other Isotope	
		6 Neutron Capture	**Z** None	
		7 Contact Radiation		
		8 Hyperthermia		
		9 High Dose Rate (HDR)		
		B Low Dose Rate (LDR)		
		C Intraoperative Radiation Therapy (IORT)		
		D Stereotactic Other Photon Radiosurgery		
		F Plaque Radiation		
		H Stereotactic Particulate Radiosurgery		
		J Stereotactic Gamma Beam Radiosurgery		

D: Radiation Therapy
U: Female Reproductive System

Modality-Character 3	Treatment Site -Character 4	Modality Qualifier-Character 5	Isotope -Character 6	Qualifier-Character 7
0 Beam Radiation	**0** Ovary	**0** Photons <1 MeV	**7** Cesium 137 (Cs-137)	**0** Intraoperative
1 Brachytherapy	**1** Cervix	**1** Photons 1 - 10 MeV	**8** Iridium 192 (Ir-192)	**1** Unidirectional Source
2 Stereotactic Radiosurgery	**2** Uterus	**2** Photons >10 MeV	**9** Iodine 125 (I-125)	**Z** None
Y Other Radiation		**3** Electrons	**B** Palladium 103 (Pd-103)	
		4 Heavy Particles (Protons, Ions)	**C** Californium 252 (Cf-252)	
		5 Neutrons	**Y** Other Isotope	
		6 Neutron Capture	**Z** None	
		7 Contact Radiation		
		8 Hyperthermia		
		9 High Dose Rate (HDR)		
		B Low Dose Rate (LDR)		
		C Intraoperative Radiation Therapy (IORT)		
		D Stereotactic Other Photon Radiosurgery		
		F Plaque Radiation		
		H Stereotactic Particulate Radiosurgery		
		J Stereotactic Gamma Beam Radiosurgery		

D: Radiation Therapy
V: Male Reproductive System

Modality-Character 3	Treatment Site -Character 4	Modality Qualifier-Character 5	Isotope -Character 6	Qualifier-Character 7
0 Beam Radiation	**0** Prostate	**0** Photons <1 MeV	**7** Cesium 137 (Cs-137)	**0** Intraoperative
1 Brachytherapy	**1** Testis	**1** Photons 1 - 10 MeV	**8** Iridium 192 (Ir-192)	**1** Unidirectional Source
2 Stereotactic Radiosurgery		**2** Photons >10 MeV	**9** Iodine 125 (I-125)	**Z** None
Y Other Radiation		**3** Electrons	**B** Palladium 103 (Pd-103)	
		4 Heavy Particles (Protons, Ions)	**C** Californium 252 (Cf-252)	
		5 Neutrons	**Y** Other Isotope	
		6 Neutron Capture	**Z** None	
		7 Contact Radiation		
		8 Hyperthermia		
		9 High Dose Rate (HDR)		
		B Low Dose Rate (LDR)		
		C Intraoperative Radiation Therapy (IORT)		
		D Stereotactic Other Photon Radiosurgery		
		F Plaque Radiation		
		H Stereotactic Particulate Radiosurgery		
		J Stereotactic Gamma Beam Radiosurgery		

D: Radiation Therapy
W: Anatomical Regions

Modality-Character 3	Treatment Site -Character 4	Modality Qualifier-Character 5	Isotope -Character 6	Qualifier-Character 7
0 Beam Radiation	**1** Head and Neck	**0** Photons <1 MeV	**7** Cesium 137 (Cs-137)	**0** Intraoperative
1 Brachytherapy	**2** Chest	**1** Photons 1 - 10 MeV	**8** Iridium 192 (Ir-192)	**1** Unidirectional Source
2 Stereotactic Radiosurgery	**3** Abdomen	**2** Photons >10 MeV	**9** Iodine 125 (I-125)	**Z** None
Y Other Radiation	**4** Hemibody	**3** Electrons	**B** Palladium 103 (Pd-103)	
	5 Whole Body	**4** Heavy Particles (Protons, Ions)	**C** Californium 252 (Cf-252)	
	6 Pelvic Region	**5** Neutrons	**D** Iodine 131 (I-131)	
		6 Neutron Capture	**F** Phosphorus 32 (P-32)	
		7 Contact Radiation	**G** Strontium 89 (Sr-89)	
		8 Hyperthermia	**H** Strontium 90 (Sr-90)	
		9 High Dose Rate (HDR)	**Y** Other Isotope	
		B Low Dose Rate (LDR)	**Z** None	
		D Stereotactic Other Photon Radiosurgery		
		F Plaque Radiation		
		G Isotope Administration		
		H Stereotactic Particulate Radiosurgery		
		J Stereotactic Gamma Beam Radiosurgery		

F: Physical Rehabilitation and Diagnostic Audiology
0: Rehabilitation

Type-Character 3	Body System/Region-Character 4	Type Qualifier-Character 5	Equipment-Character 6	Qualifier-Character 7
0 Speech Assessment	**0** Neurological System - Head and Neck	**0** Bathing/Showering	**1** Audiometer	**Z** None
1 Motor and/or Nerve Function Assessment	**1** Neurological System - Upper Back / Upper Extremity	**0** Bathing/Showering Technique	**2** Sound Field / Booth	
2 Activities of Daily Living Assessment	**2** Neurological System - Lower Back / Lower Extremity	**0** Bathing/Showering Techniques	**4** Electroacoustic Immittance / Acoustic Reflex	
6 Speech Treatment	**3** Neurological System - Whole Body	**0** Cochlear Implant Rehabilitation	**5** Hearing Aid Selection / Fitting / Test	
7 Motor Treatment	**4** Circulatory System - Head and Neck	**0** Filtered Speech	**7** Electrophysiologic	
8 Activities of Daily Living Treatment	**5** Circulatory System - Upper Back / Upper Extremity	**0** Hearing and Related Disorders Counseling	**8** Vestibular / Balance	
9 Hearing Treatment	**6** Circulatory System - Lower Back / Lower Extremity	**0** Muscle Performance	**9** Cochlear Implant	
B Cochlear Implant Treatment	**7** Circulatory System - Whole Body	**0** Nonspoken Language	**B** Physical Agents	
C Vestibular Treatment	**8** Respiratory System - Head and Neck	**0** Range of Motion and Joint Mobility	**C** Mechanical	
D Device Fitting	**9** Respiratory System - Upper Back / Upper Extremity	**0** Tinnitus Masker	**D** Electrotherapeutic	
F Caregiver Training	**B** Respiratory System - Lower Back / Lower Extremity	**0** Vestibular	**E** Orthosis	
	C Respiratory System - Whole Body	**1** Dressing	**F** Assistive, Adaptive, Supportive or Protective	
	D Integumentary System - Head and Neck	**1** Dressing Techniques	**G** Aerobic Endurance and Conditioning	
	F Integumentary System - Upper Back / Upper Extremity	**1** Hearing and Related Disorders Prevention	**H** Mechanical or Electromechanical	
	G Integumentary System -Lower Back / Lower Extremity	**1** Integumentary Integrity	**J** Somatosensory	
	H Integumentary System - Whole Body	**1** Monaural Hearing Aid	**K** Audiovisual	
	J Musculoskeletal System - Head and Neck	**1** Muscle Performance	**L** Assistive Listening	
	K Musculoskeletal System - Upper Back / Upper Extremity	**1** Perceptual Processing	**M** Augmentative / Alternative Communication	
	L Musculoskeletal System - Lower Back / Lower Extremity	**1** Speech Threshold	**N** Biosensory Feedback	
	M Musculoskeletal System - Whole Body	**1** Speech-Language Pathology and Related Disorders Counseling	**P** Computer	
	N Genitourinary System	**2** Auditory Processing	**Q** Speech Analysis	
	Z None	**2** Binaural Hearing Aid	**S** Voice Analysis	
		2 Coordination/Dexterity	**T** Aerodynamic Function	
		2 Feeding and Eating	**U** Prosthesis	
		2 Feeding/Eating	**V** Speech Prosthesis	
		2 Grooming/Personal Hygiene	**W** Swallowing	
		2 Speech/Word Recognition	**X** Cerumen Management	
		2 Speech-Language Pathology and Related Disorders Prevention	**Y** Other Equipment	
		2 Visual Motor Integration	**Z** None	
		3 Aphasia		
		3 Augmentative/Alternative Communication System		
		3 Cerumen Management		
		3 Coordination/Dexterity		

Table continued on next page

Table continued from previous page

Type-Character 3	Body System/Region-Character 4	Type Qualifier-Character 5	Equipment-Character 6	Qualifier-Character 7
		3 Feeding/Eating		
		3 Grooming/Personal Hygiene		
		3 Motor Function		
		3 Postural Control		
		3 Staggered Spondaic Word		
		4 Articulation/Phonology		
		4 Bed Mobility		
		4 Home Management		
		4 Motor Function		
		4 Sensorineural Acuity Level		
		4 Voice Prosthetic		
		4 Wheelchair Mobility		
		5 Assistive Listening Device		
		5 Aural Rehabilitation		
		5 Bed Mobility		
		5 Perceptual Processing		
		5 Range of Motion and Joint Integrity		
		5 Synthetic Sentence Identification		
		5 Transfer		
		5 Wound Management		
		6 Communicative/Cognitive Integration Skills		
		6 Dynamic Orthosis		
		6 Psychosocial Skills		
		6 Sensory Awareness/Processing/Integrity		
		6 Speech and/or Language Screening		
		6 Therapeutic Exercise		
		6 Wheelchair Mobility		
		7 Aerobic Capacity and Endurance		
		7 Facial Nerve Function		
		7 Fluency		
		7 Manual Therapy Techniques		
		7 Nonspoken Language		
		7 Static Orthosis		
		7 Therapeutic Exercise		
		7 Vocational Activities and Functional Community or Work Reintegration Skills		
		8 Airway Clearance Techniques		
		8 Anthropometric Characteristics		
		8 Motor Speech		
		8 Prosthesis		
		8 Receptive/Expressive Language		
		8 Transfer Training		
		9 Articulation/Phonology		
		9 Assistive, Adaptive, Supportive or Protective Devices		
		9 Cranial Nerve Integrity		
		9 Gait Training/Functional Ambulation		
		9 Orofacial Myofunctional		
		9 Somatosensory Evoked Potentials		

Table continued on next page

Table continued from previous page

Type-Character 3	Body System/Region-Character 4	Type Qualifier-Character 5	Equipment-Character 6	Qualifier-Character 7
		9 Wound Management		
		B Bed Mobility		
		B Environmental, Home and Work Barriers		
		B Motor Speech		
		B Receptive/Expressive Language		
		B Vocational Activities and Functional Community or Work Reintegration Skills		
		C Aphasia		
		C Ergonomics and Body Mechanics		
		C Gait Training/Functional Ambulation		
		C Transfer		
		C Voice		
		D Application, Proper Use and Care of Devices		
		D Fluency		
		D Gait and/or Balance		
		D Neuromotor Development		
		D Swallowing Dysfunction		
		F Application, Proper Use and Care of Orthoses		
		F Pain		
		F Voice		
		F Wheelchair Mobility		
		G Application, Proper Use and Care of Prosthesis		
		G Communicative/Cognitive Integration Skills		
		G Reflex Integrity		
		G Ventilation, Respiration and Circulation		
		H Bedside Swallowing and Oral Function		
		H Home Management		
		H Vocational Activities and Functional Community or Work Reintegration Skills		
		J Communication Skills		
		J Instrumental Swallowing and Oral Function		
		K Orofacial Myofunctional		
		L Augmentative/Alternative Communication System		
		M Voice Prosthetic		
		N Non-invasive Instrumental Status		
		P Oral Peripheral Mechanism		
		Q Performance Intensity Phonetically Balanced Speech Discrimination		
		R Brief Tone Stimuli		
		S Distorted Speech		
		T Dichotic Stimuli		
		V Temporal Ordering of Stimuli		
		W Masking Patterns		
		X Other Specified Central Auditory Processing		

F: Physical Rehabilitation and Diagnostic Audiology
1: Diagnostic Audiology

Type-Character 3	Body System/Region-Character 4	Type Qualifier-Character 5	Equipment-Character 6	Qualifier-Character 7
3 Hearing Assessment	**Z** None	**0** Bithermal, Binaural Caloric Irrigation	**0** Occupational Hearing	**Z** None
4 Hearing Aid Assessment		**0** Cochlear Implant	**1** Audiometer	
5 Vestibular Assessment		**0** Hearing Screening	**2** Sound Field / Booth	
		1 Bithermal, Monaural Caloric Irrigation	**3** Tympanometer	
		1 Ear Canal Probe Microphone	**4** Electroacoustic Immittance / Acoustic Reflex	
		1 Pure Tone Audiometry, Air	**5** Hearing Aid Selection / Fitting / Test	
		2 Monaural Hearing Aid	**6** Otoacoustic Emission (OAE)	
		2 Pure Tone Audiometry, Air and Bone	**7** Electrophysiologic	
		2 Unithermal Binaural Screen	**8** Vestibular / Balance	
		3 Bekesy Audiometry	**9** Cochlear Implant	
		3 Binaural Hearing Aid	**K** Audiovisual	
		3 Oscillating Tracking	**L** Assistive Listening	
		4 Assistive Listening System/Device Selection	**P** Computer	
		4 Conditioned Play Audiometry	**Y** Other Equipment	
		4 Sinusoidal Vertical Axis Rotational	**Z** None	
		5 Dix-Hallpike Dynamic		
		5 Select Picture Audiometry		
		5 Sensory Aids		
		6 Binaural Electroacoustic Hearing Aid Check		
		6 Computerized Dynamic Posturography		
		6 Visual Reinforcement Audiometry		
		7 Alternate Binaural or Monaural Loudness Balance		
		7 Ear Protector Attenuation		
		7 Tinnitus Masker		
		8 Monaural Electroacoustic Hearing Aid Check		
		8 Tone Decay		
		9 Short Increment Sensitivity Index		
		B Stenger		
		C Pure Tone Stenger		
		D Tympanometry		
		F Eustachian Tube Function		
		G Acoustic Reflex Patterns		
		H Acoustic Reflex Threshold		
		J Acoustic Reflex Decay		
		K Electrocochleography		
		L Auditory Evoked Potentials		
		M Evoked Otoacoustic Emissions, Screening		
		N Evoked Otoacoustic Emissions, Diagnostic		
		P Aural Rehabilitation Status		
		Q Auditory Processing		

G: Mental Health
Z: None

Type-Character 3	Qualifier-Character 4	Qualifier-Character 5	Qualifier-Character 6	Qualifier-Character 7
1 Psychological Tests	**0** Developmental	**Z** None	**Z** None	**Z** None
2 Crisis Intervention	**0** Educational			
3 Medication Management	**0** Interactive			
5 Individual Psychotherapy	**0** Unilateral-Single Seizure			
6 Counseling	**1** Behavioral			
7 Family Psychotherapy	**1** Personality and Behavioral			
B Electroconvulsive Therapy	**1** Unilateral-Multiple Seizure			
C Biofeedback	**1** Vocational			
F Hypnosis	**2** Bilateral-Single Seizure			
G Narcosynthesis	**2** Cognitive			
H Group Psychotherapy	**2** Intellectual and Psychoeducational			
J Light Therapy	**2** Other Family Psychotherapy			
	3 Bilateral-Multiple Seizure			
	3 Interpersonal			
	3 Neuropsychological			
	3 Other Counseling			
	4 Neurobehavioral and Cognitive Status			
	4 Other Electroconvulsive Therapy			
	4 Psychoanalysis			
	5 Psychodynamic			
	6 Supportive			
	8 Cognitive-Behavioral			
	9 Other Biofeedback			
	9 Psychophysiological			
	Z None			

H: Substance Abuse Treatment
Z: None

Type-Character 3	Qualifier-Character 4	Qualifier-Character 5	Qualifier-Character 6	Qualifier-Character 7
2 Detoxification Services	**0** Cognitive	**Z** None	**Z** None	**Z** None
3 Individual Counseling	**0** Nicotine Replacement			
4 Group Counseling	**1** Behavioral			
5 Individual Psychotherapy	**1** Methadone Maintenance			
6 Family Counseling	**2** Cognitive-Behavioral			
8 Medication Management	**2** Levo-alpha-acetylmethadol (LAAM)			
9 Pharmacotherapy	**3** 12-Step			
	3 Antabuse			
	3 Other Family Counseling			
	4 Interpersonal			
	4 Naltrexone			
	5 Interactive			
	5 Naloxone			
	5 Vocational			
	6 Clonidine			
	6 Psychoeducation			
	7 Bupropion			
	7 Motivational Enhancement			
	8 Confrontational			
	8 Psychiatric Medication			
	9 Continuing Care			
	9 Other Replacement Medication			
	9 Supportive			
	B Psychoanalysis			
	B Spiritual			
	C Pre/Post-Test Infectious Disease			
	C Psychodynamic			
	D Psychophysiological			
	Z None			

X: New Technology
2: Cardiovascular System

Operation-Character 3	Body Part-Character 4	Approach-Character 5	Device-Character 6	Qualifier-Character 7
7 Dilation	**0** Coronary Artery, One Artery	**0** Open	**1** Cerebral Embolic Filtration, Dual Filter	**1** New Technology Group 1
A Assistance	**1** Coronary Artery, Two Arteries	**3** Percutaneous	**3** Zooplastic Tissue, Rapid Deployment Technique	**2** New Technology Group 2
C Extirpation	**2** Coronary Artery, Three Arteries	**4** Percutaneous Endoscopic	**6** Orbital Atherectomy Technology	**5** New Technology Group 5
R Replacement	**3** Coronary Artery, Four or More Arteries		**8** Intraluminal Device, Sustained Release Drug-eluting	
	5 Innominate Artery and Left Common Carotid Artery		**9** Intraluminal Device, Sustained Release Drug-eluting, Two	
	6 Aortic Arch		**B** Intraluminal Device, Sustained Release Drug-eluting, Three	
	F Aortic Valve		**C** Intraluminal Device, Sustained Release Drug-eluting, Four or More	
	H Femoral Artery, Right			
	J Femoral Artery, Left			
	K Popliteal Artery, Proximal Right			
	L Popliteal Artery, Proximal Left			
	M Popliteal Artery, Distal Right			
	N Popliteal Artery, Distal Left			
	P Anterior Tibial Artery, Right			
	Q Anterior Tibial Artery, Left			
	R Posterior Tibial Artery, Right			
	S Posterior Tibial Artery, Left			
	T Peroneal Artery, Right			
	U Peroneal Artery, Left			

X: New Technology
H: Skin, Subcutaneous Tissue, Fascia and Breast

Operation-Character 3	Body Part-Character 4	Approach-Character 5	Device-Character 6	Qualifier-Character 7
R Replacement	**P** Skin	**X** External	**L** Skin Substitute, Porcine Liver Derived	**2** New Technology Group 2

X: New Technology
K: Muscles, Tendons, Bursae and Ligaments

Operation-Character 3	Body Part-Character 4	Approach-Character 5	Device-Character 6	Qualifier-Character 7
0 Introduction	**2** Muscle	**3** Percutaneous	**0** Concentrated Bone Marrow Aspirate	**3** New Technology Group 3

X: New Technology
N: Bones

Operation-Character 3	Body Part-Character 4	Approach-Character 5	Device-Character 6	Qualifier-Character 7
S Reposition	**0** Lumbar Vertebra	**0** Open	**3** Magnetically Controlled Growth Rod(s)	**2** New Technology Group 2
	3 Cervical Vertebra	**3** Percutaneous		
	4 Thoracic Vertebra			

X: New Technology
R: Joints

Operation-Character 3	Body Part-Character 4	Approach-Character 5	Device-Character 6	Qualifier-Character 7
2 Monitoring	**0** Occipital-cervical Joint	**0** Open	**2** Intraoperative Knee Replacement Sensor	**1** New Technology Group 1
G Fusion	**1** Cervical Vertebral Joint		**9** Interbody Fusion Device, Nanotextured Surface	**2** New Technology Group 2
	2 Cervical Vertebral Joints, 2 or more		**F** Interbody Fusion Device, Radiolucent Porous	**3** New Technology Group 3
	4 Cervicothoracic Vertebral Joint			
	6 Thoracic Vertebral Joint			
	7 Thoracic Vertebral Joints, 2 to 7			
	8 Thoracic Vertebral Joints, 8 or more			
	A Thoracolumbar Vertebral Joint			
	B Lumbar Vertebral Joint			
	C Lumbar Vertebral Joints, 2 or more			
	D Lumbosacral Joint			
	G Knee Joint, Right			
	H Knee Joint, Left			

X: New Technology
T: Urinary System

Operation-Character 3	Body Part-Character 4	Approach-Character 5	Device-Character 6	Qualifier-Character 7
2 Monitoring	**5** Kidney	**X** External	**E** Fluorescent Pyrazine	**5** New Technology Group 5

X: New Technology
V: Male Reproductive System

Operation-Character 3	Body Part-Character 4	Approach-Character 5	Device-Character 6	Qualifier-Character 7
5 Destruction	**0** Prostate	**8** Via Natural or Artificial Opening Endoscopic	**A** Robotic Waterjet Ablation	**4** New Technology Group 4

X: New Technology
W: Anatomical Regions

Operation-Character 3	Body Part-Character 4	Approach-Character 5	Device-Character 6	Qualifier-Character 7
0 Introduction	**1** Subcutaneous Tissue	**3** Percutaneous	**2** Ceftazidime-Avibactam Anti-infective	**1** New Technology Group 1
	3 Peripheral Vein	**X** External	**3** Idarucizumab, Dabigatran Reversal Agent	**2** New Technology Group 2
	4 Central Vein		**4** Isavuconazole Antiinfective	**3** New Technology Group 3
	D Mouth and Pharynx		**5** Blinatumomab Antineoplastic Immunotherapy	**4** New Technology Group 4
			7 Coagulation Factor Xa, Inactivated	**5** New Technology Group 5
			8 Uridine Triacetate	
			9 Defibrotide Sodium Anticoagulant	
			A Bezlotoxumab Monoclonal Antibody	
			B Cytarabine and Daunorubicin Liposome Antineoplastic	
			C Engineered Autologous Chimeric Antigen Receptor T-cell Immunotherapy	
			F Other New Technology Therapeutic Substance	
			G Plazomicin Anti-infective	
			H Synthetic Human Angiotensin II	
			J Apalutamide Antineoplastic	
			K Fosfomycin Anti-infective	
			L Erdafitinib Antineoplastic	
			N Meropenem-vaborbactam Anti-infective	
			R Venetoclax Antineoplastic	
			Q Tagraxofusp-erzs Antineoplastic	
			S Iobenguane I-131 Antineoplastic	
			T Ruxolitinib	
			U Imipenem-cilastatin-relebactam Anti-infective	
			V Gilteritinib Antineoplastic	
			W Caplacizumab	

X: New Technology
X: Physiological Systems

Operation-Character 3	Body Part-Character 4	Approach-Character 5	Device-Character 6	Qualifier-Character 7
E Measurement	**5** Circulatory	**X** External	**M** Infection, Whole Blood Nucleic Acid-base Microbial Detection	**5** New Technology Group 5

X: New Technology
Y: Extracorporeal

Operation-Character 3	Body Part-Character 4	Approach-Character 5	Device-Character 6	Qualifier-Character 7
0 Introduction	**V** Vein Graft	**X** External	**8** Endothelial Damage Inhibitor	**3** New Technology Group 3

Appendix F: Substance Key

Substance Term	ICD-10-PCS Value
AIGISRx® Antibacterial Envelope	Anti-Infective Envelope
Andexanet Alfa, Factor Xa Inhibitor Reversal Agent	Coagulation Factor Xa, Inactivated
Andexxa®	Coagulation Factor Xa, Inactivated
Angiotensin II	Synthetic Human Angiotensin II
Antibacterial Envelope (TYRX™) (AIGISRx™)	Anti-Infective Envelope
Antimicrobial Envelope	Anti-Infective Envelope
Axicabtagene Ciloeucel	Engineered Autologous Chimeric Antigen Receptor T-cell Immunotherapy
AZEDRA®	Iobenguane I-131 Antineoplastic
Bone morphogenetic protein 2 (BMP 2)	Recombinant Bone Morphogenetic Protein
CBMA (Concentrated Bone Marrow Aspirate)	Concentrated Bone Marrow Aspirate
Clolar®	Clofarabine
Coagulation Factor Xa, (Recombinant) Inactivated	Coagulation Factor Xa, Inactivated
CONTEPO™	Fosfomycin Anti-infective
Defitelio®	Defibrotide Sodium Anticoagulant
DuraGraft® Endothelial Damage Inhibitor	Endothelial Damage Inhibitor
ELZONRIS™	Tagraxofusp-erzs Antineoplastic
ERLEADA™	Apalutamide Antineoplastic
Factor Xa Inhibitor Reversal Agent, Andexanet Alfa	Coagulation Factor Xa, Inactivated
Fosfomycin injection	Fosfomycin Anti-infective
GIAPREZA™	Synthetic Human Angiotensin II
Human angiotensin II, synthetic	Synthetic Human Angiotensin II
IMI/REL	Imipenem-cilastatin-relebactam Anti-infective
Iobenguane I-131, High Specific Activity (HSA)	Iobenguane I-131 Antineoplastic
Jakafi®	Ruxolitinib
Kcentra®	4-Factor Prothrombin Complex Concentrate
KYMRIAH®	Engineered Autologous Chimeric Antigen Receptor T-cell Immunotherapy
Nesiritide®	Human B-type Natriuretic Peptide
rhBMP-2	Recombinant Bone Morphogenetic Protein
Seprafilm®	Adhesion Barrier S
STELARA®	Other New Technology Therapeutic Substance
Tisagenlecleucel	Engineered Autologous Chimeric Antigen Receptor T-cell Immunotherapy
Tissue Plasminogen Activator (tPA)(r- tPA)	Other Thrombolytic
TYRX™ Antibacterial Envelope	Anti-Infective Envelope
Ustekinumab	Other New Technology Therapeutic Substance
Vabomere™	Meropenem-vaborbactam Anti-infective
Venclexta®	Venetoclax Antineoplastic
Vistogard®	Uridine Triacetate
Voraxaze®	Glucarpidase
VYXEOS™	Cytarabine and Daunorubicin Liposome Antineoplastic
XOSPATA®	Gilteritinib Antineoplastic
ZINPLAVA™	Bezlotoxumab Monoclonal Antibody
Zyvox®	Oxazolidinones

This page intentionally left blank

TDS When more than one PCS code is needed to code procedure

Appendix G: Combination Clusters

Due to the nature of a specific procedure, the first code in the cluster needs to be reported with one or more of the additional codes listed for all codes to be considered valid. The example below is for insertion of a cardiac defibrillator lead into the right ventricle (highlighted code). The additional procedure describes the exact location of where the lead is inserted, which is required for correct reporting:

02HK0KZ
and 0JH609Z

You would need to review the first procedure in the combination/cluster to determine whether you need to report the additional code.

The CMS site also provides additional information on combinations/clusters.

02H60KZ
and 0JH608Z

02H60KZ
and 0JH638Z

02H60KZ
and 0JH808Z

02H60KZ
and 0JH838Z

02H63KZ
and 0JH608Z

02H63KZ
and 0JH638Z

02H63KZ
and 0JH808Z

02H63KZ
and 0JH838Z

02H64KZ
and 0JH608Z

02H64KZ
and 0JH638Z

02H64KZ
and 0JH808Z

02H64KZ
and 0JH838Z

02H70KZ
and 0JH608Z

02H70KZ
and 0JH638Z

02H70KZ
and 0JH808Z

02H70KZ
and 0JH838Z

02H73KZ
and 0JH608Z

02H73KZ
and 0JH638Z

02H73KZ
and 0JH808Z

02H73KZ
and 0JH838Z

02H74KZ
and 0JH608Z

02H74KZ
and 0JH638Z

02H74KZ
and 0JH808Z

02H74KZ
and 0JH838Z

02HA0RS
and 02PA0RZ

02HA0RS
and 02PA3RZ

02HA0RS
and 02PA4RZ

02HA0RZ
and 02PA0RZ

02HA0RZ
and 02PA3RZ

02HA0RZ
and 02PA4RZ

02HA3RS
and 02PA0RZ

02HA3RS
and 02PA3RZ

02HA3RS
and 02PA4RZ

02HA4RS
and 02PA0RZ

02HA4RS
and 02PA3RZ

02HA4RS
and 02PA4RZ

02HA4RZ
and 02PA0RZ

02HA4RZ
and 02PA3RZ

02HA4RZ
and 02PA4RZ

02HK0KZ
and 0JH608Z

02HK0KZ
and 0JH609Z

02HK0KZ
and 0JH638Z

02HK0KZ
and 0JH639Z

02HK0KZ
and 0JH808Z

02HK0KZ
and 0JH809Z

02HK0KZ
and 0JH838Z

02HK0KZ
and 0JH839Z

02HK3KZ
and 0JH608Z

02HK3KZ
and 0JH609Z

02HK3KZ
and 0JH638Z

02HK3KZ
and 0JH639Z

02HK3KZ
and 0JH808Z

02HK3KZ
and 0JH809Z

02HK3KZ
and 0JH838Z

02HK3KZ
and 0JH839Z

02HK4KZ
and 0JH608Z

02HK4KZ
and 0JH609Z

02HK4KZ
and 0JH638Z

02HK4KZ
and 0JH639Z

02HK4KZ
and 0JH808Z

02HK4KZ
and 0JH809Z

02HK4KZ
and 0JH838Z

02HK4KZ
and 0JH839Z

02HL0KZ
and 0JH608Z

02HL0KZ
and 0JH609Z

02HL0KZ
and 0JH638Z

02HL0KZ
and 0JH639Z

02HL0KZ
and 0JH808Z

02HL0KZ
and 0JH809Z

02HL0KZ
and 0JH838Z

02HL0KZ
and 0JH839Z

02HL0MZ
and 0JH60AZ

02HL0MZ
and 0JH63AZ

02HL0MZ
and 0JH80AZ

02HL0MZ
and 0JH83AZ

02HL3KZ
and 0JH608Z

02HL3KZ
and 0JH609Z

02HL3KZ
and 0JH638Z

02HL3KZ
and 0JH639Z

02HL3KZ
and 0JH808Z

02HL3KZ
and 0JH809Z

02HL3KZ
and 0JH838Z

02HL3KZ
and 0JH839Z

02HL3MZ
and 0JH60AZ

02HL3MZ
and 0JH63AZ

02HL3MZ
and 0JH80AZ

02HL3MZ
and 0JH83AZ

02HL4KZ
and 0JH608Z

02HL4KZ
and 0JH609Z

02HL4KZ
and 0JH638Z

02HL4KZ
and 0JH639Z

02HL4KZ
and 0JH808Z

02HL4KZ
and 0JH809Z

02HL4KZ
and 0JH838Z

02HL4KZ
and 0JH839Z

02HL4MZ
and 0JH60AZ

02HL4MZ
and 0JH63AZ

02HL4MZ
and 0JH80AZ

02HL4MZ
and 0JH83AZ

02RK0JZ
and 02RL0JZ

02WA0QZ
and 02PA0RZ

02WA0QZ
and 02PA3RZ

02WA0QZ
and 02PA4RZ

02WA0RZ
and 02PA0RZ

02WA0RZ
and 02PA3RZ

02WA0RZ
and 02PA4RZ

02WA3QZ
and 02PA0RZ

02WA3QZ
and 02PA3RZ

02WA3QZ
and 02PA4RZ

02WA3RZ
and 02PA0RZ

02WA3RZ
and 02PA3RZ

02WA3RZ
and 02PA4RZ

02WA4QZ
and 02PA0RZ

02WA4QZ
and 02PA3RZ

02WA4QZ
and 02PA4RZ

02WA4RZ
and 02PA0RZ

02WA4RZ
and 02PA3RZ

02WA4RZ
and 02PA4RZ

07BH0ZZ
and 0UTM0ZZ

07BH0ZZ
and 0UTMXZZ

07BH4ZZ
and 0UTM0ZZ

07BH4ZZ
and 0UTMXZZ

07BJ0ZZ
and 0UTM0ZZ

07BJ0ZZ
and 0UTMXZZ

07BJ4ZZ
and 0UTM0ZZ

07BJ4ZZ
and 0UTMXZZ

07T50ZZ
and 07T60ZZ
and 07T70ZZ
and 07T80ZZ
and 07T90ZZ
and 0HTV0ZZ
and 0KTH0ZZ
and 0KTJ0ZZ

07T50ZZ
and 07T60ZZ
and 0HTV0ZZ

07T50ZZ
and 07T60ZZ
and 0HTV0ZZ
and 0KTH0ZZ
and 0KTJ0ZZ

07T50ZZ
and 07T70ZZ
and 07T80ZZ
and 0HTT0ZZ
and 0KTH0ZZ

07T50ZZ
and 0HTT0ZZ

07T50ZZ
and 0HTT0ZZ
and 0KTH0ZZ

07T60ZZ
and 07T70ZZ
and 07T90ZZ
and 0HTU0ZZ
and 0KTJ0ZZ

07T60ZZ
and 0HTU0ZZ

07T60ZZ
and 0HTU0ZZ
and 0KTJ0ZZ

0DQ80ZZ
and 0WQFXZ2

0DQ90ZZ
and 0WQFXZ2

0DQA0ZZ
and 0WQFXZ2

0DQB0ZZ
and 0WQFXZ2

0DQE0ZZ
and 0WQFXZ2

0DQF0ZZ
and 0WQFXZ2

0DQG0ZZ
and 0WQFXZ2

0DQH0ZZ
and 0WQFXZ2

0DQK0ZZ
and 0WQFXZ2

0DQL0ZZ
and 0WQFXZ2

0DQM0ZZ
and 0WQFXZ2

0DQN0ZZ
and 0WQFXZ2

0DT90ZZ
and 0FTG0ZZ

0HRT37Z
and 0JD63ZZ

0HRT37Z
and 0JD73ZZ

0HRT37Z
and 0JD83ZZ

0HRT37Z
and 0JD93ZZ

0HRT37Z
and 0JDL3ZZ

0HRT37Z
and 0JDM3ZZ

0HRU37Z
and 0JD63ZZ

0HRU37Z
and 0JD73ZZ

0HRU37Z
and 0JD83ZZ

0HRU37Z
and 0JD93ZZ

0HRU37Z
and 0JDL3ZZ

0HRU37Z
and 0JDM3ZZ

0HRV37Z
and 0JD63ZZ

0HRV37Z
and 0JD73ZZ

0HRV37Z
and 0JD83ZZ

0HRV37Z
and 0JD93ZZ

0HRV37Z
and 0JDL3ZZ

0HRV37Z
and 0JDM3ZZ

0JH604Z
and 02H40JZ

0JH604Z
and 02H40MZ

0JH604Z
and 02H43JZ

0JH604Z
and 02H43MZ

0JH604Z
and 02H44JZ

0JH604Z
and 02H44MZ

0JH604Z
and 02H60JZ

0JH604Z
and 02H60MZ

0JH604Z
and 02H63JZ

0JH604Z
and 02H63MZ

0JH604Z
and 02H64JZ

0JH604Z
and 02H64MZ

0JH604Z
and 02H70JZ

0JH604Z
and 02H70MZ

0JH604Z
and 02H73JZ

0JH604Z
and 02H73MZ

0JH604Z
and 02H74JZ

0JH604Z
and 02H74MZ

0JH604Z
and 02HK0JZ

0JH604Z
and 02HK0MZ

0JH604Z
and 02HK3JZ

0JH604Z
and 02HK3MZ

0JH604Z
and 02HK4JZ

0JH604Z
and 02HK4MZ

0JH604Z
and 02HL0JZ

0JH604Z
and 02HL0MZ

0JH604Z
and 02HL3JZ

0JH604Z
and 02HL3MZ

0JH604Z
and 02HL4JZ

0JH604Z
and 02HL4MZ

0JH604Z
and 02HN0JZ

0JH604Z
and 02HN0MZ

0JH604Z
and 02HN3JZ

0JH604Z
and 02HN3MZ

0JH604Z
and 02HN4JZ

0JH604Z
and 02HN4MZ

0JH605Z
and 02H40JZ

0JH605Z
and 02H40MZ

0JH605Z
and 02H43JZ

0JH605Z
and 02H43MZ

0JH605Z
and 02H44JZ

0JH605Z
and 02H44MZ

0JH605Z
and 02H60JZ

0JH605Z
and 02H60MZ

0JH605Z
and 02H63JZ

0JH605Z
and 02H63MZ

0JH605Z
and 02H64JZ

0JH605Z
and 02H64MZ

0JH605Z
and 02H70JZ

0JH605Z
and 02H70MZ

0JH605Z
and 02H73JZ

0JH605Z
and 02H73MZ

0JH605Z
and 02H74JZ

0JH605Z
and 02H74MZ

0JH605Z
and 02HK0JZ

0JH605Z
and 02HK0MZ

0JH605Z
and 02HK3JZ

0JH605Z
and 02HK3MZ

0JH605Z
and 02HK4JZ

0JH605Z
and 02HK4MZ

0JH605Z
and 02HL0JZ

0JH605Z
and 02HL0MZ

0JH605Z
and 02HL3JZ

0JH605Z
and 02HL3MZ

0JH605Z
and 02HL4JZ

0JH605Z
and 02HL4MZ

0JH605Z
and 02HN0JZ

0JH605Z
and 02HN0MZ

0JH605Z
and 02HN3JZ

0JH605Z
and 02HN3MZ

0JH605Z
and 02HN4JZ

0JH605Z
and 02HN4MZ

0JH606Z
and 02H40JZ

0JH606Z
and 02H40MZ

0JH606Z
and 02H43JZ

0JH606Z
and 02H43MZ

0JH606Z
and 02H44JZ

0JH606Z
and 02H44MZ

0JH606Z
and 02H60JZ

0JH606Z
and 02H60MZ

0JH606Z
and 02H63JZ

0JH606Z
and 02H63MZ

0JH606Z
and 02H64JZ

0JH606Z
and 02H64MZ

0JH606Z
and 02H70JZ

0JH606Z
and 02H70MZ

0JH606Z
and 02H73JZ

0JH606Z
and 02H73MZ

0JH606Z
and 02H74JZ

0JH606Z
and 02H74MZ

0JH606Z
and 02HK0JZ

0JH606Z
and 02HK0MZ

0JH606Z
and 02HK3JZ

0JH606Z
and 02HK3MZ

0JH606Z
and 02HK4JZ

0JH606Z
and 02HK4MZ

0JH606Z
and 02HL0JZ

0JH606Z
and 02HL0MZ

0JH606Z
and 02HL3JZ

0JH606Z
and 02HL3MZ

0JH606Z
and 02HL4JZ

0JH606Z and 02HL4MZ

0JH606Z and 02HN0JZ

0JH606Z and 02HN0MZ

0JH606Z and 02HN3JZ

0JH606Z and 02HN3MZ

0JH606Z and 02HN4JZ

0JH606Z and 02HN4MZ

0JH607Z and 02H40JZ

0JH607Z and 02H40MZ

0JH607Z and 02H43JZ

0JH607Z and 02H43MZ

0JH607Z and 02H44JZ

0JH607Z and 02H44MZ

0JH607Z and 02H60JZ

0JH607Z and 02H60MZ

0JH607Z and 02H63JZ

0JH607Z and 02H63MZ

0JH607Z and 02H64JZ

0JH607Z and 02H64MZ

0JH607Z and 02H70JZ

0JH607Z and 02H70MZ

0JH607Z and 02H73JZ

0JH607Z and 02H73MZ

0JH607Z and 02H74JZ

0JH607Z and 02H74MZ

0JH607Z and 02HK0JZ

0JH607Z and 02HK0MZ

0JH607Z and 02HK3JZ

0JH607Z and 02HK3MZ

0JH607Z and 02HK4JZ

0JH607Z and 02HK4MZ

0JH607Z and 02HL0JZ

0JH607Z and 02HL0MZ

0JH607Z and 02HL3JZ

0JH607Z and 02HL3MZ

0JH607Z and 02HL4JZ

0JH607Z and 02HL4MZ

0JH607Z and 02HN0JZ

0JH607Z and 02HN0MZ

0JH607Z and 02HN3JZ

0JH607Z and 02HN3MZ

0JH607Z and 02HN4JZ

0JH607Z and 02HN4MZ

0JH608Z and 02H40KZ

0JH608Z and 02H44KZ

0JH608Z and 02HN0JZ

0JH608Z and 02HN0KZ

0JH608Z and 02HN0MZ

0JH608Z and 02HN3JZ

0JH608Z and 02HN3KZ

0JH608Z and 02HN3MZ

0JH608Z and 02HN4JZ

0JH608Z and 02HN4KZ

0JH608Z and 02HN4MZ

0JH609Z and 02H40KZ

0JH609Z and 02H43JZ

0JH609Z and 02H43KZ

0JH609Z and 02H43MZ

0JH609Z and 02H44KZ

0JH609Z and 02H60KZ

0JH609Z and 02H63KZ

0JH609Z and 02H64KZ

0JH609Z and 02H70KZ

0JH609Z and 02H73KZ

0JH609Z and 02H74KZ

0JH609Z and 02HN0JZ

0JH609Z and 02HN0KZ

0JH609Z and 02HN0MZ

0JH609Z and 02HN3JZ

0JH609Z and 02HN3KZ

0JH609Z and 02HN3MZ

0JH609Z and 02HN4JZ

0JH609Z and 02HN4KZ

0JH609Z and 02HN4MZ

0JH60BZ and 00HE0MZ

0JH60BZ and 00HE3MZ

0JH60BZ and 00HE4MZ

0JH60BZ and 00HU0MZ

0JH60BZ and 00HU3MZ

0JH60BZ and 00HU4MZ

0JH60BZ and 00HV0MZ

0JH60BZ and 00HV3MZ

0JH60BZ and 00HV4MZ

0JH60BZ and 01HY0MZ

0JH60BZ and 01HY3MZ

0JH60BZ and 01HY4MZ

0JH60BZ and 05H00MZ

0JH60BZ and 05H03MZ

0JH60BZ and 05H04MZ

0JH60BZ and 05H30MZ

0JH60BZ and 05H33MZ

0JH60BZ and 05H34MZ

0JH60BZ and 05H40MZ

0JH60BZ and 05H43MZ

0JH60BZ and 05H44MZ

0JH60BZ and 0DH60MZ

0JH60BZ and 0DH63MZ

0JH60BZ and 0DH64MZ

0JH60CZ and 00HE0MZ

0JH60CZ and 00HE3MZ

0JH60CZ and 00HE4MZ

0JH60CZ and 00HU0MZ

0JH60CZ and 00HU3MZ

0JH60CZ and 00HU4MZ

0JH60CZ and 00HV0MZ

0JH60CZ and 00HV3MZ

0JH60CZ and 00HV4MZ

0JH60CZ and 01HY0MZ

0JH60CZ and 01HY3MZ

0JH60CZ and 01HY4MZ

0JH60CZ and 05H00MZ

0JH60CZ and 05H03MZ

0JH60CZ and 05H04MZ

0JH60CZ and 05H30MZ

0JH60CZ and 05H33MZ

0JH60CZ and 05H34MZ

0JH60CZ and 05H40MZ

0JH60CZ and 05H43MZ

0JH60CZ and 05H44MZ

0JH60CZ and 0DH60MZ

0JH60CZ and 0DH63MZ

0JH60CZ and 0DH64MZ

0JH60DZ and 00H00MZ

0JH60DZ and 00H03MZ

0JH60DZ and 00H04MZ

0JH60DZ and 00H60MZ

0JH60DZ and 00H63MZ

0JH60DZ and 00H64MZ

0JH60DZ and 00HE0MZ

0JH60DZ and 00HE3MZ

0JH60DZ and 00HE4MZ

0JH60DZ and 00HU0MZ

0JH60DZ and 00HU3MZ

0JH60DZ and 00HU4MZ

0JH60DZ and 00HV0MZ

0JH60DZ and 00HV3MZ

0JH60DZ and 00HV4MZ

0JH60DZ and 01HY0MZ

0JH60DZ and 01HY3MZ

0JH60DZ and 01HY4MZ

0JH60DZ and 05H00MZ

0JH60DZ and 05H03MZ

0JH60DZ and 05H04MZ

0JH60DZ and 05H30MZ

0JH60DZ and 05H33MZ

0JH60DZ and 05H34MZ

0JH60DZ and 05H40MZ

0JH60DZ and 05H43MZ

0JH60DZ and 05H44MZ

0JH60DZ and 0DH60MZ

0JH60DZ and 0DH63MZ

0JH60DZ and 0DH64MZ

0JH60EZ and 00H00MZ

0JH60EZ and 00H03MZ

0JH60EZ and 00H04MZ
0JH60EZ and 00H60MZ
0JH60EZ and 00H63MZ
0JH60EZ and 00H64MZ
0JH60EZ and 00HE0MZ
0JH60EZ and 00HE3MZ
0JH60EZ and 00HE4MZ
0JH60EZ and 00HU0MZ
0JH60EZ and 00HU3MZ
0JH60EZ and 00HU4MZ
0JH60EZ and 00HV0MZ
0JH60EZ and 00HV3MZ
0JH60EZ and 00HV4MZ
0JH60EZ and 01HY0MZ
0JH60EZ and 01HY3MZ
0JH60EZ and 01HY4MZ
0JH60EZ and 05H00MZ
0JH60EZ and 05H03MZ
0JH60EZ and 05H04MZ
0JH60EZ and 05H30MZ
0JH60EZ and 05H33MZ
0JH60EZ and 05H34MZ
0JH60EZ and 05H40MZ
0JH60EZ and 05H43MZ
0JH60EZ and 05H44MZ
0JH60EZ and 0DH60MZ
0JH60EZ and 0DH63MZ
0JH60EZ and 0DH64MZ
0JH60PZ and 02H40JZ
0JH60PZ and 02H40MZ
0JH60PZ and 02H43JZ
0JH60PZ and 02H43MZ
0JH60PZ and 02H44JZ
0JH60PZ and 02H44MZ
0JH60PZ and 02H60JZ
0JH60PZ and 02H60MZ
0JH60PZ and 02H63JZ
0JH60PZ and 02H63MZ
0JH60PZ and 02H64JZ
0JH60PZ and 02H64MZ
0JH60PZ and 02H70JZ
0JH60PZ and 02H70MZ
0JH60PZ and 02H73JZ
0JH60PZ and 02H73MZ
0JH60PZ and 02H74JZ
0JH60PZ and 02H74MZ
0JH60PZ and 02HK0JZ
0JH60PZ and 02HK0MZ
0JH60PZ and 02HK3JZ
0JH60PZ and 02HK3MZ
0JH60PZ and 02HK4JZ
0JH60PZ and 02HK4MZ
0JH60PZ and 02HL0JZ
0JH60PZ and 02HL0MZ
0JH60PZ and 02HL3JZ
0JH60PZ and 02HL3MZ
0JH60PZ and 02HL4JZ
0JH60PZ and 02HL4MZ
0JH60PZ and 02HN0JZ
0JH60PZ and 02HN0MZ
0JH60PZ and 02HN3JZ
0JH60PZ and 02HN3MZ
0JH60PZ and 02HN4JZ
0JH60PZ and 02HN4MZ
0JH634Z and 02H40JZ
0JH634Z and 02H40MZ
0JH634Z and 02H43JZ
0JH634Z and 02H43MZ
0JH634Z and 02H44JZ
0JH634Z and 02H44MZ
0JH634Z and 02H60JZ
0JH634Z and 02H60MZ
0JH634Z and 02H63JZ
0JH634Z and 02H63MZ
0JH634Z and 02H64JZ
0JH634Z and 02H64MZ
0JH634Z and 02H70JZ
0JH634Z and 02H70MZ
0JH634Z and 02H73JZ
0JH634Z and 02H73MZ
0JH634Z and 02H74JZ
0JH634Z and 02H74MZ
0JH634Z and 02HK0JZ
0JH634Z and 02HK0MZ
0JH634Z and 02HK3JZ
0JH634Z and 02HK3MZ
0JH634Z and 02HK4JZ
0JH634Z and 02HK4MZ
0JH634Z and 02HL0JZ
0JH634Z and 02HL0MZ
0JH634Z and 02HL3JZ
0JH634Z and 02HL3MZ
0JH634Z and 02HL4JZ
0JH634Z and 02HL4MZ
0JH634Z and 02HN0JZ
0JH634Z and 02HN0MZ
0JH634Z and 02HN3JZ
0JH634Z and 02HN3MZ
0JH634Z and 02HN4JZ
0JH634Z and 02HN4MZ
0JH635Z and 02H40JZ
0JH635Z and 02H40MZ
0JH635Z and 02H43JZ
0JH635Z and 02H43MZ
0JH635Z and 02H44JZ
0JH635Z and 02H44MZ
0JH635Z and 02H60JZ
0JH635Z and 02H60MZ
0JH635Z and 02H63JZ
0JH635Z and 02H63MZ
0JH635Z and 02H64JZ
0JH635Z and 02H64MZ
0JH635Z and 02H70JZ
0JH635Z and 02H70MZ
0JH635Z and 02H73JZ
0JH635Z and 02H73MZ
0JH635Z and 02H74JZ
0JH635Z and 02H74MZ
0JH635Z and 02HK0JZ
0JH635Z and 02HK0MZ
0JH635Z and 02HK3JZ
0JH635Z and 02HK3MZ
0JH635Z and 02HK4JZ
0JH635Z and 02HK4MZ
0JH635Z and 02HL0JZ
0JH635Z and 02HL0MZ
0JH635Z and 02HL3JZ
0JH635Z and 02HL3MZ
0JH635Z and 02HL4JZ
0JH635Z and 02HL4MZ
0JH635Z and 02HN0JZ
0JH635Z and 02HN0MZ
0JH635Z and 02HN3JZ
0JH635Z and 02HN3MZ
0JH635Z and 02HN4JZ
0JH635Z and 02HN4MZ
0JH636Z and 02H40JZ
0JH636Z and 02H40MZ
0JH636Z and 02H43JZ
0JH636Z and 02H43MZ
0JH636Z and 02H44JZ
0JH636Z and 02H44MZ
0JH636Z and 02H60JZ
0JH636Z and 02H60MZ
0JH636Z and 02H63JZ
0JH636Z and 02H63MZ
0JH636Z and 02H64JZ
0JH636Z and 02H64MZ
0JH636Z and 02H70JZ
0JH636Z and 02H70MZ
0JH636Z and 02H73JZ
0JH636Z and 02H73MZ
0JH636Z and 02H74JZ
0JH636Z and 02H74MZ

0JH636Z and 02HK0JZ
0JH636Z and 02HK0MZ
0JH636Z and 02HK3JZ
0JH636Z and 02HK3MZ
0JH636Z and 02HK4JZ
0JH636Z and 02HK4MZ
0JH636Z and 02HL0JZ
0JH636Z and 02HL0MZ
0JH636Z and 02HL3JZ
0JH636Z and 02HL3MZ
0JH636Z and 02HL4JZ
0JH636Z and 02HL4MZ
0JH636Z and 02HN0JZ
0JH636Z and 02HN0MZ
0JH636Z and 02HN3JZ
0JH636Z and 02HN3MZ
0JH636Z and 02HN4JZ
0JH636Z and 02HN4MZ
0JH637Z and 02H40JZ
0JH637Z and 02H40MZ
0JH637Z and 02H43JZ
0JH637Z and 02H43MZ
0JH637Z and 02H44JZ
0JH637Z and 02H44MZ
0JH637Z and 02H60JZ
0JH637Z and 02H60MZ
0JH637Z and 02H63JZ
0JH637Z and 02H63MZ
0JH637Z and 02H64JZ
0JH637Z and 02H64MZ
0JH637Z and 02H70JZ
0JH637Z and 02H70MZ
0JH637Z and 02H73JZ
0JH637Z and 02H73MZ
0JH637Z and 02H74JZ
0JH637Z and 02H74MZ
0JH637Z and 02HK0JZ
0JH637Z and 02HK0MZ
0JH637Z and 02HK3JZ
0JH637Z and 02HK3MZ
0JH637Z and 02HK4JZ
0JH637Z and 02HK4MZ
0JH637Z and 02HL0JZ
0JH637Z and 02HL0MZ
0JH637Z and 02HL3JZ
0JH637Z and 02HL3MZ
0JH637Z and 02HL4JZ
0JH637Z and 02HL4MZ
0JH637Z and 02HN0JZ
0JH637Z and 02HN0MZ
0JH637Z and 02HN3JZ
0JH637Z and 02HN3MZ
0JH637Z and 02HN4JZ
0JH637Z and 02HN4MZ
0JH638Z and 02H40KZ
0JH638Z and 02H44KZ
0JH638Z and 02HN0JZ
0JH638Z and 02HN0KZ
0JH638Z and 02HN0MZ
0JH638Z and 02HN3JZ
0JH638Z and 02HN3KZ
0JH638Z and 02HN3MZ
0JH638Z and 02HN4JZ
0JH638Z and 02HN4KZ
0JH638Z and 02HN4MZ
0JH639Z and 02H40KZ
0JH639Z and 02H43JZ
0JH639Z and 02H43KZ
0JH639Z and 02H43MZ
0JH639Z and 02H44KZ
0JH639Z and 02H60KZ
0JH639Z and 02H63KZ
0JH639Z and 02H64KZ
0JH639Z and 02H70KZ
0JH639Z and 02H73KZ
0JH639Z and 02H74KZ
0JH639Z and 02HN0JZ
0JH639Z and 02HN0KZ
0JH639Z and 02HN0MZ
0JH639Z and 02HN3JZ
0JH639Z and 02HN3KZ
0JH639Z and 02HN3MZ
0JH639Z and 02HN4JZ
0JH639Z and 02HN4KZ
0JH639Z and 02HN4MZ
0JH63BZ and 00HE0MZ
0JH63BZ and 00HE3MZ
0JH63BZ and 00HE4MZ
0JH63BZ and 00HU0MZ
0JH63BZ and 00HU3MZ
0JH63BZ and 00HU4MZ
0JH63BZ and 00HV0MZ
0JH63BZ and 00HV3MZ
0JH63BZ and 00HV4MZ
0JH63BZ and 01HY0MZ
0JH63BZ and 01HY3MZ
0JH63BZ and 01HY4MZ
0JH63BZ and 05H00MZ
0JH63BZ and 05H03MZ
0JH63BZ and 05H04MZ
0JH63BZ and 05H30MZ
0JH63BZ and 05H33MZ
0JH63BZ and 05H34MZ
0JH63BZ and 05H40MZ
0JH63BZ and 05H43MZ
0JH63BZ and 05H44MZ
0JH63BZ and 0DH60MZ
0JH63BZ and 0DH63MZ
0JH63BZ and 0DH64MZ
0JH63CZ and 00HE0MZ
0JH63CZ and 00HE3MZ
0JH63CZ and 00HE4MZ
0JH63CZ and 00HU0MZ
0JH63CZ and 00HU3MZ
0JH63CZ and 00HU4MZ
0JH63CZ and 00HV0MZ
0JH63CZ and 00HV3MZ
0JH63CZ and 00HV4MZ
0JH63CZ and 01HY0MZ
0JH63CZ and 01HY3MZ
0JH63CZ and 01HY4MZ
0JH63CZ and 05H00MZ
0JH63CZ and 05H03MZ
0JH63CZ and 05H04MZ
0JH63CZ and 05H30MZ
0JH63CZ and 05H33MZ
0JH63CZ and 05H34MZ
0JH63CZ and 05H40MZ
0JH63CZ and 05H43MZ
0JH63CZ and 05H44MZ
0JH63CZ and 0DH60MZ
0JH63CZ and 0DH63MZ
0JH63CZ and 0DH64MZ
0JH63DZ and 00H00MZ
0JH63DZ and 00H03MZ
0JH63DZ and 00H04MZ
0JH63DZ and 00H60MZ
0JH63DZ and 00H63MZ
0JH63DZ and 00H64MZ
0JH63DZ and 00HE0MZ
0JH63DZ and 00HE3MZ
0JH63DZ and 00HE4MZ
0JH63DZ and 00HU0MZ
0JH63DZ and 00HU3MZ
0JH63DZ and 00HU4MZ
0JH63DZ and 00HV0MZ
0JH63DZ and 00HV3MZ
0JH63DZ and 00HV4MZ
0JH63DZ and 01HY0MZ
0JH63DZ and 01HY3MZ
0JH63DZ and 01HY4MZ
0JH63DZ and 05H00MZ
0JH63DZ and 05H03MZ
0JH63DZ and 05H04MZ

0JH63DZ and 05H30MZ

0JH63DZ and 05H33MZ

0JH63DZ and 05H34MZ

0JH63DZ and 05H40MZ

0JH63DZ and 05H43MZ

0JH63DZ and 05H44MZ

0JH63DZ and 0DH60MZ

0JH63DZ and 0DH63MZ

0JH63DZ and 0DH64MZ

0JH63EZ and 00H00MZ

0JH63EZ and 00H03MZ

0JH63EZ and 00H04MZ

0JH63EZ and 00H60MZ

0JH63EZ and 00H63MZ

0JH63EZ and 00H64MZ

0JH63EZ and 00HE0MZ

0JH63EZ and 00HE3MZ

0JH63EZ and 00HE4MZ

0JH63EZ and 00HU0MZ

0JH63EZ and 00HU3MZ

0JH63EZ and 00HU4MZ

0JH63EZ and 00HV0MZ

0JH63EZ and 00HV3MZ

0JH63EZ and 00HV4MZ

0JH63EZ and 01HY0MZ

0JH63EZ and 01HY3MZ

0JH63EZ and 01HY4MZ

0JH63EZ and 05H00MZ

0JH63EZ and 05H03MZ

0JH63EZ and 05H04MZ

0JH63EZ and 05H30MZ

0JH63EZ and 05H33MZ

0JH63EZ and 05H34MZ

0JH63EZ and 05H40MZ

0JH63EZ and 05H43MZ

0JH63EZ and 05H44MZ

0JH63EZ and 0DH60MZ

0JH63EZ and 0DH63MZ

0JH63EZ and 0DH64MZ

0JH63PZ and 02H40JZ

0JH63PZ and 02H40MZ

0JH63PZ and 02H43JZ

0JH63PZ and 02H43MZ

0JH63PZ and 02H44JZ

0JH63PZ and 02H44MZ

0JH63PZ and 02H60JZ

0JH63PZ and 02H60MZ

0JH63PZ and 02H63JZ

0JH63PZ and 02H63MZ

0JH63PZ and 02H64JZ

0JH63PZ and 02H64MZ

0JH63PZ and 02H70JZ

0JH63PZ and 02H70MZ

0JH63PZ and 02H73JZ

0JH63PZ and 02H73MZ

0JH63PZ and 02H74JZ

0JH63PZ and 02H74MZ

0JH63PZ and 02HK0JZ

0JH63PZ and 02HK0MZ

0JH63PZ and 02HK3JZ

0JH63PZ and 02HK3MZ

0JH63PZ and 02HK4JZ

0JH63PZ and 02HK4MZ

0JH63PZ and 02HL0JZ

0JH63PZ and 02HL0MZ

0JH63PZ and 02HL3JZ

0JH63PZ and 02HL3MZ

0JH63PZ and 02HL4JZ

0JH63PZ and 02HL4MZ

0JH63PZ and 02HN0JZ

0JH63PZ and 02HN0MZ

0JH63PZ and 02HN3JZ

0JH63PZ and 02HN3MZ

0JH63PZ and 02HN4JZ

0JH63PZ and 02HN4MZ

0JH70BZ and 00HE0MZ

0JH70BZ and 00HE3MZ

0JH70BZ and 00HE4MZ

0JH70BZ and 00HU0MZ

0JH70BZ and 00HU3MZ

0JH70BZ and 00HU4MZ

0JH70BZ and 00HV0MZ

0JH70BZ and 00HV3MZ

0JH70BZ and 00HV4MZ

0JH70BZ and 01HY0MZ

0JH70BZ and 01HY3MZ

0JH70BZ and 01HY4MZ

0JH70BZ and 05H00MZ

0JH70BZ and 05H03MZ

0JH70BZ and 05H04MZ

0JH70BZ and 05H30MZ

0JH70BZ and 05H33MZ

0JH70BZ and 05H34MZ

0JH70BZ and 05H40MZ

0JH70BZ and 05H43MZ

0JH70BZ and 05H44MZ

0JH70BZ and 0DH60MZ

0JH70BZ and 0DH63MZ

0JH70BZ and 0DH64MZ

0JH70CZ and 00HE0MZ

0JH70CZ and 00HE3MZ

0JH70CZ and 00HE4MZ

0JH70CZ and 00HU0MZ

0JH70CZ and 00HU3MZ

0JH70CZ and 00HU4MZ

0JH70CZ and 00HV0MZ

0JH70CZ and 00HV3MZ

0JH70CZ and 00HV4MZ

0JH70CZ and 01HY0MZ

0JH70CZ and 01HY3MZ

0JH70CZ and 01HY4MZ

0JH70CZ and 05H00MZ

0JH70CZ and 05H03MZ

0JH70CZ and 05H04MZ

0JH70CZ and 05H30MZ

0JH70CZ and 05H33MZ

0JH70CZ and 05H34MZ

0JH70CZ and 05H40MZ

0JH70CZ and 05H43MZ

0JH70CZ and 05H44MZ

0JH70CZ and 0DH60MZ

0JH70CZ and 0DH63MZ

0JH70CZ and 0DH64MZ

0JH70DZ and 00H00MZ

0JH70DZ and 00H03MZ

0JH70DZ and 00H04MZ

0JH70DZ and 00H60MZ

0JH70DZ and 00H63MZ

0JH70DZ and 00H64MZ

0JH70DZ and 00HE0MZ

0JH70DZ and 00HE3MZ

0JH70DZ and 00HE4MZ

0JH70DZ and 00HU0MZ

0JH70DZ and 00HU3MZ

0JH70DZ and 00HU4MZ

0JH70DZ and 00HV0MZ

0JH70DZ and 00HV3MZ

0JH70DZ and 00HV4MZ

0JH70DZ and 01HY0MZ

0JH70DZ and 01HY3MZ

0JH70DZ and 01HY4MZ

0JH70DZ and 05H00MZ

0JH70DZ and 05H03MZ

0JH70DZ and 05H04MZ

0JH70DZ and 05H30MZ

0JH70DZ and 05H33MZ

0JH70DZ and 05H34MZ

0JH70DZ and 05H40MZ

0JH70DZ and 05H43MZ

0JH70DZ and 05H44MZ

0JH70DZ and 0DH60MZ

0JH70DZ and 0DH63MZ

0JH70DZ and 0DH64MZ

0JH70EZ and 00H00MZ

0JH70EZ and 00H03MZ
0JH70EZ and 00H04MZ
0JH70EZ and 00H60MZ
0JH70EZ and 00H63MZ
0JH70EZ and 00H64MZ
0JH70EZ and 00HE0MZ
0JH70EZ and 00HE3MZ
0JH70EZ and 00HE4MZ
0JH70EZ and 00HU0MZ
0JH70EZ and 00HU3MZ
0JH70EZ and 00HU4MZ
0JH70EZ and 00HV0MZ
0JH70EZ and 00HV3MZ
0JH70EZ and 00HV4MZ
0JH70EZ and 01HY0MZ
0JH70EZ and 01HY3MZ
0JH70EZ and 01HY4MZ
0JH70EZ and 05H00MZ
0JH70EZ and 05H03MZ
0JH70EZ and 05H04MZ
0JH70EZ and 05H30MZ
0JH70EZ and 05H33MZ
0JH70EZ and 05H34MZ
0JH70EZ and 05H40MZ
0JH70EZ and 05H43MZ
0JH70EZ and 05H44MZ
0JH70EZ and 0DH60MZ
0JH70EZ and 0DH63MZ
0JH70EZ and 0DH64MZ
0JH73BZ and 00HE0MZ
0JH73BZ and 00HE3MZ
0JH73BZ and 00HE4MZ
0JH73BZ and 00HU0MZ
0JH73BZ and 00HU3MZ
0JH73BZ and 00HU4MZ
0JH73BZ and 00HV0MZ
0JH73BZ and 00HV3MZ
0JH73BZ and 00HV4MZ
0JH73BZ and 01HY0MZ
0JH73BZ and 01HY3MZ
0JH73BZ and 01HY4MZ
0JH73BZ and 05H00MZ
0JH73BZ and 05H03MZ
0JH73BZ and 05H04MZ
0JH73BZ and 05H30MZ
0JH73BZ and 05H33MZ
0JH73BZ and 05H34MZ
0JH73BZ and 05H40MZ
0JH73BZ and 05H43MZ
0JH73BZ and 05H44MZ
0JH73BZ and 0DH60MZ
0JH73BZ and 0DH63MZ
0JH73BZ and 0DH64MZ
0JH73CZ and 00HE0MZ
0JH73CZ and 00HE3MZ
0JH73CZ and 00HE4MZ
0JH73CZ and 00HU0MZ
0JH73CZ and 00HU3MZ
0JH73CZ and 00HU4MZ
0JH73CZ and 00HV0MZ
0JH73CZ and 00HV3MZ
0JH73CZ and 00HV4MZ
0JH73CZ and 01HY0MZ
0JH73CZ and 01HY3MZ
0JH73CZ and 01HY4MZ
0JH73CZ and 05H00MZ
0JH73CZ and 05H03MZ
0JH73CZ and 05H04MZ
0JH73CZ and 05H30MZ
0JH73CZ and 05H33MZ
0JH73CZ and 05H34MZ
0JH73CZ and 05H40MZ
0JH73CZ and 05H43MZ
0JH73CZ and 05H44MZ
0JH73CZ and 0DH60MZ
0JH73CZ and 0DH63MZ
0JH73CZ and 0DH64MZ
0JH73DZ and 00H00MZ
0JH73DZ and 00H03MZ
0JH73DZ and 00H04MZ
0JH73DZ and 00H60MZ
0JH73DZ and 00H63MZ
0JH73DZ and 00H64MZ
0JH73DZ and 00HE0MZ
0JH73DZ and 00HE3MZ
0JH73DZ and 00HE4MZ
0JH73DZ and 00HU0MZ
0JH73DZ and 00HU3MZ
0JH73DZ and 00HU4MZ
0JH73DZ and 00HV0MZ
0JH73DZ and 00HV3MZ
0JH73DZ and 00HV4MZ
0JH73DZ and 01HY0MZ
0JH73DZ and 01HY3MZ
0JH73DZ and 01HY4MZ
0JH73DZ and 05H00MZ
0JH73DZ and 05H03MZ
0JH73DZ and 05H04MZ
0JH73DZ and 05H30MZ
0JH73DZ and 05H33MZ
0JH73DZ and 05H34MZ
0JH73DZ and 05H40MZ
0JH73DZ and 05H43MZ
0JH73DZ and 05H44MZ
0JH73DZ and 0DH60MZ
0JH73DZ and 0DH63MZ
0JH73DZ and 0DH64MZ
0JH73EZ and 00H00MZ
0JH73EZ and 00H03MZ
0JH73EZ and 00H04MZ
0JH73EZ and 00H60MZ
0JH73EZ and 00H63MZ
0JH73EZ and 00H64MZ
0JH73EZ and 00HE0MZ
0JH73EZ and 00HE3MZ
0JH73EZ and 00HE4MZ
0JH73EZ and 00HU0MZ
0JH73EZ and 00HU3MZ
0JH73EZ and 00HU4MZ
0JH73EZ and 00HV0MZ
0JH73EZ and 00HV3MZ
0JH73EZ and 00HV4MZ
0JH73EZ and 01HY0MZ
0JH73EZ and 01HY3MZ
0JH73EZ and 01HY4MZ
0JH73EZ and 05H00MZ
0JH73EZ and 05H03MZ
0JH73EZ and 05H04MZ
0JH73EZ and 05H30MZ
0JH73EZ and 05H33MZ
0JH73EZ and 05H34MZ
0JH73EZ and 05H40MZ
0JH73EZ and 05H43MZ
0JH73EZ and 05H44MZ
0JH73EZ and 0DH60MZ
0JH73EZ and 0DH63MZ
0JH73EZ and 0DH64MZ
0JH804Z and 02H40JZ
0JH804Z and 02H40MZ
0JH804Z and 02H43JZ
0JH804Z and 02H43MZ
0JH804Z and 02H44JZ
0JH804Z and 02H44MZ
0JH804Z and 02H60JZ
0JH804Z and 02H60MZ
0JH804Z and 02H63JZ
0JH804Z and 02H63MZ
0JH804Z and 02H64JZ
0JH804Z and 02H64MZ
0JH804Z and 02H70JZ
0JH804Z and 02H70MZ
0JH804Z and 02H73JZ
0JH804Z and 02H73MZ
0JH804Z and 02H74JZ

0JH804Z and 02H74MZ
0JH804Z and 02HK0JZ
0JH804Z and 02HK0MZ
0JH804Z and 02HK3JZ
0JH804Z and 02HK3MZ
0JH804Z and 02HK4JZ
0JH804Z and 02HK4MZ
0JH804Z and 02HL0JZ
0JH804Z and 02HL0MZ
0JH804Z and 02HL3JZ
0JH804Z and 02HL3MZ
0JH804Z and 02HL4JZ
0JH804Z and 02HL4MZ
0JH804Z and 02HN0JZ
0JH804Z and 02HN0MZ
0JH804Z and 02HN3JZ
0JH804Z and 02HN3MZ
0JH804Z and 02HN4JZ
0JH804Z and 02HN4MZ
0JH805Z and 02H40JZ
0JH805Z and 02H40MZ
0JH805Z and 02H43JZ
0JH805Z and 02H43MZ
0JH805Z and 02H44JZ
0JH805Z and 02H44MZ
0JH805Z and 02H60JZ
0JH805Z and 02H60MZ
0JH805Z and 02H63JZ
0JH805Z and 02H63MZ
0JH805Z and 02H64JZ
0JH805Z and 02H64MZ
0JH805Z and 02H70JZ
0JH805Z and 02H70MZ
0JH805Z and 02H73JZ
0JH805Z and 02H73MZ
0JH805Z and 02H74JZ
0JH805Z and 02H74MZ
0JH805Z and 02HK0JZ
0JH805Z and 02HK0MZ
0JH805Z and 02HK3JZ
0JH805Z and 02HK3MZ
0JH805Z and 02HK4JZ
0JH805Z and 02HK4MZ
0JH805Z and 02HL0JZ
0JH805Z and 02HL0MZ
0JH805Z and 02HL3JZ
0JH805Z and 02HL3MZ
0JH805Z and 02HL4JZ
0JH805Z and 02HL4MZ
0JH805Z and 02HN0JZ
0JH805Z and 02HN0MZ
0JH805Z and 02HN3JZ
0JH805Z and 02HN3MZ
0JH805Z and 02HN4JZ
0JH805Z and 02HN4MZ
0JH806Z and 02H40JZ
0JH806Z and 02H40MZ
0JH806Z and 02H43JZ
0JH806Z and 02H43MZ
0JH806Z and 02H44JZ
0JH806Z and 02H44MZ
0JH806Z and 02H60JZ
0JH806Z and 02H60MZ
0JH806Z and 02H63JZ
0JH806Z and 02H63MZ
0JH806Z and 02H64JZ
0JH806Z and 02H64MZ
0JH806Z and 02H70JZ
0JH806Z and 02H70MZ
0JH806Z and 02H73JZ
0JH806Z and 02H73MZ
0JH806Z and 02H74JZ
0JH806Z and 02H74MZ
0JH806Z and 02HK0JZ
0JH806Z and 02HK0MZ
0JH806Z and 02HK3JZ
0JH806Z and 02HK3MZ
0JH806Z and 02HK4JZ
0JH806Z and 02HK4MZ
0JH806Z and 02HL0JZ
0JH806Z and 02HL0MZ
0JH806Z and 02HL3JZ
0JH806Z and 02HL3MZ
0JH806Z and 02HL4JZ
0JH806Z and 02HL4MZ
0JH806Z and 02HN0JZ
0JH806Z and 02HN0MZ
0JH806Z and 02HN3JZ
0JH806Z and 02HN3MZ
0JH806Z and 02HN4JZ
0JH806Z and 02HN4MZ
0JH807Z and 02H40JZ
0JH807Z and 02H40MZ
0JH807Z and 02H43JZ
0JH807Z and 02H43MZ
0JH807Z and 02H44JZ
0JH807Z and 02H44MZ
0JH807Z and 02H60JZ
0JH807Z and 02H60MZ
0JH807Z and 02H63JZ
0JH807Z and 02H63MZ
0JH807Z and 02H64JZ
0JH807Z and 02H64MZ
0JH807Z and 02H70JZ
0JH807Z and 02H70MZ
0JH807Z and 02H73JZ
0JH807Z and 02H73MZ
0JH807Z and 02H74JZ
0JH807Z and 02H74MZ
0JH807Z and 02HK0JZ
0JH807Z and 02HK0MZ
0JH807Z and 02HK3JZ
0JH807Z and 02HK3MZ
0JH807Z and 02HK4JZ
0JH807Z and 02HK4MZ
0JH807Z and 02HL0JZ
0JH807Z and 02HL0MZ
0JH807Z and 02HL3JZ
0JH807Z and 02HL3MZ
0JH807Z and 02HL4JZ
0JH807Z and 02HL4MZ
0JH807Z and 02HN0JZ
0JH807Z and 02HN0MZ
0JH807Z and 02HN3JZ
0JH807Z and 02HN3MZ
0JH807Z and 02HN4JZ
0JH807Z and 02HN4MZ
0JH808Z and 02H40KZ
0JH808Z and 02H44KZ
0JH808Z and 02HN0JZ
0JH808Z and 02HN0KZ
0JH808Z and 02HN0MZ
0JH808Z and 02HN3JZ
0JH808Z and 02HN3KZ
0JH808Z and 02HN3MZ
0JH808Z and 02HN4JZ
0JH808Z and 02HN4KZ
0JH808Z and 02HN4MZ
0JH809Z and 02H40KZ
0JH809Z and 02H43JZ
0JH809Z and 02H43KZ
0JH809Z and 02H43MZ
0JH809Z and 02H44KZ
0JH809Z and 02H60KZ
0JH809Z and 02H63KZ
0JH809Z and 02H64KZ
0JH809Z and 02H70KZ
0JH809Z and 02H73KZ
0JH809Z and 02H74KZ
0JH809Z and 02HN0JZ
0JH809Z and 02HN0KZ
0JH809Z and 02HN0MZ
0JH809Z and 02HN3JZ
0JH809Z and 02HN3KZ

0JH809Z and 02HN3MZ
0JH809Z and 02HN4JZ
0JH809Z and 02HN4KZ
0JH809Z and 02HN4MZ
0JH80BZ and 00HE0MZ
0JH80BZ and 00HE3MZ
0JH80BZ and 00HE4MZ
0JH80BZ and 00HU0MZ
0JH80BZ and 00HU3MZ
0JH80BZ and 00HU4MZ
0JH80BZ and 00HV0MZ
0JH80BZ and 00HV3MZ
0JH80BZ and 00HV4MZ
0JH80BZ and 01HY0MZ
0JH80BZ and 01HY3MZ
0JH80BZ and 01HY4MZ
0JH80BZ and 05H00MZ
0JH80BZ and 05H03MZ
0JH80BZ and 05H04MZ
0JH80BZ and 05H30MZ
0JH80BZ and 05H33MZ
0JH80BZ and 05H34MZ

0JH80BZ and 05H40MZ
0JH80BZ and 05H43MZ
0JH80BZ and 05H44MZ
0JH80BZ and 0DH60MZ
0JH80BZ and 0DH63MZ
0JH80BZ and 0DH64MZ
0JH80CZ and 00HE0MZ
0JH80CZ and 00HE3MZ
0JH80CZ and 00HE4MZ
0JH80CZ and 00HU0MZ
0JH80CZ and 00HU3MZ
0JH80CZ and 00HU4MZ
0JH80CZ and 00HV0MZ
0JH80CZ and 00HV3MZ
0JH80CZ and 00HV4MZ
0JH80CZ and 01HY0MZ
0JH80CZ and 01HY3MZ
0JH80CZ and 01HY4MZ
0JH80CZ and 05H00MZ
0JH80CZ and 05H03MZ
0JH80CZ and 05H04MZ
0JH80CZ and 05H30MZ

0JH80CZ and 05H33MZ
0JH80CZ and 05H34MZ
0JH80CZ and 05H40MZ
0JH80CZ and 05H43MZ
0JH80CZ and 05H44MZ
0JH80CZ and 0DH60MZ
0JH80CZ and 0DH63MZ
0JH80CZ and 0DH64MZ
0JH80DZ and 00H00MZ
0JH80DZ and 00H03MZ
0JH80DZ and 00H04MZ
0JH80DZ and 00H60MZ
0JH80DZ and 00H63MZ
0JH80DZ and 00H64MZ
0JH80DZ and 00HE0MZ
0JH80DZ and 00HE3MZ
0JH80DZ and 00HE4MZ
0JH80DZ and 00HU0MZ
0JH80DZ and 00HU3MZ
0JH80DZ and 00HU4MZ
0JH80DZ and 00HV0MZ
0JH80DZ and 00HV3MZ

0JH80DZ and 00HV4MZ
0JH80DZ and 01HY0MZ
0JH80DZ and 01HY3MZ
0JH80DZ and 01HY4MZ
0JH80DZ and 05H00MZ
0JH80DZ and 05H03MZ
0JH80DZ and 05H04MZ
0JH80DZ and 05H30MZ
0JH80DZ and 05H33MZ
0JH80DZ and 05H34MZ
0JH80DZ and 05H40MZ
0JH80DZ and 05H43MZ
0JH80DZ and 05H44MZ
0JH80DZ and 0DH60MZ
0JH80DZ and 0DH63MZ
0JH80DZ and 0DH64MZ
0JH80EZ and 00H00MZ
0JH80EZ and 00H03MZ
0JH80EZ and 00H04MZ
0JH80EZ and 00H60MZ
0JH80EZ and 00H63MZ
0JH80EZ and 00H64MZ

0JH80EZ and 00HE0MZ
0JH80EZ and 00HE3MZ
0JH80EZ and 00HE4MZ
0JH80EZ and 00HU0MZ
0JH80EZ and 00HU3MZ
0JH80EZ and 00HU4MZ
0JH80EZ and 00HV0MZ
0JH80EZ and 00HV3MZ
0JH80EZ and 00HV4MZ
0JH80EZ and 01HY0MZ
0JH80EZ and 01HY3MZ
0JH80EZ and 01HY4MZ
0JH80EZ and 05H00MZ
0JH80EZ and 05H03MZ
0JH80EZ and 05H04MZ
0JH80EZ and 05H30MZ
0JH80EZ and 05H33MZ
0JH80EZ and 05H34MZ
0JH80EZ and 05H40MZ
0JH80EZ and 05H43MZ
0JH80EZ and 05H44MZ
0JH80EZ and 0DH60MZ

0JH80EZ and 0DH63MZ
0JH80EZ and 0DH64MZ
0JH80PZ and 02H40JZ
0JH80PZ and 02H40MZ
0JH80PZ and 02H43JZ
0JH80PZ and 02H43MZ
0JH80PZ and 02H44JZ
0JH80PZ and 02H44MZ
0JH80PZ and 02H60JZ
0JH80PZ and 02H60MZ
0JH80PZ and 02H63JZ
0JH80PZ and 02H63MZ
0JH80PZ and 02H64JZ
0JH80PZ and 02H64MZ
0JH80PZ and 02H70JZ
0JH80PZ and 02H70MZ
0JH80PZ and 02H73JZ
0JH80PZ and 02H73MZ
0JH80PZ and 02H74JZ
0JH80PZ and 02H74MZ
0JH80PZ and 02HK0JZ
0JH80PZ and 02HK0MZ

0JH80PZ and 02HK3JZ
0JH80PZ and 02HK3MZ
0JH80PZ and 02HK4JZ
0JH80PZ and 02HK4MZ
0JH80PZ and 02HL0JZ
0JH80PZ and 02HL0MZ
0JH80PZ and 02HL3JZ
0JH80PZ and 02HL3MZ
0JH80PZ and 02HL4JZ
0JH80PZ and 02HL4MZ
0JH80PZ and 02HN0JZ
0JH80PZ and 02HN0MZ
0JH80PZ and 02HN3JZ
0JH80PZ and 02HN3MZ
0JH80PZ and 02HN4JZ
0JH80PZ and 02HN4MZ
0JH834Z and 02H40JZ
0JH834Z and 02H40MZ
0JH834Z and 02H43JZ
0JH834Z and 02H43MZ
0JH834Z and 02H44JZ
0JH834Z and 02H44MZ

0JH834Z and 02H60JZ
0JH834Z and 02H60MZ
0JH834Z and 02H63JZ
0JH834Z and 02H63MZ
0JH834Z and 02H64JZ
0JH834Z and 02H64MZ
0JH834Z and 02H70JZ
0JH834Z and 02H70MZ
0JH834Z and 02H73JZ
0JH834Z and 02H73MZ
0JH834Z and 02H74JZ
0JH834Z and 02H74MZ
0JH834Z and 02HK0JZ
0JH834Z and 02HK0MZ
0JH834Z and 02HK3JZ
0JH834Z and 02HK3MZ
0JH834Z and 02HK4JZ
0JH834Z and 02HK4MZ
0JH834Z and 02HL0JZ
0JH834Z and 02HL0MZ
0JH834Z and 02HL3JZ
0JH834Z and 02HL3MZ

0JH834Z and 02HL4JZ
0JH834Z and 02HL4MZ
0JH834Z and 02HN0JZ
0JH834Z and 02HN0MZ
0JH834Z and 02HN3JZ
0JH834Z and 02HN3MZ
0JH834Z and 02HN4JZ
0JH834Z and 02HN4MZ
0JH835Z and 02H40JZ
0JH835Z and 02H40MZ
0JH835Z and 02H43JZ
0JH835Z and 02H43MZ
0JH835Z and 02H44JZ
0JH835Z and 02H44MZ
0JH835Z and 02H60JZ
0JH835Z and 02H60MZ
0JH835Z and 02H63JZ
0JH835Z and 02H63MZ
0JH835Z and 02H64JZ
0JH835Z and 02H64MZ
0JH835Z and 02H70JZ
0JH835Z and 02H70MZ

0JH835Z and 02H73JZ
0JH835Z and 02H73MZ
0JH835Z and 02H74JZ
0JH835Z and 02H74MZ
0JH835Z and 02HK0JZ
0JH835Z and 02HK0MZ
0JH835Z and 02HK3JZ
0JH835Z and 02HK3MZ
0JH835Z and 02HK4JZ
0JH835Z and 02HK4MZ
0JH835Z and 02HL0JZ
0JH835Z and 02HL0MZ
0JH835Z and 02HL3JZ
0JH835Z and 02HL3MZ
0JH835Z and 02HL4JZ
0JH835Z and 02HL4MZ
0JH835Z and 02HN0JZ
0JH835Z and 02HN0MZ
0JH835Z and 02HN3JZ
0JH835Z and 02HN3MZ
0JH835Z and 02HN4JZ
0JH835Z and 02HN4MZ

0JH836Z and 02H40JZ
0JH836Z and 02H40MZ
0JH836Z and 02H43JZ
0JH836Z and 02H43MZ
0JH836Z and 02H44JZ
0JH836Z and 02H44MZ
0JH836Z and 02H60JZ
0JH836Z and 02H60MZ
0JH836Z and 02H63JZ
0JH836Z and 02H63MZ
0JH836Z and 02H64JZ
0JH836Z and 02H64MZ
0JH836Z and 02H70JZ
0JH836Z and 02H70MZ
0JH836Z and 02H73JZ
0JH836Z and 02H73MZ
0JH836Z and 02H74JZ
0JH836Z and 02H74MZ
0JH836Z and 02HK0JZ
0JH836Z and 02HK0MZ
0JH836Z and 02HK3JZ
0JH836Z and 02HK3MZ

0JH836Z and 02HK4JZ
0JH836Z and 02HK4MZ
0JH836Z and 02HL0JZ
0JH836Z and 02HL0MZ
0JH836Z and 02HL3JZ
0JH836Z and 02HL3MZ
0JH836Z and 02HL4JZ
0JH836Z and 02HL4MZ
0JH836Z and 02HN0JZ
0JH836Z and 02HN0MZ
0JH836Z and 02HN3JZ
0JH836Z and 02HN3MZ
0JH836Z and 02HN4JZ
0JH836Z and 02HN4MZ
0JH837Z and 02H40JZ
0JH837Z and 02H40MZ
0JH837Z and 02H43JZ
0JH837Z and 02H43MZ
0JH837Z and 02H44JZ
0JH837Z and 02H44MZ
0JH837Z and 02H60JZ
0JH837Z and 02H60MZ

0JH837Z and 02H63JZ
0JH837Z and 02H63MZ
0JH837Z and 02H64JZ
0JH837Z and 02H64MZ
0JH837Z and 02H70JZ
0JH837Z and 02H70MZ
0JH837Z and 02H73JZ
0JH837Z and 02H73MZ
0JH837Z and 02H74JZ
0JH837Z and 02H74MZ
0JH837Z and 02HK0JZ
0JH837Z and 02HK0MZ
0JH837Z and 02HK3JZ
0JH837Z and 02HK3MZ
0JH837Z and 02HK4JZ
0JH837Z and 02HK4MZ
0JH837Z and 02HL0JZ
0JH837Z and 02HL0MZ
0JH837Z and 02HL3JZ
0JH837Z and 02HL3MZ
0JH837Z and 02HL4JZ
0JH837Z and 02HL4MZ

0JH837Z and 02HN0JZ
0JH837Z and 02HN0MZ
0JH837Z and 02HN3JZ
0JH837Z and 02HN3MZ
0JH837Z and 02HN4JZ
0JH837Z and 02HN4MZ
0JH838Z and 02H40KZ
0JH838Z and 02H44KZ
0JH838Z and 02HN0JZ
0JH838Z and 02HN0KZ
0JH838Z and 02HN0MZ
0JH838Z and 02HN3JZ
0JH838Z and 02HN3KZ
0JH838Z and 02HN3MZ
0JH838Z and 02HN4JZ
0JH838Z and 02HN4KZ
0JH838Z and 02HN4MZ
0JH839Z and 02H40KZ
0JH839Z and 02H43JZ
0JH839Z and 02H43KZ
0JH839Z and 02H43MZ
0JH839Z and 02H44KZ

0JH839Z and 02H60KZ

0JH839Z and 02H63KZ

0JH839Z and 02H64KZ

0JH839Z and 02H70KZ

0JH839Z and 02H73KZ

0JH839Z and 02H74KZ

0JH839Z and 02HN0JZ

0JH839Z and 02HN0KZ

0JH839Z and 02HN0MZ

0JH839Z and 02HN3JZ

0JH839Z and 02HN3KZ

0JH839Z and 02HN3MZ

0JH839Z and 02HN4JZ

0JH839Z and 02HN4KZ

0JH839Z and 02HN4MZ

0JH83BZ and 00HE0MZ

0JH83BZ and 00HE3MZ

0JH83BZ and 00HE4MZ

0JH83BZ and 00HU0MZ

0JH83BZ and 00HU3MZ

0JH83BZ and 00HU4MZ

0JH83BZ and 00HV0MZ

0JH83BZ and 00HV3MZ

0JH83BZ and 00HV4MZ

0JH83BZ and 01HY0MZ

0JH83BZ and 01HY3MZ

0JH83BZ and 01HY4MZ

0JH83BZ and 05H00MZ

0JH83BZ and 05H03MZ

0JH83BZ and 05H04MZ

0JH83BZ and 05H30MZ

0JH83BZ and 05H33MZ

0JH83BZ and 05H34MZ

0JH83BZ and 05H40MZ

0JH83BZ and 05H43MZ

0JH83BZ and 05H44MZ

0JH83BZ and 0DH60MZ

0JH83BZ and 0DH63MZ

0JH83BZ and 0DH64MZ

0JH83CZ and 00HE0MZ

0JH83CZ and 00HE3MZ

0JH83CZ and 00HE4MZ

0JH83CZ and 00HU0MZ

0JH83CZ and 00HU3MZ

0JH83CZ and 00HU4MZ

0JH83CZ and 00HV0MZ

0JH83CZ and 00HV3MZ

0JH83CZ and 00HV4MZ

0JH83CZ and 01HY0MZ

0JH83CZ and 01HY3MZ

0JH83CZ and 01HY4MZ

0JH83CZ and 05H00MZ

0JH83CZ and 05H03MZ

0JH83CZ and 05H04MZ

0JH83CZ and 05H30MZ

0JH83CZ and 05H33MZ

0JH83CZ and 05H34MZ

0JH83CZ and 05H40MZ

0JH83CZ and 05H43MZ

0JH83CZ and 05H44MZ

0JH83CZ and 0DH60MZ

0JH83CZ and 0DH63MZ

0JH83CZ and 0DH64MZ

0JH83DZ and 00H00MZ

0JH83DZ and 00H03MZ

0JH83DZ and 00H04MZ

0JH83DZ and 00H60MZ

0JH83DZ and 00H63MZ

0JH83DZ and 00H64MZ

0JH83DZ and 00HE0MZ

0JH83DZ and 00HE3MZ

0JH83DZ and 00HE4MZ

0JH83DZ and 00HU0MZ

0JH83DZ and 00HU3MZ

0JH83DZ and 00HU4MZ

0JH83DZ and 00HV0MZ

0JH83DZ and 00HV3MZ

0JH83DZ and 00HV4MZ

0JH83DZ and 01HY0MZ

0JH83DZ and 01HY3MZ

0JH83DZ and 01HY4MZ

0JH83DZ and 05H00MZ

0JH83DZ and 05H03MZ

0JH83DZ and 05H04MZ

0JH83DZ and 05H30MZ

0JH83DZ and 05H33MZ

0JH83DZ and 05H34MZ

0JH83DZ and 05H40MZ

0JH83DZ and 05H43MZ

0JH83DZ and 05H44MZ

0JH83DZ and 0DH60MZ

0JH83DZ and 0DH63MZ

0JH83DZ and 0DH64MZ

0JH83EZ and 00H00MZ

0JH83EZ and 00H03MZ

0JH83EZ and 00H04MZ

0JH83EZ and 00H60MZ

0JH83EZ and 00H63MZ

0JH83EZ and 00H64MZ

0JH83EZ and 00HE0MZ

0JH83EZ and 00HE3MZ

0JH83EZ and 00HE4MZ

0JH83EZ and 00HU0MZ

0JH83EZ and 00HU3MZ

0JH83EZ and 00HU4MZ

0JH83EZ and 00HV0MZ

0JH83EZ and 00HV3MZ

0JH83EZ and 00HV4MZ

0JH83EZ and 01HY0MZ

0JH83EZ and 01HY3MZ

0JH83EZ and 01HY4MZ

0JH83EZ and 05H00MZ

0JH83EZ and 05H03MZ

0JH83EZ and 05H04MZ

0JH83EZ and 05H30MZ

0JH83EZ and 05H33MZ

0JH83EZ and 05H34MZ

0JH83EZ and 05H40MZ

0JH83EZ and 05H43MZ

0JH83EZ and 05H44MZ

0JH83EZ and 0DH60MZ

0JH83EZ and 0DH63MZ

0JH83EZ and 0DH64MZ

0JH83PZ and 02H40JZ

0JH83PZ and 02H40MZ

0JH83PZ and 02H43JZ

0JH83PZ and 02H43MZ

0JH83PZ and 02H44JZ

0JH83PZ and 02H44MZ

0JH83PZ and 02H60JZ

0JH83PZ and 02H60MZ

0JH83PZ and 02H63JZ

0JH83PZ and 02H63MZ

0JH83PZ and 02H64JZ

0JH83PZ and 02H64MZ

0JH83PZ and 02H70JZ

0JH83PZ and 02H70MZ

0JH83PZ and 02H73JZ

0JH83PZ and 02H73MZ

0JH83PZ and 02H74JZ

0JH83PZ and 02H74MZ

0JH83PZ and 02HK0JZ

0JH83PZ and 02HK0MZ

0JH83PZ and 02HK3JZ

0JH83PZ and 02HK3MZ

0JH83PZ and 02HK4JZ

0JH83PZ and 02HK4MZ

0JH83PZ and 02HL0JZ

0JH83PZ and 02HL0MZ

0JH83PZ and 02HL3JZ

0JH83PZ and 02HL3MZ

0JH83PZ and 02HL4JZ

0JH83PZ and 02HL4MZ

0JH83PZ and 02HN0JZ

0JH83PZ
and 02HN0MZ

0JH83PZ
and 02HN3JZ

0JH83PZ
and 02HN3MZ

0JH83PZ
and 02HN4JZ

0JH83PZ
and 02HN4MZ

0NH00NZ
and 00H00MZ

0NH00NZ
and 00H03MZ

0NH00NZ
and 00H04MZ

0NH00NZ
and 00H60MZ

0NH00NZ
and 00H63MZ

0NH00NZ
and 00H64MZ

0PS33ZZ
and 0PU33JZ

0PS43ZZ
and 0PU43JZ

0QS03ZZ
and 0QU03JZ

0QS13ZZ
and 0QU13JZ

0QSS3ZZ
and 0QUS3JZ

One of
0RG7070
0RG70A0
0RG70J0
0RG70K0
0RG7370
0RG73A0
0RG73J0
0RG73K0
0RG7470
0RG74A0
0RG74J0
0RG74K0
XRG70F3

with one of
0SG1070
0SG10A0
0SG10J0
0SG10K0
0SG1370
0SG13A0
0SG13J0
0SG13K0
0SG1470
0SG14A0
0SG14J0
0SG14K0
XRGC0F3

One of
0RG7071
0RG707J
0RG70AJ
0RG70J1
0RG70JJ
0RG70K1
0RG70KJ
0RG7371
0RG737J
0RG73AJ
0RG73J1
0RG73JJ
0RG73K1
0RG73KJ
0RG7471
0RG747J
0RG74AJ
0RG74J1
0RG74JJ
0RG74K1
0RG74KJ
XRG7092
XRG70F3

with one of
0SG1071
0SG107J
0SG10AJ
0SG10J1
0SG10JJ
0SG10K1
0SG10KJ
0SG1371
0SG137J
0SG13AJ
0SG13J1
0SG13JJ
0SG13K1
0SG13KJ
0SG1471
0SG147J
0SG14AJ
0SG14J1
0SG14JJ
0SG14K1
0SG14KJ
XRGC092
XRGC0F3

0SP908Z
and 0SR9019

0SP908Z
and 0SR901A

0SP908Z
and 0SR901Z

0SP908Z
and 0SR9029

0SP908Z
and 0SR902A

0SP908Z
and 0SR902Z

0SP908Z
and 0SR9039

0SP908Z
and 0SR903A

0SP908Z
and 0SR903Z

0SP908Z
and 0SR9049

0SP908Z
and 0SR904A

0SP908Z
and 0SR904Z

0SP908Z
and 0SR9069

0SP908Z
and 0SR906A

0SP908Z
and 0SR906Z

0SP908Z
and 0SR90J9

0SP908Z
and 0SR90JA

0SP908Z
and 0SR90JZ

0SP908Z
and 0SRA009

0SP908Z
and 0SRA00A

0SP908Z
and 0SRA00Z

0SP908Z
and 0SRA019

0SP908Z
and 0SRA01A

0SP908Z
and 0SRA01Z

0SP908Z
and 0SRA039

0SP908Z
and 0SRA03A

0SP908Z
and 0SRA03Z

0SP908Z
and 0SRA0J9

0SP908Z
and 0SRA0JA

0SP908Z
and 0SRA0JZ

0SP908Z
and 0SRR019

0SP908Z
and 0SRR01A

0SP908Z
and 0SRR01Z

0SP908Z
and 0SRR039

0SP908Z
and 0SRR03A

0SP908Z
and 0SRR03Z

0SP908Z
and 0SRR0J9

0SP908Z
and 0SRR0JA

0SP908Z
and 0SRR0JZ

0SP908Z
and 0SU909Z

0SP908Z
and 0SUA09Z

0SP908Z
and 0SUR09Z

0SP909Z
and 0SR9019

0SP909Z
and 0SR901A

0SP909Z
and 0SR901Z

0SP909Z
and 0SR9029

0SP909Z
and 0SR902A

0SP909Z
and 0SR902Z

0SP909Z
and 0SR9039

0SP909Z
and 0SR903A

0SP909Z
and 0SR903Z

0SP909Z
and 0SR9049

0SP909Z
and 0SR904A

0SP909Z
and 0SR904Z

0SP909Z
and 0SR9069

0SP909Z
and 0SR906A

0SP909Z
and 0SR906Z

0SP909Z
and 0SR90J9

0SP909Z
and 0SR90JA

0SP909Z
and 0SR90JZ

0SP909Z
and 0SRA009

0SP909Z
and 0SRA00A

0SP909Z
and 0SRA00Z

0SP909Z
and 0SRA019

0SP909Z
and 0SRA01A

0SP909Z
and 0SRA01Z

0SP909Z
and 0SRA039

0SP909Z
and 0SRA03A

0SP909Z
and 0SRA03Z

0SP909Z
and 0SRA0J9

0SP909Z
and 0SRA0JA

0SP909Z
and 0SRA0JZ

0SP909Z
and 0SRR019

0SP909Z
and 0SRR01A

0SP909Z
and 0SRR01Z

0SP909Z
and 0SRR039

0SP909Z
and 0SRR03A

0SP909Z
and 0SRR03Z

0SP909Z
and 0SRR0J9

0SP909Z
and 0SRR0JA

0SP909Z
and 0SRR0JZ

0SP909Z
and 0SU909Z

0SP909Z
and 0SUA09Z

0SP909Z
and 0SUR09Z

0SP90BZ
and 0SR9019

0SP90BZ
and 0SR901A

0SP90BZ
and 0SR901Z

0SP90BZ
and 0SR9029

0SP90BZ
and 0SR902A

0SP90BZ
and 0SR902Z

0SP90BZ
and 0SR9039

0SP90BZ
and 0SR903A

0SP90BZ
and 0SR903Z

0SP90BZ
and 0SR9049

0SP90BZ
and 0SR904A

0SP90BZ
and 0SR904Z

0SP90BZ
and 0SR9069

0SP90BZ
and 0SR906A

0SP90BZ
and 0SR906Z

0SP90BZ
and 0SR90J9

0SP90BZ
and 0SR90JA

0SP90BZ
and 0SR90JZ

0SP90BZ
and 0SRA009

0SP90BZ
and 0SRA00A

0SP90BZ
and 0SRA00Z

0SP90BZ and 0SRA019	0SP90EZ and 0SR902A	0SP90JZ and 0SR901A	0SP90JZ and 0SRA01Z	0SP948Z and 0SR9039	0SP948Z and 0SRA0JA	0SP94JZ and 0SR903Z
0SP90BZ and 0SRA01A	0SP90EZ and 0SR9039	0SP90JZ and 0SR901Z	0SP90JZ and 0SRA039	0SP948Z and 0SR903A	0SP948Z and 0SRA0JZ	0SP94JZ and 0SR9049
0SP90BZ and 0SRA01Z	0SP90EZ and 0SR903A	0SP90JZ and 0SR9029	0SP90JZ and 0SRA03A	0SP948Z and 0SR903Z	0SP948Z and 0SRR019	0SP94JZ and 0SR904A
0SP90BZ and 0SRA039	0SP90EZ and 0SR904A	0SP90JZ and 0SR902A	0SP90JZ and 0SRA03Z	0SP948Z and 0SR9049	0SP948Z and 0SRR01A	0SP94JZ and 0SR904Z
0SP90BZ and 0SRA03A	0SP90EZ and 0SR904Z	0SP90JZ and 0SR902Z	0SP90JZ and 0SRA0J9	0SP948Z and 0SR904A	0SP948Z and 0SRR01Z	0SP94JZ and 0SR9069
0SP90BZ and 0SRA03Z	0SP90EZ and 0SR906A	0SP90JZ and 0SR9039	0SP90JZ and 0SRA0JA	0SP948Z and 0SR904Z	0SP948Z and 0SRR039	0SP94JZ and 0SR906A
0SP90BZ and 0SRA0J9	0SP90EZ and 0SR90J9	0SP90JZ and 0SR903A	0SP90JZ and 0SRA0JZ	0SP948Z and 0SR9069	0SP948Z and 0SRR03A	0SP94JZ and 0SR906Z
0SP90BZ and 0SRA0JA	0SP90EZ and 0SR90JZ	0SP90JZ and 0SR903Z	0SP90JZ and 0SRR019	0SP948Z and 0SR906A	0SP948Z and 0SRR03Z	0SP94JZ and 0SR90J9
0SP90BZ and 0SRA0JZ	0SP90EZ and 0SRA009	0SP90JZ and 0SR9049	0SP90JZ and 0SRR01A	0SP948Z and 0SR906Z	0SP948Z and 0SRR0J9	0SP94JZ and 0SR90JA
0SP90BZ and 0SRR019	0SP90EZ and 0SRA00Z	0SP90JZ and 0SR904A	0SP90JZ and 0SRR01Z	0SP948Z and 0SR90J9	0SP948Z and 0SRR0JA	0SP94JZ and 0SR90JZ
0SP90BZ and 0SRR01A	0SP90EZ and 0SRA019	0SP90JZ and 0SR904Z	0SP90JZ and 0SRR039	0SP948Z and 0SR90JA	0SP948Z and 0SRR0JZ	0SP94JZ and 0SRA009
0SP90BZ and 0SRR01Z	0SP90EZ and 0SRA01Z	0SP90JZ and 0SR9069	0SP90JZ and 0SRR03A	0SP948Z and 0SR90JZ	0SP948Z and 0SU909Z	0SP94JZ and 0SRA00A
0SP90BZ and 0SRR039	0SP90EZ and 0SRA039	0SP90JZ and 0SR906A	0SP90JZ and 0SRR03Z	0SP948Z and 0SRA009	0SP948Z and 0SUA09Z	0SP94JZ and 0SRA00Z
0SP90BZ and 0SRR03A	0SP90EZ and 0SRA03Z	0SP90JZ and 0SR906Z	0SP90JZ and 0SRR0J9	0SP948Z and 0SRA00A	0SP948Z and 0SUR09Z	0SP94JZ and 0SRA019
0SP90BZ and 0SRR03Z	0SP90EZ and 0SRA0JA	0SP90JZ and 0SR90J9	0SP90JZ and 0SRR0JA	0SP948Z and 0SRA00Z	0SP94JZ and 0SR9019	0SP94JZ and 0SRA01A
0SP90BZ and 0SRR0J9	0SP90EZ and 0SRR01A	0SP90JZ and 0SR90JA	0SP90JZ and 0SRR0JZ	0SP948Z and 0SRA019	0SP94JZ and 0SR901A	0SP94JZ and 0SRA01Z
0SP90BZ and 0SRR0JA	0SP90EZ and 0SRR03A	0SP90JZ and 0SR90JZ	0SP948Z and 0SR9019	0SP948Z and 0SRA01A	0SP94JZ and 0SR901Z	0SP94JZ and 0SRA039
0SP90BZ and 0SRR0JZ	0SP90EZ and 0SRR0J9	0SP90JZ and 0SRA009	0SP948Z and 0SR901A	0SP948Z and 0SRA01Z	0SP94JZ and 0SR9029	0SP94JZ and 0SRA03A
0SP90BZ and 0SU909Z	0SP90EZ and 0SRR0JZ	0SP90JZ and 0SRA00A	0SP948Z and 0SR901Z	0SP948Z and 0SRA039	0SP94JZ and 0SR902A	0SP94JZ and 0SRA03Z
0SP90BZ and 0SUA09Z	0SP90EZ and 0SU909Z	0SP90JZ and 0SRA00Z	0SP948Z and 0SR9029	0SP948Z and 0SRA03A	0SP94JZ and 0SR902Z	0SP94JZ and 0SRA0J9
0SP90BZ and 0SUR09Z	0SP90EZ and 0SUA09Z	0SP90JZ and 0SRA019	0SP948Z and 0SR902A	0SP948Z and 0SRA03Z	0SP94JZ and 0SR9039	0SP94JZ and 0SRA0JA
0SP90EZ and 0SR901A	0SP90JZ and 0SR9019	0SP90JZ and 0SRA01A	0SP948Z and 0SR902Z	0SP948Z and 0SRA0J9	0SP94JZ and 0SR903A	0SP94JZ and 0SRA0JZ

0SP94JZ and 0SRR019
0SP94JZ and 0SRR01A
0SP94JZ and 0SRR01Z
0SP94JZ and 0SRR039
0SP94JZ and 0SRR03A
0SP94JZ and 0SRR03Z
0SP94JZ and 0SRR0J9
0SP94JZ and 0SRR0JA
0SP94JZ and 0SRR0JZ
0SP94JZ and 0SU909Z
0SP94JZ and 0SUA09Z
0SP94JZ and 0SUR09Z
0SPA0JZ and 0SR9019
0SPA0JZ and 0SR901A
0SPA0JZ and 0SR901Z
0SPA0JZ and 0SR9029
0SPA0JZ and 0SR902A
0SPA0JZ and 0SR902Z
0SPA0JZ and 0SR9039
0SPA0JZ and 0SR903A
0SPA0JZ and 0SR903Z
0SPA0JZ and 0SR9049
0SPA0JZ and 0SR904A
0SPA0JZ and 0SR904Z
0SPA0JZ and 0SR9069
0SPA0JZ and 0SR906A
0SPA0JZ and 0SR906Z
0SPA0JZ and 0SR90J9
0SPA0JZ and 0SR90JA
0SPA0JZ and 0SR90JZ
0SPA0JZ and 0SRA009
0SPA0JZ and 0SRA00A
0SPA0JZ and 0SRA00Z
0SPA0JZ and 0SRA019
0SPA0JZ and 0SRA01A
0SPA0JZ and 0SRA01Z
0SPA0JZ and 0SRA039
0SPA0JZ and 0SRA03A
0SPA0JZ and 0SRA03Z
0SPA0JZ and 0SRA0J9
0SPA0JZ and 0SRA0JA
0SPA0JZ and 0SRA0JZ
0SPA0JZ and 0SRR019
0SPA0JZ and 0SRR01A
0SPA0JZ and 0SRR01Z
0SPA0JZ and 0SRR039
0SPA0JZ and 0SRR03A
0SPA0JZ and 0SRR03Z
0SPA0JZ and 0SRR0J9
0SPA0JZ and 0SRR0JA
0SPA0JZ and 0SRR0JZ
0SPA4JZ and 0SR9019
0SPA4JZ and 0SR901A
0SPA4JZ and 0SR901Z
0SPA4JZ and 0SR9029
0SPA4JZ and 0SR902A
0SPA4JZ and 0SR902Z
0SPA4JZ and 0SR9039
0SPA4JZ and 0SR903A
0SPA4JZ and 0SR903Z
0SPA4JZ and 0SR9049
0SPA4JZ and 0SR904A
0SPA4JZ and 0SR904Z
0SPA4JZ and 0SR9069
0SPA4JZ and 0SR906A
0SPA4JZ and 0SR906Z
0SPA4JZ and 0SR90J9
0SPA4JZ and 0SR90JA
0SPA4JZ and 0SR90JZ
0SPA4JZ and 0SRA009
0SPA4JZ and 0SRA00A
0SPA4JZ and 0SRA00Z
0SPA4JZ and 0SRA019
0SPA4JZ and 0SRA01A
0SPA4JZ and 0SRA01Z
0SPA4JZ and 0SRA039
0SPA4JZ and 0SRA03A
0SPA4JZ and 0SRA03Z
0SPA4JZ and 0SRA0J9
0SPA4JZ and 0SRA0JA
0SPA4JZ and 0SRA0JZ
0SPA4JZ and 0SRR019
0SPA4JZ and 0SRR01A
0SPA4JZ and 0SRR01Z
0SPA4JZ and 0SRR039
0SPA4JZ and 0SRR03A
0SPA4JZ and 0SRR03Z
0SPA4JZ and 0SRR0J9
0SPA4JZ and 0SRR0JA
0SPA4JZ and 0SRR0JZ
0SPA4JZ and 0SU909Z
0SPA4JZ and 0SUA09Z
0SPA4JZ and 0SUR09Z
0SPB08Z and 0SRB019
0SPB08Z and 0SRB01A
0SPB08Z and 0SRB01Z
0SPB08Z and 0SRB029
0SPB08Z and 0SRB02A
0SPB08Z and 0SRB02Z
0SPB08Z and 0SRB039
0SPB08Z and 0SRB03A
0SPB08Z and 0SRB03Z
0SPB08Z and 0SRB049
0SPB08Z and 0SRB04A
0SPB08Z and 0SRB04Z
0SPB08Z and 0SRB069
0SPB08Z and 0SRB06A
0SPB08Z and 0SRB06Z
0SPB08Z and 0SRB0J9
0SPB08Z and 0SRB0JA
0SPB08Z and 0SRB0JZ
0SPB08Z and 0SRE009
0SPB08Z and 0SRE00A
0SPB08Z and 0SRE00Z
0SPB08Z and 0SRE019
0SPB08Z and 0SRE01A
0SPB08Z and 0SRE01Z
0SPB08Z and 0SRE039
0SPB08Z and 0SRE03A
0SPB08Z and 0SRE03Z
0SPB08Z and 0SRE0J9
0SPB08Z and 0SRE0JA
0SPB08Z and 0SRE0JZ
0SPB08Z and 0SRS019
0SPB08Z and 0SRS01A
0SPB08Z and 0SRS01Z
0SPB08Z and 0SRS039
0SPB08Z and 0SRS03A
0SPB08Z and 0SRS03Z
0SPB08Z and 0SRS0J9
0SPB08Z and 0SRS0JA
0SPB08Z and 0SRS0JZ
0SPB08Z and 0SUB09Z
0SPB08Z and 0SUE09Z
0SPB08Z and 0SUS09Z
0SPB09Z and 0SRB019
0SPB09Z and 0SRB01A
0SPB09Z and 0SRB01Z
0SPB09Z and 0SRB029
0SPB09Z and 0SRB02A
0SPB09Z and 0SRB02Z
0SPB09Z and 0SRB039
0SPB09Z and 0SRB03A
0SPB09Z and 0SRB03Z
0SPB09Z and 0SRB049
0SPB09Z and 0SRB04A
0SPB09Z and 0SRB04Z
0SPB09Z and 0SRB069
0SPB09Z and 0SRB06A
0SPB09Z and 0SRB06Z
0SPB09Z and 0SRB0J9
0SPB09Z and 0SRB0JA
0SPB09Z and 0SRB0JZ
0SPB09Z and 0SRE009

0SPB09Z and 0SRE00A
0SPB09Z and 0SRE00Z
0SPB09Z and 0SRE019
0SPB09Z and 0SRE01A
0SPB09Z and 0SRE01Z
0SPB09Z and 0SRE039
0SPB09Z and 0SRE03A
0SPB09Z and 0SRE03Z
0SPB09Z and 0SRE0J9
0SPB09Z and 0SRE0JA
0SPB09Z and 0SRE0JZ
0SPB09Z and 0SRS019
0SPB09Z and 0SRS01A
0SPB09Z and 0SRS01Z
0SPB09Z and 0SRS039
0SPB09Z and 0SRS03A
0SPB09Z and 0SRS03Z
0SPB09Z and 0SRS0J9
0SPB09Z and 0SRS0JA
0SPB09Z and 0SRS0JZ
0SPB09Z and 0SUB09Z
0SPB09Z and 0SUE09Z

0SPB09Z and 0SUS09Z
0SPB0BZ and 0SRB019
0SPB0BZ and 0SRB01A
0SPB0BZ and 0SRB01Z
0SPB0BZ and 0SRB029
0SPB0BZ and 0SRB02A
0SPB0BZ and 0SRB02Z
0SPB0BZ and 0SRB039
0SPB0BZ and 0SRB03A
0SPB0BZ and 0SRB03Z
0SPB0BZ and 0SRB049
0SPB0BZ and 0SRB04A
0SPB0BZ and 0SRB04Z
0SPB0BZ and 0SRB069
0SPB0BZ and 0SRB06A
0SPB0BZ and 0SRB06Z
0SPB0BZ and 0SRB0EZ
0SPB0BZ and 0SRB0J9
0SPB0BZ and 0SRB0JA
0SPB0BZ and 0SRB0JZ
0SPB0BZ and 0SRE009
0SPB0BZ and 0SRE00A

0SPB0BZ and 0SRE00Z
0SPB0BZ and 0SRE019
0SPB0BZ and 0SRE01A
0SPB0BZ and 0SRE01Z
0SPB0BZ and 0SRE039
0SPB0BZ and 0SRE03A
0SPB0BZ and 0SRE03Z
0SPB0BZ and 0SRE0J9
0SPB0BZ and 0SRE0JA
0SPB0BZ and 0SRE0JZ
0SPB0BZ and 0SRS019
0SPB0BZ and 0SRS01A
0SPB0BZ and 0SRS01Z
0SPB0BZ and 0SRS039
0SPB0BZ and 0SRS03A
0SPB0BZ and 0SRS03Z
0SPB0BZ and 0SRS0J9
0SPB0BZ and 0SRS0JA
0SPB0BZ and 0SRS0JZ
0SPB0BZ and 0SUB09Z
0SPB0BZ and 0SUE09Z
0SPB0BZ and 0SUS09Z

0SPB0EZ and 0SRB019
0SPB0EZ and 0SRB01Z
0SPB0EZ and 0SRB029
0SPB0EZ and 0SRB02Z
0SPB0EZ and 0SRB039
0SPB0EZ and 0SRB03A
0SPB0EZ and 0SRB03Z
0SPB0EZ and 0SRB049
0SPB0EZ and 0SRB04A
0SPB0EZ and 0SRB04Z
0SPB0EZ and 0SRB069
0SPB0EZ and 0SRB06A
0SPB0EZ and 0SRB06Z
0SPB0EZ and 0SRB0JA
0SPB0EZ and 0SRE00A
0SPB0EZ and 0SRE00Z
0SPB0EZ and 0SRE01A
0SPB0EZ and 0SRE03A
0SPB0EZ and 0SRE0J9
0SPB0EZ and 0SRE0JZ
0SPB0EZ and 0SRS01A
0SPB0EZ and 0SRS039

0SPB0EZ and 0SRS03A
0SPB0EZ and 0SRS03Z
0SPB0EZ and 0SRS0J9
0SPB0EZ and 0SRS0JA
0SPB0EZ and 0SRS0JZ
0SPB0EZ and 0SUB09Z
0SPB0EZ and 0SUE09Z
0SPB0JZ and 0SRB019
0SPB0JZ and 0SRB01A
0SPB0JZ and 0SRB01Z
0SPB0JZ and 0SRB029
0SPB0JZ and 0SRB02A
0SPB0JZ and 0SRB02Z
0SPB0JZ and 0SRB039
0SPB0JZ and 0SRB03A
0SPB0JZ and 0SRB03Z
0SPB0JZ and 0SRB049
0SPB0JZ and 0SRB04A
0SPB0JZ and 0SRB04Z
0SPB0JZ and 0SRB069
0SPB0JZ and 0SRB06A
0SPB0JZ and 0SRB06Z

0SPB0JZ and 0SRB0EZ
0SPB0JZ and 0SRB0J9
0SPB0JZ and 0SRB0JA
0SPB0JZ and 0SRB0JZ
0SPB0JZ and 0SRE009
0SPB0JZ and 0SRE00A
0SPB0JZ and 0SRE00Z
0SPB0JZ and 0SRE019
0SPB0JZ and 0SRE01A
0SPB0JZ and 0SRE01Z
0SPB0JZ and 0SRE039
0SPB0JZ and 0SRE03A
0SPB0JZ and 0SRE03Z
0SPB0JZ and 0SRE0J9
0SPB0JZ and 0SRE0JA
0SPB0JZ and 0SRE0JZ
0SPB0JZ and 0SRS019
0SPB0JZ and 0SRS01A
0SPB0JZ and 0SRS01Z
0SPB0JZ and 0SRS039
0SPB0JZ and 0SRS03A
0SPB0JZ and 0SRS03Z

0SPB0JZ and 0SRS0J9
0SPB0JZ and 0SRS0JA
0SPB0JZ and 0SRS0JZ
0SPB48Z and 0SRB019
0SPB48Z and 0SRB01A
0SPB48Z and 0SRB01Z
0SPB48Z and 0SRB029
0SPB48Z and 0SRB02A
0SPB48Z and 0SRB02Z
0SPB48Z and 0SRB039
0SPB48Z and 0SRB03A
0SPB48Z and 0SRB03Z
0SPB48Z and 0SRB049
0SPB48Z and 0SRB04A
0SPB48Z and 0SRB04Z
0SPB48Z and 0SRB069
0SPB48Z and 0SRB06A
0SPB48Z and 0SRB06Z
0SPB48Z and 0SRB0EZ
0SPB48Z and 0SRB0J9
0SPB48Z and 0SRB0JA
0SPB48Z and 0SRB0JZ

0SPB48Z and 0SRE009
0SPB48Z and 0SRE00A
0SPB48Z and 0SRE00Z
0SPB48Z and 0SRE019
0SPB48Z and 0SRE01A
0SPB48Z and 0SRE01Z
0SPB48Z and 0SRE039
0SPB48Z and 0SRE03A
0SPB48Z and 0SRE03Z
0SPB48Z and 0SRE0J9
0SPB48Z and 0SRE0JA
0SPB48Z and 0SRE0JZ
0SPB48Z and 0SRS019
0SPB48Z and 0SRS01A
0SPB48Z and 0SRS01Z
0SPB48Z and 0SRS039
0SPB48Z and 0SRS03A
0SPB48Z and 0SRS03Z
0SPB48Z and 0SRS0J9
0SPB48Z and 0SRS0JA
0SPB48Z and 0SRS0JZ
0SPB48Z and 0SUB09Z
0SPB48Z and 0SUE09Z
0SPB48Z and 0SUS09Z
0SPB4JZ and 0SRB019
0SPB4JZ and 0SRB01A
0SPB4JZ and 0SRB01Z
0SPB4JZ and 0SRB029
0SPB4JZ and 0SRB02A
0SPB4JZ and 0SRB02Z
0SPB4JZ and 0SRB039
0SPB4JZ and 0SRB03A
0SPB4JZ and 0SRB03Z
0SPB4JZ and 0SRB049
0SPB4JZ and 0SRB04A
0SPB4JZ and 0SRB04Z
0SPB4JZ and 0SRB069
0SPB4JZ and 0SRB06A
0SPB4JZ and 0SRB06Z
0SPB4JZ and 0SRB0EZ
0SPB4JZ and 0SRB0J9
0SPB4JZ and 0SRB0JA
0SPB4JZ and 0SRB0JZ
0SPB4JZ and 0SRE009
0SPB4JZ and 0SRE00A
0SPB4JZ and 0SRE00Z
0SPB4JZ and 0SRE019
0SPB4JZ and 0SRE01A
0SPB4JZ and 0SRE01Z
0SPB4JZ and 0SRE039
0SPB4JZ and 0SRE03A
0SPB4JZ and 0SRE03Z
0SPB4JZ and 0SRE0J9
0SPB4JZ and 0SRE0JA
0SPB4JZ and 0SRE0JZ
0SPB4JZ and 0SRS019
0SPB4JZ and 0SRS01A
0SPB4JZ and 0SRS01Z
0SPB4JZ and 0SRS039
0SPB4JZ and 0SRS03A
0SPB4JZ and 0SRS03Z
0SPB4JZ and 0SRS0J9
0SPB4JZ and 0SRS0JA
0SPB4JZ and 0SRS0JZ
0SPB4JZ and 0SUB09Z
0SPB4JZ and 0SUE09Z
0SPB4JZ and 0SUS09Z
0SPC08Z and 0SRC069
0SPC08Z and 0SRC06A
0SPC08Z and 0SRC06Z
0SPC08Z and 0SRC0J9
0SPC08Z and 0SRC0JA
0SPC08Z and 0SRC0JZ
0SPC08Z and 0SRC0NA
0SPC08Z and 0SRT0J9
0SPC08Z and 0SRT0JA
0SPC08Z and 0SRT0JZ
0SPC08Z and 0SRV0J9
0SPC08Z and 0SRV0JA
0SPC08Z and 0SRV0JZ
0SPC09Z and 0SRC069
0SPC09Z and 0SRC06A
0SPC09Z and 0SRC06Z
0SPC09Z and 0SRC0J9
0SPC09Z and 0SRC0JA
0SPC09Z and 0SRC0JZ
0SPC09Z and 0SRC0L9
0SPC09Z and 0SRC0LA
0SPC09Z and 0SRC0LZ
0SPC09Z and 0SRC0M9
0SPC09Z and 0SRC0MZ
0SPC09Z and 0SRC0NA
0SPC09Z and 0SRC0NZ
0SPC09Z and 0SRT0J9
0SPC09Z and 0SRT0JA
0SPC09Z and 0SRT0JZ
0SPC09Z and 0SRV0J9
0SPC09Z and 0SRV0JA
0SPC09Z and 0SRV0JZ
0SPC09Z and 0SUV09Z
0SPC0EZ and 0SRC069
0SPC0EZ and 0SRT0J9
0SPC0JC and 0SRC069
0SPC0JC and 0SRC06A
0SPC0JC and 0SRC06Z
0SPC0JC and 0SRC0EZ
0SPC0JC and 0SRC0J9
0SPC0JC and 0SRC0JA
0SPC0JC and 0SRC0JZ
0SPC0JC and 0SRC0N9
0SPC0JC and 0SRC0NA
0SPC0JC and 0SRC0NZ
0SPC0JC and 0SRT0J9
0SPC0JC and 0SRT0JA
0SPC0JC and 0SRT0JZ
0SPC0JC and 0SRV0J9
0SPC0JC and 0SRV0JA
0SPC0JC and 0SRV0JZ
0SPC0JZ and 0SRC069
0SPC0JZ and 0SRC06A
0SPC0JZ and 0SRC06Z
0SPC0JZ and 0SRC0J9
0SPC0JZ and 0SRC0JA
0SPC0JZ and 0SRC0JZ
0SPC0JZ and 0SRC0L9
0SPC0JZ and 0SRC0LA
0SPC0JZ and 0SRC0LZ
0SPC0JZ and 0SRC0MZ
0SPC0JZ and 0SRC0NA
0SPC0JZ and 0SRT0J9
0SPC0JZ and 0SRT0JA
0SPC0JZ and 0SRT0JZ
0SPC0JZ and 0SRV0J9
0SPC0JZ and 0SRV0JA
0SPC0JZ and 0SRV0JZ
0SPC0LZ and 0SRC069
0SPC0LZ and 0SRC0JZ
0SPC0LZ and 0SRT0J9
0SPC0LZ and 0SRT0JZ
0SPC0MZ and 0SRC069
0SPC0MZ and 0SRC06A
0SPC0MZ and 0SRC0J9
0SPC0MZ and 0SRC0JZ
0SPC0MZ and 0SRC0L9
0SPC0MZ and 0SRC0LZ
0SPC0MZ and 0SRT0J9
0SPC0MZ and 0SRT0JA
0SPC0MZ and 0SRT0JZ
0SPC0MZ and 0SRV0JA
0SPC0NZ and 0SRC069
0SPC0NZ and 0SRC06A
0SPC0NZ and 0SRC0J9
0SPC0NZ and 0SRC0JZ
0SPC0NZ and 0SRC0L9

0SPC0NZ and 0SRC0LZ

0SPC0NZ and 0SRT0J9

0SPC0NZ and 0SRT0JZ

0SPC0NZ and 0SRV0JA

0SPC38Z and 0SRC069

0SPC38Z and 0SRC06A

0SPC38Z and 0SRC06Z

0SPC38Z and 0SRC0J9

0SPC38Z and 0SRC0JA

0SPC38Z and 0SRC0JZ

0SPC38Z and 0SRC0NA

0SPC38Z and 0SRT0J9

0SPC38Z and 0SRT0JA

0SPC38Z and 0SRT0JZ

0SPC38Z and 0SRV0J9

0SPC38Z and 0SRV0JA

0SPC38Z and 0SRV0JZ

0SPC48Z and 0SRC069

0SPC48Z and 0SRC06A

0SPC48Z and 0SRC06Z

0SPC48Z and 0SRC0J9

0SPC48Z and 0SRC0JA

0SPC48Z and 0SRC0JZ

0SPC48Z and 0SRC0N9

0SPC48Z and 0SRC0NA

0SPC48Z and 0SRC0NZ

0SPC48Z and 0SRT0J9

0SPC48Z and 0SRT0JA

0SPC48Z and 0SRT0JZ

0SPC48Z and 0SRV0J9

0SPC48Z and 0SRV0JA

0SPC48Z and 0SRV0JZ

0SPC4JC and 0SRC069

0SPC4JC and 0SRC06A

0SPC4JC and 0SRC06Z

0SPC4JC and 0SRC0J9

0SPC4JC and 0SRC0JA

0SPC4JC and 0SRC0JZ

0SPC4JC and 0SRC0N9

0SPC4JC and 0SRC0NA

0SPC4JC and 0SRC0NZ

0SPC4JC and 0SRT0J9

0SPC4JC and 0SRT0JA

0SPC4JC and 0SRV0J9

0SPC4JC and 0SRV0JA

0SPC4JZ and 0SRC069

0SPC4JZ and 0SRC06A

0SPC4JZ and 0SRC06Z

0SPC4JZ and 0SRC0J9

0SPC4JZ and 0SRC0JA

0SPC4JZ and 0SRC0JZ

0SPC4JZ and 0SRC0L9

0SPC4JZ and 0SRC0LA

0SPC4JZ and 0SRC0LZ

0SPC4JZ and 0SRC0NA

0SPC4JZ and 0SRT0J9

0SPC4JZ and 0SRT0JA

0SPC4JZ and 0SRT0JZ

0SPC4JZ and 0SRV0J9

0SPC4JZ and 0SRV0JA

0SPC4JZ and 0SRV0JZ

0SPC4MZ and 0SRC069

0SPC4MZ and 0SRC0J9

0SPC4MZ and 0SRC0JZ

0SPC4MZ and 0SRC0L9

0SPC4MZ and 0SRC0LZ

0SPC4MZ and 0SRT0J9

0SPC4MZ and 0SRT0JZ

0SPC4NZ and 0SRC069

0SPC4NZ and 0SRC0J9

0SPC4NZ and 0SRC0JZ

0SPC4NZ and 0SRC0LZ

0SPC4NZ and 0SRT0J9

0SPC4NZ and 0SRT0JZ

0SPD08Z and 0SRD069

0SPD08Z and 0SRD06A

0SPD08Z and 0SRD06Z

0SPD08Z and 0SRD0J9

0SPD08Z and 0SRD0JA

0SPD08Z and 0SRD0JZ

0SPD08Z and 0SRU0J9

0SPD08Z and 0SRU0JA

0SPD08Z and 0SRU0JZ

0SPD08Z and 0SRW0J9

0SPD08Z and 0SRW0JA

0SPD08Z and 0SRW0JZ

0SPD09Z and 0SRD069

0SPD09Z and 0SRD06A

0SPD09Z and 0SRD06Z

0SPD09Z and 0SRD0J9

0SPD09Z and 0SRD0JA

0SPD09Z and 0SRD0JZ

0SPD09Z and 0SRD0L9

0SPD09Z and 0SRD0LA

0SPD09Z and 0SRD0LZ

0SPD09Z and 0SRD0MA

0SPD09Z and 0SRD0NA

0SPD09Z and 0SRU0J9

0SPD09Z and 0SRU0JA

0SPD09Z and 0SRU0JZ

0SPD09Z and 0SRW0J9

0SPD09Z and 0SRW0JA

0SPD09Z and 0SRW0JZ

0SPD09Z and 0SUW09Z

0SPD0EZ and 0SRD069

0SPD0EZ and 0SRD06Z

0SPD0EZ and 0SRD0JZ

0SPD0EZ and 0SRW0J9

0SPD0JC and 0SRD069

0SPD0JC and 0SRD06A

0SPD0JC and 0SRD06Z

0SPD0JC and 0SRD0J9

0SPD0JC and 0SRD0JA

0SPD0JC and 0SRD0JZ

0SPD0JC and 0SRD0N9

0SPD0JC and 0SRD0NA

0SPD0JC and 0SRD0NZ

0SPD0JC and 0SRU0J9

0SPD0JC and 0SRU0JA

0SPD0JC and 0SRU0JZ

0SPD0JC and 0SRW0J9

0SPD0JC and 0SRW0JA

0SPD0JC and 0SRW0JZ

0SPD0JZ and 0SRD069

0SPD0JZ and 0SRD06A

0SPD0JZ and 0SRD06Z

0SPD0JZ and 0SRD0J9

0SPD0JZ and 0SRD0JA

0SPD0JZ and 0SRD0JZ

0SPD0JZ and 0SRD0L9

0SPD0JZ and 0SRD0LA

0SPD0JZ and 0SRD0LZ

0SPD0JZ and 0SRD0MA

0SPD0JZ and 0SRD0NA

0SPD0JZ and 0SRU0J9

0SPD0JZ and 0SRU0JA

0SPD0JZ and 0SRU0JZ

0SPD0JZ and 0SRW0J9

0SPD0JZ and 0SRW0JA

0SPD0JZ and 0SRW0JZ

0SPD0LZ and 0SRD069

0SPD0LZ and 0SRD06A

0SPD0LZ and 0SRD06Z

0SPD0LZ and 0SRD0J9

0SPD0LZ and 0SRD0JZ

0SPD0LZ and 0SRD0L9

0SPD0LZ and 0SRD0LZ

0SPD0LZ and 0SRU0JA

0SPD0LZ and 0SRW0J9

0SPD0LZ and 0SRW0JA

0SPD0MZ and 0SRD069

0SPD0MZ and 0SRD06A

0SPD0MZ and 0SRD06Z

0SPD0MZ and 0SRD0J9

0SPD0MZ and 0SRD0JZ
0SPD0MZ and 0SRD0L9
0SPD0MZ and 0SRD0LZ
0SPD0MZ and 0SRU0JA
0SPD0MZ and 0SRW0J9
0SPD0MZ and 0SRW0JA
0SPD0NZ and 0SRD069
0SPD0NZ and 0SRD06A
0SPD0NZ and 0SRD06Z
0SPD0NZ and 0SRD0J9
0SPD0NZ and 0SRD0JA
0SPD0NZ and 0SRD0JZ
0SPD0NZ and 0SRD0L9
0SPD0NZ and 0SRD0LZ
0SPD0NZ and 0SRU0JA
0SPD0NZ and 0SRU0JZ
0SPD0NZ and 0SRW0J9
0SPD0NZ and 0SRW0JA
0SPD38Z and 0SRD069
0SPD38Z and 0SRD06A
0SPD38Z and 0SRD06Z
0SPD38Z and 0SRD0J9
0SPD38Z and 0SRD0JA
0SPD38Z and 0SRD0JZ
0SPD38Z and 0SRD0NA
0SPD38Z and 0SRU0J9
0SPD38Z and 0SRU0JA
0SPD38Z and 0SRU0JZ
0SPD38Z and 0SRW0J9
0SPD38Z and 0SRW0JA
0SPD38Z and 0SRW0JZ
0SPD48Z and 0SRD069
0SPD48Z and 0SRD06A
0SPD48Z and 0SRD06Z
0SPD48Z and 0SRD0J9
0SPD48Z and 0SRD0JA
0SPD48Z and 0SRD0JZ
0SPD48Z and 0SRD0NA
0SPD48Z and 0SRU0J9
0SPD48Z and 0SRU0JA
0SPD48Z and 0SRU0JZ
0SPD48Z and 0SRW0J9
0SPD48Z and 0SRW0JA
0SPD48Z and 0SRW0JZ
0SPD4JC and 0SRD069
0SPD4JC and 0SRD06A
0SPD4JC and 0SRD06Z
0SPD4JC and 0SRD0J9
0SPD4JC and 0SRD0JA
0SPD4JC and 0SRD0JZ
0SPD4JC and 0SRD0N9
0SPD4JC and 0SRD0NA
0SPD4JC and 0SRD0NZ
0SPD4JC and 0SRU0J9
0SPD4JC and 0SRU0JA
0SPD4JC and 0SRW0J9
0SPD4JC and 0SRW0JA
0SPD4JC and 0SRW0JZ
0SPD4JZ and 0SRD069
0SPD4JZ and 0SRD06A
0SPD4JZ and 0SRD06Z
0SPD4JZ and 0SRD0J9
0SPD4JZ and 0SRD0JA
0SPD4JZ and 0SRD0JZ
0SPD4JZ and 0SRD0L9
0SPD4JZ and 0SRD0LA
0SPD4JZ and 0SRD0LZ
0SPD4JZ and 0SRD0MA
0SPD4JZ and 0SRD0NA
0SPD4JZ and 0SRU0J9
0SPD4JZ and 0SRU0JA
0SPD4JZ and 0SRU0JZ
0SPD4JZ and 0SRW0J9
0SPD4JZ and 0SRW0JA
0SPD4JZ and 0SRW0JZ
0SPD4MZ and 0SRD06Z
0SPD4NZ and 0SRD069
0SPD4NZ and 0SRD06Z
0SPD4NZ and 0SRW0J9
0SPE0JZ and 0SRB019
0SPE0JZ and 0SRB01A
0SPE0JZ and 0SRB01Z
0SPE0JZ and 0SRB029
0SPE0JZ and 0SRB02A
0SPE0JZ and 0SRB02Z
0SPE0JZ and 0SRB039
0SPE0JZ and 0SRB03A
0SPE0JZ and 0SRB03Z
0SPE0JZ and 0SRB049
0SPE0JZ and 0SRB04A
0SPE0JZ and 0SRB04Z
0SPE0JZ and 0SRB069
0SPE0JZ and 0SRB06A
0SPE0JZ and 0SRB06Z
0SPE0JZ and 0SRB0EZ
0SPE0JZ and 0SRB0J9
0SPE0JZ and 0SRB0JA
0SPE0JZ and 0SRB0JZ
0SPE0JZ and 0SRE009
0SPE0JZ and 0SRE00A
0SPE0JZ and 0SRE00Z
0SPE0JZ and 0SRE019
0SPE0JZ and 0SRE01A
0SPE0JZ and 0SRE01Z
0SPE0JZ and 0SRE039
0SPE0JZ and 0SRE03A
0SPE0JZ and 0SRE03Z
0SPE0JZ and 0SRE0J9
0SPE0JZ and 0SRE0JA
0SPE0JZ and 0SRE0JZ
0SPE0JZ and 0SRS019
0SPE0JZ and 0SRS01A
0SPE0JZ and 0SRS01Z
0SPE0JZ and 0SRS039
0SPE0JZ and 0SRS03A
0SPE0JZ and 0SRS03Z
0SPE0JZ and 0SRS0J9
0SPE0JZ and 0SRS0JA
0SPE0JZ and 0SRS0JZ
0SPE4JZ and 0SRB019
0SPE4JZ and 0SRB01A
0SPE4JZ and 0SRB01Z
0SPE4JZ and 0SRB029
0SPE4JZ and 0SRB02A
0SPE4JZ and 0SRB02Z
0SPE4JZ and 0SRB039
0SPE4JZ and 0SRB03A
0SPE4JZ and 0SRB03Z
0SPE4JZ and 0SRB049
0SPE4JZ and 0SRB04A
0SPE4JZ and 0SRB04Z
0SPE4JZ and 0SRB069
0SPE4JZ and 0SRB06A
0SPE4JZ and 0SRB06Z
0SPE4JZ and 0SRB0EZ
0SPE4JZ and 0SRB0J9
0SPE4JZ and 0SRB0JA
0SPE4JZ and 0SRB0JZ
0SPE4JZ and 0SRE009
0SPE4JZ and 0SRE00A
0SPE4JZ and 0SRE00Z
0SPE4JZ and 0SRE019
0SPE4JZ and 0SRE01A
0SPE4JZ and 0SRE01Z
0SPE4JZ and 0SRE039
0SPE4JZ and 0SRE03A
0SPE4JZ and 0SRE03Z
0SPE4JZ and 0SRE0J9
0SPE4JZ and 0SRE0JA
0SPE4JZ and 0SRE0JZ
0SPE4JZ and 0SRS019
0SPE4JZ and 0SRS01A
0SPE4JZ and 0SRS01Z
0SPE4JZ and 0SRS039

0SPE4JZ and 0SRS03A
0SPE4JZ and 0SRS03Z
0SPE4JZ and 0SRS0J9
0SPE4JZ and 0SRS0JA
0SPE4JZ and 0SRS0JZ
0SPE4JZ and 0SUB09Z
0SPE4JZ and 0SUE09Z
0SPE4JZ and 0SUS09Z
0SPR0JZ and 0SR9019
0SPR0JZ and 0SR901A
0SPR0JZ and 0SR901Z
0SPR0JZ and 0SR9029
0SPR0JZ and 0SR902A
0SPR0JZ and 0SR902Z
0SPR0JZ and 0SR9039
0SPR0JZ and 0SR903A
0SPR0JZ and 0SR903Z
0SPR0JZ and 0SR9049
0SPR0JZ and 0SR904A
0SPR0JZ and 0SR904Z
0SPR0JZ and 0SR9069
0SPR0JZ and 0SR906A

0SPR0JZ and 0SR906Z
0SPR0JZ and 0SR90J9
0SPR0JZ and 0SR90JA
0SPR0JZ and 0SR90JZ
0SPR0JZ and 0SRA009
0SPR0JZ and 0SRA00A
0SPR0JZ and 0SRA00Z
0SPR0JZ and 0SRA019
0SPR0JZ and 0SRA01A
0SPR0JZ and 0SRA01Z
0SPR0JZ and 0SRA039
0SPR0JZ and 0SRA03A
0SPR0JZ and 0SRA03Z
0SPR0JZ and 0SRA0J9
0SPR0JZ and 0SRA0JA
0SPR0JZ and 0SRA0JZ
0SPR0JZ and 0SRR019
0SPR0JZ and 0SRR01A
0SPR0JZ and 0SRR01Z
0SPR0JZ and 0SRR039
0SPR0JZ and 0SRR03A
0SPR0JZ and 0SRR03Z

0SPR0JZ and 0SRR0J9
0SPR0JZ and 0SRR0JA
0SPR0JZ and 0SRR0JZ
0SPR4JZ and 0SR9019
0SPR4JZ and 0SR901A
0SPR4JZ and 0SR901Z
0SPR4JZ and 0SR9029
0SPR4JZ and 0SR902A
0SPR4JZ and 0SR902Z
0SPR4JZ and 0SR9039
0SPR4JZ and 0SR903A
0SPR4JZ and 0SR903Z
0SPR4JZ and 0SR9049
0SPR4JZ and 0SR904A
0SPR4JZ and 0SR904Z
0SPR4JZ and 0SR9069
0SPR4JZ and 0SR906A
0SPR4JZ and 0SR906Z
0SPR4JZ and 0SR90J9
0SPR4JZ and 0SR90JA
0SPR4JZ and 0SR90JZ
0SPR4JZ and 0SRA009

0SPR4JZ and 0SRA00A
0SPR4JZ and 0SRA00Z
0SPR4JZ and 0SRA019
0SPR4JZ and 0SRA01A
0SPR4JZ and 0SRA01Z
0SPR4JZ and 0SRA039
0SPR4JZ and 0SRA03A
0SPR4JZ and 0SRA03Z
0SPR4JZ and 0SRA0J9
0SPR4JZ and 0SRA0JA
0SPR4JZ and 0SRA0JZ
0SPR4JZ and 0SRR019
0SPR4JZ and 0SRR01A
0SPR4JZ and 0SRR01Z
0SPR4JZ and 0SRR039
0SPR4JZ and 0SRR03A
0SPR4JZ and 0SRR03Z
0SPR4JZ and 0SRR0J9
0SPR4JZ and 0SRR0JA
0SPR4JZ and 0SRR0JZ
0SPR4JZ and 0SU909Z
0SPR4JZ and 0SUA09Z

0SPR4JZ and 0SUR09Z
0SPS0JZ and 0SRB019
0SPS0JZ and 0SRB01A
0SPS0JZ and 0SRB01Z
0SPS0JZ and 0SRB029
0SPS0JZ and 0SRB02A
0SPS0JZ and 0SRB02Z
0SPS0JZ and 0SRB039
0SPS0JZ and 0SRB03A
0SPS0JZ and 0SRB03Z
0SPS0JZ and 0SRB049
0SPS0JZ and 0SRB04A
0SPS0JZ and 0SRB04Z
0SPS0JZ and 0SRB069
0SPS0JZ and 0SRB06A
0SPS0JZ and 0SRB06Z
0SPS0JZ and 0SRB0EZ
0SPS0JZ and 0SRB0J9
0SPS0JZ and 0SRB0JA
0SPS0JZ and 0SRB0JZ
0SPS0JZ and 0SRE009
0SPS0JZ and 0SRE00A

0SPS0JZ and 0SRE00Z
0SPS0JZ and 0SRE019
0SPS0JZ and 0SRE01A
0SPS0JZ and 0SRE01Z
0SPS0JZ and 0SRE039
0SPS0JZ and 0SRE03A
0SPS0JZ and 0SRE03Z
0SPS0JZ and 0SRE0J9
0SPS0JZ and 0SRE0JA
0SPS0JZ and 0SRE0JZ
0SPS0JZ and 0SRS019
0SPS0JZ and 0SRS01A
0SPS0JZ and 0SRS01Z
0SPS0JZ and 0SRS039
0SPS0JZ and 0SRS03A
0SPS0JZ and 0SRS03Z
0SPS0JZ and 0SRS0J9
0SPS0JZ and 0SRS0JA
0SPS0JZ and 0SRS0JZ
0SPS4JZ and 0SRB019
0SPS4JZ and 0SRB01A
0SPS4JZ and 0SRB01Z

0SPS4JZ and 0SRB029
0SPS4JZ and 0SRB02A
0SPS4JZ and 0SRB02Z
0SPS4JZ and 0SRB039
0SPS4JZ and 0SRB03A
0SPS4JZ and 0SRB03Z
0SPS4JZ and 0SRB049
0SPS4JZ and 0SRB04A
0SPS4JZ and 0SRB04Z
0SPS4JZ and 0SRB069
0SPS4JZ and 0SRB06A
0SPS4JZ and 0SRB06Z
0SPS4JZ and 0SRB0EZ
0SPS4JZ and 0SRB0J9
0SPS4JZ and 0SRB0JA
0SPS4JZ and 0SRB0JZ
0SPS4JZ and 0SRE009
0SPS4JZ and 0SRE00A
0SPS4JZ and 0SRE00Z
0SPS4JZ and 0SRE019
0SPS4JZ and 0SRE01A
0SPS4JZ and 0SRE01Z

0SPS4JZ and 0SRE039
0SPS4JZ and 0SRE03A
0SPS4JZ and 0SRE03Z
0SPS4JZ and 0SRE0J9
0SPS4JZ and 0SRE0JA
0SPS4JZ and 0SRE0JZ
0SPS4JZ and 0SRS019
0SPS4JZ and 0SRS01A
0SPS4JZ and 0SRS01Z
0SPS4JZ and 0SRS039
0SPS4JZ and 0SRS03A
0SPS4JZ and 0SRS03Z
0SPS4JZ and 0SRS0J9
0SPS4JZ and 0SRS0JA
0SPS4JZ and 0SRS0JZ
0SPS4JZ and 0SUB09Z
0SPS4JZ and 0SUE09Z
0SPS4JZ and 0SUS09Z
0SPT0JZ and 0SRC069
0SPT0JZ and 0SRC06A
0SPT0JZ and 0SRC06Z
0SPT0JZ and 0SRC0J9
0SPT0JZ and 0SRC0JA
0SPT0JZ and 0SRC0JZ
0SPT0JZ and 0SRC0N9
0SPT0JZ and 0SRC0NA
0SPT0JZ and 0SRC0NZ
0SPT0JZ and 0SRT0J9
0SPT0JZ and 0SRT0JA
0SPT0JZ and 0SRT0JZ
0SPT0JZ and 0SRV0J9
0SPT0JZ and 0SRV0JA
0SPT0JZ and 0SRV0JZ
0SPT4JZ and 0SRC069
0SPT4JZ and 0SRC06A
0SPT4JZ and 0SRC06Z
0SPT4JZ and 0SRC0J9
0SPT4JZ and 0SRC0JA
0SPT4JZ and 0SRC0JZ
0SPT4JZ and 0SRC0N9
0SPT4JZ and 0SRC0NA
0SPT4JZ and 0SRC0NZ
0SPT4JZ and 0SRT0J9
0SPT4JZ and 0SRT0JA
0SPT4JZ and 0SRV0J9
0SPT4JZ and 0SRV0JA
0SPU0JZ and 0SRD069
0SPU0JZ and 0SRD06A
0SPU0JZ and 0SRD06Z
0SPU0JZ and 0SRD0J9
0SPU0JZ and 0SRD0JA
0SPU0JZ and 0SRD0JZ
0SPU0JZ and 0SRD0N9
0SPU0JZ and 0SRD0NA
0SPU0JZ and 0SRD0NZ
0SPU0JZ and 0SRU0J9
0SPU0JZ and 0SRU0JA
0SPU0JZ and 0SRU0JZ
0SPU0JZ and 0SRW0J9
0SPU0JZ and 0SRW0JA
0SPU0JZ and 0SRW0JZ
0SPU4JZ and 0SRD069
0SPU4JZ and 0SRD06A
0SPU4JZ and 0SRD06Z
0SPU4JZ and 0SRD0EZ
0SPU4JZ and 0SRD0J9
0SPU4JZ and 0SRD0JA
0SPU4JZ and 0SRD0JZ
0SPU4JZ and 0SRD0N9
0SPU4JZ and 0SRD0NA
0SPU4JZ and 0SRD0NZ
0SPU4JZ and 0SRU0J9
0SPU4JZ and 0SRU0JA
0SPU4JZ and 0SRW0J9
0SPU4JZ and 0SRW0JA
0SPU4JZ and 0SRW0JZ
0SPV0JZ and 0SRC069
0SPV0JZ and 0SRC06A
0SPV0JZ and 0SRC06Z
0SPV0JZ and 0SRC0J9
0SPV0JZ and 0SRC0JA
0SPV0JZ and 0SRC0JZ
0SPV0JZ and 0SRC0NA
0SPV0JZ and 0SRT0J9
0SPV0JZ and 0SRT0JA
0SPV0JZ and 0SRT0JZ
0SPV0JZ and 0SRV0J9
0SPV0JZ and 0SRV0JA
0SPV0JZ and 0SRV0JZ
0SPV4JZ and 0SRC069
0SPV4JZ and 0SRC06A
0SPV4JZ and 0SRC06Z
0SPV4JZ and 0SRC0J9
0SPV4JZ and 0SRC0JA
0SPV4JZ and 0SRC0JZ
0SPV4JZ and 0SRC0N9
0SPV4JZ and 0SRC0NA
0SPV4JZ and 0SRC0NZ
0SPV4JZ and 0SRT0J9
0SPV4JZ and 0SRT0JA
0SPV4JZ and 0SRV0J9
0SPV4JZ and 0SRV0JA
0SPW0JZ and 0SRD069
0SPW0JZ and 0SRD06A
0SPW0JZ and 0SRD06Z
0SPW0JZ and 0SRD0J9
0SPW0JZ and 0SRD0JA
0SPW0JZ and 0SRD0JZ
0SPW0JZ and 0SRD0NA
0SPW0JZ and 0SRU0J9
0SPW0JZ and 0SRU0JA
0SPW0JZ and 0SRU0JZ
0SPW0JZ and 0SRW0J9
0SPW0JZ and 0SRW0JA
0SPW0JZ and 0SRW0JZ
0SPW4JZ and 0SRD069
0SPW4JZ and 0SRD06A
0SPW4JZ and 0SRD06Z
0SPW4JZ and 0SRD0J9
0SPW4JZ and 0SRD0JA
0SPW4JZ and 0SRD0JZ
0SPW4JZ and 0SRD0NA
0SPW4JZ and 0SRD0NZ
0SPW4JZ and 0SRU0J9
0SPW4JZ and 0SRU0JA
0SPW4JZ and 0SRW0J9
0SPW4JZ and 0SRW0JA
0SPW4JZ and 0SRW0JZ
0SR9019 and 0SP90EZ
0SR901Z and 0SP90EZ
0SR9029 and 0SP90EZ
0SR902Z and 0SP90EZ
0SR903Z and 0SP90EZ
0SR9049 and 0SP90EZ
0SR9069 and 0SP90EZ
0SR906Z and 0SP90EZ
0SR90EZ and 0SP908Z
0SR90EZ and 0SP909Z
0SR90EZ and 0SP90BZ
0SR90EZ and 0SP90JZ
0SR90EZ and 0SP948Z
0SR90EZ and 0SP94JZ
0SR90EZ and 0SPA0JZ
0SR90EZ and 0SPA4JZ
0SR90EZ and 0SPR0JZ
0SR90EZ and 0SPR4JZ
0SR90JA and 0SP90EZ
0SRA00A and 0SP90EZ
0SRA01A and 0SP90EZ
0SRA03A and 0SP90EZ
0SRA0J9 and 0SP90EZ
0SRA0JZ and 0SP90EZ
0SRB01A and 0SPB0EZ
0SRB02A and 0SPB0EZ

0SRB0EZ and 0SPB08Z
0SRB0EZ and 0SPB09Z
0SRB0J9 and 0SPB0EZ
0SRB0JZ and 0SPB0EZ
0SRC069 and 0SPC4LZ
0SRC06A and 0SPC0EZ
0SRC06A and 0SPC0LZ
0SRC06A and 0SPC4LZ
0SRC06A and 0SPC4MZ
0SRC06A and 0SPC4NZ
0SRC06Z and 0SPC0EZ
0SRC06Z and 0SPC0LZ
0SRC06Z and 0SPC0MZ
0SRC06Z and 0SPC0NZ
0SRC06Z and 0SPC4LZ
0SRC06Z and 0SPC4MZ
0SRC06Z and 0SPC4NZ
0SRC0EZ and 0SPC08Z
0SRC0EZ and 0SPC09Z
0SRC0EZ and 0SPC0JZ
0SRC0EZ and 0SPC38Z
0SRC0EZ and 0SPC48Z
0SRC0EZ and 0SPC4JC
0SRC0EZ and 0SPC4JZ
0SRC0EZ and 0SPT0JZ
0SRC0EZ and 0SPT4JZ
0SRC0EZ and 0SPV0JZ
0SRC0EZ and 0SPV4JZ
0SRC0J9 and 0SPC0EZ
0SRC0J9 and 0SPC0LZ
0SRC0J9 and 0SPC4LZ
0SRC0JA and 0SPC0EZ
0SRC0JA and 0SPC0LZ
0SRC0JA and 0SPC0MZ
0SRC0JA and 0SPC0NZ
0SRC0JA and 0SPC4LZ
0SRC0JA and 0SPC4MZ
0SRC0JA and 0SPC4NZ
0SRC0JZ and 0SPC0EZ
0SRC0JZ and 0SPC4LZ
0SRC0L9 and 0SPC0LZ
0SRC0L9 and 0SPC4LZ
0SRC0L9 and 0SPC4NZ
0SRC0LA and 0SPC0LZ
0SRC0LA and 0SPC0MZ
0SRC0LA and 0SPC0NZ
0SRC0LA and 0SPC4LZ
0SRC0LA and 0SPC4MZ
0SRC0LA and 0SPC4NZ
0SRC0LZ and 0SPC0LZ
0SRC0LZ and 0SPC4LZ
0SRC0M9 and 0SPC0JZ
0SRC0M9 and 0SPC4JZ
0SRC0MA and 0SPC09Z
0SRC0MA and 0SPC0JZ
0SRC0MA and 0SPC4JZ
0SRC0MZ and 0SPC4JZ
0SRC0N9 and 0SPC08Z
0SRC0N9 and 0SPC09Z
0SRC0N9 and 0SPC0JZ
0SRC0N9 and 0SPC38Z
0SRC0N9 and 0SPC4JZ
0SRC0N9 and 0SPV0JZ
0SRC0NZ and 0SPC08Z
0SRC0NZ and 0SPC0JZ
0SRC0NZ and 0SPC38Z
0SRC0NZ and 0SPC4JZ
0SRC0NZ and 0SPV0JZ
0SRD069 and 0SPD4LZ
0SRD069 and 0SPD4MZ
0SRD06A and 0SPD0EZ
0SRD06A and 0SPD4LZ
0SRD06A and 0SPD4MZ
0SRD06A and 0SPD4NZ
0SRD06Z and 0SPD4LZ
0SRD0EZ and 0SPD08Z
0SRD0EZ and 0SPD09Z
0SRD0EZ and 0SPD0JC
0SRD0EZ and 0SPD0JZ
0SRD0EZ and 0SPD38Z
0SRD0EZ and 0SPD48Z
0SRD0EZ and 0SPD4JC
0SRD0EZ and 0SPD4JZ
0SRD0EZ and 0SPU0JZ
0SRD0EZ and 0SPW0JZ
0SRD0EZ and 0SPW4JZ
0SRD0J9 and 0SPD0EZ
0SRD0J9 and 0SPD4LZ
0SRD0J9 and 0SPD4MZ
0SRD0J9 and 0SPD4NZ
0SRD0JA and 0SPD0EZ
0SRD0JA and 0SPD0LZ
0SRD0JA and 0SPD0MZ
0SRD0JA and 0SPD4LZ
0SRD0JA and 0SPD4MZ
0SRD0JA and 0SPD4NZ
0SRD0JZ and 0SPD4LZ
0SRD0JZ and 0SPD4MZ
0SRD0JZ and 0SPD4NZ
0SRD0L9 and 0SPD4LZ
0SRD0L9 and 0SPD4MZ
0SRD0L9 and 0SPD4NZ
0SRD0LA and 0SPD0LZ
0SRD0LA and 0SPD0MZ
0SRD0LA and 0SPD0NZ
0SRD0LA and 0SPD4LZ
0SRD0LA and 0SPD4MZ
0SRD0LA and 0SPD4NZ
0SRD0LZ and 0SPD4LZ
0SRD0LZ and 0SPD4MZ
0SRD0LZ and 0SPD4NZ
0SRD0M9 and 0SPD09Z
0SRD0M9 and 0SPD0JZ
0SRD0M9 and 0SPD4JZ
0SRD0MZ and 0SPD09Z
0SRD0MZ and 0SPD0JZ
0SRD0MZ and 0SPD4JZ
0SRD0N9 and 0SPD08Z
0SRD0N9 and 0SPD09Z
0SRD0N9 and 0SPD0JZ
0SRD0N9 and 0SPD38Z
0SRD0N9 and 0SPD48Z
0SRD0N9 and 0SPD4JZ
0SRD0N9 and 0SPW0JZ
0SRD0N9 and 0SPW4JZ
0SRD0NA and 0SPD08Z
0SRD0NZ and 0SPD08Z
0SRD0NZ and 0SPD09Z
0SRD0NZ and 0SPD0JZ
0SRD0NZ and 0SPD38Z
0SRD0NZ and 0SPD48Z
0SRD0NZ and 0SPD4JZ
0SRD0NZ and 0SPW0JZ
0SRE009 and 0SPB0EZ
0SRE019 and 0SPB0EZ
0SRE01Z and 0SPB0EZ
0SRE039 and 0SPB0EZ
0SRE03Z and 0SPB0EZ
0SRE0JA and 0SPB0EZ
0SRR019 and 0SP90EZ
0SRR01Z and 0SP90EZ
0SRR039 and 0SP90EZ
0SRR03Z and 0SP90EZ
0SRR0JA and 0SP90EZ
0SRS019 and 0SPB0EZ
0SRS01Z and 0SPB0EZ
0SRT0J9 and 0SPC4LZ
0SRT0JA and 0SPC0EZ
0SRT0JA and 0SPC0LZ
0SRT0JA and 0SPC0NZ
0SRT0JA and 0SPC4LZ
0SRT0JA and 0SPC4MZ
0SRT0JA and 0SPC4NZ
0SRT0JZ and 0SPC0EZ

0SRT0JZ
and 0SPC4LZ

0SRU0J9
and 0SPD0EZ

0SRU0J9
and 0SPD0LZ

0SRU0J9
and 0SPD0MZ

0SRU0J9
and 0SPD0NZ

0SRU0J9
and 0SPD4LZ

0SRU0J9
and 0SPD4MZ

0SRU0J9
and 0SPD4NZ

0SRU0JA
and 0SPD0EZ

0SRU0JA
and 0SPD4LZ

0SRU0JA
and 0SPD4MZ

0SRU0JA
and 0SPD4NZ

0SRU0JZ
and 0SPD0EZ

0SRU0JZ
and 0SPD0LZ

0SRU0JZ
and 0SPD0MZ

0SRU0JZ
and 0SPD4LZ

0SRU0JZ
and 0SPD4MZ

0SRU0JZ
and 0SPD4NZ

0SRV0J9
and 0SPC0EZ

0SRV0J9
and 0SPC0LZ

0SRV0J9
and 0SPC0MZ

0SRV0J9
and 0SPC0NZ

0SRV0J9
and 0SPC4LZ

0SRV0J9
and 0SPC4MZ

0SRV0J9
and 0SPC4NZ

0SRV0JA
and 0SPC0EZ

0SRV0JA
and 0SPC0LZ

0SRV0JA
and 0SPC4LZ

0SRV0JA
and 0SPC4MZ

0SRV0JA
and 0SPC4NZ

0SRV0JZ
and 0SPC0EZ

0SRV0JZ
and 0SPC0LZ

0SRV0JZ
and 0SPC0MZ

0SRV0JZ
and 0SPC0NZ

0SRV0JZ
and 0SPC4LZ

0SRV0JZ
and 0SPC4MZ

0SRV0JZ
and 0SPC4NZ

0SRW0J9
and 0SPD4LZ

0SRW0J9
and 0SPD4MZ

0SRW0JA
and 0SPD0EZ

0SRW0JA
and 0SPD4LZ

0SRW0JA
and 0SPD4MZ

0SRW0JA
and 0SPD4NZ

0SRW0JZ
and 0SPD0EZ

0SRW0JZ
and 0SPD0LZ

0SRW0JZ
and 0SPD0MZ

0SRW0JZ
and 0SPD0NZ

0SRW0JZ
and 0SPD4LZ

0SRW0JZ
and 0SPD4MZ
0SRW0JZ
and 0SPD4NZ

0SUR09Z
and 0SP90EZ

0SUS09Z
and 0SPB0EZ

0TQB0ZZ
and 0WQFXZ2

0TQB0ZZ
and 0WQFXZZ

0TQB3ZZ
and 0WQFXZ2

0TQB3ZZ
and 0WQFXZZ

0TQB4ZZ
and 0WQFXZ2

0TQB4ZZ
and 0WQFXZZ

0TTB0ZZ
and 0TTD0ZZ
and 0UT20ZZ
and 0UT70ZZ
and 0UT90ZZ
and 0UTC0ZZ
and 0UTG0ZZ

0TY00Z0
and 0FYG0Z0

0TY00Z0
and 0FYG0Z1

0TY00Z0
and 0FYG0Z2

0TY00Z1
and 0FYG0Z0

0TY00Z1
and 0FYG0Z1

0TY00Z1
and 0FYG0Z2

0TY00Z2
and 0FYG0Z0

0TY00Z2
and 0FYG0Z1

0TY00Z2
and 0FYG0Z2

0TY10Z0
and 0FYG0Z0

0TY10Z0
and 0FYG0Z1

0TY10Z0
and 0FYG0Z2

0TY10Z1
and 0FYG0Z0

0TY10Z1
and 0FYG0Z1

0TY10Z1
and 0FYG0Z2

0TY10Z2
and 0FYG0Z0

0TY10Z2
and 0FYG0Z1

0TY10Z2
and 0FYG0Z2

0UT40ZZ
and 0UT90ZZ
and 0UTC0ZZ

0UT44ZZ
and 0UT94ZZ
and 0UTC4ZZ

0UT44ZZ
and 0UT9FZZ
and 0UTC4ZZ

0UT47ZZ
and 0UT97ZZ
and 0UTC7ZZ

0UT47ZZ
and 0UT97ZZ
and 0UTC8ZZ

0UT47ZZ
and 0UT98ZZ
and 0UTC7ZZ

0UT47ZZ
and 0UT98ZZ
and 0UTC8ZZ

0UT48ZZ
and 0UT97ZZ
and 0UTC7ZZ

0UT48ZZ
and 0UT97ZZ
and 0UTC8ZZ

0UT48ZZ
and 0UT98ZZ
and 0UTC7ZZ

0UT48ZZ
and 0UT98ZZ
and 0UTC8ZZ

0VT00ZZ
and 0VT30ZZ

0VT00ZZ
and 0VT34ZZ

0VT04ZZ
and 0VT30ZZ

0VT04ZZ
and 0VT34ZZ

0VT07ZZ
and 0VT30ZZ

0VT07ZZ
and 0VT34ZZ

0VT08ZZ
and 0VT30ZZ

0VT08ZZ
and 0VT34ZZ

APPENDIX G: COMBINATION CLUSTERS

no expected impact on MS-DRG payment, may be included in procedure
procedures typically not done in OR
at lowest level of resource utilization

Appendix H: Non-OR Procedure Not Affecting MS-DRG Assignment

001607A
00160JA
00160KA
001637A
00163JA
00163KA
001647A
00164JA
00164KA
0020X0Z
0020XYZ
002EX0Z
002EXYZ
002UX0Z
002UXYZ
005F0ZZ
005F3ZZ
005F4ZZ
005G0ZZ
005G3ZZ
005G4ZZ
005H0ZZ
005H3ZZ
005H4ZZ
005J0ZZ
005J3ZZ
005J4ZZ
005K0ZZ
005K3ZZ
005K4ZZ
005L0ZZ
005L3ZZ
005L4ZZ
005M0ZZ
005M3ZZ
005M4ZZ
005N0ZZ
005N3ZZ
005N4ZZ
005P0ZZ
005P3ZZ
005P4ZZ
005Q0ZZ
005Q3ZZ
005Q4ZZ
005R0ZZ
005R3ZZ
005R4ZZ
005S0ZZ
005S3ZZ
005S4ZZ
00903ZX
00904ZX
00913ZX
00914ZX
00923ZX
00924ZX
00933ZX
00934ZX
00943ZX
00944ZX
00953ZX
00954ZX
00963ZX
00964ZX
00973ZX
00974ZX
00983ZX
00984ZX
00993ZX
00994ZX
009A3ZX
009A4ZX
009B3ZX
009B4ZX
009C3ZX
009C4ZX
009D3ZX
009D4ZX
009F3ZX
009F4ZX
009G3ZX
009G4ZX
009H3ZX
009H4ZX
009J3ZX
009J4ZX
009K3ZX
009K4ZX
009L3ZX
009L4ZX
009M3ZX
009M4ZX
009N3ZX
009N4ZX
009P3ZX
009P4ZX
009Q3ZX
009Q4ZX
009R3ZX
009R4ZX
009S3ZX
009S4ZX
009T30Z
009T3ZX
009T3ZZ
009U30Z
009U3ZX
009U3ZZ
009U40Z
009U4ZX
009U4ZZ
009W30Z
009W3ZX
009W3ZZ
009X30Z
009X3ZX
009X3ZZ
009Y30Z
009Y3ZX
009Y3ZZ
00BF3ZX
00BF4ZX
00BG3ZX
00BG4ZX
00BH3ZX
00BH4ZX
00BJ3ZX
00BJ4ZX
00BK3ZX
00BK4ZX
00BL3ZX
00BL4ZX
00BM3ZX
00BM4ZX
00BN3ZX
00BN4ZX
00BP3ZX
00BP4ZX
00BQ3ZX
00BQ4ZX
00BR3ZX
00BR4ZX
00BS3ZX
00BS4ZX
00F3XZZ
00F4XZZ
00F5XZZ
00F6XZZ
00HE32Z
00HE3YZ
00HE4YZ
00HU03Z
00HU32Z
00HU33Z
00HU3YZ
00HU43Z
00HU4YZ
00HV03Z
00HV32Z
00HV33Z
00HV43Z
00J03ZZ
00JE3ZZ
00JU3ZZ
00JV3ZZ
00P030Z
00P032Z
00P033Z
00P03YZ
00P04YZ
00P0X0Z
00P0X2Z
00P0X3Z
00P0XMZ
00P630Z
00P632Z
00P633Z
00P63YZ
00P64YZ
00P6X0Z
00P6X2Z
00P6X3Z
00P6XMZ
00PE30Z
00PE32Z
00PE33Z
00PE3YZ
00PE4YZ
00PEX0Z
00PEX2Z
00PEX3Z
00PEXMZ
00PU30Z
00PU32Z
00PU33Z
00PU3YZ
00PU4YZ
00PUX0Z
00PUX2Z
00PUX3Z
00PUXMZ
00PV30Z
00PV32Z
00PV33Z
00PV3YZ
00PV4YZ
00PVX0Z
00PVX2Z
00PVX3Z
00PVXMZ
00W03YZ
00W04YZ
00W0X0Z
00W0X2Z
00W0X3Z
00W0X7Z
00W0XJZ
00W0XKZ
00W0XMZ
00W63YZ
00W64YZ
00W6X0Z
00W6X2Z
00W6X3Z
00W6XJZ
00W6XMZ
00WE3YZ
00WE4YZ
00WEX0Z
00WEX2Z
00WEX3Z
00WEX7Z
00WEXMZ
00WU3YZ
00WU4YZ
00WUX0Z
00WUX2Z
00WUX3Z
00WUXJZ
00WUXMZ
00WV3YZ
00WV4YZ
00WVX0Z
00WVX2Z
00WVX3Z
00WVX7Z
00WVXJZ
00WVXKZ
00WVXMZ
012YX0Z
012YXYZ
01500ZZ
01503ZZ
01504ZZ
01513ZZ
01520ZZ
01523ZZ
01524ZZ
01530ZZ
01533ZZ
01534ZZ
01540ZZ
01543ZZ
01544ZZ
01550ZZ
01553ZZ
01554ZZ
01560ZZ
01563ZZ
01564ZZ
01583ZZ
01590ZZ
01593ZZ
01594ZZ
015A0ZZ
015A3ZZ
015A4ZZ
015B3ZZ
015C0ZZ
015C3ZZ
015C4ZZ
015D0ZZ
015D3ZZ
015D4ZZ
015F0ZZ
015F3ZZ
015F4ZZ
015G0ZZ
015G3ZZ
015G4ZZ
015H0ZZ
015H3ZZ
015H4ZZ
015Q0ZZ
015Q3ZZ
015Q4ZZ
015R3ZZ
019030Z
01903ZX
01903ZZ
01904ZX
019130Z
01913ZX
01913ZZ
01914ZX
019230Z
01923ZX
01923ZZ
01924ZX
019330Z
01933ZX
01933ZZ
01934ZX
019430Z
01943ZX
01943ZZ
01944ZX
019530Z
01953ZX
01953ZZ
01954ZX
019630Z
01963ZX
01963ZZ
01964ZX
019830Z
01983ZX
01983ZZ
01984ZX
019930Z
01993ZX
01993ZZ
01994ZX
019A30Z
019A3ZX
019A3ZZ
019A4ZX
019B30Z
019B3ZX
019B3ZZ
019B4ZX
019C30Z
019C3ZX
019C3ZZ
019C4ZX
019D30Z
019D3ZX
019D3ZZ
019D4ZX
019F30Z
019F3ZX
019F3ZZ
019F4ZX
019G30Z
019G3ZX
019G3ZZ
019G4ZX
019H30Z
019H3ZX
019H3ZZ
019H4ZX
019K30Z
019K3ZZ
019L30Z
019L3ZZ
019M30Z
019M3ZZ
019N30Z
019N3ZZ
019P30Z
019P3ZZ
019Q30Z
019Q3ZX
019Q3ZZ
019Q4ZX
019R30Z
019R3ZX
019R3ZZ
019R4ZX
01B03ZX
01B04ZX
01B13ZX
01B14ZX
01B23ZX
01B24ZX
01B33ZX
01B34ZX
01B43ZX
01B44ZX
01B53ZX
01B54ZX
01B63ZX
01B64ZX
01B83ZX
01B84ZX
01B93ZX
01B94ZX
01BA3ZX
01BA4ZX
01BB3ZX
01BB4ZX
01BC3ZX
01BC4ZX
01BD3ZX
01BD4ZX
01BF3ZX
01BF4ZX
01BG3ZX
01BG4ZX
01BH3ZX
01BH4ZX
01BQ3ZX
01BQ4ZX
01BR3ZX
01BR4ZX
01HY3YZ
01HY4YZ
01JY3ZZ
01PY30Z
01PY32Z
01PY3YZ
01PY4YZ
01PYX0Z
01PYX2Z
01PYXMZ
01WY3YZ
01WY4YZ
01WYX0Z
01WYX2Z
01WYX7Z
01WYXMZ
021W08A
021W09A
021W0AA
021W0JA
021W0KA
021W0ZA
021W48A
021W49A
021W4AA
021W4JA
021W4KA
021W4ZA
021X08A
021X09A
021X0AA
021X0JA
021X0KA
021X0ZA
021X48A
021X49A
021X4AA
021X4JA
021X4KA
021X4ZA
02B40ZX
02B43ZX
02B44ZX
02B50ZX
02B53ZX
02B54ZX
02B60ZX
02B63ZX
02B64ZX
02B70ZX
02B73ZX
02B74ZX
02B80ZX
02B83ZX
02B84ZX
02B90ZX
02B93ZX
02B94ZX
02BD0ZX
02BD3ZX
02BD4ZX
02BF0ZX
02BF3ZX
02BF4ZX
02BG0ZX
02BG3ZX
02BG4ZX
02BH0ZX
02BH3ZX
02BH4ZX
02BJ0ZX
02BJ3ZX
02BJ4ZX
02BK0ZX
02BK3ZX
02BK4ZX
02BL0ZX
02BL3ZX
02BL4ZX
02BM0ZX
02BM3ZX
02BM4ZX
02FNXZZ
02H00DZ
02H00YZ
02H03DZ
02H03YZ
02H04DZ
02H04YZ
02H10DZ
02H10YZ
02H13DZ
02H13YZ
02H14DZ
02H14YZ
02H20DZ
02H20YZ

02H23DZ	02HW43Z	02U24JZ	031509W	03950ZZ	039D40Z	039P30Z	03H203Z	03HP03Z
02H23YZ	02HX00Z	02U24KZ	03150AW	039530Z	039D4ZZ	039P3ZX	03H233Z	03HP33Z
02H24DZ	02HX03Z	02U307Z	03150JW	03953ZX	039F00Z	039P3ZZ	03H243Z	03HP43Z
02H24YZ	02HX30Z	02U308Z	03150KW	03953ZZ	039F0ZZ	039P40Z	03H303Z	03HQ03Z
02H30DZ	02HX33Z	02U30JZ	03150ZW	039540Z	039F30Z	039P4ZZ	03H333Z	03HQ33Z
02H30YZ	02HX40Z	02U30KZ	031609W	03954ZZ	039F3ZX	039Q00Z	03H343Z	03HQ43Z
02H33DZ	02HX43Z	02U337Z	03160AW	039600Z	039F3ZZ	039Q0ZZ	03H403Z	03HR03Z
02H33YZ	02JA3ZZ	02U338Z	03160JW	03960ZZ	039F40Z	039Q30Z	03H433Z	03HR33Z
02H34DZ	02JY3ZZ	02U33JZ	03160KW	039630Z	039F4ZZ	039Q3ZX	03H443Z	03HR43Z
02H34YZ	02PA32Z	02U33KZ	03160ZW	03963ZX	039G00Z	039Q3ZZ	03H503Z	03HS03Z
02H432Z	02PA33Z	02U347Z	031709W	03963ZZ	039G0ZZ	039Q40Z	03H533Z	03HS33Z
02H433Z	02PA3DZ	02U348Z	03170AW	039640Z	039G30Z	039Q4ZZ	03H543Z	03HS43Z
02H632Z	02PA3YZ	02U34JZ	03170JW	03964ZZ	039G3ZX	039R00Z	03H603Z	03HT03Z
02H633Z	02PA4YZ	02U34KZ	03170KW	039700Z	039G3ZZ	039R0ZZ	03H633Z	03HT33Z
02H732Z	02PAX2Z	02WA32Z	03170ZW	03970ZZ	039G40Z	039R30Z	03H643Z	03HT43Z
02H733Z	02PAX3Z	02WA33Z	031809W	039730Z	039G4ZZ	039R3ZX	03H703Z	03HU03Z
02HK30Z	02PAXDZ	02WA3DZ	03180AW	03973ZX	039H00Z	039R3ZZ	03H733Z	03HU33Z
02HK33Z	02PAXMZ	02WA3YZ	03180JW	03973ZZ	039H0ZZ	039R40Z	03H743Z	03HU43Z
02HL32Z	02PY32Z	02WA4YZ	03180KW	039740Z	039H30Z	039R4ZZ	03H803Z	03HV03Z
02HL33Z	02PY33Z	02WAX2Z	03180ZW	03974ZZ	039H3ZX	039S00Z	03H833Z	03HV33Z
02HN32Z	02PY3DZ	02WAX3Z	03193ZF	039800Z	039H3ZZ	039S0ZZ	03H843Z	03HV43Z
02HP00Z	02PY3YZ	02WAX7Z	031A3ZF	03980ZZ	039H40Z	039S30Z	03H903Z	03HY03Z
02HP02Z	02PY4YZ	02WAX8Z	031B3ZF	039830Z	039H4ZZ	039S3ZX	03H933Z	03HY32Z
02HP03Z	02PYX2Z	02WAXCZ	031C3ZF	03983ZX	039J00Z	039S3ZZ	03H943Z	03HY33Z
02HP30Z	02PYX3Z	02WAXDZ	039000Z	03983ZZ	039J0ZZ	039S40Z	03HA03Z	03HY3YZ
02HP32Z	02PYXDZ	02WAXJZ	03900ZZ	039840Z	039J30Z	039S4ZZ	03HA33Z	03HY43Z
02HP33Z	02U007Z	02WAXKZ	039030Z	03984ZZ	039J3ZX	039T00Z	03HA43Z	03HY4YZ
02HP40Z	02U008Z	02WAXMZ	03903ZX	039900Z	039J3ZZ	039T0ZZ	03HB03Z	03JY3ZZ
02HP42Z	02U00JZ	02WAXNZ	03903ZZ	03990ZZ	039J40Z	039T30Z	03HB33Z	03JY4ZZ
02HP43Z	02U00KZ	02WAXQZ	039040Z	039930Z	039J4ZZ	039T3ZX	03HB43Z	03JYXZZ
02HQ02Z	02U037Z	02WAXRS	03904ZZ	03993ZX	039K00Z	039T3ZZ	03HC03Z	03PY30Z
02HQ03Z	02U038Z	02WAXRZ	039100Z	03993ZZ	039K0ZZ	039T40Z	03HC33Z	03PY32Z
02HQ32Z	02U03JZ	02WY32Z	03910ZZ	039940Z	039K30Z	039T4ZZ	03HC43Z	03PY33Z
02HQ33Z	02U03KZ	02WY33Z	039130Z	03994ZZ	039K3ZX	039U00Z	03HD03Z	03PY3DZ
02HQ42Z	02U047Z	02WY3DZ	03913ZX	039A00Z	039K3ZZ	039U0ZZ	03HD33Z	03PY3YZ
02HQ43Z	02U048Z	02WY3YZ	03913ZZ	039A0ZZ	039K40Z	039U30Z	03HD43Z	03PY4YZ
02HR02Z	02U04JZ	02WY4YZ	039140Z	039A30Z	039K4ZZ	039U3ZX	03HF03Z	03PYX0Z
02HR03Z	02U04KZ	02WYX2Z	03914ZZ	039A3ZX	039L00Z	039U3ZZ	03HF33Z	03PYX2Z
02HR32Z	02U107Z	02WYX3Z	039200Z	039A3ZZ	039L0ZZ	039U40Z	03HF43Z	03PYX3Z
02HR33Z	02U108Z	02WYX7Z	03920ZZ	039A40Z	039L30Z	039U4ZZ	03HG03Z	03PYXDZ
02HR42Z	02U10JZ	02WYX8Z	039230Z	039A4ZZ	039L3ZX	039V00Z	03HG33Z	03PYXMZ
02HR43Z	02U10KZ	02WYXCZ	03923ZX	039B00Z	039L3ZZ	039V0ZZ	03HG43Z	03VG0HZ
02HS03Z	02U137Z	02WYXDZ	03923ZZ	039B0ZZ	039L40Z	039V30Z	03HH03Z	03VG3HZ
02HS32Z	02U138Z	02WYXJZ	039240Z	039B30Z	039L4ZZ	039V3ZX	03HH33Z	03VG4HZ
02HS33Z	02U13JZ	02WYXKZ	03924ZZ	039B3ZX	039M00Z	039V3ZZ	03HH43Z	03VH0HZ
02HS43Z	02U13KZ	031209W	039300Z	039B3ZZ	039M0ZZ	039V40Z	03HJ03Z	03VH3HZ
02HT03Z	02U147Z	03120AW	03930ZZ	039B40Z	039M30Z	039V4ZZ	03HJ33Z	03VH4HZ
02HT32Z	02U148Z	03120JW	039330Z	039B4ZZ	039M3ZX	039Y00Z	03HJ43Z	03VJ0HZ
02HT33Z	02U14JZ	03120KW	03933ZX	039C00Z	039M3ZZ	039Y0ZZ	03HK03Z	03VJ3HZ
02HT43Z	02U14KZ	03120ZW	03933ZZ	039C0ZZ	039M40Z	039Y30Z	03HK33Z	03VJ4HZ
02HV03Z	02U207Z	031309W	039340Z	039C30Z	039M4ZZ	039Y3ZX	03HK43Z	03VK0HZ
02HV32Z	02U208Z	03130AW	03934ZZ	039C3ZX	039N00Z	039Y3ZZ	03HL03Z	03VK3HZ
02HV33Z	02U20JZ	03130JW	039400Z	039C3ZZ	039N0ZZ	039Y40Z	03HL33Z	03VK4HZ
02HV43Z	02U20KZ	03130KW	03940ZZ	039C40Z	039N30Z	039Y4ZZ	03HL43Z	03VL0HZ
02HW00Z	02U237Z	03130ZW	039430Z	039C4ZZ	039N3ZX	03H003Z	03HM03Z	03VL3HZ
02HW03Z	02U238Z	031409W	03943ZX	039D00Z	039N3ZZ	03H033Z	03HM33Z	03VL4HZ
02HW30Z	02U23JZ	03140AW	03943ZZ	039D0ZZ	039N40Z	03H043Z	03HM43Z	03VM0HZ
02HW32Z	02U23KZ	03140JW	039440Z	039D30Z	039N4ZZ	03H103Z	03HN03Z	03VM3HZ
02HW33Z	02U247Z	03140KW	03944ZZ	039D3ZX	039P00Z	03H133Z	03HN33Z	03VM4HZ
02HW40Z	02U248Z	03140ZW	039500Z	039D3ZZ	039P0ZZ	03H143Z	03HN43Z	03VN0HZ

03VN3HZ
03VN4HZ
03VP0HZ
03VP3HZ
03VP4HZ
03VQ0HZ
03VQ3HZ
03VQ4HZ
03WY30Z
03WY32Z
03WY33Z
03WY3DZ
03WY3YZ
03WY4YZ
03WYX0Z
03WYX2Z
03WYX3Z
03WYX7Z
03WYXCZ
03WYXDZ
03WYXJZ
03WYXKZ
03WYXMZ
049000Z
04900ZZ
049030Z
04903ZX
04903ZZ
049040Z
04904ZZ
049100Z
04910ZZ
049130Z
04913ZX
04913ZZ
049140Z
04914ZZ
049200Z
04920ZZ
049230Z
04923ZX
04923ZZ
049240Z
04924ZZ
049300Z
04930ZZ
049330Z
04933ZX
04933ZZ
049340Z
04934ZZ
049400Z
04940ZZ
049430Z
04943ZX
04943ZZ
049440Z
04944ZZ
049500Z
04950ZZ
049530Z
04953ZX
04953ZZ
049540Z
04954ZZ
049600Z
04960ZZ
049630Z
04963ZX
04963ZZ
049640Z
04964ZZ
049700Z
04970ZZ
049730Z
04973ZX
04973ZZ
049740Z
04974ZZ
049800Z
04980ZZ
049830Z
04983ZX
04983ZZ
049840Z
04984ZZ
049900Z
04990ZZ
049930Z
04993ZX
04993ZZ
049940Z
04994ZZ
049A00Z
049A0ZZ
049A30Z
049A3ZX
049A3ZZ
049A40Z
049A4ZZ
049B00Z
049B0ZZ
049B30Z
049B3ZX
049B3ZZ
049B40Z
049B4ZZ
049C00Z
049C0ZZ
049C30Z
049C3ZX
049C3ZZ
049C40Z
049C4ZZ
049D00Z
049D0ZZ
049D30Z
049D3ZX
049D3ZZ
049D40Z
049D4ZZ
049E00Z
049E0ZZ
049E30Z
049E3ZX
049E3ZZ
049E40Z
049E4ZZ
049F00Z
049F0ZZ
049F30Z
049F3ZX
049F3ZZ
049F40Z
049F4ZZ
049H00Z
049H0ZZ
049H30Z
049H3ZX
049H3ZZ
049H40Z
049H4ZZ
049J00Z
049J0ZZ
049J30Z
049J3ZX
049J3ZZ
049J40Z
049J4ZZ
049K00Z
049K0ZZ
049K30Z
049K3ZX
049K3ZZ
049K40Z
049K4ZZ
049L00Z
049L0ZZ
049L30Z
049L3ZX
049L3ZZ
049L40Z
049L4ZZ
049M00Z
049M0ZZ
049M30Z
049M3ZX
049M3ZZ
049M40Z
049M4ZZ
049N00Z
049N0ZZ
049N30Z
049N3ZX
049N3ZZ
049N40Z
049N4ZZ
049P00Z
049P0ZZ
049P30Z
049P3ZX
049P3ZZ
049P40Z
049P4ZZ
049Q00Z
049Q0ZZ
049Q30Z
049Q3ZX
049Q3ZZ
049Q40Z
049Q4ZZ
049R00Z
049R0ZZ
049R30Z
049R3ZX
049R3ZZ
049R40Z
049R4ZZ
049S00Z
049S0ZZ
049S30Z
049S3ZX
049S3ZZ
049S40Z
049S4ZZ
049T00Z
049T0ZZ
049T30Z
049T3ZX
049T3ZZ
049T40Z
049T4ZZ
049U00Z
049U0ZZ
049U30Z
049U3ZX
049U3ZZ
049U40Z
049U4ZZ
049V00Z
049V0ZZ
049V30Z
049V3ZX
049V3ZZ
049V40Z
049V4ZZ
049W00Z
049W0ZZ
049W30Z
049W3ZX
049W3ZZ
049W40Z
049W4ZZ
049Y00Z
049Y0ZZ
049Y30Z
049Y3ZX
049Y3ZZ
049Y40Z
049Y4ZZ
04H002Z
04H003Z
04H032Z
04H033Z
04H042Z
04H043Z
04H103Z
04H133Z
04H143Z
04H203Z
04H233Z
04H243Z
04H303Z
04H333Z
04H343Z
04H403Z
04H433Z
04H443Z
04H503Z
04H533Z
04H543Z
04H603Z
04H633Z
04H643Z
04H703Z
04H733Z
04H743Z
04H803Z
04H833Z
04H843Z
04H903Z
04H933Z
04H943Z
04HA03Z
04HA33Z
04HA43Z
04HB03Z
04HB33Z
04HB43Z
04HC03Z
04HC33Z
04HC43Z
04HD03Z
04HD33Z
04HD43Z
04HE03Z
04HE33Z
04HE43Z
04HF03Z
04HF33Z
04HF43Z
04HH03Z
04HH33Z
04HH43Z
04HJ03Z
04HJ33Z
04HJ43Z
04HK03Z
04HK33Z
04HK43Z
04HL03Z
04HL33Z
04HL43Z
04HM03Z
04HM33Z
04HM43Z
04HN03Z
04HN33Z
04HN43Z
04HP03Z
04HP33Z
04HP43Z
04HQ03Z
04HQ33Z
04HQ43Z
04HR03Z
04HR33Z
04HR43Z
04HS03Z
04HS33Z
04HS43Z
04HT03Z
04HT33Z
04HT43Z
04HU03Z
04HU33Z
04HU43Z
04HV03Z
04HV33Z
04HV43Z
04HW03Z
04HW33Z
04HW43Z
04HY03Z
04HY32Z
04HY33Z
04HY3YZ
04HY43Z
04HY4YZ
04JY3ZZ
04JY4ZZ
04JYXZZ
04L23DZ
04PY30Z
04PY32Z
04PY33Z
04PY3DZ
04PY3YZ
04PY4YZ
04PYX0Z
04PYX1Z
04PYX2Z
04PYX3Z
04PYXDZ
04WY30Z
04WY32Z
04WY33Z
04WY3DZ
04WY3YZ
04WY4YZ
04WYX0Z
04WYX2Z
04WYX3Z
04WYX7Z
04WYXCZ
04WYXDZ
04WYXJZ
04WYXKZ
059000Z
05900ZZ
059030Z
05903ZX
05903ZZ
059040Z
05904ZZ
059100Z
05910ZZ
059130Z
05913ZX
05913ZZ
059140Z
05914ZZ
059300Z
05930ZZ
059330Z
05933ZX
05933ZZ
059340Z
05934ZZ
059400Z
05940ZZ
059430Z
05943ZX
05943ZZ
059440Z
05944ZZ
059500Z
05950ZZ
059530Z
05953ZX
05953ZZ
059540Z
05954ZZ
059600Z
05960ZZ
059630Z
05963ZX
05963ZZ
059640Z
05964ZZ
059700Z
05970ZZ
059730Z
05973ZX
05973ZZ
059740Z
05974ZZ
059800Z
05980ZZ
059830Z
05983ZX
05983ZZ
059840Z
05984ZZ
059900Z
05990ZZ
059930Z
05993ZX
05993ZZ
059940Z
05994ZZ
059A00Z
059A0ZZ
059A30Z
059A3ZX
059A3ZZ
059A40Z
059A4ZZ
059B00Z
059B0ZZ
059B30Z
059B3ZX
059B3ZZ
059B40Z
059B4ZZ
059C00Z
059C0ZZ
059C30Z
059C3ZX
059C3ZZ
059C40Z
059C4ZZ
059D00Z
059D0ZZ
059D30Z
059D3ZX
059D3ZZ
059D40Z
059D4ZZ
059F00Z
059F0ZZ
059F30Z
059F3ZX
059F3ZZ
059F40Z
059F4ZZ
059G00Z
059G0ZZ
059G30Z
059G3ZX
059G3ZZ
059G40Z
059G4ZZ
059H00Z
059H0ZZ
059H30Z
059H3ZX
059H3ZZ
059H40Z
059H4ZZ
059L00Z
059L0ZZ
059L30Z
059L3ZX
059L3ZZ
059L40Z
059L4ZZ
059M00Z
059M0ZZ
059M30Z
059M3ZX
059M3ZZ
059M40Z
059M4ZZ
059N00Z
059N0ZZ
059N30Z
059N3ZX
059N3ZZ
059N40Z
059N4ZZ
059P00Z
059P0ZZ
059P30Z
059P3ZX
059P3ZZ
059P40Z
059P4ZZ
059Q00Z
059Q0ZZ
059Q30Z
059Q3ZX
059Q3ZZ
059Q40Z
059Q4ZZ
059R00Z
059R0ZZ
059R30Z
059R3ZX
059R3ZZ
059R40Z
059R4ZZ
059S00Z
059S0ZZ
059S30Z
059S3ZX
059S3ZZ
059S40Z
059S4ZZ
059T00Z
059T0ZZ
059T30Z
059T3ZX
059T3ZZ
059T40Z
059T4ZZ
059V00Z
059V0ZZ
059V30Z
059V3ZX

059V3ZZ
059V40Z
059V4ZZ
059Y00Z
059Y0ZZ
059Y30Z
059Y3ZX
059Y3ZZ
059Y40Z
059Y4ZZ
05H003Z
05H033Z
05H043Z
05H103Z
05H133Z
05H143Z
05H303Z
05H333Z
05H343Z
05H403Z
05H433Z
05H443Z
05H503Z
05H533Z
05H543Z
05H603Z
05H633Z
05H643Z
05H703Z
05H733Z
05H743Z
05H803Z
05H833Z
05H843Z
05H903Z
05H933Z
05H943Z
05HA03Z
05HA33Z
05HA43Z
05HB03Z
05HB33Z
05HB43Z
05HC03Z
05HC33Z
05HC43Z
05HD03Z
05HD33Z
05HD43Z
05HF03Z
05HF33Z
05HF43Z
05HG03Z
05HG33Z
05HG43Z
05HH03Z
05HH33Z
05HH43Z
05HL03Z
05HL33Z
05HL43Z
05HM03Z
05HM33Z
05HM43Z
05HN03Z
05HN33Z
05HN43Z
05HP03Z
05HP33Z
05HP43Z
05HQ03Z
05HQ33Z
05HQ43Z
05HR03Z
05HR33Z
05HR43Z
05HS03Z
05HS33Z
05HS43Z
05HT03Z
05HT33Z
05HT43Z
05HV03Z
05HV33Z
05HV43Z
05HY03Z
05HY32Z
05HY33Z
05HY3YZ
05HY43Z
05HY4YZ
05JY3ZZ
05JYXZZ
05P002Z
05P032Z
05P042Z
05P0X2Z
05PY30Z
05PY32Z
05PY33Z
05PY3DZ
05PY3YZ
05PY4YZ
05PYX0Z
05PYX2Z
05PYX3Z
05PYXDZ
05W0XMZ
05W3XMZ
05W4XMZ
05WY30Z
05WY32Z
05WY33Z
05WY3DZ
05WY3YZ
05WY4YZ
05WYX0Z
05WYX2Z
05WYX3Z
05WYX7Z
05WYXCZ
05WYXDZ
05WYXJZ
05WYXKZ
069000Z
06900ZZ
069030Z
06903ZX
06903ZZ
069040Z
06904ZZ
069100Z
06910ZZ
069130Z
06913ZX
06913ZZ
069140Z
06914ZZ
069200Z
06920ZZ
069230Z
06923ZX
06923ZZ
069240Z
06924ZZ
069330Z
06933ZX
06933ZZ
069400Z
06940ZZ
069430Z
06943ZX
06943ZZ
069440Z
06944ZZ
069500Z
06950ZZ
069530Z
06953ZX
06953ZZ
069540Z
06954ZZ
069600Z
06960ZZ
069630Z
06963ZX
06963ZZ
069640Z
06964ZZ
069700Z
06970ZZ
069730Z
06973ZX
06973ZZ
069740Z
06974ZZ
069800Z
06980ZZ
069830Z
06983ZX
06983ZZ
069840Z
06984ZZ
069900Z
06990ZZ
069930Z
06993ZX
06993ZZ
069940Z
06994ZZ
069B00Z
069B0ZZ
069B30Z
069B3ZX
069B3ZZ
069B40Z
069B4ZZ
069C00Z
069C0ZZ
069C30Z
069C3ZX
069C3ZZ
069C40Z
069C4ZZ
069D00Z
069D0ZZ
069D30Z
069D3ZX
069D3ZZ
069D40Z
069D4ZZ
069F00Z
069F0ZZ
069F30Z
069F3ZX
069F3ZZ
069F40Z
069F4ZZ
069G00Z
069G0ZZ
069G30Z
069G3ZX
069G3ZZ
069G40Z
069G4ZZ
069H00Z
069H0ZZ
069H30Z
069H3ZX
069H3ZZ
069H40Z
069H4ZZ
069J00Z
069J0ZZ
069J30Z
069J3ZX
069J3ZZ
069J40Z
069J4ZZ
069M00Z
069M0ZZ
069M30Z
069M3ZX
069M3ZZ
069M40Z
069M4ZZ
069N00Z
069N0ZZ
069N30Z
069N3ZX
069N3ZZ
069N40Z
069N4ZZ
069P00Z
069P0ZZ
069P30Z
069P3ZX
069P3ZZ
069P40Z
069P4ZZ
069Q00Z
069Q0ZZ
069Q30Z
069Q3ZX
069Q3ZZ
069Q40Z
069Q4ZZ
069T00Z
069T0ZZ
069T30Z
069T3ZX
069T3ZZ
069T40Z
069T4ZZ
069V00Z
069V0ZZ
069V30Z
069V3ZX
069V3ZZ
069V40Z
069V4ZZ
069Y00Z
069Y0ZZ
069Y30Z
069Y3ZX
069Y3ZZ
069Y40Z
069Y4ZZ
06H003T
06H003Z
06H033T
06H033Z
06H043Z
06H103Z
06H133Z
06H143Z
06H203Z
06H233Z
06H243Z
06H303Z
06H333Z
06H343Z
06H403Z
06H433Z
06H443Z
06H503Z
06H533Z
06H543Z
06H603Z
06H633Z
06H643Z
06H703Z
06H733Z
06H743Z
06H803Z
06H833Z
06H843Z
06H903Z
06H933Z
06H943Z
06HB03Z
06HB33Z
06HB43Z
06HC03Z
06HC33Z
06HC43Z
06HD03Z
06HD33Z
06HD43Z
06HF03Z
06HF33Z
06HF43Z
06HG03Z
06HG33Z
06HG43Z
06HH03Z
06HH33Z
06HH43Z
06HJ03Z
06HJ33Z
06HJ43Z
06HM03Z
06HM33Z
06HM43Z
06HN03Z
06HN33Z
06HN43Z
06HP03Z
06HP33Z
06HP43Z
06HQ03Z
06HQ33Z
06HQ43Z
06HT03Z
06HT33Z
06HT43Z
06HV03Z
06HV33Z
06HV43Z
06HY03Z
06HY32Z
06HY33Z
06HY3YZ
06HY43Z
06HY4YZ
06JY3ZZ
06JYXZZ
06L27CZ
06L27DZ
06L27ZZ
06L28CZ
06L28DZ
06L28ZZ
06L33CZ
06L33DZ
06L33ZZ
06L34CZ
06L34DZ
06L34ZZ
06L37CZ
06L37DZ
06L37ZZ
06L38CZ
06L38DZ
06L38ZZ
06PY30Z
06PY32Z
06PY33Z
06PY3DZ
06PY3YZ
06PY4YZ
06PYX0Z
06PYX2Z
06PYX3Z
06PYXDZ
06WY30Z
06WY32Z
06WY33Z
06WY3DZ
06WY3YZ
06WY4YZ
06WYX0Z
06WYX2Z
06WYX3Z
06WYX7Z
06WYXCZ
06WYXDZ
06WYXJZ
06WYXKZ
072KX0Z
072KXYZ
072LX0Z
072LXYZ
072MX0Z
072MXYZ
072NX0Z
072NXYZ
072PX0Z
072PXYZ
072TX0Z
072TXYZ
079030Z
07903ZZ
079080Z
07908ZX
07908ZZ
079130Z
07913ZZ
079180Z
07918ZX
07918ZZ
079230Z
07923ZZ
079280Z
07928ZX
07928ZZ
079330Z
07933ZZ
079380Z
07938ZX
07938ZZ
079430Z
07943ZZ
079480Z
07948ZX
07948ZZ
079530Z
07953ZZ
079580Z
07958ZX
07958ZZ
079630Z
07963ZZ
079680Z
07968ZX
07968ZZ
079730Z
07973ZZ
079780Z
07978ZX
07978ZZ
079830Z
07983ZZ
079880Z
07988ZX
07988ZZ
079930Z
07993ZZ
079980Z
07998ZX
07998ZZ
079B30Z
079B3ZZ
079B80Z
079B8ZX
079B8ZZ
079C30Z
079C3ZZ
079C80Z
079C8ZX
079C8ZZ
079D30Z
079D3ZZ
079D80Z
079D8ZX
079D8ZZ
079F30Z
079F3ZZ
079F80Z
079F8ZX
079F8ZZ
079G30Z
079G3ZZ
079G80Z
079G8ZX
079G8ZZ
079H30Z
079H3ZZ
079H80Z
079H8ZX
079H8ZZ
079J30Z
079J3ZZ
079J80Z
079J8ZX
079J8ZZ
079K30Z
079K3ZZ
079K80Z
079K8ZX
079K8ZZ
079L30Z
079L3ZZ
079L80Z
079L8ZX
079L8ZZ
079M30Z
079M3ZZ
079P30Z
079P3ZX
079P3ZZ
079P40Z
079P4ZX
079P4ZZ
079T00Z
079T0ZX
079T0ZZ
079T30Z
079T3ZX
079T3ZZ
079T40Z
079T4ZX
079T4ZZ
07BP3ZX
07BP4ZX
07CP3ZZ
07CP4ZZ
07D03ZX
07D04ZX
07D08ZX

07D13ZX
07D14ZX
07D18ZX
07D23ZX
07D24ZX
07D28ZX
07D33ZX
07D34ZX
07D38ZX
07D43ZX
07D44ZX
07D48ZX
07D53ZX
07D54ZX
07D58ZX
07D63ZX
07D64ZX
07D68ZX
07D73ZX
07D74ZX
07D78ZX
07D83ZX
07D84ZX
07D88ZX
07D93ZX
07D94ZX
07D98ZX
07DB3ZX
07DB4ZX
07DB8ZX
07DC3ZX
07DC4ZX
07DC8ZX
07DD3ZX
07DD4ZX
07DD8ZX
07DF3ZX
07DF4ZX
07DF8ZX
07DG3ZX
07DG4ZX
07DG8ZX
07DH3ZX
07DH4ZX
07DH8ZX
07DJ3ZX
07DJ4ZX
07DJ8ZX
07DK3ZX
07DK4ZX
07DK8ZX
07DL3ZX
07DL4ZX
07DL8ZX
07DM3ZX
07DM4ZX
07DP3ZX
07DP4ZX
07DQ0ZX
07DQ0ZZ
07DQ3ZX
07DQ3ZZ
07DR0ZX
07DR0ZZ
07DR3ZX
07DR3ZZ
07DS0ZX
07DS0ZZ
07DS3ZX
07DS3ZZ
07HK03Z
07HK33Z
07HK3YZ
07HK43Z
07HL03Z
07HL33Z
07HL3YZ
07HL43Z
07HM03Z
07HM33Z
07HM3YZ
07HM43Z
07HN03Z
07HN33Z
07HN3YZ
07HN43Z
07HN4YZ
07HP03Z
07HP33Z
07HP3YZ
07HP43Z
07HP4YZ
07JK3ZZ
07JL3ZZ
07JM3ZZ
07JN3ZZ
07JN8ZZ
07JNXZZ
07JP3ZZ
07JP4ZZ
07JPXZZ
07JT0ZZ
07JT3ZZ
07JT4ZZ
07PK3YZ
07PK4YZ
07PKX0Z
07PKX3Z
07PKXDZ
07PL3YZ
07PL4YZ
07PLX0Z
07PLX3Z
07PLXDZ
07PM3YZ
07PM4YZ
07PMX0Z
07PMX3Z
07PN3YZ
07PN4YZ
07PNX0Z
07PNX3Z
07PNXDZ
07PP3YZ
07PP4YZ
07PPX0Z
07PPX3Z
07PT00Z
07PT30Z
07PT40Z
07PTX0Z
07WK3YZ
07WK4YZ
07WKX0Z
07WKX3Z
07WKX7Z
07WKXCZ
07WKXDZ
07WKXJZ
07WKXKZ
07WL3YZ
07WL4YZ
07WLX0Z
07WLX3Z
07WLX7Z
07WLXCZ
07WLXDZ
07WLXJZ
07WLXKZ
07WM3YZ
07WM4YZ
07WMX0Z
07WMX3Z
07WN3YZ
07WN4YZ
07WNX0Z
07WNX3Z
07WNX7Z
07WNXCZ
07WNXDZ
07WNXJZ
07WNXKZ
07WP3YZ
07WP4YZ
07WPX0Z
07WPX3Z
07WT00Z
07WT30Z
07WT40Z
07WTX0Z
080N07Z
080N0JZ
080N0KZ
080N0ZZ
080N37Z
080N3JZ
080N3KZ
080N3ZZ
080NX7Z
080NXJZ
080NXKZ
080NXZZ
080P07Z
080P0JZ
080P0KZ
080P0ZZ
080P37Z
080P3JZ
080P3KZ
080P3ZZ
080PX7Z
080PXJZ
080PXKZ
080PXZZ
080Q07Z
080Q0JZ
080Q0KZ
080Q0ZZ
080Q37Z
080Q3JZ
080Q3KZ
080Q3ZZ
080QX7Z
080QXJZ
080QXKZ
080QXZZ
080R07Z
080R0JZ
080R0KZ
080R0ZZ
080R37Z
080R3JZ
080R3KZ
080R3ZZ
080RX7Z
080RXJZ
080RXKZ
080RXZZ
0820X0Z
0820XYZ
0821X0Z
0821XYZ
085E3ZZ
085F3ZZ
0890XZX
0890XZZ
0891XZX
0891XZZ
0896XZX
0896XZZ
0897XZX
0897XZZ
0898XZX
0898XZZ
0899XZX
0899XZZ
089N00Z
089N0ZZ
089N30Z
089N3ZX
089N3ZZ
089NX0Z
089NXZX
089NXZZ
089P00Z
089P0ZZ
089P30Z
089P3ZX
089P3ZZ
089PX0Z
089PXZX
089PXZZ
089Q00Z
089Q0ZZ
089Q30Z
089Q3ZX
089Q3ZZ
089QX0Z
089QXZX
089QXZZ
089R00Z
089R0ZZ
089R30Z
089R3ZX
089R3ZZ
089RX0Z
089RXZX
089RXZZ
089SXZX
089SXZZ
089TXZX
089TXZZ
08C0XZZ
08C1XZZ
08C2XZZ
08C3XZZ
08C6XZZ
08C7XZZ
08CN0ZZ
08CN3ZZ
08CNXZZ
08CP0ZZ
08CP3ZZ
08CPXZZ
08CQ0ZZ
08CQ3ZZ
08CQXZZ
08CR0ZZ
08CR3ZZ
08CRXZZ
08CSXZZ
08CTXZZ
08F4XZZ
08F5XZZ
08H03YZ
08H07YZ
08H08YZ
08H13YZ
08H17YZ
08H18YZ
08J0XZZ
08J1XZZ
08JJXZZ
08JKXZZ
08JLXZZ
08JMXZZ
08P03YZ
08P070Z
08P073Z
08P07DZ
08P07YZ
08P080Z
08P083Z
08P08DZ
08P08YZ
08P0X0Z
08P0X1Z
08P0X3Z
08P0XCZ
08P0XDZ
08P0XJZ
08P13YZ
08P170Z
08P173Z
08P17DZ
08P17YZ
08P180Z
08P183Z
08P18DZ
08P18YZ
08P1X0Z
08P1X1Z
08P1X3Z
08P1XCZ
08P1XDZ
08P1XJZ
08PJ3YZ
08PK3YZ
08PL3YZ
08PM3YZ
08QN0ZZ
08QN3ZZ
08QNXZZ
08QP0ZZ
08QP3ZZ
08QPXZZ
08QQ0ZZ
08QQ3ZZ
08QQXZZ
08QR0ZZ
08QR3ZZ
08QRXZZ
08W03YZ
08W07YZ
08W08YZ
08W0X0Z
08W0X3Z
08W0X7Z
08W0XCZ
08W0XDZ
08W0XJZ
08W0XKZ
08W13YZ
08W17YZ
08W18YZ
08W1X0Z
08W1X3Z
08W1X7Z
08W1XCZ
08W1XDZ
08W1XJZ
08W1XKZ
08WJ3YZ
08WJXJZ
08WK3YZ
08WKXJZ
08WL3YZ
08WM3YZ
092HX0Z
092HXYZ
092JX0Z
092JXYZ
092KX0Z
092KXYZ
092YX0Z
092YXYZ
093K7ZZ
093K8ZZ
09500ZZ
09503ZZ
09504ZZ
0950XZZ
09510ZZ
09513ZZ
09514ZZ
0951XZZ
09530ZZ
09533ZZ
09534ZZ
09537ZZ
09538ZZ
0953XZZ
09540ZZ
09543ZZ
09544ZZ
09547ZZ
09548ZZ
0954XZZ
095F0ZZ
095F3ZZ
095F4ZZ
095F7ZZ
095F8ZZ
095G0ZZ
095G3ZZ
095G4ZZ
095G7ZZ
095G8ZZ
095K0ZZ
095K3ZZ
095K4ZZ
095K8ZZ
095KXZZ
095M0ZZ
095M3ZZ
095M4ZZ
095M8ZZ
097F0DZ
097F0ZZ
097F3ZZ
097F4ZZ
097F7DZ
097F7ZZ
097F8DZ
097F8ZZ
097G0DZ
097G0ZZ
097G3ZZ
097G4ZZ
097G7DZ
097G7ZZ
097G8DZ
097G8ZZ
099000Z
09900ZX
09900ZZ
099030Z
09903ZX
09903ZZ
099040Z
09904ZX
09904ZZ
0990X0Z
0990XZX
0990XZZ
099100Z
09910ZX
09910ZZ
099130Z
09913ZX
09913ZZ
099140Z
09914ZX
09914ZZ
0991X0Z
0991XZX
0991XZZ
099300Z
09930ZX
09930ZZ
099330Z
09933ZX
09933ZZ
099340Z
09934ZX
09934ZZ
099370Z
09937ZX
09937ZZ
099380Z
09938ZX
09938ZZ
0993X0Z
0993XZX
0993XZZ
099400Z
09940ZX
09940ZZ
099430Z
09943ZX
09943ZZ
099440Z
09944ZX
09944ZZ
099470Z
09947ZX
09947ZZ
099480Z
09948ZX
09948ZZ
0994X0Z
0994XZX
0994XZZ
09950ZZ
09957ZX
09957ZZ
099580Z
09958ZX
09958ZZ
09960ZZ
099670Z
09967ZX
09967ZZ
099680Z
09968ZX
09968ZZ
09970ZZ
09973ZZ
09974ZZ
09977ZX
09977ZZ
09978ZX
09978ZZ
09980ZZ
09983ZZ
09984ZZ
09987ZX
09987ZZ
09988ZX
09988ZZ
099970Z
09997ZX
09997ZZ
099980Z
09998ZX
09998ZZ
099A70Z
099A7ZX
099A7ZZ
099A80Z

099A8ZX
099A8ZZ
099B30Z
099B3ZZ
099B70Z
099B7ZX
099B7ZZ
099B80Z
099B8ZX
099B8ZZ
099C30Z
099C3ZZ
099C70Z
099C7ZX
099C7ZZ
099C80Z
099C8ZX
099C8ZZ
099D70Z
099D7ZX
099D7ZZ
099D80Z
099D8ZX
099D8ZZ
099E70Z
099E7ZX
099E7ZZ
099E80Z
099E8ZX
099E8ZZ
099F00Z
099F0ZZ
099F30Z
099F3ZZ
099F40Z
099F4ZZ
099F70Z
099F7ZX
099F7ZZ
099F80Z
099F8ZX
099F8ZZ
099G00Z
099G0ZZ
099G30Z
099G3ZZ
099G40Z
099G4ZZ
099G70Z
099G7ZX
099G7ZZ
099G80Z
099G8ZX
099G8ZZ
099K00Z
099K0ZX
099K0ZZ
099K30Z
099K3ZX
099K3ZZ
099K40Z
099K4ZX
099K4ZZ
099K70Z
099K7ZX
099K7ZZ
099K80Z
099K8ZX
099K8ZZ
099KX0Z
099KXZX
099KXZZ
099L00Z
099L0ZX
099L0ZZ
099L30Z
099L3ZX
099L3ZZ
099L40Z
099L4ZX
099L4ZZ
099L70Z
099L7ZX
099L7ZZ
099L80Z
099L8ZX
099L8ZZ
099M00Z
099M0ZX
099M0ZZ
099M30Z
099M3ZX
099M3ZZ
099M40Z
099M4ZX
099M4ZZ
099M70Z
099M7ZX
099M7ZZ
099M80Z
099M8ZX
099M8ZZ
099N0ZX
099N30Z
099N3ZX
099N3ZZ
099N4ZX
099N7ZX
099N8ZX
099P30Z
099P3ZX
099P3ZZ
099P40Z
099P4ZX
099P4ZZ
099P70Z
099P7ZX
099P7ZZ
099P80Z
099P8ZX
099P8ZZ
099Q30Z
099Q3ZX
099Q3ZZ
099Q40Z
099Q4ZX
099Q4ZZ
099Q70Z
099Q7ZX
099Q7ZZ
099Q80Z
099Q8ZX
099Q8ZZ
099R30Z
099R3ZX
099R3ZZ
099R40Z
099R4ZX
099R4ZZ
099R70Z
099R7ZX
099R7ZZ
099R80Z
099R8ZX
099R8ZZ
099S30Z
099S3ZX
099S3ZZ
099S40Z
099S4ZX
099S4ZZ
099S70Z
099S7ZX
099S7ZZ
099S80Z
099S8ZX
099S8ZZ
099T30Z
099T3ZX
099T3ZZ
099T40Z
099T4ZX
099T4ZZ
099T70Z
099T7ZX
099T7ZZ
099T80Z
099T8ZX
099T8ZZ
099U30Z
099U3ZX
099U3ZZ
099U40Z
099U4ZX
099U4ZZ
099U70Z
099U7ZX
099U7ZZ
099U80Z
099U8ZX
099U8ZZ
099V30Z
099V3ZX
099V3ZZ
099V40Z
099V4ZX
099V4ZZ
099V70Z
099V7ZX
099V7ZZ
099V80Z
099V8ZX
099V8ZZ
099W30Z
099W3ZX
099W3ZZ
099W40Z
099W4ZX
099W4ZZ
099W70Z
099W7ZX
099W7ZZ
099W80Z
099W8ZX
099W8ZZ
099X30Z
099X3ZX
099X3ZZ
099X40Z
099X4ZX
099X4ZZ
099X70Z
099X7ZX
099X7ZZ
099X80Z
099X8ZX
099X8ZZ
09B00ZX
09B00ZZ
09B03ZX
09B03ZZ
09B04ZX
09B04ZZ
09B0XZX
09B0XZZ
09B10ZX
09B10ZZ
09B13ZX
09B13ZZ
09B14ZX
09B14ZZ
09B1XZX
09B1XZZ
09B30ZX
09B30ZZ
09B33ZX
09B33ZZ
09B34ZX
09B34ZZ
09B37ZX
09B37ZZ
09B38ZX
09B38ZZ
09B3XZX
09B3XZZ
09B40ZX
09B40ZZ
09B43ZX
09B43ZZ
09B44ZX
09B44ZZ
09B47ZX
09B47ZZ
09B48ZX
09B48ZZ
09B4XZX
09B4XZZ
09BF0ZX
09BF0ZZ
09BF3ZX
09BF3ZZ
09BF4ZX
09BF4ZZ
09BF7ZX
09BF7ZZ
09BF8ZX
09BF8ZZ
09BG0ZX
09BG0ZZ
09BG3ZX
09BG3ZZ
09BG4ZX
09BG4ZZ
09BG7ZX
09BG7ZZ
09BG8ZX
09BG8ZZ
09BK0ZX
09BK0ZZ
09BK3ZX
09BK3ZZ
09BK4ZX
09BK4ZZ
09BK8ZX
09BK8ZZ
09BKXZX
09BKXZZ
09BL0ZX
09BL3ZX
09BL4ZX
09BL7ZX
09BL8ZX
09BM0ZX
09BM3ZX
09BM4ZX
09BM8ZX
09BN0ZX
09BN3ZX
09BN4ZX
09BN7ZX
09BN8ZX
09BP3ZX
09BP4ZX
09BP8ZX
09BQ3ZX
09BQ4ZX
09BQ8ZX
09BR3ZX
09BR4ZX
09BR8ZX
09BS3ZX
09BS4ZX
09BS8ZX
09BT3ZX
09BT4ZX
09BT8ZX
09BU3ZX
09BU4ZX
09BU8ZX
09BV3ZX
09BV4ZX
09BV8ZX
09BW3ZX
09BW4ZX
09BW8ZX
09BX3ZX
09BX4ZX
09BX8ZX
09C00ZZ
09C03ZZ
09C04ZZ
09C0XZZ
09C10ZZ
09C13ZZ
09C14ZZ
09C1XZZ
09C30ZZ
09C33ZZ
09C34ZZ
09C37ZZ
09C38ZZ
09C3XZZ
09C40ZZ
09C43ZZ
09C44ZZ
09C47ZZ
09C48ZZ
09C4XZZ
09C70ZZ
09C73ZZ
09C74ZZ
09C77ZZ
09C78ZZ
09C80ZZ
09C83ZZ
09C84ZZ
09C87ZZ
09C88ZZ
09CF0ZZ
09CF3ZZ
09CF4ZZ
09CF7ZZ
09CF8ZZ
09CG0ZZ
09CG3ZZ
09CG4ZZ
09CG7ZZ
09CG8ZZ
09CK0ZZ
09CK3ZZ
09CK4ZZ
09CK8ZZ
09CKXZZ
09CL0ZZ
09CL3ZZ
09CL4ZZ
09CL7ZZ
09CL8ZZ
09CM0ZZ
09CM3ZZ
09CM4ZZ
09CM8ZZ
09HH3YZ
09HH4YZ
09HH7YZ
09HH8YZ
09HJ3YZ
09HJ4YZ
09HJ7YZ
09HJ8YZ
09HK0YZ
09HK3YZ
09HK4YZ
09HK7YZ
09HK8YZ
09HN7BZ
09HN8BZ
09HY3YZ
09HY4YZ
09HY7YZ
09HY8YZ
09J73ZZ
09J77ZZ
09J78ZZ
09J7XZZ
09J83ZZ
09J87ZZ
09J88ZZ
09J8XZZ
09JD3ZZ
09JD8ZZ
09JDXZZ
09JE3ZZ
09JE8ZZ
09JEXZZ
09JH0ZZ
09JH3ZZ
09JH4ZZ
09JH7ZZ
09JH8ZZ
09JHXZZ
09JJ0ZZ
09JJ3ZZ
09JJ4ZZ
09JJ7ZZ
09JJ8ZZ
09JJXZZ
09JK0ZZ
09JK3ZZ
09JK4ZZ
09JK8ZZ
09JKXZZ
09JY0ZZ
09JY3ZZ
09JY4ZZ
09JY8ZZ
09JYXZZ
09N0XZZ
09N1XZZ
09N3XZZ
09N4XZZ
09NF0ZZ
09NF3ZZ
09NF4ZZ
09NF7ZZ
09NF8ZZ
09NG0ZZ
09NG3ZZ
09NG4ZZ
09NG7ZZ
09NG8ZZ
09NK0ZZ
09NK3ZZ
09NK4ZZ
09NK8ZZ
09NKXZZ
09NL0ZZ
09NL3ZZ
09NL4ZZ
09NL7ZZ
09NL8ZZ
09NM0ZZ
09NM3ZZ
09NM4ZZ
09NM8ZZ
09P700Z
09P770Z
09P780Z
09P7X0Z
09P800Z
09P870Z
09P880Z
09P8X0Z
09PH30Z
09PH3JZ
09PH3KZ
09PH3YZ
09PH40Z
09PH4JZ
09PH4KZ
09PH4YZ
09PH70Z
09PH7DZ
09PH7YZ
09PH80Z
09PH8DZ
09PH8YZ
09PHX0Z
09PHX7Z
09PHXDZ
09PHXJZ
09PHXKZ
09PJ30Z
09PJ3JZ
09PJ3KZ
09PJ3YZ
09PJ40Z
09PJ4JZ
09PJ4KZ
09PJ4YZ
09PJ70Z
09PJ7DZ
09PJ7YZ
09PJ80Z
09PJ8DZ
09PJ8YZ
09PJX0Z
09PJX7Z
09PJXDZ
09PJXJZ
09PJXKZ
09PK00Z
09PK07Z
09PK0DZ
09PK0JZ
09PK0KZ
09PK0YZ
09PK30Z
09PK37Z
09PK3DZ
09PK3JZ
09PK3KZ
09PK3YZ
09PK40Z
09PK47Z
09PK4DZ
09PK4JZ
09PK4KZ
09PK4YZ
09PK70Z
09PK77Z
09PK7DZ
09PK7JZ
09PK7KZ
09PK7YZ
09PK80Z
09PK87Z
09PK8DZ
09PK8JZ
09PK8KZ

09PK8YZ	09UC07Z	09US07Z	09UW07Z	09WK00Z	0B584ZZ	0B778DZ	0B947ZZ	0B9F3ZX
09PKX0Z	09UC0JZ	09US0JZ	09UW0JZ	09WK07Z	0B594ZZ	0B778ZZ	0B9480Z	0B9F4ZX
09PKX7Z	09UC0KZ	09US0KZ	09UW0KZ	09WK0DZ	0B5B4ZZ	0B780DZ	0B948ZX	0B9F7ZX
09PKXDZ	09UC37Z	09US37Z	09UW37Z	09WK0JZ	0B5C8ZZ	0B780ZZ	0B948ZZ	0B9F8ZX
09PKXJZ	09UC3JZ	09US3JZ	09UW3JZ	09WK0KZ	0B5D8ZZ	0B783DZ	0B953ZX	0B9G3ZX
09PKXKZ	09UC3KZ	09US3KZ	09UW3KZ	09WK0YZ	0B5F8ZZ	0B783ZZ	0B954ZX	0B9G4ZX
09PY3YZ	09UC47Z	09US47Z	09UW47Z	09WK30Z	0B5G8ZZ	0B784DZ	0B9570Z	0B9G7ZX
09PY4YZ	09UC4JZ	09US4JZ	09UW4JZ	09WK37Z	0B5H8ZZ	0B784ZZ	0B957ZX	0B9G8ZX
09PY7YZ	09UC4KZ	09US4KZ	09UW4KZ	09WK3DZ	0B5J8ZZ	0B787DZ	0B957ZZ	0B9H3ZX
09PY8YZ	09UC77Z	09US77Z	09UW77Z	09WK3JZ	0B5K8ZZ	0B787ZZ	0B9580Z	0B9H4ZX
09PYX0Z	09UC7JZ	09US7JZ	09UW7JZ	09WK3KZ	0B5L8ZZ	0B788DZ	0B958ZX	0B9H7ZX
09Q0XZZ	09UC7KZ	09US7KZ	09UW7KZ	09WK3YZ	0B5M8ZZ	0B788ZZ	0B958ZZ	0B9J3ZX
09Q1XZZ	09UC87Z	09US87Z	09UW87Z	09WK40Z	0B730DZ	0B790DZ	0B963ZX	0B9J4ZX
09Q2XZZ	09UC8JZ	09US8JZ	09UW8JZ	09WK47Z	0B730ZZ	0B790ZZ	0B964ZX	0B9J7ZX
09Q3XZZ	09UC8KZ	09US8KZ	09UW8KZ	09WK4DZ	0B733DZ	0B793DZ	0B9670Z	0B9J8ZX
09Q4XZZ	09UP07Z	09UT07Z	09UX07Z	09WK4JZ	0B733ZZ	0B793ZZ	0B967ZX	0B9K3ZX
09QF0ZZ	09UP0JZ	09UT0JZ	09UX0JZ	09WK4KZ	0B734DZ	0B794DZ	0B967ZZ	0B9K4ZX
09QF3ZZ	09UP0KZ	09UT0KZ	09UX0KZ	09WK4YZ	0B734ZZ	0B794ZZ	0B9680Z	0B9K7ZX
09QF4ZZ	09UP37Z	09UT37Z	09UX37Z	09WK70Z	0B737DZ	0B797DZ	0B968ZX	0B9L3ZX
09QF7ZZ	09UP3JZ	09UT3JZ	09UX3JZ	09WK77Z	0B737ZZ	0B797ZZ	0B968ZZ	0B9L4ZX
09QF8ZZ	09UP3KZ	09UT3KZ	09UX3KZ	09WK7DZ	0B738DZ	0B798DZ	0B973ZX	0B9L7ZX
09QFXZZ	09UP47Z	09UT47Z	09UX47Z	09WK7JZ	0B738ZZ	0B798ZZ	0B974ZX	0B9M3ZX
09QG0ZZ	09UP4JZ	09UT4JZ	09UX4JZ	09WK7KZ	0B740DZ	0B7B0DZ	0B9770Z	0B9M4ZX
09QG3ZZ	09UP4KZ	09UT4KZ	09UX4KZ	09WK7YZ	0B740ZZ	0B7B0ZZ	0B977ZX	0B9M7ZX
09QG4ZZ	09UP77Z	09UT77Z	09UX77Z	09WK80Z	0B743DZ	0B7B3DZ	0B977ZZ	0B9N00Z
09QG7ZZ	09UP7JZ	09UT7JZ	09UX7JZ	09WK87Z	0B743ZZ	0B7B3ZZ	0B9780Z	0B9N0ZX
09QG8ZZ	09UP7KZ	09UT7KZ	09UX7KZ	09WK8DZ	0B744DZ	0B7B4DZ	0B978ZX	0B9N0ZZ
09QGXZZ	09UP87Z	09UT87Z	09UX87Z	09WK8JZ	0B744ZZ	0B7B4ZZ	0B978ZZ	0B9N30Z
09QKXZZ	09UP8JZ	09UT8JZ	09UX8JZ	09WK8KZ	0B747DZ	0B7B7DZ	0B983ZX	0B9N3ZX
09SF0ZZ	09UP8KZ	09UT8KZ	09UX8KZ	09WK8YZ	0B747ZZ	0B7B7ZZ	0B984ZX	0B9N3ZZ
09SF4ZZ	09UQ07Z	09UU07Z	09WH3JZ	09WKX0Z	0B748DZ	0B7B8DZ	0B9870Z	0B9N4ZX
09SF7ZZ	09UQ0JZ	09UU0JZ	09WH3KZ	09WKX7Z	0B748ZZ	0B7B8ZZ	0B987ZX	0B9N80Z
09SF8ZZ	09UQ0KZ	09UU0KZ	09WH3YZ	09WKXDZ	0B750DZ	0B913ZX	0B987ZZ	0B9N8ZX
09SG0ZZ	09UQ37Z	09UU37Z	09WH4JZ	09WKXJZ	0B750ZZ	0B914ZX	0B9880Z	0B9N8ZZ
09SG4ZZ	09UQ3JZ	09UU3JZ	09WH4KZ	09WKXKZ	0B753DZ	0B9170Z	0B988ZX	0B9P00Z
09SG7ZZ	09UQ3KZ	09UU3KZ	09WH4YZ	09WY3YZ	0B753ZZ	0B917ZX	0B988ZZ	0B9P0ZX
09SG8ZZ	09UQ47Z	09UU47Z	09WH7DZ	09WY4YZ	0B754DZ	0B917ZZ	0B993ZX	0B9P0ZZ
09TF0ZZ	09UQ4JZ	09UU4JZ	09WH7YZ	09WY7YZ	0B754ZZ	0B9180Z	0B994ZX	0B9P30Z
09TF4ZZ	09UQ4KZ	09UU4KZ	09WH8DZ	09WY8YZ	0B757DZ	0B918ZX	0B9970Z	0B9P3ZX
09TF7ZZ	09UQ77Z	09UU77Z	09WH8YZ	09WYX0Z	0B757ZZ	0B918ZZ	0B997ZX	0B9P3ZZ
09TF8ZZ	09UQ7JZ	09UU7JZ	09WHX0Z	0B110D6	0B758DZ	0B923ZX	0B997ZZ	0B9P4ZX
09TG0ZZ	09UQ7KZ	09UU7KZ	09WHX7Z	0B20X0Z	0B758ZZ	0B924ZX	0B9980Z	0B9P80Z
09TG4ZZ	09UQ87Z	09UU87Z	09WHXDZ	0B20XYZ	0B760DZ	0B9270Z	0B998ZX	0B9P8ZX
09TG7ZZ	09UQ8JZ	09UU8JZ	09WHXJZ	0B21X0Z	0B760ZZ	0B927ZX	0B998ZZ	0B9P8ZZ
09TG8ZZ	09UQ8KZ	09UU8KZ	09WHXKZ	0B21XEZ	0B763DZ	0B927ZZ	0B9B3ZX	0B9T30Z
09UB07Z	09UR07Z	09UV07Z	09WJ3JZ	0B21XFZ	0B763ZZ	0B9280Z	0B9B4ZX	0B9T3ZX
09UB0JZ	09UR0JZ	09UV0JZ	09WJ3KZ	0B21XYZ	0B764DZ	0B928ZX	0B9B70Z	0B9T3ZZ
09UB0KZ	09UR0KZ	09UV0KZ	09WJ3YZ	0B2KX0Z	0B764ZZ	0B928ZZ	0B9B7ZX	0B9T40Z
09UB37Z	09UR37Z	09UV37Z	09WJ4JZ	0B2KXYZ	0B767DZ	0B933ZX	0B9B7ZZ	0B9T4ZX
09UB3JZ	09UR3JZ	09UV3JZ	09WJ4KZ	0B2LX0Z	0B767ZZ	0B934ZX	0B9B80Z	0B9T4ZZ
09UB3KZ	09UR3KZ	09UV3KZ	09WJ4YZ	0B2LXYZ	0B768DZ	0B9370Z	0B9B8ZX	0BB13ZX
09UB47Z	09UR47Z	09UV47Z	09WJ7DZ	0B2QX0Z	0B768ZZ	0B937ZX	0B9B8ZZ	0BB14ZX
09UB4JZ	09UR4JZ	09UV4JZ	09WJ7YZ	0B2QXYZ	0B770DZ	0B937ZZ	0B9C3ZX	0BB17ZX
09UB4KZ	09UR4KZ	09UV4KZ	09WJ8DZ	0B2TX0Z	0B770ZZ	0B9380Z	0B9C4ZX	0BB18ZX
09UB77Z	09UR77Z	09UV77Z	09WJ8YZ	0B2TXYZ	0B773DZ	0B938ZX	0B9C7ZX	0BB23ZX
09UB7JZ	09UR7JZ	09UV7JZ	09WJX0Z	0B534ZZ	0B773ZZ	0B938ZZ	0B9C8ZX	0BB24ZX
09UB7KZ	09UR7KZ	09UV7KZ	09WJX7Z	0B544ZZ	0B774DZ	0B943ZX	0B9D3ZX	0BB27ZX
09UB87Z	09UR87Z	09UV87Z	09WJXDZ	0B554ZZ	0B774ZZ	0B944ZX	0B9D4ZX	0BB28ZX
09UB8JZ	09UR8JZ	09UV8JZ	09WJXJZ	0B564ZZ	0B777DZ	0B9470Z	0B9D7ZX	0BB33ZX
09UB8KZ	09UR8KZ	09UV8KZ	09WJXKZ	0B574ZZ	0B777ZZ	0B947ZX	0B9D8ZX	0BB34ZX

0BB34ZZ
0BB37ZX
0BB38ZX
0BB38ZZ
0BB43ZX
0BB44ZX
0BB44ZZ
0BB47ZX
0BB48ZX
0BB48ZZ
0BB53ZX
0BB54ZX
0BB54ZZ
0BB57ZX
0BB58ZX
0BB58ZZ
0BB63ZX
0BB64ZX
0BB64ZZ
0BB67ZX
0BB68ZX
0BB68ZZ
0BB73ZX
0BB74ZX
0BB74ZZ
0BB77ZX
0BB78ZX
0BB78ZZ
0BB83ZX
0BB84ZX
0BB84ZZ
0BB87ZX
0BB88ZX
0BB88ZZ
0BB93ZX
0BB94ZX
0BB94ZZ
0BB97ZX
0BB98ZX
0BB98ZZ
0BBB3ZX
0BBB4ZX
0BBB4ZZ
0BBB7ZX
0BBB8ZX
0BBB8ZZ
0BBC3ZX
0BBC8ZZ
0BBD3ZX
0BBD8ZZ
0BBF3ZX
0BBF8ZZ
0BBG3ZX
0BBG8ZZ
0BBH3ZX
0BBH8ZZ
0BBJ3ZX
0BBJ8ZZ
0BBK3ZX
0BBK8ZZ
0BBL3ZX
0BBL8ZZ
0BBM3ZX
0BBM4ZZ
0BBM8ZZ
0BBN0ZX
0BBN3ZX
0BBP0ZX
0BBP3ZX
0BC17ZZ
0BC18ZZ
0BC27ZZ
0BC28ZZ
0BC37ZZ
0BC38ZZ
0BC47ZZ
0BC48ZZ
0BC57ZZ
0BC58ZZ
0BC67ZZ
0BC68ZZ
0BC77ZZ
0BC78ZZ
0BC87ZZ
0BC88ZZ
0BC97ZZ
0BC98ZZ
0BCB7ZZ
0BCB8ZZ
0BCN3ZZ
0BCP3ZZ
0BD14ZX
0BD18ZX
0BD24ZX
0BD28ZX
0BD34ZX
0BD38ZX
0BD44ZX
0BD48ZX
0BD54ZX
0BD58ZX
0BD64ZX
0BD68ZX
0BD74ZX
0BD78ZX
0BD84ZX
0BD88ZX
0BD94ZX
0BD98ZX
0BDB4ZX
0BDB8ZX
0BDC4ZX
0BDC8ZX
0BDD4ZX
0BDD8ZX
0BDF4ZX
0BDF8ZX
0BDG4ZX
0BDG8ZX
0BDH4ZX
0BDH8ZX
0BDJ4ZX
0BDJ8ZX
0BDK4ZX
0BDK8ZX
0BDL4ZX
0BDL8ZX
0BDM4ZX
0BDM8ZX
0BF1XZZ
0BF2XZZ
0BF37ZZ
0BF38ZZ
0BF3XZZ
0BF47ZZ
0BF48ZZ
0BF4XZZ
0BF57ZZ
0BF58ZZ
0BF5XZZ
0BF67ZZ
0BF68ZZ
0BF6XZZ
0BF77ZZ
0BF78ZZ
0BF7XZZ
0BF87ZZ
0BF88ZZ
0BF8XZZ
0BF97ZZ
0BF98ZZ
0BF9XZZ
0BFB7ZZ
0BFB8ZZ
0BFBXZZ
0BH03YZ
0BH072Z
0BH073Z
0BH07DZ
0BH07YZ
0BH082Z
0BH083Z
0BH08DZ
0BH08YZ
0BH13EZ
0BH13YZ
0BH172Z
0BH17DZ
0BH17EZ
0BH17YZ
0BH182Z
0BH18DZ
0BH18EZ
0BH18YZ
0BH38GZ
0BH48GZ
0BH58GZ
0BH68GZ
0BH78GZ
0BH88GZ
0BH98GZ
0BHB8GZ
0BHK3YZ
0BHK72Z
0BHK73Z
0BHK7YZ
0BHK82Z
0BHK83Z
0BHL3YZ
0BHL72Z
0BHL73Z
0BHL7YZ
0BHL82Z
0BHL83Z
0BHQ3YZ
0BHQ7YZ
0BHT3YZ
0BHT7YZ
0BHT8YZ
0BJ03ZZ
0BJ07ZZ
0BJ08ZZ
0BJ0XZZ
0BJ13ZZ
0BJ14ZZ
0BJ17ZZ
0BJ18ZZ
0BJ1XZZ
0BJK3ZZ
0BJK7ZZ
0BJK8ZZ
0BJKXZZ
0BJL3ZZ
0BJL7ZZ
0BJL8ZZ
0BJLXZZ
0BJQ3ZZ
0BJQ7ZZ
0BJQ8ZZ
0BJQXZZ
0BJT3ZZ
0BJT7ZZ
0BJT8ZZ
0BJTXZZ
0BP03YZ
0BP04YZ
0BP070Z
0BP072Z
0BP073Z
0BP07DZ
0BP07YZ
0BP080Z
0BP082Z
0BP083Z
0BP08DZ
0BP08YZ
0BP0X0Z
0BP0X1Z
0BP0X2Z
0BP0X3Z
0BP0XDZ
0BP10FZ
0BP13FZ
0BP14FZ
0BP170Z
0BP172Z
0BP17DZ
0BP17FZ
0BP180Z
0BP182Z
0BP18DZ
0BP18FZ
0BP1X0Z
0BP1X2Z
0BP1XDZ
0BP1XFZ
0BPK3YZ
0BPK70Z
0BPK71Z
0BPK72Z
0BPK73Z
0BPK7YZ
0BPK80Z
0BPK81Z
0BPK82Z
0BPK83Z
0BPKX0Z
0BPKX1Z
0BPKX2Z
0BPKX3Z
0BPL3YZ
0BPL70Z
0BPL72Z
0BPL73Z
0BPL7YZ
0BPL80Z
0BPL82Z
0BPL83Z
0BPLX0Z
0BPLX1Z
0BPLX2Z
0BPLX3Z
0BPQ00Z
0BPQ01Z
0BPQ02Z
0BPQ30Z
0BPQ31Z
0BPQ32Z
0BPQ3YZ
0BPQ40Z
0BPQ41Z
0BPQ42Z
0BPQ70Z
0BPQ71Z
0BPQ72Z
0BPQ7YZ
0BPQ80Z
0BPQ81Z
0BPQ82Z
0BPQX0Z
0BPQX1Z
0BPQX2Z
0BPT3YZ
0BPT70Z
0BPT72Z
0BPT7YZ
0BPT80Z
0BPT82Z
0BPT8YZ
0BPTX0Z
0BPTX2Z
0BPTXMZ
0BW03YZ
0BW04YZ
0BW072Z
0BW073Z
0BW07DZ
0BW07YZ
0BW082Z
0BW083Z
0BW08DZ
0BW08YZ
0BW0X0Z
0BW0X2Z
0BW0X3Z
0BW0X7Z
0BW0XCZ
0BW0XDZ
0BW0XJZ
0BW0XKZ
0BW1X0Z
0BW1X2Z
0BW1X7Z
0BW1XCZ
0BW1XDZ
0BW1XFZ
0BW1XJZ
0BW1XKZ
0BWK3YZ
0BWK70Z
0BWK72Z
0BWK73Z
0BWK7YZ
0BWK80Z
0BWK82Z
0BWK83Z
0BWKX0Z
0BWKX2Z
0BWKX3Z
0BWL3YZ
0BWL70Z
0BWL72Z
0BWL73Z
0BWL7YZ
0BWL80Z
0BWL82Z
0BWL83Z
0BWLX0Z
0BWLX2Z
0BWLX3Z
0BWQ00Z
0BWQ02Z
0BWQ0YZ
0BWQ30Z
0BWQ32Z
0BWQ3YZ
0BWQ40Z
0BWQ42Z
0BWQ70Z
0BWQ72Z
0BWQ7YZ
0BWQ80Z
0BWQ82Z
0BWQX0Z
0BWQX2Z
0BWT3YZ
0BWT7YZ
0BWT8YZ
0BWTX0Z
0BWTX2Z
0BWTX7Z
0BWTXJZ
0BWTXKZ
0BWTXMZ
0C2AX0Z
0C2AXYZ
0C2SX0Z
0C2SXYZ
0C2YX0Z
0C2YXYZ
0C550ZZ
0C553ZZ
0C55XZZ
0C560ZZ
0C563ZZ
0C56XZZ
0C5W0Z0
0C5W0Z1
0C5W0Z2
0C5WXZ0
0C5WXZ1
0C5WXZ2
0C5X0Z0
0C5X0Z1
0C5X0Z2
0C5XXZ0
0C5XXZ1
0C5XXZ2
0C7B0DZ
0C7B0ZZ
0C7B3DZ
0C7B3ZZ
0C7B7DZ
0C7B7ZZ
0C7C0DZ
0C7C0ZZ
0C7C3DZ
0C7C3ZZ
0C7C7DZ
0C7C7ZZ
0C7M7DZ
0C7M7ZZ
0C7M8DZ
0C7M8ZZ
0C900ZX
0C9030Z
0C903ZX
0C903ZZ
0C90XZX
0C910ZX
0C9130Z
0C913ZX
0C913ZZ
0C91XZX
0C9230Z
0C923ZZ
0C9330Z
0C933ZZ
0C940ZX
0C9430Z
0C943ZX
0C943ZZ
0C94XZX
0C9500Z
0C950ZX
0C950ZZ
0C9530Z
0C953ZX
0C953ZZ
0C95X0Z
0C95XZX
0C95XZZ
0C9600Z
0C960ZX
0C960ZZ
0C9630Z
0C963ZX
0C963ZZ
0C96X0Z
0C96XZX
0C96XZZ
0C9730Z
0C973ZX
0C973ZZ
0C97XZX
0C9800Z
0C9830Z
0C983ZX
0C983ZZ
0C9900Z
0C9930Z
0C993ZX
0C993ZZ
0C9B00Z
0C9B0ZZ
0C9B30Z
0C9B3ZX
0C9B3ZZ
0C9C00Z
0C9C0ZZ
0C9C30Z
0C9C3ZX
0C9C3ZZ
0C9D00Z
0C9D0ZZ
0C9D30Z
0C9D3ZX
0C9D3ZZ
0C9F00Z
0C9F0ZZ
0C9F30Z
0C9F3ZX
0C9F3ZZ
0C9G00Z
0C9G30Z
0C9G3ZX
0C9G3ZZ
0C9H00Z
0C9H30Z
0C9H3ZX
0C9H3ZZ
0C9J00Z
0C9J0ZZ
0C9J30Z
0C9J3ZX
0C9J3ZZ
0C9M0ZX
0C9M30Z
0C9M3ZX
0C9M3ZZ
0C9M4ZX
0C9M7ZX
0C9M8ZX
0C9N30Z
0C9N3ZZ
0C9P30Z
0C9P3ZZ
0C9Q30Z
0C9Q3ZZ
0C9R30Z
0C9R3ZX
0C9R3ZZ
0C9R4ZX
0C9R7ZX
0C9R8ZX
0C9S30Z
0C9S3ZX
0C9S3ZZ
0C9S4ZX
0C9S7ZX
0C9S8ZX
0C9T30Z
0C9T3ZX
0C9T3ZZ
0C9T4ZX
0C9T7ZX
0C9T8ZX
0C9V30Z
0C9V3ZX
0C9V3ZZ

0C9V4ZX
0C9V7ZX
0C9V8ZX
0C9W000
0C9W001
0C9W002
0C9W0Z0
0C9W0Z1
0C9W0Z2
0C9WX00
0C9WX01
0C9WX02
0C9WXZ0
0C9WXZ1
0C9WXZ2
0C9X000
0C9X001
0C9X002
0C9X0Z0
0C9X0Z1
0C9X0Z2
0C9XX00
0C9XX01
0C9XX02
0C9XXZ0
0C9XXZ1
0C9XXZ2
0CB00ZX
0CB03ZX
0CB0XZX
0CB10ZX
0CB13ZX
0CB1XZX
0CB40ZX
0CB43ZX
0CB4XZX
0CB50ZX
0CB50ZZ
0CB53ZX
0CB53ZZ
0CB5XZX
0CB5XZZ
0CB60ZX
0CB60ZZ
0CB63ZX
0CB63ZZ
0CB6XZX
0CB6XZZ
0CB73ZX
0CB7XZX
0CB83ZX
0CB93ZX
0CBB3ZX
0CBC3ZX
0CBD3ZX
0CBF3ZX
0CBG3ZX
0CBH3ZX
0CBJ3ZX
0CBM0ZX
0CBM3ZX
0CBM4ZX
0CBM7ZX
0CBM8ZX
0CBR3ZX
0CBR4ZX
0CBR7ZX
0CBR8ZX
0CBS3ZX
0CBS4ZX
0CBS7ZX
0CBS8ZX
0CBT3ZX
0CBT4ZX
0CBT7ZX
0CBT8ZX
0CBV3ZX
0CBV4ZX
0CBV7ZX
0CBV8ZX
0CBW0Z0
0CBW0Z1
0CBW0Z2
0CBWXZ0
0CBWXZ1
0CBWXZ2
0CBX0Z0
0CBX0Z1
0CBX0Z2
0CBXXZ0
0CBXXZ1
0CBXXZ2
0CC0XZZ
0CC1XZZ
0CC2XZZ
0CC3XZZ
0CC4XZZ
0CC50ZZ
0CC53ZZ
0CC5XZZ
0CC60ZZ
0CC63ZZ
0CC6XZZ
0CC7XZZ
0CC83ZZ
0CC93ZZ
0CCB0ZZ
0CCB3ZZ
0CCC0ZZ
0CCC3ZZ
0CCD0ZZ
0CCD3ZZ
0CCF0ZZ
0CCF3ZZ
0CCG3ZZ
0CCH3ZZ
0CCJ0ZZ
0CCJ3ZZ
0CCM7ZZ
0CCM8ZZ
0CCNXZZ
0CCPXZZ
0CCQXZZ
0CCS7ZZ
0CCS8ZZ
0CCW0Z0
0CCW0Z1
0CCW0Z2
0CCWXZ0
0CCWXZ1
0CCWXZ2
0CCX0Z0
0CCX0Z1
0CCX0Z2
0CCXXZ0
0CCXXZ1
0CCXXZ2
0CDWXZ0
0CDWXZ1
0CDWXZ2
0CDXXZ0
0CDXXZ1
0CDXXZ2
0CFB0ZZ
0CFB3ZZ
0CFB7ZZ
0CFBXZZ
0CFC0ZZ
0CFC3ZZ
0CFC7ZZ
0CFCXZZ
0CHA3YZ
0CHA7YZ
0CHA8YZ
0CHS0YZ
0CHS3YZ
0CHS7YZ
0CHS8YZ
0CHY0YZ
0CHY3YZ
0CHY7BZ
0CHY7YZ
0CHY8BZ
0CHY8YZ
0CJA0ZZ
0CJA3ZZ
0CJAXZZ
0CJS0ZZ
0CJS3ZZ
0CJS4ZZ
0CJS7ZZ
0CJS8ZZ
0CJSXZZ
0CJY0ZZ
0CJY3ZZ
0CJY4ZZ
0CJY7ZZ
0CJY8ZZ
0CJYXZZ
0CMW0Z0
0CMW0Z1
0CMW0Z2
0CMWXZ0
0CMWXZ1
0CMWXZ2
0CMX0Z0
0CMX0Z1
0CMX0Z2
0CMXXZ0
0CMXXZ1
0CMXXZ2
0CN00ZZ
0CN03ZZ
0CN0XZZ
0CN10ZZ
0CN13ZZ
0CN1XZZ
0CN4XZZ
0CN50ZZ
0CN53ZZ
0CN5XZZ
0CN60ZZ
0CN63ZZ
0CN6XZZ
0CN70ZZ
0CN73ZZ
0CN7XZZ
0CNW0Z0
0CNW0Z1
0CNW0Z2
0CNWXZ0
0CNWXZ1
0CNWXZ2
0CNX0Z0
0CNX0Z1
0CNX0Z2
0CNXXZ0
0CNXXZ1
0CNXXZ2
0CPA00Z
0CPA0CZ
0CPA0YZ
0CPA30Z
0CPA3CZ
0CPA3YZ
0CPA7YZ
0CPA8YZ
0CPS3YZ
0CPS70Z
0CPS7DZ
0CPS7YZ
0CPS80Z
0CPS8DZ
0CPS8YZ
0CPSX0Z
0CPSX7Z
0CPSXDZ
0CPSXJZ
0CPSXKZ
0CPY3YZ
0CPY70Z
0CPY7DZ
0CPY7YZ
0CPY80Z
0CPY8DZ
0CPY8YZ
0CPYX0Z
0CPYX1Z
0CPYX7Z
0CPYXDZ
0CPYXJZ
0CPYXKZ
0CQ0XZZ
0CQ1XZZ
0CQ4XZZ
0CQ50ZZ
0CQ53ZZ
0CQ5XZZ
0CQ60ZZ
0CQ63ZZ
0CQ6XZZ
0CQ7XZZ
0CQW0Z0
0CQW0Z1
0CQW0Z2
0CQWXZ0
0CQWXZ1
0CQWXZ2
0CQX0Z0
0CQX0Z1
0CQX0Z2
0CQXXZ0
0CQXXZ1
0CQXXZ2
0CRW070
0CRW071
0CRW072
0CRW0J0
0CRW0J1
0CRW0J2
0CRW0K0
0CRW0K1
0CRW0K2
0CRWX70
0CRWX71
0CRWX72
0CRWXJ0
0CRWXJ1
0CRWXJ2
0CRWXK0
0CRWXK1
0CRWXK2
0CRX070
0CRX071
0CRX072
0CRX0J0
0CRX0J1
0CRX0J2
0CRX0K0
0CRX0K1
0CRX0K2
0CRXX70
0CRXX71
0CRXX72
0CRXXJ0
0CRXXJ1
0CRXXJ2
0CRXXK0
0CRXXK1
0CRXXK2
0CSW050
0CSW051
0CSW052
0CSW0Z0
0CSW0Z1
0CSW0Z2
0CSWX50
0CSWX51
0CSWX52
0CSWXZ0
0CSWXZ1
0CSWXZ2
0CSX050
0CSX051
0CSX052
0CSX0Z0
0CSX0Z1
0CSX0Z2
0CSXX50
0CSXX51
0CSXX52
0CSXXZ0
0CSXXZ1
0CSXXZ2
0CTW0Z0
0CTW0Z1
0CTW0Z2
0CTX0Z0
0CTX0Z1
0CTX0Z2
0CU20JZ
0CU23JZ
0CWA00Z
0CWA0CZ
0CWA0YZ
0CWA30Z
0CWA3CZ
0CWA3YZ
0CWA7YZ
0CWA8YZ
0CWAX0Z
0CWAXCZ
0CWS3YZ
0CWS7YZ
0CWS8YZ
0CWSX0Z
0CWSX7Z
0CWSXDZ
0CWSXJZ
0CWSXKZ
0CWY07Z
0CWY3YZ
0CWY7YZ
0CWY8YZ
0CWYX0Z
0CWYX1Z
0CWYX7Z
0CWYXDZ
0CWYXJZ
0CWYXKZ
0D16074
0D160J4
0D160K4
0D160Z4
0D163J4
0D16474
0D164J4
0D164K4
0D164Z4
0D16874
0D168J4
0D168K4
0D168Z4
0D18074
0D18078
0D1807H
0D1807K
0D1807L
0D1807M
0D1807N
0D1807P
0D1807Q
0D180J4
0D180J8
0D180JH
0D180JK
0D180JL
0D180JM
0D180JN
0D180JP
0D180JQ
0D180K4
0D180K8
0D180KH
0D180KK
0D180KL
0D180KM
0D180KN
0D180KP
0D180KQ
0D180Z4
0D180Z8
0D180ZH
0D180ZK
0D180ZL
0D180ZM
0D180ZN
0D180ZP
0D180ZQ
0D18474
0D18478
0D1847H
0D1847K
0D1847L
0D1847M
0D1847N
0D1847P
0D1847Q
0D184J4
0D184J8
0D184JH
0D184JK
0D184JL
0D184JM
0D184JN
0D184JP
0D184JQ
0D184K4
0D184K8
0D184KH
0D184KK
0D184KL
0D184KM
0D184KN
0D184KP
0D184KQ
0D184Z4
0D184Z8
0D184ZH
0D184ZK
0D184ZL
0D184ZM
0D184ZN
0D184ZP
0D184ZQ
0D18874
0D18878
0D1887H
0D1887K
0D1887L
0D1887M
0D1887N
0D1887P
0D1887Q
0D188J4
0D188J8
0D188JH
0D188JK
0D188JL
0D188JM
0D188JN
0D188JP
0D188JQ
0D188K4
0D188K8
0D188KH
0D188KK
0D188KL
0D188KM
0D188KN
0D188KP
0D188KQ
0D188Z4
0D188Z8
0D188ZH
0D188ZK
0D188ZL
0D188ZM
0D188ZN
0D188ZP
0D188ZQ
0D1E074
0D1E07E
0D1E07P
0D1E0J4
0D1E0JE
0D1E0JP
0D1E0K4
0D1E0KE
0D1E0KP
0D1E0Z4
0D1E0ZE
0D1E0ZP
0D1E474
0D1E47E
0D1E47P
0D1E4J4
0D1E4JE
0D1E4JP
0D1E4K4
0D1E4KE
0D1E4KP
0D1E4Z4
0D1E4ZE
0D1E4ZP
0D1E874
0D1E87E
0D1E87P
0D1E8J4
0D1E8JE
0D1E8JP
0D1E8K4
0D1E8KE
0D1E8KP
0D1E8Z4
0D1E8ZE
0D1E8ZP
0D20X0Z
0D20XUZ
0D20XYZ
0D2DX0Z
0D2DXUZ
0D2DXYZ
0D2UX0Z
0D2UXYZ
0D2VX0Z
0D2VXYZ
0D2WX0Z
0D2WXYZ
0D514ZZ

0D518ZZ	0D757ZZ	0D7F8ZZ	0D924ZX	0D9A8ZX	0D9L4ZX	0DB17ZX	0DBE3ZX	0DBW4ZX
0D524ZZ	0D758DZ	0D7G0DZ	0D927ZX	0D9B30Z	0D9L70Z	0DB18ZX	0DBE4ZX	0DC17ZZ
0D528ZZ	0D758ZZ	0D7G3DZ	0D928ZX	0D9B3ZX	0D9L7ZX	0DB18ZZ	0DBE7ZX	0DC18ZZ
0D534ZZ	0D767DZ	0D7G4DZ	0D9330Z	0D9B3ZZ	0D9L80Z	0DB23ZX	0DBE8ZX	0DC27ZZ
0D538ZZ	0D767ZZ	0D7G7DZ	0D933ZX	0D9B4ZX	0D9L8ZX	0DB24ZX	0DBE8ZZ	0DC28ZZ
0D544ZZ	0D768DZ	0D7G7ZZ	0D933ZZ	0D9B70Z	0D9M30Z	0DB24ZZ	0DBF3ZX	0DC37ZZ
0D548ZZ	0D768ZZ	0D7G8DZ	0D934ZX	0D9B7ZX	0D9M3ZX	0DB27ZX	0DBF4ZX	0DC38ZZ
0D554ZZ	0D774DZ	0D7G8ZZ	0D937ZX	0D9B80Z	0D9M3ZZ	0DB28ZX	0DBF7ZX	0DC47ZZ
0D558ZZ	0D777DZ	0D7H0DZ	0D938ZX	0D9B8ZX	0D9M4ZX	0DB28ZZ	0DBF8ZX	0DC48ZZ
0D564ZZ	0D777ZZ	0D7H3DZ	0D9430Z	0D9C30Z	0D9M70Z	0DB33ZX	0DBF8ZZ	0DC57ZZ
0D568ZZ	0D778DZ	0D7H4DZ	0D943ZX	0D9C3ZX	0D9M7ZX	0DB34ZX	0DBG3ZX	0DC58ZZ
0D574ZZ	0D778ZZ	0D7H7DZ	0D943ZZ	0D9C3ZZ	0D9M80Z	0DB34ZZ	0DBG4ZX	0DC67ZZ
0D578ZZ	0D780DZ	0D7H7ZZ	0D944ZX	0D9C4ZX	0D9M8ZX	0DB37ZX	0DBG7ZX	0DC68ZZ
0D588ZZ	0D783DZ	0D7H8DZ	0D947ZX	0D9C7ZX	0D9N30Z	0DB38ZX	0DBG8ZX	0DC77ZZ
0D594ZZ	0D784DZ	0D7H8ZZ	0D948ZX	0D9C8ZX	0D9N3ZX	0DB38ZZ	0DBG8ZZ	0DC78ZZ
0D598ZZ	0D787DZ	0D7K0DZ	0D9530Z	0D9E30Z	0D9N3ZZ	0DB43ZX	0DBH3ZX	0DC87ZZ
0D5A8ZZ	0D787ZZ	0D7K3DZ	0D953ZX	0D9E3ZX	0D9N4ZX	0DB44ZX	0DBH4ZX	0DC88ZZ
0D5B8ZZ	0D788DZ	0D7K4DZ	0D953ZZ	0D9E3ZZ	0D9N70Z	0DB47ZX	0DBH7ZX	0DC97ZZ
0D5C8ZZ	0D788ZZ	0D7K7DZ	0D954ZX	0D9E4ZX	0D9N7ZX	0DB48ZX	0DBH8ZX	0DC98ZZ
0D5E4ZZ	0D790DZ	0D7K7ZZ	0D957ZX	0D9E70Z	0D9N80Z	0DB48ZZ	0DBH8ZZ	0DCA7ZZ
0D5E8ZZ	0D793DZ	0D7K8DZ	0D958ZX	0D9E7ZX	0D9N8ZX	0DB53ZX	0DBK3ZX	0DCA8ZZ
0D5F4ZZ	0D794DZ	0D7K8ZZ	0D9630Z	0D9E80Z	0D9P30Z	0DB54ZX	0DBK4ZX	0DCB7ZZ
0D5F8ZZ	0D797DZ	0D7L0DZ	0D963ZX	0D9E8ZX	0D9P3ZX	0DB54ZZ	0DBK7ZX	0DCB8ZZ
0D5G4ZZ	0D797ZZ	0D7L3DZ	0D963ZZ	0D9F30Z	0D9P3ZZ	0DB57ZX	0DBK8ZX	0DCC7ZZ
0D5G8ZZ	0D798DZ	0D7L4DZ	0D964ZX	0D9F3ZX	0D9P4ZX	0DB58ZX	0DBK8ZZ	0DCC8ZZ
0D5H4ZZ	0D798ZZ	0D7L7DZ	0D9670Z	0D9F3ZZ	0D9P70Z	0DB58ZZ	0DBL3ZX	0DCE7ZZ
0D5H8ZZ	0D7A0DZ	0D7L7ZZ	0D967ZX	0D9F4ZX	0D9P7ZX	0DB63ZX	0DBL4ZX	0DCE8ZZ
0D5K4ZZ	0D7A3DZ	0D7L8DZ	0D9680Z	0D9F70Z	0D9P80Z	0DB64ZX	0DBL7ZX	0DCF7ZZ
0D5K8ZZ	0D7A4DZ	0D7L8ZZ	0D968ZX	0D9F7ZX	0D9P8ZX	0DB64ZZ	0DBL8ZX	0DCF8ZZ
0D5L4ZZ	0D7A7DZ	0D7M0DZ	0D9730Z	0D9F80Z	0D9Q0ZX	0DB67ZX	0DBL8ZZ	0DCG7ZZ
0D5L8ZZ	0D7A7ZZ	0D7M3DZ	0D973ZX	0D9F8ZX	0D9Q30Z	0DB68ZX	0DBM3ZX	0DCG8ZZ
0D5M4ZZ	0D7A8DZ	0D7M4DZ	0D973ZZ	0D9G30Z	0D9Q3ZX	0DB68ZZ	0DBM4ZX	0DCH7ZZ
0D5M8ZZ	0D7A8ZZ	0D7M7DZ	0D974ZX	0D9G3ZX	0D9Q3ZZ	0DB73ZX	0DBM7ZX	0DCH8ZZ
0D5N4ZZ	0D7B0DZ	0D7M7ZZ	0D9770Z	0D9G3ZZ	0D9Q4ZX	0DB74ZX	0DBM8ZX	0DCK7ZZ
0D5N8ZZ	0D7B3DZ	0D7M8DZ	0D977ZX	0D9G4ZX	0D9Q7ZX	0DB74ZZ	0DBM8ZZ	0DCK8ZZ
0D5P0ZZ	0D7B4DZ	0D7M8ZZ	0D9780Z	0D9G70Z	0D9Q8ZX	0DB77ZX	0DBN3ZX	0DCL7ZZ
0D5P3ZZ	0D7B7DZ	0D7N0DZ	0D978ZX	0D9G7ZX	0D9QXZX	0DB78ZX	0DBN4ZX	0DCL8ZZ
0D5P4ZZ	0D7B7ZZ	0D7N3DZ	0D9830Z	0D9G80Z	0D9R0ZX	0DB78ZZ	0DBN7ZX	0DCM7ZZ
0D5P7ZZ	0D7B8DZ	0D7N4DZ	0D983ZX	0D9G8ZX	0D9R30Z	0DB83ZX	0DBN8ZX	0DCM8ZZ
0D5P8ZZ	0D7B8ZZ	0D7N7DZ	0D983ZZ	0D9H30Z	0D9R3ZX	0DB84ZX	0DBN8ZZ	0DCN7ZZ
0D5Q4ZZ	0D7C0DZ	0D7N7ZZ	0D984ZX	0D9H3ZX	0D9R3ZZ	0DB87ZX	0DBP3ZX	0DCN8ZZ
0D5Q8ZZ	0D7C3DZ	0D7N8DZ	0D9870Z	0D9H3ZZ	0D9R4ZX	0DB88ZX	0DBP4ZX	0DCP7ZZ
0D5R4ZZ	0D7C4DZ	0D7N8ZZ	0D987ZX	0D9H4ZX	0D9U30Z	0DB93ZX	0DBP7ZX	0DCP8ZZ
0D717DZ	0D7C7DZ	0D7P7DZ	0D9880Z	0D9H70Z	0D9U3ZX	0DB94ZX	0DBP8ZX	0DCQ7ZZ
0D717ZZ	0D7C7ZZ	0D7P7ZZ	0D988ZX	0D9H7ZX	0D9U3ZZ	0DB94ZZ	0DBP8ZZ	0DCQ8ZZ
0D718DZ	0D7C8DZ	0D7P8DZ	0D9930Z	0D9H80Z	0D9U40Z	0DB97ZX	0DBQ0ZX	0DCQXZZ
0D718ZZ	0D7C8ZZ	0D7P8ZZ	0D993ZX	0D9H8ZX	0D9U4ZZ	0DB98ZX	0DBQ3ZX	0DD13ZX
0D727DZ	0D7E0DZ	0D7Q7DZ	0D993ZZ	0D9J30Z	0D9V30Z	0DB98ZZ	0DBQ4ZX	0DD14ZX
0D727ZZ	0D7E3DZ	0D7Q7ZZ	0D994ZX	0D9J3ZZ	0D9V3ZX	0DBA3ZX	0DBQ7ZX	0DD18ZX
0D728DZ	0D7E4DZ	0D7Q8DZ	0D9970Z	0D9K30Z	0D9V3ZZ	0DBA4ZX	0DBQ8ZX	0DD23ZX
0D728ZZ	0D7E7DZ	0D7Q8ZZ	0D997ZX	0D9K3ZX	0D9V40Z	0DBA7ZX	0DBQ8ZZ	0DD24ZX
0D737DZ	0D7E7ZZ	0D9130Z	0D9980Z	0D9K3ZZ	0D9V4ZZ	0DBA8ZX	0DBQXZX	0DD28ZX
0D737ZZ	0D7E8DZ	0D913ZX	0D998ZX	0D9K4ZX	0D9W30Z	0DBB3ZX	0DBR0ZX	0DD33ZX
0D738DZ	0D7E8ZZ	0D913ZZ	0D9A30Z	0D9K70Z	0D9W3ZX	0DBB4ZX	0DBR3ZX	0DD34ZX
0D738ZZ	0D7F0DZ	0D914ZX	0D9A3ZX	0D9K7ZX	0D9W3ZZ	0DBB7ZX	0DBR4ZX	0DD38ZX
0D747DZ	0D7F3DZ	0D917ZX	0D9A3ZZ	0D9K80Z	0D9W40Z	0DBB8ZX	0DBU3ZX	0DD43ZX
0D747ZZ	0D7F4DZ	0D918ZX	0D9A4ZX	0D9K8ZX	0D9W4ZZ	0DBC3ZX	0DBU4ZX	0DD44ZX
0D748DZ	0D7F7DZ	0D9230Z	0D9A70Z	0D9L30Z	0DB13ZX	0DBC4ZX	0DBV3ZX	0DD48ZX
0D748ZZ	0D7F7ZZ	0D923ZX	0D9A7ZX	0D9L3ZX	0DB14ZX	0DBC7ZX	0DBV4ZX	0DD53ZX
0D757DZ	0D7F8DZ	0D923ZZ	0D9A80Z	0D9L3ZZ	0DB14ZZ	0DBC8ZX	0DBW3ZX	0DD54ZX

0DD58ZX
0DD63ZX
0DD64ZX
0DD68ZX
0DD73ZX
0DD74ZX
0DD78ZX
0DD83ZX
0DD84ZX
0DD88ZX
0DD93ZX
0DD94ZX
0DD98ZX
0DDA3ZX
0DDA4ZX
0DDA8ZX
0DDB3ZX
0DDB4ZX
0DDB8ZX
0DDC3ZX
0DDC4ZX
0DDC8ZX
0DDE3ZX
0DDE4ZX
0DDE8ZX
0DDF3ZX
0DDF4ZX
0DDF8ZX
0DDG3ZX
0DDG4ZX
0DDG8ZX
0DDH3ZX
0DDH4ZX
0DDH8ZX
0DDK3ZX
0DDK4ZX
0DDK8ZX
0DDL3ZX
0DDL4ZX
0DDL8ZX
0DDM3ZX
0DDM4ZX
0DDM8ZX
0DDN3ZX
0DDN4ZX
0DDN8ZX
0DDP3ZX
0DDP4ZX
0DDP8ZX
0DDQ3ZX
0DDQ4ZX
0DDQ8ZX
0DDQXZX
0DF5XZZ
0DF6XZZ
0DF8XZZ
0DF9XZZ
0DFAXZZ
0DFBXZZ
0DFEXZZ
0DFFXZZ
0DFGXZZ
0DFHXZZ
0DFJXZZ
0DFKXZZ
0DFLXZZ
0DFMXZZ
0DFNXZZ
0DFPXZZ
0DFQXZZ
0DH00YZ
0DH03YZ
0DH04YZ
0DH07YZ
0DH08YZ
0DH50DZ
0DH50UZ
0DH53DZ
0DH53UZ
0DH53YZ
0DH54DZ
0DH54UZ
0DH54YZ
0DH572Z
0DH573Z
0DH57BZ
0DH57DZ
0DH57UZ
0DH57YZ
0DH582Z
0DH583Z
0DH58BZ
0DH58DZ
0DH58UZ
0DH58YZ
0DH63UZ
0DH63YZ
0DH64UZ
0DH64YZ
0DH672Z
0DH673Z
0DH67DZ
0DH67UZ
0DH67YZ
0DH682Z
0DH683Z
0DH68DZ
0DH68UZ
0DH68YZ
0DH80DZ
0DH80UZ
0DH83DZ
0DH83UZ
0DH84DZ
0DH84UZ
0DH872Z
0DH873Z
0DH87DZ
0DH87UZ
0DH882Z
0DH883Z
0DH88DZ
0DH88UZ
0DH90DZ
0DH90UZ
0DH93DZ
0DH93UZ
0DH94DZ
0DH94UZ
0DH972Z
0DH973Z
0DH97DZ
0DH97UZ
0DH982Z
0DH983Z
0DH98DZ
0DH98UZ
0DHA0DZ
0DHA0UZ
0DHA3DZ
0DHA3UZ
0DHA4DZ
0DHA4UZ
0DHA72Z
0DHA73Z
0DHA7DZ
0DHA7UZ
0DHA82Z
0DHA83Z
0DHA8DZ
0DHA8UZ
0DHB0DZ
0DHB0UZ
0DHB3DZ
0DHB3UZ
0DHB4DZ
0DHB4UZ
0DHB72Z
0DHB73Z
0DHB7DZ
0DHB7UZ
0DHB82Z
0DHB83Z
0DHB8DZ
0DHB8UZ
0DHD0YZ
0DHD3YZ
0DHD4YZ
0DHD7YZ
0DHD8YZ
0DHE0DZ
0DHE3DZ
0DHE4DZ
0DHE7DZ
0DHE8DZ
0DHP0DZ
0DHP3DZ
0DHP4DZ
0DHP7DZ
0DHP8DZ
0DJ03ZZ
0DJ07ZZ
0DJ08ZZ
0DJ0XZZ
0DJ63ZZ
0DJ67ZZ
0DJ68ZZ
0DJ6XZZ
0DJD3ZZ
0DJD7ZZ
0DJD8ZZ
0DJDXZZ
0DJU3ZZ
0DJUXZZ
0DJV3ZZ
0DJVXZZ
0DJW3ZZ
0DJWXZZ
0DL10CZ
0DL10DZ
0DL10ZZ
0DL13CZ
0DL13DZ
0DL13ZZ
0DL14CZ
0DL14DZ
0DL14ZZ
0DL17DZ
0DL17ZZ
0DL18DZ
0DL18ZZ
0DL20CZ
0DL20DZ
0DL20ZZ
0DL23CZ
0DL23DZ
0DL23ZZ
0DL24CZ
0DL24DZ
0DL24ZZ
0DL27DZ
0DL27ZZ
0DL28DZ
0DL28ZZ
0DL30CZ
0DL30DZ
0DL30ZZ
0DL33CZ
0DL33DZ
0DL33ZZ
0DL34CZ
0DL34DZ
0DL34ZZ
0DL37DZ
0DL37ZZ
0DL38DZ
0DL38ZZ
0DL40CZ
0DL40DZ
0DL40ZZ
0DL43CZ
0DL43DZ
0DL43ZZ
0DL44CZ
0DL44DZ
0DL44ZZ
0DL47DZ
0DL47ZZ
0DL48DZ
0DL48ZZ
0DL50CZ
0DL50DZ
0DL50ZZ
0DL53CZ
0DL53DZ
0DL53ZZ
0DL54CZ
0DL54DZ
0DL54ZZ
0DL57DZ
0DL57ZZ
0DL58DZ
0DL58ZZ
0DN87ZZ
0DN88ZZ
0DN97ZZ
0DN98ZZ
0DNA7ZZ
0DNA8ZZ
0DNB7ZZ
0DNB8ZZ
0DNE7ZZ
0DNE8ZZ
0DNF7ZZ
0DNF8ZZ
0DNG7ZZ
0DNG8ZZ
0DNH7ZZ
0DNH8ZZ
0DNK7ZZ
0DNK8ZZ
0DNL7ZZ
0DNL8ZZ
0DNM7ZZ
0DNM8ZZ
0DNN7ZZ
0DNN8ZZ
0DP03YZ
0DP04YZ
0DP070Z
0DP072Z
0DP073Z
0DP07DZ
0DP07UZ
0DP07YZ
0DP080Z
0DP082Z
0DP083Z
0DP08DZ
0DP08UZ
0DP08YZ
0DP0X0Z
0DP0X2Z
0DP0X3Z
0DP0XDZ
0DP0XUZ
0DP53YZ
0DP54YZ
0DP571Z
0DP57DZ
0DP57YZ
0DP581Z
0DP58DZ
0DP58YZ
0DP5X1Z
0DP5X2Z
0DP5X3Z
0DP5XDZ
0DP5XUZ
0DP63YZ
0DP64YZ
0DP670Z
0DP672Z
0DP673Z
0DP67DZ
0DP67UZ
0DP67YZ
0DP680Z
0DP682Z
0DP683Z
0DP68DZ
0DP68UZ
0DP68YZ
0DP6X0Z
0DP6X2Z
0DP6X3Z
0DP6XDZ
0DP6XUZ
0DPD3YZ
0DPD4YZ
0DPD70Z
0DPD72Z
0DPD73Z
0DPD7DZ
0DPD7UZ
0DPD7YZ
0DPD80Z
0DPD82Z
0DPD83Z
0DPD8DZ
0DPD8UZ
0DPD8YZ
0DPDX0Z
0DPDX2Z
0DPDX3Z
0DPDXDZ
0DPDXUZ
0DPP71Z
0DPP81Z
0DPPX1Z
0DQU0ZZ
0DQU3ZZ
0DQU4ZZ
0DS5XZZ
0DS6XZZ
0DS9XZZ
0DSAXZZ
0DSBXZZ
0DSHXZZ
0DSKXZZ
0DSLXZZ
0DSMXZZ
0DSNXZZ
0DSPXZZ
0DSQXZZ
0DV67DZ
0DV68DZ
0DW03YZ
0DW04YZ
0DW07YZ
0DW08YZ
0DW0X0Z
0DW0X2Z
0DW0X3Z
0DW0X7Z
0DW0XCZ
0DW0XDZ
0DW0XJZ
0DW0XKZ
0DW0XUZ
0DW50YZ
0DW53YZ
0DW54YZ
0DW57YZ
0DW58YZ
0DW5XDZ
0DW63YZ
0DW64YZ
0DW67YZ
0DW68YZ
0DW6X0Z
0DW6X2Z
0DW6X3Z
0DW6X7Z
0DW6XCZ
0DW6XDZ
0DW6XJZ
0DW6XKZ
0DW6XUZ
0DWD3YZ
0DWD4YZ
0DWD7YZ
0DWD8YZ
0DWDX0Z
0DWDX2Z
0DWDX3Z
0DWDX7Z
0DWDXCZ
0DWDXDZ
0DWDXJZ
0DWDXKZ
0DWDXUZ
0DWU00Z
0DWU30Z
0DWU40Z
0DWV00Z
0DWV30Z
0DWV40Z
0DWW00Z
0DWW30Z
0DWW40Z
0DXE0Z7
0DXE4Z7
0DY50Z0
0DY50Z1
0DY50Z2
0F20X0Z
0F20XYZ
0F24X0Z
0F24XYZ
0F2BX0Z
0F2BXYZ
0F2DX0Z
0F2DXYZ
0F2GX0Z
0F2GXYZ
0F554ZZ
0F558ZZ
0F564ZZ
0F568ZZ
0F574ZZ
0F578ZZ
0F584ZZ
0F588ZZ
0F594ZZ
0F598ZZ
0F5C4ZZ
0F5C8ZZ
0F5D4ZZ
0F5D8ZZ
0F5F4ZZ
0F5F8ZZ
0F5G4ZF
0F5G4ZZ
0F5G8ZZ
0F753DZ
0F753ZZ
0F754DZ
0F754ZZ
0F757DZ
0F758DZ
0F758ZZ
0F763DZ
0F763ZZ
0F764DZ
0F764ZZ
0F767DZ
0F768DZ
0F768ZZ
0F773DZ
0F773ZZ
0F774DZ
0F774ZZ
0F777DZ
0F778DZ
0F778ZZ
0F783DZ
0F783ZZ
0F784DZ
0F784ZZ
0F787DZ
0F788DZ
0F788ZZ
0F793DZ
0F793ZZ
0F794DZ
0F794ZZ
0F797DZ
0F798DZ
0F798ZZ
0F7C8DZ
0F7C8ZZ
0F7D4DZ
0F7D4ZZ
0F7D7DZ
0F7D8DZ
0F7D8ZZ
0F7F4DZ
0F7F4ZZ
0F7F8DZ
0F7F8ZZ
0F9030Z
0F903ZX
0F903ZZ
0F9040Z
0F904ZX
0F904ZZ
0F9130Z
0F913ZX
0F913ZZ
0F9140Z
0F914ZX
0F914ZZ
0F9230Z
0F923ZX
0F923ZZ
0F9240Z
0F924ZX
0F924ZZ
0F9430Z
0F943ZX
0F943ZZ
0F9440Z
0F944ZX
0F944ZZ
0F9480Z
0F948ZX
0F948ZZ
0F9530Z
0F953ZX

0F953ZZ
0F954ZX
0F957ZX
0F9580Z
0F958ZX
0F958ZZ
0F9630Z
0F963ZX
0F963ZZ
0F964ZX
0F967ZX
0F9680Z
0F968ZX
0F968ZZ
0F9730Z
0F973ZX
0F973ZZ
0F9740Z
0F974ZX
0F974ZZ
0F9770Z
0F977ZX
0F977ZZ
0F9780Z
0F978ZX
0F978ZZ
0F9830Z
0F983ZX
0F983ZZ
0F984ZX
0F987ZX
0F9880Z
0F988ZX
0F988ZZ
0F9930Z
0F993ZX
0F993ZZ
0F994ZX
0F994ZZ
0F997ZX
0F997ZZ
0F9980Z
0F998ZX
0F998ZZ
0F9C30Z
0F9C3ZX
0F9C3ZZ
0F9C40Z
0F9C4ZX
0F9C4ZZ
0F9C7ZX
0F9C80Z
0F9C8ZX
0F9C8ZZ
0F9D30Z
0F9D3ZX
0F9D3ZZ
0F9D4ZX
0F9D7ZX
0F9D80Z
0F9D8ZX
0F9D8ZZ
0F9F30Z
0F9F3ZX
0F9F3ZZ
0F9F4ZX
0F9F7ZX
0F9F80Z
0F9F8ZX
0F9F8ZZ
0F9G30Z
0F9G3ZX
0F9G3ZZ
0F9G4ZX
0F9G80Z
0F9G8ZX
0F9G8ZZ
0FB03ZX
0FB13ZX
0FB23ZX
0FB43ZX
0FB44ZX
0FB48ZX
0FB53ZX
0FB54ZX
0FB54ZZ
0FB57ZX
0FB58ZX
0FB58ZZ
0FB63ZX
0FB64ZX
0FB64ZZ
0FB67ZX
0FB68ZX
0FB68ZZ
0FB73ZX
0FB74ZX
0FB74ZZ
0FB77ZX
0FB78ZX
0FB78ZZ
0FB83ZX
0FB84ZX
0FB84ZZ
0FB87ZX
0FB88ZX
0FB88ZZ
0FB93ZX
0FB94ZX
0FB94ZZ
0FB97ZX
0FB98ZX
0FB98ZZ
0FBC3ZX
0FBC4ZX
0FBC4ZZ
0FBC7ZX
0FBC8ZX
0FBC8ZZ
0FBD3ZX
0FBD4ZX
0FBD4ZZ
0FBD7ZX
0FBD8ZX
0FBD8ZZ
0FBF3ZX
0FBF4ZX
0FBF4ZZ
0FBF7ZX
0FBF8ZX
0FBF8ZZ
0FBG3ZX
0FBG4ZX
0FBG8ZX
0FC53ZZ
0FC54ZZ
0FC57ZZ
0FC58ZZ
0FC63ZZ
0FC64ZZ
0FC67ZZ
0FC68ZZ
0FC73ZZ
0FC74ZZ
0FC77ZZ
0FC78ZZ
0FC83ZZ
0FC84ZZ
0FC87ZZ
0FC88ZZ
0FC93ZZ
0FC94ZZ
0FC97ZZ
0FC98ZZ
0FCC4ZZ
0FCC8ZZ
0FCD3ZZ
0FCD4ZZ
0FCD8ZZ
0FCF3ZZ
0FCF4ZZ
0FCF8ZZ
0FD03ZX
0FD13ZX
0FD23ZX
0FD43ZX
0FD44ZX
0FD48ZX
0FD53ZX
0FD54ZX
0FD58ZX
0FD63ZX
0FD64ZX
0FD68ZX
0FD73ZX
0FD74ZX
0FD78ZX
0FD83ZX
0FD84ZX
0FD88ZX
0FD93ZX
0FD94ZX
0FD98ZX
0FDC3ZX
0FDC4ZX
0FDC8ZX
0FDD3ZX
0FDD4ZX
0FDD8ZX
0FDF3ZX
0FDF4ZX
0FDF8ZX
0FDG3ZX
0FDG4ZX
0FDG8ZX
0FF48ZZ
0FF4XZZ
0FF58ZZ
0FF5XZZ
0FF68ZZ
0FF6XZZ
0FF78ZZ
0FF7XZZ
0FF88ZZ
0FF8XZZ
0FF98ZZ
0FF9XZZ
0FFC8ZZ
0FFCXZZ
0FFD8ZZ
0FFDXZZ
0FFF8ZZ
0FFFXZZ
0FH003Z
0FH033Z
0FH03YZ
0FH043Z
0FH04YZ
0FH103Z
0FH133Z
0FH143Z
0FH203Z
0FH233Z
0FH243Z
0FH403Z
0FH433Z
0FH43YZ
0FH443Z
0FH44YZ
0FHB03Z
0FHB33Z
0FHB3YZ
0FHB43Z
0FHB4DZ
0FHB4YZ
0FHB72Z
0FHB73Z
0FHB7YZ
0FHB82Z
0FHB83Z
0FHB8DZ
0FHB8YZ
0FHD03Z
0FHD33Z
0FHD3YZ
0FHD43Z
0FHD4DZ
0FHD4YZ
0FHD72Z
0FHD73Z
0FHD7YZ
0FHD82Z
0FHD83Z
0FHD8DZ
0FHD8YZ
0FHG03Z
0FHG33Z
0FHG3YZ
0FHG43Z
0FHG4YZ
0FJ03ZZ
0FJ0XZZ
0FJ43ZZ
0FJ48ZZ
0FJ4XZZ
0FJB3ZZ
0FJB7ZZ
0FJB8ZZ
0FJD3ZZ
0FJD7ZZ
0FJD8ZZ
0FJG3ZZ
0FJG8ZZ
0FJGXZZ
0FL53CZ
0FL53DZ
0FL53ZZ
0FL54CZ
0FL54DZ
0FL54ZZ
0FL57DZ
0FL57ZZ
0FL58DZ
0FL58ZZ
0FL63CZ
0FL63DZ
0FL63ZZ
0FL64CZ
0FL64DZ
0FL64ZZ
0FL67DZ
0FL67ZZ
0FL68DZ
0FL68ZZ
0FL73CZ
0FL73DZ
0FL73ZZ
0FL74CZ
0FL74DZ
0FL74ZZ
0FL77DZ
0FL77ZZ
0FL78DZ
0FL78ZZ
0FL83CZ
0FL83DZ
0FL83ZZ
0FL84CZ
0FL84DZ
0FL84ZZ
0FL87DZ
0FL87ZZ
0FL88DZ
0FL88ZZ
0FL93CZ
0FL93DZ
0FL93ZZ
0FL94CZ
0FL94DZ
0FL94ZZ
0FL97DZ
0FL97ZZ
0FL98DZ
0FL98ZZ
0FM44ZZ
0FM54ZZ
0FM64ZZ
0FM74ZZ
0FM84ZZ
0FM94ZZ
0FP03YZ
0FP04YZ
0FP0X0Z
0FP0X2Z
0FP0X3Z
0FP43YZ
0FP44YZ
0FP4X0Z
0FP4X2Z
0FP4X3Z
0FP4XDZ
0FPB3YZ
0FPB4YZ
0FPB70Z
0FPB72Z
0FPB73Z
0FPB7DZ
0FPB7YZ
0FPB80Z
0FPB82Z
0FPB83Z
0FPB8DZ
0FPB8YZ
0FPBX0Z
0FPBX1Z
0FPBX2Z
0FPBX3Z
0FPBXDZ
0FPD3YZ
0FPD4YZ
0FPD70Z
0FPD72Z
0FPD73Z
0FPD7DZ
0FPD7YZ
0FPD80Z
0FPD82Z
0FPD83Z
0FPD8DZ
0FPD8YZ
0FPDX0Z
0FPDX1Z
0FPDX2Z
0FPDX3Z
0FPDXDZ
0FPG3YZ
0FPG4YZ
0FPGX0Z
0FPGX2Z
0FPGX3Z
0FTD4ZZ
0FTD8ZZ
0FTF4ZZ
0FTF8ZZ
0FV53CZ
0FV53DZ
0FV53ZZ
0FV54CZ
0FV54DZ
0FV54ZZ
0FV57DZ
0FV57ZZ
0FV58DZ
0FV58ZZ
0FV63CZ
0FV63DZ
0FV63ZZ
0FV64CZ
0FV64DZ
0FV64ZZ
0FV67DZ
0FV67ZZ
0FV68DZ
0FV68ZZ
0FV73CZ
0FV73DZ
0FV73ZZ
0FV74CZ
0FV74DZ
0FV74ZZ
0FV77DZ
0FV77ZZ
0FV78DZ
0FV78ZZ
0FV83CZ
0FV83DZ
0FV83ZZ
0FV84CZ
0FV84DZ
0FV84ZZ
0FV87DZ
0FV87ZZ
0FV88DZ
0FV88ZZ
0FV93CZ
0FV93DZ
0FV93ZZ
0FV94CZ
0FV94DZ
0FV94ZZ
0FV97DZ
0FV97ZZ
0FV98DZ
0FV98ZZ
0FW03YZ
0FW04YZ
0FW0X0Z
0FW0X2Z
0FW0X3Z
0FW43YZ
0FW44YZ
0FW4X0Z
0FW4X2Z
0FW4X3Z
0FW4XDZ
0FWB3YZ
0FWB4YZ
0FWB7YZ
0FWB80Z
0FWB82Z
0FWB8DZ
0FWB8YZ
0FWBX0Z
0FWBX2Z
0FWBX3Z
0FWBX7Z
0FWBXCZ
0FWBXDZ
0FWBXJZ
0FWBXKZ
0FWD3YZ
0FWD4YZ
0FWD7YZ
0FWD80Z
0FWD82Z
0FWD8DZ
0FWD8YZ
0FWDX0Z
0FWDX2Z
0FWDX3Z
0FWDX7Z
0FWDXCZ
0FWDXDZ
0FWDXJZ
0FWDXKZ
0FWG3YZ
0FWG4YZ
0FWGX0Z
0FWGX2Z
0FWGX3Z
0FWGXDZ
0G20X0Z
0G20XYZ
0G21X0Z
0G21XYZ
0G25X0Z
0G25XYZ
0G2KX0Z
0G2KXYZ
0G2RX0Z
0G2RXYZ
0G2SX0Z
0G2SXYZ
0G9030Z
0G903ZZ
0G9130Z
0G913ZZ
0G9230Z
0G923ZX
0G923ZZ
0G924ZX
0G9330Z
0G933ZX
0G933ZZ
0G934ZX
0G9430Z
0G943ZX
0G943ZZ
0G944ZX
0G9630Z
0G963ZZ
0G9730Z
0G973ZZ
0G9830Z
0G983ZZ
0G9930Z
0G993ZZ
0G9B30Z
0G9B3ZZ
0G9C30Z
0G9C3ZZ
0G9D30Z
0G9D3ZZ
0G9F30Z
0G9F3ZZ
0G9G30Z
0G9G3ZX
0G9G3ZZ
0G9G40Z
0G9G4ZX
0G9G4ZZ
0G9H30Z
0G9H3ZX
0G9H3ZZ
0G9H40Z
0G9H4ZX
0G9H4ZZ
0G9K30Z
0G9K3ZX
0G9K3ZZ

0G9K40Z	0GWKX0Z	0H95XZZ	0H9T70Z	0HB4XZX	0HBY8ZX	0HDHXZZ	0HPT7JZ	0HR4X72
0G9K4ZX	0GWRX0Z	0H96X0Z	0H9T7ZX	0HB4XZZ	0HC0XZZ	0HDJXZZ	0HPT7KZ	0HR5X72
0G9K4ZZ	0GWS3YZ	0H96XZX	0H9T7ZZ	0HB5XZX	0HC1XZZ	0HDKXZZ	0HPT7NZ	0HR6X72
0G9L30Z	0GWS4YZ	0H96XZZ	0H9T80Z	0HB5XZZ	0HC2XZZ	0HDLXZZ	0HPT7YZ	0HR7X72
0G9L3ZZ	0GWSX0Z	0H97X0Z	0H9T8ZX	0HB6XZX	0HC3XZZ	0HDMXZZ	0HPT80Z	0HR8X72
0G9L40Z	0GWSX2Z	0H97XZX	0H9T8ZZ	0HB6XZZ	0HC4XZZ	0HDNXZZ	0HPT81Z	0HR9X72
0G9L4ZZ	0GWSX3Z	0H97XZZ	0H9U00Z	0HB7XZX	0HC5XZZ	0HDQXZZ	0HPT87Z	0HRAX72
0G9M30Z	0H0T3JZ	0H98X0Z	0H9U30Z	0HB7XZZ	0HC6XZZ	0HDRXZZ	0HPT8JZ	0HRBX72
0G9M3ZZ	0H0U3JZ	0H98XZX	0H9U3ZX	0HB8XZX	0HC7XZZ	0HDSXZZ	0HPT8KZ	0HRCX72
0G9M40Z	0H0V3JZ	0H98XZZ	0H9U3ZZ	0HB8XZZ	0HC8XZZ	0HDT0ZZ	0HPT8NZ	0HRDX72
0G9M4ZZ	0H2PX0Z	0H99XZX	0H9U70Z	0HB9XZX	0HC9XZZ	0HDU0ZZ	0HPT8YZ	0HREX72
0G9N30Z	0H2PXYZ	0H9AX0Z	0H9U7ZX	0HBAXZX	0HCAXZZ	0HDV0ZZ	0HPU00Z	0HRFX72
0G9N3ZZ	0H2TX0Z	0H9AXZX	0H9U7ZZ	0HBAXZZ	0HCBXZZ	0HDY0ZZ	0HPU01Z	0HRGX72
0G9N40Z	0H2TXYZ	0H9AXZZ	0H9U80Z	0HBBXZX	0HCCXZZ	0HHPXYZ	0HPU07Z	0HRHX72
0G9N4ZZ	0H2UX0Z	0H9BX0Z	0H9U8ZX	0HBBXZZ	0HCDXZZ	0HHT3YZ	0HPU0KZ	0HRJX72
0G9P30Z	0H2UXYZ	0H9BXZX	0H9U8ZZ	0HBCXZX	0HCEXZZ	0HHT7YZ	0HPU30Z	0HRKX72
0G9P3ZZ	0H52XZD	0H9BXZZ	0H9V00Z	0HBCXZZ	0HCFXZZ	0HHT8YZ	0HPU31Z	0HRLX72
0G9P40Z	0H52XZZ	0H9CX0Z	0H9V30Z	0HBDXZX	0HCGXZZ	0HHU3YZ	0HPU37Z	0HRMX72
0G9P4ZZ	0H53XZD	0H9CXZX	0H9V3ZX	0HBDXZZ	0HCHXZZ	0HHU7YZ	0HPU3KZ	0HRNX72
0G9Q30Z	0H53XZZ	0H9CXZZ	0H9V3ZZ	0HBEXZX	0HCJXZZ	0HHU8YZ	0HPU3YZ	0HRSX7Z
0G9Q3ZZ	0H80XZZ	0H9DX0Z	0H9V70Z	0HBEXZZ	0HCKXZZ	0HJPXZZ	0HPU70Z	0HSSXZZ
0G9Q40Z	0H81XZZ	0H9DXZX	0H9V7ZX	0HBFXZX	0HCLXZZ	0HJQXZZ	0HPU71Z	0HTQXZZ
0G9Q4ZZ	0H82XZZ	0H9DXZZ	0H9V7ZZ	0HBFXZZ	0HCMXZZ	0HJRXZZ	0HPU77Z	0HTRXZZ
0G9R30Z	0H83XZZ	0H9EX0Z	0H9V80Z	0HBGXZX	0HCNXZZ	0HJT0ZZ	0HPU7JZ	0HUT3JZ
0G9R3ZZ	0H84XZZ	0H9EXZX	0H9V8ZX	0HBGXZZ	0HCQXZZ	0HJT3ZZ	0HPU7KZ	0HUU3JZ
0G9R40Z	0H85XZZ	0H9EXZZ	0H9V8ZZ	0HBHXZX	0HCRXZZ	0HJT7ZZ	0HPU7NZ	0HUV3JZ
0G9R4ZZ	0H86XZZ	0H9FX0Z	0H9W00Z	0HBHXZZ	0HCT3ZZ	0HJT8ZZ	0HPU7YZ	0HWPX0Z
0GB23ZX	0H87XZZ	0H9FXZX	0H9W30Z	0HBJXZX	0HCT7ZZ	0HJU0ZZ	0HPU80Z	0HWPX7Z
0GB24ZX	0H88XZZ	0H9FXZZ	0H9W3ZX	0HBJXZZ	0HCT8ZZ	0HJU3ZZ	0HPU81Z	0HWPXJZ
0GB33ZX	0H89XZZ	0H9GX0Z	0H9W3ZZ	0HBKXZX	0HCU3ZZ	0HJU7ZZ	0HPU87Z	0HWPXKZ
0GB34ZX	0H8AXZZ	0H9GXZX	0H9W70Z	0HBKXZZ	0HCU7ZZ	0HJU8ZZ	0HPU8JZ	0HWPXYZ
0GB43ZX	0H8BXZZ	0H9GXZZ	0H9W7ZX	0HBLXZX	0HCU8ZZ	0HM0XZZ	0HPU8KZ	0HWQX0Z
0GB44ZX	0H8CXZZ	0H9HX0Z	0H9W7ZZ	0HBLXZZ	0HCV3ZZ	0HPPX0Z	0HPU8NZ	0HWQX7Z
0GBG3ZX	0H8DXZZ	0H9HXZX	0H9W80Z	0HBMXZX	0HCV7ZZ	0HPPX7Z	0HPU8YZ	0HWQXJZ
0GBG4ZX	0H8EXZZ	0H9HXZZ	0H9W8ZX	0HBMXZZ	0HCV8ZZ	0HPPXJZ	0HQ0XZZ	0HWQXKZ
0GBH3ZX	0H8FXZZ	0H9JX0Z	0H9W8ZZ	0HBNXZX	0HCW3ZZ	0HPPXKZ	0HQ1XZZ	0HWRX0Z
0GBH4ZX	0H8GXZZ	0H9JXZX	0H9WX0Z	0HBNXZZ	0HCW7ZZ	0HPPXYZ	0HQ2XZZ	0HWRX7Z
0GBJ3ZX	0H8HXZZ	0H9JXZZ	0H9WXZX	0HBQXZX	0HCW8ZZ	0HPQX0Z	0HQ3XZZ	0HWRXJZ
0GBJ4ZX	0H8JXZZ	0H9KX0Z	0H9WXZZ	0HBQXZZ	0HCWXZZ	0HPQX7Z	0HQ4XZZ	0HWRXKZ
0GHS3YZ	0H8KXZZ	0H9KXZX	0H9X00Z	0HBRXZX	0HCX3ZZ	0HPQXJZ	0HQ5XZZ	0HWSX7Z
0GHS4YZ	0H8LXZZ	0H9KXZZ	0H9X30Z	0HBRXZZ	0HCX7ZZ	0HPQXKZ	0HQ6XZZ	0HWSXJZ
0GJ03ZZ	0H8MXZZ	0H9LX0Z	0H9X3ZX	0HBT3ZX	0HCX8ZZ	0HPRX0Z	0HQ7XZZ	0HWSXKZ
0GJ13ZZ	0H8NXZZ	0H9LXZX	0H9X3ZZ	0HBT7ZX	0HCXXZZ	0HPRX7Z	0HQ8XZZ	0HWT00Z
0GJ53ZZ	0H90X0Z	0H9LXZZ	0H9X70Z	0HBT8ZX	0HD0XZZ	0HPRXJZ	0HQAXZZ	0HWT07Z
0GJK3ZZ	0H90XZX	0H9MX0Z	0H9X7ZX	0HBU3ZX	0HD1XZZ	0HPRXKZ	0HQBXZZ	0HWT0KZ
0GJR3ZZ	0H90XZZ	0H9MXZX	0H9X7ZZ	0HBU7ZX	0HD2XZZ	0HPSX7Z	0HQCXZZ	0HWT0NZ
0GJS3ZZ	0H91X0Z	0H9MXZZ	0H9X80Z	0HBU8ZX	0HD3XZZ	0HPSXJZ	0HQDXZZ	0HWT30Z
0GP0X0Z	0H91XZX	0H9NX0Z	0H9X8ZX	0HBV3ZX	0HD4XZZ	0HPSXKZ	0HQEXZZ	0HWT37Z
0GP1X0Z	0H91XZZ	0H9NXZX	0H9X8ZZ	0HBV7ZX	0HD5XZZ	0HPT00Z	0HQFXZZ	0HWT3KZ
0GP5X0Z	0H92X0Z	0H9NXZZ	0H9XX0Z	0HBV8ZX	0HD6XZZ	0HPT01Z	0HQGXZZ	0HWT3NZ
0GPKX0Z	0H92XZX	0H9QX0Z	0H9XXZX	0HBW3ZX	0HD7XZZ	0HPT07Z	0HQHXZZ	0HWT3YZ
0GPRX0Z	0H92XZZ	0H9QXZX	0H9XXZZ	0HBW7ZX	0HD8XZZ	0HPT0KZ	0HQJXZZ	0HWT70Z
0GPS3YZ	0H93X0Z	0H9QXZZ	0HB0XZX	0HBW8ZX	0HD9XZZ	0HPT30Z	0HQKXZZ	0HWT77Z
0GPS4YZ	0H93XZX	0H9RX0Z	0HB0XZZ	0HBWXZX	0HDAXZZ	0HPT31Z	0HQLXZZ	0HWT7JZ
0GPSX0Z	0H93XZZ	0H9RXZX	0HB1XZX	0HBX3ZX	0HDBXZZ	0HPT37Z	0HQMXZZ	0HWT7KZ
0GPSX2Z	0H94X0Z	0H9RXZZ	0HB1XZZ	0HBX7ZX	0HDCXZZ	0HPT3KZ	0HQNXZZ	0HWT7NZ
0GPSX3Z	0H94XZX	0H9T00Z	0HB2XZX	0HBX8ZX	0HDDXZZ	0HPT3YZ	0HR0X72	0HWT7YZ
0GW0X0Z	0H94XZZ	0H9T30Z	0HB2XZZ	0HBXXZX	0HDEXZZ	0HPT70Z	0HR1X72	0HWT80Z
0GW1X0Z	0H95X0Z	0H9T3ZX	0HB3XZX	0HBY3ZX	0HDFXZZ	0HPT71Z	0HR2X72	0HWT87Z
0GW5X0Z	0H95XZX	0H9T3ZZ	0HB3XZZ	0HBY7ZX	0HDGXZZ	0HPT77Z	0HR3X72	0HWT8JZ

0HWT8KZ	0J973ZX	0J9M3ZX	0JBP0ZX	0JDJ3ZZ	0JNKXZZ	0JPTXHZ	0JPWXHZ	0JWWXHZ
0HWT8NZ	0J973ZZ	0J9M3ZZ	0JBP3ZX	0JDK3ZZ	0JNLXZZ	0JPTXVZ	0JPWXVZ	0JWWXJZ
0HWT8YZ	0J9800Z	0J9N00Z	0JBQ0ZX	0JDN3ZZ	0JNMXZZ	0JPTXXZ	0JPWXXZ	0JWWXKZ
0HWU00Z	0J980ZX	0J9N0ZX	0JBQ3ZX	0JDP3ZZ	0JNNXZZ	0JPV00Z	0JQ03ZZ	0JWWXNZ
0HWU07Z	0J9830Z	0J9N30Z	0JBR0ZX	0JDQ3ZZ	0JNPXZZ	0JPV01Z	0JQ13ZZ	0JWWXVZ
0HWU0KZ	0J983ZX	0J9N3ZX	0JBR3ZX	0JDR3ZZ	0JNQXZZ	0JPV03Z	0JQ43ZZ	0JWWXWZ
0HWU0NZ	0J983ZZ	0J9N3ZZ	0JC00ZZ	0JH60FZ	0JNRXZZ	0JPV07Z	0JQ53ZZ	0JWWXXZ
0HWU30Z	0J9900Z	0J9P00Z	0JC03ZZ	0JH63FZ	0JPS00Z	0JPV0HZ	0JQ63ZZ	0K2XX0Z
0HWU37Z	0J990ZX	0J9P0ZX	0JC10ZZ	0JHD0HZ	0JPS01Z	0JPV0JZ	0JQ73ZZ	0K2XXYZ
0HWU3KZ	0J9930Z	0J9P30Z	0JC13ZZ	0JHD3HZ	0JPS03Z	0JPV0KZ	0JQ83ZZ	0K2YX0Z
0HWU3NZ	0J993ZX	0J9P3ZX	0JC40ZZ	0JHF0HZ	0JPS07Z	0JPV0NZ	0JQ93ZZ	0K2YXYZ
0HWU3YZ	0J993ZZ	0J9P3ZZ	0JC43ZZ	0JHF3HZ	0JPS0JZ	0JPV0VZ	0JQB3ZZ	0K9030Z
0HWU70Z	0J9B00Z	0J9Q00Z	0JC50ZZ	0JHG0HZ	0JPS0KZ	0JPV0WZ	0JQC3ZZ	0K903ZZ
0HWU77Z	0J9B0ZX	0J9Q0ZX	0JC53ZZ	0JHG3HZ	0JPS0NZ	0JPV0XZ	0JQD3ZZ	0K9130Z
0HWU7JZ	0J9B30Z	0J9Q30Z	0JC60ZZ	0JHH0HZ	0JPS0YZ	0JPV0YZ	0JQF3ZZ	0K913ZZ
0HWU7KZ	0J9B3ZX	0J9Q3ZX	0JC63ZZ	0JHH3HZ	0JPS30Z	0JPV30Z	0JQG3ZZ	0K9230Z
0HWU7NZ	0J9B3ZZ	0J9Q3ZZ	0JC70ZZ	0JHL0HZ	0JPS31Z	0JPV31Z	0JQH3ZZ	0K923ZZ
0HWU7YZ	0J9C00Z	0J9R00Z	0JC73ZZ	0JHL3HZ	0JPS33Z	0JPV33Z	0JQJ3ZZ	0K9330Z
0HWU80Z	0J9C0ZX	0J9R0ZX	0JC80ZZ	0JHM0HZ	0JPS37Z	0JPV37Z	0JQK3ZZ	0K933ZZ
0HWU87Z	0J9C30Z	0J9R30Z	0JC83ZZ	0JHM3HZ	0JPS3JZ	0JPV3HZ	0JQL3ZZ	0K9430Z
0HWU8JZ	0J9C3ZX	0J9R3ZX	0JC90ZZ	0JHN0HZ	0JPS3KZ	0JPV3JZ	0JQM3ZZ	0K943ZZ
0HWU8KZ	0J9C3ZZ	0J9R3ZZ	0JC93ZZ	0JHS03Z	0JPS3NZ	0JPV3KZ	0JQN3ZZ	0K9530Z
0HWU8NZ	0J9D00Z	0JB00ZX	0JCB0ZZ	0JHS33Z	0JPS3YZ	0JPV3NZ	0JQP3ZZ	0K953ZZ
0HWU8YZ	0J9D0ZX	0JB03ZX	0JCB3ZZ	0JHS3YZ	0JPSX0Z	0JPV3VZ	0JQQ3ZZ	0K9630Z
0J2SX0Z	0J9D30Z	0JB10ZX	0JCC0ZZ	0JHT03Z	0JPSX1Z	0JPV3WZ	0JQR3ZZ	0K963ZZ
0J2SXYZ	0J9D3ZX	0JB13ZX	0JCC3ZZ	0JHT33Z	0JPSX3Z	0JPV3XZ	0JWSX0Z	0K9730Z
0J2TX0Z	0J9D3ZZ	0JB40ZX	0JCD0ZZ	0JHT3YZ	0JPT00Z	0JPV3YZ	0JWSX3Z	0K973ZZ
0J2TXYZ	0J9F00Z	0JB43ZX	0JCD3ZZ	0JHV03Z	0JPT01Z	0JPVX0Z	0JWSX7Z	0K9830Z
0J2VX0Z	0J9F0ZX	0JB50ZX	0JCF0ZZ	0JHV33Z	0JPT02Z	0JPVX1Z	0JWSXJZ	0K983ZZ
0J2VXYZ	0J9F30Z	0JB53ZX	0JCF3ZZ	0JHV3YZ	0JPT03Z	0JPVX3Z	0JWSXKZ	0K9930Z
0J2WX0Z	0J9F3ZX	0JB60ZX	0JCG0ZZ	0JHW03Z	0JPT07Z	0JPVXHZ	0JWSXNZ	0K993ZZ
0J2WXYZ	0J9F3ZZ	0JB63ZX	0JCG3ZZ	0JHW33Z	0JPT0FZ	0JPVXVZ	0JWT0FZ	0K9B30Z
0J9000Z	0J9G00Z	0JB70ZX	0JCH0ZZ	0JHW3YZ	0JPT0HZ	0JPVXXZ	0JWT3FZ	0K9B3ZZ
0J900ZX	0J9G0ZX	0JB73ZX	0JCH3ZZ	0JJS0ZZ	0JPT0JZ	0JPW00Z	0JWT3YZ	0K9C30Z
0J9030Z	0J9G30Z	0JB80ZX	0JCJ0ZZ	0JJS3ZZ	0JPT0KZ	0JPW01Z	0JWTX0Z	0K9C3ZZ
0J903ZX	0J9G3ZX	0JB83ZX	0JCJ3ZZ	0JJSXZZ	0JPT0MZ	0JPW03Z	0JWTX2Z	0K9C4ZZ
0J903ZZ	0J9G3ZZ	0JB90ZX	0JCK0ZZ	0JJT0ZZ	0JPT0NZ	0JPW07Z	0JWTX3Z	0K9D30Z
0J9100Z	0J9H00Z	0JB93ZX	0JCK3ZZ	0JJT3ZZ	0JPT0VZ	0JPW0HZ	0JWTX7Z	0K9D3ZZ
0J910ZX	0J9H0ZX	0JBB0ZX	0JCL0ZZ	0JJTXZZ	0JPT0WZ	0JPW0JZ	0JWTXFZ	0K9D4ZZ
0J9130Z	0J9H30Z	0JBB3ZX	0JCL3ZZ	0JJV0ZZ	0JPT0XZ	0JPW0KZ	0JWTXHZ	0K9F30Z
0J913ZX	0J9H3ZX	0JBC0ZX	0JCM0ZZ	0JJV3ZZ	0JPT0YZ	0JPW0NZ	0JWTXJZ	0K9F3ZZ
0J913ZZ	0J9H3ZZ	0JBC3ZX	0JCM3ZZ	0JJVXZZ	0JPT30Z	0JPW0VZ	0JWTXKZ	0K9G30Z
0J9400Z	0J9J00Z	0JBD0ZX	0JCN0ZZ	0JJW0ZZ	0JPT31Z	0JPW0WZ	0JWTXNZ	0K9G3ZZ
0J940ZX	0J9J0ZX	0JBD3ZX	0JCN3ZZ	0JJW3ZZ	0JPT32Z	0JPW0XZ	0JWTXPZ	0K9H30Z
0J9430Z	0J9J30Z	0JBF0ZX	0JCP0ZZ	0JJWXZZ	0JPT33Z	0JPW0YZ	0JWTXVZ	0K9H3ZZ
0J943ZX	0J9J3ZX	0JBF3ZX	0JCP3ZZ	0JN0XZZ	0JPT37Z	0JPW30Z	0JWTXWZ	0K9J30Z
0J943ZZ	0J9J3ZZ	0JBG0ZX	0JCQ0ZZ	0JN1XZZ	0JPT3FZ	0JPW31Z	0JWTXXZ	0K9J3ZZ
0J9500Z	0J9K00Z	0JBG3ZX	0JCQ3ZZ	0JN4XZZ	0JPT3HZ	0JPW33Z	0JWVX0Z	0K9K30Z
0J950ZX	0J9K0ZX	0JBH0ZX	0JCR0ZZ	0JN5XZZ	0JPT3JZ	0JPW37Z	0JWVX3Z	0K9K3ZZ
0J9530Z	0J9K30Z	0JBH3ZX	0JCR3ZZ	0JN6XZZ	0JPT3KZ	0JPW3HZ	0JWVX7Z	0K9L30Z
0J953ZX	0J9K3ZX	0JBJ0ZX	0JD03ZZ	0JN7XZZ	0JPT3MZ	0JPW3JZ	0JWVXHZ	0K9L3ZZ
0J953ZZ	0J9K3ZZ	0JBJ3ZX	0JD13ZZ	0JN8XZZ	0JPT3NZ	0JPW3KZ	0JWVXJZ	0K9M30Z
0J9600Z	0J9L00Z	0JBK0ZX	0JD43ZZ	0JN9XZZ	0JPT3VZ	0JPW3NZ	0JWVXKZ	0K9M3ZZ
0J960ZX	0J9L0ZX	0JBK3ZX	0JD53ZZ	0JNBXZZ	0JPT3WZ	0JPW3VZ	0JWVXNZ	0K9N30Z
0J9630Z	0J9L30Z	0JBL0ZX	0JDB3ZZ	0JNCXZZ	0JPT3XZ	0JPW3WZ	0JWVXVZ	0K9N3ZZ
0J963ZX	0J9L3ZX	0JBL3ZX	0JDC3ZZ	0JNDXZZ	0JPT3YZ	0JPW3XZ	0JWVXWZ	0K9P30Z
0J963ZZ	0J9L3ZZ	0JBM0ZX	0JDD3ZZ	0JNFXZZ	0JPTX0Z	0JPW3YZ	0JWVXXZ	0K9P3ZZ
0J9700Z	0J9M00Z	0JBM3ZX	0JDF3ZZ	0JNGXZZ	0JPTX1Z	0JPWX0Z	0JWWX0Z	0K9Q30Z
0J970ZX	0J9M0ZX	0JBN0ZX	0JDG3ZZ	0JNHXZZ	0JPTX2Z	0JPWX1Z	0JWWX3Z	0K9Q3ZZ
0J9730Z	0J9M30Z	0JBN3ZX	0JDH3ZZ	0JNJXZZ	0JPTX3Z	0JPWX3Z	0JWWX7Z	0K9R30Z

0K9R3ZZ-0N9V0ZZ
APPENDIX H: NON-OR PROCEDURE NOT AFFECTING MS-DRG ASSIGNMENT

0K9R3ZZ
0K9S30Z
0K9S3ZZ
0K9T30Z
0K9T3ZZ
0K9V30Z
0K9V3ZZ
0K9W30Z
0K9W3ZZ
0KHX3YZ
0KHX4YZ
0KHY3YZ
0KHY4YZ
0KJX3ZZ
0KJXXZZ
0KJY3ZZ
0KJYXZZ
0KN0XZZ
0KN1XZZ
0KN2XZZ
0KN3XZZ
0KN4XZZ
0KN5XZZ
0KN6XZZ
0KN7XZZ
0KN8XZZ
0KN9XZZ
0KNBXZZ
0KNCXZZ
0KNDXZZ
0KNFXZZ
0KNGXZZ
0KNHXZZ
0KNJXZZ
0KNKXZZ
0KNLXZZ
0KNMXZZ
0KNNXZZ
0KNPXZZ
0KNQXZZ
0KNRXZZ
0KNSXZZ
0KNTXZZ
0KNVXZZ
0KNWXZZ
0KPX3YZ
0KPX4YZ
0KPXX0Z
0KPXXMZ
0KPY3YZ
0KPY4YZ
0KPYX0Z
0KPYXMZ
0KWX3YZ
0KWX4YZ
0KWXX0Z
0KWXX7Z
0KWXXJZ
0KWXXKZ
0KWXXMZ
0KWY3YZ
0KWY4YZ
0KWYX0Z
0KWYX7Z
0KWYXJZ
0KWYXKZ
0KWYXMZ
0L2XX0Z
0L2XXYZ
0L2YX0Z
0L2YXYZ
0L9030Z
0L903ZZ
0L9130Z
0L913ZZ
0L9230Z
0L923ZZ
0L9330Z
0L933ZZ
0L9430Z
0L943ZZ
0L9530Z
0L953ZZ
0L9630Z
0L963ZZ
0L9730Z
0L973ZZ
0L974ZZ
0L9830Z
0L983ZZ
0L984ZZ
0L9930Z
0L993ZZ
0L9B30Z
0L9B3ZZ
0L9C30Z
0L9C3ZZ
0L9D30Z
0L9D3ZZ
0L9F30Z
0L9F3ZZ
0L9G30Z
0L9G3ZZ
0L9H30Z
0L9H3ZZ
0L9J30Z
0L9J3ZZ
0L9K30Z
0L9K3ZZ
0L9L30Z
0L9L3ZZ
0L9M30Z
0L9M3ZZ
0L9N30Z
0L9N3ZZ
0L9P30Z
0L9P3ZZ
0L9Q30Z
0L9Q3ZZ
0L9R30Z
0L9R3ZZ
0L9S30Z
0L9S3ZZ
0L9T30Z
0L9T3ZZ
0L9V30Z
0L9V3ZZ
0L9W30Z
0L9W3ZZ
0LHX3YZ
0LHX4YZ
0LHY3YZ
0LHY4YZ
0LJX3ZZ
0LJXXZZ
0LJY3ZZ
0LJYXZZ
0LN0XZZ
0LN1XZZ
0LN2XZZ
0LN3XZZ
0LN4XZZ
0LN5XZZ
0LN6XZZ
0LN7XZZ
0LN8XZZ
0LN9XZZ
0LNBXZZ
0LNCXZZ
0LNDXZZ
0LNFXZZ
0LNGXZZ
0LNHXZZ
0LNJXZZ
0LNKXZZ
0LNLXZZ
0LNMXZZ
0LNNXZZ
0LNPXZZ
0LNQXZZ
0LNRXZZ
0LNSXZZ
0LNTXZZ
0LNVXZZ
0LNWXZZ
0LPX30Z
0LPX3YZ
0LPX4YZ
0LPXX0Z
0LPY30Z
0LPY3YZ
0LPY4YZ
0LPYX0Z
0LWX3YZ
0LWX4YZ
0LWXX0Z
0LWXX7Z
0LWXXJZ
0LWXXKZ
0LWY3YZ
0LWY4YZ
0LWYX0Z
0LWYX7Z
0LWYXJZ
0LWYXKZ
0M2XX0Z
0M2XXYZ
0M2YX0Z
0M2YXYZ
0M900ZX
0M9030Z
0M903ZX
0M903ZZ
0M904ZX
0M904ZZ
0M910ZX
0M9130Z
0M913ZX
0M913ZZ
0M9140Z
0M914ZX
0M920ZX
0M9230Z
0M923ZX
0M923ZZ
0M9240Z
0M924ZX
0M930ZX
0M9330Z
0M933ZX
0M933ZZ
0M9340Z
0M934ZX
0M940ZX
0M9430Z
0M943ZX
0M943ZZ
0M9440Z
0M944ZX
0M950ZX
0M9530Z
0M953ZX
0M953ZZ
0M954ZX
0M954ZZ
0M960ZX
0M9630Z
0M963ZX
0M963ZZ
0M964ZX
0M964ZZ
0M970ZX
0M9730Z
0M973ZX
0M973ZZ
0M9740Z
0M974ZX
0M974ZZ
0M980ZX
0M9830Z
0M983ZX
0M983ZZ
0M9840Z
0M984ZX
0M984ZZ
0M9930Z
0M993ZZ
0M9940Z
0M994ZZ
0M9B30Z
0M9B3ZZ
0M9B40Z
0M9B4ZZ
0M9C0ZX
0M9C30Z
0M9C3ZX
0M9C3ZZ
0M9C40Z
0M9C4ZX
0M9C4ZZ
0M9D0ZX
0M9D30Z
0M9D3ZX
0M9D3ZZ
0M9D40Z
0M9D4ZX
0M9D4ZZ
0M9F0ZX
0M9F30Z
0M9F3ZX
0M9F3ZZ
0M9F40Z
0M9F4ZX
0M9F4ZZ
0M9G0ZX
0M9G30Z
0M9G3ZX
0M9G3ZZ
0M9G40Z
0M9G4ZX
0M9G4ZZ
0M9H30Z
0M9H3ZZ
0M9H40Z
0M9H4ZZ
0M9J30Z
0M9J3ZZ
0M9J40Z
0M9J4ZZ
0M9K30Z
0M9K3ZZ
0M9K40Z
0M9K4ZZ
0M9L0ZX
0M9L30Z
0M9L3ZX
0M9L3ZZ
0M9L40Z
0M9L4ZX
0M9M0ZX
0M9M30Z
0M9M3ZX
0M9M3ZZ
0M9M40Z
0M9M4ZX
0M9N0ZX
0M9N30Z
0M9N3ZX
0M9N3ZZ
0M9N4ZX
0M9N4ZZ
0M9P0ZX
0M9P30Z
0M9P3ZX
0M9P3ZZ
0M9P4ZX
0M9P4ZZ
0M9Q0ZX
0M9Q30Z
0M9Q3ZX
0M9Q3ZZ
0M9Q4ZX
0M9Q4ZZ
0M9R0ZX
0M9R30Z
0M9R3ZX
0M9R3ZZ
0M9R4ZX
0M9R4ZZ
0M9S0ZX
0M9S30Z
0M9S3ZX
0M9S3ZZ
0M9S4ZX
0M9S4ZZ
0M9T0ZX
0M9T30Z
0M9T3ZX
0M9T3ZZ
0M9T4ZX
0M9T4ZZ
0M9V30Z
0M9V3ZZ
0M9V40Z
0M9V4ZZ
0M9W30Z
0M9W3ZZ
0M9W40Z
0M9W4ZZ
0MB00ZX
0MB03ZX
0MB04ZX
0MB10ZX
0MB13ZX
0MB14ZX
0MB20ZX
0MB23ZX
0MB24ZX
0MB30ZX
0MB33ZX
0MB34ZX
0MB40ZX
0MB43ZX
0MB44ZX
0MB50ZX
0MB53ZX
0MB54ZX
0MB60ZX
0MB63ZX
0MB64ZX
0MB70ZX
0MB73ZX
0MB74ZX
0MB80ZX
0MB83ZX
0MB84ZX
0MB94ZX
0MBB0ZX
0MBB3ZX
0MBB4ZX
0MBC0ZX
0MBC3ZX
0MBC4ZX
0MBD0ZX
0MBD3ZX
0MBD4ZX
0MBF0ZX
0MBF3ZX
0MBF4ZX
0MBG0ZX
0MBG3ZX
0MBG4ZX
0MBL0ZX
0MBL3ZX
0MBL4ZX
0MBM0ZX
0MBM3ZX
0MBM4ZX
0MBN0ZX
0MBN3ZX
0MBN4ZX
0MBP0ZX
0MBP3ZX
0MBP4ZX
0MBQ0ZX
0MBQ3ZX
0MBQ4ZX
0MBR0ZX
0MBR3ZX
0MBR4ZX
0MBS0ZX
0MBS3ZX
0MBS4ZX
0MBT0ZX
0MBT3ZX
0MBT4ZX
0MHX3YZ
0MHX4YZ
0MHY3YZ
0MHY4YZ
0MJX3ZZ
0MJXXZZ
0MJY3ZZ
0MJYXZZ
0MN0XZZ
0MN1XZZ
0MN2XZZ
0MN3XZZ
0MN4XZZ
0MN5XZZ
0MN6XZZ
0MN7XZZ
0MN8XZZ
0MN9XZZ
0MNBXZZ
0MNCXZZ
0MNDXZZ
0MNFXZZ
0MNGXZZ
0MNHXZZ
0MNJXZZ
0MNKXZZ
0MNLXZZ
0MNMXZZ
0MNNXZZ
0MNPXZZ
0MNQXZZ
0MNRXZZ
0MNSXZZ
0MNTXZZ
0MNVXZZ
0MNWXZZ
0MPX30Z
0MPX3YZ
0MPX4YZ
0MPXX0Z
0MPY30Z
0MPY3YZ
0MPY4YZ
0MPYX0Z
0MWX3YZ
0MWX4YZ
0MWXX0Z
0MWXX7Z
0MWXXJZ
0MWXXKZ
0MWY3YZ
0MWY4YZ
0MWYX0Z
0MWYX7Z
0MWYXJZ
0MWYXKZ
0N20X0Z
0N20XYZ
0N2BX0Z
0N2BXYZ
0N2WX0Z
0N2WXYZ
0N8B0ZZ
0N8B3ZZ
0N8B4ZZ
0N9030Z
0N903ZZ
0N9130Z
0N913ZZ
0N9330Z
0N933ZZ
0N9430Z
0N943ZZ
0N9530Z
0N953ZZ
0N9630Z
0N963ZZ
0N9730Z
0N973ZZ
0N9B00Z
0N9B0ZX
0N9B0ZZ
0N9B30Z
0N9B3ZX
0N9B3ZZ
0N9B40Z
0N9B4ZX
0N9B4ZZ
0N9C30Z
0N9C3ZZ
0N9F30Z
0N9F3ZZ
0N9G30Z
0N9G3ZZ
0N9H30Z
0N9H3ZZ
0N9J30Z
0N9J3ZZ
0N9K30Z
0N9K3ZZ
0N9L30Z
0N9L3ZZ
0N9M30Z
0N9M3ZZ
0N9N30Z
0N9N3ZZ
0N9P30Z
0N9P3ZZ
0N9Q30Z
0N9Q3ZZ
0N9R00Z
0N9R0ZZ
0N9R30Z
0N9R3ZZ
0N9R40Z
0N9R4ZZ
0N9T00Z
0N9T0ZZ
0N9T30Z
0N9T3ZZ
0N9T40Z
0N9T4ZZ
0N9V00Z
0N9V0ZZ

0N9V30Z	0NPB37Z	0NSG34Z	0NSV35Z	0P943ZZ	0PHG38Z	0PPY30Z	0PSC4ZZ	0PW3X7Z
0N9V3ZZ	0NPB3JZ	0NSG3ZZ	0NSV3ZZ	0P9530Z	0PHG47Z	0PPYX0Z	0PSCXZZ	0PW3XJZ
0N9V40Z	0NPB3KZ	0NSG44Z	0NSV44Z	0P953ZZ	0PHG48Z	0PPYXMZ	0PSD3ZZ	0PW3XKZ
0N9V4ZZ	0NPB3MZ	0NSG4ZZ	0NSV45Z	0P9630Z	0PHH08Z	0PQ0XZZ	0PSD4ZZ	0PW4X4Z
0N9X30Z	0NPB40Z	0NSGXZZ	0NSV4ZZ	0P963ZZ	0PHH38Z	0PQ1XZZ	0PSDXZZ	0PW4X7Z
0N9X3ZZ	0NPB44Z	0NSH34Z	0NSVXZZ	0P9730Z	0PHH48Z	0PQ2XZZ	0PSF3ZZ	0PW4XJZ
0NBB0ZX	0NPB47Z	0NSH3ZZ	0NSX34Z	0P973ZZ	0PHJ08Z	0PQ3XZZ	0PSF4ZZ	0PW4XKZ
0NBB3ZX	0NPB4JZ	0NSH44Z	0NSX3ZZ	0P9830Z	0PHJ38Z	0PQ4XZZ	0PSFXZZ	0PW5X4Z
0NBB4ZX	0NPB4KZ	0NSH4ZZ	0NSX44Z	0P983ZZ	0PHJ48Z	0PQ5XZZ	0PSG3ZZ	0PW5X7Z
0NBR0ZX	0NPB4MZ	0NSHXZZ	0NSX4ZZ	0P9930Z	0PHK08Z	0PQ6XZZ	0PSG4ZZ	0PW5XJZ
0NBR3ZX	0NPBX0Z	0NSJ34Z	0NSXXZZ	0P993ZZ	0PHK38Z	0PQ7XZZ	0PSGXZZ	0PW5XKZ
0NBR4ZX	0NPBX4Z	0NSJ3ZZ	0NW0X0Z	0P9B30Z	0PHK48Z	0PQ8XZZ	0PSH3ZZ	0PW6X4Z
0NBT0ZX	0NPBXMZ	0NSJ44Z	0NW0X4Z	0P9B3ZZ	0PHL08Z	0PQ9XZZ	0PSH4ZZ	0PW6X7Z
0NBT3ZX	0NPWX0Z	0NSJ4ZZ	0NW0X5Z	0P9C30Z	0PHL38Z	0PQBXZZ	0PSHXZZ	0PW6XJZ
0NBT4ZX	0NPWXMZ	0NSJXZZ	0NW0X7Z	0P9C3ZZ	0PHL48Z	0PQCXZZ	0PSJ3ZZ	0PW6XKZ
0NBV0ZX	0NQ0XZZ	0NSK34Z	0NW0XJZ	0P9D30Z	0PJY3ZZ	0PQDXZZ	0PSJ4ZZ	0PW7X4Z
0NBV3ZX	0NQ1XZZ	0NSK3ZZ	0NW0XKZ	0P9D3ZZ	0PJYXZZ	0PQFXZZ	0PSJXZZ	0PW7X7Z
0NBV4ZX	0NQ3XZZ	0NSK44Z	0NW0XMZ	0P9F30Z	0PP0X4Z	0PQGXZZ	0PSK3ZZ	0PW7XJZ
0NCB0ZZ	0NQ4XZZ	0NSK4ZZ	0NW0XSZ	0P9F3ZZ	0PP1X4Z	0PQHXZZ	0PSK4ZZ	0PW7XKZ
0NCB3ZZ	0NQ5XZZ	0NSKXZZ	0NWB00Z	0P9G30Z	0PP2X4Z	0PQJXZZ	0PSKXZZ	0PW8X4Z
0NCB4ZZ	0NQ6XZZ	0NSL34Z	0NWB04Z	0P9G3ZZ	0PP3X4Z	0PQKXZZ	0PSL3ZZ	0PW8X7Z
0NCR0ZZ	0NQ7XZZ	0NSL3ZZ	0NWB07Z	0P9H30Z	0PP4X4Z	0PQLXZZ	0PSL4ZZ	0PW8XJZ
0NCR3ZZ	0NQBXZZ	0NSL44Z	0NWB0JZ	0P9H3ZZ	0PP5X4Z	0PQMXZZ	0PSLXZZ	0PW8XKZ
0NCR4ZZ	0NQCXZZ	0NSL4ZZ	0NWB0KZ	0P9J30Z	0PP6X4Z	0PQNXZZ	0PSM3ZZ	0PW9X4Z
0NCT0ZZ	0NQFXZZ	0NSLXZZ	0NWB0MZ	0P9J3ZZ	0PP7X4Z	0PQPXZZ	0PSM4ZZ	0PW9X7Z
0NCT3ZZ	0NQGXZZ	0NSM34Z	0NWB30Z	0P9K30Z	0PP8X4Z	0PQQXZZ	0PSMXZZ	0PW9XJZ
0NCT4ZZ	0NQHXZZ	0NSM3ZZ	0NWB34Z	0P9K3ZZ	0PP9X4Z	0PQRXZZ	0PSN3ZZ	0PW9XKZ
0NCV0ZZ	0NQJXZZ	0NSM44Z	0NWB37Z	0P9L30Z	0PPBX4Z	0PQSXZZ	0PSN4ZZ	0PWBX4Z
0NCV3ZZ	0NQKXZZ	0NSM4ZZ	0NWB3JZ	0P9L3ZZ	0PPCX4Z	0PQTXZZ	0PSNXZZ	0PWBX7Z
0NCV4ZZ	0NQLXZZ	0NSMXZZ	0NWB3KZ	0P9M30Z	0PPCX5Z	0PQVXZZ	0PSP3ZZ	0PWBXJZ
0NH005Z	0NQMXZZ	0NSN34Z	0NWB3MZ	0P9M3ZZ	0PPDX4Z	0PS03ZZ	0PSP4ZZ	0PWBXKZ
0NH035Z	0NQNXZZ	0NSN3ZZ	0NWB40Z	0P9N30Z	0PPDX5Z	0PS04ZZ	0PSPXZZ	0PWCX4Z
0NH045Z	0NQPXZZ	0NSN44Z	0NWB44Z	0P9N3ZZ	0PPFX4Z	0PS0XZZ	0PSQ3ZZ	0PWCX5Z
0NHB04Z	0NQQXZZ	0NSN4ZZ	0NWB47Z	0P9P30Z	0PPFX5Z	0PS13ZZ	0PSQ4ZZ	0PWCX7Z
0NHB0MZ	0NQRXZZ	0NSNXZZ	0NWB4JZ	0P9P3ZZ	0PPGX4Z	0PS14ZZ	0PSQXZZ	0PWCXJZ
0NHB34Z	0NQTXZZ	0NSP34Z	0NWB4KZ	0P9Q30Z	0PPGX5Z	0PS1XZZ	0PSR3ZZ	0PWCXKZ
0NHB3MZ	0NQVXZZ	0NSP3ZZ	0NWB4MZ	0P9Q3ZZ	0PPHX4Z	0PS23ZZ	0PSR4ZZ	0PWDX4Z
0NHB44Z	0NQXXZZ	0NSP44Z	0NWBX0Z	0P9R30Z	0PPHX5Z	0PS24ZZ	0PSRXZZ	0PWDX5Z
0NHB4MZ	0NS0XZZ	0NSP4ZZ	0NWBX4Z	0P9R3ZZ	0PPJX4Z	0PS2XZZ	0PSS3ZZ	0PWDX7Z
0NJ03ZZ	0NS1XZZ	0NSPXZZ	0NWBX7Z	0P9S30Z	0PPJX5Z	0PS3XZZ	0PSS4ZZ	0PWDXJZ
0NJ0XZZ	0NS3XZZ	0NSQ34Z	0NWBXJZ	0P9S3ZZ	0PPKX4Z	0PS4XZZ	0PSSXZZ	0PWDXKZ
0NJB3ZZ	0NS4XZZ	0NSQ3ZZ	0NWBXKZ	0P9T30Z	0PPKX5Z	0PS53ZZ	0PST3ZZ	0PWFX4Z
0NJBXZZ	0NS5XZZ	0NSQ44Z	0NWBXMZ	0P9T3ZZ	0PPLX4Z	0PS54ZZ	0PST4ZZ	0PWFX5Z
0NJW3ZZ	0NS6XZZ	0NSQ4ZZ	0NWWX0Z	0P9V30Z	0PPLX5Z	0PS5XZZ	0PSTXZZ	0PWFX7Z
0NJWXZZ	0NS7XZZ	0NSQXZZ	0NWWX4Z	0P9V3ZZ	0PPMX4Z	0PS63ZZ	0PSV3ZZ	0PWFXJZ
0NNB0ZZ	0NSB34Z	0NSR34Z	0NWWX7Z	0PHC08Z	0PPMX5Z	0PS64ZZ	0PSV4ZZ	0PWFXKZ
0NNB3ZZ	0NSB3ZZ	0NSR35Z	0NWWXJZ	0PHC38Z	0PPNX4Z	0PS6XZZ	0PSVXZZ	0PWGX4Z
0NNB4ZZ	0NSB44Z	0NSR3ZZ	0NWWXKZ	0PHC48Z	0PPNX5Z	0PS73ZZ	0PW0X4Z	0PWGX5Z
0NP035Z	0NSB4ZZ	0NSR44Z	0NWWXMZ	0PHD08Z	0PPPX4Z	0PS74ZZ	0PW0X7Z	0PWGX7Z
0NP045Z	0NSBXZZ	0NSR45Z	0P2YX0Z	0PHD38Z	0PPPX5Z	0PS7XZZ	0PW0XJZ	0PWGXJZ
0NP0X0Z	0NSC34Z	0NSR4ZZ	0P2YXYZ	0PHD48Z	0PPQX4Z	0PS83ZZ	0PW0XKZ	0PWGXKZ
0NP0X5Z	0NSC3ZZ	0NSRXZZ	0P9030Z	0PHF07Z	0PPQX5Z	0PS84ZZ	0PW1X4Z	0PWHX4Z
0NPB00Z	0NSC44Z	0NST34Z	0P903ZZ	0PHF08Z	0PPRX4Z	0PS8XZZ	0PW1X7Z	0PWHX5Z
0NPB04Z	0NSC4ZZ	0NST35Z	0P9130Z	0PHF37Z	0PPRX5Z	0PS93ZZ	0PW1XJZ	0PWHX7Z
0NPB07Z	0NSCXZZ	0NST3ZZ	0P913ZZ	0PHF38Z	0PPSX4Z	0PS94ZZ	0PW1XKZ	0PWHXJZ
0NPB0JZ	0NSF34Z	0NST44Z	0P9230Z	0PHF47Z	0PPSX5Z	0PS9XZZ	0PW2X4Z	0PWHXKZ
0NPB0KZ	0NSF3ZZ	0NST45Z	0P923ZZ	0PHF48Z	0PPTX4Z	0PSB3ZZ	0PW2X7Z	0PWJX4Z
0NPB0MZ	0NSF44Z	0NST4ZZ	0P9330Z	0PHG07Z	0PPTX5Z	0PSB4ZZ	0PW2XJZ	0PWJX5Z
0NPB30Z	0NSF4ZZ	0NSTXZZ	0P933ZZ	0PHG08Z	0PPVX4Z	0PSBXZZ	0PW2XKZ	0PWJX7Z
0NPB34Z	0NSFXZZ	0NSV34Z	0P9430Z	0PHG37Z	0PPVX5Z	0PSC3ZZ	0PW3X4Z	0PWJXJZ

0PWJXKZ
0PWKX4Z
0PWKX5Z
0PWKX7Z
0PWKXJZ
0PWKXKZ
0PWLX4Z
0PWLX5Z
0PWLX7Z
0PWLXJZ
0PWLXKZ
0PWMX4Z
0PWMX5Z
0PWMX7Z
0PWMXJZ
0PWMXKZ
0PWNX4Z
0PWNX5Z
0PWNX7Z
0PWNXJZ
0PWNXKZ
0PWPX4Z
0PWPX5Z
0PWPX7Z
0PWPXJZ
0PWPXKZ
0PWQX4Z
0PWQX5Z
0PWQX7Z
0PWQXJZ
0PWQXKZ
0PWRX4Z
0PWRX5Z
0PWRX7Z
0PWRXJZ
0PWRXKZ
0PWSX4Z
0PWSX5Z
0PWSX7Z
0PWSXJZ
0PWSXKZ
0PWTX4Z
0PWTX5Z
0PWTX7Z
0PWTXJZ
0PWTXKZ
0PWVX4Z
0PWVX5Z
0PWVX7Z
0PWVXJZ
0PWVXKZ
0PWYX0Z
0PWYXMZ
0Q2YX0Z
0Q2YXYZ
0Q9030Z
0Q903ZZ
0Q9130Z
0Q913ZZ
0Q9230Z
0Q923ZZ
0Q9330Z
0Q933ZZ
0Q9430Z
0Q943ZZ
0Q9530Z
0Q953ZZ
0Q9630Z
0Q963ZZ
0Q9730Z
0Q973ZZ
0Q9830Z
0Q983ZZ
0Q9930Z
0Q993ZZ
0Q9B30Z
0Q9B3ZZ
0Q9C30Z
0Q9C3ZZ
0Q9D30Z
0Q9D3ZZ
0Q9F30Z
0Q9F3ZZ
0Q9G30Z
0Q9G3ZZ
0Q9H30Z
0Q9H3ZZ
0Q9J30Z
0Q9J3ZZ
0Q9K30Z
0Q9K3ZZ
0Q9L30Z
0Q9L3ZZ
0Q9M30Z
0Q9M3ZZ
0Q9N30Z
0Q9N3ZZ
0Q9P30Z
0Q9P3ZZ
0Q9Q30Z
0Q9Q3ZZ
0Q9R30Z
0Q9R3ZZ
0Q9S30Z
0Q9S3ZZ
0QH608Z
0QH638Z
0QH648Z
0QH708Z
0QH738Z
0QH748Z
0QH807Z
0QH808Z
0QH837Z
0QH838Z
0QH847Z
0QH848Z
0QH907Z
0QH908Z
0QH937Z
0QH938Z
0QH947Z
0QH948Z
0QHB08Z
0QHB38Z
0QHB48Z
0QHC08Z
0QHC38Z
0QHC48Z
0QHG07Z
0QHG08Z
0QHG37Z
0QHG38Z
0QHG47Z
0QHG48Z
0QHH07Z
0QHH08Z
0QHH37Z
0QHH38Z
0QHH47Z
0QHH48Z
0QHJ08Z
0QHJ38Z
0QHJ48Z
0QHK08Z
0QHK38Z
0QHK48Z
0QJY3ZZ
0QJYXZZ
0QP0X4Z
0QP1X4Z
0QP2X4Z
0QP2X5Z
0QP3X4Z
0QP3X5Z
0QP4X4Z
0QP5X4Z
0QP6X4Z
0QP6X5Z
0QP7X4Z
0QP7X5Z
0QP8X4Z
0QP8X5Z
0QP9X4Z
0QP9X5Z
0QPBX4Z
0QPBX5Z
0QPCX4Z
0QPCX5Z
0QPDX4Z
0QPDX5Z
0QPFX4Z
0QPFX5Z
0QPGX4Z
0QPGX5Z
0QPHX4Z
0QPHX5Z
0QPJX4Z
0QPJX5Z
0QPKX4Z
0QPKX5Z
0QPLX4Z
0QPLX5Z
0QPMX4Z
0QPMX5Z
0QPNX4Z
0QPNX5Z
0QPPX4Z
0QPPX5Z
0QPQX4Z
0QPQX5Z
0QPRX4Z
0QPRX5Z
0QPSX4Z
0QPY30Z
0QPYX0Z
0QPYXMZ
0QQ0XZZ
0QQ1XZZ
0QQ2XZZ
0QQ3XZZ
0QQ4XZZ
0QQ5XZZ
0QQ6XZZ
0QQ7XZZ
0QQ8XZZ
0QQ9XZZ
0QQBXZZ
0QQCXZZ
0QQDXZZ
0QQFXZZ
0QQGXZZ
0QQHXZZ
0QQJXZZ
0QQKXZZ
0QQLXZZ
0QQMXZZ
0QQNXZZ
0QQPXZZ
0QQQXZZ
0QQRXZZ
0QQSXZZ
0QS0XZZ
0QS1XZZ
0QS23ZZ
0QS24ZZ
0QS2XZZ
0QS33ZZ
0QS34ZZ
0QS3XZZ
0QS43ZZ
0QS44ZZ
0QS4XZZ
0QS53ZZ
0QS54ZZ
0QS5XZZ
0QS63ZZ
0QS64ZZ
0QS6XZZ
0QS73ZZ
0QS74ZZ
0QS7XZZ
0QS83ZZ
0QS84ZZ
0QS8XZZ
0QS93ZZ
0QS94ZZ
0QS9XZZ
0QSB3ZZ
0QSB4ZZ
0QSBXZZ
0QSC3ZZ
0QSC4ZZ
0QSCXZZ
0QSD3ZZ
0QSD4ZZ
0QSDXZZ
0QSF3ZZ
0QSF4ZZ
0QSFXZZ
0QSG3ZZ
0QSG4ZZ
0QSGXZZ
0QSH3ZZ
0QSH4ZZ
0QSHXZZ
0QSJ3ZZ
0QSJ4ZZ
0QSJXZZ
0QSK3ZZ
0QSK4ZZ
0QSKXZZ
0QSL3ZZ
0QSL4ZZ
0QSLXZZ
0QSM3ZZ
0QSM4ZZ
0QSMXZZ
0QSN3Z2
0QSN3ZZ
0QSN4Z2
0QSN4ZZ
0QSNXZ2
0QSNXZZ
0QSP3Z2
0QSP3ZZ
0QSP4Z2
0QSP4ZZ
0QSPXZ2
0QSPXZZ
0QSQ3ZZ
0QSQ4ZZ
0QSQXZZ
0QSR3ZZ
0QSR4ZZ
0QSRXZZ
0QSSXZZ
0QW0X4Z
0QW0X7Z
0QW0XJZ
0QW0XKZ
0QW1X4Z
0QW1X7Z
0QW1XJZ
0QW1XKZ
0QW2X4Z
0QW2X5Z
0QW2X7Z
0QW2XJZ
0QW2XKZ
0QW3X4Z
0QW3X5Z
0QW3X7Z
0QW3XJZ
0QW3XKZ
0QW4X4Z
0QW4X7Z
0QW4XJZ
0QW4XKZ
0QW5X4Z
0QW5X7Z
0QW5XJZ
0QW5XKZ
0QW6X4Z
0QW6X5Z
0QW6X7Z
0QW6XJZ
0QW6XKZ
0QW7X4Z
0QW7X5Z
0QW7X7Z
0QW7XJZ
0QW7XKZ
0QW8X4Z
0QW8X5Z
0QW8X7Z
0QW8XJZ
0QW8XKZ
0QW9X4Z
0QW9X5Z
0QW9X7Z
0QW9XJZ
0QW9XKZ
0QWBX4Z
0QWBX5Z
0QWBX7Z
0QWBXJZ
0QWBXKZ
0QWCX4Z
0QWCX5Z
0QWCX7Z
0QWCXJZ
0QWCXKZ
0QWDX4Z
0QWDX5Z
0QWDX7Z
0QWDXJZ
0QWDXKZ
0QWFX4Z
0QWFX5Z
0QWFX7Z
0QWFXJZ
0QWFXKZ
0QWGX4Z
0QWGX5Z
0QWGX7Z
0QWGXJZ
0QWGXKZ
0QWHX4Z
0QWHX5Z
0QWHX7Z
0QWHXJZ
0QWHXKZ
0QWJX4Z
0QWJX5Z
0QWJX7Z
0QWJXJZ
0QWJXKZ
0QWKX4Z
0QWKX5Z
0QWKX7Z
0QWKXJZ
0QWKXKZ
0QWLX4Z
0QWLX5Z
0QWLX7Z
0QWLXJZ
0QWLXKZ
0QWMX4Z
0QWMX5Z
0QWMX7Z
0QWMXJZ
0QWMXKZ
0QWNX4Z
0QWNX5Z
0QWNX7Z
0QWNXJZ
0QWNXKZ
0QWPX4Z
0QWPX5Z
0QWPX7Z
0QWPXJZ
0QWPXKZ
0QWQX4Z
0QWQX5Z
0QWQX7Z
0QWQXJZ
0QWQXKZ
0QWRX4Z
0QWRX5Z
0QWRX7Z
0QWRXJZ
0QWRXKZ
0QWSX4Z
0QWSX7Z
0QWSXJZ
0QWSXKZ
0QWYX0Z
0QWYXMZ
0R2YX0Z
0R2YXYZ
0R533ZZ
0R534ZZ
0R553ZZ
0R554ZZ
0R593ZZ
0R594ZZ
0R5B3ZZ
0R5B4ZZ
0R900ZX
0R9030Z
0R903ZX
0R903ZZ
0R9040Z
0R904ZX
0R904ZZ
0R910ZX
0R9130Z
0R913ZX
0R913ZZ
0R9140Z
0R914ZX
0R914ZZ
0R930ZX
0R9330Z
0R933ZX
0R933ZZ
0R9340Z
0R934ZX
0R934ZZ
0R940ZX
0R9430Z
0R943ZX
0R943ZZ
0R9440Z
0R944ZX
0R944ZZ
0R950ZX
0R9530Z
0R953ZX
0R953ZZ
0R9540Z
0R954ZX
0R954ZZ
0R960ZX
0R9630Z
0R963ZX
0R963ZZ
0R9640Z
0R964ZX
0R964ZZ
0R990ZX
0R9930Z
0R993ZX
0R993ZZ
0R9940Z
0R994ZX
0R994ZZ
0R9A0ZX
0R9A30Z
0R9A3ZX
0R9A3ZZ
0R9A40Z
0R9A4ZX
0R9A4ZZ
0R9B0ZX
0R9B30Z
0R9B3ZX
0R9B3ZZ
0R9B40Z
0R9B4ZX
0R9B4ZZ
0R9C30Z
0R9C3ZZ
0R9D30Z
0R9D3ZZ
0R9E0ZX
0R9E30Z
0R9E3ZX
0R9E3ZZ
0R9E40Z
0R9E4ZX
0R9E4ZZ
0R9F0ZX
0R9F30Z
0R9F3ZX
0R9F3ZZ
0R9F40Z
0R9F4ZX
0R9F4ZZ
0R9G0ZX
0R9G30Z
0R9G3ZX
0R9G3ZZ
0R9G40Z
0R9G4ZX
0R9G4ZZ
0R9H0ZX
0R9H30Z
0R9H3ZX
0R9H3ZZ
0R9H40Z
0R9H4ZX
0R9H4ZZ
0R9J0ZX
0R9J30Z
0R9J3ZX
0R9J3ZZ
0R9J40Z
0R9J4ZX
0R9J4ZZ
0R9K0ZX
0R9K30Z
0R9K3ZX
0R9K3ZZ
0R9K40Z
0R9K4ZX
0R9K4ZZ
0R9L0ZX
0R9L30Z

0R9L3ZX
0R9L3ZZ
0R9L40Z
0R9L4ZX
0R9L4ZZ
0R9M0ZX
0R9M30Z
0R9M3ZX
0R9M3ZZ
0R9M40Z
0R9M4ZX
0R9M4ZZ
0R9N0ZX
0R9N30Z
0R9N3ZX
0R9N3ZZ
0R9N40Z
0R9N4ZX
0R9N4ZZ
0R9P0ZX
0R9P30Z
0R9P3ZX
0R9P3ZZ
0R9P40Z
0R9P4ZX
0R9P4ZZ
0R9Q0ZX
0R9Q30Z
0R9Q3ZX
0R9Q3ZZ
0R9Q40Z
0R9Q4ZX
0R9Q4ZZ
0R9R0ZX
0R9R30Z
0R9R3ZX
0R9R3ZZ
0R9R40Z
0R9R4ZX
0R9R4ZZ
0R9S0ZX
0R9S30Z
0R9S3ZX
0R9S3ZZ
0R9S40Z
0R9S4ZX
0R9S4ZZ
0R9T0ZX
0R9T30Z
0R9T3ZX
0R9T3ZZ
0R9T40Z
0R9T4ZX
0R9T4ZZ
0R9U0ZX
0R9U30Z
0R9U3ZX
0R9U3ZZ
0R9U40Z
0R9U4ZX
0R9U4ZZ
0R9V0ZX
0R9V30Z
0R9V3ZX
0R9V3ZZ
0R9V40Z
0R9V4ZX
0R9V4ZZ
0R9W0ZX
0R9W30Z
0R9W3ZX
0R9W3ZZ
0R9W40Z
0R9W4ZX
0R9W4ZZ
0R9X0ZX
0R9X30Z
0R9X3ZX
0R9X3ZZ
0R9X40Z
0R9X4ZX
0R9X4ZZ
0RB00ZX
0RB03ZX
0RB04ZX
0RB10ZX
0RB13ZX
0RB14ZX
0RB30ZX
0RB33ZX
0RB34ZX
0RB40ZX
0RB43ZX
0RB44ZX
0RB50ZX
0RB53ZX
0RB54ZX
0RB60ZX
0RB63ZX
0RB64ZX
0RB90ZX
0RB93ZX
0RB94ZX
0RBA0ZX
0RBA3ZX
0RBA4ZX
0RBB0ZX
0RBB3ZX
0RBB4ZX
0RBE0ZX
0RBE3ZX
0RBE4ZX
0RBF0ZX
0RBF3ZX
0RBF4ZX
0RBG0ZX
0RBG3ZX
0RBG4ZX
0RBH0ZX
0RBH3ZX
0RBH4ZX
0RBJ0ZX
0RBJ3ZX
0RBJ4ZX
0RBK0ZX
0RBK3ZX
0RBK4ZX
0RBL0ZX
0RBL3ZX
0RBL4ZX
0RBM0ZX
0RBM3ZX
0RBM4ZX
0RBN0ZX
0RBN3ZX
0RBN4ZX
0RBP0ZX
0RBP3ZX
0RBP4ZX
0RBQ0ZX
0RBQ3ZX
0RBQ4ZX
0RBR0ZX
0RBR3ZX
0RBR4ZX
0RBS0ZX
0RBS3ZX
0RBS4ZX
0RBT0ZX
0RBT3ZX
0RBT4ZX
0RBU0ZX
0RBU3ZX
0RBU4ZX
0RBV0ZX
0RBV3ZX
0RBV4ZX
0RBW0ZX
0RBW3ZX
0RBW4ZX
0RBX0ZX
0RBX3ZX
0RBX4ZX
0RH003Z
0RH008Z
0RH033Z
0RH038Z
0RH043Z
0RH048Z
0RH103Z
0RH108Z
0RH133Z
0RH138Z
0RH143Z
0RH148Z
0RH303Z
0RH333Z
0RH343Z
0RH403Z
0RH408Z
0RH433Z
0RH438Z
0RH443Z
0RH448Z
0RH503Z
0RH533Z
0RH543Z
0RH603Z
0RH608Z
0RH633Z
0RH638Z
0RH643Z
0RH648Z
0RH903Z
0RH933Z
0RH943Z
0RHA03Z
0RHA08Z
0RHA33Z
0RHA38Z
0RHA43Z
0RHA48Z
0RHB03Z
0RHB33Z
0RHB43Z
0RHC08Z
0RHC33Z
0RHC38Z
0RHC48Z
0RHD08Z
0RHD33Z
0RHD38Z
0RHD48Z
0RHE03Z
0RHE08Z
0RHE33Z
0RHE38Z
0RHE43Z
0RHE48Z
0RHF03Z
0RHF08Z
0RHF33Z
0RHF38Z
0RHF43Z
0RHF48Z
0RHG03Z
0RHG08Z
0RHG33Z
0RHG38Z
0RHG43Z
0RHG48Z
0RHH03Z
0RHH08Z
0RHH33Z
0RHH38Z
0RHH43Z
0RHH48Z
0RHJ03Z
0RHJ08Z
0RHJ33Z
0RHJ38Z
0RHJ43Z
0RHJ48Z
0RHK03Z
0RHK08Z
0RHK33Z
0RHK38Z
0RHK43Z
0RHK48Z
0RHL03Z
0RHL08Z
0RHL33Z
0RHL38Z
0RHL43Z
0RHL48Z
0RHM03Z
0RHM08Z
0RHM33Z
0RHM38Z
0RHM43Z
0RHM48Z
0RHN03Z
0RHN08Z
0RHN33Z
0RHN38Z
0RHN43Z
0RHN48Z
0RHP03Z
0RHP08Z
0RHP33Z
0RHP38Z
0RHP43Z
0RHP48Z
0RHQ03Z
0RHQ08Z
0RHQ33Z
0RHQ38Z
0RHQ43Z
0RHQ48Z
0RHR03Z
0RHR08Z
0RHR33Z
0RHR38Z
0RHR43Z
0RHR48Z
0RHS03Z
0RHS08Z
0RHS33Z
0RHS38Z
0RHS43Z
0RHS48Z
0RHT03Z
0RHT08Z
0RHT33Z
0RHT38Z
0RHT43Z
0RHT48Z
0RHU03Z
0RHU08Z
0RHU33Z
0RHU38Z
0RHU43Z
0RHU48Z
0RHV03Z
0RHV08Z
0RHV33Z
0RHV38Z
0RHV43Z
0RHV48Z
0RHW03Z
0RHW08Z
0RHW33Z
0RHW38Z
0RHW43Z
0RHW48Z
0RHX03Z
0RHX08Z
0RHX33Z
0RHX38Z
0RHX43Z
0RHX48Z
0RJ03ZZ
0RJ0XZZ
0RJ13ZZ
0RJ1XZZ
0RJ33ZZ
0RJ3XZZ
0RJ43ZZ
0RJ4XZZ
0RJ53ZZ
0RJ5XZZ
0RJ63ZZ
0RJ6XZZ
0RJ93ZZ
0RJ9XZZ
0RJA3ZZ
0RJAXZZ
0RJB3ZZ
0RJBXZZ
0RJC3ZZ
0RJCXZZ
0RJD3ZZ
0RJDXZZ
0RJE3ZZ
0RJEXZZ
0RJF3ZZ
0RJFXZZ
0RJG3ZZ
0RJGXZZ
0RJH3ZZ
0RJHXZZ
0RJJ3ZZ
0RJJXZZ
0RJK3ZZ
0RJKXZZ
0RJL3ZZ
0RJLXZZ
0RJM3ZZ
0RJMXZZ
0RJN3ZZ
0RJNXZZ
0RJP3ZZ
0RJPXZZ
0RJQ3ZZ
0RJQXZZ
0RJR3ZZ
0RJRXZZ
0RJS3ZZ
0RJSXZZ
0RJT3ZZ
0RJTXZZ
0RJU3ZZ
0RJUXZZ
0RJV3ZZ
0RJVXZZ
0RJW3ZZ
0RJWXZZ
0RJX3ZZ
0RJXXZZ
0RN0XZZ
0RN1XZZ
0RN3XZZ
0RN4XZZ
0RN5XZZ
0RN6XZZ
0RN9XZZ
0RNAXZZ
0RNBXZZ
0RNCXZZ
0RNDXZZ
0RNEXZZ
0RNFXZZ
0RNGXZZ
0RNHXZZ
0RNJXZZ
0RNKXZZ
0RNLXZZ
0RNMXZZ
0RNNXZZ
0RNPXZZ
0RNQXZZ
0RNRXZZ
0RNSXZZ
0RNTXZZ
0RNUXZZ
0RNVXZZ
0RNWXZZ
0RNXXZZ
0RP008Z
0RP030Z
0RP033Z
0RP038Z
0RP048Z
0RP0X0Z
0RP0X3Z
0RP0X4Z
0RP108Z
0RP130Z
0RP133Z
0RP138Z
0RP148Z
0RP1X0Z
0RP1X3Z
0RP1X4Z
0RP330Z
0RP333Z
0RP3X0Z
0RP3X3Z
0RP408Z
0RP430Z
0RP433Z
0RP438Z
0RP448Z
0RP4X0Z
0RP4X3Z
0RP4X4Z
0RP530Z
0RP533Z
0RP5X0Z
0RP5X3Z
0RP608Z
0RP630Z
0RP633Z
0RP638Z
0RP648Z
0RP6X0Z
0RP6X3Z
0RP6X4Z
0RP930Z
0RP933Z
0RP9X0Z
0RP9X3Z
0RPA08Z
0RPA30Z
0RPA33Z
0RPA38Z
0RPA48Z
0RPAX0Z
0RPAX3Z
0RPAX4Z
0RPB30Z
0RPB33Z
0RPBX0Z
0RPBX3Z
0RPC08Z
0RPC30Z
0RPC33Z
0RPC38Z
0RPC48Z
0RPCX0Z
0RPCX3Z
0RPD08Z
0RPD30Z
0RPD33Z
0RPD38Z
0RPD48Z
0RPDX0Z
0RPDX3Z
0RPE08Z
0RPE30Z
0RPE33Z
0RPE38Z
0RPE48Z
0RPEX0Z
0RPEX3Z
0RPEX4Z
0RPF08Z
0RPF30Z
0RPF33Z
0RPF38Z
0RPF48Z
0RPFX0Z
0RPFX3Z
0RPFX4Z
0RPG08Z
0RPG30Z
0RPG33Z
0RPG38Z
0RPG48Z
0RPGX0Z
0RPGX3Z
0RPGX4Z
0RPH08Z
0RPH30Z
0RPH33Z
0RPH38Z
0RPH48Z
0RPHX0Z
0RPHX3Z
0RPHX4Z
0RPJ08Z
0RPJ30Z
0RPJ33Z
0RPJ38Z
0RPJ48Z
0RPJX0Z
0RPJX3Z
0RPJX4Z
0RPK08Z
0RPK30Z
0RPK33Z
0RPK38Z
0RPK48Z
0RPKX0Z
0RPKX3Z
0RPKX4Z
0RPL08Z
0RPL30Z
0RPL33Z
0RPL38Z
0RPL48Z
0RPLX0Z
0RPLX3Z
0RPLX4Z
0RPLX5Z
0RPM08Z
0RPM30Z
0RPM33Z
0RPM38Z
0RPM48Z

0RPMX0Z
0RPMX3Z
0RPMX4Z
0RPMX5Z
0RPN08Z
0RPN30Z
0RPN33Z
0RPN38Z
0RPN48Z
0RPNX0Z
0RPNX3Z
0RPNX4Z
0RPNX5Z
0RPP08Z
0RPP30Z
0RPP33Z
0RPP38Z
0RPP48Z
0RPPX0Z
0RPPX3Z
0RPPX4Z
0RPPX5Z
0RPQ08Z
0RPQ30Z
0RPQ33Z
0RPQ38Z
0RPQ48Z
0RPQX0Z
0RPQX3Z
0RPQX4Z
0RPQX5Z
0RPR08Z
0RPR30Z
0RPR33Z
0RPR38Z
0RPR48Z
0RPRX0Z
0RPRX3Z
0RPRX4Z
0RPRX5Z
0RPS08Z
0RPS30Z
0RPS33Z
0RPS38Z
0RPS48Z
0RPSX0Z
0RPSX3Z
0RPSX4Z
0RPSX5Z
0RPT08Z
0RPT30Z
0RPT33Z
0RPT38Z
0RPT48Z
0RPTX0Z
0RPTX3Z
0RPTX4Z
0RPTX5Z
0RPU08Z
0RPU30Z
0RPU33Z
0RPU38Z
0RPU48Z
0RPUX0Z
0RPUX3Z
0RPUX4Z
0RPUX5Z
0RPV08Z
0RPV30Z
0RPV33Z
0RPV38Z
0RPV48Z
0RPVX0Z
0RPVX3Z
0RPVX4Z
0RPVX5Z
0RPW08Z
0RPW30Z
0RPW33Z
0RPW38Z
0RPW48Z
0RPWX0Z
0RPWX3Z
0RPWX4Z
0RPWX5Z
0RPX08Z
0RPX30Z
0RPX33Z
0RPX38Z
0RPX48Z
0RPXX0Z
0RPXX3Z
0RPXX4Z
0RPXX5Z
0RQ0XZZ
0RQ1XZZ
0RQ3XZZ
0RQ4XZZ
0RQ5XZZ
0RQ6XZZ
0RQ9XZZ
0RQAXZZ
0RQBXZZ
0RQCXZZ
0RQDXZZ
0RQEXZZ
0RQFXZZ
0RQGXZZ
0RQHXZZ
0RQJXZZ
0RQKXZZ
0RQLXZZ
0RQMXZZ
0RQNXZZ
0RQPXZZ
0RQQXZZ
0RQRXZZ
0RQSXZZ
0RQTXZZ
0RQUXZZ
0RQVXZZ
0RQWXZZ
0RQXXZZ
0RS034Z
0RS03ZZ
0RS044Z
0RS04ZZ
0RS0X4Z
0RS0XZZ
0RS134Z
0RS13ZZ
0RS144Z
0RS14ZZ
0RS1X4Z
0RS1XZZ
0RS434Z
0RS43ZZ
0RS444Z
0RS44ZZ
0RS4X4Z
0RS4XZZ
0RS634Z
0RS63ZZ
0RS644Z
0RS64ZZ
0RS6X4Z
0RS6XZZ
0RSA34Z
0RSA3ZZ
0RSA44Z
0RSA4ZZ
0RSAX4Z
0RSAXZZ
0RSC34Z
0RSC3ZZ
0RSC44Z
0RSC4ZZ
0RSCX4Z
0RSCXZZ
0RSD34Z
0RSD3ZZ
0RSD44Z
0RSD4ZZ
0RSDX4Z
0RSDXZZ
0RSE34Z
0RSE3ZZ
0RSE44Z
0RSE4ZZ
0RSEX4Z
0RSEXZZ
0RSF34Z
0RSF3ZZ
0RSF44Z
0RSF4ZZ
0RSFX4Z
0RSFXZZ
0RSG34Z
0RSG3ZZ
0RSG44Z
0RSG4ZZ
0RSGX4Z
0RSGXZZ
0RSH34Z
0RSH3ZZ
0RSH44Z
0RSH4ZZ
0RSHX4Z
0RSHXZZ
0RSJ34Z
0RSJ3ZZ
0RSJ44Z
0RSJ4ZZ
0RSJX4Z
0RSJXZZ
0RSK34Z
0RSK3ZZ
0RSK44Z
0RSK4ZZ
0RSKX4Z
0RSKXZZ
0RSL34Z
0RSL35Z
0RSL3ZZ
0RSL44Z
0RSL45Z
0RSL4ZZ
0RSLX4Z
0RSLX5Z
0RSLXZZ
0RSM34Z
0RSM35Z
0RSM3ZZ
0RSM44Z
0RSM45Z
0RSM4ZZ
0RSMX4Z
0RSMX5Z
0RSMXZZ
0RSN34Z
0RSN35Z
0RSN3ZZ
0RSN44Z
0RSN45Z
0RSN4ZZ
0RSNX4Z
0RSNX5Z
0RSNXZZ
0RSP34Z
0RSP35Z
0RSP3ZZ
0RSP44Z
0RSP45Z
0RSP4ZZ
0RSPX4Z
0RSPX5Z
0RSPXZZ
0RSQ34Z
0RSQ35Z
0RSQ3ZZ
0RSQ44Z
0RSQ45Z
0RSQ4ZZ
0RSQX4Z
0RSQX5Z
0RSQXZZ
0RSR34Z
0RSR35Z
0RSR3ZZ
0RSR44Z
0RSR45Z
0RSR4ZZ
0RSRX4Z
0RSRX5Z
0RSRXZZ
0RSS34Z
0RSS35Z
0RSS3ZZ
0RSS44Z
0RSS45Z
0RSS4ZZ
0RSSX4Z
0RSSX5Z
0RSSXZZ
0RST34Z
0RST35Z
0RST3ZZ
0RST44Z
0RST45Z
0RST4ZZ
0RSTX4Z
0RSTX5Z
0RSTXZZ
0RSU34Z
0RSU35Z
0RSU3ZZ
0RSU44Z
0RSU45Z
0RSU4ZZ
0RSUX4Z
0RSUX5Z
0RSUXZZ
0RSV34Z
0RSV35Z
0RSV3ZZ
0RSV44Z
0RSV45Z
0RSV4ZZ
0RSVX4Z
0RSVX5Z
0RSVXZZ
0RSW34Z
0RSW35Z
0RSW3ZZ
0RSW44Z
0RSW45Z
0RSW4ZZ
0RSWX4Z
0RSWX5Z
0RSWXZZ
0RSX34Z
0RSX35Z
0RSX3ZZ
0RSX44Z
0RSX45Z
0RSX4ZZ
0RSXX4Z
0RSXX5Z
0RSXXZZ
0RW0X0Z
0RW0X3Z
0RW0X4Z
0RW0X7Z
0RW0X8Z
0RW0XAZ
0RW0XJZ
0RW0XKZ
0RW1X0Z
0RW1X3Z
0RW1X4Z
0RW1X7Z
0RW1X8Z
0RW1XAZ
0RW1XJZ
0RW1XKZ
0RW3X0Z
0RW3X3Z
0RW3X7Z
0RW3XJZ
0RW3XKZ
0RW4X0Z
0RW4X3Z
0RW4X4Z
0RW4X7Z
0RW4X8Z
0RW4XAZ
0RW4XJZ
0RW4XKZ
0RW5X0Z
0RW5X3Z
0RW5X7Z
0RW5XJZ
0RW5XKZ
0RW6X0Z
0RW6X3Z
0RW6X4Z
0RW6X7Z
0RW6X8Z
0RW6XAZ
0RW6XJZ
0RW6XKZ
0RW9X0Z
0RW9X3Z
0RW9X7Z
0RW9XJZ
0RW9XKZ
0RWAX0Z
0RWAX3Z
0RWAX4Z
0RWAX7Z
0RWAX8Z
0RWAXAZ
0RWAXJZ
0RWAXKZ
0RWBX0Z
0RWBX3Z
0RWBX7Z
0RWBXJZ
0RWBXKZ
0RWCX0Z
0RWCX3Z
0RWCX4Z
0RWCX7Z
0RWCX8Z
0RWCXJZ
0RWCXKZ
0RWDX0Z
0RWDX3Z
0RWDX4Z
0RWDX7Z
0RWDX8Z
0RWDXJZ
0RWDXKZ
0RWEX0Z
0RWEX3Z
0RWEX4Z
0RWEX7Z
0RWEX8Z
0RWEXJZ
0RWEXKZ
0RWFX0Z
0RWFX3Z
0RWFX4Z
0RWFX7Z
0RWFX8Z
0RWFXJZ
0RWFXKZ
0RWGX0Z
0RWGX3Z
0RWGX4Z
0RWGX7Z
0RWGX8Z
0RWGXJZ
0RWGXKZ
0RWHX0Z
0RWHX3Z
0RWHX4Z
0RWHX7Z
0RWHX8Z
0RWHXJZ
0RWHXKZ
0RWJX0Z
0RWJX3Z
0RWJX4Z
0RWJX7Z
0RWJX8Z
0RWJXJZ
0RWJXKZ
0RWKX0Z
0RWKX3Z
0RWKX4Z
0RWKX7Z
0RWKX8Z
0RWKXJZ
0RWKXKZ
0RWLX0Z
0RWLX3Z
0RWLX4Z
0RWLX5Z
0RWLX7Z
0RWLX8Z
0RWLXJZ
0RWLXKZ
0RWMX0Z
0RWMX3Z
0RWMX4Z
0RWMX5Z
0RWMX7Z
0RWMX8Z
0RWMXJZ
0RWMXKZ
0RWNX0Z
0RWNX3Z
0RWNX4Z
0RWNX5Z
0RWNX7Z
0RWNX8Z
0RWNXJZ
0RWNXKZ
0RWPX0Z
0RWPX3Z
0RWPX4Z
0RWPX5Z
0RWPX7Z
0RWPX8Z
0RWPXJZ
0RWPXKZ
0RWQX0Z
0RWQX3Z
0RWQX4Z
0RWQX5Z
0RWQX7Z
0RWQX8Z
0RWQXJZ
0RWQXKZ
0RWRX0Z
0RWRX3Z
0RWRX4Z
0RWRX5Z
0RWRX7Z
0RWRX8Z
0RWRXJZ
0RWRXKZ
0RWSX0Z
0RWSX3Z
0RWSX4Z
0RWSX5Z
0RWSX7Z
0RWSX8Z
0RWSXJZ
0RWSXKZ
0RWTX0Z
0RWTX3Z
0RWTX4Z
0RWTX5Z
0RWTX7Z
0RWTX8Z
0RWTXJZ
0RWTXKZ
0RWUX0Z
0RWUX3Z
0RWUX4Z
0RWUX5Z
0RWUX7Z
0RWUX8Z
0RWUXJZ
0RWUXKZ
0RWVX0Z
0RWVX3Z
0RWVX4Z
0RWVX5Z
0RWVX7Z
0RWVX8Z
0RWVXJZ
0RWVXKZ
0RWWX0Z
0RWWX3Z
0RWWX4Z
0RWWX5Z
0RWWX7Z
0RWWX8Z
0RWWXJZ
0RWWXKZ
0RWXX0Z
0RWXX3Z
0RWXX4Z
0RWXX5Z
0RWXX7Z
0RWXX8Z
0RWXXJZ
0RWXXKZ
0S2YX0Z
0S2YXYZ
0S900ZX
0S9030Z
0S903ZX
0S903ZZ
0S9040Z
0S904ZX
0S904ZZ
0S920ZX
0S9230Z
0S923ZX
0S923ZZ
0S9240Z
0S924ZX
0S924ZZ
0S930ZX
0S9330Z
0S933ZX

0S933ZZ
0S9340Z
0S934ZX
0S934ZZ
0S940ZX
0S9430Z
0S943ZX
0S943ZZ
0S9440Z
0S944ZX
0S944ZZ
0S950ZX
0S9530Z
0S953ZX
0S953ZZ
0S9540Z
0S954ZX
0S954ZZ
0S960ZX
0S9630Z
0S963ZX
0S963ZZ
0S9640Z
0S964ZX
0S964ZZ
0S970ZX
0S9730Z
0S973ZX
0S973ZZ
0S9740Z
0S974ZX
0S974ZZ
0S980ZX
0S9830Z
0S983ZX
0S983ZZ
0S9840Z
0S984ZX
0S984ZZ
0S990ZX
0S9930Z
0S993ZX
0S993ZZ
0S9940Z
0S994ZX
0S994ZZ
0S9B0ZX
0S9B30Z
0S9B3ZX
0S9B3ZZ
0S9B40Z
0S9B4ZX
0S9B4ZZ
0S9C0ZX
0S9C30Z
0S9C3ZX
0S9C3ZZ
0S9C40Z
0S9C4ZX
0S9C4ZZ
0S9D0ZX
0S9D30Z
0S9D3ZX
0S9D3ZZ
0S9D40Z
0S9D4ZX
0S9D4ZZ
0S9F0ZX
0S9F30Z
0S9F3ZX
0S9F3ZZ
0S9F40Z
0S9F4ZX
0S9F4ZZ
0S9G0ZX
0S9G30Z
0S9G3ZX
0S9G3ZZ
0S9G40Z
0S9G4ZX
0S9G4ZZ
0S9H0ZX
0S9H30Z
0S9H3ZX
0S9H3ZZ
0S9H40Z
0S9H4ZX
0S9H4ZZ
0S9J0ZX
0S9J30Z
0S9J3ZX
0S9J3ZZ
0S9J40Z
0S9J4ZX
0S9J4ZZ
0S9K0ZX
0S9K30Z
0S9K3ZX
0S9K3ZZ
0S9K40Z
0S9K4ZX
0S9K4ZZ
0S9L0ZX
0S9L30Z
0S9L3ZX
0S9L3ZZ
0S9L40Z
0S9L4ZX
0S9L4ZZ
0S9M0ZX
0S9M30Z
0S9M3ZX
0S9M3ZZ
0S9M40Z
0S9M4ZX
0S9M4ZZ
0S9N0ZX
0S9N30Z
0S9N3ZX
0S9N3ZZ
0S9N40Z
0S9N4ZX
0S9N4ZZ
0S9P0ZX
0S9P30Z
0S9P3ZX
0S9P3ZZ
0S9P40Z
0S9P4ZX
0S9P4ZZ
0S9Q0ZX
0S9Q30Z
0S9Q3ZX
0S9Q3ZZ
0S9Q40Z
0S9Q4ZX
0S9Q4ZZ
0SB00ZX
0SB03ZX
0SB04ZX
0SB20ZX
0SB23ZX
0SB24ZX
0SB30ZX
0SB33ZX
0SB34ZX
0SB40ZX
0SB43ZX
0SB44ZX
0SB50ZX
0SB53ZX
0SB54ZX
0SB60ZX
0SB63ZX
0SB64ZX
0SB70ZX
0SB73ZX
0SB74ZX
0SB80ZX
0SB83ZX
0SB84ZX
0SB90ZX
0SB93ZX
0SB94ZX
0SBB0ZX
0SBB3ZX
0SBB4ZX
0SBC0ZX
0SBC3ZX
0SBC4ZX
0SBD0ZX
0SBD3ZX
0SBD4ZX
0SBF0ZX
0SBF3ZX
0SBF4ZX
0SBG0ZX
0SBG3ZX
0SBG4ZX
0SBH0ZX
0SBH3ZX
0SBH4ZX
0SBJ0ZX
0SBJ3ZX
0SBJ4ZX
0SBK0ZX
0SBK3ZX
0SBK4ZX
0SBL0ZX
0SBL3ZX
0SBL4ZX
0SBM0ZX
0SBM3ZX
0SBM4ZX
0SBN0ZX
0SBN3ZX
0SBN4ZX
0SBP0ZX
0SBP3ZX
0SBP4ZX
0SBQ0ZX
0SBQ3ZX
0SBQ4ZX
0SH003Z
0SH008Z
0SH033Z
0SH038Z
0SH043Z
0SH048Z
0SH203Z
0SH208Z
0SH233Z
0SH238Z
0SH243Z
0SH248Z
0SH303Z
0SH308Z
0SH333Z
0SH338Z
0SH343Z
0SH348Z
0SH403Z
0SH408Z
0SH433Z
0SH438Z
0SH443Z
0SH448Z
0SH503Z
0SH508Z
0SH533Z
0SH538Z
0SH543Z
0SH548Z
0SH603Z
0SH608Z
0SH633Z
0SH638Z
0SH643Z
0SH648Z
0SH703Z
0SH708Z
0SH733Z
0SH738Z
0SH743Z
0SH748Z
0SH803Z
0SH808Z
0SH833Z
0SH838Z
0SH843Z
0SH848Z
0SH903Z
0SH933Z
0SH938Z
0SH943Z
0SH948Z
0SHB03Z
0SHB33Z
0SHB38Z
0SHB43Z
0SHB48Z
0SHC03Z
0SHC33Z
0SHC38Z
0SHC43Z
0SHC48Z
0SHD03Z
0SHD33Z
0SHD38Z
0SHD43Z
0SHD48Z
0SHF03Z
0SHF08Z
0SHF33Z
0SHF38Z
0SHF43Z
0SHF48Z
0SHG03Z
0SHG08Z
0SHG33Z
0SHG38Z
0SHG43Z
0SHG48Z
0SHH03Z
0SHH08Z
0SHH33Z
0SHH38Z
0SHH43Z
0SHH48Z
0SHJ03Z
0SHJ08Z
0SHJ33Z
0SHJ38Z
0SHJ43Z
0SHJ48Z
0SHK03Z
0SHK08Z
0SHK33Z
0SHK38Z
0SHK43Z
0SHK48Z
0SHL03Z
0SHL08Z
0SHL33Z
0SHL38Z
0SHL43Z
0SHL48Z
0SHM03Z
0SHM08Z
0SHM33Z
0SHM38Z
0SHM43Z
0SHM48Z
0SHN03Z
0SHN08Z
0SHN33Z
0SHN38Z
0SHN43Z
0SHN48Z
0SHP03Z
0SHP08Z
0SHP33Z
0SHP38Z
0SHP43Z
0SHP48Z
0SHQ03Z
0SHQ08Z
0SHQ33Z
0SHQ38Z
0SHQ43Z
0SHQ48Z
0SJ03ZZ
0SJ0XZZ
0SJ23ZZ
0SJ2XZZ
0SJ33ZZ
0SJ3XZZ
0SJ43ZZ
0SJ4XZZ
0SJ53ZZ
0SJ5XZZ
0SJ63ZZ
0SJ6XZZ
0SJ73ZZ
0SJ7XZZ
0SJ83ZZ
0SJ8XZZ
0SJ93ZZ
0SJ9XZZ
0SJB3ZZ
0SJBXZZ
0SJC3ZZ
0SJCXZZ
0SJD3ZZ
0SJDXZZ
0SJF3ZZ
0SJFXZZ
0SJG3ZZ
0SJGXZZ
0SJH3ZZ
0SJHXZZ
0SJJ3ZZ
0SJJXZZ
0SJK3ZZ
0SJKXZZ
0SJL3ZZ
0SJLXZZ
0SJM3ZZ
0SJMXZZ
0SJN3ZZ
0SJNXZZ
0SJP3ZZ
0SJPXZZ
0SJQ3ZZ
0SJQXZZ
0SN0XZZ
0SN2XZZ
0SN3XZZ
0SN4XZZ
0SN5XZZ
0SN6XZZ
0SN7XZZ
0SN8XZZ
0SN9XZZ
0SNBXZZ
0SNCXZZ
0SNDXZZ
0SNFXZZ
0SNGXZZ
0SNHXZZ
0SNJXZZ
0SNKXZZ
0SNLXZZ
0SNMXZZ
0SNNXZZ
0SNPXZZ
0SNQXZZ
0SP008Z
0SP030Z
0SP033Z
0SP038Z
0SP048Z
0SP0X0Z
0SP0X3Z
0SP0X4Z
0SP230Z
0SP233Z
0SP2X0Z
0SP2X3Z
0SP308Z
0SP330Z
0SP333Z
0SP338Z
0SP348Z
0SP3X0Z
0SP3X3Z
0SP3X4Z
0SP430Z
0SP433Z
0SP4X0Z
0SP4X3Z
0SP508Z
0SP530Z
0SP533Z
0SP538Z
0SP548Z
0SP5X0Z
0SP5X3Z
0SP5X4Z
0SP608Z
0SP630Z
0SP633Z
0SP638Z
0SP648Z
0SP6X0Z
0SP6X3Z
0SP6X4Z
0SP708Z
0SP730Z
0SP733Z
0SP738Z
0SP748Z
0SP7X0Z
0SP7X3Z
0SP7X4Z
0SP808Z
0SP830Z
0SP833Z
0SP838Z
0SP848Z
0SP8X0Z
0SP8X3Z
0SP8X4Z
0SP930Z
0SP933Z
0SP938Z
0SP9X0Z
0SP9X3Z
0SP9X4Z
0SP9X5Z
0SPB30Z
0SPB33Z
0SPB38Z
0SPBX0Z
0SPBX3Z
0SPBX4Z
0SPBX5Z
0SPC30Z
0SPC33Z
0SPCX0Z
0SPCX3Z
0SPCX4Z
0SPCX5Z
0SPD30Z
0SPD33Z
0SPDX0Z
0SPDX3Z
0SPDX4Z
0SPDX5Z
0SPF08Z
0SPF30Z
0SPF33Z
0SPF38Z
0SPF48Z
0SPFX0Z
0SPFX3Z
0SPFX4Z
0SPFX5Z
0SPG08Z
0SPG30Z
0SPG33Z
0SPG38Z
0SPG48Z
0SPGX0Z
0SPGX3Z
0SPGX4Z
0SPGX5Z
0SPH08Z
0SPH30Z
0SPH33Z
0SPH38Z
0SPH48Z
0SPHX0Z
0SPHX3Z
0SPHX4Z
0SPHX5Z
0SPJ08Z
0SPJ30Z
0SPJ33Z
0SPJ38Z
0SPJ48Z
0SPJX0Z
0SPJX3Z
0SPJX4Z
0SPJX5Z
0SPK08Z
0SPK30Z
0SPK33Z
0SPK38Z
0SPK48Z
0SPKX0Z
0SPKX3Z
0SPKX4Z
0SPKX5Z
0SPL08Z
0SPL30Z
0SPL33Z
0SPL38Z
0SPL48Z
0SPLX0Z
0SPLX3Z
0SPLX4Z
0SPLX5Z
0SPM08Z
0SPM30Z
0SPM33Z
0SPM38Z
0SPM48Z
0SPMX0Z
0SPMX3Z

0SPMX4Z
0SPMX5Z
0SPN08Z
0SPN30Z
0SPN33Z
0SPN38Z
0SPN48Z
0SPNX0Z
0SPNX3Z
0SPNX4Z
0SPNX5Z
0SPP08Z
0SPP30Z
0SPP33Z
0SPP38Z
0SPP48Z
0SPPX0Z
0SPPX3Z
0SPPX4Z
0SPPX5Z
0SPQ08Z
0SPQ30Z
0SPQ33Z
0SPQ38Z
0SPQ48Z
0SPQX0Z
0SPQX3Z
0SPQX4Z
0SPQX5Z
0SQ0XZZ
0SQ2XZZ
0SQ3XZZ
0SQ4XZZ
0SQ5XZZ
0SQ6XZZ
0SQ7XZZ
0SQ8XZZ
0SQ9XZZ
0SQBXZZ
0SQCXZZ
0SQDXZZ
0SQFXZZ
0SQGXZZ
0SQHXZZ
0SQJXZZ
0SQKXZZ
0SQLXZZ
0SQMXZZ
0SQNXZZ
0SQPXZZ
0SQQXZZ
0SS034Z
0SS03ZZ
0SS044Z
0SS04ZZ
0SS0X4Z
0SS0XZZ
0SS334Z
0SS33ZZ
0SS344Z
0SS34ZZ
0SS3X4Z
0SS3XZZ
0SS534Z
0SS53ZZ
0SS544Z
0SS54ZZ
0SS5X4Z
0SS5XZZ
0SS634Z
0SS63ZZ
0SS644Z
0SS64ZZ
0SS6X4Z
0SS6XZZ
0SS734Z
0SS73ZZ
0SS744Z
0SS74ZZ
0SS7X4Z
0SS7XZZ
0SS834Z
0SS83ZZ
0SS844Z
0SS84ZZ
0SS8X4Z
0SS8XZZ
0SS934Z
0SS935Z
0SS93ZZ
0SS944Z
0SS945Z
0SS94ZZ
0SS9X4Z
0SS9X5Z
0SS9XZZ
0SSB34Z
0SSB35Z
0SSB3ZZ
0SSB44Z
0SSB45Z
0SSB4ZZ
0SSBX4Z
0SSBX5Z
0SSBXZZ
0SSC34Z
0SSC35Z
0SSC3ZZ
0SSC44Z
0SSC45Z
0SSC4ZZ
0SSCX4Z
0SSCX5Z
0SSCXZZ
0SSD34Z
0SSD35Z
0SSD3ZZ
0SSD44Z
0SSD45Z
0SSD4ZZ
0SSDX4Z
0SSDX5Z
0SSDXZZ
0SSF34Z
0SSF35Z
0SSF3ZZ
0SSF44Z
0SSF45Z
0SSF4ZZ
0SSFX4Z
0SSFX5Z
0SSFXZZ
0SSG34Z
0SSG35Z
0SSG3ZZ
0SSG44Z
0SSG45Z
0SSG4ZZ
0SSGX4Z
0SSGX5Z
0SSGXZZ
0SSH34Z
0SSH35Z
0SSH3ZZ
0SSH44Z
0SSH45Z
0SSH4ZZ
0SSHX4Z
0SSHX5Z
0SSHXZZ
0SSJ34Z
0SSJ35Z
0SSJ3ZZ
0SSJ44Z
0SSJ45Z
0SSJ4ZZ
0SSJX4Z
0SSJX5Z
0SSJXZZ
0SSK34Z
0SSK35Z
0SSK3ZZ
0SSK44Z
0SSK45Z
0SSK4ZZ
0SSKX4Z
0SSKX5Z
0SSKXZZ
0SSL34Z
0SSL35Z
0SSL3ZZ
0SSL44Z
0SSL45Z
0SSL4ZZ
0SSLX4Z
0SSLX5Z
0SSLXZZ
0SSM34Z
0SSM35Z
0SSM3ZZ
0SSM44Z
0SSM45Z
0SSM4ZZ
0SSMX4Z
0SSMX5Z
0SSMXZZ
0SSN34Z
0SSN35Z
0SSN3ZZ
0SSN44Z
0SSN45Z
0SSN4ZZ
0SSNX4Z
0SSNX5Z
0SSNXZZ
0SSP34Z
0SSP35Z
0SSP3ZZ
0SSP44Z
0SSP45Z
0SSP4ZZ
0SSPX4Z
0SSPX5Z
0SSPXZZ
0SSQ34Z
0SSQ35Z
0SSQ3ZZ
0SSQ44Z
0SSQ45Z
0SSQ4ZZ
0SSQX4Z
0SSQX5Z
0SSQXZZ
0SW0X0Z
0SW0X3Z
0SW0X4Z
0SW0X7Z
0SW0X8Z
0SW0XAZ
0SW0XJZ
0SW0XKZ
0SW2X0Z
0SW2X3Z
0SW2X7Z
0SW2XJZ
0SW2XKZ
0SW3X0Z
0SW3X3Z
0SW3X4Z
0SW3X7Z
0SW3X8Z
0SW3XAZ
0SW3XJZ
0SW3XKZ
0SW4X0Z
0SW4X3Z
0SW4X7Z
0SW4XJZ
0SW4XKZ
0SW5X0Z
0SW5X3Z
0SW5X4Z
0SW5X7Z
0SW5X8Z
0SW5XJZ
0SW5XKZ
0SW6X0Z
0SW6X3Z
0SW6X4Z
0SW6X7Z
0SW6X8Z
0SW6XJZ
0SW6XKZ
0SW7X0Z
0SW7X3Z
0SW7X4Z
0SW7X7Z
0SW7X8Z
0SW7XJZ
0SW7XKZ
0SW8X0Z
0SW8X3Z
0SW8X4Z
0SW8X7Z
0SW8X8Z
0SW8XJZ
0SW8XKZ
0SW9X0Z
0SW9X3Z
0SW9X4Z
0SW9X5Z
0SW9X7Z
0SW9X8Z
0SW9XJZ
0SW9XKZ
0SWAXJZ
0SWBX0Z
0SWBX3Z
0SWBX4Z
0SWBX5Z
0SWBX7Z
0SWBX8Z
0SWBXJZ
0SWBXKZ
0SWCX0Z
0SWCX3Z
0SWCX4Z
0SWCX5Z
0SWCX7Z
0SWCX8Z
0SWCXJC
0SWCXJZ
0SWCXKZ
0SWDX0Z
0SWDX3Z
0SWDX4Z
0SWDX5Z
0SWDX7Z
0SWDX8Z
0SWDXJC
0SWDXJZ
0SWDXKZ
0SWEXJZ
0SWFX0Z
0SWFX3Z
0SWFX4Z
0SWFX5Z
0SWFX7Z
0SWFX8Z
0SWFXJZ
0SWFXKZ
0SWGX0Z
0SWGX3Z
0SWGX4Z
0SWGX5Z
0SWGX7Z
0SWGX8Z
0SWGXJZ
0SWGXKZ
0SWHX0Z
0SWHX3Z
0SWHX4Z
0SWHX5Z
0SWHX7Z
0SWHX8Z
0SWHXJZ
0SWHXKZ
0SWJX0Z
0SWJX3Z
0SWJX4Z
0SWJX5Z
0SWJX7Z
0SWJX8Z
0SWJXJZ
0SWJXKZ
0SWKX0Z
0SWKX3Z
0SWKX4Z
0SWKX5Z
0SWKX7Z
0SWKX8Z
0SWKXJZ
0SWKXKZ
0SWLX0Z
0SWLX3Z
0SWLX4Z
0SWLX5Z
0SWLX7Z
0SWLX8Z
0SWLXJZ
0SWLXKZ
0SWMX0Z
0SWMX3Z
0SWMX4Z
0SWMX5Z
0SWMX7Z
0SWMX8Z
0SWMXJZ
0SWMXKZ
0SWNX0Z
0SWNX3Z
0SWNX4Z
0SWNX5Z
0SWNX7Z
0SWNX8Z
0SWNXJZ
0SWNXKZ
0SWPX0Z
0SWPX3Z
0SWPX4Z
0SWPX5Z
0SWPX7Z
0SWPX8Z
0SWPXJZ
0SWPXKZ
0SWQX0Z
0SWQX3Z
0SWQX4Z
0SWQX5Z
0SWQX7Z
0SWQX8Z
0SWQXJZ
0SWQXKZ
0SWRXJZ
0SWSXJZ
0SWTXJZ
0SWUXJZ
0SWVXJZ
0SWWXJZ
0T25X0Z
0T25XYZ
0T29X0Z
0T29XYZ
0T2BX0Z
0T2BXYZ
0T2DX0Z
0T2DXYZ
0T5D0ZZ
0T5D3ZZ
0T5D4ZZ
0T5D7ZZ
0T5D8ZZ
0T5DXZZ
0T760DZ
0T763DZ
0T764DZ
0T767DZ
0T767ZZ
0T770DZ
0T773DZ
0T774DZ
0T777DZ
0T777ZZ
0T780DZ
0T783DZ
0T784DZ
0T787DZ
0T787ZZ
0T788ZZ
0T7B7DZ
0T7B7ZZ
0T7C0DZ
0T7C0ZZ
0T7C3DZ
0T7C3ZZ
0T7C4DZ
0T7C4ZZ
0T7C7DZ
0T7C7ZZ
0T7C8DZ
0T7C8ZZ
0T7D0DZ
0T7D3DZ
0T7D4DZ
0T7D7DZ
0T7D7ZZ
0T7D8DZ
0T7D8ZZ
0T9030Z
0T903ZX
0T903ZZ
0T904ZX
0T904ZZ
0T907ZX
0T908ZX
0T9130Z
0T913ZX
0T913ZZ
0T914ZX
0T914ZZ
0T917ZX
0T918ZX
0T9330Z
0T933ZX
0T933ZZ
0T934ZX
0T934ZZ
0T937ZX
0T938ZX
0T9430Z
0T943ZX
0T943ZZ
0T944ZX
0T944ZZ
0T947ZX
0T948ZX
0T9600Z
0T9630Z
0T963ZX
0T963ZZ
0T9640Z
0T964ZX
0T9670Z
0T967ZX
0T9680Z
0T968ZX
0T9700Z
0T9730Z
0T973ZX
0T973ZZ
0T9740Z
0T974ZX
0T9770Z
0T977ZX
0T9780Z
0T978ZX
0T9800Z
0T9830Z
0T983ZX
0T983ZZ
0T9840Z
0T984ZX
0T9870Z
0T987ZX
0T9880Z
0T988ZX
0T9B30Z
0T9B3ZZ
0T9B40Z
0T9B4ZZ
0T9B70Z
0T9B7ZZ
0T9B80Z
0T9B8ZZ
0T9C30Z
0T9C3ZZ
0T9C40Z
0T9C4ZZ
0T9C70Z
0T9C7ZZ
0T9C80Z
0T9C8ZZ
0T9D0ZX
0T9D30Z
0T9D3ZX
0T9D3ZZ
0T9D4ZX
0T9D7ZX
0T9D8ZX
0T9DXZX
0TB03ZX
0TB04ZX
0TB07ZX
0TB08ZX
0TB13ZX
0TB14ZX
0TB17ZX
0TB18ZX
0TB33ZX
0TB34ZX
0TB37ZX
0TB38ZX
0TB43ZX
0TB44ZX
0TB47ZX
0TB48ZX
0TB63ZX
0TB64ZX
0TB67ZX
0TB68ZX

0SPMX4Z-0TB68ZX
APPENDIX H: NON-OR PROCEDURE NOT AFFECTING MS-DRG ASSIGNMENT

0TB73ZX	0TH933Z	0TP58DZ	0TW5X3Z	0U7C4DZ	0U9K30Z	0UHD7YZ	0UPD8CZ	0UWH8YZ
0TB74ZX	0TH93YZ	0TP5X0Z	0TW5X7Z	0U7C4ZZ	0U9K3ZZ	0UHD83Z	0UPD8DZ	0UWHX0Z
0TB77ZX	0TH943Z	0TP5X2Z	0TW5XCZ	0U7C7DZ	0U9K40Z	0UHD8YZ	0UPD8HZ	0UWHX3Z
0TB78ZX	0TH94YZ	0TP5X3Z	0TW5XDZ	0U7C7ZZ	0U9K4ZZ	0UHF7GZ	0UPD8YZ	0UWHX7Z
0TBD0ZX	0TH972Z	0TP5XDZ	0TW5XJZ	0U7C8DZ	0U9K70Z	0UHF8GZ	0UPDX0Z	0UWHXDZ
0TBD3ZX	0TH973Z	0TP93YZ	0TW5XKZ	0U7C8ZZ	0U9K7ZZ	0UHG7GZ	0UPDX3Z	0UWHXJZ
0TBD4ZX	0TH97YZ	0TP94YZ	0TW93YZ	0U7G7DZ	0U9K80Z	0UHG8GZ	0UPDXDZ	0UWHXKZ
0TBD7ZX	0TH982Z	0TP970Z	0TW94YZ	0U7G7ZZ	0U9K8ZZ	0UHH3YZ	0UPDXHZ	0UWMX0Z
0TBD8ZX	0TH983Z	0TP972Z	0TW97YZ	0U7G8DZ	0U9KX0Z	0UHH4YZ	0UPH3YZ	0UWMX7Z
0TBDXZX	0THB03Z	0TP973Z	0TW9X0Z	0U7G8ZZ	0U9KXZZ	0UHH73Z	0UPH4YZ	0UWMXJZ
0TCB7ZZ	0THB33Z	0TP97DZ	0TW9X2Z	0U8K7ZZ	0U9L00Z	0UHH7YZ	0UPH70Z	0UWMXKZ
0TCB8ZZ	0THB3YZ	0TP97YZ	0TW9X3Z	0U8K8ZZ	0U9L0ZZ	0UHH83Z	0UPH73Z	0V24X0Z
0TCC7ZZ	0THB43Z	0TP980Z	0TW9X7Z	0U8KXZZ	0U9LX0Z	0UHH8YZ	0UPH7DZ	0V24XYZ
0TCC8ZZ	0THB4YZ	0TP982Z	0TW9XCZ	0U9030Z	0U9LXZZ	0UJ33ZZ	0UPH7YZ	0V28X0Z
0TCD7ZZ	0THB72Z	0TP983Z	0TW9XDZ	0U903ZZ	0UC97ZZ	0UJ38ZZ	0UPH80Z	0V28XYZ
0TCD8ZZ	0THB73Z	0TP98DZ	0TW9XJZ	0U9080Z	0UC98ZZ	0UJ3XZZ	0UPH83Z	0V2DX0Z
0TCDXZZ	0THB7YZ	0TP9X0Z	0TW9XKZ	0U908ZX	0UCG7ZZ	0UJ83ZZ	0UPH8DZ	0V2DXYZ
0TF30ZZ	0THB82Z	0TP9X2Z	0TW9XMZ	0U908ZZ	0UCG8ZZ	0UJ87ZZ	0UPH8YZ	0V2MX0Z
0TF37ZZ	0THB83Z	0TP9X3Z	0TWB3YZ	0U9130Z	0UCGXZZ	0UJ88ZZ	0UPHX0Z	0V2MXYZ
0TF38ZZ	0THD03Z	0TP9XDZ	0TWB4YZ	0U913ZZ	0UCK0ZZ	0UJ8XZZ	0UPHX1Z	0V2RX0Z
0TF40ZZ	0THD33Z	0TPB3YZ	0TWB7YZ	0U9180Z	0UCK3ZZ	0UJD3ZZ	0UPHX3Z	0V2RXYZ
0TF47ZZ	0THD3YZ	0TPB4YZ	0TWBX0Z	0U918ZX	0UCK4ZZ	0UJD7ZZ	0UPHXDZ	0V2SX0Z
0TF48ZZ	0THD43Z	0TPB70Z	0TWBX2Z	0U918ZZ	0UCK7ZZ	0UJD8ZZ	0UPMX0Z	0V2SXYZ
0TF60ZZ	0THD4YZ	0TPB72Z	0TWBX3Z	0U9230Z	0UCK8ZZ	0UJDXZZ	0UQG7ZZ	0V550ZZ
0TF63ZZ	0THD72Z	0TPB73Z	0TWBX7Z	0U923ZZ	0UCKXZZ	0UJH3ZZ	0UQGXZZ	0V553ZZ
0TF64ZZ	0THD73Z	0TPB7DZ	0TWBXCZ	0U9280Z	0UCMXZZ	0UJH7ZZ	0UQKXZZ	0V554ZZ
0TF67ZZ	0THD7YZ	0TPB7YZ	0TWBXDZ	0U928ZX	0UF5XZZ	0UJH8ZZ	0UQMXZZ	0V55XZZ
0TF68ZZ	0THD82Z	0TPB80Z	0TWBXJZ	0U928ZZ	0UF6XZZ	0UJHXZZ	0US9XZZ	0V5N0ZZ
0TF70ZZ	0THD83Z	0TPB82Z	0TWBXKZ	0U9430Z	0UF7XZZ	0UJMXZZ	0UW33YZ	0V5N3ZZ
0TF73ZZ	0THD8YZ	0TPB83Z	0TWBXLZ	0U943ZZ	0UF9XZZ	0UP33YZ	0UW34YZ	0V5N4ZZ
0TF74ZZ	0THDX3Z	0TPB8DZ	0TWBXMZ	0U9480Z	0UH303Z	0UP34YZ	0UW37YZ	0V5N8ZZ
0TF77ZZ	0TJ53ZZ	0TPBX0Z	0TWD3YZ	0U948ZX	0UH30YZ	0UP37YZ	0UW38YZ	0V5P0ZZ
0TF78ZZ	0TJ54ZZ	0TPBX2Z	0TWD4YZ	0U948ZZ	0UH333Z	0UP38YZ	0UW3X0Z	0V5P3ZZ
0TFB0ZZ	0TJ57ZZ	0TPBX3Z	0TWD7YZ	0U9530Z	0UH33YZ	0UP3X0Z	0UW3X3Z	0V5P4ZZ
0TFB3ZZ	0TJ58ZZ	0TPBXDZ	0TWD8YZ	0U953ZZ	0UH343Z	0UP3X3Z	0UW83YZ	0V5P8ZZ
0TFB4ZZ	0TJ5XZZ	0TPBXLZ	0TWDX0Z	0U954ZZ	0UH34YZ	0UP83YZ	0UW84YZ	0V5Q0ZZ
0TFB7ZZ	0TJ93ZZ	0TPD3YZ	0TWDX2Z	0U957ZZ	0UH37YZ	0UP84YZ	0UW87YZ	0V5Q3ZZ
0TFB8ZZ	0TJ94ZZ	0TPD4YZ	0TWDX3Z	0U958ZZ	0UH38YZ	0UP870Z	0UW88YZ	0V5Q4ZZ
0TFC0ZZ	0TJ97ZZ	0TPD70Z	0TWDX7Z	0U9630Z	0UH803Z	0UP873Z	0UW8X0Z	0V5Q8ZZ
0TFC3ZZ	0TJ98ZZ	0TPD72Z	0TWDXCZ	0U963ZZ	0UH80YZ	0UP87DZ	0UW8X3Z	0V9030Z
0TFC4ZZ	0TJ9XZZ	0TPD73Z	0TWDXDZ	0U964ZZ	0UH833Z	0UP87YZ	0UW8X7Z	0V903ZX
0TFC7ZZ	0TJB3ZZ	0TPD7DZ	0TWDXJZ	0U967ZZ	0UH83YZ	0UP880Z	0UW8XCZ	0V903ZZ
0TFC8ZZ	0TJB7ZZ	0TPD7YZ	0TWDXKZ	0U968ZZ	0UH843Z	0UP883Z	0UW8XDZ	0V9040Z
0TFD0ZZ	0TJB8ZZ	0TPD80Z	0TWDXLZ	0U9730Z	0UH84YZ	0UP88DZ	0UW8XJZ	0V904ZX
0TFD3ZZ	0TJBXZZ	0TPD82Z	0U23X0Z	0U973ZZ	0UH873Z	0UP88YZ	0UW8XKZ	0V904ZZ
0TFD4ZZ	0TJD3ZZ	0TPD83Z	0U23XYZ	0U974ZZ	0UH87YZ	0UP8X0Z	0UWD3YZ	0V907ZX
0TFD7ZZ	0TJD4ZZ	0TPD8DZ	0U28X0Z	0U977ZZ	0UH883Z	0UP8X3Z	0UWD4YZ	0V908ZX
0TFD8ZZ	0TJD7ZZ	0TPD8YZ	0U28XYZ	0U978ZZ	0UH88YZ	0UP8XDZ	0UWD7YZ	0V9130Z
0TFDXZZ	0TJD8ZZ	0TPDX0Z	0U2DX0Z	0U9930Z	0UH90HZ	0UPD3CZ	0UWD8YZ	0V913ZX
0TH503Z	0TJDXZZ	0TPDX2Z	0U2DXHZ	0U993ZZ	0UH97HZ	0UPD3YZ	0UWDX0Z	0V913ZZ
0TH533Z	0TP53YZ	0TPDX3Z	0U2DXYZ	0U9C30Z	0UH98HZ	0UPD4CZ	0UWDX3Z	0V9140Z
0TH53YZ	0TP54YZ	0TPDXDZ	0U2HX0Z	0U9C3ZZ	0UHC7HZ	0UPD4YZ	0UWDX7Z	0V914ZX
0TH543Z	0TP570Z	0TTD4ZZ	0U2HXGZ	0U9F30Z	0UHC8HZ	0UPD70Z	0UWDXCZ	0V914ZZ
0TH54YZ	0TP572Z	0TTD7ZZ	0U2HXYZ	0U9F3ZZ	0UHD03Z	0UPD73Z	0UWDXDZ	0V9230Z
0TH572Z	0TP573Z	0TTD8ZZ	0U2MX0Z	0U9F40Z	0UHD0YZ	0UPD7CZ	0UWDXHZ	0V923ZX
0TH573Z	0TP57DZ	0TW53YZ	0U2MXYZ	0U9F4ZZ	0UHD33Z	0UPD7DZ	0UWDXJZ	0V923ZZ
0TH57YZ	0TP57YZ	0TW54YZ	0U7C0DZ	0U9G30Z	0UHD3YZ	0UPD7HZ	0UWDXKZ	0V9240Z
0TH582Z	0TP580Z	0TW57YZ	0U7C0ZZ	0U9G3ZZ	0UHD43Z	0UPD7YZ	0UWH3YZ	0V924ZX
0TH583Z	0TP582Z	0TW5X0Z	0U7C3DZ	0U9K00Z	0UHD4YZ	0UPD80Z	0UWH4YZ	0V924ZZ
0TH903Z	0TP583Z	0TW5X2Z	0U7C3ZZ	0U9K0ZZ	0UHD73Z	0UPD83Z	0UWH7YZ	0V9330Z

0V933ZX
0V933ZZ
0V9340Z
0V934ZX
0V934ZZ
0V9500Z
0V950ZX
0V9530Z
0V953ZX
0V953ZZ
0V9540Z
0V954ZX
0V954ZZ
0V95X0Z
0V95XZX
0V95XZZ
0V9600Z
0V960ZX
0V960ZZ
0V9630Z
0V963ZX
0V963ZZ
0V9640Z
0V964ZX
0V964ZZ
0V9700Z
0V970ZX
0V970ZZ
0V9730Z
0V973ZX
0V973ZZ
0V9740Z
0V974ZX
0V974ZZ
0V9930Z
0V993ZX
0V993ZZ
0V9940Z
0V994ZX
0V994ZZ
0V9B30Z
0V9B3ZX
0V9B3ZZ
0V9B40Z
0V9B4ZX
0V9B4ZZ
0V9C30Z
0V9C3ZX
0V9C3ZZ
0V9C40Z
0V9C4ZX
0V9C4ZZ
0V9F00Z
0V9F0ZX
0V9F0ZZ
0V9F30Z
0V9F3ZX
0V9F3ZZ
0V9F40Z
0V9F4ZX
0V9F4ZZ
0V9G0CZ
0V9G0ZX
0V9G0ZZ
0V9G30Z
0V9G3ZX
0V9G3ZZ
0V9G40Z
0V9G4ZX
0V9G4ZZ
0V9H00Z
0V9H0ZX
0V9H0ZZ
0V9H30Z
0V9H3ZX
0V9H3ZZ
0V9H40Z
0V9H4ZX
0V9H4ZZ
0V9J0ZX
0V9J30Z
0V9J3ZX
0V9J3ZZ
0V9J4ZX
0V9K0ZX
0V9K30Z
0V9K3ZX
0V9K3ZZ
0V9K4ZX
0V9L0ZX
0V9L30Z
0V9L3ZX
0V9L3ZZ
0V9L4ZX
0V9N00Z
0V9N0ZX
0V9N0ZZ
0V9N30Z
0V9N3ZX
0V9N3ZZ
0V9N40Z
0V9N4ZX
0V9N4ZZ
0V9P00Z
0V9P0ZX
0V9P0ZZ
0V9P30Z
0V9P3ZX
0V9P3ZZ
0V9P40Z
0V9P4ZX
0V9P4ZZ
0V9Q00Z
0V9Q0ZX
0V9Q0ZZ
0V9Q30Z
0V9Q3ZX
0V9Q3ZZ
0V9Q40Z
0V9Q4ZX
0V9Q4ZZ
0V9S30Z
0V9S3ZZ
0V9T30Z
0V9T3ZZ
0VB03ZX
0VB04ZX
0VB07ZX
0VB08ZX
0VB13ZX
0VB14ZX
0VB23ZX
0VB24ZX
0VB33ZX
0VB34ZX
0VB50ZX
0VB53ZX
0VB53ZZ
0VB54ZX
0VB54ZZ
0VB5XZX
0VB5XZZ
0VB60ZX
0VB63ZX
0VB64ZX
0VB70ZX
0VB73ZX
0VB74ZX
0VB93ZX
0VB94ZX
0VBB3ZX
0VBB4ZX
0VBC3ZX
0VBC4ZX
0VBF0ZX
0VBF3ZX
0VBF4ZX
0VBF8ZX
0VBG0ZX
0VBG3ZX
0VBG4ZX
0VBG8ZX
0VBH0ZX
0VBH3ZX
0VBH4ZX
0VBH8ZX
0VBJ0ZX
0VBJ3ZX
0VBJ4ZX
0VBJ8ZX
0VBK0ZX
0VBK3ZX
0VBK4ZX
0VBK8ZX
0VBL0ZX
0VBL3ZX
0VBL4ZX
0VBL8ZX
0VBN0ZX
0VBN0ZZ
0VBN3ZX
0VBN3ZZ
0VBN4ZX
0VBN4ZZ
0VBN8ZX
0VBN8ZZ
0VBP0ZX
0VBP0ZZ
0VBP3ZX
0VBP3ZZ
0VBP4ZX
0VBP4ZZ
0VBP8ZX
0VBP8ZZ
0VBQ0ZX
0VBQ0ZZ
0VBQ3ZX
0VBQ3ZZ
0VBQ4ZX
0VBQ4ZZ
0VBQ8ZX
0VBQ8ZZ
0VC53ZZ
0VC54ZZ
0VC5XZZ
0VC60ZZ
0VC63ZZ
0VC64ZZ
0VC70ZZ
0VC73ZZ
0VC74ZZ
0VCN0ZZ
0VCN3ZZ
0VCN4ZZ
0VCP0ZZ
0VCP3ZZ
0VCP4ZZ
0VCQ0ZZ
0VCQ3ZZ
0VCQ4ZZ
0VCSXZZ
0VH403Z
0VH40YZ
0VH433Z
0VH43YZ
0VH443Z
0VH44YZ
0VH473Z
0VH47YZ
0VH483Z
0VH48YZ
0VH803Z
0VH80YZ
0VH833Z
0VH83YZ
0VH843Z
0VH84YZ
0VH873Z
0VH87YZ
0VH883Z
0VH88YZ
0VHD03Z
0VHD0YZ
0VHD33Z
0VHD3YZ
0VHD43Z
0VHD4YZ
0VHD73Z
0VHD7YZ
0VHD83Z
0VHD8YZ
0VHM03Z
0VHM0YZ
0VHM33Z
0VHM3YZ
0VHM43Z
0VHM4YZ
0VHM73Z
0VHM7YZ
0VHM83Z
0VHM8YZ
0VHR03Z
0VHR0YZ
0VHR33Z
0VHR3YZ
0VHR43Z
0VHR4YZ
0VHR73Z
0VHR7YZ
0VHR83Z
0VHR8YZ
0VHS03Z
0VHS0YZ
0VHS33Z
0VHS3YZ
0VHS43Z
0VHS4YZ
0VHS7YZ
0VHS8YZ
0VHSX3Z
0VJ43ZZ
0VJ4XZZ
0VJ80ZZ
0VJ83ZZ
0VJ84ZZ
0VJ8XZZ
0VJD3ZZ
0VJDXZZ
0VJM3ZZ
0VJMXZZ
0VJR3ZZ
0VJRXZZ
0VJS0ZZ
0VJS3ZZ
0VJS4ZZ
0VJSXZZ
0VLF0CZ
0VLF0DZ
0VLF0ZZ
0VLF3CZ
0VLF3DZ
0VLF3ZZ
0VLF4CZ
0VLF4DZ
0VLF4ZZ
0VLF8CZ
0VLF8DZ
0VLF8ZZ
0VLG0CZ
0VLG0DZ
0VLG0ZZ
0VLG3CZ
0VLG3DZ
0VLG3ZZ
0VLG4CZ
0VLG4DZ
0VLG4ZZ
0VLG8CZ
0VLG8DZ
0VLG8ZZ
0VLH0CZ
0VLH0DZ
0VLH0ZZ
0VLH3CZ
0VLH3DZ
0VLH3ZZ
0VLH4CZ
0VLH4DZ
0VLH4ZZ
0VLH8CZ
0VLH8DZ
0VLH8ZZ
0VLN0CZ
0VLN0ZZ
0VLN3CZ
0VLN3ZZ
0VLN4CZ
0VLN4ZZ
0VLN8CZ
0VLN8ZZ
0VLP0CZ
0VLP0ZZ
0VLP3CZ
0VLP3ZZ
0VLP4CZ
0VLP4ZZ
0VLP8CZ
0VLP8ZZ
0VLQ0CZ
0VLQ0ZZ
0VLQ3CZ
0VLQ3ZZ
0VLQ4CZ
0VLQ4ZZ
0VLQ8CZ
0VLQ8ZZ
0VN90ZZ
0VN93ZZ
0VN94ZZ
0VNB0ZZ
0VNB3ZZ
0VNB4ZZ
0VNC0ZZ
0VNC3ZZ
0VNC4ZZ
0VNT0ZZ
0VNT3ZZ
0VNT4ZZ
0VNTXZZ
0VP43YZ
0VP44YZ
0VP470Z
0VP473Z
0VP47YZ
0VP480Z
0VP483Z
0VP48YZ
0VP4X0Z
0VP4X1Z
0VP4X3Z
0VP800Z
0VP803Z
0VP807Z
0VP80JZ
0VP80KZ
0VP80YZ
0VP830Z
0VP833Z
0VP837Z
0VP83JZ
0VP83KZ
0VP83YZ
0VP840Z
0VP843Z
0VP847Z
0VP84JZ
0VP84KZ
0VP84YZ
0VP870Z
0VP873Z
0VP877Z
0VP87JZ
0VP87KZ
0VP87YZ
0VP880Z
0VP883Z
0VP887Z
0VP88JZ
0VP88KZ
0VP88YZ
0VP8X0Z
0VP8X3Z
0VPD3YZ
0VPD4YZ
0VPD70Z
0VPD73Z
0VPD7YZ
0VPD80Z
0VPD83Z
0VPD8YZ
0VPDX0Z
0VPDX3Z
0VPM3YZ
0VPM4YZ
0VPM70Z
0VPM73Z
0VPM7YZ
0VPM80Z
0VPM83Z
0VPM8YZ
0VPMX0Z
0VPMX3Z
0VPR00Z
0VPR03Z
0VPR07Z
0VPR0CZ
0VPR0JZ
0VPR0KZ
0VPR0YZ
0VPR30Z
0VPR33Z
0VPR37Z
0VPR3CZ
0VPR3JZ
0VPR3KZ
0VPR3YZ
0VPR40Z
0VPR43Z
0VPR47Z
0VPR4CZ
0VPR4JZ
0VPR4KZ
0VPR4YZ
0VPR70Z
0VPR73Z
0VPR77Z
0VPR7CZ
0VPR7DZ
0VPR7JZ
0VPR7KZ
0VPR7YZ
0VPR80Z
0VPR83Z
0VPR87Z
0VPR8CZ
0VPR8DZ
0VPR8JZ
0VPR8KZ
0VPR8YZ
0VPRX0Z
0VPRX3Z
0VPRXDZ
0VPS3YZ
0VPS4YZ
0VPS70Z
0VPS73Z
0VPS7YZ
0VPS80Z
0VPS83Z
0VPS8YZ
0VPSX0Z
0VPSX3Z
0VQ50ZZ
0VQ53ZZ
0VQ54ZZ
0VQ5XZZ
0VQ60ZZ
0VQ63ZZ
0VQ64ZZ
0VQ70ZZ
0VQ73ZZ
0VQ74ZZ
0VT50ZZ
0VT54ZZ
0VT5XZZ
0VTN0ZZ
0VTN4ZZ
0VTP0ZZ
0VTP4ZZ
0VTQ0ZZ
0VTQ4ZZ
0VTT0ZZ
0VTT4ZZ
0VTTXZZ
0VUSX7Z
0VUSXJZ
0VUSXKZ
0VW43YZ
0VW44YZ
0VW47YZ
0VW48YZ
0VW4X0Z
0VW4X3Z
0VW4X7Z
0VW4XJZ
0VW4XKZ
0VW800Z
0VW803Z
0VW807Z
0VW80JZ
0VW80KZ
0VW80YZ
0VW830Z
0VW833Z
0VW837Z
0VW83JZ
0VW83KZ
0VW83YZ
0VW840Z
0VW843Z
0VW847Z
0VW84JZ
0VW84KZ
0VW84YZ
0VW870Z
0VW873Z
0VW877Z
0VW87JZ
0VW87KZ
0VW87YZ

0VW880Z	0VWR7KZ	0W1G4JG	0W904ZZ	0W9F30Z	0WB5XZX	0WFCXZZ	0WHR4YZ	0WP00KZ
0VW883Z	0VWR7YZ	0W1G4JJ	0W9130Z	0W9F3ZZ	0WB60ZX	0WFGXZZ	0WHR73Z	0WP00YZ
0VW887Z	0VWR80Z	0W1J0J4	0W913ZX	0W9F40Z	0WB63ZX	0WFJ0ZZ	0WHR7YZ	0WP030Z
0VW88JZ	0VWR83Z	0W1J0JW	0W913ZZ	0W9F4ZZ	0WB64ZX	0WFJ3ZZ	0WHR83Z	0WP031Z
0VW88KZ	0VWR87Z	0W1J0JY	0W9140Z	0W9G30Z	0WB6XZX	0WFJ4ZZ	0WHR8YZ	0WP033Z
0VW88YZ	0VWR8CZ	0W1J3J4	0W914ZX	0W9G3ZX	0WB80ZX	0WFJXZZ	0WJ03ZZ	0WP037Z
0VW8X0Z	0VWR8DZ	0W1J3JW	0W914ZZ	0W9G3ZZ	0WB83ZX	0WFP0ZZ	0WJ04ZZ	0WP03JZ
0VW8X3Z	0VWR8JZ	0W1J3JY	0W920ZX	0W9G40Z	0WB84ZX	0WFP3ZZ	0WJ0XZZ	0WP03KZ
0VW8X7Z	0VWR8KZ	0W1J4J4	0W9230Z	0W9G4ZZ	0WB8XZX	0WFP4ZZ	0WJ13ZZ	0WP03YZ
0VW8XJZ	0VWR8YZ	0W1J4JW	0W923ZX	0W9H30Z	0WBC3ZX	0WFP7ZZ	0WJ23ZZ	0WP040Z
0VW8XKZ	0VWRX0Z	0W1J4JY	0W923ZZ	0W9H3ZZ	0WBC4ZX	0WFP8ZZ	0WJ24ZZ	0WP041Z
0VWD3YZ	0VWRX3Z	0W20X0Z	0W924ZX	0W9J30Z	0WBH3ZX	0WFPXZZ	0WJ2XZZ	0WP043Z
0VWD4YZ	0VWRX7Z	0W20XYZ	0W930ZX	0W9J3ZZ	0WBH4ZX	0WFQXZZ	0WJ30ZZ	0WP047Z
0VWD7YZ	0VWRXCZ	0W21X0Z	0W9330Z	0W9K00Z	0WBK0ZX	0WFR0ZZ	0WJ33ZZ	0WP04JZ
0VWD8YZ	0VWRXDZ	0W21XYZ	0W933ZX	0W9K0ZX	0WBK3ZX	0WFR3ZZ	0WJ34ZZ	0WP04KZ
0VWDX0Z	0VWRXJZ	0W22X0Z	0W933ZZ	0W9K0ZZ	0WBK4ZX	0WFR4ZZ	0WJ3XZZ	0WP04YZ
0VWDX3Z	0VWRXKZ	0W22XYZ	0W934ZX	0W9K30Z	0WBKXZX	0WFR7ZZ	0WJ43ZZ	0WP0X0Z
0VWDX7Z	0VWS3YZ	0W24X0Z	0W940ZX	0W9K3ZX	0WBL0ZX	0WFR8ZZ	0WJ44ZZ	0WP0X1Z
0VWDXJZ	0VWS4YZ	0W24XYZ	0W9430Z	0W9K3ZZ	0WBL3ZX	0WH103Z	0WJ4XZZ	0WP0X3Z
0VWDXKZ	0VWS7YZ	0W25X0Z	0W943ZX	0W9K40Z	0WBL4ZX	0WH133Z	0WJ53ZZ	0WP0X7Z
0VWM3YZ	0VWS8YZ	0W25XYZ	0W943ZZ	0W9K4ZX	0WBLXZX	0WH143Z	0WJ54ZZ	0WP0XJZ
0VWM4YZ	0VWSX0Z	0W26X0Z	0W944ZX	0W9K4ZZ	0WBM0ZX	0WH803Z	0WJ5XZZ	0WP0XKZ
0VWM7YZ	0VWSX3Z	0W26XYZ	0W950ZX	0W9L00Z	0WBM3ZX	0WH80YZ	0WJ63ZZ	0WP0XYZ
0VWM8YZ	0VWSX7Z	0W28X0Z	0W9530Z	0W9L0ZX	0WBM4ZX	0WH833Z	0WJ6XZZ	0WP103Z
0VWMX0Z	0VWSXJZ	0W28XYZ	0W953ZX	0W9L0ZZ	0WBMXZX	0WH83YZ	0WJ83ZZ	0WP133Z
0VWMX3Z	0VWSXKZ	0W29X0Z	0W953ZZ	0W9L30Z	0WC1XZZ	0WH843Z	0WJ8XZZ	0WP143Z
0VWMX7Z	0W190J4	0W29XYZ	0W954ZX	0W9L3ZX	0WC3XZZ	0WH84YZ	0WJ93ZZ	0WP1X0Z
0VWMXCZ	0W190JG	0W2BX0Z	0W960ZX	0W9L3ZZ	0WC40ZZ	0WH903Z	0WJB3ZZ	0WP1X1Z
0VWMXJZ	0W190JW	0W2BXYZ	0W9630Z	0W9L40Z	0WC43ZZ	0WH90YZ	0WJC3ZZ	0WP1X3Z
0VWMXKZ	0W190JY	0W2CX0Z	0W963ZX	0W9L4ZX	0WC44ZZ	0WH933Z	0WJD0ZZ	0WP200Z
0VWR00Z	0W193J4	0W2CXYZ	0W963ZZ	0W9L4ZZ	0WC50ZZ	0WH93YZ	0WJD3ZZ	0WP201Z
0VWR03Z	0W193JG	0W2DX0Z	0W964ZX	0W9M00Z	0WC53ZZ	0WH943Z	0WJF3ZZ	0WP203Z
0VWR07Z	0W193JW	0W2DXYZ	0W9800Z	0W9M0ZX	0WC54ZZ	0WH94YZ	0WJFXZZ	0WP207Z
0VWR0CZ	0W193JY	0W2FX0Z	0W980ZX	0W9M0ZZ	0WC90ZZ	0WHB03Z	0WJG3ZZ	0WP20JZ
0VWR0DZ	0W194J4	0W2FXYZ	0W980ZZ	0W9M30Z	0WC93ZZ	0WHB0YZ	0WJH3ZZ	0WP20KZ
0VWR0JZ	0W194JG	0W2GX0Z	0W9830Z	0W9M3ZX	0WC94ZZ	0WHB33Z	0WJJ3ZZ	0WP20YZ
0VWR0KZ	0W194JW	0W2GXYZ	0W983ZX	0W9M3ZZ	0WC9XZZ	0WHB3YZ	0WJK3ZZ	0WP230Z
0VWR0YZ	0W194JY	0W2HX0Z	0W983ZZ	0W9M40Z	0WCB0ZZ	0WHB43Z	0WJK4ZZ	0WP231Z
0VWR30Z	0W1B0J4	0W2HXYZ	0W9840Z	0W9M4ZX	0WCB3ZZ	0WHB4YZ	0WJKXZZ	0WP233Z
0VWR33Z	0W1B0JG	0W2JX0Z	0W984ZX	0W9M4ZZ	0WCB4ZZ	0WHG33Z	0WJL3ZZ	0WP237Z
0VWR37Z	0W1B0JW	0W2JXYZ	0W984ZZ	0W9N0ZX	0WCBXZZ	0WHP0YZ	0WJL4ZZ	0WP23JZ
0VWR3CZ	0W1B0JY	0W2KX0Z	0W9900Z	0W9N30Z	0WCCXZZ	0WHP33Z	0WJLXZZ	0WP23KZ
0VWR3DZ	0W1B3J4	0W2KXYZ	0W990ZX	0W9N3ZX	0WCDXZZ	0WHP3YZ	0WJM3ZZ	0WP23YZ
0VWR3JZ	0W1B3JG	0W2LX0Z	0W990ZZ	0W9N3ZZ	0WCGXZZ	0WHP43Z	0WJMXZZ	0WP240Z
0VWR3KZ	0W1B3JW	0W2LXYZ	0W9930Z	0W9N4ZX	0WCHXZZ	0WHP4YZ	0WJN3ZZ	0WP241Z
0VWR3YZ	0W1B3JY	0W2MX0Z	0W993ZX	0WB00ZX	0WCJXZZ	0WHP73Z	0WJNXZZ	0WP243Z
0VWR40Z	0W1B4J4	0W2MXYZ	0W993ZZ	0WB03ZX	0WCP7ZZ	0WHP7YZ	0WJP3ZZ	0WP247Z
0VWR43Z	0W1B4JG	0W2NX0Z	0W9B00Z	0WB04ZX	0WCP8ZZ	0WHP83Z	0WJP7ZZ	0WP24JZ
0VWR47Z	0W1B4JW	0W2NXYZ	0W9B0ZX	0WB0XZX	0WCPXZZ	0WHP8YZ	0WJP8ZZ	0WP24KZ
0VWR4CZ	0W1B4JY	0W3G0ZZ	0W9B0ZZ	0WB20ZX	0WCQ0ZZ	0WHQ03Z	0WJQ3ZZ	0WP24YZ
0VWR4DZ	0W1G0J9	0W3P8ZZ	0W9B30Z	0WB23ZX	0WCQ3ZZ	0WHQ0YZ	0WJQ7ZZ	0WP2X0Z
0VWR4JZ	0W1G0JB	0W8NXZZ	0W9B3ZX	0WB24ZX	0WCQ4ZZ	0WHQ73Z	0WJQ8ZZ	0WP2X1Z
0VWR4KZ	0W1G0JG	0W9000Z	0W9B3ZZ	0WB2XZX	0WCQXZZ	0WHQ7YZ	0WJR3ZZ	0WP2X3Z
0VWR4YZ	0W1G0JJ	0W900ZX	0W9C30Z	0WB40ZX	0WCR7ZZ	0WHQ83Z	0WJR7ZZ	0WP2X7Z
0VWR70Z	0W1G3J9	0W900ZZ	0W9C3ZX	0WB43ZX	0WCR8ZZ	0WHQ8YZ	0WJR8ZZ	0WP2XJZ
0VWR73Z	0W1G3JB	0W9030Z	0W9C3ZZ	0WB44ZX	0WCRXZZ	0WHR03Z	0WP000Z	0WP2XKZ
0VWR77Z	0W1G3JG	0W903ZX	0W9C4ZX	0WB4XZX	0WF1XZZ	0WHR0YZ	0WP001Z	0WP2XYZ
0VWR7CZ	0W1G3JJ	0W903ZZ	0W9D30Z	0WB50ZX	0WF3XZZ	0WHR33Z	0WP003Z	0WP400Z
0VWR7DZ	0W1G4J9	0W9040Z	0W9D3ZX	0WB53ZX	0WF9XZZ	0WHR3YZ	0WP007Z	0WP401Z
0VWR7JZ	0W1G4JB	0W904ZX	0W9D3ZZ	0WB54ZX	0WFBXZZ	0WHR43Z	0WP00JZ	0WP403Z

0WP407Z
0WP40JZ
0WP40KZ
0WP40YZ
0WP430Z
0WP431Z
0WP433Z
0WP437Z
0WP43JZ
0WP43KZ
0WP43YZ
0WP440Z
0WP441Z
0WP443Z
0WP447Z
0WP44JZ
0WP44KZ
0WP44YZ
0WP4X0Z
0WP4X1Z
0WP4X3Z
0WP4X7Z
0WP4XJZ
0WP4XKZ
0WP4XYZ
0WP500Z
0WP501Z
0WP503Z
0WP507Z
0WP50JZ
0WP50KZ
0WP50YZ
0WP530Z
0WP531Z
0WP533Z
0WP537Z
0WP53JZ
0WP53KZ
0WP53YZ
0WP540Z
0WP541Z
0WP543Z
0WP547Z
0WP54JZ
0WP54KZ
0WP54YZ
0WP5X0Z
0WP5X1Z
0WP5X3Z
0WP5X7Z
0WP5XJZ
0WP5XKZ
0WP5XYZ
0WP600Z
0WP601Z
0WP603Z
0WP607Z
0WP60JZ
0WP60KZ
0WP60YZ
0WP630Z
0WP631Z
0WP633Z
0WP637Z
0WP63JZ
0WP63KZ
0WP63YZ
0WP640Z
0WP641Z
0WP643Z
0WP647Z
0WP64JZ
0WP64KZ
0WP64YZ
0WP6X0Z
0WP6X1Z
0WP6X3Z
0WP6X7Z
0WP6XJZ
0WP6XKZ
0WP6XYZ
0WP800Z
0WP801Z
0WP803Z
0WP807Z
0WP80JZ
0WP80KZ
0WP80YZ
0WP830Z
0WP831Z
0WP833Z
0WP837Z
0WP83JZ
0WP83KZ
0WP83YZ
0WP840Z
0WP841Z
0WP843Z
0WP847Z
0WP84JZ
0WP84KZ
0WP84YZ
0WP8X0Z
0WP8X1Z
0WP8X3Z
0WP8X7Z
0WP8XJZ
0WP8XKZ
0WP8XYZ
0WP900Z
0WP901Z
0WP903Z
0WP90JZ
0WP90YZ
0WP930Z
0WP931Z
0WP933Z
0WP93JZ
0WP93YZ
0WP940Z
0WP941Z
0WP943Z
0WP94JZ
0WP94YZ
0WP9X0Z
0WP9X1Z
0WP9X3Z
0WPB00Z
0WPB01Z
0WPB03Z
0WPB0JZ
0WPB0YZ
0WPB30Z
0WPB31Z
0WPB33Z
0WPB3JZ
0WPB3YZ
0WPB40Z
0WPB41Z
0WPB43Z
0WPB4JZ
0WPB4YZ
0WPBX0Z
0WPBX1Z
0WPBX3Z
0WPCX0Z
0WPCX1Z
0WPCX3Z
0WPCX7Z
0WPCXJZ
0WPCXKZ
0WPCXYZ
0WPDX0Z
0WPDX1Z
0WPDX3Z
0WPFX0Z
0WPFX1Z
0WPFX3Z
0WPFX7Z
0WPFXJZ
0WPFXKZ
0WPFXYZ
0WPGX0Z
0WPGX1Z
0WPGX3Z
0WPHX0Z
0WPHX1Z
0WPHX3Z
0WPJ00Z
0WPJ01Z
0WPJ03Z
0WPJ0JZ
0WPJ0YZ
0WPJ30Z
0WPJ31Z
0WPJ33Z
0WPJ3JZ
0WPJ3YZ
0WPJ40Z
0WPJ41Z
0WPJ43Z
0WPJ4JZ
0WPJ4YZ
0WPJX0Z
0WPJX1Z
0WPJX3Z
0WPK00Z
0WPK01Z
0WPK03Z
0WPK07Z
0WPK0JZ
0WPK0KZ
0WPK0YZ
0WPK30Z
0WPK31Z
0WPK33Z
0WPK37Z
0WPK3JZ
0WPK3KZ
0WPK3YZ
0WPK40Z
0WPK41Z
0WPK43Z
0WPK47Z
0WPK4JZ
0WPK4KZ
0WPK4YZ
0WPKX0Z
0WPKX1Z
0WPKX3Z
0WPKX7Z
0WPKXJZ
0WPKXKZ
0WPKXYZ
0WPL00Z
0WPL01Z
0WPL03Z
0WPL07Z
0WPL0JZ
0WPL0KZ
0WPL0YZ
0WPL30Z
0WPL31Z
0WPL33Z
0WPL37Z
0WPL3JZ
0WPL3KZ
0WPL3YZ
0WPL40Z
0WPL41Z
0WPL43Z
0WPL47Z
0WPL4JZ
0WPL4KZ
0WPL4YZ
0WPLX0Z
0WPLX1Z
0WPLX3Z
0WPLX7Z
0WPLXJZ
0WPLXKZ
0WPLXYZ
0WPM00Z
0WPM01Z
0WPM03Z
0WPM0JZ
0WPM0YZ
0WPM30Z
0WPM31Z
0WPM33Z
0WPM3JZ
0WPM3YZ
0WPM40Z
0WPM41Z
0WPM43Z
0WPM4JZ
0WPM4YZ
0WPMX0Z
0WPMX1Z
0WPMX3Z
0WPMXYZ
0WPNX0Z
0WPNX1Z
0WPNX3Z
0WPNX7Z
0WPNXJZ
0WPNXKZ
0WPNXYZ
0WPP31Z
0WPP33Z
0WPP3YZ
0WPP41Z
0WPP43Z
0WPP4YZ
0WPP71Z
0WPP73Z
0WPP7YZ
0WPP81Z
0WPP83Z
0WPP8YZ
0WPPX1Z
0WPPX3Z
0WPPXYZ
0WPQ01Z
0WPQ03Z
0WPQ0YZ
0WPQ73Z
0WPQ83Z
0WPQ8YZ
0WPQX1Z
0WPQX3Z
0WPQXYZ
0WPR01Z
0WPR03Z
0WPR0YZ
0WPR31Z
0WPR33Z
0WPR3YZ
0WPR41Z
0WPR43Z
0WPR4YZ
0WPR71Z
0WPR73Z
0WPR7YZ
0WPR81Z
0WPR83Z
0WPR8YZ
0WPRX1Z
0WPRX3Z
0WPRXYZ
0WQNXZZ
0WW0X0Z
0WW0X1Z
0WW0X3Z
0WW0X7Z
0WW0XJZ
0WW0XKZ
0WW0XYZ
0WW1X0Z
0WW1X1Z
0WW1X3Z
0WW1XJZ
0WW1XYZ
0WW2X0Z
0WW2X1Z
0WW2X3Z
0WW2X7Z
0WW2XJZ
0WW2XKZ
0WW2XYZ
0WW4X0Z
0WW4X1Z
0WW4X3Z
0WW4X7Z
0WW4XJZ
0WW4XKZ
0WW4XYZ
0WW5X0Z
0WW5X1Z
0WW5X3Z
0WW5X7Z
0WW5XJZ
0WW5XKZ
0WW5XYZ
0WW6X0Z
0WW6X1Z
0WW6X3Z
0WW6X7Z
0WW6XJZ
0WW6XKZ
0WW6XYZ
0WW800Z
0WW801Z
0WW803Z
0WW807Z
0WW80JZ
0WW80KZ
0WW80YZ
0WW830Z
0WW831Z
0WW833Z
0WW837Z
0WW83JZ
0WW83KZ
0WW83YZ
0WW840Z
0WW841Z
0WW843Z
0WW847Z
0WW84JZ
0WW84KZ
0WW84YZ
0WW8X0Z
0WW8X1Z
0WW8X3Z
0WW8X7Z
0WW8XJZ
0WW8XKZ
0WW8XYZ
0WW900Z
0WW901Z
0WW903Z
0WW90JZ
0WW90YZ
0WW930Z
0WW931Z
0WW933Z
0WW93JZ
0WW93YZ
0WW940Z
0WW941Z
0WW943Z
0WW94JZ
0WW94YZ
0WW9X0Z
0WW9X1Z
0WW9X3Z
0WW9XJZ
0WW9XYZ
0WWB00Z
0WWB01Z
0WWB03Z
0WWB0JZ
0WWB0YZ
0WWB30Z
0WWB31Z
0WWB33Z
0WWB3JZ
0WWB3YZ
0WWB40Z
0WWB41Z
0WWB43Z
0WWB4JZ
0WWB4YZ
0WWBX0Z
0WWBX1Z
0WWBX3Z
0WWBXJZ
0WWBXYZ
0WWCX0Z
0WWCX1Z
0WWCX3Z
0WWCX7Z
0WWCXJZ
0WWCXKZ
0WWCXYZ
0WWDX0Z
0WWDX1Z
0WWDX3Z
0WWDXYZ
0WWFX0Z
0WWFX1Z
0WWFX3Z
0WWFX7Z
0WWFXJZ
0WWFXKZ
0WWFXYZ
0WWGX0Z
0WWGX1Z
0WWGX3Z
0WWGXJZ
0WWGXYZ
0WWHX0Z
0WWHX1Z
0WWHX3Z
0WWHXYZ
0WWJX0Z
0WWJX1Z
0WWJX3Z
0WWJXJZ
0WWJXYZ
0WWKX0Z
0WWKX1Z
0WWKX3Z
0WWKX7Z
0WWKXJZ
0WWKXKZ
0WWKXYZ
0WWLX0Z
0WWLX1Z
0WWLX3Z
0WWLX7Z
0WWLXJZ
0WWLXKZ
0WWLXYZ
0WWMX0Z
0WWMX1Z
0WWMX3Z
0WWMX7Z
0WWMXJZ
0WWMXKZ
0WWMXYZ
0WWNX0Z
0WWNX1Z
0WWNX3Z
0WWNX7Z
0WWNXJZ
0WWNXKZ
0WWNXYZ
0WWP31Z
0WWP33Z
0WWP3YZ
0WWP41Z
0WWP43Z
0WWP4YZ
0WWP71Z
0WWP73Z
0WWP7YZ
0WWP81Z
0WWP83Z
0WWP8YZ
0WWPX1Z
0WWPX3Z
0WWPXYZ
0WWQ01Z
0WWQ03Z
0WWQ0YZ
0WWQX1Z
0WWQX3Z
0WWQXYZ
0WWR01Z
0WWR03Z
0WWR0YZ
0WWR31Z
0WWR33Z
0WWR3YZ
0WWR41Z
0WWR43Z
0WWR4YZ
0WWR71Z
0WWR73Z
0WWR7YZ
0WWR81Z
0WWR83Z
0WWR8YZ
0WWRX1Z
0WWRX3Z
0WWRXYZ
0X26X0Z
0X26XYZ
0X27X0Z
0X27XYZ
0X9200Z
0X920ZX
0X920ZZ
0X9230Z
0X923ZX
0X923ZZ
0X9240Z
0X924ZX
0X924ZZ
0X9300Z
0X930ZX
0X930ZZ
0X9330Z
0X933ZX
0X933ZZ
0X9340Z
0X934ZX
0X934ZZ

APPENDIX H: NON-OR PROCEDURE NOT AFFECTING MS-DRG ASSIGNMENT

0X9400Z
0X940ZX
0X940ZZ
0X9430Z
0X943ZX
0X943ZZ
0X9440Z
0X944ZX
0X944ZZ
0X9500Z
0X950ZX
0X950ZZ
0X9530Z
0X953ZX
0X953ZZ
0X9540Z
0X954ZX
0X954ZZ
0X9600Z
0X960ZX
0X960ZZ
0X9630Z
0X963ZX
0X963ZZ
0X9640Z
0X964ZX
0X964ZZ
0X9700Z
0X970ZX
0X970ZZ
0X9730Z
0X973ZX
0X973ZZ
0X9740Z
0X974ZX
0X974ZZ
0X9800Z
0X980ZX
0X980ZZ
0X9830Z
0X983ZX
0X983ZZ
0X9840Z
0X984ZX
0X984ZZ
0X9900Z
0X990ZX
0X990ZZ
0X9930Z
0X993ZX
0X993ZZ
0X9940Z
0X994ZX
0X994ZZ
0X9B00Z
0X9B0ZX
0X9B0ZZ
0X9B30Z
0X9B3ZX
0X9B3ZZ
0X9B40Z
0X9B4ZX
0X9B4ZZ
0X9C00Z
0X9C0ZX
0X9C0ZZ
0X9C30Z
0X9C3ZX
0X9C3ZZ
0X9C40Z
0X9C4ZX
0X9C4ZZ
0X9D00Z
0X9D0ZX
0X9D0ZZ
0X9D30Z
0X9D3ZX
0X9D3ZZ
0X9D40Z
0X9D4ZX
0X9D4ZZ
0X9F00Z
0X9F0ZX
0X9F0ZZ
0X9F30Z
0X9F3ZX
0X9F3ZZ
0X9F40Z
0X9F4ZX
0X9F4ZZ
0X9G00Z
0X9G0ZX
0X9G0ZZ
0X9G30Z
0X9G3ZX
0X9G3ZZ
0X9G40Z
0X9G4ZX
0X9G4ZZ
0X9H00Z
0X9H0ZX
0X9H0ZZ
0X9H30Z
0X9H3ZX
0X9H3ZZ
0X9H40Z
0X9H4ZX
0X9H4ZZ
0X9J00Z
0X9J0ZX
0X9J0ZZ
0X9J30Z
0X9J3ZX
0X9J3ZZ
0X9J40Z
0X9J4ZX
0X9J4ZZ
0X9K00Z
0X9K0ZX
0X9K0ZZ
0X9K30Z
0X9K3ZX
0X9K3ZZ
0X9K40Z
0X9K4ZX
0X9K4ZZ
0XB20ZX
0XB23ZX
0XB24ZX
0XB30ZX
0XB33ZX
0XB34ZX
0XB40ZX
0XB43ZX
0XB44ZX
0XB50ZX
0XB53ZX
0XB54ZX
0XB60ZX
0XB63ZX
0XB64ZX
0XB70ZX
0XB73ZX
0XB74ZX
0XB80ZX
0XB83ZX
0XB84ZX
0XB90ZX
0XB93ZX
0XB94ZX
0XBB0ZX
0XBB3ZX
0XBB4ZX
0XBC0ZX
0XBC3ZX
0XBC4ZX
0XBD0ZX
0XBD3ZX
0XBD4ZX
0XBF0ZX
0XBF3ZX
0XBF4ZX
0XBG0ZX
0XBG3ZX
0XBG4ZX
0XBH0ZX
0XBH3ZX
0XBH4ZX
0XBJ0ZX
0XBJ3ZX
0XBJ4ZX
0XBK0ZX
0XBK3ZX
0XBK4ZX
0XJ23ZZ
0XJ24ZZ
0XJ2XZZ
0XJ33ZZ
0XJ34ZZ
0XJ3XZZ
0XJ43ZZ
0XJ44ZZ
0XJ4XZZ
0XJ53ZZ
0XJ54ZZ
0XJ5XZZ
0XJ63ZZ
0XJ64ZZ
0XJ6XZZ
0XJ73ZZ
0XJ74ZZ
0XJ7XZZ
0XJ83ZZ
0XJ84ZZ
0XJ8XZZ
0XJ93ZZ
0XJ94ZZ
0XJ9XZZ
0XJB3ZZ
0XJB4ZZ
0XJBXZZ
0XJC3ZZ
0XJC4ZZ
0XJCXZZ
0XJD3ZZ
0XJD4ZZ
0XJDXZZ
0XJF3ZZ
0XJF4ZZ
0XJFXZZ
0XJG3ZZ
0XJG4ZZ
0XJGXZZ
0XJH3ZZ
0XJH4ZZ
0XJHXZZ
0XJJ3ZZ
0XJJXZZ
0XJK3ZZ
0XJKXZZ
0XP600Z
0XP601Z
0XP603Z
0XP607Z
0XP60JZ
0XP60KZ
0XP60YZ
0XP630Z
0XP631Z
0XP633Z
0XP637Z
0XP63JZ
0XP63KZ
0XP63YZ
0XP640Z
0XP641Z
0XP643Z
0XP647Z
0XP64JZ
0XP64KZ
0XP64YZ
0XP6X0Z
0XP6X1Z
0XP6X3Z
0XP6X7Z
0XP6XJZ
0XP6XKZ
0XP6XYZ
0XP700Z
0XP701Z
0XP703Z
0XP707Z
0XP70JZ
0XP70KZ
0XP70YZ
0XP730Z
0XP731Z
0XP733Z
0XP737Z
0XP73JZ
0XP73KZ
0XP73YZ
0XP740Z
0XP741Z
0XP743Z
0XP747Z
0XP74JZ
0XP74KZ
0XP74YZ
0XP7X0Z
0XP7X1Z
0XP7X3Z
0XP7X7Z
0XP7XJZ
0XP7XKZ
0XP7XYZ
0XW6X0Z
0XW6X3Z
0XW6X7Z
0XW6XJZ
0XW6XKZ
0XW6XYZ
0XW7X0Z
0XW7X3Z
0XW7X7Z
0XW7XJZ
0XW7XKZ
0XW7XYZ
0Y29X0Z
0Y29XYZ
0Y2BX0Z
0Y2BXYZ
0Y9000Z
0Y900ZX
0Y900ZZ
0Y9030Z
0Y903ZX
0Y903ZZ
0Y9040Z
0Y904ZX
0Y904ZZ
0Y9100Z
0Y910ZX
0Y910ZZ
0Y9130Z
0Y913ZX
0Y913ZZ
0Y9140Z
0Y914ZX
0Y914ZZ
0Y9530Z
0Y953ZZ
0Y9630Z
0Y963ZZ
0Y9700Z
0Y970ZX
0Y970ZZ
0Y9730Z
0Y973ZX
0Y973ZZ
0Y9740Z
0Y974ZX
0Y974ZZ
0Y9800Z
0Y980ZX
0Y980ZZ
0Y9830Z
0Y983ZX
0Y983ZZ
0Y9840Z
0Y984ZX
0Y984ZZ
0Y9900Z
0Y990ZX
0Y990ZZ
0Y9930Z
0Y993ZX
0Y993ZZ
0Y9940Z
0Y994ZX
0Y994ZZ
0Y9B00Z
0Y9B0ZX
0Y9B0ZZ
0Y9B30Z
0Y9B3ZX
0Y9B3ZZ
0Y9B40Z
0Y9B4ZX
0Y9B4ZZ
0Y9C00Z
0Y9C0ZX
0Y9C0ZZ
0Y9C30Z
0Y9C3ZX
0Y9C3ZZ
0Y9C40Z
0Y9C4ZX
0Y9C4ZZ
0Y9D00Z
0Y9D0ZX
0Y9D0ZZ
0Y9D30Z
0Y9D3ZX
0Y9D3ZZ
0Y9D40Z
0Y9D4ZX
0Y9D4ZZ
0Y9F00Z
0Y9F0ZX
0Y9F0ZZ
0Y9F30Z
0Y9F3ZX
0Y9F3ZZ
0Y9F40Z
0Y9F4ZX
0Y9F4ZZ
0Y9G00Z
0Y9G0ZX
0Y9G0ZZ
0Y9G30Z
0Y9G3ZX
0Y9G3ZZ
0Y9G40Z
0Y9G4ZX
0Y9G4ZZ
0Y9H00Z
0Y9H0ZX
0Y9H0ZZ
0Y9H30Z
0Y9H3ZX
0Y9H3ZZ
0Y9H40Z
0Y9H4ZX
0Y9H4ZZ
0Y9J00Z
0Y9J0ZX
0Y9J0ZZ
0Y9J30Z
0Y9J3ZX
0Y9J3ZZ
0Y9J40Z
0Y9J4ZX
0Y9J4ZZ
0Y9K00Z
0Y9K0ZX
0Y9K0ZZ
0Y9K30Z
0Y9K3ZX
0Y9K3ZZ
0Y9K40Z
0Y9K4ZX
0Y9K4ZZ
0Y9L00Z
0Y9L0ZX
0Y9L0ZZ
0Y9L30Z
0Y9L3ZX
0Y9L3ZZ
0Y9L40Z
0Y9L4ZX
0Y9L4ZZ
0Y9M00Z
0Y9M0ZX
0Y9M0ZZ
0Y9M30Z
0Y9M3ZX
0Y9M3ZZ
0Y9M40Z
0Y9M4ZX
0Y9M4ZZ
0Y9N00Z
0Y9N0ZX
0Y9N0ZZ
0Y9N30Z
0Y9N3ZX
0Y9N3ZZ
0Y9N40Z
0Y9N4ZX
0Y9N4ZZ
0YB00ZX
0YB03ZX
0YB04ZX
0YB10ZX
0YB13ZX
0YB14ZX
0YB90ZX
0YB93ZX
0YB94ZX
0YBB0ZX
0YBB3ZX
0YBB4ZX
0YBC0ZX
0YBC3ZX
0YBC4ZX
0YBD0ZX
0YBD3ZX
0YBD4ZX
0YBF0ZX
0YBF3ZX
0YBF4ZX
0YBG0ZX
0YBG3ZX
0YBG4ZX
0YBH0ZX
0YBH3ZX
0YBH4ZX
0YBJ0ZX
0YBJ3ZX
0YBJ4ZX
0YBK0ZX
0YBK3ZX
0YBK4ZX
0YBL0ZX
0YBL3ZX
0YBL4ZX
0YBM0ZX
0YBM3ZX
0YBM4ZX
0YBN0ZX
0YBN3ZX
0YBN4ZX
0YJ03ZZ
0YJ04ZZ
0YJ0XZZ
0YJ13ZZ
0YJ14ZZ
0YJ1XZZ
0YJ53ZZ
0YJ5XZZ
0YJ63ZZ
0YJ6XZZ
0YJ73ZZ
0YJ7XZZ
0YJ83ZZ
0YJ8XZZ
0YJ93ZZ
0YJ94ZZ
0YJ9XZZ
0YJA3ZZ
0YJAXZZ
0YJB3ZZ
0YJB4ZZ
0YJBXZZ
0YJC3ZZ
0YJC4ZZ
0YJCXZZ
0YJD3ZZ
0YJD4ZZ
0YJDXZZ
0YJE3ZZ
0YJEXZZ
0YJF3ZZ
0YJF4ZZ
0YJFXZZ
0YJG3ZZ
0YJG4ZZ
0YJGXZZ
0YJH3ZZ
0YJH4ZZ
0YJHXZZ
0YJJ3ZZ
0YJJ4ZZ
0YJJXZZ
0YJK3ZZ
0YJK4ZZ
0YJKXZZ
0YJL3ZZ
0YJL4ZZ
0YJLXZZ
0YJM3ZZ
0YJM4ZZ
0YJMXZZ
0YJN3ZZ
0YJN4ZZ
0YJNXZZ
0YP900Z
0YP901Z
0YP903Z
0YP907Z

0YP90JZ	0YW9X7Z	10J1XZZ	10Q03ZF	10Q07YT	10Y03ZM	2W02X0Z	2W08X6Z	2W0FX3Z
0YP90KZ	0YW9XJZ	10J20ZZ	10Q03ZG	10Q07YV	10Y03ZN	2W02X1Z	2W08X7Z	2W0FX4Z
0YP90YZ	0YW9XKZ	10J23ZZ	10Q03ZH	10Q07YY	10Y03ZP	2W02X2Z	2W08XYZ	2W0FX5Z
0YP930Z	0YW9XYZ	10J24ZZ	10Q03ZJ	10Q07ZE	10Y03ZQ	2W02X3Z	2W09X0Z	2W0FX6Z
0YP931Z	0YWBX0Z	10J27ZZ	10Q03ZK	10Q07ZF	10Y03ZR	2W02X4Z	2W09X1Z	2W0FX7Z
0YP933Z	0YWBX3Z	10J28ZZ	10Q03ZL	10Q07ZG	10Y03ZS	2W02X5Z	2W09X2Z	2W0FXYZ
0YP937Z	0YWBX7Z	10J2XZZ	10Q03ZM	10Q07ZH	10Y03ZT	2W02X6Z	2W09X3Z	2W0GX0Z
0YP93JZ	0YWBXJZ	10P003Z	10Q03ZN	10Q07ZJ	10Y03ZV	2W02X7Z	2W09X4Z	2W0GX1Z
0YP93KZ	0YWBXKZ	10P00YZ	10Q03ZP	10Q07ZK	10Y03ZY	2W02XYZ	2W09X5Z	2W0GX2Z
0YP93YZ	0YWBXYZ	10P073Z	10Q03ZQ	10Q07ZL	10Y04ZE	2W03X0Z	2W09X6Z	2W0GX3Z
0YP940Z	102073Z	10P07YZ	10Q03ZR	10Q07ZM	10Y04ZF	2W03X1Z	2W09X7Z	2W0GX4Z
0YP941Z	10207YZ	10Q00YE	10Q03ZS	10Q07ZN	10Y04ZG	2W03X2Z	2W09XYZ	2W0GX5Z
0YP943Z	10900Z9	10Q00YF	10Q03ZT	10Q07ZP	10Y04ZH	2W03X3Z	2W0AX0Z	2W0GX6Z
0YP947Z	10900ZA	10Q00YG	10Q03ZV	10Q07ZQ	10Y04ZJ	2W03X4Z	2W0AX1Z	2W0GX7Z
0YP94JZ	10900ZB	10Q00YH	10Q03ZY	10Q07ZR	10Y04ZK	2W03X5Z	2W0AX2Z	2W0GXYZ
0YP94KZ	10900ZC	10Q00YJ	10Q04YE	10Q07ZS	10Y04ZL	2W03X6Z	2W0AX3Z	2W0HX0Z
0YP94YZ	10900ZD	10Q00YK	10Q04YF	10Q07ZT	10Y04ZM	2W03X7Z	2W0AX4Z	2W0HX1Z
0YP9X0Z	10900ZU	10Q00YL	10Q04YG	10Q07ZV	10Y04ZN	2W03XYZ	2W0AX5Z	2W0HX2Z
0YP9X1Z	10903Z9	10Q00YM	10Q04YH	10Q07ZY	10Y04ZP	2W04X0Z	2W0AX6Z	2W0HX3Z
0YP9X3Z	10903ZA	10Q00YN	10Q04YJ	10Q08YE	10Y04ZQ	2W04X1Z	2W0AX7Z	2W0HX4Z
0YP9X7Z	10903ZB	10Q00YP	10Q04YK	10Q08YF	10Y04ZR	2W04X2Z	2W0AXYZ	2W0HX5Z
0YP9XJZ	10903ZC	10Q00YQ	10Q04YL	10Q08YG	10Y04ZS	2W04X3Z	2W0BX0Z	2W0HX6Z
0YP9XKZ	10903ZD	10Q00YR	10Q04YM	10Q08YH	10Y04ZT	2W04X4Z	2W0BX1Z	2W0HX7Z
0YP9XYZ	10903ZU	10Q00YS	10Q04YN	10Q08YJ	10Y04ZV	2W04X5Z	2W0BX2Z	2W0HXYZ
0YPB00Z	10904Z9	10Q00YT	10Q04YP	10Q08YK	10Y04ZY	2W04X6Z	2W0BX3Z	2W0JX0Z
0YPB01Z	10904ZA	10Q00YV	10Q04YQ	10Q08YL	10Y07ZE	2W04X7Z	2W0BX4Z	2W0JX1Z
0YPB03Z	10904ZB	10Q00YY	10Q04YR	10Q08YM	10Y07ZF	2W04XYZ	2W0BX5Z	2W0JX2Z
0YPB07Z	10904ZC	10Q00ZE	10Q04YS	10Q08YN	10Y07ZG	2W05X0Z	2W0BX6Z	2W0JX3Z
0YPB0JZ	10904ZD	10Q00ZF	10Q04YT	10Q08YP	10Y07ZH	2W05X1Z	2W0BX7Z	2W0JX4Z
0YPB0KZ	10904ZU	10Q00ZG	10Q04YV	10Q08YQ	10Y07ZJ	2W05X2Z	2W0BXYZ	2W0JX5Z
0YPB0YZ	10907Z9	10Q00ZH	10Q04YY	10Q08YR	10Y07ZK	2W05X3Z	2W0CX0Z	2W0JX6Z
0YPB30Z	10907ZA	10Q00ZJ	10Q04ZE	10Q08YS	10Y07ZL	2W05X4Z	2W0CX1Z	2W0JX7Z
0YPB31Z	10907ZB	10Q00ZK	10Q04ZF	10Q08YT	10Y07ZM	2W05X5Z	2W0CX2Z	2W0JXYZ
0YPB33Z	10907ZC	10Q00ZL	10Q04ZG	10Q08YV	10Y07ZN	2W05X6Z	2W0CX3Z	2W0KX0Z
0YPB37Z	10907ZD	10Q00ZM	10Q04ZH	10Q08YY	10Y07ZP	2W05X7Z	2W0CX4Z	2W0KX1Z
0YPB3JZ	10907ZU	10Q00ZN	10Q04ZJ	10Q08ZE	10Y07ZQ	2W05XYZ	2W0CX5Z	2W0KX2Z
0YPB3KZ	10908Z9	10Q00ZP	10Q04ZK	10Q08ZF	10Y07ZR	2W06X0Z	2W0CX6Z	2W0KX3Z
0YPB3YZ	10908ZA	10Q00ZQ	10Q04ZL	10Q08ZG	10Y07ZS	2W06X1Z	2W0CX7Z	2W0KX4Z
0YPB40Z	10908ZB	10Q00ZR	10Q04ZM	10Q08ZH	10Y07ZT	2W06X2Z	2W0CXYZ	2W0KX5Z
0YPB41Z	10908ZC	10Q00ZS	10Q04ZN	10Q08ZJ	10Y07ZV	2W06X3Z	2W0DX0Z	2W0KX6Z
0YPB43Z	10908ZD	10Q00ZT	10Q04ZP	10Q08ZK	10Y07ZY	2W06X4Z	2W0DX1Z	2W0KX7Z
0YPB47Z	10908ZU	10Q00ZV	10Q04ZQ	10Q08ZL	2W00X0Z	2W06X5Z	2W0DX2Z	2W0KXYZ
0YPB4JZ	10A07Z6	10Q00ZY	10Q04ZR	10Q08ZM	2W00X1Z	2W06X6Z	2W0DX3Z	2W0LX0Z
0YPB4KZ	10A07ZW	10Q03YE	10Q04ZS	10Q08ZN	2W00X2Z	2W06X7Z	2W0DX4Z	2W0LX1Z
0YPB4YZ	10A07ZX	10Q03YF	10Q04ZT	10Q08ZP	2W00X3Z	2W06XYZ	2W0DX5Z	2W0LX2Z
0YPBX0Z	10H003Z	10Q03YG	10Q04ZV	10Q08ZQ	2W00X4Z	2W07X0Z	2W0DX6Z	2W0LX3Z
0YPBX1Z	10H00YZ	10Q03YH	10Q04ZY	10Q08ZR	2W00X5Z	2W07X1Z	2W0DX7Z	2W0LX4Z
0YPBX3Z	10H073Z	10Q03YJ	10Q07YE	10Q08ZS	2W00X6Z	2W07X2Z	2W0DXYZ	2W0LX5Z
0YPBX7Z	10H07YZ	10Q03YK	10Q07YF	10Q08ZT	2W00X7Z	2W07X3Z	2W0EX0Z	2W0LX6Z
0YPBXJZ	10J00ZZ	10Q03YL	10Q07YG	10Q08ZV	2W00XYZ	2W07X4Z	2W0EX1Z	2W0LX7Z
0YPBXKZ	10J03ZZ	10Q03YM	10Q07YH	10Q08ZY	2W01X0Z	2W07X5Z	2W0EX2Z	2W0LXYZ
0YPBXYZ	10J04ZZ	10Q03YN	10Q07YJ	10S07ZZ	2W01X1Z	2W07X6Z	2W0EX3Z	2W0MX0Z
0YQ5XZZ	10J07ZZ	10Q03YP	10Q07YK	10S0XZZ	2W01X2Z	2W07X7Z	2W0EX4Z	2W0MX1Z
0YQ6XZZ	10J08ZZ	10Q03YQ	10Q07YL	10Y03ZE	2W01X3Z	2W07XYZ	2W0EX5Z	2W0MX2Z
0YQ7XZZ	10J0XZZ	10Q03YR	10Q07YM	10Y03ZF	2W01X4Z	2W08X0Z	2W0EX6Z	2W0MX3Z
0YQ8XZZ	10J10ZZ	10Q03YS	10Q07YN	10Y03ZG	2W01X5Z	2W08X1Z	2W0EX7Z	2W0MX4Z
0YQAXZZ	10J13ZZ	10Q03YT	10Q07YP	10Y03ZH	2W01X6Z	2W08X2Z	2W0EXYZ	2W0MX5Z
0YQEXZZ	10J14ZZ	10Q03YV	10Q07YQ	10Y03ZJ	2W01X7Z	2W08X3Z	2W0FX0Z	2W0MX6Z
0YW9X0Z	10J17ZZ	10Q03YY	10Q07YR	10Y03ZK	2W01X9Z	2W08X4Z	2W0FX1Z	2W0MX7Z
0YW9X3Z	10J18ZZ	10Q03ZE	10Q07YS	10Y03ZL	2W01XYZ	2W08X5Z	2W0FX2Z	2W0MXYZ

0YP90JZ-2W0MXYZ
APPENDIX H: NON-OR PROCEDURE NOT AFFECTING MS-DRG ASSIGNMENT

2W0NX0Z
2W0NX1Z
2W0NX2Z
2W0NX3Z
2W0NX4Z
2W0NX5Z
2W0NX6Z
2W0NX7Z
2W0NXYZ
2W0PX0Z
2W0PX1Z
2W0PX2Z
2W0PX3Z
2W0PX4Z
2W0PX5Z
2W0PX6Z
2W0PX7Z
2W0PXYZ
2W0QX0Z
2W0QX1Z
2W0QX2Z
2W0QX3Z
2W0QX4Z
2W0QX5Z
2W0QX6Z
2W0QX7Z
2W0QXYZ
2W0RX0Z
2W0RX1Z
2W0RX2Z
2W0RX3Z
2W0RX4Z
2W0RX5Z
2W0RX6Z
2W0RX7Z
2W0RXYZ
2W0SX0Z
2W0SX1Z
2W0SX2Z
2W0SX3Z
2W0SX4Z
2W0SX5Z
2W0SX6Z
2W0SX7Z
2W0SXYZ
2W0TX0Z
2W0TX1Z
2W0TX2Z
2W0TX3Z
2W0TX4Z
2W0TX5Z
2W0TX6Z
2W0TX7Z
2W0TXYZ
2W0UX0Z
2W0UX1Z
2W0UX2Z
2W0UX3Z
2W0UX4Z
2W0UX5Z
2W0UX6Z
2W0UX7Z
2W0UXYZ
2W0VX0Z
2W0VX1Z
2W0VX2Z
2W0VX3Z
2W0VX4Z
2W0VX5Z
2W0VX6Z
2W0VX7Z
2W0VXYZ
2W10X6Z
2W10X7Z
2W11X6Z
2W11X7Z
2W12X6Z
2W12X7Z
2W13X6Z
2W13X7Z
2W14X6Z
2W14X7Z
2W15X6Z
2W15X7Z
2W16X6Z
2W16X7Z
2W17X6Z
2W17X7Z
2W18X6Z
2W18X7Z
2W19X6Z
2W19X7Z
2W1AX6Z
2W1AX7Z
2W1BX6Z
2W1BX7Z
2W1CX6Z
2W1CX7Z
2W1DX6Z
2W1DX7Z
2W1EX6Z
2W1EX7Z
2W1FX6Z
2W1FX7Z
2W1GX6Z
2W1GX7Z
2W1HX6Z
2W1HX7Z
2W1JX6Z
2W1JX7Z
2W1KX6Z
2W1KX7Z
2W1LX6Z
2W1LX7Z
2W1MX6Z
2W1MX7Z
2W1NX6Z
2W1NX7Z
2W1PX6Z
2W1PX7Z
2W1QX6Z
2W1QX7Z
2W1RX6Z
2W1RX7Z
2W1SX6Z
2W1SX7Z
2W1TX6Z
2W1TX7Z
2W1UX6Z
2W1UX7Z
2W1VX6Z
2W1VX7Z
2W20X4Z
2W21X4Z
2W22X4Z
2W23X4Z
2W24X4Z
2W25X4Z
2W26X4Z
2W27X4Z
2W28X4Z
2W29X4Z
2W2AX4Z
2W2BX4Z
2W2CX4Z
2W2DX4Z
2W2EX4Z
2W2FX4Z
2W2GX4Z
2W2HX4Z
2W2JX4Z
2W2KX4Z
2W2LX4Z
2W2MX4Z
2W2NX4Z
2W2PX4Z
2W2QX4Z
2W2RX4Z
2W2SX4Z
2W2TX4Z
2W2UX4Z
2W2VX4Z
2W30X1Z
2W30X2Z
2W30X3Z
2W30XYZ
2W31X1Z
2W31X2Z
2W31X3Z
2W31X9Z
2W31XYZ
2W32X1Z
2W32X2Z
2W32X3Z
2W32XYZ
2W33X1Z
2W33X2Z
2W33X3Z
2W33XYZ
2W34X1Z
2W34X2Z
2W34X3Z
2W34XYZ
2W35X1Z
2W35X2Z
2W35X3Z
2W35XYZ
2W36X1Z
2W36X2Z
2W36X3Z
2W36XYZ
2W37X1Z
2W37X2Z
2W37X3Z
2W37XYZ
2W38X1Z
2W38X2Z
2W38X3Z
2W38XYZ
2W39X1Z
2W39X2Z
2W39X3Z
2W39XYZ
2W3AX1Z
2W3AX2Z
2W3AX3Z
2W3AXYZ
2W3BX1Z
2W3BX2Z
2W3BX3Z
2W3BXYZ
2W3CX1Z
2W3CX2Z
2W3CX3Z
2W3CXYZ
2W3DX1Z
2W3DX2Z
2W3DX3Z
2W3DXYZ
2W3EX1Z
2W3EX2Z
2W3EX3Z
2W3EXYZ
2W3FX1Z
2W3FX2Z
2W3FX3Z
2W3FXYZ
2W3GX1Z
2W3GX2Z
2W3GX3Z
2W3GXYZ
2W3HX1Z
2W3HX2Z
2W3HX3Z
2W3HXYZ
2W3JX1Z
2W3JX2Z
2W3JX3Z
2W3JXYZ
2W3KX1Z
2W3KX2Z
2W3KX3Z
2W3KXYZ
2W3LX1Z
2W3LX2Z
2W3LX3Z
2W3LXYZ
2W3MX1Z
2W3MX2Z
2W3MX3Z
2W3MXYZ
2W3NX1Z
2W3NX2Z
2W3NX3Z
2W3NXYZ
2W3PX1Z
2W3PX2Z
2W3PX3Z
2W3PXYZ
2W3QX1Z
2W3QX2Z
2W3QX3Z
2W3QXYZ
2W3RX1Z
2W3RX2Z
2W3RX3Z
2W3RXYZ
2W3SX1Z
2W3SX2Z
2W3SX3Z
2W3SXYZ
2W3TX1Z
2W3TX2Z
2W3TX3Z
2W3TXYZ
2W3UX1Z
2W3UX2Z
2W3UX3Z
2W3UXYZ
2W3VX1Z
2W3VX2Z
2W3VX3Z
2W3VXYZ
2W40X5Z
2W41X5Z
2W42X5Z
2W43X5Z
2W44X5Z
2W45X5Z
2W46X5Z
2W47X5Z
2W48X5Z
2W49X5Z
2W4AX5Z
2W4BX5Z
2W4CX5Z
2W4DX5Z
2W4EX5Z
2W4FX5Z
2W4GX5Z
2W4HX5Z
2W4JX5Z
2W4KX5Z
2W4LX5Z
2W4MX5Z
2W4NX5Z
2W4PX5Z
2W4QX5Z
2W4RX5Z
2W4SX5Z
2W4TX5Z
2W4UX5Z
2W4VX5Z
2W50X0Z
2W50X1Z
2W50X2Z
2W50X3Z
2W50X4Z
2W50X5Z
2W50X6Z
2W50X7Z
2W50XYZ
2W51X0Z
2W51X1Z
2W51X2Z
2W51X3Z
2W51X4Z
2W51X5Z
2W51X6Z
2W51X7Z
2W51X9Z
2W51XYZ
2W52X0Z
2W52X1Z
2W52X2Z
2W52X3Z
2W52X4Z
2W52X5Z
2W52X6Z
2W52X7Z
2W52XYZ
2W53X0Z
2W53X1Z
2W53X2Z
2W53X3Z
2W53X4Z
2W53X5Z
2W53X6Z
2W53X7Z
2W53XYZ
2W54X0Z
2W54X1Z
2W54X2Z
2W54X3Z
2W54X4Z
2W54X5Z
2W54X6Z
2W54X7Z
2W54XYZ
2W55X0Z
2W55X1Z
2W55X2Z
2W55X3Z
2W55X4Z
2W55X5Z
2W55X6Z
2W55X7Z
2W55XYZ
2W56X0Z
2W56X1Z
2W56X2Z
2W56X3Z
2W56X4Z
2W56X5Z
2W56X6Z
2W56X7Z
2W56XYZ
2W57X0Z
2W57X1Z
2W57X2Z
2W57X3Z
2W57X4Z
2W57X5Z
2W57X6Z
2W57X7Z
2W57XYZ
2W58X0Z
2W58X1Z
2W58X2Z
2W58X3Z
2W58X4Z
2W58X5Z
2W58X6Z
2W58X7Z
2W58XYZ
2W59X0Z
2W59X1Z
2W59X2Z
2W59X3Z
2W59X4Z
2W59X5Z
2W59X6Z
2W59X7Z
2W59XYZ
2W5AX0Z
2W5AX1Z
2W5AX2Z
2W5AX3Z
2W5AX4Z
2W5AX5Z
2W5AX6Z
2W5AX7Z
2W5AXYZ
2W5BX0Z
2W5BX1Z
2W5BX2Z
2W5BX3Z
2W5BX4Z
2W5BX5Z
2W5BX6Z
2W5BX7Z
2W5BXYZ
2W5CX0Z
2W5CX1Z
2W5CX2Z
2W5CX3Z
2W5CX4Z
2W5CX5Z
2W5CX6Z
2W5CX7Z
2W5CXYZ
2W5DX0Z
2W5DX1Z
2W5DX2Z
2W5DX3Z
2W5DX4Z
2W5DX5Z
2W5DX6Z
2W5DX7Z
2W5DXYZ
2W5EX0Z
2W5EX1Z
2W5EX2Z
2W5EX3Z
2W5EX4Z
2W5EX5Z
2W5EX6Z
2W5EX7Z
2W5EXYZ
2W5FX0Z
2W5FX1Z
2W5FX2Z
2W5FX3Z
2W5FX4Z
2W5FX5Z
2W5FX6Z
2W5FX7Z
2W5FXYZ
2W5GX0Z
2W5GX1Z
2W5GX2Z
2W5GX3Z
2W5GX4Z
2W5GX5Z
2W5GX6Z
2W5GX7Z
2W5GXYZ
2W5HX0Z
2W5HX1Z
2W5HX2Z
2W5HX3Z
2W5HX4Z
2W5HX5Z
2W5HX6Z
2W5HX7Z
2W5HXYZ
2W5JX0Z
2W5JX1Z
2W5JX2Z
2W5JX3Z
2W5JX4Z
2W5JX5Z
2W5JX6Z
2W5JX7Z
2W5JXYZ
2W5KX0Z
2W5KX1Z
2W5KX2Z
2W5KX3Z
2W5KX4Z
2W5KX5Z
2W5KX6Z
2W5KX7Z
2W5KXYZ
2W5LX0Z
2W5LX1Z
2W5LX2Z
2W5LX3Z
2W5LX4Z
2W5LX5Z
2W5LX6Z
2W5LX7Z
2W5LXYZ
2W5MX0Z
2W5MX1Z
2W5MX2Z
2W5MX3Z
2W5MX4Z
2W5MX5Z
2W5MX6Z
2W5MX7Z
2W5MXYZ
2W5NX0Z
2W5NX1Z
2W5NX2Z
2W5NX3Z
2W5NX4Z
2W5NX5Z
2W5NX6Z
2W5NX7Z
2W5NXYZ
2W5PX0Z
2W5PX1Z
2W5PX2Z
2W5PX3Z
2W5PX4Z
2W5PX5Z
2W5PX6Z
2W5PX7Z
2W5PXYZ
2W5QX0Z
2W5QX1Z
2W5QX2Z
2W5QX3Z
2W5QX4Z
2W5QX5Z
2W5QX6Z
2W5QX7Z
2W5QXYZ
2W5RX0Z

2W5RX1Z
2W5RX2Z
2W5RX3Z
2W5RX4Z
2W5RX5Z
2W5RX6Z
2W5RX7Z
2W5RXYZ
2W5SX0Z
2W5SX1Z
2W5SX2Z
2W5SX3Z
2W5SX4Z
2W5SX5Z
2W5SX6Z
2W5SX7Z
2W5SXYZ
2W5TX0Z
2W5TX1Z
2W5TX2Z
2W5TX3Z
2W5TX4Z
2W5TX5Z
2W5TX6Z
2W5TX7Z
2W5TXYZ
2W5UX0Z
2W5UX1Z
2W5UX2Z
2W5UX3Z
2W5UX4Z
2W5UX5Z
2W5UX6Z
2W5UX7Z
2W5UXYZ
2W5VX0Z
2W5VX1Z
2W5VX2Z
2W5VX3Z
2W5VX4Z
2W5VX5Z
2W5VX6Z
2W5VX7Z
2W5VXYZ
2W60X0Z
2W60XZZ
2W61X0Z
2W61XZZ
2W62X0Z
2W62XZZ
2W63X0Z
2W63XZZ
2W64X0Z
2W64XZZ
2W65X0Z
2W65XZZ
2W66X0Z
2W66XZZ
2W67X0Z
2W67XZZ
2W68X0Z
2W68XZZ
2W69X0Z
2W69XZZ
2W6AX0Z
2W6AXZZ
2W6BX0Z
2W6BXZZ
2W6CX0Z
2W6CXZZ
2W6DX0Z
2W6DXZZ
2W6EX0Z
2W6EXZZ
2W6FX0Z
2W6FXZZ
2W6GX0Z
2W6GXZZ
2W6HX0Z
2W6HXZZ
2W6JX0Z
2W6JXZZ
2W6KX0Z
2W6KXZZ
2W6LX0Z
2W6LXZZ
2W6MX0Z
2W6MXZZ
2W6NX0Z
2W6NXZZ
2W6PX0Z
2W6PXZZ
2W6QX0Z
2W6QXZZ
2W6RX0Z
2W6RXZZ
2W6SX0Z
2W6SXZZ
2W6TX0Z
2W6TXZZ
2W6UX0Z
2W6UXZZ
2W6VX0Z
2W6VXZZ
2Y00X5Z
2Y01X5Z
2Y02X5Z
2Y03X5Z
2Y04X5Z
2Y05X5Z
2Y40X5Z
2Y41X5Z
2Y42X5Z
2Y43X5Z
2Y44X5Z
2Y45X5Z
2Y50X5Z
2Y51X5Z
2Y52X5Z
2Y53X5Z
2Y54X5Z
2Y55X5Z
30230AZ
30230G0
30230G2
30230G3
30230G4
30230H0
30230H1
30230J0
30230J1
30230K0
30230K1
30230L0
30230L1
30230M0
30230M1
30230N0
30230N1
30230P0
30230P1
30230Q0
30230Q1
30230R0
30230R1
30230S0
30230S1
30230T0
30230T1
30230U2
30230U3
30230U4
30230V0
30230V1
30230W0
30230W1
30230X0
30230X2
30230X3
30230X4
30230Y0
30230Y2
30230Y3
30230Y4
30233G2
30233G3
30233G4
30233H0
30233H1
30233J0
30233J1
30233K0
30233K1
30233L0
30233L1
30233M0
30233M1
30233N0
30233N1
30233P0
30233P1
30233Q0
30233Q1
30233R0
30233R1
30233S0
30233S1
30233T0
30233T1
30233U2
30233U3
30233U4
30233V0
30233V1
30233W0
30233W1
30233X2
30233X3
30233X4
30233Y2
30233Y3
30233Y4
30240AZ
30240G0
30240G2
30240G3
30240G4
30240H0
30240H1
30240J0
30240J1
30240K0
30240K1
30240L0
30240L1
30240M0
30240M1
30240N0
30240N1
30240P0
30240P1
30240Q0
30240Q1
30240R0
30240R1
30240S0
30240S1
30240T0
30240T1
30240U2
30240U3
30240U4
30240V0
30240V1
30240W0
30240W1
30240X0
30240X2
30240X3
30240X4
30240Y0
30240Y2
30240Y3
30240Y4
30243G2
30243G3
30243G4
30243H0
30243H1
30243J0
30243J1
30243K0
30243K1
30243L0
30243L1
30243M0
30243M1
30243N0
30243N1
30243P0
30243P1
30243Q0
30243Q1
30243R0
30243R1
30243S0
30243S1
30243T0
30243T1
30243U2
30243U3
30243U4
30243V0
30243V1
30243W0
30243W1
30243X2
30243X3
30243X4
30243Y2
30243Y3
30243Y4
30273H1
30273J1
30273K1
30273L1
30273M1
30273N1
30273P1
30273Q1
30273R1
30273S1
30273T1
30273V1
30273W1
30277H1
30277J1
30277K1
30277L1
30277M1
30277N1
30277P1
30277Q1
30277R1
30277S1
30277T1
30277V1
30277W1
30280B1
30283B1
3C1ZX8Z
3E00X05
3E00X0M
3E00X28
3E00X29
3E00X3Z
3E00X4Z
3E00XBZ
3E00XGC
3E00XKZ
3E00XMZ
3E00XNZ
3E00XTZ
3E0102A
3E01305
3E0130M
3E01328
3E01329
3E0132A
3E0133Z
3E01340
3E0134Z
3E0136Z
3E0137Z
3E013BZ
3E013GC
3E013HZ
3E013KZ
3E013NZ
3E013TZ
3E013VG
3E013VJ
3E02305
3E0230M
3E02328
3E02329
3E0233Z
3E02340
3E0234Z
3E0236Z
3E0237Z
3E023BZ
3E023GC
3E023HZ
3E023KZ
3E023NZ
3E023TZ
3E03003
3E03005
3E0300M
3E0300P
3E03016
3E03028
3E03029
3E0303Z
3E0304Z
3E0306Z
3E0307Z
3E030FZ
3E030GC
3E030GN
3E030HZ
3E030KZ
3E030NZ
3E030PZ
3E030RZ
3E030TZ
3E030VG
3E030VH
3E030VJ
3E030WK
3E030WL
3E030XZ
3E03303
3E03305
3E0330M
3E0330P
3E03316
3E03328
3E03329
3E0333Z
3E0334Z
3E0336Z
3E0337Z
3E033FZ
3E033GC
3E033GN
3E033GQ
3E033HZ
3E033KZ
3E033NZ
3E033PZ
3E033RZ
3E033TZ
3E033VG
3E033VH
3E033VJ
3E033WK
3E033WL
3E033XZ
3E04003
3E04005
3E0400M
3E0400P
3E04016
3E04028
3E04029
3E0403Z
3E0404Z
3E0406Z
3E0407Z
3E040FZ
3E040GC
3E040GN
3E040HZ
3E040KZ
3E040NZ
3E040PZ
3E040RZ
3E040TZ
3E040VG
3E040VH
3E040VJ
3E040WK
3E040WL
3E040XZ
3E04303
3E04305
3E0430M
3E0430P
3E04316
3E04328
3E04329
3E0433Z
3E0434Z
3E0436Z
3E0437Z
3E043FZ
3E043GC
3E043GN
3E043GQ
3E043HZ
3E043KZ
3E043NZ
3E043PZ
3E043RZ
3E043TZ
3E043VG
3E043VH
3E043VJ
3E043WK
3E043WL
3E043XZ
3E05003
3E05005
3E0500M
3E0500P
3E05016
3E05028
3E05029
3E0503Z
3E0504Z
3E0506Z
3E0507Z
3E050FZ
3E050GC
3E050GN
3E050HZ
3E050KZ
3E050NZ
3E050PZ
3E050RZ
3E050TZ
3E050VG
3E050VH
3E050VJ
3E050WK
3E050WL
3E050XZ
3E05303
3E05305
3E0530M
3E0530P
3E05316
3E05328
3E05329
3E0533Z
3E0534Z
3E0536Z
3E0537Z
3E053FZ
3E053GC
3E053GN
3E053HZ
3E053KZ
3E053NZ
3E053PZ
3E053RZ
3E053TZ
3E053VG
3E053VH
3E053VJ
3E053WK
3E053WL
3E053XZ
3E06003
3E06005
3E0600M
3E0600P
3E06016
3E06028
3E06029
3E0603Z
3E0604Z
3E0606Z
3E0607Z
3E060FZ
3E060GC
3E060GN
3E060HZ
3E060KZ
3E060NZ
3E060PZ
3E060RZ
3E060TZ
3E060VG
3E060VH
3E060VJ
3E060WK
3E060WL

3E060XZ
3E06303
3E06305
3E0630M
3E0630P
3E06316
3E06328
3E06329
3E0633Z
3E0634Z
3E0636Z
3E0637Z
3E063FZ
3E063GC
3E063GN
3E063HZ
3E063KZ
3E063NZ
3E063PZ
3E063RZ
3E063TZ
3E063VG
3E063VH
3E063VJ
3E063WK
3E063WL
3E063XZ
3E07016
3E07017
3E070GC
3E070KZ
3E070PZ
3E07316
3E07317
3E073GC
3E073KZ
3E073PZ
3E074GC
3E08016
3E080GC
3E080KZ
3E080PZ
3E08316
3E083GC
3E083KZ
3E083PZ
3E084GC
3E09305
3E0930M
3E09328
3E09329
3E0933Z
3E0934Z
3E093BZ
3E093GC
3E093HZ
3E093KZ
3E093NZ
3E093TZ
3E09705
3E0970M
3E09728
3E09729
3E0973Z
3E0974Z
3E097BZ
3E097GC
3E097HZ
3E097KZ
3E097NZ
3E097TZ
3E09X05
3E09X0M
3E09X28
3E09X29
3E09X3Z
3E09X4Z
3E09XBZ
3E09XGC
3E09XHZ
3E09XKZ
3E09XNZ
3E09XTZ
3E0A305
3E0A30M
3E0A3GC
3E0B304
3E0B305
3E0B30M
3E0B328
3E0B329
3E0B33Z
3E0B3BZ
3E0B3GC
3E0B3HZ
3E0B3KZ
3E0B3NZ
3E0B3TZ
3E0B704
3E0B705
3E0B70M
3E0B728
3E0B729
3E0B73Z
3E0B7BZ
3E0B7GC
3E0B7HZ
3E0B7KZ
3E0B7NZ
3E0B7TZ
3E0BX04
3E0BX05
3E0BX0M
3E0BX28
3E0BX29
3E0BX3Z
3E0BXBZ
3E0BXGC
3E0BXHZ
3E0BXKZ
3E0BXNZ
3E0BXTZ
3E0C304
3E0C305
3E0C30M
3E0C328
3E0C329
3E0C33Z
3E0C3BZ
3E0C3GC
3E0C3HZ
3E0C3KZ
3E0C3MZ
3E0C3NZ
3E0C3SF
3E0C3TZ
3E0C704
3E0C705
3E0C70M
3E0C728
3E0C729
3E0C73Z
3E0C7BZ
3E0C7GC
3E0C7HZ
3E0C7KZ
3E0C7MZ
3E0C7NZ
3E0C7SF
3E0C7TZ
3E0CX04
3E0CX05
3E0CX0M
3E0CX28
3E0CX29
3E0CX3Z
3E0CXBZ
3E0CXGC
3E0CXHZ
3E0CXKZ
3E0CXMZ
3E0CXNZ
3E0CXSF
3E0CXTZ
3E0D304
3E0D305
3E0D30M
3E0D328
3E0D329
3E0D33Z
3E0D34Z
3E0D36Z
3E0D37Z
3E0D3BZ
3E0D3GC
3E0D3HZ
3E0D3KZ
3E0D3NZ
3E0D3RZ
3E0D3TZ
3E0D704
3E0D705
3E0D70M
3E0D728
3E0D729
3E0D73Z
3E0D74Z
3E0D76Z
3E0D77Z
3E0D7BZ
3E0D7GC
3E0D7HZ
3E0D7KZ
3E0D7NZ
3E0D7RZ
3E0D7TZ
3E0DX04
3E0DX05
3E0DX0M
3E0DX28
3E0DX29
3E0DX3Z
3E0DX4Z
3E0DX6Z
3E0DX7Z
3E0DXBZ
3E0DXGC
3E0DXHZ
3E0DXKZ
3E0DXNZ
3E0DXRZ
3E0DXTZ
3E0E304
3E0E305
3E0E30M
3E0E328
3E0E329
3E0E33Z
3E0E36Z
3E0E37Z
3E0E3BZ
3E0E3GC
3E0E3HZ
3E0E3KZ
3E0E3NZ
3E0E3SF
3E0E3TZ
3E0E4GC
3E0E704
3E0E705
3E0E70M
3E0E728
3E0E729
3E0E73Z
3E0E76Z
3E0E77Z
3E0E7BZ
3E0E7GC
3E0E7HZ
3E0E7KZ
3E0E7NZ
3E0E7SF
3E0E7TZ
3E0E804
3E0E805
3E0E80M
3E0E828
3E0E829
3E0E83Z
3E0E86Z
3E0E87Z
3E0E8BZ
3E0E8GC
3E0E8HZ
3E0E8KZ
3E0E8NZ
3E0E8SF
3E0E8TZ
3E0F304
3E0F305
3E0F30M
3E0F328
3E0F329
3E0F33Z
3E0F36Z
3E0F37Z
3E0F3BZ
3E0F3GC
3E0F3HZ
3E0F3KZ
3E0F3NZ
3E0F3SD
3E0F3SF
3E0F3TZ
3E0F4GC
3E0F704
3E0F705
3E0F70M
3E0F728
3E0F729
3E0F73Z
3E0F76Z
3E0F77Z
3E0F7BZ
3E0F7GC
3E0F7HZ
3E0F7KZ
3E0F7NZ
3E0F7SD
3E0F7SF
3E0F7TZ
3E0F804
3E0F805
3E0F80M
3E0F828
3E0F829
3E0F83Z
3E0F86Z
3E0F87Z
3E0F8BZ
3E0F8GC
3E0F8HZ
3E0F8KZ
3E0F8NZ
3E0F8SD
3E0F8SF
3E0F8TZ
3E0G304
3E0G305
3E0G30M
3E0G328
3E0G329
3E0G33Z
3E0G36Z
3E0G37Z
3E0G3BZ
3E0G3GC
3E0G3HZ
3E0G3KZ
3E0G3NZ
3E0G3SF
3E0G3TZ
3E0G4GC
3E0G704
3E0G705
3E0G70M
3E0G728
3E0G729
3E0G73Z
3E0G76Z
3E0G77Z
3E0G7BZ
3E0G7GC
3E0G7HZ
3E0G7KZ
3E0G7NZ
3E0G7SF
3E0G7TZ
3E0G804
3E0G805
3E0G80M
3E0G828
3E0G829
3E0G83Z
3E0G86Z
3E0G87Z
3E0G8BZ
3E0G8GC
3E0G8HZ
3E0G8KZ
3E0G8NZ
3E0G8SF
3E0G8TZ
3E0H304
3E0H305
3E0H30M
3E0H328
3E0H329
3E0H33Z
3E0H36Z
3E0H37Z
3E0H3BZ
3E0H3GC
3E0H3HZ
3E0H3KZ
3E0H3NZ
3E0H3SF
3E0H3TZ
3E0H4GC
3E0H704
3E0H705
3E0H70M
3E0H728
3E0H729
3E0H73Z
3E0H76Z
3E0H77Z
3E0H7BZ
3E0H7GC
3E0H7HZ
3E0H7KZ
3E0H7NZ
3E0H7SF
3E0H7TZ
3E0H804
3E0H805
3E0H80M
3E0H828
3E0H829
3E0H83Z
3E0H86Z
3E0H87Z
3E0H8BZ
3E0H8GC
3E0H8HZ
3E0H8KZ
3E0H8NZ
3E0H8SF
3E0H8TZ
3E0J304
3E0J305
3E0J30M
3E0J328
3E0J329
3E0J33Z
3E0J36Z
3E0J37Z
3E0J3BZ
3E0J3GC
3E0J3HZ
3E0J3KZ
3E0J3NZ
3E0J3SF
3E0J3TZ
3E0J4GC
3E0J704
3E0J705
3E0J70M
3E0J728
3E0J729
3E0J73Z
3E0J76Z
3E0J77Z
3E0J7BZ
3E0J7GC
3E0J7HZ
3E0J7KZ
3E0J7NZ
3E0J7SF
3E0J7TZ
3E0J804
3E0J805
3E0J80M
3E0J828
3E0J829
3E0J83Z
3E0J86Z
3E0J87Z
3E0J8BZ
3E0J8GC
3E0J8HZ
3E0J8KZ
3E0J8NZ
3E0J8SF
3E0J8TZ
3E0K304
3E0K305
3E0K30M
3E0K328
3E0K329
3E0K33Z
3E0K36Z
3E0K37Z
3E0K3BZ
3E0K3GC
3E0K3HZ
3E0K3KZ
3E0K3NZ
3E0K3SF
3E0K3TZ
3E0K4GC
3E0K704
3E0K705
3E0K70M
3E0K728
3E0K729
3E0K73Z
3E0K76Z
3E0K77Z
3E0K7BZ
3E0K7GC
3E0K7HZ
3E0K7KZ
3E0K7NZ
3E0K7SF
3E0K7TZ
3E0K804
3E0K805
3E0K80M
3E0K828
3E0K829
3E0K83Z
3E0K86Z
3E0K87Z
3E0K8BZ
3E0K8GC
3E0K8HZ
3E0K8KZ
3E0K8NZ
3E0K8SF
3E0K8TZ
3E0L05Z
3E0L304
3E0L305
3E0L30M
3E0L328
3E0L329
3E0L33Z
3E0L35Z
3E0L36Z
3E0L37Z
3E0L3BZ
3E0L3GC
3E0L3HZ
3E0L3KZ
3E0L3NZ
3E0L3SF
3E0L3TZ
3E0L45Z
3E0L4GC
3E0L704
3E0L705
3E0L70M
3E0L7SF
3E0M05Z
3E0M304
3E0M305
3E0M30M
3E0M30Y
3E0M328
3E0M329
3E0M33Z
3E0M35Z
3E0M36Z
3E0M37Z
3E0M3BZ
3E0M3GC
3E0M3HZ
3E0M3KZ
3E0M3NZ
3E0M3SF
3E0M3TZ
3E0M45Z
3E0M4GC
3E0M704
3E0M705
3E0M70M
3E0M7SF
3E0N304
3E0N305

3E0N30M
3E0N328
3E0N329
3E0N33Z
3E0N36Z
3E0N37Z
3E0N3BZ
3E0N3GC
3E0N3HZ
3E0N3KZ
3E0N3NZ
3E0N3SF
3E0N3TZ
3E0N4GC
3E0N704
3E0N705
3E0N70M
3E0N728
3E0N729
3E0N73Z
3E0N76Z
3E0N77Z
3E0N7BZ
3E0N7GC
3E0N7HZ
3E0N7KZ
3E0N7NZ
3E0N7SF
3E0N7TZ
3E0N804
3E0N805
3E0N80M
3E0N828
3E0N829
3E0N83Z
3E0N86Z
3E0N87Z
3E0N8BZ
3E0N8GC
3E0N8HZ
3E0N8KZ
3E0N8NZ
3E0N8SF
3E0N8TZ
3E0P05Z
3E0P304
3E0P305
3E0P30M
3E0P328
3E0P329
3E0P33Z
3E0P35Z
3E0P36Z
3E0P37Z
3E0P3BZ
3E0P3GC
3E0P3HZ
3E0P3KZ
3E0P3LZ
3E0P3NZ
3E0P3Q0
3E0P3Q1
3E0P3SF
3E0P3TZ
3E0P3VZ
3E0P45Z
3E0P4GC
3E0P704
3E0P705
3E0P70M
3E0P728
3E0P729
3E0P73Z
3E0P76Z
3E0P77Z
3E0P7BZ
3E0P7GC
3E0P7HZ
3E0P7KZ
3E0P7LZ
3E0P7NZ
3E0P7Q0
3E0P7Q1
3E0P7SF
3E0P7TZ
3E0P7VZ
3E0P804
3E0P805
3E0P80M
3E0P828
3E0P829
3E0P83Z
3E0P86Z
3E0P87Z
3E0P8BZ
3E0P8GC
3E0P8HZ
3E0P8KZ
3E0P8NZ
3E0P8SF
3E0P8TZ
3E0Q004
3E0Q00M
3E0Q028
3E0Q029
3E0Q03Z
3E0Q06Z
3E0Q07Z
3E0Q0AZ
3E0Q0BZ
3E0Q0E0
3E0Q0E1
3E0Q0GC
3E0Q0HZ
3E0Q0KZ
3E0Q0NZ
3E0Q0SF
3E0Q0TZ
3E0Q304
3E0Q30M
3E0Q328
3E0Q329
3E0Q33Z
3E0Q36Z
3E0Q37Z
3E0Q3AZ
3E0Q3BZ
3E0Q3E0
3E0Q3E1
3E0Q3GC
3E0Q3HZ
3E0Q3KZ
3E0Q3NZ
3E0Q3SF
3E0Q3TZ
3E0Q704
3E0Q70M
3E0Q7SF
3E0R0AZ
3E0R0E0
3E0R0E1
3E0R303
3E0R304
3E0R305
3E0R30M
3E0R328
3E0R329
3E0R33Z
3E0R36Z
3E0R37Z
3E0R3AZ
3E0R3BZ
3E0R3E0
3E0R3E1
3E0R3GC
3E0R3HZ
3E0R3KZ
3E0R3NZ
3E0R3SF
3E0R3TZ
3E0R7SF
3E0S303
3E0S304
3E0S305
3E0S30M
3E0S328
3E0S329
3E0S33Z
3E0S36Z
3E0S37Z
3E0S3BZ
3E0S3GC
3E0S3HZ
3E0S3KZ
3E0S3NZ
3E0S3SF
3E0S3TZ
3E0S7SF
3E0T33Z
3E0T3BZ
3E0T3GC
3E0T3TZ
3E0U028
3E0U029
3E0U0GB
3E0U304
3E0U305
3E0U30M
3E0U328
3E0U329
3E0U33Z
3E0U36Z
3E0U37Z
3E0U3BZ
3E0U3GB
3E0U3GC
3E0U3HZ
3E0U3KZ
3E0U3NZ
3E0U3SF
3E0U3TZ
3E0U4GC
3E0V0GB
3E0V305
3E0V30M
3E0V328
3E0V329
3E0V33Z
3E0V36Z
3E0V37Z
3E0V3BZ
3E0V3GB
3E0V3GC
3E0V3HZ
3E0V3KZ
3E0V3NZ
3E0V3TZ
3E0W305
3E0W30M
3E0W328
3E0W329
3E0W33Z
3E0W36Z
3E0W37Z
3E0W3BZ
3E0W3GC
3E0W3HZ
3E0W3KZ
3E0W3NZ
3E0W3TZ
3E0X33Z
3E0X3BZ
3E0X3GC
3E0X3TZ
3E0Y304
3E0Y305
3E0Y30M
3E0Y328
3E0Y329
3E0Y33Z
3E0Y36Z
3E0Y37Z
3E0Y3BZ
3E0Y3GC
3E0Y3HZ
3E0Y3KZ
3E0Y3NZ
3E0Y3SF
3E0Y3TZ
3E0Y4GC
3E0Y704
3E0Y705
3E0Y70M
3E0Y7SF
3E1038X
3E1038Z
3E10X8X
3E10X8Z
3E1938X
3E1938Z
3E1978X
3E1978Z
3E1988X
3E1988Z
3E1B38X
3E1B38Z
3E1B78X
3E1B78Z
3E1B88X
3E1B88Z
3E1C38X
3E1C38Z
3E1CX8X
3E1CX8Z
3E1F38X
3E1F38Z
3E1F78X
3E1F78Z
3E1F88X
3E1F88Z
3E1G38X
3E1G38Z
3E1G78X
3E1G78Z
3E1G88X
3E1G88Z
3E1H38X
3E1H38Z
3E1H78X
3E1H78Z
3E1H88X
3E1H88Z
3E1J38X
3E1J38Z
3E1J78X
3E1J78Z
3E1J88X
3E1J88Z
3E1K38X
3E1K38Z
3E1K78X
3E1K78Z
3E1K88X
3E1K88Z
3E1L38X
3E1L38Z
3E1M38X
3E1M38Z
3E1M39Z
3E1N38X
3E1N38Z
3E1N78X
3E1N78Z
3E1N88X
3E1N88Z
3E1P38X
3E1P38Z
3E1P78X
3E1P78Z
3E1P88X
3E1P88Z
3E1Q38X
3E1Q38Z
3E1R38X
3E1R38Z
3E1S38X
3E1S38Z
3E1U38X
3E1U38Z
3E1U48X
3E1U48Z
3E1Y38X
3E1Y38Z
4A0002Z
4A0004Z
4A000BZ
4A0034Z
4A003BD
4A003KD
4A003RD
4A0074Z
4A007BD
4A007KD
4A007RD
4A0084Z
4A008BD
4A008KD
4A008RD
4A00X2Z
4A00X4Z
4A01029
4A0102B
4A0104Z
4A01329
4A0132B
4A0134Z
4A01729
4A0172B
4A0174Z
4A01829
4A0182B
4A0184Z
4A01X29
4A01X2B
4A01X4Z
4A0204Z
4A0209Z
4A020CZ
4A020FZ
4A020HZ
4A020PZ
4A0234Z
4A0239Z
4A023CZ
4A023HZ
4A023PZ
4A0274Z
4A0279Z
4A027CZ
4A027HZ
4A027PZ
4A0284Z
4A0289Z
4A028CZ
4A028HZ
4A028PZ
4A02X4A
4A02X4Z
4A02X9Z
4A02XCZ
4A02XFZ
4A02XHZ
4A02XM4
4A02XPZ
4A03051
4A03053
4A0305C
4A030B1
4A030B3
4A030BC
4A030BF
4A030H1
4A030J1
4A030J3
4A030JC
4A030R1
4A03351
4A03353
4A0335C
4A033B1
4A033B3
4A033BC
4A033BF
4A033H1
4A033J1
4A033J3
4A033JC
4A033R1
4A03X51
4A03XB1
4A03XH1
4A03XJ1
4A03XR1
4A04050
4A04051
4A04052
4A04053
4A040B0
4A040B1
4A040B2
4A040B3
4A040J0
4A040J1
4A040J2
4A040J3
4A040R1
4A04350
4A04351
4A04352
4A04353
4A043B0
4A043B1
4A043B2
4A043B3
4A043J0
4A043J1
4A043J2
4A043J3
4A043R1
4A04X51
4A04XB1
4A04XJ1
4A04XR1
4A05XLZ
4A0605Z
4A060BZ
4A0635Z
4A063BZ
4A0675Z
4A067BZ
4A0685Z
4A068BZ
4A07X0Z
4A07X7Z
4A07XBZ
4A08X0Z
4A0971Z
4A0975Z
4A097CZ
4A097DZ
4A097LZ
4A097MZ
4A0981Z
4A0985Z
4A098CZ
4A098DZ
4A098LZ
4A098MZ
4A09X1Z
4A09X5Z
4A09XCZ
4A09XDZ
4A09XLZ
4A09XMZ
4A0B78Z
4A0B7BZ
4A0B7GZ
4A0B88Z
4A0B8BZ
4A0B8GZ
4A0C35Z
4A0C3BZ
4A0C45Z
4A0C4BZ
4A0C75Z
4A0C7BZ
4A0C85Z
4A0C8BZ
4A0D73Z
4A0D75Z
4A0D7BZ
4A0D7DZ
4A0D7LZ
4A0D83Z
4A0D85Z
4A0D8BZ
4A0D8DZ
4A0D8LZ
4A0F33Z
4A0FX3Z
4A0H74Z
4A0H7CZ
4A0H7FZ
4A0H7HZ
4A0H84Z
4A0H8CZ
4A0H8FZ
4A0H8HZ
4A0HX4Z
4A0HXCZ
4A0HXFZ
4A0HXHZ
4A0J72Z
4A0J74Z
4A0J7BZ
4A0J82Z
4A0J84Z
4A0J8BZ
4A0JX2Z
4A0JX4Z
4A0JXBZ
4A0Z76Z
4A0Z7KZ
4A0ZX6Z
4A0ZXKZ
4A0ZXQZ
4A1002Z
4A1004G
4A1004Z
4A100BZ

4A1034G	4A12X9Z	4A143R0	4A1J7BZ	6A0Z1ZZ	7W01X5Z	7W07X5Z	8E0W3CZ	9WB2XBZ
4A1034Z	4A12XCZ	4A143R2	4A1J82Z	6A150ZZ	7W01X6Z	7W07X6Z	8E0W3EZ	9WB2XCZ
4A103BD	4A12XFZ	4A143R3	4A1J84Z	6A151ZZ	7W01X7Z	7W07X7Z	8E0W4CZ	9WB2XDZ
4A103KD	4A12XHZ	4A14X51	4A1J8BZ	6A210ZZ	7W01X8Z	7W07X8Z	8E0W4EZ	9WB2XFZ
4A103RD	4A12XM4	4A14XB1	4A1JX2Z	6A211ZZ	7W01X9Z	7W07X9Z	8E0W7CZ	9WB2XGZ
4A1074G	4A12XSH	4A14XJ1	4A1JX4Z	6A220ZZ	7W02X0Z	7W08X0Z	8E0W7EZ	9WB2XHZ
4A1074Z	4A13051	4A1605H	4A1JXBZ	6A221ZZ	7W02X1Z	7W08X1Z	8E0W8CZ	9WB2XJZ
4A107BD	4A13053	4A1605Z	4A1Z7KZ	6A3Z0ZZ	7W02X2Z	7W08X2Z	8E0W8EZ	9WB2XKZ
4A107KD	4A1305C	4A160BZ	4A1ZXKZ	6A3Z1ZZ	7W02X3Z	7W08X3Z	8E0WXBF	9WB2XLZ
4A107RD	4A130B1	4A1635H	4A1ZXQZ	6A4Z0ZZ	7W02X4Z	7W08X4Z	8E0WXBG	9WB3XBZ
4A1084G	4A130B3	4A1635Z	4B00XVZ	6A4Z1ZZ	7W02X5Z	7W08X5Z	8E0WXBH	9WB3XCZ
4A1084Z	4A130BC	4A163BZ	4B01XVZ	6A550Z0	7W02X6Z	7W08X6Z	8E0WXBZ	9WB3XDZ
4A108BD	4A130H1	4A1675H	4B02XSZ	6A550Z1	7W02X7Z	7W08X7Z	8E0WXCZ	9WB3XFZ
4A108KD	4A130J1	4A1675Z	4B02XTZ	6A550Z2	7W02X8Z	7W08X8Z	8E0WXY8	9WB3XGZ
4A108RD	4A130J3	4A167BZ	4B09XSZ	6A550Z3	7W02X9Z	7W08X9Z	8E0X0CZ	9WB3XHZ
4A10X2Z	4A130JC	4A1685H	4B0FXVZ	6A550ZT	7W03X0Z	7W09X0Z	8E0X0EZ	9WB3XJZ
4A10X4G	4A130R1	4A1685Z	5A02110	6A550ZV	7W03X1Z	7W09X1Z	8E0X3CZ	9WB3XKZ
4A10X4Z	4A13351	4A168BZ	5A02115	6A551Z0	7W03X2Z	7W09X2Z	8E0X3EZ	9WB3XLZ
4A11029	4A13353	4A1971Z	5A02116	6A551Z1	7W03X3Z	7W09X3Z	8E0X4CZ	9WB4XBZ
4A1102B	4A1335C	4A1975Z	5A0211D	6A551Z2	7W03X4Z	7W09X4Z	8E0X4EZ	9WB4XCZ
4A1104G	4A133B1	4A197CZ	5A02210	6A551Z3	7W03X5Z	7W09X5Z	8E0XXBF	9WB4XDZ
4A1104Z	4A133B3	4A197DZ	5A02215	6A551ZT	7W03X6Z	7W09X6Z	8E0XXBG	9WB4XFZ
4A11329	4A133BC	4A197LZ	5A02216	6A551ZV	7W03X7Z	7W09X7Z	8E0XXBH	9WB4XGZ
4A1132B	4A133H1	4A19X1Z	5A0221D	6A600ZZ	7W03X8Z	7W09X8Z	8E0XXBZ	9WB4XHZ
4A1134G	4A133J1	4A19X5Z	5A05121	6A601ZZ	7W03X9Z	7W09X9Z	8E0XXCZ	9WB4XJZ
4A1134Z	4A133J3	4A19XCZ	5A0512C	6A650ZZ	7W04X0Z	8C01X6J	8E0XXY8	9WB4XKZ
4A11729	4A133JC	4A19XDZ	5A05221	6A651ZZ	7W04X1Z	8C01X6L	8E0Y0CZ	9WB4XLZ
4A1172B	4A133R1	4A19XLZ	5A0522C	6A750Z4	7W04X2Z	8C02X6K	8E0Y0EZ	9WB5XBZ
4A1174G	4A13X51	4A1B78Z	5A0920Z	6A750Z5	7W04X3Z	8C02X6L	8E0Y3CZ	9WB5XCZ
4A1174Z	4A13XB1	4A1B7BZ	5A09357	6A750Z6	7W04X4Z	8E01XY7	8E0Y3EZ	9WB5XDZ
4A11829	4A13XH1	4A1B7GZ	5A09358	6A750Z7	7W04X5Z	8E023DZ	8E0Y4CZ	9WB5XFZ
4A1182B	4A13XJ1	4A1B88Z	5A09359	6A750ZZ	7W04X6Z	8E090CZ	8E0Y4EZ	9WB5XGZ
4A1184G	4A13XR1	4A1B8BZ	5A0935B	6A751Z4	7W04X7Z	8E090EM	8E0YXBF	9WB5XHZ
4A1184Z	4A14050	4A1B8GZ	5A0935Z	6A751Z5	7W04X8Z	8E090EZ	8E0YXBG	9WB5XJZ
4A11X29	4A14051	4A1BXSH	5A09457	6A751Z6	7W04X9Z	8E093CZ	8E0YXBH	9WB5XKZ
4A11X2B	4A14052	4A1D73Z	5A09458	6A751Z7	7W05X0Z	8E093EZ	8E0YXBZ	9WB5XLZ
4A11X4G	4A14053	4A1D75Z	5A09459	6A751ZZ	7W05X1Z	8E094CZ	8E0YXCZ	9WB6XBZ
4A11X4Z	4A140B0	4A1D7BZ	5A0945B	6A800ZZ	7W05X2Z	8E094EZ	8E0YXY8	9WB6XCZ
4A1204Z	4A140B1	4A1D7DZ	5A0945Z	6A801ZZ	7W05X3Z	8E097CZ	8E0ZXY1	9WB6XDZ
4A1209Z	4A140B2	4A1D7LZ	5A09557	6A930ZZ	7W05X4Z	8E097EZ	8E0ZXY4	9WB6XFZ
4A120CZ	4A140B3	4A1D83Z	5A09558	6A931ZZ	7W05X5Z	8E098CZ	8E0ZXY5	9WB6XGZ
4A120FZ	4A140J0	4A1D85Z	5A09559	6AB50BZ	7W05X6Z	8E098EZ	8E0ZXY6	9WB6XHZ
4A120HZ	4A140J1	4A1D8BZ	5A0955B	6ABB0BZ	7W05X7Z	8E09XBF	9WB0XBZ	9WB6XJZ
4A1234Z	4A140J2	4A1D8DZ	5A0955Z	6ABF0BZ	7W05X8Z	8E09XBG	9WB0XCZ	9WB6XKZ
4A1239Z	4A140J3	4A1D8LZ	5A12012	6ABT0BZ	7W05X9Z	8E09XBH	9WB0XDZ	9WB6XLZ
4A123CZ	4A140R0	4A1GXSH	5A1213Z	7W00X0Z	7W06X0Z	8E09XBZ	9WB0XFZ	9WB7XBZ
4A123FZ	4A140R2	4A1H74Z	5A1221Z	7W00X1Z	7W06X1Z	8E09XCZ	9WB0XGZ	9WB7XCZ
4A123HZ	4A140R3	4A1H7CZ	5A1223Z	7W00X2Z	7W06X2Z	8E09XY8	9WB0XHZ	9WB7XDZ
4A1274Z	4A14350	4A1H7FZ	5A1522F	7W00X3Z	7W06X3Z	8E0H300	9WB0XJZ	9WB7XFZ
4A1279Z	4A14351	4A1H7HZ	5A15A2F	7W00X4Z	7W06X4Z	8E0H30Z	9WB0XKZ	9WB7XGZ
4A127CZ	4A14352	4A1H84Z	5A15A2G	7W00X5Z	7W06X5Z	8E0HX62	9WB0XLZ	9WB7XHZ
4A127FZ	4A14353	4A1H8CZ	5A15A2H	7W00X6Z	7W06X6Z	8E0HXY9	9WB1XBZ	9WB7XJZ
4A127HZ	4A143B0	4A1H8FZ	5A19054	7W00X7Z	7W06X7Z	8E0KX1Z	9WB1XCZ	9WB7XKZ
4A1284Z	4A143B1	4A1H8HZ	5A1C00Z	7W00X8Z	7W06X8Z	8E0KXY7	9WB1XDZ	9WB7XLZ
4A1289Z	4A143B2	4A1HX4Z	5A1C60Z	7W00X9Z	7W06X9Z	8E0UXY7	9WB1XFZ	9WB8XBZ
4A128CZ	4A143B3	4A1HXCZ	5A1D70Z	7W01X0Z	7W07X0Z	8E0VX1C	9WB1XGZ	9WB8XCZ
4A128FZ	4A143J0	4A1HXFZ	5A1D80Z	7W01X1Z	7W07X1Z	8E0VX1D	9WB1XHZ	9WB8XDZ
4A128HZ	4A143J1	4A1HXHZ	5A1D90Z	7W01X2Z	7W07X2Z	8E0VX63	9WB1XJZ	9WB8XFZ
4A12X45	4A143J2	4A1J72Z	5A2204Z	7W01X3Z	7W07X3Z	8E0W0CZ	9WB1XKZ	9WB8XGZ
4A12X4Z	4A143J3	4A1J74Z	6A0Z0ZZ	7W01X4Z	7W07X4Z	8E0W0EZ	9WB1XLZ	9WB8XHZ

9WB8XJZ
9WB8XKZ
9WB8XLZ
9WB9XBZ
9WB9XCZ
9WB9XDZ
9WB9XFZ
9WB9XGZ
9WB9XHZ
9WB9XJZ
9WB9XKZ
9WB9XLZ
B00B0ZZ
B00B1ZZ
B00BYZZ
B00BZZZ
B01B0ZZ
B01B1ZZ
B01BYZZ
B01BZZZ
B02000Z
B0200ZZ
B02010Z
B0201ZZ
B020Y0Z
B020YZZ
B020ZZZ
B02700Z
B0270ZZ
B02710Z
B0271ZZ
B027Y0Z
B027YZZ
B027ZZZ
B02800Z
B0280ZZ
B02810Z
B0281ZZ
B028Y0Z
B028YZZ
B028ZZZ
B02900Z
B0290ZZ
B02910Z
B0291ZZ
B029Y0Z
B029YZZ
B029ZZZ
B02B00Z
B02B0ZZ
B02B10Z
B02B1ZZ
B02BY0Z
B02BYZZ
B02BZZZ
B030Y0Z
B030YZZ
B030ZZZ
B039Y0Z
B039YZZ
B039ZZZ
B03BY0Z
B03BYZZ
B03BZZZ
B03CY0Z
B03CYZZ
B03CZZZ
B040ZZZ
B04BZZZ
B210010
B210110
B210Y10
B211010
B211110
B211Y10
B212010
B212110
B212Y10
B213010
B213110
B213Y10
B22100Z
B2210ZZ
B22110Z
B2211ZZ
B221Y0Z
B221YZZ
B221Z2Z
B221ZZZ
B22300Z
B2230ZZ
B22310Z
B2231ZZ
B223Y0Z
B223YZZ
B223Z2Z
B223ZZZ
B22600Z
B2260ZZ
B22610Z
B2261ZZ
B226Y0Z
B226YZZ
B226Z2Z
B226ZZZ
B231Y0Z
B231YZZ
B231ZZZ
B233Y0Z
B233YZZ
B233ZZZ
B236Y0Z
B236YZZ
B236ZZZ
B240YZZ
B240ZZ3
B240ZZ4
B240ZZZ
B241YZZ
B241ZZ3
B241ZZ4
B241ZZZ
B244YZZ
B244ZZ3
B244ZZ4
B244ZZZ
B245YZZ
B245ZZ3
B245ZZ4
B245ZZZ
B246YZZ
B246ZZ3
B246ZZ4
B246ZZZ
B24BYZZ
B24BZZ3
B24BZZ4
B24BZZZ
B24CYZZ
B24CZZ3
B24CZZ4
B24CZZZ
B24DYZZ
B24DZZ3
B24DZZ4
B24DZZZ
B3000ZZ
B3001ZZ
B300YZZ
B300ZZZ
B3010ZZ
B3011ZZ
B301YZZ
B301ZZZ
B3020ZZ
B3021ZZ
B302YZZ
B302ZZZ
B3030ZZ
B3031ZZ
B303YZZ
B303ZZZ
B3040ZZ
B3041ZZ
B304YZZ
B304ZZZ
B3050ZZ
B3051ZZ
B305YZZ
B305ZZZ
B3060ZZ
B3061ZZ
B306YZZ
B306ZZZ
B3070ZZ
B3071ZZ
B307YZZ
B307ZZZ
B3080ZZ
B3081ZZ
B308YZZ
B308ZZZ
B3090ZZ
B3091ZZ
B309YZZ
B309ZZZ
B30B0ZZ
B30B1ZZ
B30BYZZ
B30BZZZ
B30C0ZZ
B30C1ZZ
B30CYZZ
B30CZZZ
B30D0ZZ
B30D1ZZ
B30DYZZ
B30DZZZ
B30F0ZZ
B30F1ZZ
B30FYZZ
B30FZZZ
B30G0ZZ
B30G1ZZ
B30GYZZ
B30GZZZ
B30H0ZZ
B30H1ZZ
B30HYZZ
B30HZZZ
B30J0ZZ
B30J1ZZ
B30JYZZ
B30JZZZ
B30K0ZZ
B30K1ZZ
B30KYZZ
B30KZZZ
B30L0ZZ
B30L1ZZ
B30LYZZ
B30LZZZ
B30M0ZZ
B30M1ZZ
B30MYZZ
B30MZZZ
B30N0ZZ
B30N1ZZ
B30NYZZ
B30NZZZ
B30P0ZZ
B30P1ZZ
B30PYZZ
B30PZZZ
B30Q0ZZ
B30Q1ZZ
B30QYZZ
B30QZZZ
B30R0ZZ
B30R1ZZ
B30RYZZ
B30RZZZ
B30S0ZZ
B30S1ZZ
B30SYZZ
B30SZZZ
B30T0ZZ
B30T1ZZ
B30TYZZ
B30TZZZ
B310010
B3100ZZ
B310110
B3101ZZ
B310Y10
B310YZZ
B310ZZZ
B311010
B3110ZZ
B311110
B3111ZZ
B311Y10
B311YZZ
B311ZZZ
B312010
B3120ZZ
B312110
B3121ZZ
B312Y10
B312YZZ
B312ZZZ
B313010
B3130ZZ
B313110
B3131ZZ
B313Y10
B313YZZ
B313ZZZ
B314010
B3140ZZ
B314110
B3141ZZ
B314Y10
B314YZZ
B314ZZZ
B315010
B3150ZZ
B315110
B3151ZZ
B315Y10
B315YZZ
B315ZZZ
B316010
B3160ZZ
B316110
B3161ZZ
B316Y10
B316YZZ
B316ZZZ
B317010
B3170ZZ
B317110
B3171ZZ
B317Y10
B317YZZ
B317ZZZ
B318010
B3180ZZ
B318110
B3181ZZ
B318Y10
B318YZZ
B318ZZZ
B319010
B3190ZZ
B319110
B3191ZZ
B319Y10
B319YZZ
B319ZZZ
B31B010
B31B0ZZ
B31B110
B31B1ZZ
B31BY10
B31BYZZ
B31BZZZ
B31C010
B31C0ZZ
B31C110
B31C1ZZ
B31CY10
B31CYZZ
B31CZZZ
B31D010
B31D0ZZ
B31D110
B31D1ZZ
B31DY10
B31DYZZ
B31DZZZ
B31F010
B31F0ZZ
B31F110
B31F1ZZ
B31FY10
B31FYZZ
B31FZZZ
B31G010
B31G0ZZ
B31G110
B31G1ZZ
B31GY10
B31GYZZ
B31GZZZ
B31H010
B31H0ZZ
B31H110
B31H1ZZ
B31HY10
B31HYZZ
B31HZZZ
B31J010
B31J0ZZ
B31J110
B31J1ZZ
B31JY10
B31JYZZ
B31JZZZ
B31K010
B31K0ZZ
B31K110
B31K1ZZ
B31KY10
B31KYZZ
B31KZZZ
B31L010
B31L0ZZ
B31L110
B31L1ZZ
B31LY10
B31LYZZ
B31LZZZ
B31M010
B31M0ZZ
B31M110
B31M1ZZ
B31MY10
B31MYZZ
B31MZZZ
B31N010
B31N0ZZ
B31N110
B31N1ZZ
B31NY10
B31NYZZ
B31NZZZ
B31P010
B31P0ZZ
B31P110
B31P1ZZ
B31PY10
B31PYZZ
B31PZZZ
B31Q010
B31Q0ZZ
B31Q110
B31Q1ZZ
B31QY10
B31QYZZ
B31QZZZ
B31R010
B31R0ZZ
B31R110
B31R1ZZ
B31RY10
B31RYZZ
B31RZZZ
B31S010
B31S0ZZ
B31S110
B31S1ZZ
B31SY10
B31SYZZ
B31SZZZ
B31T010
B31T0ZZ
B31T110
B31T1ZZ
B31TY10
B31TYZZ
B31TZZZ
B31U010
B31U0ZZ
B31U110
B31U1ZZ
B31UY10
B31UYZZ
B31UZZZ
B3200ZZ
B3201ZZ
B320YZZ
B320Z2Z
B320ZZZ
B3250ZZ
B3251ZZ
B325YZZ
B325Z2Z
B325ZZZ
B3280ZZ
B3281ZZ
B328YZZ
B328Z2Z
B328ZZZ
B32G0ZZ
B32G1ZZ
B32GYZZ
B32GZ2Z
B32GZZZ
B32R0ZZ
B32R1ZZ
B32RYZZ
B32RZ2Z
B32RZZZ
B32S0ZZ
B32S1ZZ
B32SYZZ
B32SZ2Z
B32SZZZ
B32T0ZZ
B32T1ZZ
B32TYZZ
B32TZ2Z
B32TZZZ
B330Y0Z
B330YZZ
B330ZZZ
B335Y0Z
B335YZZ
B335ZZZ
B338Y0Z
B338YZZ
B338ZZZ
B33GY0Z
B33GYZZ
B33GZZZ
B33HY0Z
B33HYZZ
B33HZZZ
B33JY0Z
B33JYZZ
B33JZZZ
B33KY0Z
B33KYZZ
B33KZZZ
B33MY0Z
B33MYZZ
B33MZZZ
B33QY0Z
B33QYZZ
B33QZZZ
B33RY0Z
B33RYZZ
B33RZZZ
B340ZZ3
B340ZZZ
B341ZZ3
B341ZZZ
B342ZZ3
B342ZZZ
B343ZZ3
B343ZZZ
B344ZZ3
B344ZZZ
B345ZZ3
B345ZZZ
B346ZZ3
B346ZZZ
B347ZZ3
B347ZZZ
B348ZZ3
B348ZZZ
B34HZZ3
B34HZZZ
B34JZZ3
B34JZZZ
B34KZZ3
B34KZZZ
B34RZZ3
B34RZZZ
B34SZZ3
B34SZZZ
B34TZZ3
B34TZZZ
B34VZZ3
B34VZZZ
B4000ZZ
B4001ZZ
B400YZZ
B4020ZZ

B4021ZZ
B402YZZ
B4030ZZ
B4031ZZ
B403YZZ
B4040ZZ
B4041ZZ
B404YZZ
B4050ZZ
B4051ZZ
B405YZZ
B4060ZZ
B4061ZZ
B406YZZ
B4070ZZ
B4071ZZ
B407YZZ
B4080ZZ
B4081ZZ
B408YZZ
B4090ZZ
B4091ZZ
B409YZZ
B40B0ZZ
B40B1ZZ
B40BYZZ
B40C0ZZ
B40C1ZZ
B40CYZZ
B40D0ZZ
B40D1ZZ
B40DYZZ
B40F0ZZ
B40F1ZZ
B40FYZZ
B40G0ZZ
B40G1ZZ
B40GYZZ
B40J0ZZ
B40J1ZZ
B40JYZZ
B40M0ZZ
B40M1ZZ
B40MYZZ
B410010
B4100ZZ
B410110
B4101ZZ
B410Y10
B410YZZ
B410ZZZ
B412010
B4120ZZ
B412110
B4121ZZ
B412Y10
B412YZZ
B412ZZZ
B413010
B4130ZZ
B413110
B4131ZZ
B413Y10
B413YZZ
B413ZZZ
B414010
B4140ZZ
B414110
B4141ZZ
B414Y10
B414YZZ
B414ZZZ
B415010
B4150ZZ
B415110
B4151ZZ
B415Y10
B415YZZ
B415ZZZ
B416010
B4160ZZ
B416110
B4161ZZ
B416Y10
B416YZZ
B416ZZZ
B417010
B4170ZZ
B417110
B4171ZZ
B417Y10
B417YZZ
B417ZZZ
B418010
B4180ZZ
B418110
B4181ZZ
B418Y10
B418YZZ
B418ZZZ
B419010
B4190ZZ
B419110
B4191ZZ
B419Y10
B419YZZ
B419ZZZ
B41B010
B41B0ZZ
B41B110
B41B1ZZ
B41BY10
B41BYZZ
B41BZZZ
B41C010
B41C0ZZ
B41C110
B41C1ZZ
B41CY10
B41CYZZ
B41CZZZ
B41D010
B41D0ZZ
B41D110
B41D1ZZ
B41DY10
B41DYZZ
B41DZZZ
B41F010
B41F0ZZ
B41F110
B41F1ZZ
B41FY10
B41FYZZ
B41FZZZ
B41G010
B41G0ZZ
B41G110
B41G1ZZ
B41GY10
B41GYZZ
B41GZZZ
B41J010
B41J0ZZ
B41J110
B41J1ZZ
B41JY10
B41JYZZ
B41JZZZ
B4200ZZ
B4201ZZ
B420YZZ
B420Z2Z
B420ZZZ
B4210ZZ
B4211ZZ
B421YZZ
B421Z2Z
B421ZZZ
B4240ZZ
B4241ZZ
B424YZZ
B424Z2Z
B424ZZZ
B4280ZZ
B4281ZZ
B428YZZ
B428Z2Z
B428ZZZ
B42C0ZZ
B42C1ZZ
B42CYZZ
B42CZ2Z
B42CZZZ
B42F0ZZ
B42F1ZZ
B42FYZZ
B42FZ2Z
B42FZZZ
B42G0ZZ
B42G1ZZ
B42GYZZ
B42GZ2Z
B42GZZZ
B42H0ZZ
B42H1ZZ
B42HYZZ
B42HZ2Z
B42HZZZ
B42M0ZZ
B42M1ZZ
B42MYZZ
B42MZ2Z
B42MZZZ
B430Y0Z
B430YZZ
B430ZZZ
B431Y0Z
B431YZZ
B431ZZZ
B434Y0Z
B434YZZ
B434ZZZ
B438Y0Z
B438YZZ
B438ZZZ
B43CY0Z
B43CYZZ
B43CZZZ
B43FY0Z
B43FYZZ
B43FZZZ
B43GY0Z
B43GYZZ
B43GZZZ
B43HY0Z
B43HYZZ
B43HZZZ
B440ZZ3
B440ZZZ
B444ZZ3
B444ZZZ
B445ZZ3
B445ZZZ
B446ZZ3
B446ZZZ
B447ZZ3
B447ZZZ
B448ZZ3
B448ZZZ
B44BZZ3
B44BZZZ
B44FZZ3
B44FZZZ
B44GZZ3
B44GZZZ
B44HZZ3
B44HZZZ
B44KZZ3
B44KZZZ
B44LZZ3
B44LZZZ
B44NZZ3
B44NZZZ
B5000ZZ
B5001ZZ
B500YZZ
B5010ZZ
B5011ZZ
B501YZZ
B5020ZZ
B5021ZZ
B502YZZ
B5030ZZ
B5031ZZ
B503YZZ
B5040ZZ
B5041ZZ
B504YZZ
B5050ZZ
B5051ZZ
B505YZZ
B5060ZZ
B5061ZZ
B506YZZ
B5070ZZ
B5071ZZ
B507YZZ
B5080ZZ
B5081ZZ
B508YZZ
B5090ZZ
B5091ZZ
B509YZZ
B50B0ZZ
B50B1ZZ
B50BYZZ
B50C0ZZ
B50C1ZZ
B50CYZZ
B50D0ZZ
B50D1ZZ
B50DYZZ
B50F0ZZ
B50F1ZZ
B50FYZZ
B50G0ZZ
B50G1ZZ
B50GYZZ
B50H0ZZ
B50H1ZZ
B50HYZZ
B50J0ZZ
B50J1ZZ
B50JYZZ
B50K0ZZ
B50K1ZZ
B50KYZZ
B50L0ZZ
B50L1ZZ
B50LYZZ
B50M0ZZ
B50M1ZZ
B50MYZZ
B50N0ZZ
B50N1ZZ
B50NYZZ
B50P0ZZ
B50P1ZZ
B50PYZZ
B50Q0ZZ
B50Q1ZZ
B50QYZZ
B50R0ZZ
B50R1ZZ
B50RYZZ
B50S0ZZ
B50S1ZZ
B50SYZZ
B50T0ZZ
B50T1ZZ
B50TYZZ
B50V0ZZ
B50V1ZZ
B50VYZZ
B50W0ZZ
B50W1ZZ
B50WYZZ
B5100ZA
B5100ZZ
B5101ZA
B5101ZZ
B510YZA
B510YZZ
B510ZZA
B510ZZZ
B5110ZA
B5110ZZ
B5111ZA
B5111ZZ
B511YZA
B511YZZ
B511ZZA
B511ZZZ
B5120ZA
B5120ZZ
B5121ZA
B5121ZZ
B512YZA
B512YZZ
B512ZZA
B512ZZZ
B5130ZA
B5130ZZ
B5131ZA
B5131ZZ
B513YZA
B513YZZ
B513ZZA
B513ZZZ
B5140ZA
B5140ZZ
B5141ZA
B5141ZZ
B514YZA
B514YZZ
B514ZZA
B514ZZZ
B5150ZA
B5150ZZ
B5151ZA
B5151ZZ
B515YZA
B515YZZ
B515ZZA
B515ZZZ
B5160ZA
B5160ZZ
B5161ZA
B5161ZZ
B516YZA
B516YZZ
B516ZZA
B516ZZZ
B5170ZA
B5170ZZ
B5171ZA
B5171ZZ
B517YZA
B517YZZ
B517ZZA
B517ZZZ
B5180ZA
B5180ZZ
B5181ZA
B5181ZZ
B518YZA
B518YZZ
B518ZZA
B518ZZZ
B5190ZA
B5190ZZ
B5191ZA
B5191ZZ
B519YZA
B519YZZ
B519ZZA
B519ZZZ
B51B0ZA
B51B0ZZ
B51B1ZA
B51B1ZZ
B51BYZA
B51BYZZ
B51BZZA
B51BZZZ
B51C0ZA
B51C0ZZ
B51C1ZA
B51C1ZZ
B51CYZA
B51CYZZ
B51CZZA
B51CZZZ
B51D0ZA
B51D0ZZ
B51D1ZA
B51D1ZZ
B51DYZA
B51DYZZ
B51DZZA
B51DZZZ
B51F0ZA
B51F0ZZ
B51F1ZA
B51F1ZZ
B51FYZA
B51FYZZ
B51FZZA
B51FZZZ
B51G0ZA
B51G0ZZ
B51G1ZA
B51G1ZZ
B51GYZA
B51GYZZ
B51GZZA
B51GZZZ
B51H0ZA
B51H0ZZ
B51H1ZA
B51H1ZZ
B51HYZA
B51HYZZ
B51HZZA
B51HZZZ
B51J0ZA
B51J0ZZ
B51J1ZA
B51J1ZZ
B51JYZA
B51JYZZ
B51JZZA
B51JZZZ
B51K0ZA
B51K0ZZ
B51K1ZA
B51K1ZZ
B51KYZA
B51KYZZ
B51KZZA
B51KZZZ
B51L0ZA
B51L0ZZ
B51L1ZA
B51L1ZZ
B51LYZA
B51LYZZ
B51LZZA
B51LZZZ
B51M0ZA
B51M0ZZ
B51M1ZA
B51M1ZZ
B51MYZA
B51MYZZ
B51MZZA
B51MZZZ
B51N0ZA
B51N0ZZ
B51N1ZA
B51N1ZZ
B51NYZA
B51NYZZ
B51NZZA
B51NZZZ
B51P0ZA
B51P0ZZ
B51P1ZA
B51P1ZZ
B51PYZA
B51PYZZ
B51PZZA
B51PZZZ
B51Q0ZA
B51Q0ZZ
B51Q1ZA
B51Q1ZZ
B51QYZA
B51QYZZ
B51QZZA
B51QZZZ
B51R0ZA
B51R0ZZ
B51R1ZA
B51R1ZZ
B51RYZA
B51RYZZ
B51RZZA
B51RZZZ
B51S0ZA
B51S0ZZ
B51S1ZA
B51S1ZZ
B51SYZA
B51SYZZ
B51SZZA
B51SZZZ
B51T0ZA
B51T0ZZ
B51T1ZA
B51T1ZZ
B51TYZA
B51TYZZ
B51TZZA
B51TZZZ
B51V0ZA
B51V0ZZ
B51V1ZA
B51V1ZZ

B51VYZA	B52J00Z	B532YZZ	B549ZZA	B70C1ZZ	B9071ZZ	B92F10Z	BB2800Z	BF03YZZ
B51VYZZ	B52J0ZZ	B532ZZZ	B549ZZZ	B70CYZZ	B907YZZ	B92F1ZZ	BB280ZZ	BF0C0ZZ
B51VZZA	B52J10Z	B535Y0Z	B54BZZ3	B8000ZZ	B9080ZZ	B92FY0Z	BB2810Z	BF0C1ZZ
B51VZZZ	B52J1ZZ	B535YZZ	B54BZZA	B8001ZZ	B9081ZZ	B92FYZZ	BB281ZZ	BF0CYZZ
B51W0ZA	B52JY0Z	B535ZZZ	B54BZZZ	B800YZZ	B908YZZ	B92FZZZ	BB28Y0Z	BF100ZZ
B51W0ZZ	B52JYZZ	B538Y0Z	B54CZZ3	B8010ZZ	B9090ZZ	B92J00Z	BB28YZZ	BF101ZZ
B51W1ZA	B52JZ2Z	B538YZZ	B54CZZA	B8011ZZ	B9091ZZ	B92J0ZZ	BB28ZZZ	BF10YZZ
B51W1ZZ	B52JZZZ	B538ZZZ	B54CZZZ	B801YZZ	B909YZZ	B92J10Z	BB2900Z	BF110ZZ
B51WYZA	B52K00Z	B539Y0Z	B54DZZ3	B8020ZZ	B90B0ZZ	B92J1ZZ	BB290ZZ	BF111ZZ
B51WYZZ	B52K0ZZ	B539YZZ	B54DZZA	B8021ZZ	B90B1ZZ	B92JY0Z	BB2910Z	BF11YZZ
B51WZZA	B52K10Z	B539ZZZ	B54DZZZ	B802YZZ	B90BYZZ	B92JYZZ	BB291ZZ	BF120ZZ
B51WZZZ	B52K1ZZ	B53BY0Z	B54JZZ3	B803ZZZ	B90C0ZZ	B92JZZZ	BB29Y0Z	BF121ZZ
B52200Z	B52KY0Z	B53BYZZ	B54JZZA	B804ZZZ	B90C1ZZ	B930Y0Z	BB29YZZ	BF12YZZ
B5220ZZ	B52KYZZ	B53BZZZ	B54JZZZ	B805ZZZ	B90CYZZ	B930YZZ	BB29ZZZ	BF130ZZ
B52210Z	B52KZ2Z	B53CY0Z	B54KZZ3	B806ZZZ	B90D0ZZ	B930ZZZ	BB2F00Z	BF131ZZ
B5221ZZ	B52KZZZ	B53CYZZ	B54KZZA	B807ZZZ	B90D1ZZ	B932Y0Z	BB2F0ZZ	BF13YZZ
B522Y0Z	B52L00Z	B53CZZZ	B54KZZZ	B82500Z	B90DYZZ	B932YZZ	BB2F10Z	BF140ZZ
B522YZZ	B52L0ZZ	B53DY0Z	B54LZZ3	B8250ZZ	B90FZZZ	B932ZZZ	BB2F1ZZ	BF141ZZ
B522Z2Z	B52L10Z	B53DYZZ	B54LZZA	B82510Z	B90HZZZ	B935Y0Z	BB2FY0Z	BF14YZZ
B522ZZZ	B52L1ZZ	B53DZZZ	B54LZZZ	B8251ZZ	B91GYZZ	B935YZZ	BB2FYZZ	BF180ZZ
B52800Z	B52LY0Z	B53HY0Z	B54MZZ3	B825Y0Z	B91GZZZ	B936ZZZ	BB2FZZZ	BF181ZZ
B5280ZZ	B52LYZZ	B53HYZZ	B54MZZA	B825YZZ	B91JYZZ	B939Y0Z	BB3GY0Z	BF18YZZ
B52810Z	B52LZ2Z	B53HZZZ	B54MZZZ	B825ZZZ	B91JZZZ	B939YZZ	BB3GYZZ	BF2500Z
B5281ZZ	B52LZZZ	B53LY0Z	B54NZZ3	B82600Z	B92000Z	B939ZZZ	BB3GZZZ	BF250ZZ
B528Y0Z	B52Q00Z	B53LYZZ	B54NZZA	B8260ZZ	B9200ZZ	B93DY0Z	BB4BZZZ	BF2510Z
B528YZZ	B52Q0ZZ	B53LZZZ	B54NZZZ	B82610Z	B92010Z	B93DYZZ	BB4CZZZ	BF251ZZ
B528Z2Z	B52Q10Z	B53MY0Z	B54PZZ3	B8261ZZ	B9201ZZ	B93DZZZ	BD11YZZ	BF25Y0Z
B528ZZZ	B52Q1ZZ	B53MYZZ	B54PZZA	B826Y0Z	B920Y0Z	B93FY0Z	BD11ZZZ	BF25YZZ
B52900Z	B52QY0Z	B53MZZZ	B54PZZZ	B826YZZ	B920YZZ	B93FYZZ	BD12YZZ	BF25ZZZ
B5290ZZ	B52QYZZ	B53NY0Z	B54TZZ3	B826ZZZ	B920ZZZ	B93FZZZ	BD12ZZZ	BF2600Z
B52910Z	B52QZ2Z	B53NYZZ	B54TZZA	B82700Z	B92200Z	B93JY0Z	BD13YZZ	BF260ZZ
B5291ZZ	B52QZZZ	B53NZZZ	B54TZZZ	B8270ZZ	B9220ZZ	B93JYZZ	BD13ZZZ	BF2610Z
B529Y0Z	B52R00Z	B53PY0Z	B7000ZZ	B82710Z	B92210Z	B93JZZZ	BD14YZZ	BF261ZZ
B529YZZ	B52R0ZZ	B53PYZZ	B7001ZZ	B8271ZZ	B9221ZZ	BB07YZZ	BD14ZZZ	BF26Y0Z
B529Z2Z	B52R10Z	B53PZZZ	B700YZZ	B827Y0Z	B922Y0Z	BB08YZZ	BD15YZZ	BF26YZZ
B529ZZZ	B52R1ZZ	B53SY0Z	B7010ZZ	B827YZZ	B922YZZ	BB09YZZ	BD15ZZZ	BF26ZZZ
B52F00Z	B52RY0Z	B53SYZZ	B7011ZZ	B827ZZZ	B922ZZZ	BB0DZZZ	BD16YZZ	BF2700Z
B52F0ZZ	B52RYZZ	B53SZZZ	B701YZZ	B835Y0Z	B92600Z	BB12ZZZ	BD16ZZZ	BF270ZZ
B52F10Z	B52RZ2Z	B53TY0Z	B7040ZZ	B835YZZ	B9260ZZ	BB13ZZZ	BD19YZZ	BF2710Z
B52F1ZZ	B52RZZZ	B53TYZZ	B7041ZZ	B835ZZZ	B92610Z	BB14ZZZ	BD19ZZZ	BF271ZZ
B52FY0Z	B52S00Z	B53TZZZ	B704YZZ	B836Y0Z	B9261ZZ	BB16ZZZ	BD1BYZZ	BF27Y0Z
B52FYZZ	B52S0ZZ	B53VY0Z	B7050ZZ	B836YZZ	B926Y0Z	BB17YZZ	BD1BZZZ	BF27YZZ
B52FZ2Z	B52S10Z	B53VYZZ	B7051ZZ	B836ZZZ	B926YZZ	BB18YZZ	BD2400Z	BF27ZZZ
B52FZZZ	B52S1ZZ	B53VZZZ	B705YZZ	B837Y0Z	B926ZZZ	BB19YZZ	BD240ZZ	BF2C00Z
B52G00Z	B52SY0Z	B543ZZ3	B7060ZZ	B837YZZ	B92900Z	BB1CZZZ	BD2410Z	BF2C0ZZ
B52G0ZZ	B52SYZZ	B543ZZA	B7061ZZ	B837ZZZ	B9290ZZ	BB1DZZZ	BD241ZZ	BF2C10Z
B52G10Z	B52SZ2Z	B543ZZZ	B706YZZ	B845ZZZ	B92910Z	BB2400Z	BD24Y0Z	BF2C1ZZ
B52G1ZZ	B52SZZZ	B544ZZ3	B7070ZZ	B846ZZZ	B9291ZZ	BB240ZZ	BD24YZZ	BF2CY0Z
B52GY0Z	B52T00Z	B544ZZA	B7071ZZ	B847ZZZ	B929Y0Z	BB2410Z	BD24ZZZ	BF2CYZZ
B52GYZZ	B52T0ZZ	B544ZZZ	B707YZZ	B902ZZZ	B929YZZ	BB241ZZ	BD41ZZZ	BF2CZZZ
B52GZ2Z	B52T10Z	B546ZZ3	B7080ZZ	B9040ZZ	B929ZZZ	BB24Y0Z	BD42ZZZ	BF35Y0Z
B52GZZZ	B52T1ZZ	B546ZZA	B7081ZZ	B9041ZZ	B92D00Z	BB24YZZ	BD47ZZZ	BF35YZZ
B52H00Z	B52TY0Z	B546ZZZ	B708YZZ	B904YZZ	B92D0ZZ	BB24ZZZ	BD48ZZZ	BF35ZZZ
B52H0ZZ	B52TYZZ	B547ZZ3	B7090ZZ	B9050ZZ	B92D10Z	BB2700Z	BD49ZZZ	BF36Y0Z
B52H10Z	B52TZ2Z	B547ZZA	B7091ZZ	B9051ZZ	B92D1ZZ	BB270ZZ	BD4CZZZ	BF36YZZ
B52H1ZZ	B52TZZZ	B547ZZZ	B709YZZ	B905YZZ	B92DY0Z	BB2710Z	BF000ZZ	BF36ZZZ
B52HY0Z	B531Y0Z	B548ZZ3	B70B0ZZ	B9060ZZ	B92DYZZ	BB271ZZ	BF001ZZ	BF37Y0Z
B52HYZZ	B531YZZ	B548ZZA	B70B1ZZ	B9061ZZ	B92DZZZ	BB27Y0Z	BF00YZZ	BF37YZZ
B52HZ2Z	B531ZZZ	B548ZZZ	B70BYZZ	B906YZZ	B92F00Z	BB27YZZ	BF030ZZ	BF37ZZZ
B52HZZZ	B532Y0Z	B549ZZ3	B70C0ZZ	B9070ZZ	B92F0ZZ	BB27ZZZ	BF031ZZ	BF40ZZZ

BF42ZZZ
BF43ZZZ
BF45ZZZ
BF46ZZZ
BF47ZZZ
BF4CZZZ
BG2200Z
BG220ZZ
BG2210Z
BG221ZZ
BG22Y0Z
BG22YZZ
BG22ZZZ
BG2300Z
BG230ZZ
BG2310Z
BG231ZZ
BG23Y0Z
BG23YZZ
BG23ZZZ
BG2400Z
BG240ZZ
BG2410Z
BG241ZZ
BG24Y0Z
BG24YZZ
BG24ZZZ
BG32Y0Z
BG32YZZ
BG32ZZZ
BG33Y0Z
BG33YZZ
BG33ZZZ
BG34Y0Z
BG34YZZ
BG34ZZZ
BG40ZZZ
BG41ZZZ
BG42ZZZ
BG43ZZZ
BG44ZZZ
BH00ZZZ
BH01ZZZ
BH02ZZZ
BH030ZZ
BH031ZZ
BH03YZZ
BH03ZZZ
BH040ZZ
BH041ZZ
BH04YZZ
BH04ZZZ
BH050ZZ
BH051ZZ
BH05YZZ
BH05ZZZ
BH060ZZ
BH061ZZ
BH06YZZ
BH06ZZZ
BH30Y0Z
BH30YZZ
BH30ZZZ
BH31Y0Z
BH31YZZ
BH31ZZZ
BH32Y0Z
BH32YZZ
BH32ZZZ
BH3DY0Z
BH3DYZZ
BH3DZZZ
BH3FY0Z
BH3FYZZ
BH3FZZZ
BH3GY0Z
BH3GYZZ
BH3GZZZ
BH3HY0Z
BH3HYZZ
BH3HZZZ
BH3JY0Z
BH3JYZZ
BH3JZZZ
BH40ZZZ
BH41ZZZ
BH42ZZZ
BH47ZZZ
BH48ZZZ
BH49ZZZ
BH4BZZZ
BH4CZZZ
BL30Y0Z
BL30YZZ
BL30ZZZ
BL31Y0Z
BL31YZZ
BL31ZZZ
BL32Y0Z
BL32YZZ
BL32ZZZ
BL33Y0Z
BL33YZZ
BL33ZZZ
BL40ZZZ
BL41ZZZ
BL42ZZZ
BL43ZZZ
BN00ZZZ
BN01ZZZ
BN02ZZZ
BN03ZZZ
BN04ZZZ
BN05ZZZ
BN06ZZZ
BN070ZZ
BN071ZZ
BN07YZZ
BN07ZZZ
BN080ZZ
BN081ZZ
BN08YZZ
BN08ZZZ
BN090ZZ
BN091ZZ
BN09YZZ
BN09ZZZ
BN0BZZZ
BN0CZZZ
BN0DZZZ
BN0GZZZ
BN0HZZZ
BN0JZZZ
BN170ZZ
BN171ZZ
BN17YZZ
BN17ZZZ
BN180ZZ
BN181ZZ
BN18YZZ
BN18ZZZ
BN190ZZ
BN191ZZ
BN19YZZ
BN19ZZZ
BN200ZZ
BN201ZZ
BN20YZZ
BN20ZZZ
BN230ZZ
BN231ZZ
BN23YZZ
BN23ZZZ
BN250ZZ
BN251ZZ
BN25YZZ
BN25ZZZ
BN260ZZ
BN261ZZ
BN26YZZ
BN26ZZZ
BN290ZZ
BN291ZZ
BN29YZZ
BN29ZZZ
BN2F0ZZ
BN2F1ZZ
BN2FYZZ
BN2FZZZ
BN39YZZ
BN39ZZZ
BP00ZZZ
BP01ZZZ
BP02ZZZ
BP03ZZZ
BP04ZZZ
BP05ZZZ
BP06ZZZ
BP07ZZZ
BP080ZZ
BP081ZZ
BP08YZZ
BP08ZZZ
BP090ZZ
BP091ZZ
BP09YZZ
BP09ZZZ
BP0AZZZ
BP0BZZZ
BP0C0ZZ
BP0C1ZZ
BP0CYZZ
BP0CZZZ
BP0D0ZZ
BP0D1ZZ
BP0DYZZ
BP0DZZZ
BP0EZZZ
BP0FZZZ
BP0G0ZZ
BP0G1ZZ
BP0GYZZ
BP0GZZZ
BP0H0ZZ
BP0H1ZZ
BP0HYZZ
BP0HZZZ
BP0JZZZ
BP0KZZZ
BP0L0ZZ
BP0L1ZZ
BP0LYZZ
BP0LZZZ
BP0M0ZZ
BP0M1ZZ
BP0MYZZ
BP0MZZZ
BP0NZZZ
BP0PZZZ
BP0RZZZ
BP0SZZZ
BP0XZZZ
BP0YZZZ
BP10ZZZ
BP11ZZZ
BP12ZZZ
BP13ZZZ
BP14ZZZ
BP15ZZZ
BP16ZZZ
BP17ZZZ
BP180ZZ
BP181ZZ
BP18YZZ
BP18ZZZ
BP190ZZ
BP191ZZ
BP19YZZ
BP19ZZZ
BP1AZZZ
BP1BZZZ
BP1C0ZZ
BP1C1ZZ
BP1CYZZ
BP1D0ZZ
BP1D1ZZ
BP1DYZZ
BP1EZZZ
BP1FZZZ
BP1G0ZZ
BP1G1ZZ
BP1GYZZ
BP1H0ZZ
BP1H1ZZ
BP1HYZZ
BP1JZZZ
BP1KZZZ
BP1L0ZZ
BP1L1ZZ
BP1LYZZ
BP1LZZZ
BP1M0ZZ
BP1M1ZZ
BP1MYZZ
BP1MZZZ
BP1NZZZ
BP1PZZZ
BP1RZZZ
BP1SZZZ
BP1XZZZ
BP1YZZZ
BP200ZZ
BP201ZZ
BP20YZZ
BP210ZZ
BP211ZZ
BP21YZZ
BP220ZZ
BP221ZZ
BP22YZZ
BP22ZZZ
BP230ZZ
BP231ZZ
BP23YZZ
BP23ZZZ
BP240ZZ
BP241ZZ
BP24YZZ
BP24ZZZ
BP250ZZ
BP251ZZ
BP25YZZ
BP25ZZZ
BP260ZZ
BP261ZZ
BP26YZZ
BP26ZZZ
BP270ZZ
BP271ZZ
BP27YZZ
BP27ZZZ
BP280ZZ
BP281ZZ
BP28YZZ
BP28ZZZ
BP290ZZ
BP291ZZ
BP29YZZ
BP29ZZZ
BP2A0ZZ
BP2A1ZZ
BP2AYZZ
BP2AZZZ
BP2B0ZZ
BP2B1ZZ
BP2BYZZ
BP2BZZZ
BP2CZZZ
BP2DZZZ
BP2E0ZZ
BP2E1ZZ
BP2EYZZ
BP2EZZZ
BP2F0ZZ
BP2F1ZZ
BP2FYZZ
BP2FZZZ
BP2G0ZZ
BP2G1ZZ
BP2GYZZ
BP2GZZZ
BP2H0ZZ
BP2H1ZZ
BP2HYZZ
BP2HZZZ
BP2J0ZZ
BP2J1ZZ
BP2JYZZ
BP2JZZZ
BP2K0ZZ
BP2K1ZZ
BP2KYZZ
BP2KZZZ
BP2L0ZZ
BP2L1ZZ
BP2LYZZ
BP2LZZZ
BP2M0ZZ
BP2M1ZZ
BP2MYZZ
BP2MZZZ
BP2N0ZZ
BP2N1ZZ
BP2NYZZ
BP2NZZZ
BP2P0ZZ
BP2P1ZZ
BP2PYZZ
BP2PZZZ
BP2Q0ZZ
BP2Q1ZZ
BP2QYZZ
BP2QZZZ
BP2R0ZZ
BP2R1ZZ
BP2RYZZ
BP2RZZZ
BP2S0ZZ
BP2S1ZZ
BP2SYZZ
BP2SZZZ
BP2T0ZZ
BP2T1ZZ
BP2TYZZ
BP2TZZZ
BP2U0ZZ
BP2U1ZZ
BP2UYZZ
BP2UZZZ
BP2V0ZZ
BP2V1ZZ
BP2VYZZ
BP2VZZZ
BP2W0ZZ
BP2W1ZZ
BP2WYZZ
BP2X0ZZ
BP2X1ZZ
BP2XYZZ
BP2XZZZ
BP2Y0ZZ
BP2Y1ZZ
BP2YYZZ
BP2YZZZ
BP38Y0Z
BP38YZZ
BP38ZZZ
BP39Y0Z
BP39YZZ
BP39ZZZ
BP3CY0Z
BP3CYZZ
BP3CZZZ
BP3DY0Z
BP3DYZZ
BP3DZZZ
BP3EY0Z
BP3EYZZ
BP3EZZZ
BP3FY0Z
BP3FYZZ
BP3FZZZ
BP3GY0Z
BP3GYZZ
BP3GZZZ
BP3HY0Z
BP3HYZZ
BP3HZZZ
BP3JY0Z
BP3JYZZ
BP3JZZZ
BP3KY0Z
BP3KYZZ
BP3KZZZ
BP3LY0Z
BP3LYZZ
BP3LZZZ
BP3MY0Z
BP3MYZZ
BP3MZZZ
BP48ZZ1
BP48ZZZ
BP49ZZ1
BP49ZZZ
BP4GZZ1
BP4GZZZ
BP4HZZ1
BP4HZZZ
BP4LZZ1
BP4LZZZ
BP4MZZ1
BP4MZZZ
BP4NZZ1
BP4NZZZ
BP4PZZ1
BP4PZZZ
BQ000ZZ
BQ001ZZ
BQ00YZZ
BQ00ZZ1
BQ00ZZZ
BQ010ZZ
BQ011ZZ
BQ01YZZ
BQ01ZZ1
BQ01ZZZ
BQ03ZZ1
BQ03ZZZ
BQ04ZZ1
BQ04ZZZ
BQ070ZZ
BQ071ZZ
BQ07YZZ
BQ07ZZZ
BQ080ZZ
BQ081ZZ
BQ08YZZ
BQ08ZZZ
BQ0DZZZ
BQ0FZZZ
BQ0G0ZZ
BQ0G1ZZ
BQ0GYZZ
BQ0GZZZ
BQ0H0ZZ
BQ0H1ZZ
BQ0HYZZ
BQ0HZZZ
BQ0JZZZ
BQ0KZZZ
BQ0LZZZ
BQ0MZZZ
BQ0PZZZ
BQ0QZZZ
BQ0VZZZ
BQ0WZZZ
BQ0X0ZZ
BQ0X1ZZ
BQ0XYZZ
BQ0Y0ZZ
BQ0Y1ZZ
BQ0YYZZ
BQ100ZZ
BQ101ZZ
BQ10YZZ
BQ10ZZZ
BQ110ZZ
BQ111ZZ
BQ11YZZ
BQ11ZZZ
BQ13ZZZ
BQ14ZZZ
BQ170ZZ
BQ171ZZ
BQ17YZZ
BQ17ZZZ
BQ180ZZ
BQ181ZZ
BQ18YZZ
BQ18ZZZ
BQ1DZZZ
BQ1FZZZ
BQ1G0ZZ
BQ1G1ZZ
BQ1GYZZ
BQ1GZZZ
BQ1H0ZZ
BQ1H1ZZ
BQ1HYZZ
BQ1HZZZ
BQ1JZZZ
BQ1KZZZ
BQ1LZZZ
BQ1MZZZ
BQ1PZZZ
BQ1QZZZ
BQ1VZZZ
BQ1WZZZ
BQ1X0ZZ
BQ1X1ZZ
BQ1XYZZ
BQ1XZZZ
BQ1Y0ZZ
BQ1Y1ZZ
BQ1YYZZ
BQ1YZZZ
BQ200ZZ
BQ201ZZ
BQ20YZZ
BQ20ZZZ

BQ210ZZ
BQ211ZZ
BQ21YZZ
BQ21ZZZ
BQ230ZZ
BQ231ZZ
BQ23YZZ
BQ23ZZZ
BQ240ZZ
BQ241ZZ
BQ24YZZ
BQ24ZZZ
BQ270ZZ
BQ271ZZ
BQ27YZZ
BQ27ZZZ
BQ280ZZ
BQ281ZZ
BQ28YZZ
BQ28ZZZ
BQ2B0ZZ
BQ2B1ZZ
BQ2BYZZ
BQ2C0ZZ
BQ2C1ZZ
BQ2CYZZ
BQ2D0ZZ
BQ2D1ZZ
BQ2DYZZ
BQ2DZZZ
BQ2F0ZZ
BQ2F1ZZ
BQ2FYZZ
BQ2FZZZ
BQ2G0ZZ
BQ2G1ZZ
BQ2GYZZ
BQ2GZZZ
BQ2H0ZZ
BQ2H1ZZ
BQ2HYZZ
BQ2HZZZ
BQ2J0ZZ
BQ2J1ZZ
BQ2JYZZ
BQ2JZZZ
BQ2K0ZZ
BQ2K1ZZ
BQ2KYZZ
BQ2KZZZ
BQ2L0ZZ
BQ2L1ZZ
BQ2LYZZ
BQ2LZZZ
BQ2M0ZZ
BQ2M1ZZ
BQ2MYZZ
BQ2MZZZ
BQ2P0ZZ
BQ2P1ZZ
BQ2PYZZ
BQ2PZZZ
BQ2Q0ZZ
BQ2Q1ZZ
BQ2QYZZ
BQ2QZZZ
BQ2R0ZZ
BQ2R1ZZ
BQ2RYZZ
BQ2RZZZ
BQ2S0ZZ
BQ2S1ZZ
BQ2SYZZ
BQ2SZZZ
BQ2V0ZZ
BQ2V1ZZ
BQ2VYZZ
BQ2VZZZ
BQ2W0ZZ
BQ2W1ZZ
BQ2WYZZ
BQ2WZZZ
BQ2X0ZZ
BQ2X1ZZ
BQ2XYZZ
BQ2XZZZ
BQ2Y0ZZ
BQ2Y1ZZ
BQ2YYZZ
BQ2YZZZ
BQ30Y0Z
BQ30YZZ
BQ30ZZZ
BQ31Y0Z
BQ31YZZ
BQ31ZZZ
BQ33Y0Z
BQ33YZZ
BQ33ZZZ
BQ34Y0Z
BQ34YZZ
BQ34ZZZ
BQ37Y0Z
BQ37YZZ
BQ37ZZZ
BQ38Y0Z
BQ38YZZ
BQ38ZZZ
BQ3DY0Z
BQ3DYZZ
BQ3DZZZ
BQ3FY0Z
BQ3FYZZ
BQ3FZZZ
BQ3GY0Z
BQ3GYZZ
BQ3GZZZ
BQ3HY0Z
BQ3HYZZ
BQ3HZZZ
BQ3JY0Z
BQ3JYZZ
BQ3JZZZ
BQ3KY0Z
BQ3KYZZ
BQ3KZZZ
BQ3LY0Z
BQ3LYZZ
BQ3LZZZ
BQ3MY0Z
BQ3MYZZ
BQ3MZZZ
BQ3PY0Z
BQ3PYZZ
BQ3PZZZ
BQ3QY0Z
BQ3QYZZ
BQ3QZZZ
BQ3VY0Z
BQ3VYZZ
BQ3VZZZ
BQ3WY0Z
BQ3WYZZ
BQ3WZZZ
BQ40ZZZ
BQ41ZZZ
BQ42ZZZ
BQ47ZZZ
BQ48ZZZ
BQ49ZZZ
BR00ZZ1
BR00ZZZ
BR010ZZ
BR011ZZ
BR01YZZ
BR01ZZZ
BR020ZZ
BR021ZZ
BR02YZZ
BR02ZZZ
BR030ZZ
BR031ZZ
BR03YZZ
BR03ZZZ
BR040ZZ
BR041ZZ
BR04YZZ
BR04ZZZ
BR050ZZ
BR051ZZ
BR05YZZ
BR05ZZZ
BR060ZZ
BR061ZZ
BR06YZZ
BR06ZZZ
BR07ZZ1
BR07ZZZ
BR08ZZZ
BR09ZZ1
BR09ZZZ
BR0BZZZ
BR0CZZZ
BR0D0ZZ
BR0D1ZZ
BR0DYZZ
BR0DZZZ
BR0FZZZ
BR0GZZ1
BR0GZZZ
BR0HZZZ
BR100ZZ
BR101ZZ
BR10YZZ
BR10ZZZ
BR110ZZ
BR111ZZ
BR11YZZ
BR11ZZZ
BR120ZZ
BR121ZZ
BR12YZZ
BR12ZZZ
BR130ZZ
BR131ZZ
BR13YZZ
BR13ZZZ
BR140ZZ
BR141ZZ
BR14YZZ
BR14ZZZ
BR150ZZ
BR151ZZ
BR15YZZ
BR15ZZZ
BR160ZZ
BR161ZZ
BR16YZZ
BR16ZZZ
BR170ZZ
BR171ZZ
BR17YZZ
BR17ZZZ
BR180ZZ
BR181ZZ
BR18YZZ
BR18ZZZ
BR190ZZ
BR191ZZ
BR19YZZ
BR19ZZZ
BR1B0ZZ
BR1B1ZZ
BR1BYZZ
BR1BZZZ
BR1C0ZZ
BR1C1ZZ
BR1CYZZ
BR1CZZZ
BR1D0ZZ
BR1D1ZZ
BR1DYZZ
BR1DZZZ
BR1F0ZZ
BR1F1ZZ
BR1FYZZ
BR1FZZZ
BR1G0ZZ
BR1G1ZZ
BR1GYZZ
BR1GZZZ
BR1H0ZZ
BR1H1ZZ
BR1HYZZ
BR1HZZZ
BR200ZZ
BR201ZZ
BR20YZZ
BR20ZZZ
BR270ZZ
BR271ZZ
BR27YZZ
BR27ZZZ
BR290ZZ
BR291ZZ
BR29YZZ
BR29ZZZ
BR2C0ZZ
BR2C1ZZ
BR2CYZZ
BR2CZZZ
BR2D0ZZ
BR2D1ZZ
BR2DYZZ
BR2DZZZ
BR2F0ZZ
BR2F1ZZ
BR2FYZZ
BR2FZZZ
BR30Y0Z
BR30YZZ
BR30ZZZ
BR31Y0Z
BR31YZZ
BR31ZZZ
BR32Y0Z
BR32YZZ
BR32ZZZ
BR33Y0Z
BR33YZZ
BR33ZZZ
BR37Y0Z
BR37YZZ
BR37ZZZ
BR39Y0Z
BR39YZZ
BR39ZZZ
BR3CY0Z
BR3CYZZ
BR3CZZZ
BR3FY0Z
BR3FYZZ
BR3FZZZ
BR40ZZZ
BR47ZZZ
BR49ZZZ
BR4FZZZ
BT000ZZ
BT001ZZ
BT00YZZ
BT00ZZZ
BT010ZZ
BT011ZZ
BT01YZZ
BT01ZZZ
BT020ZZ
BT021ZZ
BT02YZZ
BT02ZZZ
BT030ZZ
BT031ZZ
BT03YZZ
BT03ZZZ
BT040ZZ
BT041ZZ
BT04YZZ
BT04ZZZ
BT050ZZ
BT051ZZ
BT05YZZ
BT05ZZZ
BT060ZZ
BT061ZZ
BT06YZZ
BT06ZZZ
BT070ZZ
BT071ZZ
BT07YZZ
BT07ZZZ
BT080ZZ
BT081ZZ
BT08YZZ
BT08ZZZ
BT0B0ZZ
BT0B1ZZ
BT0BYZZ
BT0BZZZ
BT0C0ZZ
BT0C1ZZ
BT0CYZZ
BT0CZZZ
BT100ZZ
BT101ZZ
BT10YZZ
BT10ZZZ
BT110ZZ
BT111ZZ
BT11YZZ
BT11ZZZ
BT120ZZ
BT121ZZ
BT12YZZ
BT12ZZZ
BT130ZZ
BT131ZZ
BT13YZZ
BT13ZZZ
BT140ZZ
BT141ZZ
BT14YZZ
BT14ZZZ
BT150ZZ
BT151ZZ
BT15YZZ
BT15ZZZ
BT160ZZ
BT161ZZ
BT16YZZ
BT16ZZZ
BT170ZZ
BT171ZZ
BT17YZZ
BT17ZZZ
BT1B0ZZ
BT1B1ZZ
BT1BYZZ
BT1BZZZ
BT1C0ZZ
BT1C1ZZ
BT1CYZZ
BT1CZZZ
BT1D0ZZ
BT1D1ZZ
BT1DYZZ
BT1DZZZ
BT1F0ZZ
BT1F1ZZ
BT1FYZZ
BT1FZZZ
BT1G0ZZ
BT1G1ZZ
BT1GYZZ
BT1GZZZ
BT2000Z
BT200ZZ
BT2010Z
BT201ZZ
BT20Y0Z
BT20YZZ
BT20ZZZ
BT2100Z
BT210ZZ
BT2110Z
BT211ZZ
BT21Y0Z
BT21YZZ
BT21ZZZ
BT2200Z
BT220ZZ
BT2210Z
BT221ZZ
BT22Y0Z
BT22YZZ
BT22ZZZ
BT2300Z
BT230ZZ
BT2310Z
BT231ZZ
BT23Y0Z
BT23YZZ
BT23ZZZ
BT2900Z
BT290ZZ
BT2910Z
BT291ZZ
BT29Y0Z
BT29YZZ
BT29ZZZ
BT30Y0Z
BT30YZZ
BT30ZZZ
BT31Y0Z
BT31YZZ
BT31ZZZ
BT32Y0Z
BT32YZZ
BT32ZZZ
BT33Y0Z
BT33YZZ
BT33ZZZ
BT39Y0Z
BT39YZZ
BT39ZZZ
BT40ZZZ
BT41ZZZ
BT42ZZZ
BT43ZZZ
BT45ZZZ
BT46ZZZ
BT47ZZZ
BT48ZZZ
BT49ZZZ
BT4JZZZ
BU000ZZ
BU001ZZ
BU00YZZ
BU010ZZ
BU011ZZ
BU01YZZ
BU020ZZ
BU021ZZ
BU02YZZ
BU060ZZ
BU061ZZ
BU06YZZ
BU080ZZ
BU081ZZ
BU08YZZ
BU090ZZ
BU091ZZ
BU09YZZ
BU100ZZ
BU101ZZ
BU10YZZ
BU10ZZZ
BU110ZZ
BU111ZZ
BU11YZZ
BU11ZZZ
BU120ZZ
BU121ZZ
BU12YZZ
BU12ZZZ
BU160ZZ
BU161ZZ
BU16YZZ
BU16ZZZ
BU180ZZ
BU181ZZ
BU18YZZ
BU18ZZZ
BU190ZZ
BU191ZZ
BU19YZZ
BU19ZZZ
BU33Y0Z
BU33YZZ
BU33ZZZ
BU34Y0Z
BU34YZZ
BU34ZZZ
BU35Y0Z
BU35YZZ
BU35ZZZ
BU36Y0Z
BU36YZZ
BU36ZZZ
BU39Y0Z
BU39YZZ
BU39ZZZ
BU3BY0Z
BU3BYZZ
BU3BZZZ
BU3CY0Z
BU3CYZZ
BU3CZZZ
BU40YZZ
BU40ZZZ
BU41YZZ
BU41ZZZ
BU42YZZ
BU42ZZZ
BU43YZZ
BU43ZZZ
BU44YZZ
BU44ZZZ
BU45YZZ
BU45ZZZ
BU46YZZ
BU46ZZZ

BU4CYZZ
BU4CZZZ
BV000ZZ
BV001ZZ
BV00YZZ
BV010ZZ
BV011ZZ
BV01YZZ
BV020ZZ
BV021ZZ
BV02YZZ
BV030ZZ
BV031ZZ
BV03YZZ
BV050ZZ
BV051ZZ
BV05YZZ
BV060ZZ
BV061ZZ
BV06YZZ
BV080ZZ
BV081ZZ
BV08YZZ
BV100ZZ
BV101ZZ
BV10YZZ
BV10ZZZ
BV180ZZ
BV181ZZ
BV18YZZ
BV18ZZZ
BV2300Z
BV230ZZ
BV2310Z
BV231ZZ
BV23Y0Z
BV23YZZ
BV23ZZZ
BV30Y0Z
BV30YZZ
BV30ZZZ
BV33Y0Z
BV33YZZ
BV33ZZZ
BV34Y0Z
BV34YZZ
BV34ZZZ
BV35Y0Z
BV35YZZ
BV35ZZZ
BV36Y0Z
BV36YZZ
BV36ZZZ
BV37Y0Z
BV37YZZ
BV37ZZZ
BV44ZZZ
BV49ZZZ
BV4BZZZ
BW00ZZZ
BW01ZZZ
BW03ZZZ
BW0BZZZ
BW0CZZZ
BW0JZZZ
BW0KZZZ
BW0LZZZ
BW0MZZZ
BW110ZZ
BW111ZZ
BW11YZZ
BW11ZZZ
BW190ZZ
BW191ZZ
BW19YZZ
BW19ZZZ
BW1C0ZZ
BW1C1ZZ
BW1CYZZ
BW1CZZZ
BW1J0ZZ
BW1J1ZZ
BW1JYZZ
BW1JZZZ
BW2000Z
BW200ZZ
BW2010Z
BW201ZZ
BW20Y0Z
BW20YZZ
BW20ZZZ
BW2100Z
BW210ZZ
BW2110Z
BW211ZZ
BW21Y0Z
BW21YZZ
BW21ZZZ
BW2400Z
BW240ZZ
BW2410Z
BW241ZZ
BW24Y0Z
BW24YZZ
BW24ZZZ
BW2500Z
BW250ZZ
BW2510Z
BW251ZZ
BW25Y0Z
BW25YZZ
BW25ZZZ
BW2800Z
BW280ZZ
BW2810Z
BW281ZZ
BW28Y0Z
BW28YZZ
BW28ZZZ
BW2900Z
BW290ZZ
BW2910Z
BW291ZZ
BW29Y0Z
BW29YZZ
BW29ZZZ
BW2F00Z
BW2F0ZZ
BW2F10Z
BW2F1ZZ
BW2FY0Z
BW2FYZZ
BW2FZZZ
BW2G00Z
BW2G0ZZ
BW2G10Z
BW2G1ZZ
BW2GY0Z
BW2GYZZ
BW2GZZZ
BW30Y0Z
BW30YZZ
BW30ZZZ
BW33Y0Z
BW33YZZ
BW38Y0Z
BW38YZZ
BW38ZZZ
BW3FY0Z
BW3FYZZ
BW3FZZZ
BW3GY0Z
BW3GYZZ
BW3GZZZ
BW3HY0Z
BW3HYZZ
BW3HZZZ
BW3PY0Z
BW3PYZZ
BW3PZZZ
BW40ZZZ
BW41ZZZ
BW4FZZZ
BW4GZZZ
BY30Y0Z
BY30YZZ
BY30ZZZ
BY31Y0Z
BY31YZZ
BY31ZZZ
BY32Y0Z
BY32YZZ
BY32ZZZ
BY33Y0Z
BY33YZZ
BY33ZZZ
BY34Y0Z
BY34YZZ
BY34ZZZ
BY35Y0Z
BY35YZZ
BY35ZZZ
BY36Y0Z
BY36YZZ
BY36ZZZ
BY47ZZZ
BY48ZZZ
BY49ZZZ
BY4BZZZ
BY4CZZZ
BY4DZZZ
BY4FZZZ
BY4GZZZ
C0101ZZ
C010YZZ
C015DZZ
C015YZZ
C01YYZZ
C0201ZZ
C020FZZ
C020SZZ
C020YZZ
C025DZZ
C025YZZ
C02YYZZ
C030BZZ
C030KZZ
C030MZZ
C030YZZ
C03YYZZ
C050VZZ
C050YZZ
C05YYZZ
C2161ZZ
C216YZZ
C21G1ZZ
C21GDZZ
C21GSZZ
C21GYZZ
C21GZZZ
C21YYZZ
C2261ZZ
C226YZZ
C22G1ZZ
C22GDZZ
C22GKZZ
C22GSZZ
C22GYZZ
C22GZZZ
C22YYZZ
C23GKZZ
C23GMZZ
C23GQZZ
C23GRZZ
C23GYZZ
C23YYZZ
C2561ZZ
C256YZZ
C25YYZZ
C51B1ZZ
C51BYZZ
C51C1ZZ
C51CYZZ
C51D1ZZ
C51DYZZ
C51N1ZZ
C51NYZZ
C51P1ZZ
C51PYZZ
C51Q1ZZ
C51QYZZ
C51R1ZZ
C51RYZZ
C51YYZZ
C7101ZZ
C710DZZ
C710YZZ
C7121ZZ
C712YZZ
C713DZZ
C713YZZ
C7151ZZ
C715YZZ
C71D1ZZ
C71DYZZ
C71J1ZZ
C71JYZZ
C71K1ZZ
C71KYZZ
C71L1ZZ
C71LYZZ
C71M1ZZ
C71MYZZ
C71N1ZZ
C71NYZZ
C71P1ZZ
C71PYZZ
C71YYZZ
C7221ZZ
C722YZZ
C72YYZZ
C7551ZZ
C755YZZ
C75D1ZZ
C75DYZZ
C75J1ZZ
C75JYZZ
C75K1ZZ
C75KYZZ
C75L1ZZ
C75LYZZ
C75M1ZZ
C75MYZZ
C75N1ZZ
C75NYZZ
C75P1ZZ
C75PYZZ
C75YYZZ
C7631ZZ
C7637ZZ
C763CZZ
C763DZZ
C763HZZ
C763WZZ
C763YZZ
C76YYZZ
C8191ZZ
C819YZZ
C81YYZZ
C91B1ZZ
C91BYZZ
C91YYZZ
CB121ZZ
CB129ZZ
CB12TZZ
CB12VZZ
CB12YZZ
CB1YYZZ
CB221ZZ
CB229ZZ
CB22YZZ
CB2YYZZ
CB32KZZ
CB32YZZ
CB3YYZZ
CD151ZZ
CD15DZZ
CD15YZZ
CD171ZZ
CD17DZZ
CD17YZZ
CD1YYZZ
CD271ZZ
CD27DZZ
CD27YZZ
CD2YYZZ
CF141ZZ
CF14YZZ
CF151ZZ
CF15YZZ
CF161ZZ
CF16YZZ
CF1C1ZZ
CF1CYZZ
CF1YYZZ
CF241ZZ
CF24YZZ
CF251ZZ
CF25YZZ
CF261ZZ
CF26YZZ
CF2YYZZ
CG111ZZ
CG11SZZ
CG11YZZ
CG121ZZ
CG12FZZ
CG12GZZ
CG12YZZ
CG14GZZ
CG14YZZ
CG1YYZZ
CG211ZZ
CG21SZZ
CG21YZZ
CG2YYZZ
CG421ZZ
CG42FZZ
CG42GZZ
CG42YZZ
CG4YYZZ
CH101ZZ
CH10SZZ
CH10YZZ
CH111ZZ
CH11SZZ
CH11YZZ
CH121ZZ
CH12SZZ
CH12YZZ
CH1YYZZ
CH201ZZ
CH20SZZ
CH20YZZ
CH211ZZ
CH21SZZ
CH21YZZ
CH221ZZ
CH22SZZ
CH22YZZ
CH2YYZZ
CP111ZZ
CP11YZZ
CP141ZZ
CP14YZZ
CP151ZZ
CP15YZZ
CP161ZZ
CP16YZZ
CP171ZZ
CP17YZZ
CP181ZZ
CP18YZZ
CP191ZZ
CP19YZZ
CP1B1ZZ
CP1BYZZ
CP1C1ZZ
CP1CYZZ
CP1D1ZZ
CP1DYZZ
CP1F1ZZ
CP1FYZZ
CP1YYZZ
CP1Z1ZZ
CP1ZYZZ
CP211ZZ
CP21YZZ
CP221ZZ
CP22YZZ
CP231ZZ
CP23YZZ
CP241ZZ
CP24YZZ
CP261ZZ
CP26YZZ
CP271ZZ
CP27YZZ
CP281ZZ
CP28YZZ
CP291ZZ
CP29YZZ
CP2B1ZZ
CP2BYZZ
CP2C1ZZ
CP2CYZZ
CP2D1ZZ
CP2DYZZ
CP2F1ZZ
CP2FYZZ
CP2G1ZZ
CP2GYZZ
CP2H1ZZ
CP2HYZZ
CP2J1ZZ
CP2JYZZ
CP2YYZZ
CP55ZZZ
CP5NZZZ
CP5PZZZ
CP5YYZZ
CT131ZZ
CT13FZZ
CT13GZZ
CT13YZZ
CT1H1ZZ
CT1HYZZ
CT1YYZZ
CT231ZZ
CT23YZZ
CT2YYZZ
CT631ZZ
CT63FZZ
CT63GZZ
CT63HZZ
CT63YZZ
CT6YYZZ
CV191ZZ
CV19YZZ
CV1YYZZ
CW101ZZ
CW10DZZ
CW10FZZ
CW10GZZ
CW10LZZ
CW10SZZ
CW10YZZ
CW111ZZ
CW11DZZ
CW11FZZ
CW11GZZ
CW11LZZ
CW11SZZ
CW11YZZ
CW131ZZ
CW13DZZ
CW13FZZ
CW13GZZ
CW13KZZ
CW13LZZ
CW13SZZ
CW13YZZ
CW141ZZ
CW14DZZ
CW14FZZ
CW14GZZ
CW14LZZ
CW14SZZ
CW14YZZ
CW161ZZ
CW16DZZ
CW16FZZ
CW16GZZ
CW16LZZ
CW16SZZ
CW16YZZ
CW1B1ZZ
CW1BDZZ
CW1BFZZ
CW1BGZZ
CW1BLZZ
CW1BSZZ
CW1BYZZ
CW1D1ZZ
CW1DDZZ
CW1DFZZ
CW1DGZZ
CW1DLZZ
CW1DSZZ
CW1DYZZ
CW1J1ZZ
CW1JDZZ
CW1JFZZ
CW1JGZZ
CW1JLZZ
CW1JSZZ
CW1JYZZ
CW1M1ZZ
CW1MDZZ
CW1MFZZ
CW1MGZZ
CW1MLZZ
CW1MSZZ
CW1MYZZ
CW1N1ZZ
CW1NDZZ
CW1NFZZ
CW1NGZZ
CW1NLZZ
CW1NSZZ

CW1NYZZ
CW1YYZZ
CW1ZZZZ
CW201ZZ
CW20DZZ
CW20FZZ
CW20GZZ
CW20KZZ
CW20LZZ
CW20SZZ
CW20YZZ
CW211ZZ
CW21DZZ
CW21FZZ
CW21GZZ
CW21KZZ
CW21LZZ
CW21SZZ
CW21YZZ
CW231ZZ
CW23DZZ
CW23FZZ
CW23GZZ
CW23KZZ
CW23LZZ
CW23SZZ
CW23YZZ
CW241ZZ
CW24DZZ
CW24FZZ
CW24GZZ
CW24KZZ
CW24LZZ
CW24SZZ
CW24YZZ
CW261ZZ
CW26DZZ
CW26FZZ
CW26GZZ
CW26KZZ
CW26LZZ
CW26SZZ
CW26YZZ
CW2B1ZZ
CW2BDZZ
CW2BFZZ
CW2BGZZ
CW2BKZZ
CW2BLZZ
CW2BSZZ
CW2BYZZ
CW2D1ZZ
CW2DDZZ
CW2DFZZ
CW2DGZZ
CW2DKZZ
CW2DLZZ
CW2DSZZ
CW2DYZZ
CW2J1ZZ
CW2JDZZ
CW2JFZZ
CW2JGZZ
CW2JKZZ
CW2JLZZ
CW2JSZZ
CW2JYZZ
CW2M1ZZ
CW2MDZZ
CW2MFZZ
CW2MGZZ
CW2MKZZ
CW2MLZZ
CW2MSZZ
CW2MYZZ
CW2YYZZ
CW3NYZZ
CW501ZZ
CW50DZZ
CW50YZZ
CW511ZZ
CW51DZZ
CW51YZZ
CW531ZZ
CW53DZZ
CW53YZZ
CW541ZZ
CW54DZZ
CW54YZZ
CW561ZZ
CW56DZZ
CW56YZZ
CW5B1ZZ
CW5BDZZ
CW5BYZZ
CW5D1ZZ
CW5DDZZ
CW5DYZZ
CW5J1ZZ
CW5JDZZ
CW5JYZZ
CW5M1ZZ
CW5MDZZ
CW5MYZZ
CW70NZZ
CW70YZZ
CW73NZZ
CW73YZZ
CW7GGZZ
CW7GYZZ
CW7N8ZZ
CW7NGZZ
CW7NNZZ
CW7NPZZ
CW7NYZZ
CW7YYZZ
D0000ZZ
D0001ZZ
D0002ZZ
D0003Z0
D0003ZZ
D0004ZZ
D0005ZZ
D0006ZZ
D0010ZZ
D0011ZZ
D0012ZZ
D0013Z0
D0013ZZ
D0014ZZ
D0015ZZ
D0016ZZ
D0060ZZ
D0061ZZ
D0062ZZ
D0063Z0
D0063ZZ
D0064ZZ
D0065ZZ
D0066ZZ
D0070ZZ
D0071ZZ
D0072ZZ
D0073Z0
D0073ZZ
D0074ZZ
D0075ZZ
D0076ZZ
D01097Z
D01098Z
D01099Z
D0109BZ
D0109CZ
D0109YZ
D010B7Z
D010B8Z
D010B9Z
D010BB1
D010BBZ
D010BCZ
D010BYZ
D01197Z
D01198Z
D01199Z
D0119BZ
D0119CZ
D0119YZ
D011B7Z
D011B8Z
D011B9Z
D011BB1
D011BBZ
D011BCZ
D011BYZ
D01697Z
D01698Z
D01699Z
D0169BZ
D0169CZ
D0169YZ
D016B7Z
D016B8Z
D016B9Z
D016BB1
D016BBZ
D016BCZ
D016BYZ
D01797Z
D01798Z
D01799Z
D0179BZ
D0179CZ
D0179YZ
D017B7Z
D017B8Z
D017B9Z
D017BB1
D017BBZ
D017BCZ
D017BYZ
D0Y07ZZ
D0Y08ZZ
D0Y0FZZ
D0Y0KZZ
D0Y17ZZ
D0Y18ZZ
D0Y1FZZ
D0Y1KZZ
D0Y67ZZ
D0Y68ZZ
D0Y6FZZ
D0Y6KZZ
D0Y77ZZ
D0Y78ZZ
D0Y7FZZ
D0Y7KZZ
D7000ZZ
D7001ZZ
D7002ZZ
D7003Z0
D7003ZZ
D7004ZZ
D7005ZZ
D7006ZZ
D7010ZZ
D7011ZZ
D7012ZZ
D7013Z0
D7013ZZ
D7014ZZ
D7015ZZ
D7016ZZ
D7020ZZ
D7021ZZ
D7022ZZ
D7023Z0
D7023ZZ
D7024ZZ
D7025ZZ
D7026ZZ
D7030ZZ
D7031ZZ
D7032ZZ
D7033Z0
D7033ZZ
D7034ZZ
D7035ZZ
D7036ZZ
D7040ZZ
D7041ZZ
D7042ZZ
D7043Z0
D7043ZZ
D7044ZZ
D7045ZZ
D7046ZZ
D7050ZZ
D7051ZZ
D7052ZZ
D7053Z0
D7053ZZ
D7054ZZ
D7055ZZ
D7056ZZ
D7060ZZ
D7061ZZ
D7062ZZ
D7063Z0
D7063ZZ
D7064ZZ
D7065ZZ
D7066ZZ
D7070ZZ
D7071ZZ
D7072ZZ
D7073Z0
D7073ZZ
D7074ZZ
D7075ZZ
D7076ZZ
D7080ZZ
D7081ZZ
D7082ZZ
D7083Z0
D7083ZZ
D7084ZZ
D7085ZZ
D7086ZZ
D71097Z
D71098Z
D71099Z
D7109BZ
D7109CZ
D7109YZ
D710B7Z
D710B8Z
D710B9Z
D710BB1
D710BBZ
D710BCZ
D710BYZ
D71197Z
D71198Z
D71199Z
D7119BZ
D7119CZ
D7119YZ
D711B7Z
D711B8Z
D711B9Z
D711BB1
D711BBZ
D711BCZ
D711BYZ
D71297Z
D71298Z
D71299Z
D7129BZ
D7129CZ
D7129YZ
D712B7Z
D712B8Z
D712B9Z
D712BB1
D712BBZ
D712BCZ
D712BYZ
D71397Z
D71398Z
D71399Z
D7139BZ
D7139CZ
D7139YZ
D713B7Z
D713B8Z
D713B9Z
D713BB1
D713BBZ
D713BCZ
D713BYZ
D71497Z
D71498Z
D71499Z
D7149BZ
D7149CZ
D7149YZ
D714B7Z
D714B8Z
D714B9Z
D714BB1
D714BBZ
D714BCZ
D714BYZ
D71597Z
D71598Z
D71599Z
D7159BZ
D7159CZ
D7159YZ
D715B7Z
D715B8Z
D715B9Z
D715BB1
D715BBZ
D715BCZ
D715BYZ
D71697Z
D71698Z
D71699Z
D7169BZ
D7169CZ
D7169YZ
D716B7Z
D716B8Z
D716B9Z
D716BB1
D716BBZ
D716BCZ
D716BYZ
D71797Z
D71798Z
D71799Z
D7179BZ
D7179CZ
D7179YZ
D717B7Z
D717B8Z
D717B9Z
D717BB1
D717BBZ
D717BCZ
D717BYZ
D71897Z
D71898Z
D71899Z
D7189BZ
D7189CZ
D7189YZ
D718B7Z
D718B8Z
D718B9Z
D718BB1
D718BBZ
D718BCZ
D718BYZ
D7Y08ZZ
D7Y0FZZ
D7Y18ZZ
D7Y1FZZ
D7Y28ZZ
D7Y2FZZ
D7Y38ZZ
D7Y3FZZ
D7Y48ZZ
D7Y4FZZ
D7Y58ZZ
D7Y5FZZ
D7Y68ZZ
D7Y6FZZ
D7Y78ZZ
D7Y7FZZ
D7Y88ZZ
D7Y8FZZ
D80C0ZZ
D80C1ZZ
D80C2ZZ
D80C3Z0
D80C3ZZ
D80C4ZZ
D80C5ZZ
D80C6ZZ
D81097Z
D81098Z
D81099Z
D8109BZ
D8109CZ
D8109YZ
D810B7Z
D810B8Z
D810B9Z
D810BB1
D810BBZ
D810BCZ
D810BYZ
D8Y07ZZ
D8Y08ZZ
D8Y0FZZ
D9000ZZ
D9001ZZ
D9002ZZ
D9003Z0
D9003ZZ
D9004ZZ
D9005ZZ
D9006ZZ
D9010ZZ
D9011ZZ
D9012ZZ
D9013Z0
D9013ZZ
D9014ZZ
D9015ZZ
D9016ZZ
D9030ZZ
D9031ZZ
D9032ZZ
D9033Z0
D9033ZZ
D9034ZZ
D9035ZZ
D9036ZZ
D9040ZZ
D9041ZZ
D9042ZZ
D9043Z0
D9043ZZ
D9044ZZ
D9045ZZ
D9046ZZ
D9050ZZ
D9051ZZ
D9052ZZ
D9053Z0
D9053ZZ
D9054ZZ
D9055ZZ
D9056ZZ
D9060ZZ
D9061ZZ
D9062ZZ
D9063Z0
D9063ZZ
D9064ZZ
D9065ZZ
D9066ZZ
D9070ZZ
D9071ZZ
D9072ZZ
D9073Z0
D9073ZZ
D9074ZZ
D9075ZZ
D9076ZZ
D9080ZZ
D9081ZZ
D9082ZZ
D9083Z0
D9083ZZ
D9084ZZ
D9085ZZ
D9086ZZ
D9090ZZ
D9091ZZ
D9092ZZ
D9093Z0
D9093ZZ
D9094ZZ
D9095ZZ
D9096ZZ
D90B0ZZ
D90B1ZZ
D90B2ZZ
D90B3Z0
D90B3ZZ
D90B4ZZ
D90B5ZZ
D90B6ZZ
D90D0ZZ
D90D1ZZ
D90D2ZZ
D90D3Z0
D90D3ZZ
D90D4ZZ
D90D5ZZ
D90D6ZZ
D90F0ZZ
D90F1ZZ
D90F2ZZ
D90F3Z0
D90F3ZZ

D90F4ZZ
D90F5ZZ
D90F6ZZ
D91097Z
D91098Z
D91099Z
D9109BZ
D9109CZ
D9109YZ
D910B7Z
D910B8Z
D910B9Z
D910BB1
D910BBZ
D910BCZ
D910BYZ
D91197Z
D91198Z
D91199Z
D9119BZ
D9119CZ
D9119YZ
D911B7Z
D911B8Z
D911B9Z
D911BB1
D911BBZ
D911BCZ
D911BYZ
D91397Z
D91398Z
D91399Z
D9139BZ
D9139CZ
D9139YZ
D913B7Z
D913B8Z
D913B9Z
D913BB1
D913BBZ
D913BCZ
D913BYZ
D91497Z
D91498Z
D91499Z
D9149BZ
D9149CZ
D9149YZ
D914B7Z
D914B8Z
D914B9Z
D914BB1
D914BBZ
D914BCZ
D914BYZ
D91597Z
D91598Z
D91599Z
D9159BZ
D9159CZ
D9159YZ
D915B7Z
D915B8Z
D915B9Z
D915BB1
D915BBZ
D915BCZ
D915BYZ
D91697Z
D91698Z
D91699Z
D9169BZ
D9169CZ
D9169YZ
D916B7Z
D916B8Z
D916B9Z
D916BB1
D916BBZ
D916BCZ
D916BYZ
D91797Z
D91798Z
D91799Z
D9179BZ
D9179CZ
D9179YZ
D917B7Z
D917B8Z
D917B9Z
D917BB1
D917BBZ
D917BCZ
D917BYZ
D91897Z
D91898Z
D91899Z
D9189BZ
D9189CZ
D9189YZ
D918B7Z
D918B8Z
D918B9Z
D918BB1
D918BBZ
D918BCZ
D918BYZ
D91997Z
D91998Z
D91999Z
D9199BZ
D9199CZ
D9199YZ
D919B7Z
D919B8Z
D919B9Z
D919BB1
D919BBZ
D919BCZ
D919BYZ
D91B97Z
D91B98Z
D91B99Z
D91B9BZ
D91B9CZ
D91B9YZ
D91BB7Z
D91BB8Z
D91BB9Z
D91BBB1
D91BBBZ
D91BBCZ
D91BBYZ
D91D97Z
D91D98Z
D91D99Z
D91D9BZ
D91D9CZ
D91D9YZ
D91DB7Z
D91DB8Z
D91DB9Z
D91DBB1
D91DBBZ
D91DBCZ
D91DBYZ
D91F97Z
D91F98Z
D91F99Z
D91F9BZ
D91F9CZ
D91F9YZ
D91FB7Z
D91FB8Z
D91FB9Z
D91FBB1
D91FBBZ
D91FBCZ
D91FBYZ
D9Y07ZZ
D9Y08ZZ
D9Y0FZZ
D9Y17ZZ
D9Y18ZZ
D9Y1FZZ
D9Y37ZZ
D9Y38ZZ
D9Y47ZZ
D9Y48ZZ
D9Y4CZZ
D9Y4FZZ
D9Y57ZZ
D9Y58ZZ
D9Y5FZZ
D9Y67ZZ
D9Y68ZZ
D9Y6FZZ
D9Y77ZZ
D9Y78ZZ
D9Y7FZZ
D9Y87ZZ
D9Y88ZZ
D9Y8FZZ
D9Y97ZZ
D9Y98ZZ
D9Y9FZZ
D9YB7ZZ
D9YB8ZZ
D9YBCZZ
D9YBFZZ
D9YCCZZ
D9YCFZZ
D9YD7ZZ
D9YD8ZZ
D9YDCZZ
D9YDFZZ
D9YF7ZZ
D9YF8ZZ
DB000ZZ
DB001ZZ
DB002ZZ
DB003Z0
DB003ZZ
DB004ZZ
DB005ZZ
DB006ZZ
DB010ZZ
DB011ZZ
DB012ZZ
DB013Z0
DB013ZZ
DB014ZZ
DB015ZZ
DB016ZZ
DB020ZZ
DB021ZZ
DB022ZZ
DB023Z0
DB023ZZ
DB024ZZ
DB025ZZ
DB026ZZ
DB050ZZ
DB051ZZ
DB052ZZ
DB053Z0
DB053ZZ
DB054ZZ
DB055ZZ
DB056ZZ
DB060ZZ
DB061ZZ
DB062ZZ
DB063Z0
DB063ZZ
DB064ZZ
DB065ZZ
DB066ZZ
DB070ZZ
DB071ZZ
DB072ZZ
DB073Z0
DB073ZZ
DB074ZZ
DB075ZZ
DB076ZZ
DB080ZZ
DB081ZZ
DB082ZZ
DB083Z0
DB083ZZ
DB084ZZ
DB085ZZ
DB086ZZ
DB1097Z
DB1098Z
DB1099Z
DB109BZ
DB109CZ
DB109YZ
DB10B7Z
DB10B8Z
DB10B9Z
DB10BB1
DB10BBZ
DB10BCZ
DB10BYZ
DB1197Z
DB1198Z
DB1199Z
DB119BZ
DB119CZ
DB119YZ
DB11B7Z
DB11B8Z
DB11B9Z
DB11BB1
DB11BBZ
DB11BCZ
DB11BYZ
DB1297Z
DB1298Z
DB1299Z
DB129BZ
DB129CZ
DB129YZ
DB12B7Z
DB12B8Z
DB12B9Z
DB12BB1
DB12BBZ
DB12BCZ
DB12BYZ
DB1597Z
DB1598Z
DB1599Z
DB159BZ
DB159CZ
DB159YZ
DB15B7Z
DB15B8Z
DB15B9Z
DB15BB1
DB15BBZ
DB15BCZ
DB15BYZ
DB1697Z
DB1698Z
DB1699Z
DB169BZ
DB169CZ
DB169YZ
DB16B7Z
DB16B8Z
DB16B9Z
DB16BB1
DB16BBZ
DB16BCZ
DB16BYZ
DB1797Z
DB1798Z
DB1799Z
DB179BZ
DB179CZ
DB179YZ
DB17B7Z
DB17B8Z
DB17B9Z
DB17BB1
DB17BBZ
DB17BCZ
DB17BYZ
DB1897Z
DB1898Z
DB1899Z
DB189BZ
DB189CZ
DB189YZ
DB18B7Z
DB18B8Z
DB18B9Z
DB18BB1
DB18BBZ
DB18BCZ
DB18BYZ
DBY07ZZ
DBY08ZZ
DBY0FZZ
DBY0KZZ
DBY17ZZ
DBY18ZZ
DBY1FZZ
DBY1KZZ
DBY27ZZ
DBY28ZZ
DBY2FZZ
DBY2KZZ
DBY57ZZ
DBY58ZZ
DBY5FZZ
DBY5KZZ
DBY67ZZ
DBY68ZZ
DBY6FZZ
DBY6KZZ
DBY77ZZ
DBY78ZZ
DBY7FZZ
DBY7KZZ
DBY87ZZ
DBY88ZZ
DBY8FZZ
DBY8KZZ
DD000ZZ
DD001ZZ
DD002ZZ
DD003Z0
DD003ZZ
DD004ZZ
DD005ZZ
DD006ZZ
DD010ZZ
DD011ZZ
DD012ZZ
DD013Z0
DD013ZZ
DD014ZZ
DD015ZZ
DD016ZZ
DD020ZZ
DD021ZZ
DD022ZZ
DD023Z0
DD023ZZ
DD024ZZ
DD025ZZ
DD026ZZ
DD030ZZ
DD031ZZ
DD032ZZ
DD033Z0
DD033ZZ
DD034ZZ
DD035ZZ
DD036ZZ
DD040ZZ
DD041ZZ
DD042ZZ
DD043Z0
DD043ZZ
DD044ZZ
DD045ZZ
DD046ZZ
DD050ZZ
DD051ZZ
DD052ZZ
DD053Z0
DD053ZZ
DD054ZZ
DD055ZZ
DD056ZZ
DD070ZZ
DD071ZZ
DD072ZZ
DD073Z0
DD073ZZ
DD074ZZ
DD075ZZ
DD076ZZ
DD1097Z
DD1098Z
DD1099Z
DD109BZ
DD109CZ
DD109YZ
DD10B7Z
DD10B8Z
DD10B9Z
DD10BB1
DD10BBZ
DD10BCZ
DD10BYZ
DD1197Z
DD1198Z
DD1199Z
DD119BZ
DD119CZ
DD119YZ
DD11B7Z
DD11B8Z
DD11B9Z
DD11BB1
DD11BBZ
DD11BCZ
DD11BYZ
DD1297Z
DD1298Z
DD1299Z
DD129BZ
DD129CZ
DD129YZ
DD12B7Z
DD12B8Z
DD12B9Z
DD12BB1
DD12BBZ
DD12BCZ
DD12BYZ
DD1397Z
DD1398Z
DD1399Z
DD139BZ
DD139CZ
DD139YZ
DD13B7Z
DD13B8Z
DD13B9Z
DD13BB1
DD13BBZ
DD13BCZ
DD13BYZ
DD1497Z
DD1498Z
DD1499Z
DD149BZ
DD149CZ
DD149YZ
DD14B7Z
DD14B8Z
DD14B9Z
DD14BB1
DD14BBZ
DD14BCZ
DD14BYZ
DD1597Z
DD1598Z
DD1599Z
DD159BZ
DD159CZ
DD159YZ
DD15B7Z
DD15B8Z
DD15B9Z
DD15BB1
DD15BBZ
DD15BCZ
DD15BYZ
DD1797Z
DD1798Z
DD1799Z
DD179BZ
DD179CZ
DD179YZ
DD17B7Z
DD17B8Z
DD17B9Z
DD17BB1
DD17BBZ
DD17BCZ
DD17BYZ
DDY07ZZ
DDY08ZZ
DDY0FZZ
DDY0KZZ
DDY17ZZ
DDY18ZZ
DDY1CZZ
DDY1FZZ
DDY1KZZ
DDY27ZZ
DDY28ZZ
DDY2CZZ
DDY2FZZ
DDY2KZZ
DDY37ZZ
DDY38ZZ
DDY3CZZ
DDY3FZZ
DDY3KZZ
DDY47ZZ

DDY48ZZ
DDY4CZZ
DDY4FZZ
DDY4KZZ
DDY57ZZ
DDY58ZZ
DDY5CZZ
DDY5FZZ
DDY5KZZ
DDY77ZZ
DDY78ZZ
DDY7CZZ
DDY7FZZ
DDY7KZZ
DDY8CZZ
DDY8FZZ
DDY8KZZ
DF000ZZ
DF001ZZ
DF002ZZ
DF003Z0
DF003ZZ
DF004ZZ
DF005ZZ
DF006ZZ
DF010ZZ
DF011ZZ
DF012ZZ
DF013Z0
DF013ZZ
DF014ZZ
DF015ZZ
DF016ZZ
DF020ZZ
DF021ZZ
DF022ZZ
DF023Z0
DF023ZZ
DF024ZZ
DF025ZZ
DF026ZZ
DF030ZZ
DF031ZZ
DF032ZZ
DF033Z0
DF033ZZ
DF034ZZ
DF035ZZ
DF036ZZ
DF1097Z
DF1098Z
DF1099Z
DF109BZ
DF109CZ
DF109YZ
DF10B7Z
DF10B8Z
DF10B9Z
DF10BB1
DF10BBZ
DF10BCZ
DF10BYZ
DF1197Z
DF1198Z
DF1199Z
DF119BZ
DF119CZ
DF119YZ
DF11B7Z
DF11B8Z
DF11B9Z
DF11BB1
DF11BBZ
DF11BCZ
DF11BYZ
DF1297Z
DF1298Z
DF1299Z
DF129BZ
DF129CZ
DF129YZ
DF12B7Z
DF12B8Z
DF12B9Z
DF12BB1
DF12BBZ
DF12BCZ
DF12BYZ
DF1397Z
DF1398Z
DF1399Z
DF139BZ
DF139CZ
DF139YZ
DF13B7Z
DF13B8Z
DF13B9Z
DF13BB1
DF13BBZ
DF13BCZ
DF13BYZ
DFY07ZZ
DFY08ZZ
DFY0CZZ
DFY0FZZ
DFY0KZZ
DFY17ZZ
DFY18ZZ
DFY1CZZ
DFY1FZZ
DFY1KZZ
DFY27ZZ
DFY28ZZ
DFY2CZZ
DFY2FZZ
DFY2KZZ
DFY37ZZ
DFY38ZZ
DFY3CZZ
DFY3FZZ
DFY3KZZ
DG000ZZ
DG001ZZ
DG002ZZ
DG003Z0
DG003ZZ
DG005ZZ
DG006ZZ
DG010ZZ
DG011ZZ
DG012ZZ
DG013Z0
DG013ZZ
DG015ZZ
DG016ZZ
DG020ZZ
DG021ZZ
DG022ZZ
DG023Z0
DG023ZZ
DG025ZZ
DG026ZZ
DG040ZZ
DG041ZZ
DG042ZZ
DG043Z0
DG043ZZ
DG045ZZ
DG046ZZ
DG050ZZ
DG051ZZ
DG052ZZ
DG053Z0
DG053ZZ
DG055ZZ
DG056ZZ
DG1097Z
DG1098Z
DG1099Z
DG109BZ
DG109CZ
DG109YZ
DG10B7Z
DG10B8Z
DG10B9Z
DG10BB1
DG10BBZ
DG10BCZ
DG10BYZ
DG1197Z
DG1198Z
DG1199Z
DG119BZ
DG119CZ
DG119YZ
DG11B7Z
DG11B8Z
DG11B9Z
DG11BB1
DG11BBZ
DG11BCZ
DG11BYZ
DG1297Z
DG1298Z
DG1299Z
DG129BZ
DG129CZ
DG129YZ
DG12B7Z
DG12B8Z
DG12B9Z
DG12BB1
DG12BBZ
DG12BCZ
DG12BYZ
DG1497Z
DG1498Z
DG1499Z
DG149BZ
DG149CZ
DG149YZ
DG14B7Z
DG14B8Z
DG14B9Z
DG14BB1
DG14BBZ
DG14BCZ
DG14BYZ
DG1597Z
DG1598Z
DG1599Z
DG159BZ
DG159CZ
DG159YZ
DG15B7Z
DG15B8Z
DG15B9Z
DG15BB1
DG15BBZ
DG15BCZ
DG15BYZ
DGY07ZZ
DGY08ZZ
DGY0FZZ
DGY0KZZ
DGY17ZZ
DGY18ZZ
DGY1FZZ
DGY1KZZ
DGY27ZZ
DGY28ZZ
DGY2FZZ
DGY2KZZ
DGY47ZZ
DGY48ZZ
DGY4FZZ
DGY4KZZ
DGY57ZZ
DGY58ZZ
DGY5FZZ
DGY5KZZ
DH020ZZ
DH021ZZ
DH022ZZ
DH023Z0
DH023ZZ
DH024ZZ
DH025ZZ
DH026ZZ
DH030ZZ
DH031ZZ
DH032ZZ
DH033Z0
DH033ZZ
DH034ZZ
DH035ZZ
DH036ZZ
DH040ZZ
DH041ZZ
DH042ZZ
DH043Z0
DH043ZZ
DH044ZZ
DH045ZZ
DH046ZZ
DH060ZZ
DH061ZZ
DH062ZZ
DH063Z0
DH063ZZ
DH064ZZ
DH065ZZ
DH066ZZ
DH070ZZ
DH071ZZ
DH072ZZ
DH073Z0
DH073ZZ
DH074ZZ
DH075ZZ
DH076ZZ
DH080ZZ
DH081ZZ
DH082ZZ
DH083Z0
DH083ZZ
DH084ZZ
DH085ZZ
DH086ZZ
DH090ZZ
DH091ZZ
DH092ZZ
DH093Z0
DH093ZZ
DH094ZZ
DH095ZZ
DH096ZZ
DH0B0ZZ
DH0B1ZZ
DH0B2ZZ
DH0B3Z0
DH0B3ZZ
DH0B4ZZ
DH0B5ZZ
DH0B6ZZ
DHY27ZZ
DHY28ZZ
DHY2FZZ
DHY37ZZ
DHY38ZZ
DHY3FZZ
DHY47ZZ
DHY48ZZ
DHY4FZZ
DHY5FZZ
DHY67ZZ
DHY68ZZ
DHY6FZZ
DHY77ZZ
DHY78ZZ
DHY7FZZ
DHY87ZZ
DHY88ZZ
DHY8FZZ
DHY97ZZ
DHY98ZZ
DHY9FZZ
DHYB7ZZ
DHYB8ZZ
DHYBFZZ
DHYCFZZ
DM000ZZ
DM001ZZ
DM002ZZ
DM003Z0
DM003ZZ
DM004ZZ
DM005ZZ
DM006ZZ
DM010ZZ
DM011ZZ
DM012ZZ
DM013Z0
DM013ZZ
DM014ZZ
DM015ZZ
DM016ZZ
DM1097Z
DM1098Z
DM1099Z
DM109BZ
DM109CZ
DM109YZ
DM10B7Z
DM10B8Z
DM10B9Z
DM10BB1
DM10BBZ
DM10BCZ
DM10BYZ
DM1197Z
DM1198Z
DM1199Z
DM119BZ
DM119CZ
DM119YZ
DM11B7Z
DM11B8Z
DM11B9Z
DM11BB1
DM11BBZ
DM11BCZ
DM11BYZ
DMY07ZZ
DMY08ZZ
DMY0FZZ
DMY0KZZ
DMY17ZZ
DMY18ZZ
DMY1FZZ
DMY1KZZ
DP000ZZ
DP001ZZ
DP002ZZ
DP003Z0
DP003ZZ
DP004ZZ
DP005ZZ
DP006ZZ
DP020ZZ
DP021ZZ
DP022ZZ
DP023Z0
DP023ZZ
DP024ZZ
DP025ZZ
DP026ZZ
DP030ZZ
DP031ZZ
DP032ZZ
DP033Z0
DP033ZZ
DP034ZZ
DP035ZZ
DP036ZZ
DP040ZZ
DP041ZZ
DP042ZZ
DP043Z0
DP043ZZ
DP044ZZ
DP045ZZ
DP046ZZ
DP050ZZ
DP051ZZ
DP052ZZ
DP053Z0
DP053ZZ
DP054ZZ
DP055ZZ
DP056ZZ
DP060ZZ
DP061ZZ
DP062ZZ
DP063Z0
DP063ZZ
DP064ZZ
DP065ZZ
DP066ZZ
DP070ZZ
DP071ZZ
DP072ZZ
DP073Z0
DP073ZZ
DP074ZZ
DP075ZZ
DP076ZZ
DP080ZZ
DP081ZZ
DP082ZZ
DP083Z0
DP083ZZ
DP084ZZ
DP085ZZ
DP086ZZ
DP090ZZ
DP091ZZ
DP092ZZ
DP093Z0
DP093ZZ
DP094ZZ
DP095ZZ
DP096ZZ
DP0B0ZZ
DP0B1ZZ
DP0B2ZZ
DP0B3Z0
DP0B3ZZ
DP0B4ZZ
DP0B5ZZ
DP0B6ZZ
DP0C0ZZ
DP0C1ZZ
DP0C2ZZ
DP0C3Z0
DP0C3ZZ
DP0C4ZZ
DP0C5ZZ
DP0C6ZZ
DPY07ZZ
DPY08ZZ
DPY0FZZ
DPY27ZZ
DPY28ZZ
DPY2FZZ
DPY37ZZ
DPY38ZZ
DPY3FZZ
DPY47ZZ
DPY48ZZ
DPY4FZZ
DPY57ZZ
DPY58ZZ
DPY5FZZ
DPY67ZZ
DPY68ZZ
DPY6FZZ
DPY77ZZ
DPY78ZZ
DPY7FZZ
DPY87ZZ
DPY88ZZ
DPY8FZZ
DPY97ZZ
DPY98ZZ
DPY9FZZ
DPYB7ZZ
DPYB8ZZ
DPYBFZZ
DPYC7ZZ
DPYC8ZZ
DPYCFZZ
DT000ZZ
DT001ZZ
DT002ZZ
DT003Z0
DT003ZZ
DT004ZZ
DT005ZZ
DT006ZZ
DT010ZZ
DT011ZZ
DT012ZZ
DT013Z0
DT013ZZ
DT014ZZ
DT015ZZ
DT016ZZ
DT020ZZ
DT021ZZ
DT022ZZ
DT023Z0
DT023ZZ
DT024ZZ
DT025ZZ
DT026ZZ
DT030ZZ
DT031ZZ
DT032ZZ
DT033Z0
DT033ZZ
DT034ZZ
DT035ZZ
DT036ZZ
DT1097Z
DT1098Z
DT1099Z
DT109BZ
DT109CZ
DT109YZ

DT10B7Z
DT10B8Z
DT10B9Z
DT10BB1
DT10BBZ
DT10BCZ
DT10BYZ
DT1197Z
DT1198Z
DT1199Z
DT119BZ
DT119CZ
DT119YZ
DT11B7Z
DT11B8Z
DT11B9Z
DT11BB1
DT11BBZ
DT11BCZ
DT11BYZ
DT1297Z
DT1298Z
DT1299Z
DT129BZ
DT129CZ
DT129YZ
DT12B7Z
DT12B8Z
DT12B9Z
DT12BB1
DT12BBZ
DT12BCZ
DT12BYZ
DT1397Z
DT1398Z
DT1399Z
DT139BZ
DT139CZ
DT139YZ
DT13B7Z
DT13B8Z
DT13B9Z
DT13BB1
DT13BBZ
DT13BCZ
DT13BYZ
DTY07ZZ
DTY08ZZ
DTY0CZZ
DTY0FZZ
DTY17ZZ
DTY18ZZ
DTY1CZZ
DTY1FZZ
DTY27ZZ
DTY28ZZ
DTY2CZZ
DTY2FZZ
DTY37ZZ
DTY38ZZ
DTY3CZZ
DTY3FZZ
DU000ZZ
DU001ZZ
DU002ZZ
DU003Z0
DU003ZZ
DU004ZZ
DU005ZZ
DU006ZZ
DU010ZZ
DU011ZZ
DU012ZZ
DU013Z0
DU013ZZ
DU014ZZ
DU015ZZ
DU016ZZ
DU020ZZ
DU021ZZ
DU022ZZ
DU023Z0
DU023ZZ
DU024ZZ
DU025ZZ
DU026ZZ
DU1097Z
DU1098Z
DU1099Z
DU109BZ
DU109CZ
DU109YZ
DU10B7Z
DU10B8Z
DU10B9Z
DU10BB1
DU10BBZ
DU10BCZ
DU10BYZ
DU1197Z
DU1198Z
DU1199Z
DU119BZ
DU119CZ
DU119YZ
DU11B7Z
DU11B8Z
DU11B9Z
DU11BB1
DU11BBZ
DU11BCZ
DU11BYZ
DU1297Z
DU1298Z
DU1299Z
DU129BZ
DU129CZ
DU129YZ
DU12B7Z
DU12B8Z
DU12B9Z
DU12BB1
DU12BBZ
DU12BCZ
DU12BYZ
DUY07ZZ
DUY08ZZ
DUY0CZZ
DUY0FZZ
DUY17ZZ
DUY18ZZ
DUY1CZZ
DUY1FZZ
DUY27ZZ
DUY28ZZ
DUY2CZZ
DUY2FZZ
DV000ZZ
DV001ZZ
DV002ZZ
DV003Z0
DV003ZZ
DV004ZZ
DV005ZZ
DV006ZZ
DV010ZZ
DV011ZZ
DV012ZZ
DV013Z0
DV013ZZ
DV014ZZ
DV015ZZ
DV016ZZ
DV1097Z
DV1098Z
DV1099Z
DV109BZ
DV109CZ
DV109YZ
DV10B7Z
DV10B8Z
DV10B9Z
DV10BB1
DV10BBZ
DV10BCZ
DV10BYZ
DV1197Z
DV1198Z
DV1199Z
DV119BZ
DV119CZ
DV119YZ
DV11B7Z
DV11B8Z
DV11B9Z
DV11BB1
DV11BBZ
DV11BCZ
DV11BYZ
DVY07ZZ
DVY08ZZ
DVY0CZZ
DVY0FZZ
DVY0KZZ
DVY17ZZ
DVY18ZZ
DVY1FZZ
DW010ZZ
DW011ZZ
DW012ZZ
DW013Z0
DW013ZZ
DW014ZZ
DW015ZZ
DW016ZZ
DW020ZZ
DW021ZZ
DW022ZZ
DW023Z0
DW023ZZ
DW024ZZ
DW025ZZ
DW026ZZ
DW030ZZ
DW031ZZ
DW032ZZ
DW033Z0
DW033ZZ
DW034ZZ
DW035ZZ
DW036ZZ
DW040ZZ
DW041ZZ
DW042ZZ
DW043Z0
DW043ZZ
DW044ZZ
DW045ZZ
DW046ZZ
DW050ZZ
DW051ZZ
DW052ZZ
DW053Z0
DW053ZZ
DW054ZZ
DW055ZZ
DW056ZZ
DW060ZZ
DW061ZZ
DW062ZZ
DW063Z0
DW063ZZ
DW064ZZ
DW065ZZ
DW066ZZ
DW10BB1
DW10BBZ
DW1197Z
DW1198Z
DW1199Z
DW119BZ
DW119CZ
DW119YZ
DW11B7Z
DW11B8Z
DW11B9Z
DW11BB1
DW11BBZ
DW11BCZ
DW11BYZ
DW1297Z
DW1298Z
DW1299Z
DW129BZ
DW129CZ
DW129YZ
DW12B7Z
DW12B8Z
DW12B9Z
DW12BB1
DW12BBZ
DW12BCZ
DW12BYZ
DW1397Z
DW1398Z
DW1399Z
DW139BZ
DW139CZ
DW139YZ
DW13B7Z
DW13B8Z
DW13B9Z
DW13BB1
DW13BBZ
DW13BCZ
DW13BYZ
DW1697Z
DW1698Z
DW1699Z
DW169BZ
DW169CZ
DW169YZ
DW16B7Z
DW16B8Z
DW16B9Z
DW16BB1
DW16BBZ
DW16BCZ
DW16BYZ
DW1KBB1
DW1KBBZ
DW1LBB1
DW1LBBZ
DW1PBB1
DW1PBBZ
DW1QBB1
DW1QBBZ
DW1RBB1
DW1RBBZ
DW1XBB1
DW1XBBZ
DW1YBB1
DW1YBBZ
DWY17ZZ
DWY18ZZ
DWY1FZZ
DWY27ZZ
DWY28ZZ
DWY2FZZ
DWY37ZZ
DWY38ZZ
DWY3FZZ
DWY47ZZ
DWY48ZZ
DWY4FZZ
DWY57ZZ
DWY58ZZ
DWY5FZZ
DWY5GDZ
DWY5GFZ
DWY5GGZ
DWY5GHZ
DWY5GYZ
DWY67ZZ
DWY68ZZ
DWY6FZZ
F0DZ8ZZ
F0DZ9EZ
F0DZ9FZ
F0DZ9UZ
F0DZ9ZZ
F13Z00Z
F13Z01Z
F13Z02Z
F13Z03Z
F13Z08Z
F13Z09Z
F13Z0ZZ
F13Z10Z
F13Z11Z
F13Z12Z
F13Z1ZZ
F13Z20Z
F13Z21Z
F13Z22Z
F13Z2ZZ
F13Z31Z
F13Z32Z
F13Z3ZZ
F13Z41Z
F13Z42Z
F13Z4KZ
F13Z4ZZ
F13Z51Z
F13Z52Z
F13Z5KZ
F13Z5ZZ
F13Z61Z
F13Z62Z
F13Z6ZZ
F13Z71Z
F13Z7KZ
F13Z7ZZ
F13Z83Z
F13Z84Z
F13Z8ZZ
F13Z91Z
F13Z92Z
F13Z9ZZ
F13ZB1Z
F13ZB2Z
F13ZBZZ
F13ZC1Z
F13ZC2Z
F13ZCZZ
F13ZD3Z
F13ZD4Z
F13ZDZZ
F13ZF3Z
F13ZF4Z
F13ZFZZ
F13ZG3Z
F13ZG4Z
F13ZGZZ
F13ZH3Z
F13ZH4Z
F13ZHZZ
F13ZJ3Z
F13ZJ4Z
F13ZJZZ
F13ZK7Z
F13ZKZZ
F13ZL7Z
F13ZLZZ
F13ZM6Z
F13ZMZZ
F13ZN6Z
F13ZNZZ
F13ZP1Z
F13ZP2Z
F13ZP4Z
F13ZP9Z
F13ZPKZ
F13ZPLZ
F13ZPPZ
F13ZPZZ
F13ZQKZ
F13ZQPZ
F13ZQYZ
F13ZQZZ
F14Z01Z
F14Z02Z
F14Z03Z
F14Z04Z
F14Z05Z
F14Z07Z
F14Z09Z
F14Z0KZ
F14Z0LZ
F14Z0PZ
F14Z0YZ
F14Z0ZZ
F14Z15Z
F14Z1ZZ
F14Z21Z
F14Z22Z
F14Z23Z
F14Z24Z
F14Z25Z
F14Z2KZ
F14Z2LZ
F14Z2PZ
F14Z2ZZ
F14Z31Z
F14Z32Z
F14Z33Z
F14Z34Z
F14Z35Z
F14Z3KZ
F14Z3LZ
F14Z3PZ
F14Z3ZZ
F14Z41Z
F14Z42Z
F14Z43Z
F14Z44Z
F14Z4KZ
F14Z4LZ
F14Z4ZZ
F14Z51Z
F14Z52Z
F14Z53Z
F14Z54Z
F14Z55Z
F14Z5KZ
F14Z5LZ
F14Z5ZZ
F14Z65Z
F14Z6ZZ
F14Z70Z
F14Z7ZZ
F14Z85Z
F14Z8ZZ
F15Z08Z
F15Z0ZZ
F15Z18Z
F15Z1ZZ
F15Z28Z
F15Z2ZZ
F15Z38Z
F15Z3ZZ
F15Z48Z
F15Z4ZZ
F15Z58Z
F15Z5ZZ
F15Z68Z
F15Z6ZZ
F15Z75Z
F15Z7ZZ
GZ10ZZZ
GZ11ZZZ
GZ12ZZZ
GZ13ZZZ
GZ14ZZZ
GZ2ZZZZ
GZ3ZZZZ
GZ50ZZZ
GZ51ZZZ
GZ52ZZZ
GZ53ZZZ
GZ54ZZZ
GZ55ZZZ
GZ56ZZZ
GZ58ZZZ
GZ59ZZZ
GZ60ZZZ
GZ61ZZZ
GZ63ZZZ
GZ72ZZZ
GZB0ZZZ
GZB1ZZZ
GZB2ZZZ
GZB3ZZZ
GZB4ZZZ
GZC9ZZZ
GZFZZZZ
GZGZZZZ
GZHZZZZ
GZJZZZZ
HZ2ZZZZ
HZ3CZZZ
HZ4CZZZ
HZ63ZZZ
HZ80ZZZ
HZ81ZZZ
HZ82ZZZ
HZ83ZZZ
HZ84ZZZ
HZ85ZZZ
HZ86ZZZ
HZ87ZZZ
HZ88ZZZ
HZ89ZZZ
HZ90ZZZ
HZ91ZZZ
HZ92ZZZ
HZ93ZZZ
HZ94ZZZ
HZ95ZZZ
HZ96ZZZ
HZ97ZZZ
HZ98ZZZ
HZ99ZZZ
X27H385
X27H395
X27H3B5
X27H3C5
X27J385
X27J395
X27J3B5

X27J3C5
X27K385
X27K395
X27K3B5
X27K3C5
X27L385
X27L395
X27L3B5
X27L3C5
X27M385
X27M395
X27M3B5
X27M3C5
X27N385
X27N395
X27N3B5
X27N3C5
X27P385
X27P395
X27P3B5
X27P3C5
X27Q385
X27Q395
X27Q3B5
X27Q3C5
X27R385
X27R395
X27R3B5
X27R3C5
X27S385
X27S395
X27S3B5
X27S3C5
X27T385
X27T395
X27T3B5
X27T3C5
X27U385
X27U395
X27U3B5
X27U3C5
X2A5312
X2A6325
X2C0361
X2C1361
X2C2361
X2C3361
X2RF032
X2RF332
X2RF432
XHRPXL2
XK02303
XNS0032
XNS0332
XNS3032
XNS3332
XNS4032
XNS4332
XR2G021
XR2H021
XRG0092
XRG00F3
XRG1092
XRG10F3
XRG2092
XRG20F3
XRG4092
XRG40F3
XRG6092
XRG60F3
XRG7092
XRG70F3
XRG8092
XRG80F3
XRGA092
XRGA0F3
XRGB092
XRGB0F3
XRGC092
XRGC0F3
XRGD092
XRGD0F3
XT25XE5
XV508A4
XW013W5
XW03321
XW03331
XW03341
XW03351
XW03372
XW03392
XW033A3
XW033B3
XW033F3
XW033G4
XW033H4
XW033K5
XW033N5
XW033Q5
XW033S5
XW033U5
XW033W5
XW04321
XW04331
XW04341
XWC4351
XWC4372
XWC4392
XWC43A3
XWC43B3
XWC43F3
XWC43G4
XWC43H4
XWC43K5
XWC43N5
XWC43Q5
XWC43S5
XWC43U5
XWC43W5
XWCDX82
XW0DXJ5
XW0DXL5
XW0DXR5
XW0DXT5
XW0DXV5
XXE5XM5
XY0VX83

This page intentionally left blank

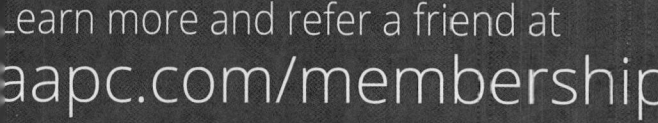

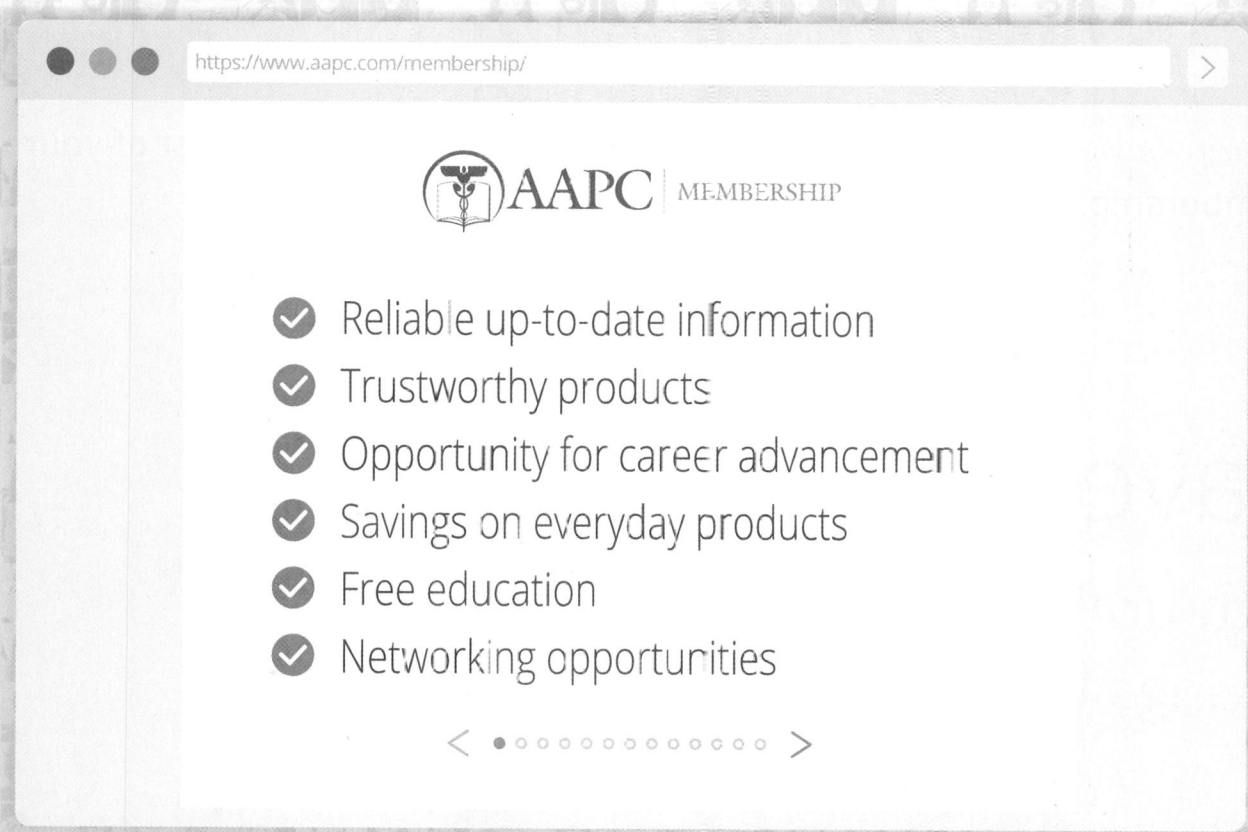

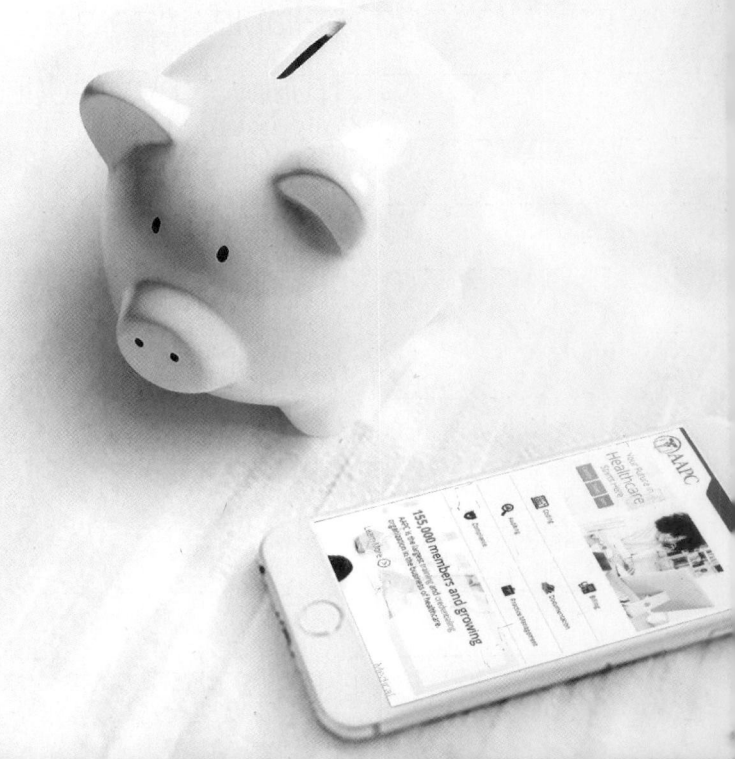

NOTES

NOTES

NOTES

NOTES

NOTES

NOTES